David Allan

David Allan received his medical training at Cambridge University and Guy's Hospital in England. He was Chief Resident in Pediatrics at Bellevue Hospital in New York City before moving to San Diego, California.

Dr. Allan has worked as a family physician in England, a pediatrician in San Diego, and Associate Dean at the University of California, San Diego School of Medicine. He has designed, written, and produced more than 100 award-winning multimedia programs with virtual reality as their conceptual base. Dr. Allan resides happily in San Diego and enjoys the warmth of the people, the weather, and the beaches.

Karen Lockyer

Karen Lockyer holds a degree in Health Information (RHIT), a national coding certification (CPC) and a BA from Rutgers University. She is also a credentialed member of AHIMA (American Health Information Management Association) and AAPC (American Academy of Professional Coders).

Mrs. Lockyer has worked in medical practice administration and the health information management fields for many years. She has taught medical terminology for high school, community college, and workforce development areas at the National Institutes of Health and the federal government's Office of Personnel Management. She has also taught billing for undergraduate and certificate programs at the community college level.

Residing in Philadelphia, Pennsylvania, Karen enjoys being back in the city of her birth and being closer to her family and friends.

BRIEF CONTENTS

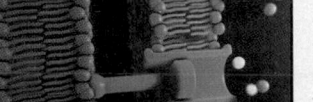
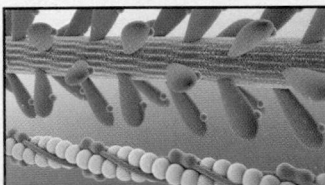
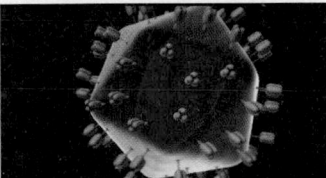
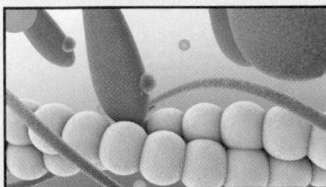

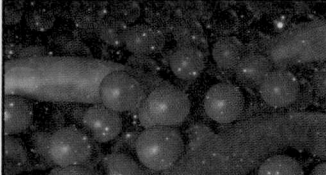
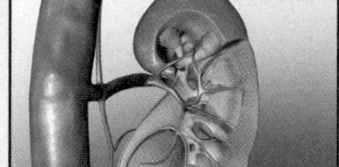
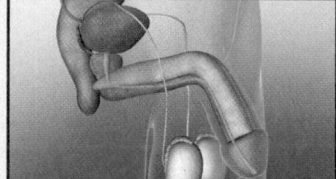
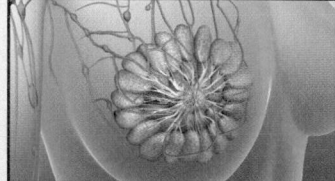
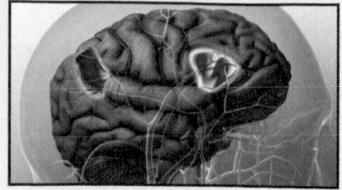

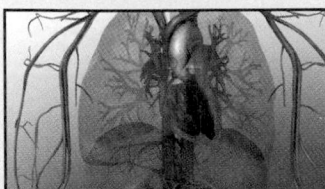
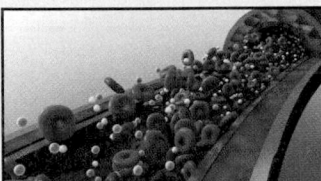
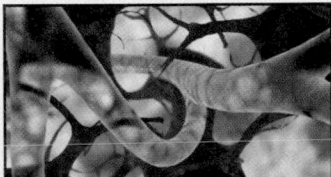
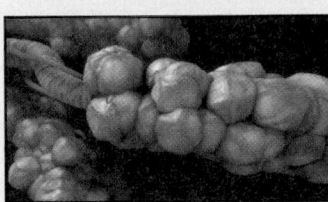
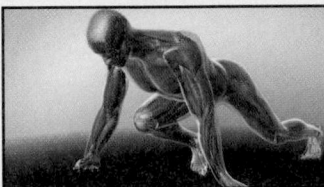

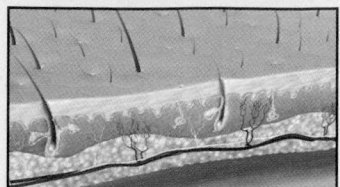
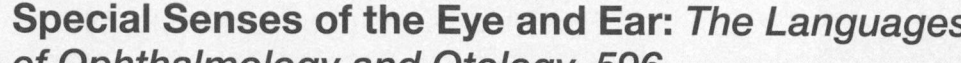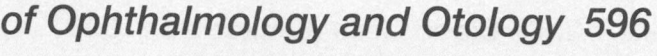
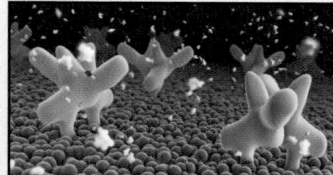
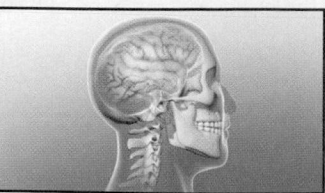

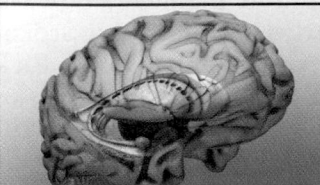
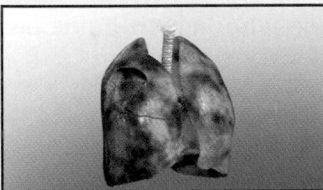
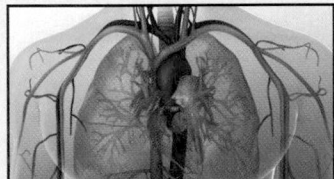
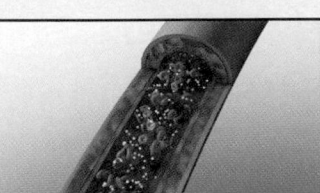

ACKNOWLEDGMENTS

We would like to thank the extraordinary efforts of a talented group of individuals at McGraw-Hill who made this textbook and its ancillaries come together: our managing director, Michael Ledbetter; Natalie Ruffatto, our executive brand manager; Edward Helmold, our developmental editor; Jessica Cannavo, our marketing manager; Srdjan Savanovic, our senior designer; Katherine Ward, our digital developmental editor; Rick Hecker, our lead project manager; Brent dela Cruz, our media producer; Carol Bielski, our senior buyer; and Jeremy Cheshareck, our photo researcher. We also thank Perrin Aikens Davis at Agate Publishing in Evanston, IL for her invaluable services in the development of this book.

We are indebted to the following individuals who helped develop, critique, and shape the ancillary package: Heather Kies, Goodwin College; Lynn Egler, Dorsey Schools; Mirella Pardee, the University of Toledo; and Veronica Zurcher, National College.

We would like to recognize the valuable contributions of those who helped guide our developmental decisions with their insightful reviews and suggestions:

Third Edition Reviewers

Theresa Louise Allyn, BS, MEd
Edmonds Community College

Rachel Curran Basco, MHS, RRT-NPS
Bossier Parish Community College

Ruth Berger, RS, RHIA
Chippewa Valley Technical College

Carole Berube, MA, MSN, BSN, RN
Bristol Community College

Jean L. Bucher, BA, MSEd
Clark College

Ruth A. Bush, PhD, MPH
San Diego Mesa College

Robin L. Cavallo, RN, BSN
Montgomery County Community College

Robert Edward Fanger, BS, MEd
Del Mar College

Mary W. Hood, MS, ARRT(R)(CT)
William Rainey Harper College

Harold N. Horn
Lincoln Land Community College

Bud W. Hunton, MA
Sinclair Community College

Judith Karls, RN, BSN, MSEd
Madison Area Technical College

Heather Kies, MHA, CMA (AAMA)
Goodwin College

Barbara Klomp, BA, RT(R)
Macomb Community College

James M. Lynch, MD
Florida Southern College

Heather Marti
Carrington College

Amie L. Mayhall, MBA, CCA
Olney Central College

David McBride, BA, MA, RT(R)(CT)(MR)
Westmoreland County Community College

Steve G. Moon, MS, FAMI, CMI
Ohio State University

Charlotte Susie Myers, MA
Kansas City Community College

Eva Oltman, Med, CPC-I, CPC, CMA, EMT
Jefferson Community and Technical College

Mirella G. Pardee, MSN, MA, RN
University of Toledo

Donna J. Slovensky, PhD, RHIA, FAHIMA
University of Alabama at Birmingham

Susan Stockmaster, MHS, CMA (AAMA)
Trident Technical College

Margaret A. Tiemann, RN, BS
St. Charles Community College

Rita F. Waller, MSN, RRT
Augusta Technical College

Carole A. Zeglin, MSEd, BS, MT, RMA
Westmoreland County Community College

Second Edition Reviewers

Dr. Irfan Akhtar
Career Institute of Health and Technology

Jessica Lynn Alexander, BS, MN
Mississippi University for Women

Suzanne Allen, RMA, RPT
Sanford-Brown Institute

Emil Asdurian, MA
Bramson ORT College

Dr. Joseph H. Balatbat
Sanford-Brown Institute

Nina Beaman, MS, RNC-AWHC,
CMA (AAMA)
Bryant & Stratton College

Jean M. Chenu, MS
Genesee Community College

Carolyn Sue Coleman, LPN, AS
National College

Lucinda A. Conley, RHIT
Ozarka College

Mary Alice Conrad, ADN
Delaware Technical and Community College

Lynn M. Egler, RMA, AHI, CPhT
Dorsey Schools

William C. Fiala, BS, MA
University of Akron, Allied Health Department

Nancy Gacke, BA
Southeast Technical Institute

Leslie Harbers, BSN, RMA
National College

Betty Hassler, RN, RMA
National College

Katherine Hawkins, BS, MS
Ivy Tech Community College

Judy Hurtt, MEd
East Central Community College

Carol Lee Jarrell, MLT, AHI
Brown Mackie College

Sherry Jones, COTA/L
Sinclair Community College

Timothy J. Jones, MA
Oklahoma City Community College

Cathy Kelley-Arney, CMA, MLTC,
BSHS
National College and National College of Business and Technology

Crystal Kitchens, CMT, MA
Richland Community College

Naomi Kupfer, CMA
Heritage College

LM Liggan, MEd, C-AHI, RMA
Director of Health Care Education, National College

Susan Long, BS
Ogeechee Technician College

Ann M. Lunde, BS, CMT
Waubonsee Community College

Loreen W. MacNichol, CMRS,
RMC
Andover College

Allan L. Markezich, PhD
Black Hawk College

Mindy S. McDonald, CMA
(AAMA)
University of Northwestern Ohio

Elizabeth L. Miller, CPC CMA
Probill PMCC

Deborah M. Mullen, CCS-P, CPC,
CPC-I
Probill PMCC

Gail P. Orr, BA
National College

Judith L. Paulsen, BA
Vatterott College

Pamela K. Roemershauser, CPC
MedVance Institute

Patricia L. Sell, AAS, BS, MSEd
National College

Shirley J. Shaw, MA
Northland Pioneer College

Gene Simon, RHIA, RMD
Florida Career College

Christine Sproles, RN, BSN, MS
Pensacola Christian College

Susan Stockmaster, MHS
Trident Technical College

Diane Swift, RHIT
State Fair Community College

Kathryn Whitley, RN, MSN, NP-C
Patrick Henry Community College

Cassandra E. Williams, MS, RHIA
Ogeechee Technical College

Kari Williams, BS, DC
Front Range Community College

Melinda J. Fernandez, AA, EMT-P,
NR-CMA, NR-RPT,
Keiser Career College

Kathie Folsom, MS, BSN, RN
Whidbey Island Campus, Skagit Valley College

Mark W. Forquer, BS
Advanced Career Training

Margaret Schell Frazier, CMA, RN, BS
Formerly of Ivy Tech State College–Northeast

Eugenia M. Fulcher, RN, BSN, EdD, CMA
Eastern New Mexico University,

Tracie Fuqua, BS, CMA
Wallace State Community College

Ron Gaines, MS, BS
Cameron University

Mary A. Harmon, BS, CMA, CPC
Med Tech College

Katherine Harper
Pellissippi State Technical Community College

Katherine Hawkins, BS
Ivy Tech Community College of Indiana

Barbara J. Hogg, MLT, RN, BSN
South Arkansas Community College

Janet R. Hunter, MBA, MS, ABD
Northland Pioneer College

Judy Hurtt, MEd
East Central Community College

Frances C. Hutson, MSN, RN
Louisiana Technical College

Sherry Jones, COTA/L
Sinclair Community College

Beverly W. Juett, MS
Midway College

Mike Kennamer, NREMT-P, MPA
Northeast Alabama Community College

Pat King, MA, RHIA
Baker College of Cass City

Crystal Kitchens, MA, CMT
Richland Community College

Judy Kronenberger, RN, CMA, MEd
Sinclair Community College

Naomi Kupfer, CMA, CMBS
Heritage College

Wei Li, MD, MSCS
North Georgia Technical College

Patricia B. Lisk, RN, BSN
Augusta Technical College

Martha Luebke, AA, BA, CPC, NIIC
High-Tech Institute

Ann M. Lunde, BS, CMT
Waubonsee Community College

Loreen W. MacNichol, CMRS, RMC
Andover College

Susan Madden, MEd, RHIT
Brown College

Alicia Mata, BS, MA
Corinthian Colleges, Inc.

Sister Sheila McGinnis, RN, BSN, CMT
Center for Human Integration

Peggy L. Meli, MS, RHIA, LHRM
Valencia College

Tanya Mercer, BS, RN, RMA
KAPLAN Higher Education Corporation

Maureen E. Russell Messier, CMA, RMA
Brandford Hall Career Institute

James J. Mizner Jr., BS Pharmacy, MBA
ACT College

Kay A. Nave, CMA, MRT
Hagerstown Business College

Laurence C. Neely, BS, MAE
EPCI College of Technology

Judith L. Neville, BA
Vatterott College

Alice M. Nolan, MBA, RHIA
University of Central Florida

Tammy O'Brien, MEd
Augusta Technical College

D.J. Overbey, RN, CCRC
Virginia College at Austin

Murray Paton Pendarvis, PhD
Southern Louisiana University

Roberta Pavy Ramont, RN, EdD
Corinthian Colleges Inc.

Brian David Riffe, BS, CMA, RMA, AHI
National College of Business and Technology

Alan Rosenberg, MS
Allied Schools

- Instructor's Manual

- **McGraw-Hill's EZ-Test Test Generator.** This flexible electronic testing program allows instructors to create tests from book-specific items. It accommodates a wide range of question types, and instructors may add their own questions. Multiple versions of a test can be created, and any test can be exported for use with course management systems such as WebCT, Blackboard, or PageOut. EZ-Test Online gives you a place online to easily administer your EZ-Test-created exams and quizzes. The program is available for Windows and Macintosh environments.

- **PowerPoint® Lecture Outlines.** PowerPoint lectures with speaking notes are available for the chapters in the textbook. Each 50-minute lesson plan in the Instructor's Manual Lesson Planning Guide dedicates approximately 20 to 25 minutes to the use of the corresponding ready-made PowerPoint presentations. The PowerPoint presentations, which combine art and lecture notes, are designed to help instructors discuss with students the important points of the lessons. The slides are customizable, allowing instructors to modify lectures to ensure that the needs of their unique students and curricula are met.

- **Image Bank.** The image bank features selected textbook images.

- **BodyAnimat3D.** Integrated 3D animations help students visualize the most difficult concepts, with pre-and post-assessment questions for every animation.

Need help? Contact the Digital Care Support Team

Visit our Digital CARE Support Website at www.mhhe.com/support . Browse the FAQs (Frequently Asked Questions) and product documentation and/or contact a sales representative. The Digital CARE Support Team is available Sunday through Friday.

HOW TO TEACH MEDICAL TERMINOLOGY

The **Online Course for Instructors to Support** *Medical Language for Modern Health Care* is found in the Instructor Resources section of the Online Learning Center, www.mhhe .com/allanmedlanguage3e.

The **How to Teach Medical Terminology online course** provides instructors with the introductory knowledge and resources they need to begin using the *Medical Language for Modern Health Care* textbook and related materials effectively. This course is designed to cover the "basics" of how to teach medical terminology effectively.

The How to Teach Medical Terminology online course allows instructors to choose for themselves which module they wish to take, or they may opt to take a self-assessment survey that will recommend one of the three modules.

- **Module 1** is designed for the inexperienced instructor.

- **Module 2** is designed for the instructor who has previous classroom experience but has never taught medical terminology.

- **Module 3** is designed for the experienced medical terminology instructor who has not previously used a contextualized approach to teaching the subject.

Upon completion of a given module, instructors will take a final assessment designed to demonstrate their understanding and achievement of the learning objectives for that module. Those who score 70% or higher on the final assessment will receive a certificate that can be printed for professional development purposes.

Learning Medical Language

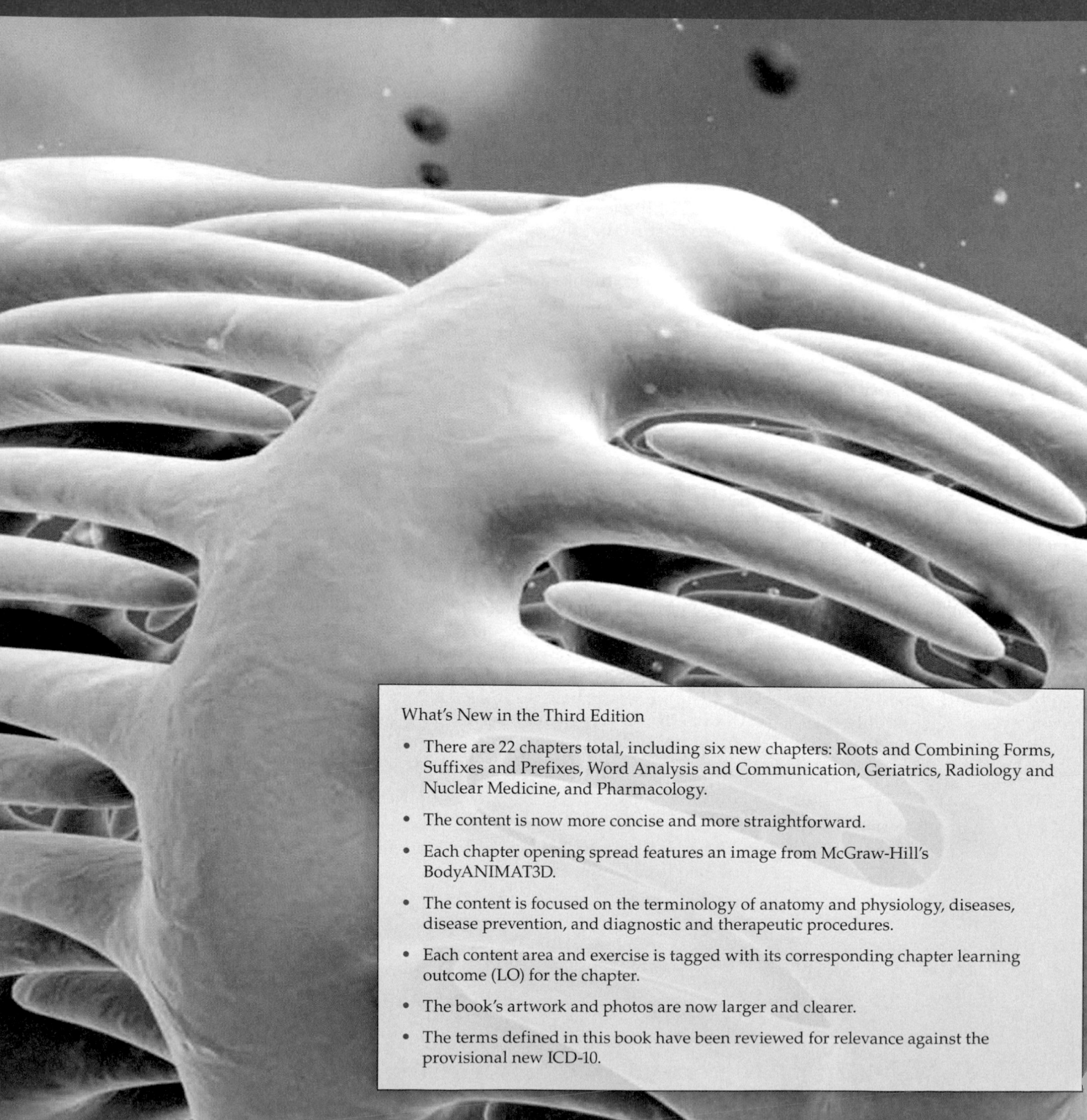

What's New in the Third Edition

- There are 22 chapters total, including six new chapters: Roots and Combining Forms, Suffixes and Prefixes, Word Analysis and Communication, Geriatrics, Radiology and Nuclear Medicine, and Pharmacology.

- The content is now more concise and more straightforward.

- Each chapter opening spread features an image from McGraw-Hill's BodyANIMAT3D.

- The content is focused on the terminology of anatomy and physiology, diseases, disease prevention, and diagnostic and therapeutic procedures.

- Each content area and exercise is tagged with its corresponding chapter learning outcome (LO) for the chapter.

- The book's artwork and photos are now larger and clearer.

- The terms defined in this book have been reviewed for relevance against the provisional new ICD-10.

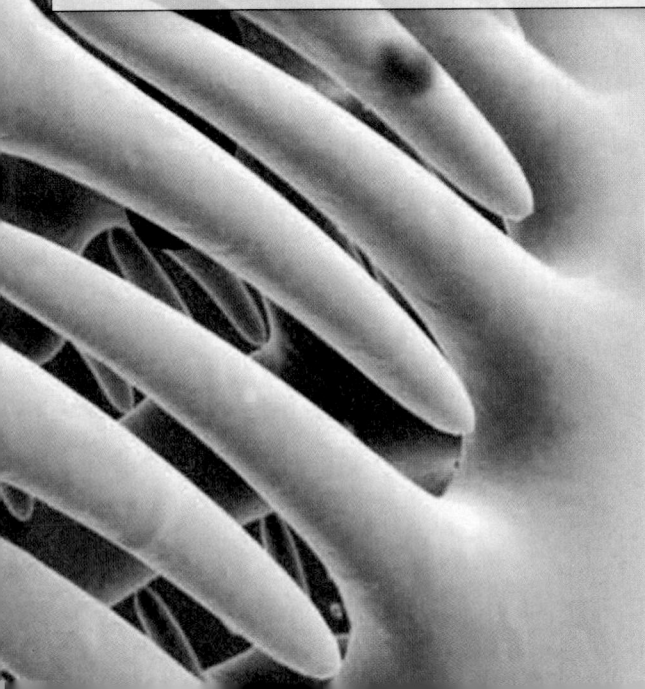

Case Report (CR) W.1

You are

. . . a student preparing for a career as a health professional. As part of your training program, you must complete a supervised **externship**. You have just arrived at Fulwood Medical Center for your first day as an **extern**. You are glad to have this opportunity: Fulwood is a busy medical center with highly skilled, compassionate staff members. Between attending classes at night, working during the day, and raising two children, you have a full schedule. However, the knowledge and skills you are learning in your studies, and at Fulwood, will prepare you for a successful future.

The abbreviation LO stands for a chapter learning outcome or goal that can be achieved by a learner during the chapter. Each LO will be linked to appropriate major headings on each page of text.

Welcome

Chapter Learning Outcomes

Your journey through this book, and your externship at Fulwood Medical Center, begins with getting to know the surroundings in which you will experience medical language.

In order to get the most out of your experience, you need to be able to:

LO W.1 Establish a commitment to learn medical terminology.

LO W.2 Recognize the knowledge and skills you will need to be an active learner.

LO W.3 Understand how the contextual approach of this book promotes active learning.

LO W.4 Differentiate the roles of the various members of a health care team in different medical specialties.

LO W.5 Utilize the pedagogic devices used in each chapter and lesson.

LO W.6 Use the vivid illustrations, photos, and tables in the book to help you understand the concepts being taught.

LO W.7 Describe the importance of effective organizational strategies and study habits.

LO W.8 Understand how a commitment to lifelong learning can enhance your professionalism.

The information in this lesson will enable you to:

W.1.1 Understand the reasons for learning medical terminology in order to communicate and document information effectively as a health professional.
W.1.2 Describe the conceptual approach used in the book and how it motivates your learning.
W.1.3 Understand the concept and structure of a health care team.
W.1.4 Determine how to be an active learner and how to actively experience medical language.

LO W.1, W.2 Why You Should Learn Medical Terminology

Medical terminology is not just another subject for which you memorize the facts and then forget them when you move on to your next course. Medical language will be used throughout your studies, as well as every day on your job. Nothing you hear or read in your studies or in a health care setting will make sense without an understanding of medical terminology. Once you learn medical language, however, the world of health care is open to you to explore—and be included as a health professional.

Even beyond your career goals, everyone becomes a patient at one time or another. You may also accompany an elderly parent, friend, or child to a doctor or emergency room. Knowing medical terminology makes it easier for you to communicate with physicians and use the Internet to research health information—and ultimately to become a proactive medical consumer.

Figure W.1 shows an electronic report of a patient's condition, which is something you must be able to understand as a health professional. Terms like **dyspnea**, **pleuritic**, **effusion**, and **neutrophils** are used every day in medical language.

Health care professionals use specific terms to describe and talk about objects and situations they encounter each day. Like every language, medical terminology changes constantly as new knowledge is discovered. For example, in the world of genetics, the terminology used today was unheard of a decade ago. Medical terms quickly become outdated as new information makes its debut. **Consumption** is now known as **tuberculosis**, **grippe** as **influenza**, and **whooping cough** as **pertussis**.

Modern medical terminology is an artificial language constructed over centuries, using words and elements from Greek and Latin origins as its building blocks. Some 15,000 or more words are formed from 1,200 Greek and Latin roots. It serves as an international language, enabling medical scientists from different countries and in different medical fields to communicate with a common understanding.

In your world as a health care professional, medical terminology enables you to communicate with your team leader, with other health care professionals on your team, and with other professionals in different disciplines outside your team. Understanding medical terminology also enables you to translate the medical terms into language your patients can understand, thus improving the quality of their care and demonstrating your professionalism.

In short, if you can't speak the language, you can't join the club *(Figure W.2)*.

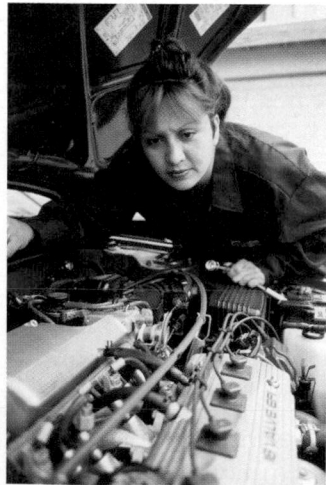

▲ **Figure W.2** Every profession has its own language. For instance, you may have difficulty understanding your auto mechanic when she tells you that the expansion valve, evaporator core, and orifice tubes in your air-conditioning system need to be replaced.

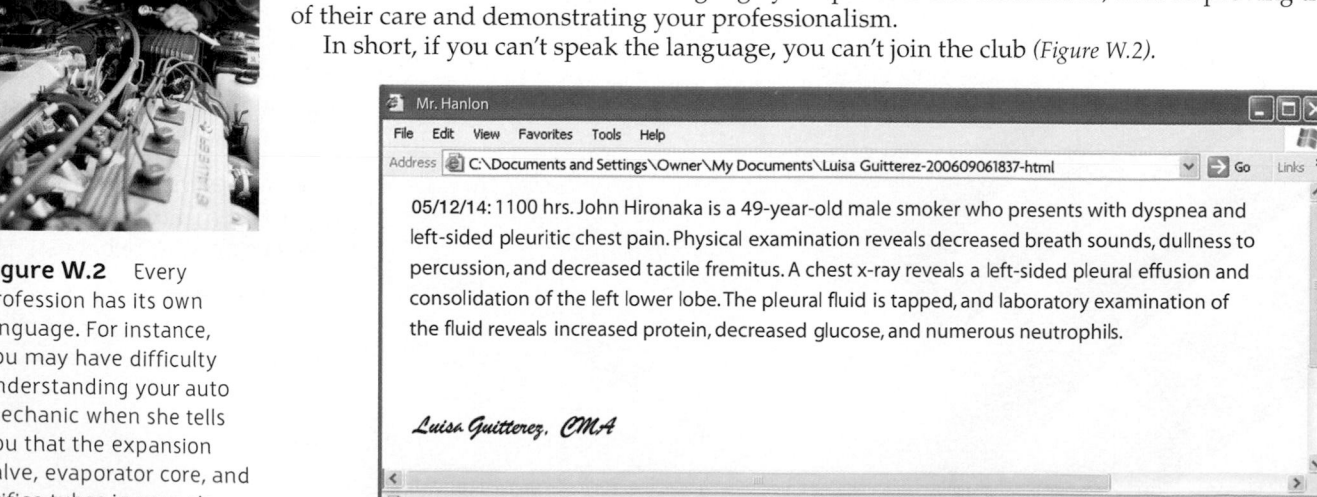

05/12/14: 1100 hrs. John Hironaka is a 49-year-old male smoker who presents with dyspnea and left-sided pleuritic chest pain. Physical examination reveals decreased breath sounds, dullness to percussion, and decreased tactile fremitus. A chest x-ray reveals a left-sided pleural effusion and consolidation of the left lower lobe. The pleural fluid is tapped, and laboratory examination of the fluid reveals increased protein, decreased glucose, and numerous neutrophils.

Luisa Guitterez, CMA

▲ **Figure W.1** Electronic Report of a Patient's Condition.

LO W.3 The Contextual Approach to Learning

When medical terms are separated from their intended context, as they are in other medical terminology textbooks, it is easy to lose sight of how important it is to use them accurately and precisely. Learning medical terminology in the context of the medical setting reinforces the importance of correct usage and precision in communication.

In every chapter and lesson in this book, the learner steps into the role of a health professional working in a situation that is relevant to the medical specialty associated with the body system being studied in that chapter. You will learn the medical terminology used in that medical specialty and body system through the context of anatomy and physiology, pathology, and therapeutic and diagnostic procedures and tests.

Patient case reports and documentation are used to illustrate the real-life application of medical terminology in modern health care, to care for and communicate with patients and to interact with other members of the health care team.

Fulwood Medical Center is the realistic health care setting in which these interactions take place. It consists of a medical office building and an attached 250-bed hospital. The office building houses physicians practicing primary care, the major medical and surgical specialties, and some complementary medicine therapies—in all, nearly 100 physicians in 25 specialty areas. The hospital and the medical offices share pharmacy, laboratory, radiology, physical therapy, health education, and cafeteria facilities, but they have separate main entrances. A directory on the wall near the hospital lobby lists all the departments and doctors and their locations *(Figure W.3)*.

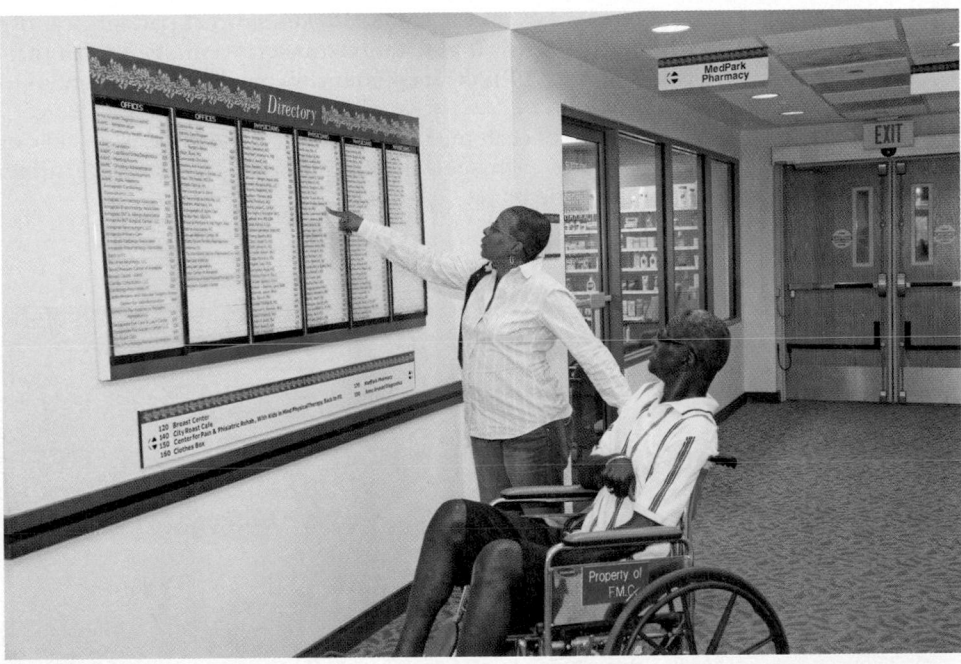

▲ **Figure W.3**   An office directory can help orient visitors within the medical office complex.

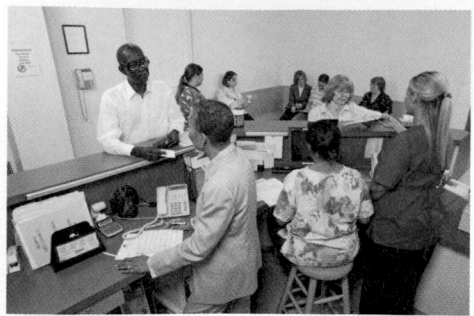

▲ **Figure W.4** A busy medical practice at Fulwood Medical Center.

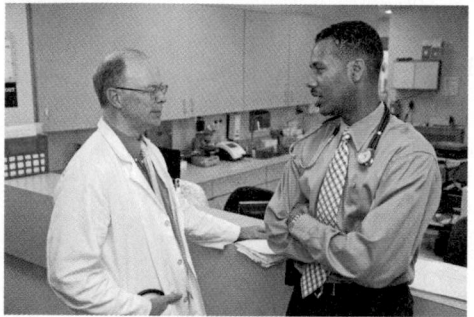

▲ **Figure W.5** A primary care physician refers patients to specialists when necessary.

LO W.4 The Health Care Team

A variety of health professionals make up the teams caring for patients in each medical specialty. As a **health professional**, you are part of a team of medical and other professionals who provide health care services designed to improve patients' health and well-being in each medical specialty and setting *(Figure W.4)*.

The team leader is a medical doctor, or physician, who can be an **MD** (doctor of medicine) or a **DO** (doctor of osteopathy). Most **managed care systems** require the patient to have a **primary care physician (PCP)** *(Figure W.5)*. This PCP, who may be a **family practitioner**, **internist**, or **pediatrician** (a doctor for children), is responsible for the overall care of the patient. In managed care delivery systems, such as Health Maintenance Organizations (HMOs) and Preferred Provider Organizations (PPOs), the PCP acts as the gatekeeper for the patient to enter the system, supervising all care the patient receives.

If needed medical care is beyond the expertise of the PCP, the patient is referred to a medical specialist *(Figure W.5)*, whose expertise is based on a specific body system or even a part of a body system. For example, a **cardiologist** has expertise in diseases of the heart and vascular system, a **dermatologist** specializes in diseases of the skin, and an **orthopedist** specializes in problems with the musculoskeletal system. A **gastroenterologist** is an expert in diseases of the whole digestive system, whereas a **colorectal surgeon** specializes only in diseases of the lower gastrointestinal tract.

Other health professionals work under the supervision of the physician and provide direct care to the patient *(Figure W.6)*. These can include a **physician assistant**, **nurse practitioner**, **medical assistant**, and, in specialty areas, different therapists, technologists, and technicians with expertise in the use of specific therapeutic and diagnostic tools.

Still other health professionals on the team provide indirect patient care *(Figure W.7)*. These include **administrative medical assistants**, **transcriptionists**, **health information technicians**, **medical insurance billers**, and **coders**, all of whom are essential to providing high-quality patient care.

As you study the language of each medical specialty at Fulwood Medical Center, you will also meet the members of each specialty's health care team and learn more about their roles in caring for the patient.

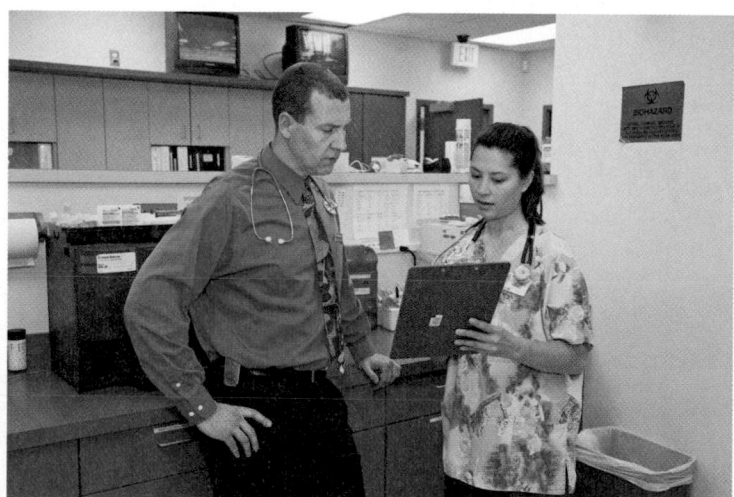

▲ **Figure W.6** Physicians, nurses, and medical assistants provide direct care to patients.

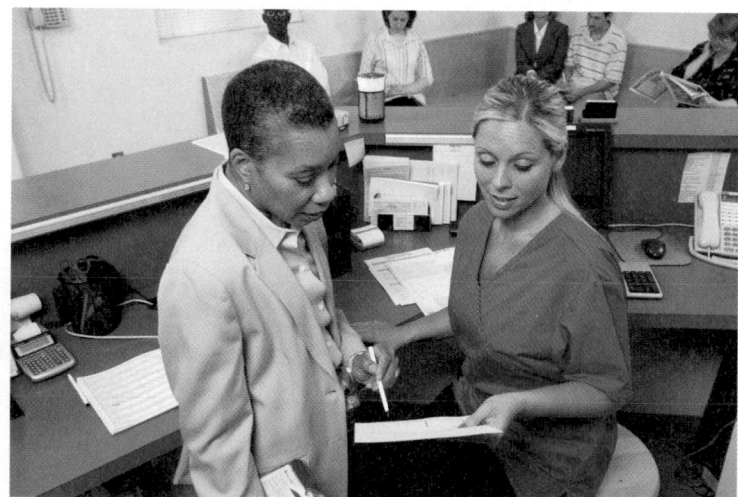

▲ **Figure W.7** Administrative medical assistants are among the health professionals who provide indirect care to patients.

LO W.2, W.3, W.5 Actively Experiencing Medical Language

Medical terms provide health care professionals a way to communicate with each other and document the care they provide. To provide effective patient care, all health care professionals must be fluent in medical language. One misused or misspelled medical term on a patient record can cause errors that can result in injury or death to patients, incorrect coding or billing of medical claims, and possible fraud charges. The patient care record is a legal document as well as a clinical document.

When the medical terms are separated from their intended context, as they are in other medical terminology textbooks, it is easy to lose sight of how important it is to use these medical terms accurately and precisely. Learning medical terminology in the context of the medical setting reinforces the importance of correct usage and precision in communication.

During your time at Fulwood Medical Center, you will *experience* medical language. Just as in a real medical center, you will encounter and apply medical terminology in a variety of ways. Actively experiencing medical language will help ensure that you are truly learning, and not simply memorizing, the medical terms in each chapter. Memorizing a term allows you to use it in the same situation (for example, repeating a definition) but doesn't help you apply it in new situations. Whether you are reading chart notes in a patient's medical record or a description of the treatment prescribed by a physician, you will see medical terms being used for the purpose they were intended.

This book goes beyond simply presenting and defining new medical terms. Fulwood Medical Center, with its wide range of patient cases and health professionals and its realistic medical environment, allows you to encounter and discover terms the way they are used in real life—in different medical settings. Experiencing medical language in this context bridges the gap between what you learn in the classroom and what really happens in the clinical setting.

As you progress through this book,

- You will encounter, and be asked to interact with, patients and health care professionals.

- You will analyze medical records and documentation.

- You will be introduced to diagnostic and therapeutic methods and the pathophysiology of disease.

- You will be able to see how all of these activities depend on effective communication, accurate comprehension, and precise use of medical language.

LO W.2, W.3, W.5 Actively Experiencing Medical Language (continued)

Below are just a few of the ways you will use medical language on your first day at Fulwood.

Listening and Speaking

You will

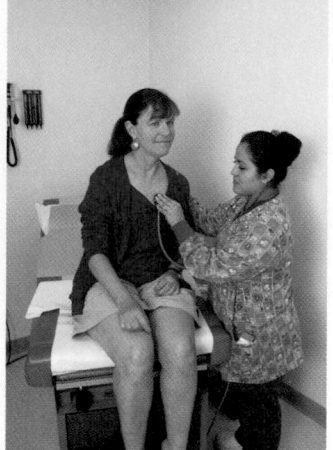

▲ **Figure W.8**   A CMA interviews a patient to learn more about her condition.

- Listen to patients as they describe their medical history and explain their symptoms *(Figure W.8)*. A conversation between Luisa Guitterez, a Certified Medical Assistant (CMA), and Mrs. Martha Jones, a patient, follows:

  Luisa Guitterez, CMA: "Mrs. Jones, I'm Luisa, an assistant to Dr. Lee. The receptionist noticed that you were looking pale and sweaty and notified Dr. Lee."

  Mrs. Jones: "In the rush to get here this morning, Luisa, I didn't have time to eat breakfast. I'm not feeling so well right now. . . . I'm diabetic, you know."

  Luisa Guitterez, CMA: "Dr. Lee has asked me to test your blood sugar level. As a diabetic, you've done this many times yourself, I'm sure."

- Listen to and carry out physicians' instructions and information concerning patient care.

- Speak to physicians and other health care professionals, report information, and ask questions.

- Talk with patients in the course of patient encounters and phone calls, including giving instructions and answering questions about the physician's prescribed treatment plans.

- Document your interaction with the patient.

Reading

You will

- Read physicians' comments and treatment plans in patient medical records and case reports.
- Read the results of physical examinations, procedures, and laboratory and diagnostic tests *(Figure W.9)*.

Writing

You will

- Document actions taken by yourself and other members of the health care team *(Figure W.10)*.
- Proofread medical documentation to ensure its accuracy.

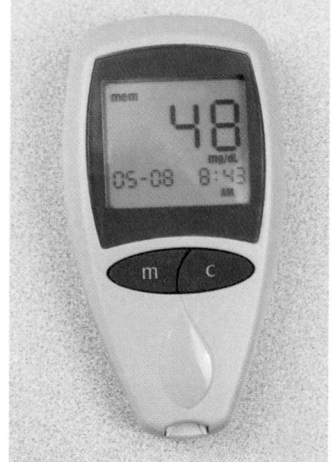

▲ **Figure W.9**   One of your responsibilities may be to read the results of diagnostic tests, such as this blood sugar reading.

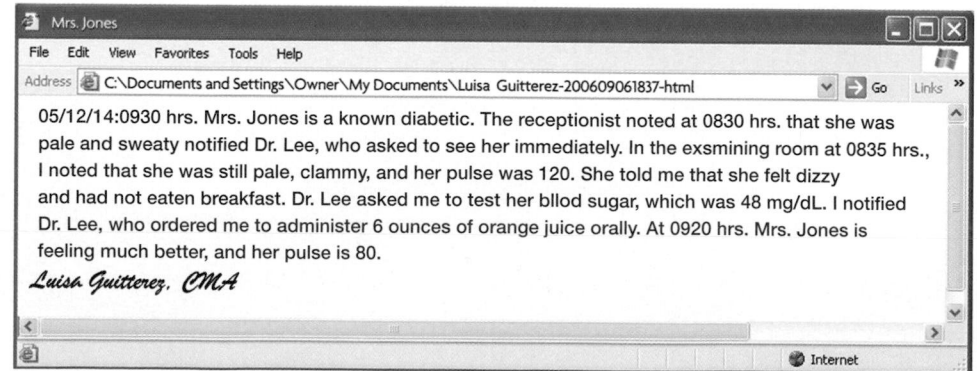

05/12/14:0930 hrs. Mrs. Jones is a known diabetic. The receptionist noted at 0830 hrs. that she was pale and sweaty notified Dr. Lee, who asked to see her immediately. In the exsmining room at 0835 hrs., I noted that she was still pale, clammy, and her pulse was 120. She told me that she felt dizzy and had not eaten breakfast. Dr. Lee asked me to test her bllod sugar, which was 48 mg/dL. I notified Dr. Lee, who ordered me to administer 6 ounces of orange juice orally. At 0920 hrs. Mrs. Jones is feeling much better, and her pulse is 80.

Luisa Guitterez, CMA

▲ **Figure W.10**   It is important to proofread documentation to ensure its accuracy.

Thinking Critically

You will

- Evaluate medical documentation for accuracy *(Figure W.11)*.
- Translate technical medical communication into words patients can understand.
- Analyze and understand unfamiliar medical terms using the strategies presented in this book.

Learning from Patient Cases

You will encounter realistic patient cases throughout this book. These cases ask you to step into the role of a health care professional *(You are . . .)* and focus on a real patient with real health care needs *(Your patient is . . .)*.

Taking full advantage of the patient cases in this book allows you to

- Experience various health care careers.
- Examine the roles you may fill to provide care for patients.
- See the types of documentation needed in these situations.
- Become acquainted with medical terminology in real-life settings.

Applying What You Learn

Throughout each chapter, you will be asked to apply and practice what you are learning. These application opportunities are designed to help you practice using medical terms in a variety of ways and for a variety of purposes. Specifically, the exercises will require you to perform tasks you would perform on the job, such as *listening and speaking, reading, writing,* and *thinking critically*. They are designed to help you move beyond simple memorization and become fluent in the language of modern health care.

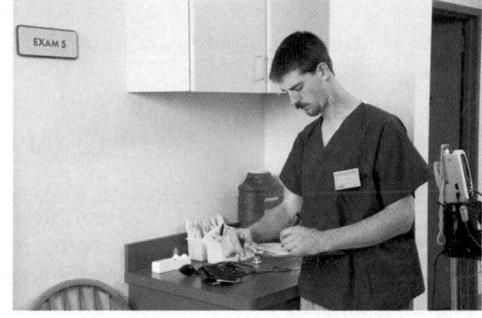

▲ **Figure W.11** Your knowledge of medical terminology will help you understand your patients' medical records.

Exercises

A. Each encounter with medical language improves your ability to (a) understand the medical terms you hear, (b) speak accurately and precisely using medical terms, (c) write accurately and precisely using the appropriate medical terms, (d) read and understand medical terms, and (e) think critically about the medical terms you experience. *These five skills are very important for all health care professionals. It is important to be able to identify experiences that build your knowledge and skill with medical language. Write the letter of the skill or skills being used in each blank below. More than one skill may be needed for each activity.* **LO W.2**

Skills:

    a. Understand spoken medical terms.

    b. Speak accurately and precisely with medical terms.

    c. Write accurately and precisely with medical terms

    d. Read and understand medical terms.

    e. Think critically about medical language.

_____   **1.** Answering a patient's questions about the physician's diagnosis and instructions.

_____   **2.** Taking a phone message when a specialist calls from another facility and has information concerning one of the patients of a physician in your facility.

_____   **3.** Proofreading an insurance claim form.

_____   **4.** Teaching a patient with special nutritional needs how to modify her diet.

_____   **5.** Using the Internet and textbooks to learn more about a disease or condition.

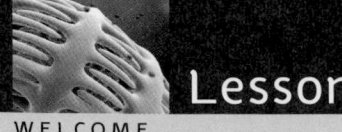

Lesson W.2 Learning Medical Language

WELCOME

LESSON OBJECTIVES

The information in this lesson will enable you to:

W.2.1 Identify the need for continual, lifelong learning among health professionals.

W.2.2 Assemble study strategies and habits to enhance your learning and test-taking capabilities.

W.2.3 Detail the pedagogic aids in the book.

W.2.4 Explain how the pedagogic aids enhance your understanding of the material.

W.2.5 Understand how to access and use the tools and features of McGraw-Hill Connect Plus.

Keynote

As novelist Lillian Smith once said, *"When you stop learning, stop listening, stop looking and asking questions, always new questions, then it is time to die."*

"I don't think much of a man who is not wiser today that he was yesterday." Abraham Lincoln

LO W.8 Lifelong Learning

No matter where you are in your life's journey—an infant trying to walk, a child beginning school, an adolescent working in your first job, a parent changing a diaper, an adult watching television, a grandparent playing with your grandchild—every day provides numerous opportunities for learning. If you actively absorb each piece of learning as it becomes available, you form a foundation on which you can build your continually increasing body of knowledge and experience *(Figure W.12)*.

Your current training in medical terminology is necessary for you to be able to continue your education in health care, but school is just one of the many places where you acquire knowledge. Each time you solve a problem in life, such as working through an argument with a friend or helping your child perform better in school, the knowledge you gain is *your own* answer to *your own* problem. This type of knowledge—discovered through experience—is genuine, real, and trustworthy for you. It is not determined by some distant authority, like what you learn in school. Your medical terminology instructor isn't likely to ask a test question on how to unclog your sink. Instead, this type of learning is driven by your needs and goals. The knowledge you gain from solving your own problems, whether by yourself or with the help of other people or resources, motivates you to learn even more and helps you grow as a person and as a professional.

When you are working as a health care professional, your ongoing education is an integral and inseparable part of your work activities. You'll need additional classroom training to keep your skills and professional knowledge up to date. You'll also continue to learn on your own through experience. As a health care professional, every time you interact with a patient, read a report, or talk with your team leader or peers, you are given another opportunity to learn.

Everything you do in life results in learning. Your own experience and judgment become your most valuable resources to make your life vivid, strong, creative, and, ultimately, what *you* want it to be. Take advantage of these resources, and use them to maximize your professional and personal success.

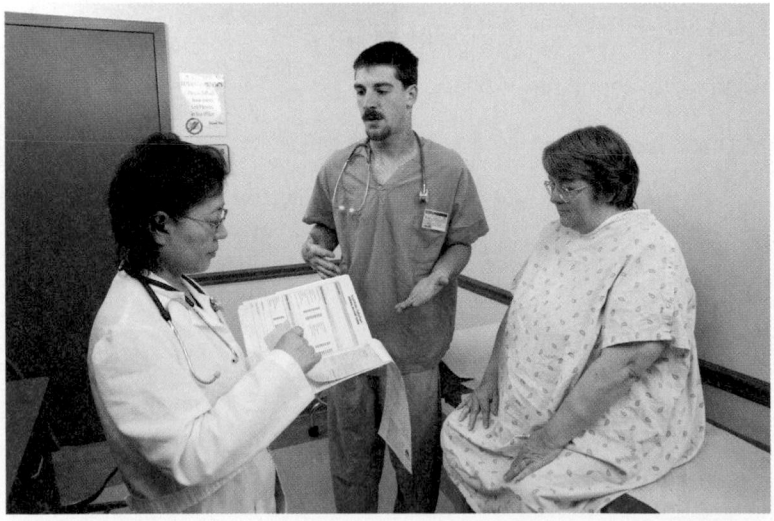

▲ **Figure W.12** Learning doesn't stop when you leave the classroom; every time you interact with other health care professionals and patients, you have the opportunity to learn something.

Case Report W.1 (continued)

Your first day at Fulwood Medical Center went very well. The supervisor, Rosana Rice, gave you a tour of the facilities and introduced you to several health care professionals with whom you will be working. Ms. Rice discussed your duties and her expectations of you, and she asked you to review your plan for keeping up with your studies. Now it's late evening, and you have yet to feed your kids and get them into bed—not to mention pick up around the house, pay bills, and, oh yes, review a whole chapter in your medical terminology textbook to prepare for a test in class tomorrow night. How are you going to get everything done?

LO W.7 Study Strategies and Habits

- Recognize the stresses you are under *(Figure W.13).*
- Determine what you can change because the situation, people, and events are making excessive demands on you.
- Prioritize your schedule in your head or on paper and handle each task in the proper order of importance.

In this case, eat a healthy meal with your kids, enjoy putting them to bed, pay the bills, and then take some deep breaths to relax (or meditate) for 10 minutes. When you feel more relaxed, settle down to review the text, and then go to bed at a reasonable hour. Picking up around the house will have to wait, since studying and sleeping are a higher priority. Sound too easy? What other choices can help you study in an effective way?

- Find ways to give yourself a break from stressful situations.

If you know you have a test every Thursday night, ask your spouse, mother, sister, or friend or someone in your support group to take care of the children on Wednesday night so you can get to a quiet place and dedicate the evening to studying. A support group of family and friends is essential to your success, so look for ways to surround yourself with people you can trust and rely on.

This lesson contains strategies that will help you get focused. It will help you learn how to manage your time and your studies to succeed—but this lesson can't do it alone. You are what you put into your studies. You have a lot of time and money invested in your education. Don't waste it by putting in half the effort. Succeeding in this class, and in life, requires the following:

- Committing with your time and perseverance to learning
- Knowing and motivating yourself
- Getting organized
- Scheduling and managing your time
- Being an active learner

The rest of this lesson will help you learn how to be effective in these areas. As you encounter new learning situations during your externship at Fulwood, you will be prepared to handle them.

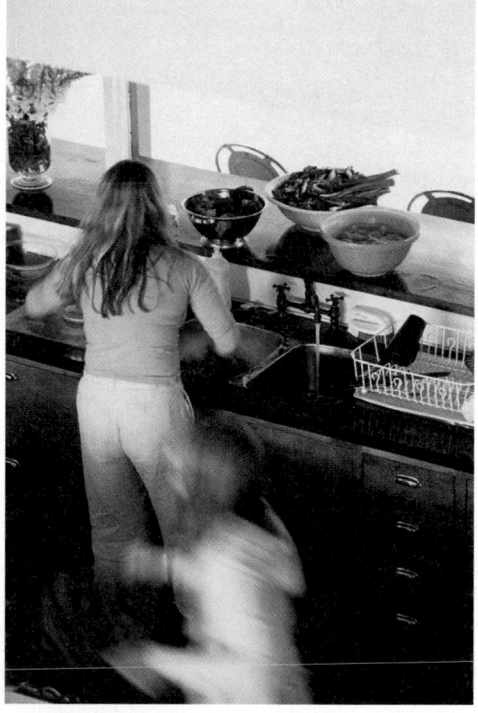

▲ **Figure W.13** An evening at home.

Keynote

A few years of committed study time now is nothing compared to the lifetime that awaits you.

Exercises

A. Reflect on the idea of lifelong learning and how you can make it work for you to enrich your life's experience. *Think about one instance in your life when something you learned (by yourself, from another person, from research, etc.) became the foundation upon which you built further learning and information. Some examples are how to paint a room, clean a fish, use a computer, and cook a meal. Briefly describe that here.* **LO W.9**

1. What I learned, and how I learned it: _____

   _____

2. Now describe why you need to be committed to learning from everyday experiences on the job, and explain how that can help you in your career.

   _____

   _____

LO W.8 Study Strategies and Habits (continued)

Committing Yourself to Learning: Your Time and Perseverance

Understanding—and mastering—what you learn in the classroom and during your externship at Fulwood Medical Center will take time and patience. Nothing worthwhile comes easily. Be committed to your studies, and you will reap the benefits in the long run. Consider this: Your training in health care is the foundation of your future career. If the foundation is poorly built, it will lead only to difficulties later.

Knowing and Motivating Yourself

What type of learner are you? When are you most productive? Know yourself and your limits, and work within them *(Figure W.14)*. Know how to motivate yourself to give your all to your studies and achieve your goals. You are the one who benefits most from your success. If you lack self-motivation and drive, you are the first person who suffers.

Know yourself. Just as there are many types of learners, there is no right or wrong way of learning. In which of the following categories do you see yourself?

Visual learner. You respond best to seeing processes and information. Take advantage of the strengths of your learning style by doing the following:

- Focus on text illustrations and charts, as well as course handouts.
- Check to see if there are animations on the course or text website to help you.
- Consider drawing diagrams in your notes to illustrate concepts.
- Use the contextual and labeling exercises at McGraw-Hill Connect Plus.

Auditory learner. You work best by listening to processes and information. Take advantage of the strengths of your learning style by doing the following:

- Listen carefully to—and possibly tape record (with instructor permission)—the lecture.
- Talk information through with a study partner.
- Listen to audio pronunciations of terms at McGraw-Hill Connect Plus.

Tactile/kinesthetic learner. Hands-on learning works best for you. Take advantage of the strengths of your learning style by doing the following:

- Apply what you have learned in a role-play or realistic scenario.
- Think of ways to apply your critical thinking skills in application-based ways.
- The Online Learning Center and McGraw-Hill Connect Plus will also help you.

In addition to these suggestions, here are a few helpful hints for students of all learning styles:

- Ask questions to make sure you understand what you hear, read, and do.
- Rephrase what you have heard in lectures and read in the text as you talk with your peers.
- Study with a partner to help you stay committed and double-check your understanding of concepts.

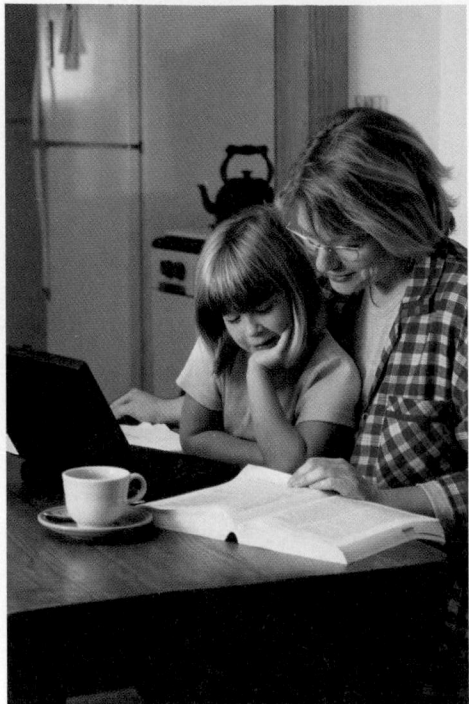

▲ **Figure W.14** Identify your own personal preferences for learning, and seek out the resources that will best help you with your studies. Recognize your weaknesses, and try to compensate for or work to improve them.

Getting Organized

It seems the more organized you are, the easier things come. This will definitely be the case as you proceed through this class and your externship at Fulwood. Take time now to look around and analyze your life and your study habits. Get organized now, and you'll find you have a little more time—and a lot less stress.

Find a calendar system that works for you. The best kind is one that you can take with you everywhere. To be truly organized, you should integrate all aspects of your life into this one calendar—school, work, family, and leisure *(Figure W.15)*. Some people also find it helpful to have an additional monthly calendar posted in a convenient place (for example, on the refrigerator) for "at a glance" dates and to have a visual of what is to come. If you do this, be sure you are consistently synchronizing both calendars so that you do not miss anything. (More tips for organizing your calendar can be found in the following Scheduling and Managing Your Time section.) Some sample entries follow:

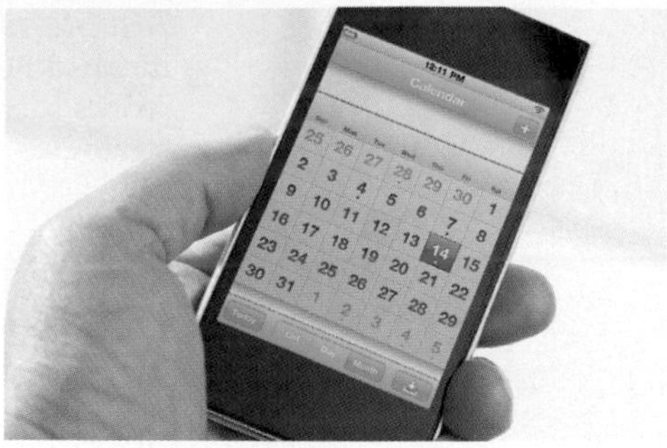

▲ **Figure W.15** Use a daily planner to help you organize school, work, family, and leisure time.

Thursday

- Work from 8:00 a.m. to 3:30 p.m.
- Doctor's appointment from 4:00 to 4:45
- Dinner from 5:15 to 6:15
- Class from 6:30 to 9:30
- Study from 10:00 to 10:30

Keep everything for your course or courses in one place—and at your fingertips. A three-ring binder works well because it allows you to add or organize handouts and notes from class in any order you prefer. Incorporating your own custom tabs helps you flip instantly to the material you need.

Find your space. Find a place that helps you be organized and focused. If it is a desk or table at home, keep it clean. Clutter adds confusion and stress, and it wastes time. If there are small children in your home, be sure your study materials are kept out of their reach. If your study space is at the library or a relative's house, keep a backpack or bag fully stocked with your text, binder or notes, pens, highlighters, sticky notes, phone numbers of study partners, and anything else you might need.

Scheduling and Managing Your Time

There is never enough time in the week to get everything done, and managing your time is one of the most difficult tasks to successfully master. Valuable time slips through your fingers so easily. Here are just a few ways time slips away unnoticed:

- **Procrastination**—putting off tasks simply because you don't feel in the mood to do them right away.
- **Distraction**—getting sidetracked by the endless variety of other things that seem easier (or more fun) to do.
- **Underestimating the value of small bits of time**—thinking it isn't worth doing any work because you have something else to do, or someplace else to be, in 20 minutes or so.

Just as you make choices about where to spend your money and how to get the best value for your dollar, you do the same with your time *(Figure W.15)*. In order to get the most out of your externship at Fulwood Medical Center and out of your life in general, you have to spend your time wisely. You may be able to save money for future use, but you *can't* store away time to use later. However, you *can* plan how you will spend your time in a way that maximizes the quality and the quantity of things you can get done in a day, week, month, or year. If you're like most people, you may not have a good idea of how your time is actually being used.

Keynote

We all lead busy lives, but we all make choices as to how we spend our time. Choose wisely, and make the most of every minute you have.

Exercises

A. Take time to assess your learning style, and use that to aid your study and classroom habits. *Identify the type of learner you are, and briefly describe which of the strengths in that style work best for you.* **LO W.5**

1. I am a _____ learner.

2. This works best for me:

_____

_____

_____

Ten Steps to a Study Schedule That Works   Making a study schedule you will actually follow means knowing yourself and your limits. Implement the following tips to develop a schedule that works for you. Or, if success in the class is not important to you, skip to the next section containing strategies for guaranteeing failure.

1. **Study when you are most productive.** When are you most productive? Are you a night owl or an early bird? Plan to study when you are most alert and can have uninterrupted segments of time. This could include a quick 5-minute review before class or a 1-hour problem-solving study session with a friend.

2. **Create a set study time for yourself daily.** Having a set schedule means making a commitment to studying. Write your study time on your calendar, and do not schedule other activities during this time.

3. **Schedule study time using shorter, focused blocks with small breaks.** Studying a little each day rather than cramming the night before a test is a much more effective use of your time. Doing this helps you learn the material and store it in your long-term memory, not just memorize it and forget it after the test. Also, you will be less fatigued and less likely to procrastinate.

4. **Plan time for family, leisure, friends, exercise, and sleep.** Studying should be your main focus, but you need to balance your time—and your life.

5. **Log your projects and homework deadlines.** Record all due dates, tests, and projects in your personal calendar so that you know what is coming. If you have a large writing project, break the assignment down into smaller targets. Set a goal for the first draft, second draft, and final copy, and record each of these deadlines in your calendar.

6. **Try to complete tasks ahead of schedule.** This will give you a chance to carefully review your work before you hand it in. You'll feel less stressed in the end.

7. **Prioritize.** In your calendar or planner, highlight or number key projects. Do them first; then cross them off when they are completed. Give yourself a pat on the back for getting them done.

8. **Review and reprioritize daily.** Check your scheduled activities each day, and adjust them if priorities have changed.

9. **Resist distractions.** Don't let unscheduled activities take you away from designated study time. The Internet is a notorious time-waster. It is easy to lose hours surfing the Web or instant messaging. It's just as easy to let a 5-minute phone call with a friend turn into a 3-hour conversation. Stick to your schedule.

10. **Multitask when possible.** You may find a lot of extra time you didn't think you had. Review material or deconstruct medical terms in your head while walking to class, while doing laundry, or during "mental down time." (*Note:* Mental down time does *not* mean in the middle of a lecture.)

LO W.7 Study Strategies and Habits (continued)

How To Set Yourself Up for success

1. Don't skip class and always be be on time.

2. Allow enough time to study. Schedule studying on your calendar so you won't run out of time right before a test or assignment.

3. Get a good night's sleep.

4. Ask questions and participate in class. If you have a question, someone else probably does, too.

5. Take advantage of instructor office hours. If you are an online student, be sure to contact your instructor when you need additional assistance.

6. Exam preparation should be an ongoing activity. Make sure you complete your homework, and take advantage of online activities that will enhance the learning process.

7. The learning outcomes at the beginning of every chapter summarize what you must understand by the end of that chapter. Use the book and digital resources to ensure you understand the chapter material.

8. Take notes in class. Your instructor will often provide tips for remembering difficult concepts or alert you to what will be on your exams.

Good luck on your journey to mastering the language of medicine!

Study Hints

Use previous quizzes and tests as study materials. Be certain you find out the correct answer for each question you answered incorrectly. Learn from your mistakes. These questions may appear on the final exam in one form or another.

As a way to review before a test, write 10 sample questions that might appear on the test. Ask your study partner or study group to write their 10 questions. Compare questions, and try to answer every question correctly. Subject matter that you have all included in a sample question is probably important enough to be on the test.

Keynotes

Additional points to remember about your study schedule:

- Be realistic when planning—know your limits and priorities.
- Be prepared for the unexpected (child's illness, your illness, overtime at work, inclement weather), which will leave any well-planned schedule in shambles.
- Reprioritize daily on the basis of schedule disruptions and other conflicts.
- Keep the overall picture in mind, and set long- and short-term goals (what you need to get done this week, this month, before the end of the semester, and so on).
- Form a support group.

Exercises

A. Be honest with yourself and self-assess. *Are you guilty of any of the self-defeating tendencies described earlier? If so, determine to change at least one bad habit before this course begins.* **LO W.7**

1. The habit I would most like to change is

_____

2. I recognize that if I change this habit, the *benefit* to me will be

_____

Remember: Your instructor puts time and effort into preparing this class and marking tests. You need to devote your time and energy to the class as well.

Being an Active Learner

As you will find out in your externship at Fulwood Medical Center, true learning is active. You can't sit back and let someone else pour knowledge into your head. You need to play the various health care professional roles you'll assume at Fulwood and work to get as much from them as you can. Simply attending your medical terminology class is another valuable thing you can do to help yourself. However, it doesn't end there. Here are more ways you can be an active learner and get the most out of your studies.

Getting the Most Out of Lectures

1. **Prepare.** You'll be amazed at how much easier it is to understand the material when you have previewed the chapter before going to class. If you find it difficult to carve out the time, simply arrive at class 5 to 15 minutes earlier than usual and skim the chapter before the lecture begins. This will at least give you an overview of what may be discussed.

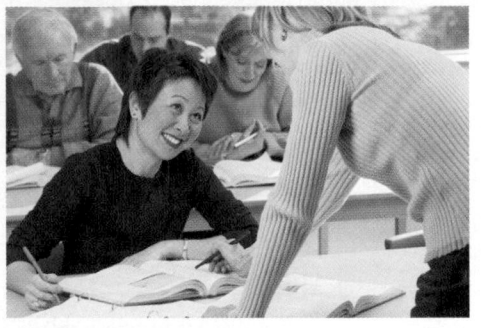

▲ **Figure W.16** Being a good listener is important to success.

2. **Be a good listener.** Most people think they are good listeners, but few really are *(Figure W.16)*. Are you?
   - You can't listen if you are talking or text messaging or looking at your cell phone.
   - You can't listen if you are daydreaming or dozing.
   - Listening and comprehending are two different things. If you don't understand something the instructor is saying, ask a question or jot a note and visit the instructor after class. Don't feel intimidated: You probably aren't the only person who "doesn't get it."

3. **Take good notes.** Here are some tips for successful note-taking:
   - Use a standard-size notebook or, better yet, a three-ring binder with loose-leaf paper. The binder will allow you to organize and integrate your notes and handouts.
   - Use a standard black or blue ink pen to take your initial notes. You can annotate later using a pencil, which can be erased if necessary.
   - Start a new page with each lecture or note-taking session.
   - Label each page of your notes with the date and a heading.
   - Focus on the main points, and try to use an outline format to take notes. This will help you capture key ideas and organize subpoints.
   - Review and edit your notes shortly after class—at least within 24 hours—to make sure they make sense. You may also want to compare your notes with those of a study partner later to make sure neither of you has missed anything.

Getting the Most Out of Reading

1. **Concentrate on what you are reading.** Survey the titles, outcomes, objectives, and headings in each chapter, and look at the visuals to identify what the chapter is all about.
2. **Use the SQ3R** (see the Study Hint) to help you read actively.
3. **Take notes on key ideas** in the reading.
4. **Write down any questions** you have.
5. **Discuss what you have read** with your study partner.

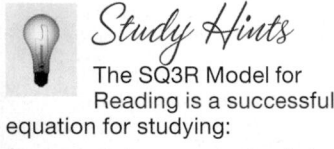

Study Hints

The SQ3R Model for Reading is a successful equation for studying:

Survey what you are going to read.

Question what you are going to learn after the preview.

Read—Read the assignment.

Recite—Stop every once in a while, look up from the book, and put what you've just read into your own words.

Review—After you've finished, review the main points.

LO W.7 Study Strategies and Habits (continued)

Performing Well on Tests

1. **Always read the directions.** If you are unsure, ask. Find out if there is a penalty for guessing. If there is not, try to answer every question on the test even if you have to guess at some.

2. **Before you begin, scan the entire test** so that you know how long it is and what types of activities and questions it contains.

3. **Answer the easy questions or sections first** so that you get as much of the exam finished as possible if difficult questions slow you down.
   - When answering multiple-choice questions, eliminate each incorrect option until you are left with the answer that seems most correct to you.
   - When answering matching questions, match all items you know first; then do your best with the ones that remain.
   - When answering essay questions, reword the question as a statement to be sure you have answered it. Give enough examples and explanation to support your points.

4. **Once you have finished the test, use any extra time to check that you have answered all questions.** If you still have time after checking for completion, reread the questions and recheck your answers.

Studying with a Partner or Group

1. **Get a study partner.** *Schedule fixed* study dates. Talk through the concepts, compare notes, and quiz each other. Studying with a partner can be fun. Think of it this way: You are multitasking, layering study time and social time. Just be sure the social time doesn't squeeze out the study time.

2. **Don't take advantage of your study partner.** If you can't make a study date or attend a class, let your partner know. You won't have a study partner—or a friend—much longer if it isn't a mutually beneficial arrangement.

3. **Establish a study group.** Choose a few students in the class, including your study partner, with whom to study on a regular basis. Having a group in addition to a study partner ensures that you will still be able to study with others if your partner has to miss a session.

Exercises

A. Budgeting your time is key to being able to take care of your priorities. *Follow these steps with the list of tasks you need to get done.* **LO W.7**

1. Rank each of the tasks in the table in order of its priority (e.g., 1 is the highest priority, 2 is next highest, and so on).

2. On a separate sheet of paper, plan a weekly schedule that will help you accomplish these tasks. Include all seven days of the week, and block off the days in hourly increments.

3. Keep in mind that while some activities have set times, others can be flexible. Also consider that activities like studying and household tasks will need to be done for a period of time *every day*, not just once a week.

   (*Note: There is no one "correct" answer to this exercise; however, it is beneficial to see how other students in the class chose to budget their time. Be creative but realistic. Don't forget to budget for travel time between tasks if needed.*)

Weekly Tasks

Studying for Medical Terminology _____	*Errands (groceries, etc.)* _____	*Leisure time* _____
Sleep _____	*Family time* _____	*Household chores* _____
Medical Terminology class (Tuesday and Thursday 6:30–9:30 p.m.) _____	*Work (8:00–3:30 daily)* _____	*Meals, including preparation & cleanup* _____
Church and/or hobbies _____	*Exercise* _____	*Grooming* _____

Now that you understand what it takes to be successful, you are ready to move through this textbook and engage in an externship at Fulwood Medical Center.

LO W.5, W.6 Innovative Learning Aids in this Book

Each chapter is structured around a consistent and unique framework of learning devices including vivid illustrations, photographs, specific content tables, Word Analysis and Definition (WAD) tables, Case Reports, and contextual placements. No matter what the subject matter of a chapter, the structure enables you to develop a consistent learning strategy, making *Medical Language for Modern Health Care 3e* a superior learning tool.

You Are . . . Your Patient Is

Each chapter opens by placing you in the role of a health professional related to the specialty and associated body systems and areas covered by the chapter. You are also introduced to a patient and given information about the patient's case.

Chapter Learning Outcomes

At the same time, **Chapter Learning Outcomes** let you know what you will learn in each chapter. This technique immediately engages you, motivating you to read on to learn how a particular patient's case (and the health care provider's role in the patient's care) relates to the medical terminology being introduced in the chapter.

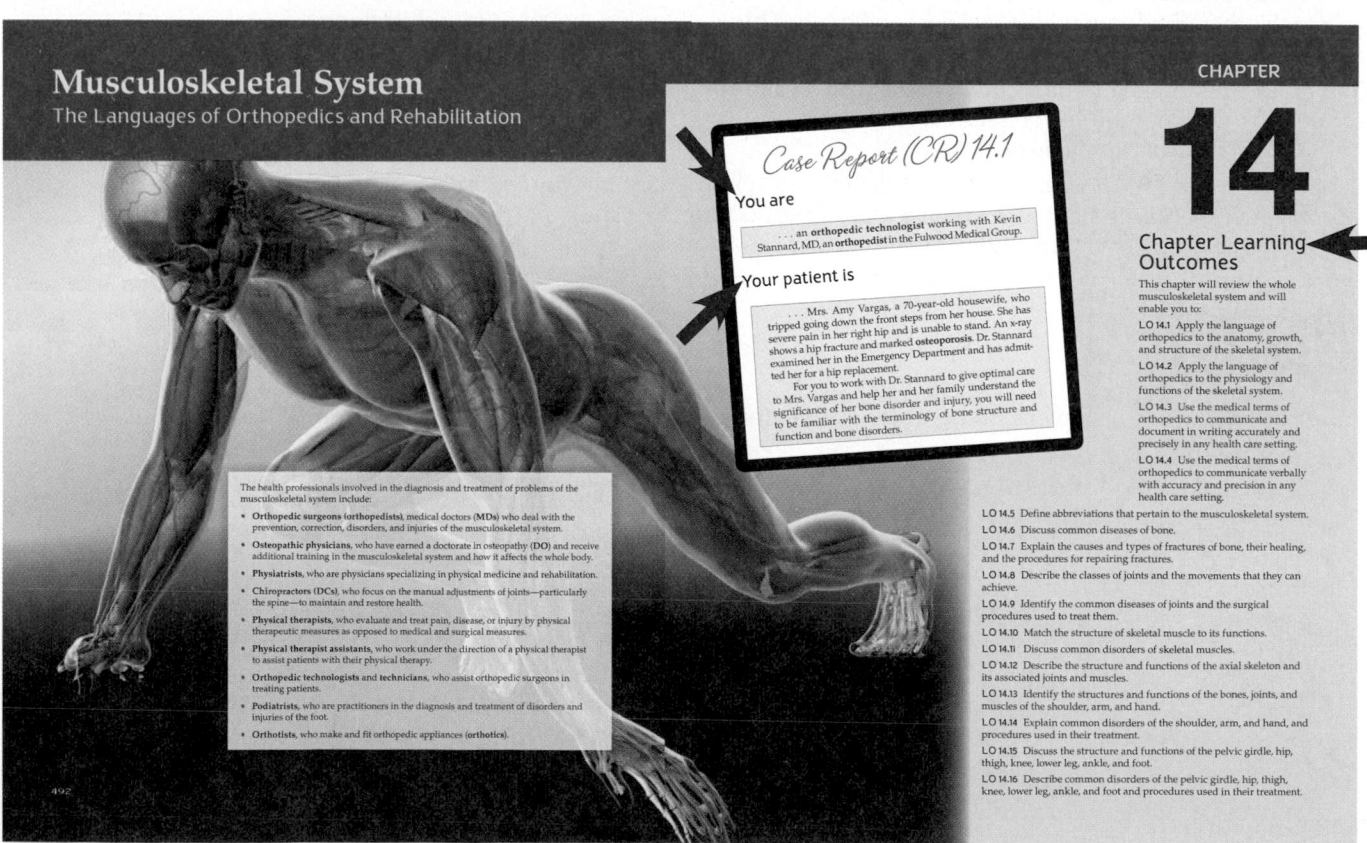

Lesson-Based Organization

The chapter content is broken down into chunks, or lessons, in order to help you digest new information and relate it to previously learned information. Rather than containing many various topics within a chapter, these lessons group the chapter material into logical, streamlined learning units designed to help you achieve the chapter outcomes. Lessons within a chapter build on one another to form a cohesive, coherent experience for the learner.

Each lesson is based on specific lesson **objectives** designed to support your achievement of the overall **chapter learning outcomes**. Each lesson in a chapter contains an introduction, lesson objectives, lesson topics, Word Analysis and Definition boxes, and lesson exercises. Within each lesson, all topics and information are presented in **self-contained two-page spreads**. This means you do not have to flip back and forth to see figures on one page that are described on another. Each section of information and every exercise are tagged with the appropriate chapter learning outcome (LO).

Word Analysis and Definition Boxes

The medical terms covered in each lesson are introduced in context, either within a patient case or in the lesson topics. To facilitate easy reference and review, the terms are also listed in boxes as a group. The **Word Analysis and Definition (WAD) boxes** list the term and its pronunciation, elements, and definition in a concise, color-coded, at-a-glance format.

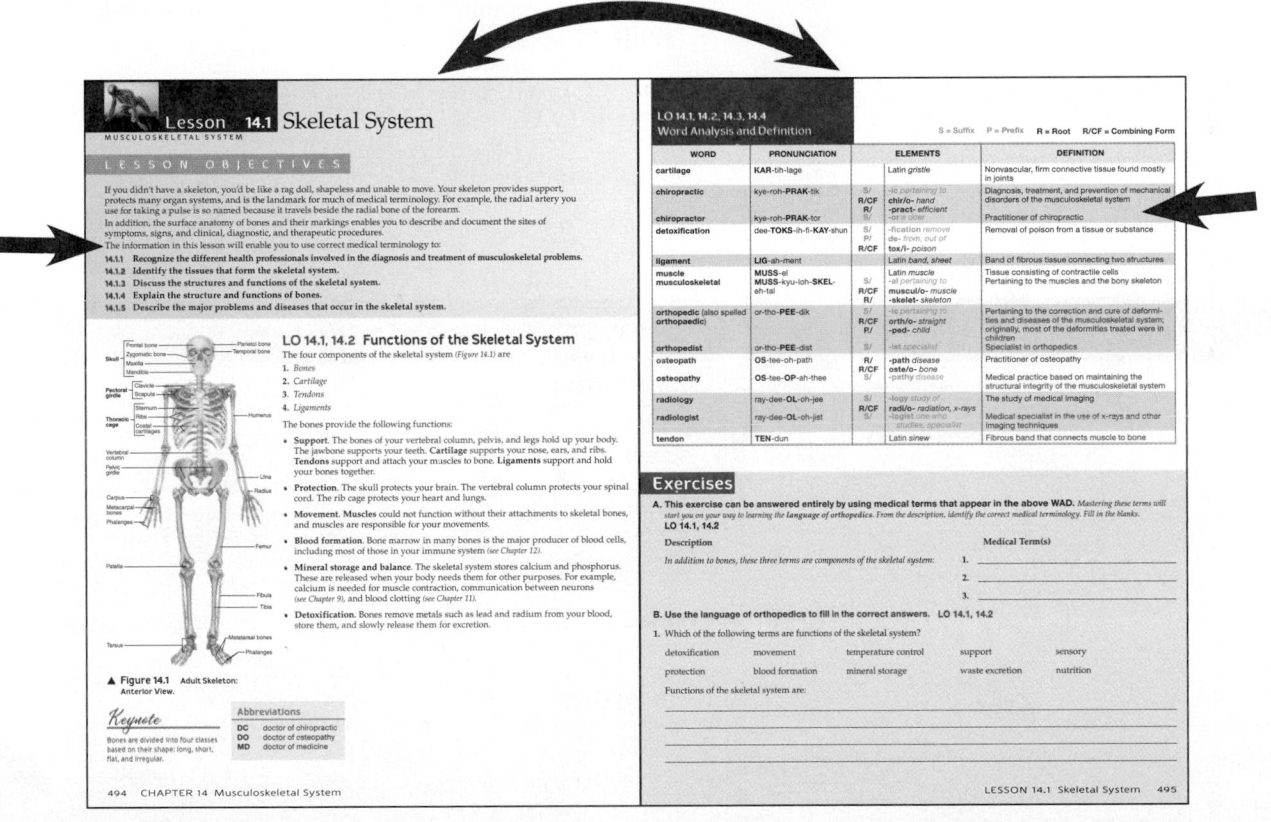

Exercises

A. Describe how lesson-based organization of the material will help you learn more efficiently.   LO W.5

1. _____

B. Detail how to use the chapter Learning Outcomes to develop a study outline for the chapter material.   LO W.5

1. _____

Exercises

A. After you deconstruct the following medical terms into their basic elements, provide a brief definition for each term. *Fill in the chart; then fill in the blanks at the end of the exercise.* The first one is done for you. **LO 14.2, 14.3, 14.7**

Medical Term	Prefix	Root/Combining Form	Suffix	Definition of Medical Term
reduction	*re*	*duct*	*ion*	*The restoration of a structure to its normal position*
alignment	1.	2.	3.	4.
malunion	5.	6.	7.	8.
hematoma	9.	10.	11.	12.

B. Demonstrate your understanding of the terms by finishing this exercise. *Refer to the chart in Exercise A for the answers to this exercise.* **LO 14.2, 14.3, 14.7**

1. Use *both* the terms **reduction** and **alignment** in *one sentence*.

   _____

   _____

2. The suffix **-oma** means *tumor* as well as *mass*. Briefly explain why a hematoma is not a tumor.

   _____

   _____

3. Explain the difference between a **malunion** and a **nonunion** of a fracture.

   malunion: _____

   _____

   nonunion: _____

   _____

LESSON 14.1 Skeletal System   501

LO W.6 Innovative Learning Aids (continued)

Spread and Chapter-End Exercises

Each spread ends with exercises designed to allow you to check your basic understanding of the terms you just learned. These checkpoints can be used by instructors as assignments or in-class activities or by students for self-evaluation.

At the end of each chapter you will find 10 to 14 pages of exercises that ask you to apply what you learned in all lessons of a chapter. These chapter-end exercises reinforce learning and help you go beyond mere memorization to think critically about the medical language you use. In addition to reviewing and recalling the definitions of terms learned in the chapter, you will be asked to use medical terms in new and different ways.

Study Hint Boxes

Study Hint boxes are found throughout the review exercises. They reinforce, and remind you to use, basic study skills.

O. Documentation. Case Report 6.3 presents all the information you need to fill out the HPI (History of Present Illness) form for the patient's medical record. *You are translating the patient's own words into medical terminology.* First read Case Report 6.3 about Mrs. Dobson; then read the questions you need to answer. This will help you to fill in the blanks in the HPI form. The last part of the exercise involves asking Mrs. Dobson additional questions you think will provide helpful information for the doctor. Use the correct medical term whenever possible, and be prepared to define each term you use. **(LO 6.3,** *Apply, Analyze)*

You are
...a medical assistant working in the office of Dr. Susan Lee, a primary care physician at Fulwood Medical Center.

Your patient is
...Mrs. Caroline Dobson, a 32-year-old housewife. You have asked her to describe the reason for her visit to the office today, 06/09/13.

Case Report 6.3
Patient Interview

Mrs. Dobson:

"Since yesterday afternoon I've had a lot of pain low down in my belly and in my lower back. I keep having to go to the bathroom every hour or so to pee. It's often difficult to start, and it burns as it comes out. I've had this problem twice before when I was pregnant with my two kids, so I've started drinking cranberry juice. I've been shivering since I woke up this morning, and the last urine I passed was pink. Was that due to the cranberry juice?"

What additional questions could you ask Mrs. Dobson that would provide helpful information for Dr. Lee?

1. _____

2. _____

P. Terminology challenge. Medical terminology is full of words that sound and look similar but have very different meanings. Think about the following terms, and explain in plain language how they are different. Notice that these two terms differ by only one letter—this is where precision comes in! Fill in the blanks. **(LO 6.3,** *Analyze)*

1. Reflex: _____

2. Reflux: _____

Q. Common denominator. Each of the following groups of terms has something in common. Your knowledge of the terminology and functional anatomy of the urinary system will help you determine the common denominator for each group. Fill in the blanks. **(LO 6.1, 6.2, 6.3, 6.11,** *Analyze)*

1. urination, micturition, voiding

   All are _____

2. ESWL, ureteroscopy, percutaneous nephrolithotomy

   All are _____

3. stress, urge, overflow, functional

   All are _____

Urinary System

R. Roots and combining forms. Form the foundation of a medical term. All these terms have the same suffix. Differentiate their meanings by analyzing the rest of the term. On the basis of the word part specify what each term means. Every one of these terms could be a diagnosis for your next patient. Fill in the blanks. **(LO 6.3, 6.7,** *Analyze)*

Medical Term	Meaning of Prefix	Meaning of Root/Combining Form	Meaning of Suffix	Meaning of Term
anuria	1.	2.	3.	4.
dysuria	5.	6.	7.	8.
glycosuria	9.	10.	11.	12.
hematuria	13.	14.	15.	16.
oliguria	17.	18.	19.	20.
proteinuria	21.	22.	23.	24.

Determine the meaning of these two terms after analyzing the rest of their elements.

25. If **py** means *pus*, then **pyuria** means _____

26. If **noct** means *night*, then **nocturia** means _____

S. Tests and procedures. Patients with urinary problems will be sent for various renal function tests and diagnostic procedures that may result in a surgical procedure. Any of the following procedures might be ordered for your patient. Do you know their purpose? Be prepared to discuss which terms are tests and which are procedures. **(LO 6.8, 6.11,** *Analyze)*

____ 1. Contrast material injected to locate stones	a. dialysis	
____ 2. Collection of bladder sample in newborns	b. transplant	
____ 3. Incision for removal of kidney stone	c. KUB	
____ 4. Crushing renal stone by sound waves	d. retrograde pyelogram	
____ 5. Assess blood flow to the kidneys	e. cystoscopy	
____ 6. Tissue bank matching of donor to recipient	f. nephrolithotomy	
____ 7. Treatment for renal cell carcinoma	g. nephrectomy	
____ 8. X-ray of the abdominal urinary organs	h. needle aspiration	
____ 9. Viewing the bladder through a scope	i. renal angiogram	
____ 10. Filtering blood through an artificial kidney machine	j. lithotripsy	

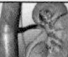

Study Hint
Create a study hint for yourself that will make it easy to remember exactly what an IVP is.

Write your hint here: _____

_____

LO W.7 Vivid Illustrations and Photos

Colorful, precise anatomical illustrations and photos lend a realistic view of body structures and correlate to the clinical context of the lessons.

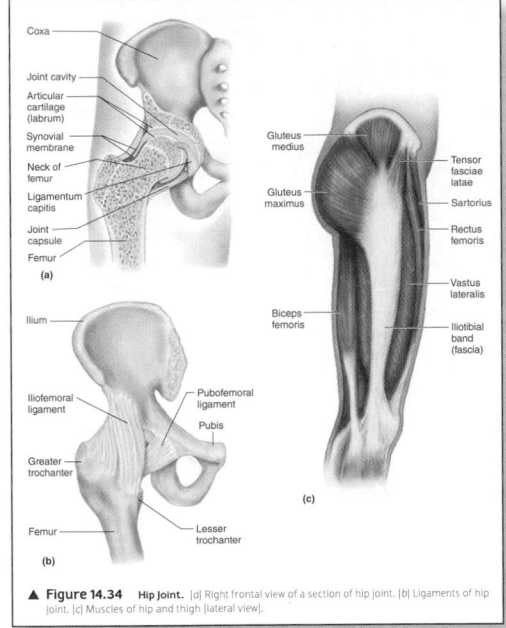

▲ **Figure 14.34** **Hip Joint.** [a] Right frontal view of a section of hip joint. [b] Ligaments of hip joint. [c] Muscles of hip and thigh (lateral view).

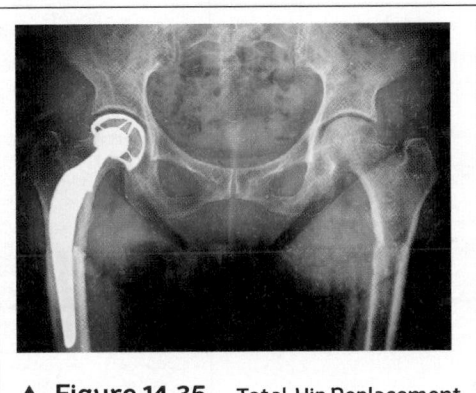

▲ **Figure 14.35** **Total-Hip Replacement.** Colored x-ray of prosthetic hip.

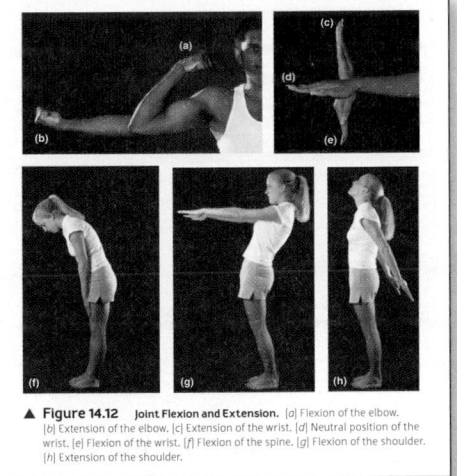

▲ **Figure 14.12** **Joint Flexion and Extension.** [a] Flexion of the elbow. [b] Extension of the elbow. [c] Extension of the wrist. [d] Neutral position of the wrist. [e] Flexion of the wrist. [f] Flexion of the spine. [g] Flexion of the shoulder. [h] Extension of the shoulder.

Exercises

A. Pick one of the photos above and explain how it helps you understand the material better. LO W.6

1. _____
_____
_____

B. Practice precision in medical terminology. *Choose any five terms in the illustration of the hip joint above. See the term, hear it, and write it down. Make sure you spell it correctly.* **LO W. 6**

1. _____

2. _____

3. _____

4. _____

5. _____

Tables

Meaningful tables aid in summarizing concepts and lesson topics.

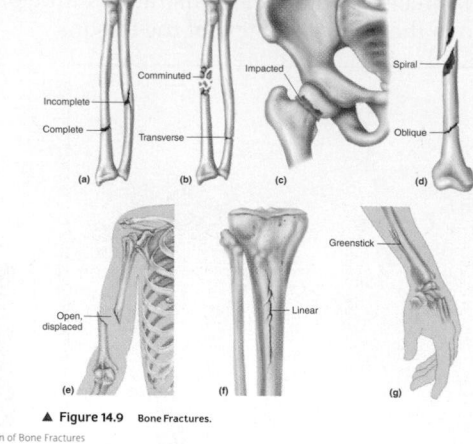

▲ Figure 14.9 Bone Fractures.

LO 14.7 **Table 14.1** Classification of Bone Fractures

Name	Description	Reference
Closed	A bone is broken, but the skin is not broken.	Figure 14.9a, b, c, d, f, and g
Open	A fragment of the fractured bone breaks the skin, or a wound extends to the site of the fracture.	Figure 14.9e
Displaced	The fractured bone parts are out of alignment.	Figure 14.9e
Complete	A bone is broken into at least two fragments.	Figure 14.9a
Incomplete	The fracture does not extend completely across the bone; it can be **hairline** (as in a stress fracture in the foot when there is no separation of the two fragments).	Figure 14.9a
Comminuted	The bone breaks into several pieces, usually two major pieces and several smaller fragments.	Figure 14.9b
Transverse	The fracture is at a right angle to the long axis of the bone.	Figure 14.9b
Impacted	One bone fragment is driven into the other, with resulting shortening of a limb.	Figure 14.9c
Spiral	The fracture spirals around the long axis of the bone.	Figure 14.9d
Oblique	A diagonal fracture runs across the long axis of the bone.	Figure 14.9d
Linear	The fracture runs parallel to the long axis of the bone.	Figure 14.9f
Greenstick (closed)	This is a partial fracture: one side breaks, the other bends.	Figure 14.9g
Pathologic	The fracture occurs in an area of bone weakened by disease (such as cancer). Also called stress fracture	—
Compression	The fracture occurs in a vertebra from trauma or pathology leading to the vertebra being crushed.	—

502   CHAPTER 14 Musculoskeletal System

Keynotes and Abbreviations

Keynote and Abbreviation boxes offer you additional information correlating with the lesson.

LO 14.1 Bone Growth and Structure

Factors that affect bone growth include:

1. **Genes.** Genes determine the size and shape of bones and the ultimate adult height.
2. **Nutrition.** Calcium and phosphorus are needed to develop good bone density.
3. **Exercise.** Exercise increases bone density and total bone mass.
4. **Mineral deposition.** Calcium and phosphate are taken from plasma and deposited in bone.
5. **Mineral resorption.** Calcium and phosphate are released from bone back into the plasma when they are needed elsewhere. For example, calcium is needed for muscle contraction, communication between neurons, and blood clotting. Phosphate is a component of deoxyribonucleic acid (DNA) and ribonucleic acid (RNA).
6. **Vitamins.** Vitamin A activates osteoblasts; vitamin C is essential for collagen synthesis; vitamin D stimulates absorption of calcium and phosphate, its transport, and its deposition into bones.
7. **Hormones.** For example, growth hormone stimulates the epiphyseal plate to calcify, and estrogen and testosterone accelerate bone growth after puberty and maintain bone density *(see Chapter 17)*.

LO 14.1, 14.2 Structure and Functions of Bones

Long bones are the most common type of bone in the body *(Figure 14.2)*.

The shaft of a long bone is called the **diaphysis**. Each end of the bone is called the **epiphysis** and is expanded to provide extra surface area for the attachment of ligaments and tendons.

Sandwiched between the diaphysis and epiphysis is a thin area called the **metaphysis**. Thin layers of cartilage cells in the **epiphyseal plate** enable the diaphysis (bone shaft) to grow in length. When growth stops, compact bone grows into the epiphyseal plate and forms the **epiphyseal line** *(Figure 14.2 b)*.

A tough connective tissue sheath called **periosteum** covers the outer surface of all bones and is attached to the compact or **cortical** bone by tough collagen fibers. The periosteum protects the bone and anchors blood vessels and nerves to the surface of the bone.

The hollow cylinder inside the diaphysis is called the **medullary cavity**. It contains bone **marrow** and is lined by a thin membrane called the **endosteum**. The marrow is a fatty tissue that contains blood cells in different stages of development *(see Chapter 11)*.

The endosteum and periosteum contain **osteoblasts**, cells that produce the matrix of new bone tissue. This process is called **osteogenesis**. Bone **matrix** consists of cells, collagen fibers, a gel that supports and suspends the fibers, and calcium phosphate crystals that give bone its hardness.

When osteoblasts are incorporated into the new bone, they become **osteocytes**. These cells, which maintain the matrix, reside in small spaces in the matrix called **lacunae**.

Osteoclasts are produced by the bone marrow. They dissolve calcium, phosphorus, and the organic components of the bone matrix. There is a continual balancing act going on as osteoclasts remove matrix and osteoblasts produce matrix. If osteoclasts outperform the osteoblasts, then **osteoporosis** occurs, as with Mrs. Vargas.

All bones are well supplied with blood *(Figure 14.3)*. The blood vessels travel through the bone in a system of small **haversian (central) canals**. Because of its good blood supply, bone heals well.

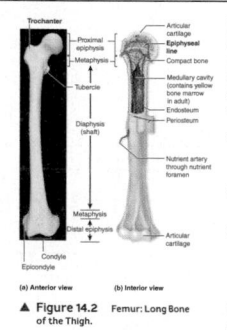

▲ Figure 14.2 Femur: Long Bone of the Thigh.

(a) Anterior view   (b) Interior view

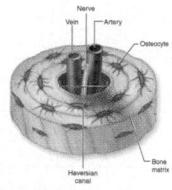

▲ Figure 14.3 Blood Supply to Bone.

Keynote

Minerals are deposited in bone when the supply is ample and released when they are needed elsewhere.

496   CHAPTER 14 Musculoskeletal System

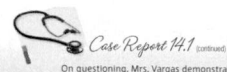

Case Report 14.1 (continued)

On questioning, Mrs. Vargas demonstrated many of the risk factors for osteoporosis, including a family history, lack of exercise, cigarette smoking, inadequate diet, postmenopause, and increasing age.

LO 14.6 Diseases of Bone

Osteoporosis results from a loss of bone density *(Figure 14.4)* when the rate of bone **resorption** exceeds the rate of bone **formation**. It is more common in women than in men, and its incidence increases with age. Ten million people in the United States already have osteoporosis, and 18 million more have low bone density **(osteopenia)** and are at risk for developing osteoporosis.

In women, production of the hormone estrogen decreases after menopause, and its protection against osteoclast activity is lost. This leads to fragile, brittle bones. In men, reduction in testosterone has a similar but less marked effect.

Women at risk for osteoporosis should have **bone mineral density (BMD)** screening using a dual-energy **x-ray absorptiometry (DEXA)** scan. Men and women over age 50 should take 1200 mg of calcium daily and 600 to 1,000 **international units (IU)** of vitamin D or expose the body to the sun for 15 minutes daily.

Several medications approved by the **U.S. Food and Drug Administration (FDA)** are available for the treatment of osteoporosis. Most inhibit osteoclast activity.

Osteomyelitis is an inflammation of an area of bone due to bacterial infection, usually with a staphylococcus. Untreated tuberculosis can spread from its original infection in the lungs to bones via the bloodstream to produce tuberculous osteomyelitis.

Osteomalacia, known as **rickets** in children, is a disease caused by vitamin D deficiency. When bones lack calcium, they become soft and flexible. They are not strong enough to bear weight and become bowed. Osteomalacia occurs in some developing nations and occasionally in this country when children drink soft drinks instead of milk fortified with vitamin D.

Achondroplasia occurs when the long bones stop growing in childhood but the bones of the axial skeleton are not affected *(Figure 14.5)*. This leads to short-stature individuals who are about 4 feet tall. Intelligence and life span are normal. It is caused by a spontaneous gene mutation that then becomes a dominant gene for succeeding generations.

Osteogenic sarcoma is the most common malignant bone tumor. Peak incidence is between 10 and 15 years of age; the tumor often occurs around the knee joint.

Osteogenesis imperfecta is a rare genetic disorder, producing very brittle bones that are easily fractured, often in utero (while inside the uterus).

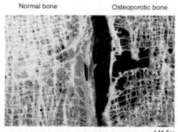

Normal bone   Osteoporotic bone

LM 5×

▲ Figure 14.4 Normal Bone and Osteoporotic Bone.

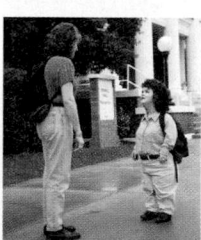

▲ Figure 14.5 Achondroplastic Dwarf with College Roommate.

Abbreviations

BMD	bone mineral density
DEXA	dual energy x-ray absorptiometry
FDA	U.S. Food and Drug Administration
IU	international unit(s)

498   CHAPTER 14 Musculoskeletal System

Notes

Roots and Combining Forms
The Language of Health Care

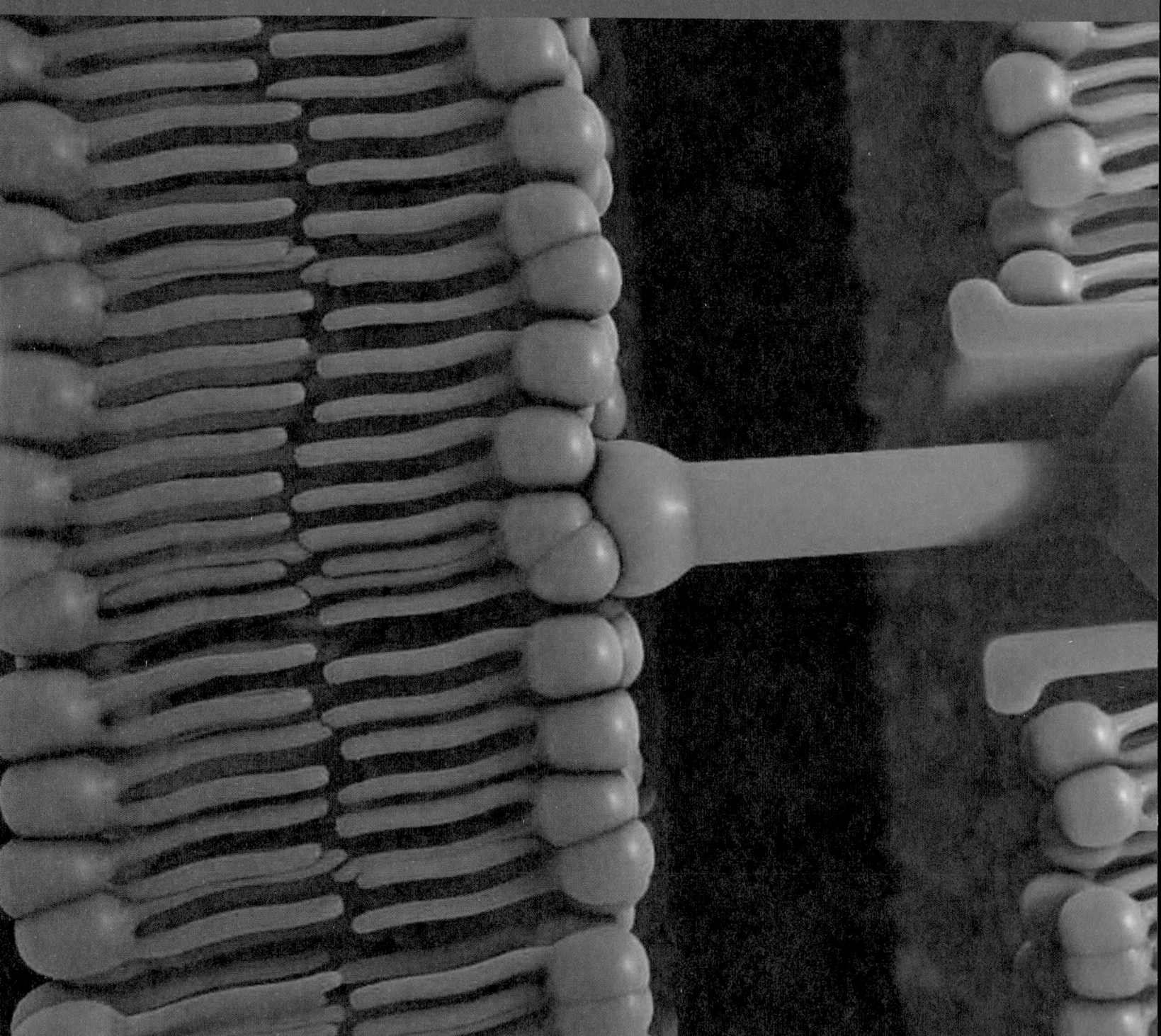

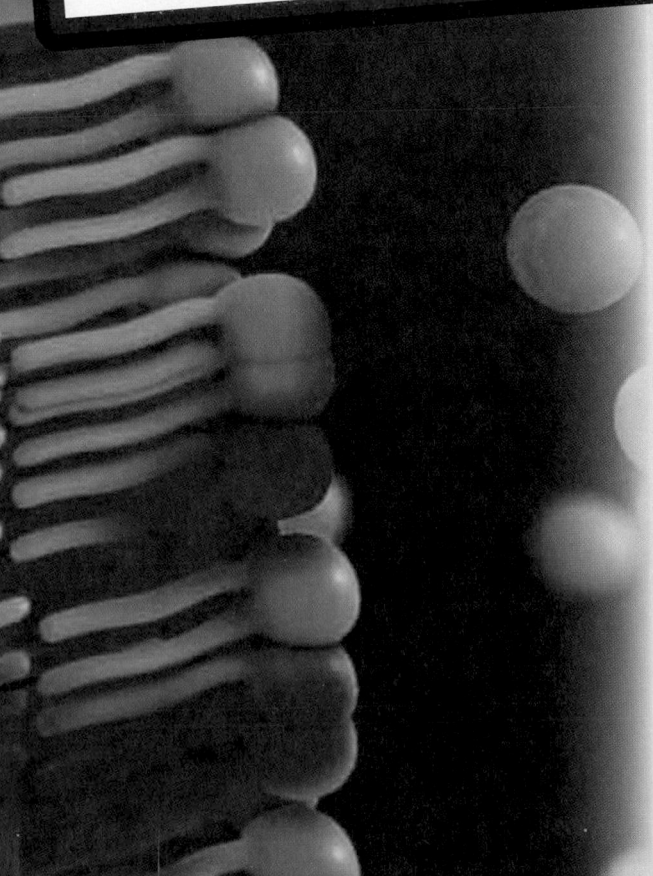

Case Report (CR) 1.1

You are

... a medical assistant working for Russell Gordon, MD, a primary care physician at Fulwood Medical Center.

Your patient is

... Mrs. Connie Bishop, a 55-year-old woman who presents with swelling in her lower abdomen, shortness of breath, and the production of clear mucus when she coughs. She has no gynecologic or gastroenterologic symptoms. Her previous medical history shows recurrent dermatitis of her hands since her teenage years and an arthroscopy for a knee injury at age 40. Physical examination reveals a circular mass 6 inches in diameter in the left lower quadrant of her abdomen. There is no abnormality in her cardiovascular system.

Your role is to maintain her medical record and document her care, assist Dr. Gordon during his examinations, explain the examination and treatment procedures to Mrs. Bishop, and enable Dr. Gordon to refer her to a specialist.

Chapter Learning Outcomes

Case Report (CR) 1.1 features several medical terms that illustrate how medicine has its own language. This language provides all the health professionals involved in the care of a patient with the ability to communicate with each other by using medical terms with precise meanings. To be a qualified health professional, you must be able to speak and write this language of medicine. If you can, you will be able to communicate with other health professionals and to document the care given to your patients. This chapter is designed to give you the information and tools you will need to:

LO 1.1 Relate the logic of the language of medicine to your practice as a health care professional.

LO 1.2 Define the terms *root, combining vowel,* and *combining form.*

LO 1.3 Recognize that **roots** and **combining forms** are the core elements of any medical term.

LO 1.4 Deconstruct medical terms into **roots** and **combining forms**.

LO 1.5 Interpret the meaning of **roots** and **combining forms** in commonly used medical terms.

LO 1.6 Use **roots** and **combining forms** to construct commonly used medical terms.

LO 1.7 Identify the medical terms taken directly from Greek or Latin words.

LO 1.8 Differentiate between medical terms that are spelled and/or pronounced similarly.

Lesson 1.1 Roots and Combining Forms

The technical language of medicine has been developed logically, mainly from Latin and Greek **roots**. The first steps to take to understand the language of medicine are to:

1.1.1 Describe the logic behind the terms used in the language of health care.

1.1.2 Select the root of each medical term.

1.1.3 Define the meanings of the roots of commonly used medical terms.

1.1.4 Define the terms *combining vowel* and *combining form*.

1.1.5 Construct combining forms for commonly used medical terms.

1.1.6 Identify the combining vowel and combining form of commonly used medical terms.

THE ELEMENTS OF A MEDICAL TERM ARE:

- prefix—the beginning of some words
- **root**—the foundation of the word that provides its meaning
- **combining vowel**—vowel that joins a **root** to another **root** or to a suffix
- **combining form**—combination of a **root** and a **combining vowel**
- suffix—the ending of some words

ROOTS:

- the constant, unchanging foundation of a medical term
- usually of Greek or Latin origin
- one or more is found in most medical terms

COMBINING VOWEL:

- has no meaning of its own
- joins a **root** to another **root**
- joins a **root** to a suffix
- makes a word easier to pronounce
- "o"—the most common **combining vowel**, with "a" as the next most common

LO 1.1, 1.2, 1.3, 1.5 Understanding the Logic of Medical Terminology

Understanding and being comfortable with the technical language of medicine are keys to a successful career as a health professional. Your ability to use language to communicate verbally and in writing is essential for patient safety, high-quality patient care, interaction with other health care professionals, and your own self-esteem as a health care professional.

Your confidence in using medical terms will increase as you understand the logic of how these terms are built from their individual parts, or **elements**. In addition, understanding the logic of this process will help you analyze, or "deconstruct," a medical term, break the term down into its elements, or its "anatomy," and also construct the elements into a whole to understand the meaning of a medical term.

The core element of any term is its **root**. You can use the following information about **roots** to help you understand Mrs. Bishop's Case Report 1.1 on the previous spread.

Nearly every medical term has at least one **root**, the element that carries the core meaning of the word. Ninety percent of all roots arise from Greek and Latin words, and many of them have been in use for over 2000 years. For example,

> **Gynecologic** uses the Greek root **gynec-**, meaning *female*.
>
> **Dermatitis** has the root **dermat-**, from the Greek word for *skin*.
>
> **Arthroscopy** has the root **arthr-**, derived from the Greek word for *joint*.
>
> **Respiratory** uses the root **respir-**, from the Latin word for *to breathe*.

Many words contain more than one **root**. For example, **gastroenterology** has the **root gastr-**, from the Greek word for *stomach* and the **root -enter-**, from the Greek word for *intestine*. The term means the medical specialty of the stomach and intestines. The term **pneumothorax** has the **root pneum-**, from the Greek word **pneuma**, meaning *air,* and the **root -thorax**, the Latin word for *chest*. The term means the *presence of air in the chest outside the lungs.*

Combining Vowels

You build medical terms on the foundation of a **root**. Adding a **combining vowel** to the end of a **root** joins that **root** to other word elements. This vowel has no meaning of its own. It is the vehicle that joins word elements to create medical terms. It also makes the word easier to pronounce. Creating medical terms is like assembling pieces of a jigsaw puzzle.

The vowel "**o**" is a **combining vowel**, as shown in gynecologist:

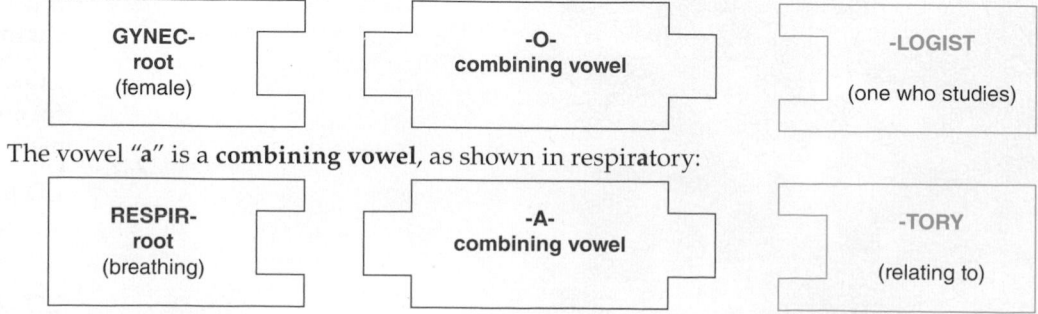

> *Study Hint*
>
> Some confusion might exist over the terms "to breathe" and "breath." *To breathe* (with the "e") is the verb/action term. When you breathe, you take a *breath* (which is the noun term). If you misspell either word in an answer, your response will be scored as incorrect.

GYNEC- root (female)	-O- combining vowel	-LOGIST (one who studies)

The vowel "**a**" is a **combining vowel**, as shown in respiratory:

RESPIR- root (breathing)	-A- combining vowel	-TORY (relating to)

"O" is the most common **combining vowel**. The vowels "a," "i," and "u" are used less frequently.

Some words have more than one **combining vowel**. Gastroenterology has two "o" **combining vowels** attached to different **roots**.

A combining vowel can be used to link two **roots** even when the second **root** begins with a vowel, as shown in gastroenterology:

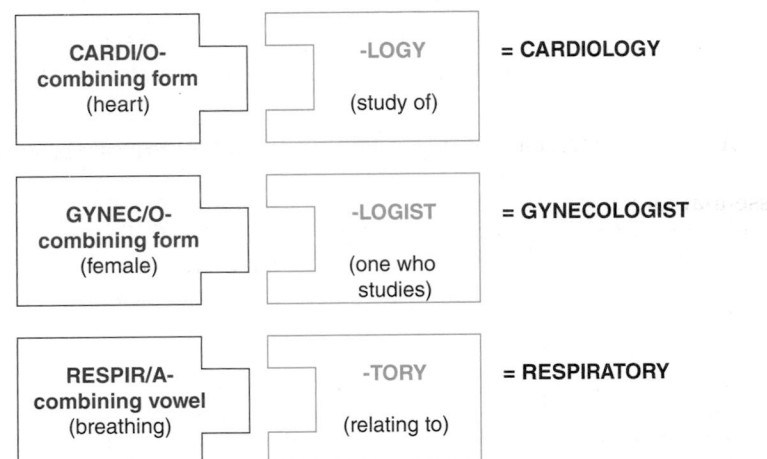

| GASTR-
root
(stomach) | -O-
combining vowel | -ENTER-
root
(intestine) | -O-
combining vowel | -LOGY
(study of) |

Combining Forms

A **root** with a **combining vowel** added to it is called a **combining form**. For example, the root **abd-**, the vowel "**o**," or **abd/o-**, meaning *belly*, is the **combining form** for the word, **abdomen (abd/o-men)**.

Examples of **combining forms** are

| CARDI/O-
combining form
(heart) | -LOGY
(study of) | = CARDIOLOGY |

| GYNEC/O-
combining form
(female) | -LOGIST
(one who studies) | = GYNECOLOGIST |

| RESPIR/A-
combining vowel
(breathing) | -TORY
(relating to) | = RESPIRATORY |

An example of a word that has two **combining forms** is **gastroenterology**, the elements of which can be pieced together like this:

| GASTR/O-
combining form
(stomach) | -ENTER/O-
combining form
(intestine) | -LOGY
(study of) | = GASTROENTEROLOGY |

Prefixes and **suffixes** are discussed in Chapter 2.

Keynote

A *gynecologist* is a medical specialist in the care of the female reproductive system. *Respiratory* means relating to respiration or breathing.

> COMBINING FORMS:
> - combines a **root** and a **combining vowel**
> - can be attached to another **root** or **combining form**
> - can precede a **suffix**

Keynote

Gastroenterology is the medical specialty concerned with the function and disorders of the stomach, intestines, and associated organs.

Keynote

When a medical term is being analyzed and broken down into its elements, a combining form will be shown with a / between the root and the combining vowel.

Exercises

A. The jigsaw pieces are your visual aid to understanding the logic of how elements form medical terms. *Number the puzzle pieces with each of the statements below that pertains to that part of the puzzle. Each puzzle piece will have several numbers. Fill in the blanks.* **LO 1.4, 1.5, 1.6**

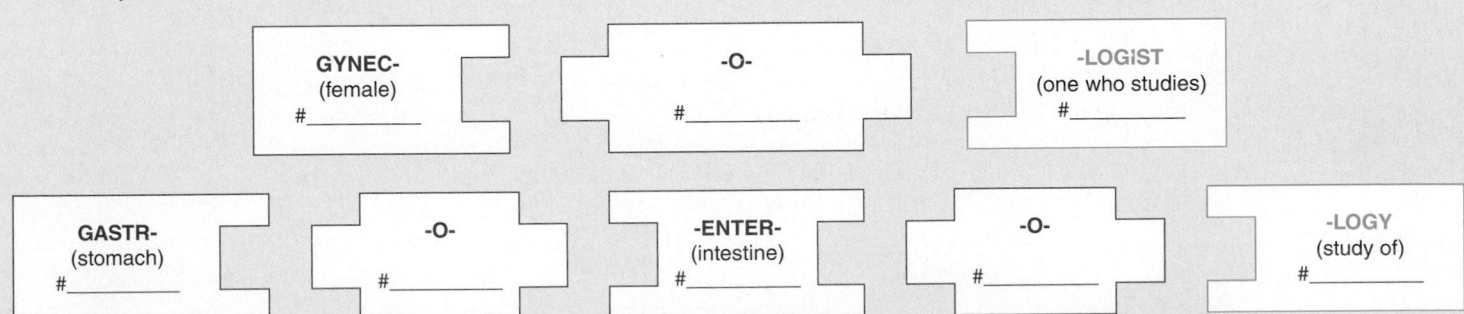

| GYNEC-
(female)
#_____ | -O-
#_____ | -LOGIST
(one who studies)
#_____ |

| GASTR-
(stomach)
#_____ | -O-
#_____ | -ENTER-
(intestine)
#_____ | -O-
#_____ | -LOGY
(study of)
#_____ |

Place the numbers of the following statements into the correct puzzle piece.

1. This piece is a root.
2. This piece is a combining vowel.
3. This piece is the end of the term, or the suffix.
4. This piece needs to be in every term.
5. This piece attaches to a root.
6. This piece comes before a suffix.
7. This piece has no meaning of its own.
8. This piece is usually of Greek or Latin origin.

LO 1.7 Greek, Latin, and Old English Words

Case Report 1.1, which describes Mrs. Connie Bishop's presentation, features several medical terms taken directly from Latin or Greek words or from Old English terms that do not break down (deconstruct) into word elements. Several of them are used in general language outside of medicine. These medical terms in Case Report 1.1 are:

- **patient,** an old English term meaning *to suffer* or *undergo*; the term refers to a person who is under medical or surgical treatment.

- **medical,** from a Latin term meaning *to heal*; it means *pertaining to the practice of medicine.*

- **breath,** an Old English word meaning *a single cycle of inhaling and exhaling.*

- **mucus,** a Latin word for *a clear, sticky secretion.*

- **knee,** an Old English word meaning *an angular shape*; today it refers to the **joint** (a Latin word for junction) between the upper and lower leg.

- **quadrant,** a Latin word meaning *a quarter*; the abdomen is divided into four *quadrants* by horizontal and vertical planes that intersect at the **umbilicus**, which is a Latin word for the navel or belly button.

- **record,** a Latin word meaning *to remember*; a medical *record* is a written account of a patient's medical history.

- **care,** an Old English word meaning *to worry*; when you care for your patients, you look after them and are concerned about them.

- **specialist,** a Latin word meaning *of a given species*; a *specialist* devotes professional attention to a particular subject area.

Other examples not used in Case Report 1.1 include:

- **apex,** a Latin word meaning *tip* or *summit* (as in Mount Everest); the apex of the heart is the downward pointing tip of the cone-shaped heart.

- **patent,** a Latin word meaning *open* or *exposed*; a *patent* blood vessel is open to the circulation of freely flowing blood.

- **toxin,** a Greek word meaning *poison*; a *toxin* is a poisonous substance formed by a cell, such as a bacterium.

- **lymph,** a Latin word meaning *clear spring water*; *lymph* is a clear, shimmering fluid collected from the body tissues.

- **breech,** an Old English word meaning *buttocks*; in obstetrics, a fetus is in a *breech* presentation when the buttocks, rather than the head, are the presenting part at delivery.

LO 1.8 Terms That Are Alike

Precision in both written and verbal communication is essential for a health professional, with great attention given to detail. There are many words in the medical language that are very similar to each other in both their spelling and pronunciation. Examples are

- **ilium**, pronounced **ill-ee-um**, a bone in the pelvis
- **ileum**, pronounced the same way, **ill-ee-um**, a segment of the small intestine

- **ureter,** the tube from the kidney to the bladder
- **urethra,** the tube from the bladder to the outside

- **trapezius,** a muscle in the back
- **trapezium,** a bone in the wrist

- **malleus,** a small bone in the middle ear
- **malleolus,** a bony protuberance at the ankle

- **neurology,** the study of diseases of the nervous system
- **urology,** the study of diseases of the kidney and bladder

Exercises

A. The following medical terms are all of Greek or Latin origin. *Match the meaning in the first column to the term in the second column.*   **LO 1.7**

_c_	1. tip or summit	a.	patent
_d_	2. buttocks	b.	mucus
_e_	3. poison	c.	apex
_b_	4. clear, sticky secretion	d.	breech
_a_	5. open	e.	toxin

B. Identify the incorrect statement about a root by circling it, and then rewrite it correctly on the line below.   LO 1.2

1. A root is the foundation of every medical term. (T) F

2. The root *dermat* means *skin*. (T) F

3. Many words contain more than one root. (T) F

4. The root *thorax* is the Latin word for *lung*. T (F)

5. Roots are usually of Latin or Greek origin. (T) F

6. Correction of incorrect statement:

   thorax ⟶ chest

   the root thorax is the Latin word for chest

Roots and Combining Forms

Challenge Your Knowledge

A. Identify the statements below as either true or false. Circle the correct answer. On the lines below, rewrite any false answer *correctly.* (**LO 1.2,** *Remember*)

1. A term never has more than one root.   T   (F)

✗ 2. Some terms will have no combining vowel.   (T)   F

3. Modification may be necessary to make a word easier to pronounce.   (T)   F

4. A vowel must always be present in a combining form.   (T)   F

5. Corrected statement:

all term could have more than one root

B. The root or combining form is the core meaning of the term and the foundation on which the term is built. Recognize the root or combining form in each of the following terms, and define it. (**LO 1.3,** *Remember*)

Term	Root/Combining form	Meaning of Root/Combining form
cardiology	cardio	heart
gynecologic	gynec	female
dermatitis	dermat	skin
arthroscopy	arthr	joint

C. Identify and underline the core foundation in each of the following terms. (**LO 1.2, 1.3,** *Remember*)

1. cardiology   study of heart

2. gastroenterology   study of stomach and intestine

3. respiratory   related to breathing

4. dermatitis

5. cardiologist

6. arthroscopy

7. cardiopathy

8. gastric

9. pneumothorax

10. gynecologist

D. **Once you have a good knowledge of roots and combining forms, you can identify what unknown terms relate to.** Below are medical terms you have not seen yet, but will recognize. Identify the root or combining form in each term and you will know the relationship it has to other terms. <u>The first one is done for you.</u> (**LO 1.3,** *Remember, Analyze*)

1. The term *hypogastric* relates to <u>under or below the stomach.</u>

2. The term *neuroglia* relates to _____.

3. The term *cardiopulmonary* relates to _____.

4. The term *subdermal* relates to _____.

5. The term *arthralgia* relates to <u>pain in joints</u> _____.

6. The term *endocarditis* relates to <u>endo→inside cardi→ c̅ "itis→inflamation</u> .

7. The term *pneumonitis* relates to <u>pneum→air</u> _____.

This is the logic of medical language.

E. **Match the Greek/Latin elements in the first column with their meanings in the second column. (LO 1.5, 1.7,** *Understand*)

_j_ **1.** pneum		a. to breathe
_i_ **2.** gynec		b. open
_k_ **3.** lymph		c. clear, sticky secretion
_f_ **4.** thorax		d. tip or summit
_h_ **5.** arthr		e. buttocks
_a_ **6.** respir		f. chest
_c_ **7.** mucus		g. skin
_b_ **8.** patent		h. joint
_l_ **9.** toxin		i. female
_d_ **10.** apex		j. air
_g_ **11.** dermat		k. clear spring water
_e_ **12.** breech		l. poison

Roots and Combining Forms

X **F.** **Spelling is most important in medical terminology.** For example, **ilium** and **ileum** may be similar in appearance and sound, but the difference of one letter makes each a different body part. Choose the correct spelling for the following terms. Fill in the blanks. (**LO 1.6, 1.8,** *Understand*)

1. A Pap smear is part of a _____ exam.

   gynecologik   gyneckologic   [gynecologic]

2. The _____ system keeps you breathing.

   respieratory   [respiratory]   resspiratory

3. Inflammation of the heart is _____.

   carditus   [carditis]   cardiitis

4. A muscle in the back is the _____.

   trapeze   trapezium   [trapezius]

5. A bony protuberance in your ankle is the _____.

   maleus   malius   [malleolus]

G. **Use your newly acquired knowledge of medical language to correctly answer the following questions.** Let the roots and combining forms be your guide. Circle the best choice. (**LO 1.5, 1.6,** *Apply*)

1. This term means one who studies the female reproductive system.

   [gynecologist]   urologist   neurologist

2. This term relates to the intestines and the stomach.

   [gastroenterology]   cardiology   dermatology

3. This term relates to the process of breathing.

   apex   toxic   [respiratory]

4. This term relates to the stomach.

   [gastritis]   gynecology   dermatitis

5. This term relates to a joint.

   [arthritis]   urethritis   neuralgia

H. **Use the correct medical term to complete the sentence.** Fill in the blanks. (**LO 1.6, 1.7,** *Apply*)

1. A __Cardilogist__ is a specialist in the care of the heart.

2. __Ureter__ is a tube from the kidney to the bladder.

3. Urology is the study of diseases of the __Kidney__ and __bladder__.

4. A segment of the small intestine is the __ileum__.

5. __beech__ means the buttocks, not the head, present first at delivery.

6. __urethra__ is the tube from the bladder to the outside.

7. __lymph__ is a fluid collected from body tissues.

8. A bone in the wrist is the __trapezium__.

9. The bony protuberance at the ankle is the __malleoIus__.

10. __ilium__ is a bone in the pelvis.

I. **Deconstruct the following medical terms by extracting their roots or combining forms.** Write root (R) or combining form (CF) on the line beside the term, to identify it as either a R or a CF. (**LO 1.4,** *Analyze*)

1. gynecologic   gynec (R)   gyneco (CF)

2. gastroenterology   _____

3. dermatitis   _____

4. arthroscopy   _____

5. respiratory   _____

6. cardiology   _____

J. **Separate the terms that have only roots from the terms that have combining forms.** Put a checkmark (√) in the appropriate column, and then answer the questions below the chart. (**LO 1.1, 1.2, 1.3,** *Analyze*)

Medical Term	Root	Combining Form
1. gynecologist	gynec	gyneco
2. urology	uri	uro
3. pneumothorax	pneum	pneumo
4. cardiac	cadi	
5. respiration	respir	respira
6. arthritis	arthr	—
7. dermatology	dermat	dermato
8. enteritis	enter	—
9. neuritis	neur	—
10. gastric	gastr	— (ic) ⟹ pertainting to *meaning*

11. Which term has more than one root? _Pneumothorax_

12. Which terms have similar endings? _8 - 9 "itis"_

13. What element changes a root into a combining form? _Combining vowel_

14. You build medical terms on the foundation of a _root_.

K. **Root + combining vowel = combining form.** Deconstruct the following terms to determine the correct combining form (CF). Finding the root(s) (Rs) first will put you on the right track. Fill in the blanks. (**LO 1.4,** *Analyze*)

Term	Root(s)	Combining Vowel	Combining Form
1. cardiology	cardi	o	cardio
2. gynecologic	gynec	o	
3. dermatology	dermat	o	dermato
4. arthroscopy	arthr	o	arthro

Roots and Combining Forms

L. **Recognizing word elements will help you "dissect," or deconstruct, a term.** The following terms have an element set in bold. Identify the type of element, and give a brief definition of its meaning. **(LO 1.3, 1.4, *Analyze*)**

Type of Element   **Meaning of Element**

1. **arthro**plasty   _root - Joint_____   2. _____

3. endo**card**itis   _(R) card - heart_____   4. _____

5. **respiratory**   _Combining form - related to breathing_   6. _____

7. hypo**tensi**on   _____   8. _____

9. hyper**gastric**   _gastr (R) stomach_____   10. _____

M. **Case report questions.** This Case Report is taken from the beginning of this chapter. You should feel more comfortable with the medical terminology now. Read the report again, and you will be able to answer the questions. Fill in the blanks. **(LO 1.5, *Analyze*)**

Case Report 1.1

You are

...a medical assistant employed by Russell Gordon, MD, a primary care physician at Fulwood Medical Center.

Your patient is

...Mrs. Connie Bishop, a 55-year-old woman who presents with a swelling in her lower abdomen and shortness of breath. She has no gynecologic or gastroenterologic symptoms. Her previous medical history shows recurrent dermatitis of her hands since a teenager and an arthroscopy for a knee injury at age 40. Physical examination reveals a circular mass 6 inches in diameter in the left lower quadrant of her abdomen. There is no abnormality in her respiratory or cardiovascular system.

Your role is to maintain her medical record and document her care, assist Dr. Gordon during his examinations, explain the examination and treatment procedures to Mrs. Bishop, and facilitate her referral for specialist care.

> *Study Hint*
> Many elements have more than one meaning. You must know the different meanings because that will make a difference in the use of the medical term.

1. What type of skin problem has Mrs. Bishop had since she was a teenager? _____

2. She "has no gynecologic or gastroenterologic symptoms."

   Define **gynecologic.** _____

   Define **gastroenterologic.** _____

3. Her knee injury required what type of procedure? _arthroscopy_____

   Describe this procedure. _____

4. She shows "no abnormality in her respiratory or cardiovascular system." Explain this in layman's terms.

   _____

5. What symptoms does Mrs. Bishop have that brought her to Dr. Gordon? _____

Congratulations! You are on your way to learning medical terminology.

CHAPTER SUMMARY EXERCISES

A. **Spelling comprehension.** Circle the correct spelling of the term. (**LO 1.5, 1.7,** *Remember*)

1. abdomin   abdumin   (abdomen)   addumen   adumen

2. cardilogist   cardelogist   (cardiologist)   cardeologist   cardiollogist

3. (respiratory)   rispiratory   risperatory   resspiratory   resperatory

4. maleum   (malleus)   malium   mallium   maileus

5. (gastroenterology)   gastricenterology   gastrioenterology   gastrology   gastraenterology

6. iillium   (ilium)   (ileum)   illeum   ellium

7. cardeopathy   cardeeopathy   cardeopathie   (cardiopathy)   cardiopethy

8. arthriscopy   (arthroscopy)   artroscopy   arterioscopy   arterioscopie

9. (trapezium)   (trapezius)   trrapezius   trapizium   trapezeum

10. gyneckologic   (gynecologic)   gynicologic   gynickologic   gynekologic

B. **Match the number of the correct spelling of the term in Exercise A with the brief description of the term below.** (**LO 1.5, 1.7,** *Apply*)

1. study of the stomach and intestines   *gynecoenterology*

2. visual examination of a joint   *arthroscopy*

3. small bone in the middle ear   *malleus*

4. specialist in treating heart problems   *Cardiologist*

5. Latin word for *belly*   *abd*

6. pertaining to breathing   *respiric*

7. bone in the pelvis   *ilium*

8. root meaning *female*   *gynec*

9. bone in the wrist   *trapezium*

10. disease of the heart   *Cardiopathy*

Roots and Combining Forms

C. Using your knowledge of terms 1–10 in Exercises A and B and their correct spelling, write a brief sentence for each of the terms as it might appear in patient documentation. **(LO 1.5, 1.7, *Apply*)**

1. _____

2. _____

3. _____

4. _____

5. _____

6. _____

7. _____

8. _____

9. _____

10. _____

D. Meet the goals of each of the Chapter Learning Outcomes and insert the correct answers to the questions. **(LO 1.1–1.8, *Analyze*)**

1. Topic: Relate the logic of the language of medicine to your practice as a health care professional. Be prepared to discuss this in class. Make a brief outline of your thoughts for this discussion. **(LO 1.1)**

   _____

   _____

   _____

2. Define the terms *root, combining vowel,* and *combining form.* **(LO 1.2)**

   a. root: _____

   b. combining vowel: _____

   c. combining form: _____

3. Recognize that roots and combining forms are the foundation of any medical term. Identify the root or combining form in each of the following terms. **(LO 1.3)**

   a. gastrologist _____

   b. gynecologist _____

   c. neurologist _____

4. Deconstruct medical terms into their roots and combining forms. Underline the root or combining form in each of the following terms. (**LO 1.4**)

   a. arthroscopy

   b. dermatome

   c. cardiogram

5. Interpret the meaning of the roots and combining forms in commonly used medical terms. (**LO 1.5**)

   a. In the term *cardiography*, the root _____ means _____.

   b. In the term *respiration*, the root _____ means _____.

   c. In the term *gastric*, the root _____ means _____.

6. Use roots and combining forms to construct commonly used medical terms. (**LO 1.6**)

   a. An operation to limit food intake is a _____ bypass.

   b. CPR is the abbreviation for _____ resuscitation.

7. Among the following medical terms, identify the ones that are taken directly from Greek or Latin words. Circle your choices. (**LO 1.7**)

   renal   mucus   hypothermic   breath   knee   popliteal   bilateral   quadrant   hyperbaric   toxin   umbilicus

8. Differentiate between medical terms that are spelled and/or pronounced similarly. What is the difference between "patient" and "patent"? (**LO 1.8**)

   a. patient _____

   b. patent _____

Suffixes and Prefixes
The Language of Health Care

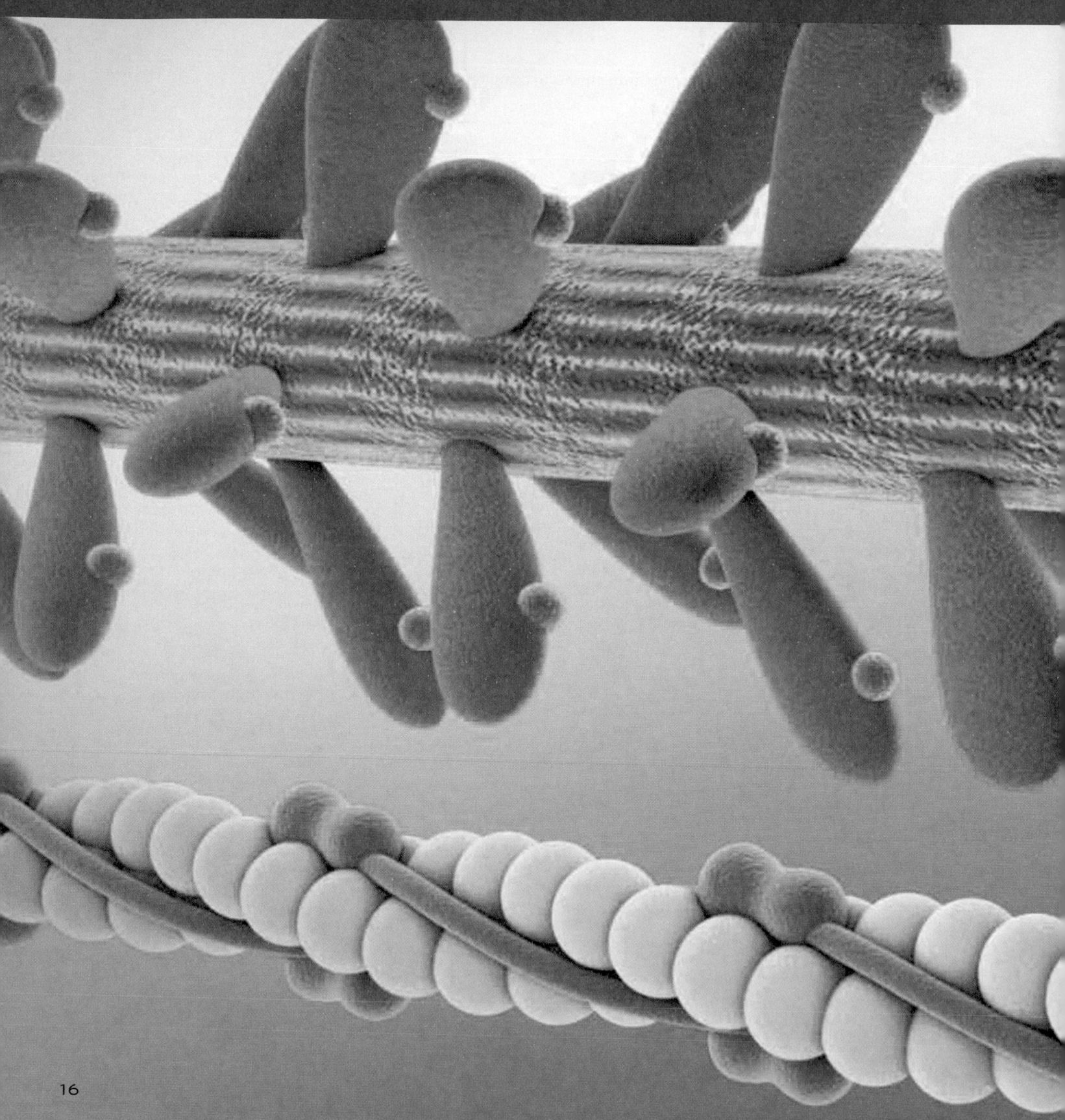

2

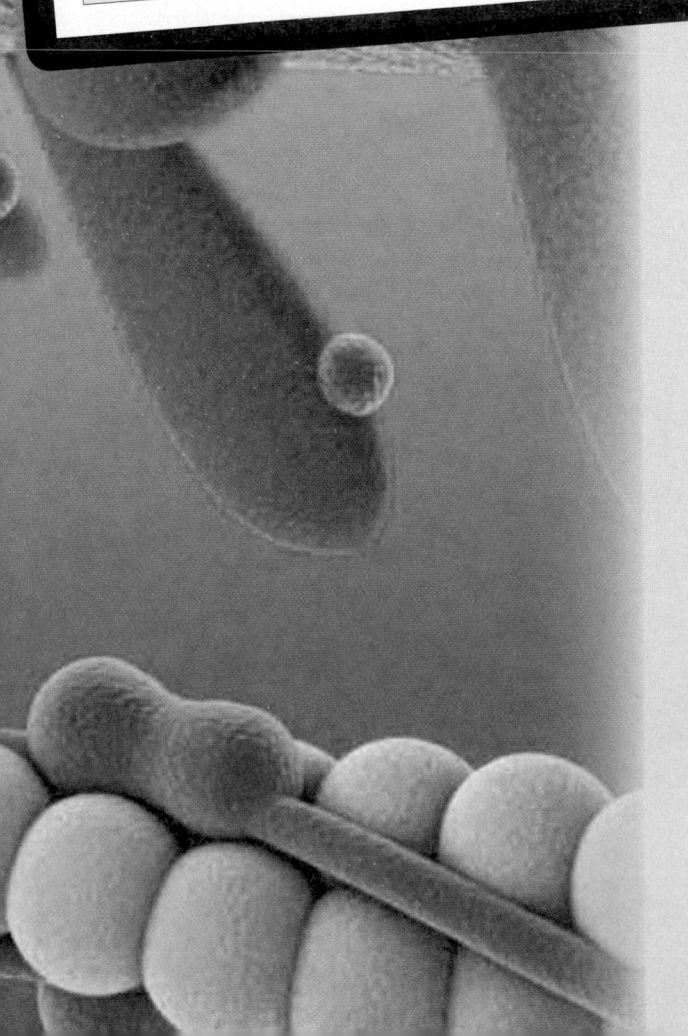

Case Report (CR) 2.1

You are

... a genetic nurse working with geneticist Ingrid Hughes, MD, PhD, in the Genetics Department at Fulwood Medical Center.

Your patient is

... Mrs. Geraldine Long, a 37-year-old administrative assistant who has been referred by primary care physician Susan Lee, MD. Mrs. Long has twin girls who are 12 years old. She is an award-winning ballroom dancer who does not smoke, drinks alcohol only occasionally, and rehearses her dance routines four or five days each week. Her mother, aged 62, is being treated for ovarian cancer. Her mother's sister is being treated for breast cancer and has been found to carry a gene mutation associated with breast cancer. Mrs. Long's mammogram is normal. She has requested genetic screening.

Chapter Learning Outcomes

Adding a different suffix to the end of the same **root (R)** or **combining form (CF)** enables you to build a whole new set of words, all with different meanings. Adding a different prefix in front of the **root** or **combining form** also helps to build more medical terms. This lesson will increase your medical word building power by enabling you to:

LO 2.1 Define the term *suffix*.

LO 2.2 Identify the suffixes of commonly used medical terms and their meanings.

LO 2.3 Establish a classification of suffixes.

LO 2.4 Define the term *prefix*.

LO 2.5 Identify the prefixes of commonly used medical terms and their meanings.

LO 2.6 Establish a classification of prefixes.

LO 2.7 Link word elements of prefixes, suffixes, **roots**, and **combining forms** together to construct medical terms.

LO 2.8 Deconstruct medical terms into their elements.

You add a suffix onto the end of a word to modify the core of the **root** or combining form and give it a new meaning.

2.1.1 Create words with different meanings by adding different suffixes to the same root and/or combining form.

2.1.2 Classify suffixes into groups with diagnostic, surgical, and pathologic meanings.

2.1.3 Classify suffixes into groups that transform roots and combining forms into adjectives or nouns.

SUFFIX:

- a group of letters
- positioned at the end of a medical term
- attaches to the end of a **root** or **combining form**
- can have more than one meaning
- if a suffix begins with a consonant, add a **combining vowel** to the **root**
- if a suffix starts with a vowel, no **combining vowel** is needed
- an occasional medical term can have two suffixes

LO 2.1, 2.2, 2.3 Suffixes

In the Case Report 2.1 on the chapter opening spread, the **root genet-**, meaning origin or gene, is teamed with the suffix -ic, which means *pertaining to,* to form the word genetic, *pertaining to a gene.* Again, the **root genet** is teamed with the suffix -ics, which means *knowledge of,* to form the word **genetics**, *the knowledge of or the science of the inheritance of characteristics.* Also, the **root genet-** can be teamed with two suffixes, -ic, *pertaining to,* and -ist, *a specialist,* to form the word geneticist, *pertaining to a specialist in genetics.* There can be more than one suffix in a single word.

Using the combining form of **cardi/o,** in the medical specialty of cardiology, a cardiologist will often diagnose a cardiopathy. The suffix -logy, which means *study of,* and the suffix -logist, which means *one who studies* or *a specialist,* and the suffix -pathy, which means *disease,* all give different meanings in the sentence, "in the specialty of cardiology, a cardiologist will often diagnose a cardiopathy."

Another example of the use of suffixes is in the medical specialty of dermatology, when a dermatologist will often diagnose a case of dermatitis (*Table 2.1, Figure 2.1*).

Table 2.1 Use of Suffixes

Complete Word	Combining Form or Root	Suffix	Meaning of Suffix	Meaning of Word
dermatitis	dermat-	-itis	inflammation	inflammation of the skin
dermatologist	dermat/o-	-logist	one who studies	one who studies the skin, specialist in dermatology
dermatology	dermat/o-	-logy	study of	study of the skin

In *dermatitis,* the suffix -itis starts with a vowel, so there is no need for a **combining vowel,** and the suffix is attached directly to the **root.**

In a different example of the use of suffixes, an orthopedic surgeon operating on a joint can perform an arthroscopy, an arthrodesis, or an arthroplasty, all different operations with different outcomes as shown in *Table 2.2.*

You always need a **combining vowel** before a suffix that begins with a consonant (e.g., dermatology, arthroplasty).

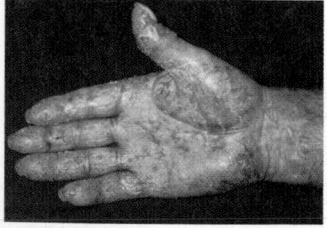

▲ **Figure 2.1** Dermatitis Due to a Latex Glove.

Table 2.2 Different Meanings of Suffixes

Complete Word	Combining Form	Suffix	Meaning of Suffix	Meaning of Word
arthroscopy	arthr/o-	-scopy	visual examination	visual examination of a joint
arthrodesis	arthr/o-	-desis	fixation	fixation of a joint
arthroplasty	arthr/o-	-plasty	surgical repair	repair of a joint

LO 2.3 Classification of Suffixes

One strategy to help you understand medical terms is to divide suffixes into different types, such as diagnostic, surgical, pathologic, and descriptive and adjectival.

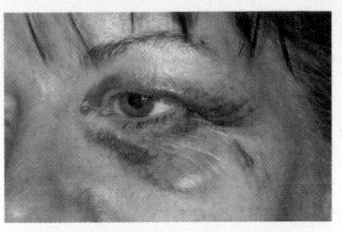

▲ **Figure 2.2** Hematoma (black eye) following a fall.

Diagnostic Suffixes

This group of suffixes, when added to a **root** or **combining form**, produce a medical term that is a diagnosis or a procedure or test to identify the nature of an illness.

The **roots/combining forms hem/o** and **hemat/o** both mean *blood*. Adding diagnostic suffixes can produce a variety of diagnostic medical terms throughout the body systems *(Table 2.3)*.

Table 2.3 Diagnostic Suffixes

Diagnostic Suffix	Meaning of Suffix	Word Example	Meaning of Surgical Procedure
-oma	tumor, mass	**hemat**oma (Figure 2.2)	collection of blood in a tissue
-uria	urine	**hemat**uria	blood in the urine
-dialysis	to separate	**hem/o**dialysis	Removal of excess waste materials from blood
-chezia	pass a stool	**hemat/o**chezia	passage of a bloody stool
-crit	to separate	**hemat/o**crit	percentage of red blood cells in the blood
-gram	record	**cardi/o**gram	record derived from the heart
-graph	instrument for recording	**cardi/o**graph	instrument for recording the heart
-lysis	destruction	**hem/o**lysis	destruction of red blood cells
-philia	attraction	**hem/o**philia	an inherited blood disease
-ptysis	spit	**hem/o**ptysis	to cough up bloody sputum
-rrhage	to flow profusely	**hem/o**rrhage	to bleed profusely
-rrhoid	to flow	**hem/o**rrhoid	painful anal swelling of venous blood

As you go through each body system in the book, there will be another 20 diagnostic suffixes you will learn in relation to the actual diagnoses made at that point in the book.

Surgical Suffixes

When added to a **root** or **combining form**, surgical suffixes produce medical terms that describe the invasive surgical procedure performed on the body *(Table 2.4)*.

Table 2.4 Surgical Suffixes

Surgical Suffix	Meaning of Suffix	Word Example	Meaning of Surgical Procedure
-centesis	surgical puncture	**arthr/o**centesis	surgical puncture of a joint space with a needle
-desis	fixation	**arthr/o**desis	surgical binding together of the bones of a joint
-ectomy	surgical removal	**append**ectomy	surgical removal of the appendix
-plasty	surgical repair	**rhin/o**plasty	surgical repair of the nose
-rrhaphy	surgical suture	**herni/o**rrhaphy	surgical suture of a hernia
-stomy	surgical formation of an opening	**trache/o**stomy	surgical formation of an artificial opening into the trachea into which a tube is inserted
-tomy	surgical incision	**trache/o**tomy	surgical incision into the trachea to enable a tracheostomy tube to be inserted
-tripsy	crushing	**lith/o**tripsy	crushing of a stone (calculus), e.g., in the ureters

LO 2.3 Classification of Suffixes (continued)

Pathologic Suffixes

When added to a root or combining form, this type of suffix produces a medical term that describes a symptom or sign of a disease process (*Table 2.5*).

Table 2.5 Pathologic Suffixes

Pathologic Suffix	Meaning of Suffix	Word Example	Meaning of Pathologic Term
-algia	pain	arthralgia	pain in a joint(s)
-ectasis	dilation	bronchiectasis	chronic dilation of bronchi
-edema	accumulation of fluid in tissues	lymphedema	swelling in tissues as a result of obstruction of lymphatic vessels
-emesis	vomiting	hematemesis	vomiting of blood
-genesis	form, produce	oste/ogenesis	formation of new bone
-itis	inflammation	cystitis	inflammation of the urinary bladder
-oma	tumor, mass	hematoma	mass of blood leaked outside blood vessels into tissues
-osis	abnormal condition	cyanosis	dark blue coloration of blood due to lack of oxygen
-pathy	disease	neur/opathy	any disease of the nervous system
-penia	deficiency, lack of	erythr/openia	decrease in red blood cells
-phobia	fear of	agoraphobia	an unfounded fear of public places that arouses a state of panic
-stenosis	narrowing	arteri/ostenosis	abnormal narrowing of an artery

Adjectival Suffixes

As you learn new medical terms in each body system chapter in this book, you will see that there are 28 suffixes that mean *pertaining to*. These suffixes are used as adjectives to describe the **root**. Examples of adjectival suffixes are:

- -ac **cardi**ac pertaining to the heart
- -ary **pulmon**ary pertaining to the lungs
- -ior **poster**ior pertaining to the back of the body

Those 28 suffixes are listed in the Keynote on this page.

Noun Suffixes

Several suffixes do not fall under any of the earlier classifications, but maintain the **root** or **combining form** as a noun (*Table 2.6*).

Table 2.6 Noun Suffixes

Noun Suffix	Meaning of Suffix	Word Example	Meaning of Medical Term
-iatry	treatment, medical specialty	psychiatry	diagnosis and treatment of mental disorders
-ician	expert, specialist	pediatrician	medical specialist in children's development and disorders
-icle	small, minute	ossicle (Figure 2.3)	small bone, relating to the three small bones in the middle ear
-ist	expert, specialist	dentist	specialist in disorders of the orofacial complex
-istry	medical specialty	dentistry	specialty in disorders of the orofacial complex
-ole	small, minute	arteriole	small artery
-ule	small, minute	venule	small vein

Note that in the above table, three suffixes mean "small," two suffixes mean "specialist," and two suffixes mean "medical specialty."

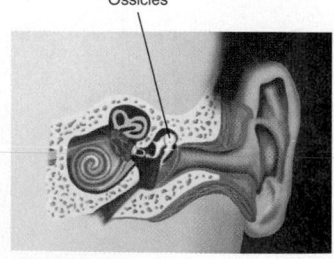

Ossicles

▲ **Figure 2.3** Ossicles of the Middle Ear.

Keynote

Adjectival suffixes meaning *pertaining to:*

-ac, -al, -ale, -alis, -ar, -aris, -ary, atic, -ative, -eal, -ent, -etic, -ial, -ic, -ica, -ical, -ine, -ior, -iosum, -ious, -istic, -ius, -nic, -ous, -tic, -tiz, -tous, -us.

Lesson 2.2 Prefixes

LESSON OBJECTIVES

To continue expanding terms derived from the core **root** of a medical term, you can place a prefix at the beginning of the **root**.

2.2.1 Define the term prefix.

2.2.2 Identify the prefixes **of commonly used medical terms.**

2.2.3 Establish a classification of prefixes.

LO 2.4, 2.5, 2.6, 2.7, 2.8 Prefixes

Prefixes are added directly to the **root** or **combining form** and do not require **combining vowels**.

For example, you can add the different prefixes peri- and endo- to the same root, **cardi-**, to produce the different words pericardium and endocardium, which have very different meanings, as shown in *Table 2.7*.

PREFIX:
- one letter or a group of letters
- precedes a **root** to give it a different meaning
- can have more than one meaning
- never requires a **combining vowel**
- can have two prefixes in an occasional medical term

Table 2.7 Use of Prefixes

Complete Word	Prefix	Meaning of Prefix	Meaning of Word
pericardium	peri-	around	structure around the heart
endocardium	endo-	inside	structure inside the heart

Note that -um is a suffix meaning *structure*.

Similarly, epigastric, hypogastric, and endogastric all have the same **root**, **gastr-**, but because of the different prefixes, epi-, hypo-, and endo-, have very different meanings, as shown in *Table 2.8*.

Table 2.8 Different Meanings of Prefixes

Complete Word	Prefix	Meaning of Prefix	Meaning of Word
epigastric	epi-	above	pertaining to above the stomach
hypogastric	hypo-	below	pertaining to below the stomach
endogastric	endo-	inside	pertaining to inside the stomach

Note that -ic is a suffix meaning *pertaining to.*

Exercises

A. Building onto the elements of roots, combining vowels, and combining forms are the prefixes and suffixes of medical terminology. *Prefixes and suffixes are additional word elements that give further meaning to a root or combining form. Develop your knowledge of more word elements with the following exercise. Circle the correct answer and then rewrite the false statement correctly on the lines below.* **LO 2.1, 2.2, 2.4, 2.7**

1. In a medical term, the suffix will always appear at the end.   (T)   F

2. Every medical term has to have a prefix.   T   (F)

3. In the terms **arthroscopy** and **arthrodesis**, the combining form is the same, but the suffix is different.   (T)   F

4. If a suffix begins with a consonant, you will need a combining vowel before it.   (T)   F

5. Corrected statement:

_____

_____

B. Terminology challenge. *Use your new knowledge of prefixes and suffixes to answer the following questions.* **LO 2.2, 2.5, 2.6**

1. *Atrium, septum,* and *myocardium* are all medical terms you have not learned yet. One element in each of the terms can give you a clue.

All of these terms have the same element ____ *u m* ____, which relates to a ____ *structure* ____.

2. The prefixes *epi, hypo,* and *endo* all relate to _____.

Your learning goal is to understand the logic of medical language.

Classification of Prefixes

Many prefixes can be classified into prefixes of position, prefixes of number or measurement, and prefixes of direction (*Tables 2.9, 2.10, 2.11*).

Table 2.9 Prefixes of Position

Position Prefix	Meaning of Prefix	Word Example	Meaning of Medical Term
ante-	*before, forward*	ante**vert**	*to tilt forward, as a uterus can*
anti-	*against*	anti**bio**tic	*an agent that can destroy bacteria and other microorganisms*
circum-	*around*	circum**cision**	*to cut around the penis to remove the foreskin*
endo-	*inside, inner*	endo**crine**	*a gland that secretes directly into the blood*
epi-	*above, over, upon*	epi**dermis**	*the top layer of the skin*
exo-	*outside, outward*	exo**crine**	*a gland that excretes outwardly through ducts*
hyper-	*above, excessive*	hyper**trophy**	*increase in size*
hypo-	*below*	hypo**dermis**	*tissue layer below the top layer of the skin*
inter-	*between*	inter**costal**	*the space between two ribs*
intra-	*inside, within*	intra**dermal** (Figure 2.4)	*within the skin*
para-	*adjacent, alongside*	para**noid**	*having delusions of persecution*
peri-	*around*	peri**nat**al	*around the time of birth*
post-	*after*	post**natal**	*after the time of birth*
pre-	*before*	pre**nat**al	*before the time of birth*
retro-	*backward*	retro**vert**	*to tilt backward, as a uterus can*
supra-	*above, excessive*	supra**pub**ic	*above the pubic bone*
trans-	*across, through*	trans**dermal**	*going across or through the skin*
ultra-	*higher, beyond*	ultra**sound** (Figure 2.5)	*very high-frequency sound waves*

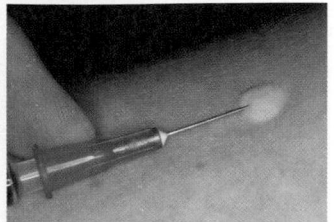

▲ **Figure 2.4** Intradermal Injection.

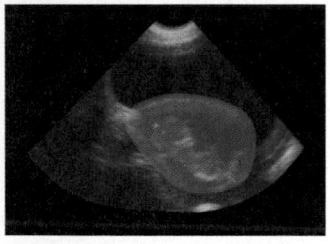

▲ **Figure 2.5** Obstetric Ultrasonography of a 22-Year Old Woman. The 12-week-old fetus (*in brown*) is in the placenta (*in green*).

Table 2.10 Prefixes of Number and Measurement

Measurement Prefix	Meaning of Prefix	Word Example	Meaning of Medical Term
bi-	two, twice, double	bi**later**al	on two sides of the body
brady-	slow	brady**cardi**a	slow heart rate
di-	two	di**pleg**ia	paralysis of corresponding parts on both sides of the body
eu-	normal	eu**pnea**	normal breathing
hemi-	half	hemi**paresis**	weakness of one side of the body
macro-	large	macro**cyte**	large red blood cell
micro-	small	micro**cyte**	small red blood cell
mono-	single, one	mono**cyte**	white blood cell with a single nucleus
multi-	many	multi**para**	woman who has given birth at least twice
pan-	all	pan**cyto**penia	deficiency of all types of blood cells
poly-	excessive	poly**uria**	excessive production of urine
primi-	first	primi**para**	woman who has given birth for the first time
quadri-	four	quadri**pleg**ia	paralysis of all four limbs
tachy-	rapid	tachy**cardi**a	rapid heart rate
tri-	three	tri**cusp**id	having three points—a tricuspid heart valve has three flaps
uni-	single, one	uni**polar**	depression

Table 2.11 Prefixes of Direction and Location

Directional Prefix	Meaning of Prefix	Medical Term Example	Meaning of Medical Term
ab-	away from	abduction	action of moving away from the midline
ad-	toward	adduction	action of moving toward the midline
ante-	coming before, in front of	antevert	to tilt forward
post-	coming after, behind	postnatal	occurring after birth
sub-	under	subdural	in the space under the dura mater
syn-	coming together	synapse	junction between two nerve cells

Exercises

A. Review the prefixes and terms in Table 2.9 and circle the correct term to complete the statement.   LO 2.5, 2.7, 2.8

1. Dr. Baker said the patient's uterus is <u>retroverted</u>, so she will need

   antibiotics   (surgery)   pain medication

2. The transdermal route of drug administration goes

   on the skin   (in an IV)   through the mouth

3. *Postpartum* occurs

   before delivery   during delivery   (after delivery)

4. *Retroverted* means

   tilted sideways   tilted forward   (tilted backward)

5. *Hyper* means the same as

   (supra)   ante   retro

B. Review the prefixes and terms in Table 2.9.   LO 2.4, 2.5

1. Which terms in Table 2.9 are opposites?

   a. ___post (after)___ and ___pre (before)___

   b. ___hyper (above)___ and ___hypo (below)___

2. Which of the following is a false statement about prefixes?

   a. They usually appear in the beginning of a term.   (T)   F

   b. They can attach to a root or combining form.   (T)   F

   c. Every term must have a prefix.   T   (F)

   d. Some terms can have more than one prefix.   (T)   F

   e. A prefix can designate number or location.   (T)   F

Suffixes and Prefixes

Challenge Your Knowledge

A. **Word elements are the building blocks of medical terminology.** Being able to define word elements will help you use them correctly. Identify the element by placing a checkmark (√) in the correct column; then define the meaning of the element. In the last column, give an example of a medical term containing that element. Fill in the chart. (**LO 2.1, 2.5,** *Remember*)

Element	Prefix	Root/Combining Form	Suffix	Meaning of Element	Medical Term
1. cardio		√		2. heart	3.
4. multi	√			5. many	6.
7. dermat		√		8. skin	9.
10. logy			√	11. study of	12.
13. mono	√			14. one	15.
16. scopy			√	17. visual examination	18.
19. itis			√	20. inflamation	21.
22. bi	√			23. two	24.
25. logist			√	26. specialist	27.

B. **The following three elements have something in common.** Fill in the blanks. (**LO 2.5. 2.6,** *Remember*)

1. *Epi* means __above__.

2. *Hypo* means __below__.

3. *Endo* means __inside__.

4. Each of these are all (circle one)   **prefixes**   roots   combining forms   suffixes

5. They can be grouped by (circle one)   color   size   **location**

C. **In this exercise, you are given definitions.** What term matches these definitions? (**LO 2.7,** *Remember*)

1. repair of a joint   __arthrodesis__

2. small red blood cell   __hem__

3. deficiency of all types of blood cells   __pancytopenia__

4. excessive production of urine   __polyuria__

5. normal breathing   __eupnea__

D. Because a lot of clinical documentation centers on surgeries, knowledge of surgical suffixes is most important— especially for coders. Test your knowledge of surgical suffixes and make the correct match of meaning and suffix. (**LO 2.2, 2.7, Remember, Understand, Apply**)

_____b_____ 1. scopy   a. surgical repair

_____c_____ 2. desis   b. visual examination

_____a_____ 3. plasty   c. surgical fixation

Combine these suffixes with the CF arthr/o and fill in the blanks with the correct medical term.

4. The surgeon wants a closer look inside Mr. Parker's knee so he is scheduled for an __arthroscopy__ tomorrow morning.

5. Mary Collins has torn her knee ligaments playing high school basketball. Her treatment plan includes scheduling a(n) __arthrodesis__ to reattach them. (fixation)

6. June Larkin had a bad skiing accident while on vacation. Her tendons and ligaments in her knee will require extensive surgery to get her walking again without crutches. She needs a(n) __arthropathy__. (repair)

E. To better retain medical language, it may be helpful to relate terms to groups. The following terms are grouped. Your knowledge of the suffixes will help to define them. (**LO 2.2, Understand**)

1. gastrology means   _____

2. gastric means   _____

3. gastrologist means   _____

4. gastritis means   _____

5. gastroscopy means   _____

6. The common root/combining form among each of these terms is __gastric__ and means __stomach__.

F. Match the correct medical term with the statement. (**LO 2.7, 2.8, Understand**)

1. specialist in disorders of the female reproductive system _c_   a. arthrodesis

2. inflammation of the skin _e_   b. cardiopathy

3. heart disease _b_   c. gynecologist

4. fixation of a joint _a_   d. pericardium

5. structure around the heart _d_   e. dermatitis

G. Below is a list of medical terms you have learned. Circle the only one that has a prefix. (**LO 2.5, Understand**)

✓ 1. endocardium

2. dermatitis

3. arthrodesis

4. gynecologist

5. cardiologist

Suffixes and Prefixes

H. Identify the only false statement about a suffix. Circle your answer, and then rewrite the false statement correctly on the lines below. (**LO 2.1**, *Understand*)

1. An occasional medical term can have two suffixes.   T   F

2. If a suffix starts with a vowel, no combining vowel is needed.   T   F

3. A suffix can appear anywhere in the term.   T   F

4. A suffix is a group of letters.   T   F

5. A suffix can have more than one meaning.   T   F

6. Rewrite correctly:

_____

I. A prefix appears at the beginning of the term, but not every term will have a prefix. Keeping the same prefix but changing the root and other elements will produce new terms. First, underline the prefix in every term. Then use your knowledge of the meaning of prefixes to fill in the blanks. (**LO 2.5, 2.7**, *Understand, Apply*)

1. An **endoscope** is an instrument for looking _____inside_____ the body.

   An **endotracheal** tube is inserted _____inside_____ the trachea.

2. The **pericardium** is the structure _____around_____ the heart.

   The **perirectal** area is the tissue _____around_____ the rectum.

3. **Epigastric** is the area _____above_____ the stomach.

   Epidermal is the layer of skin _____above_____ the dermal layer.

4. **Hypotension** is _____low_____ blood pressure.

   Hypothyroidism is a condition that occurs when the level of thyroid hormone in your blood is _____low_____.

5. **Hypertension** is _____high_____ blood pressure.

   Hyperglycemia is _____high_____ sugar content in the blood.

J. Understand your word choice to be precise. Errors in medical documentation are a threat to patient safety and a legal liability. Circle the correct answer. (**LO 2.7, 2.8**, *Understand, Apply*)

1. A visual **examination** of the stomach is a

   (gastroscopy)   gastropexy   gastrodesis   gastroplasty

2. An **abdominoplasty** would be a surgical

   fusion   fixation   (repair)   examination

3. **Endogastric** would be

   above the stomach   below the stomach   (within the stomach)   outside the stomach

4. **Arthropathy** would be a disease of

   skin   (joints)   arteries   blood vessels

5. If **rhin/o** means *nose*, what would a surgical repair of a broken nose be called?

   rhinodesis   rhinoscopy   (rhinoplasty)   rhinopexy

K. **Analyze the following medical terms on the basis of your knowledge of elements.** Put a slash (/) between each element of the terms listed below and then write the definition of each term on the line next to it. (**LO 2.8**, *Understand, Apply*)

1. dermatitis _____inflamation of skin_____

2. pericardium _____around the heart_____

3. arthroplasty _____repair of joints_____

4. epigastric _____above the stomach_____

5. arthroscopy _____visual examination of joints_____

L. **Construct any three sentences of patient documentation using any of the terms in Chapters 1 and 2.** Choose your terms from the word bank provided. You may have to deconstruct the terms for their meanings before you construct the sentences. (**LO 2.7, 2.8,** *Apply*)

Word Bank:

arthrodesis	pericardium	gastrologist	arthroscopy
cardiopathy	dermatitis	arthropathy	arthritis
endogastric	gastroenterologist	gynecologist	respiratory

1. _____

_____

_____

2. _____

_____

_____

3. _____

_____

_____

M. **Constructing terms is taking the building blocks of elements and correctly arranging them to form the term you need.** Employ your knowledge of prefixes, roots, combining forms, and suffixes to construct the term required. Fill in the chart. (**LO 2.7, 2.8,** *Apply*)

Element	Prefix	Root(s)	Combining Form	Suffix	Medical Term
1. inflammation of the stomach and intestines	—	gastr enter	gastro	itis	2. gastroenteritis
3. pertaining to the rib and spine					4.
5. inflammation of a joint	—	arthr	—	itis	6. arthritis
7. visual examination of the stomach	—	gastr	gastro	scopy	8. gastroscopy
9. blood bursting forth					10.
11. pertaining to on top of the skin	epi	dermat			12. epidermis
13. one who studies the heart	—	cardi	cardio	logist	14. cardiologist
15. visual examination within the body				scopy	16.

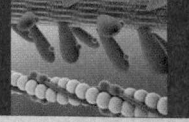

Suffixes and Prefixes

N. **A suffix appears at the end of the term.** Its purpose is to modify the core of the root or combining form and give it new meaning. Your knowledge of suffixes will help you complete this exercise. Circle the correct choice, and finish filling in the blanks. *A hint for the suffix is bolded in each statement.* (**LO 2.7, Apply**)

1. A **disease** of the heart is cardi/o _____.

   -logy   (-pathy)   -plasty

2. A **specialist** in the study of skin is a dermat/o _____.

   -itis   -logy   (-logist)

3. Visual **examination** of a joint is an arthr/o _____.

   -plasty   (-scopy)   -desis

4. A **structure** around the heart is the pericardi um _____ p _____.

   -osis   -itis   (-um)

5. An **inflammation** of the stomach is gastr _____.

   -logy   -plasty   (-itis)

6. The **study of** the skin is called dermat/o _____.

   -pathy   -tosis   (-logy)

O. **To construct the defined medical term, you may have to add a suffix and/or a prefix.** If you add a prefix, write P under the element; if you add a suffix, write S under the element. (**LO 2.7, Apply**)

1. study of the skin   _____/dermato/_____

2. visual examination of a joint   _____/arthro/_____

3. structure around the heart   _____/cardi/_____

4. above the stomach   _____/gastr/_____

5. heart disease   _____/cardio/_____

P. **Use your knowledge of elements to fill in the blanks.** (**LO 2.7, 2.8, Apply**)

1. In the term *arthroplasty*, identify the suffix.   _____

2. In the term *epigastric*, identify the prefix.   _____

3. In the term *dermatologist*, identify the suffix.   _____

4. In the term *gynecologist*, identify the root/combining form. _____

5. In the term *endocardium*, identify the prefix.   _____

Q. **Use your new knowledge of prefixes and suffixes to circle the correct medical term.** (LO 2.2, 2.5, *Analyze*)

1. Circle the term with the prefix that means *above* or *on top of.*

   hypogastric   endocardium   epigastric

2. Circle the term with the suffix that means *structure.*

   pericardium   carditis   cardiology

3. Circle the term with the prefix that means *within.*

   intracellular   bipolar   endocarditis

4. Circle the term with the suffix that means *pertaining to.*

   cardiologist   gastric   arthrodesis

5. Circle the term with the suffix that means *repair of a joint.*

   arthrodesis   gastroscopy   arthroplasty

R. **Prefixes can be grouped by size, number, location, quantity, and color.** Define the following group of medical terms. (LO 2.5, 2.6, *Analyze*)

1. Epigastric means   _____

2. Hypogastric means   _____

3. Endogastric means   _____

4. These are all prefixes of   _____

5. Next, apply these prefixes to the following terms.

   a. *above the skin* _____/derm/al   **b.** *below the tongue* _____/gloss/al   **c.** *within the heart* _____/cardi/um

S. **Extend your knowledge of prefixes and suffixes to other medical terms.** Fill in the blanks. (LO 2.2, 2.5, 2.7, 2.8, *Analyze*)

1. If *pericardium* means structure around the heart, what would *periosteum* mean? (*Hint: oste* means bone) _____

2. If *rhin/o* means nose, what is a surgical repair of the nose called? _____

3. If *arthroscopy* is a visual examination of the joint, what is a visual examination of the stomach called? _____

4. If *endocardium* is a structure inside the heart, what is a tube inside the windpipe called? (trachea = windpipe) _____

5. If a *dermatologist* is a specialist in the study of the skin, what is a specialist in the study of the heart called? _____

T. **Test your knowledge of the two new elements introduced in this chapter.** Differentiate the statements; some apply to either suffixes or prefixes. Circle P (for prefix) or S (for suffix) to identify them correctly. (LO 2.1, 2.4, *Analyze*)

1. This element can only appear at the end of the term	P	S
2. This element can identify color	P	S
3. This element can be a single letter	P	S
4. This element does not require a combining vowel	P	S
5. This element attaches to the end of an R or CF	P	S

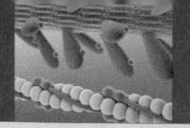

Suffixes and Prefixes

U. Deconstruct the following terms into their elements. Write the type of element (P, R, CF, S) under the line. Fill in the blanks. Remember, not every term will have a prefix. (**LO 2.8, *Analyze***)

1. arthrodesis   _____ / _____ / _____

2. gastrologist   _____ / _____ / _____

3. endocardium   _____ / _____ / _____

4. hypogastric   _____ / _____ / _____

5. dermatology   _____ / _____ / _____

6. Define any one of the terms above.

_____

_____

V. The suffix in this exercise remains the same, but changing the root will change the specialist. You are looking for a position as a medical assistant. The following practices have advertised on the County Medical Society's job hotline. What are their specialties? (Use a dictionary or glossary if needed.) (**LO 2.8, *Analyze***)

Type of Physician	Medical Specialty
urologist	1.
gynecologist	2.
gastroenterologist	3.
hematologist	4.
cardiologist	5.
dermatologist	6.

W. Recognizing word elements will help you "dissect," or deconstruct, a term. The following terms have an element set in bold. Identify the type of element, and give a brief definition of its meaning. (**LO 2.8, *Analyze***)

	Prefix, Root, Combining Form, Suffix	Medical Specialty
arthro**plasty**	1.	2.
endocarditis	3.	4.
dermato**logy**	5.	6.
hypotension	7.	8.
hypergast**ric**	9.	10.

X. Precision is the mark of an educated professional. Review these statements for accuracy, and correct where necessary. The sentence may contain a spelling or a factual error. Some sentences are correct. Rewrite the incorrect statements on the lines below. (**LO 2.8,** *Analyze*)

1. Patient has a bad rash. I referred her to a neurologist.

2. Diagnosis for Mr. Baker is resolving endocarditis.

3. Because of a possible bowel obstruction, I have asked a gastroenterologist to see the patient.

4. Patient is suffering from a topical dermatitiis.

5. Patient will be scheduled for gastrodesis of her knee on Monday.

6. Corrected statements:

_____

_____

_____

_____

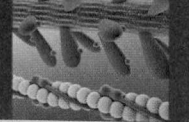
Suffixes and Prefixes

CHAPTER SUMMARY EXERCISE

A. Spelling comprehension. Circle the correct spelling of the term. (**LO 2.2, 2.5, 2.8,** *Remember*)

1. endogastrik	indogastrik	(endogastric)	endogestric	endagastrik
2. (dermatologist)	dermetologisst	dermetologist	dermitologist	dirmetologist
3. arrthroplasty	(arthroplasty)	arthroplastie	artroplasty	arthroplassty
4. (pericardium)	piricardium	pericarium	piricarddium	pericardeum
5. hypogestric	hipogastric	hyypogastric	hypogastrk	(hypogastric)
6. arthroedisis	artredesis	arthredessis	(arthrodesis)	arthridisis
7. cardeopathy	cardeeopathy	cardeopathie	(cardiopathy)	cardiopethy
8. arthriscopy	(arthroscopy)	artroscopy	arterioscopy	arterioscopie
9. dermatitiis	(dermatitis)	dermotitis	dermetitious	dermititis
10. epigastrric	epigestric	epigastrik	(epigastric)	epegastrik

B. Match the correct spelling of the term in Exercise A with the brief description of one of the following terms. (**LO 2.8,** *Apply*)

1. one who studies the skin — *dermatologist*

2. visual examination of a joint — *arthroscopy*

3. surgical repair of a joint — *arthroplasty*

4. pertaining to below the stomach — *hypogastric*

5. inflammation of the skin — *dermatitis*

6. pertaining to inside the stomach — *endogastric*

7. surgical fixation of a joint — *arthrodesis*

8. structure around the heart — *pericardium*

9. heart disease — *cardiopathy*

10. pertaining to above the stomach — *epigastric*

C. Using your knowledge of terms 1–10 in Exercises A and B and their correct spelling, write a brief sentence for each of the terms as it might appear in patient documentation. (LO 2.7, 2.8, *Apply*)

1. _____

2. _____

3. _____

4. _____

5. _____

6. _____

7. _____

8. _____

9. _____

10. _____

D. **Meet a lesson objective and list each of the building blocks of a medical term.** Describe their usual position in the term, and give an example of each type of element. Then answer question 4. (LO 2.1, 2.2, 2.4, 2.5, 2.8, *Apply*)

1. The building blocks of a medical term are _root_____, _combining V_, _suffic_____, _prefin____, _combining F_

2. The usual position of these building blocks in the term is

   a. _____ usually appears _____

   b. _____ usually appears _____

   c. _____ usually appears _____

   d. _____ usually appears _____

   e. _____ usually appears _____

3. Give an example of each type of element, and its meaning:

   a. Element: _____ Meaning: _____

   b. Element: _____ Meaning: _____

   c. Element: _____ Meaning: _____

   d. Element: _____ Meaning: _____

   e. Element: _____ Meaning: _____

4. To analyze a medical term, where should you start?

   _____

   _____

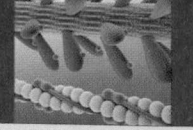

Suffixes and Prefixes

E. Meet the goals of each of the chapter outcomes and insert the correct answers to the questions. (LO 2.1–2.8, *Analyze*)

1. Define the term *suffix*. What is the function of a suffix? **(LO 2.1)**

   _____

2. Identify the suffixes of commonly used medical terms and their meanings. **(LO 2.2)**

   a. The term *gastric* has the suffix _____, and the suffix means

   _____.

   b. The term *cardiologist* has the suffix _____, and the suffix means

   _____.

   c. The term *endocardium* has the suffix _____, and the suffix means

   _____.

3. Establish a classification of suffixes. Read the answer choices below and locate the three suffixes that can be classified together. Then explain why they can be grouped. **(LO 2.3)**

   arthroplasty   dermatology   dermatitis   circumcision   arthrodesis

   epigastric   arthroscopy   hypotension

   a. These three suffixes can be grouped together: _____, _____ and _____.

   b. They can group together because they are all _____.

4. Define the term *prefix*. Where in a medical term does the prefix usually appear? **(LO 2.4)**

   _____

5. Identify the prefixes of commonly used medical terms and their meanings. Write the following prefixes and the terms' meanings below. **(LO 2.5)**

   a. *epigastric*: the prefix is _____ and means _____

   b. *hypogastric*: the prefix is _____ and means _____

   c. *endogastric*: the prefix is _____ and means _____

6. Establish a classification of prefixes. Find three prefixes that share something in common. **(LO 2.6)**

   hyper   ab   di   macro   hypo   tachy   brady   ad   epi

   a. Three prefixes with something in common are _____, _____, and _____.

   b. They can all be grouped together because they all describe _____.

7. Link word elements of prefixes, suffixes, roots, and combining forms together to construct medical terms. Construct the correct medical term using the following elements. (**LO 2.7**)

ary	ic	logist	um	itis	scopy
arthro	cardi/o	gastr	respire	dermat	

   a. Construct the term meaning *a visual examination of a joint:* _____/_____/_____

   b. Construct the term meaning *inflammation of the stomach:* _____/_____/_____

   c. Construct the term meaning *a specialist in heart problems.* _____/_____/_____

8. Deconstruct medical terms into their elements. Deconstruct the medical term *hypogastric* and then indicate whether the following statements about the term *hypogastric* are true or false. (**LO 2.8**)

   a. Deconstruct *hypogastric:* _____/_____/_____

   b. This term has no prefix.   T   F

   c. *Hypogastric* means *below the intestines.*   T   F

   d. This term has neither a prefix nor a suffix.   T   F

   e. This term means *pertaining to below the stomach.*   T   F

   f. This term has a root meaning *intestine.*   T   F

Word Analysis and Communication
The Language of Health Care

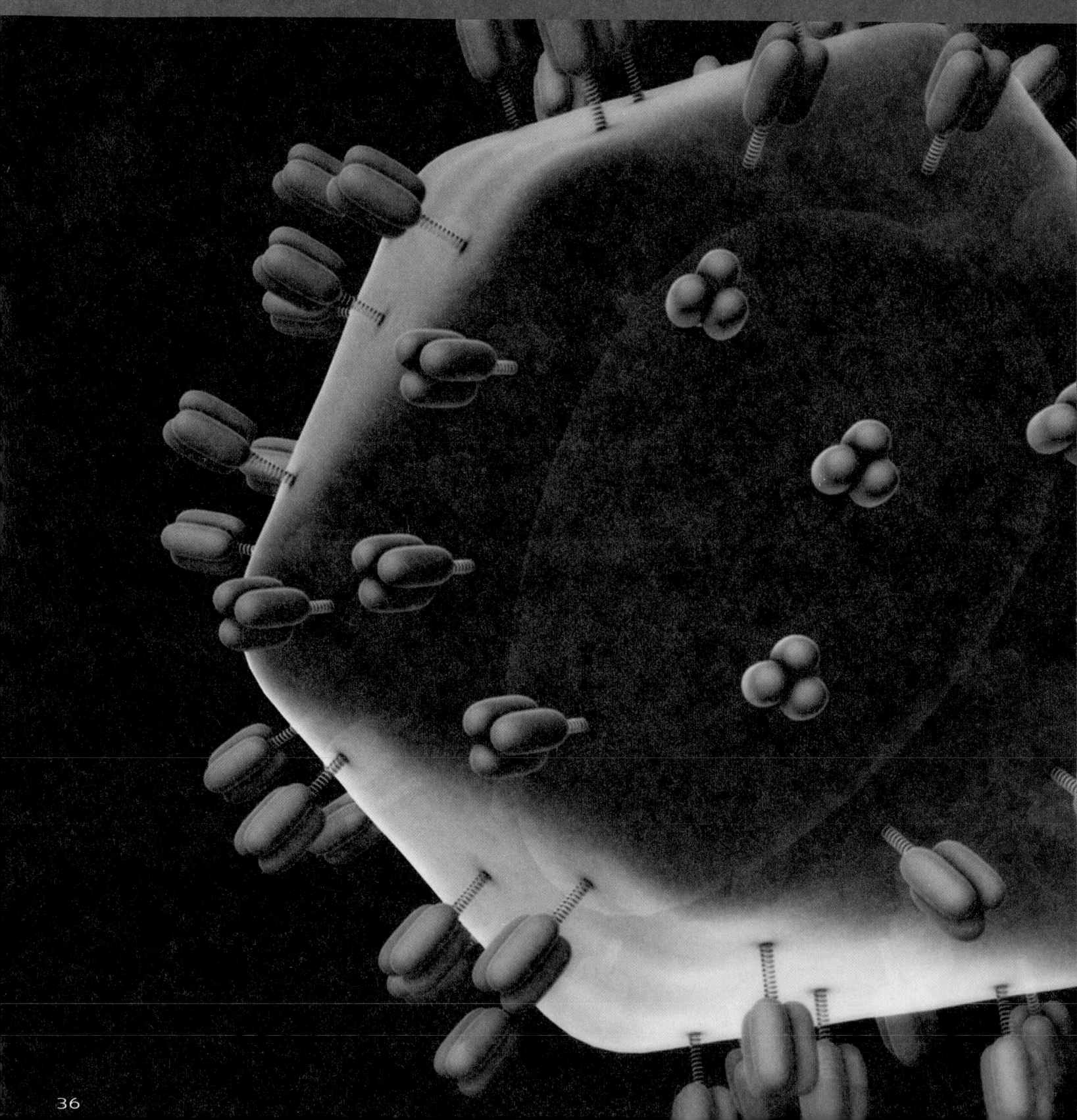

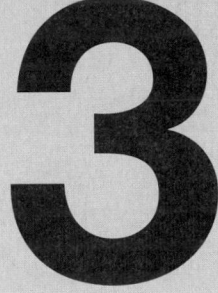

Case Report (CR) 3.1

You are

> . . . an emergency medical technician **(EMT)** employed in the Emergency Department at Fulwood Medical Center.

Your patient is

> . . . Barbara Rotelli, a 17-year-old woman, who presents with **pyrexia** and shaking chills. On her medical record, you read that her physical examination reveals splinter **hemorrhages** under her fingernails and a heart **murmur**. There is blood in her urine. She had **dental** surgery four days ago. A provisional **diagnosis** is made of acute **endocarditis**. You are to prepare her for admission to intensive care.

Chapter Learning Outcomes

LO 3.1 Deconstruct a medical term into its basic elements.

LO 3.2 Use word elements to identify or construct a medical term.

LO 3.3 Connect the singular and plural components of medical terms.

LO 3.4 Employ the phonetic system used to pronounce medical terms.

LO 3.5 Use Word Analysis and Definition Boxes to describe the phonetic pronunciation, word elements, and definition of terms used in the book.

LO 3.6 Communicate with precision in both written and verbal communication in all health care fields.

Lesson 3.1 Word Analysis and Definition

LESSON OBJECTIVES

When you see a medical term you do not understand, the first step you can take to analyze, decipher, or deconstruct the term is to break it down into its component elements, or parts. In this lesson, you will learn to:

3.1.1 Deconstruct a medical term into its word elements.

3.1.2 Use the word elements to identify the medical term.

Abbreviation	
EMT	emergency medical technician

LO 3.1, 3.2, 3.3 Word Analysis, Definition, and Pronunciation

For words you need to define, first identify the suffix.

For example, in the term **endocarditis**, the suffix at the end of the word is -itis, which means *inflammation*.

That leaves **endocard-**. You have learned that **-card-** is a **root** meaning *heart*. So now you have *inflammation of the heart*.

Card − itis = inflammation of the heart

That leaves **endo-**, a prefix meaning *inside*. So now you can assemble the pieces together to form the word meaning *inflammation of the inside of the heart*:

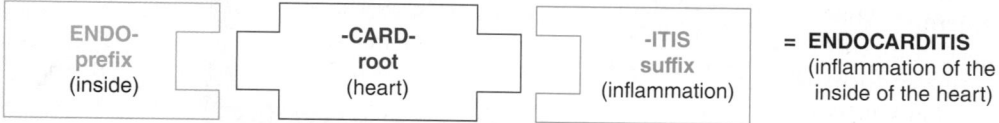

You also have learned that the suffix -um means *a structure*. So changing the suffix to **endocardium** would be the structure that lines the inside of the heart.

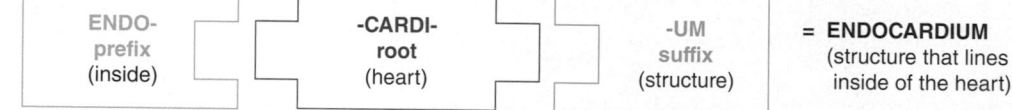

Therefore, you can understand that **endocarditis** is used to mean that the endocardium lining the heart has become inflamed or infected. Both **-card-** and **-cardi-** are **roots** meaning *heart*.

Another example is the word **hemorrhage**, used in CR 3.1 in the opening spread of this chapter. The suffix **-rrhage** following the **combining vowel "o"** is borrowed from the Greek word meaning *to flow profusely*. The **combining form hem/o-** is from the Greek word for *blood*. The elements of the medical term **hemorrhage** are assembled together and used to mean *profuse bleeding*.

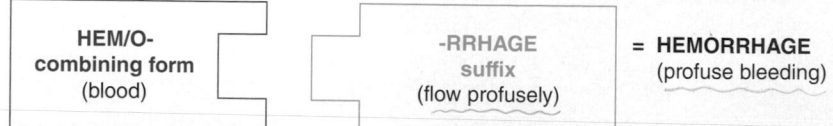

In this book, when the medical terms are broken down into their elements, a hyphen is used to isolate each major element and to identify its position in the whole word.

When a **combining form** is used, the **combining vowel** is separated from the **root** by a slash (/).

One of the key design concepts of this book is that all the textual and visual information you need for any given topic will be on the two-page spread open in front of you. As part of this, in the top right-hand quarter of the two-page spread will be a box designed to give you the elements, definition, and pronunciation of every new medical term that appears in the two pages you are reviewing. For example, the box will look like the box at the top of the next page, which refers to the medical terms used on these two pages and to the boldfaced terms in the Case Report at the beginning of the chapter. This box is a Word Analysis and Definition box, called a WAD for short.

WORD	PRONUNCIATION	ELEMENTS		DEFINITION
dental	**DEN**-tal	S/ R/	-al *pertaining to* dent- *tooth*	Pertaining to the teeth
dentist dentistry (*Note:* This word has two suffixes and one root.)	**DEN**-tist **DEN**-tis-tree	S/ S/	-ist *specialist* -ry *occupation*	Legally qualified specialist in dentistry Evaluation, diagnosis, prevention, and treatment of conditions of the oral cavity and associated structures
diagnosis (noun)	die-ag-**NO**-sis	P/ R/	dia- *complete* -gnosis *knowledge of an abnormal condition*	The determination of the cause of a disease
diagnoses (pl) diagnostic (adj) (*Note:* The "is" in gnosis is deleted to allow the word to flow.)	die-ag-**NO**-sees die-ag-**NOS**-tik	S/	-tic *pertaining to*	Pertaining to or establishing a diagnosis
diagnose (verb)	die-ag-**NOSE**	R/	-gnose *recognize an abnormal condition*	To make a diagnosis
endocarditis	**EN**-doh-kar-**DIE**-tis	S/ P/ R/	-itis *inflammation* endo- *within, inner* -card- *heart*	Inflammation of the lining of the heart
endocardium	**EN**-doh-kar-**DEE**-um	S/ P/ R/	-um *structure* endo- *within, inner* -cardi- *heart*	The inside lining of the heart
hemorrhage	**HEM**-oh-raj	S/ R/CF	-rrhage *to flow profusely* hem/o- *blood*	To bleed profusely
murmur	**MUR**-mur		Latin *murmur*	Abnormal sound heard on auscultation of the heart or blood vessels
pyrexia	pie-**REK**-see-ah	S/ R/	-ia *condition* pyrex- *fever, heat*	An abnormally high body temperature or fever

Many of the exercises at the end of each spread are based on information found in the Word Analysis and Definition box (WAD) or in the spread.

Exercises

A. To analyze a medical term, simply break the elements down (deconstruct them) into their basic forms. *To construct a new term, take the appropriate elements, put them in the correct position in the term, and build your term.* **Note:** *Remember that not every term will have all elements present at the same time.* **LO 3.1, 3.2**

1. **To deconstruct:** Take the medical term **endocarditis** and break it down into elements. / <u>endo</u> / <u>cardi</u> / <u>itis</u>

                                                                  P   R/CF   S

    The prefix <u>endo</u> means <u>inside</u>.

    The root <u>card</u> means <u>heart</u>.

    The suffix <u>itis</u> means <u>inflamation</u>.

    The term **endocarditis** means <u>inflamation inside the heart</u>.

2. **To construct:** Take the following elements and construct a new term with them. <u>endo</u> / <u>cardi</u> / <u>um</u>

                                                                    P   R/CF   S

    The element "**um**" means <u>Structure</u>. What type of word element is this? _____

    The element "**endo**" means _____. What type of word element is this? _____

    The element "**cardi**" means _____. What type of word element is this? _____

    This term is _____ and means _____.

LESSON OBJECTIVES

In your career as a health professional, the correct, precise pronunciation of medical terms is an essential part of your daily life and of your self-esteem. It is also critical for patient safety and high-quality patient care. The information in this lesson will enable you to:

3.2.1 Connect the singular and plural components of medical terms.

3.2.2 Employ the system for describing pronunciation used in the textbook.

3.2.3 Verbalize the pronunciation of common medical terms.

LO 3.4, 3.5 Plurals and Pronunciations

Plurals

When you change a medical term from singular to plural, it is not as simple as adding an *s*, as you often can in the English language. Unfortunately, in medical terms, the end of the word changes in ways that were logical in Latin and Greek but have to be learned by memory in English. This is shown in *Table 3.1*.

Table 3.1 Singular and Plural Forms

Singular Ending	Plural Ending	Examples	Singular Ending	Plural Ending	Examples
-a		axilla	-on		ganglion
	-ae	axillae		-a	ganglia
-ax		thorax	-um		septum
	-aces	thoraces		-a	septa
-en		lumen	-us		viscus
	-ina	lumina		-era	viscera
-ex		cortex	-us		villus
	-ices	cortices		-i	villi
-is		diagnosis	-us		corpus
	-es	diagnoses		-ora	corpora
-is		epididymis	-x		phalanx
	-ides	epididymides		-ges	phalanges
-ix		appendix	-y		ovary
	-ices	appendices		-ies	ovaries
-ma		carcinoma	-yx		calyx
	-mata	carcinomata		-ices	calices

Pronunciations

In your role as a health professional, pronouncing medical terms correctly and precisely is not only about understanding conversations with your peers or a physician. It is also a matter of ensuring patient safety and providing high-quality patient care.

Correct pronunciation is essential so that other health professionals with whom you are working can understand what you are saying. Throughout this textbook, the pronunciation of each medical term will be written out phonetically using modern English forms. The part(s) of the word to which you give the strongest, or primary, emphasis is (are) written in bold, uppercase letters.

For example, the term **gastroenterology** will be phonetically written **GAS**-troh-en-ter-**OL**-oh-gee, whereas the term **gastritis**, which means *inflammation of the stomach*, will be phonetically written as gas-**TRY**-tis. **Hemorrhage** will be written as **HEM**-oh-raj, whereas the term **hemostasis**, which means *the stopping of bleeding*, will be written he-moh-**STAY**-sis.

The only way you can learn how to pronounce medical terms is to say them repeatedly and have your pronunciation checked against a standard which is found in McGraw-Hill Connect Plus.

Exercises

A. Forming plurals of medical terms will be less difficult if you follow the rules and apply them correctly. *The rules are given to you in the following chart—practice changing the medical terms from singular to plural. Fill in the chart.*   **LO 3.3**

Singular	Plural	Singular Term	Plural Term	Singular	Plural	Singular Term	Plural Term
-a	-ae	axilla	1.	-on	-a	ganglion	2.
-ax	-aces	thorax	3.	-um	-a	septum	4.
-en	-ina	lumen	5.	-us**	-era	viscus	6.
-ex	-ices	cortex	7.	-us**	-i	villus	8.
-is*	-es	diagnosis	9.	-us**	-ora	corpus	10.
-is*	-ides	epididymis	11.	-x	-ges	phalanx	12.
-ix	-ices	appendix	13.	-y	-ies	ovary	14.
-ma	-mata	carcinoma	15.	-yx	-ices	calyx	16.

Note: In the case of the rules with an asterisk (*), both singular terms can end in -is. You have to know on a case-by-case basis which singular terms change to -es and which ones change to -ides.
**The same applies to the singular terms ending in -us—some will form plurals with -era, -i, or -ora.

Lesson 3.3 Precision in Communication

LESSON OBJECTIVES

This year in the United States, more than 400,000 people will die because of drug reactions and medical errors. Many of these deaths are due to inaccurate or imprecise written or verbal communications between the different members of the health care team. You can avoid making errors in your own communications, and this lesson will help you do that by enabling you to:

3.3.1 **Communicate with precision both verbally and in writing.**

3.3.2 **Use word analysis to ensure the precise use of words.**

You are

. . . a radiology technician working in the Radiology Department of Fulwood Medical Center.

Your patient is

. . . Mrs. Matilda Morones, a 38-year-old woman who presents with sudden onset of severe, **colicky** right-flank pain and pain in her **urethra** as she passes urine.

Keynotes

- Communicate verbally and in writing with attention to detail, accuracy, and precision.
- When you understand the individual word elements that make up a medical term, you are better able to understand clearly the medical terms you are using.

Abbreviation

stat immediately, at once

Case Report 3.2

The physical examination revealed that Mrs. Morones is in severe distress, with marked tenderness in the right **costovertebral** angle and in the right lower quadrant of her abdomen. Microscopy of her urine showed numerous red blood cells. The **stat abdominal** x-ray you have taken reveals a **radiopaque** stone in the right **ureter**. She has now become faint and is in **hypotension**.

How are you going to communicate Mrs. Morones' condition as you ask for help and then document her condition and your response?

LO 3.5, 3.6 Precision in Communication

In Case Report 3.2, if **hypotension** (low blood pressure) is confused with **hypertension** (high blood pressure), incorrect treatments could be prescribed. Confusing Mrs. Morones' **ureter** (the tube from the kidney to the bladder) with her **urethra** (the tube from the bladder to the outside) could lead to disastrous consequences.

Being a health professional requires the utmost attention to detail and precision, both in written documentation and in verbal communication. A patient's life could be in your hands. In addition, the medical record in which you document a patient's care and your actions is a legal document. It can be used in court as evidence in professional medical liability cases. Any incorrect spelling can reflect badly on the whole health care team.

LO 3.3, 3.5, 3.6 Use of Word Analysis

In Case Report 3.2, **ureter** (you-RET-er) and **urethra** (you-REE-thra) are both simple words with no prefix, **combining vowel**, or suffix. They are derived from the Greek word for *urine*. They are similar words but have very different anatomic locations (*Chapter 6*).

To deconstruct the word **hypotension** (high-po-TEN-shun), start with the suffix -ion, which means *a condition*. Next, the prefix hypo- means *below* or *less than normal*. The **root -tens-** is from the Latin word for *pressure*. Place the pieces together to form a word meaning *condition of below-normal pressure*, or low blood pressure.

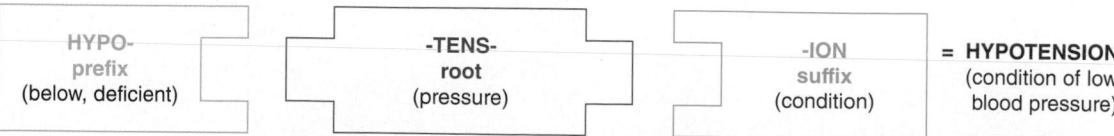

| HYPO-
prefix
(below, deficient) | -TENS-
root
(pressure) | -ION
suffix
(condition) | = HYPOTENSION
(condition of low
blood pressure) |

To deconstruct the term **costovertebral** (koss-toh-ver-TEE-bral), start with the suffix -al, which means *pertaining to*. Separated by the **combining vowel "o"** are two **roots**, cost- and -vertebr-. The **combining form cost/o-** is from the Latin word for *a rib*. -Vertebr- is from the Latin word for *backbone or spine*. So you have *pertaining to the rib and the spine*.

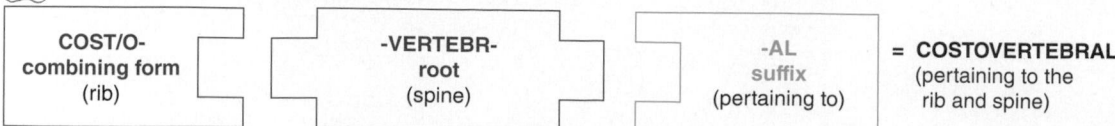

| COST/O-
combining form
(rib) | -VERTEBR-
root
(spine) | -AL
suffix
(pertaining to) | = COSTOVERTEBRAL
(pertaining to the
rib and spine) |

The **costovertebral angle** is the angle pertaining to or between the 12th rib and the spine. This angle is a surface anatomy marking for the kidney.

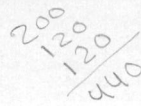

WORD	PRONUNCIATION	ELEMENTS		DEFINITION
abdomen	**AB**-doh-men		Latin *abdomen*	The part of the trunk that lies between the thorax and the pelvis
abdominal	ab-**DOM**-in-al	S/ R/	-al *pertaining to* **abdomin-** *abdomen*	Pertaining to the abdomen
colic	**KOL**-ik	S/ R/	-ic *pertaining to* **col-** *colon*	Pertaining to the colon
colicky	**KOL**-icky	S/	-icky *arising from*	Pain in the colon
costovertebral	kos-toe-**VER**-tee-bral	S/ R/CF R/	-al *pertaining to* **cost/o-** *rib* **-vertebr-** *spine*	Pertaining to the rib and spine
hypertension	**HIGH**-per-**TEN**-shun	S/ P/ R/	-ion *action, condition* **hyper-** *excessive* **-tens-** *pressure*	Persistent high arterial blood pressure
hypotension	**HIGH**-poh-**TEN**-shun	P/	**hypo-** *low, below*	Persistent low arterial blood pressure
radiopaque	ray-dee-oh-**PAKE**	S/ R/CF	-paque *shady* **radi/o-** *radiation*	Impenetrable by x-rays or other forms of radiation
ureter (***Note:*** Two "e"s = two tubes.)	you-**RET**-er		Greek *urinary canal*	Tube that connects the kidney to the urinary bladder
urethra	you-**REE**-thra		Greek *urethra*	Canal leading from the urinary bladder to the outside

Exercises

A. Precision in communication. *Verbal and written communication must always be precise and accurate for patient safety and legal requirements. Develop your eyes' and ears' ability to distinguish correct pronunciations, word choice, and spelling to ensure documentation and communication accuracy. Fill in the following blanks:*   **LO 3.6**

1. If the doctor tells you a patient's blood pressure readings are elevated, does the patient have hypertension or hypotension?

   _____

2. If the patient has a problem with his malleolus, would you send him to see an orthopedist (bone specialist) or an ENT (ear, nose and throat) specialist?

   _____

3. If a patient fell off a ladder and injured his back, would it most likely be his trapezius or his trapezium that was hurt?

   _____

4. Does a patient with a kidney infection need to see a urologist or a neurologist?

   _____

5. What is the difference in anatomic location of the ureter and the urethra?

   The ureter is _____.

   The urethra is _____.

6. Do you remember what is unusual about the elements of the words ***ureter*** and ***urethra***?

   They have no _____.

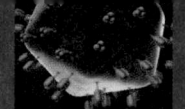

Word Analysis and Communication

Challenge Your Knowledge

A. **The answers to all these questions can be retrieved from the WAD on page 43. (LO 3.3, 3.6,** *Remember*)

1. Which two terms denote locations on the body? _____ and _____

2. What organ does the term *colic* refer to? _____

3. Which two terms in this WAD are opposites? _____ and _____

4. What is the difference between the ureter and the urethra?

   a. ureter: _____

   b. urethra: _____

5. *Costovertebral* pertains to the

   a. rib and colon

   b. heart and rib cage

   c. rib and spine

   d. lung and rib

   e. rib and kidney

B. **Recall your pronunciation.** Circle the correct answer below. **(LO 3.5,** *Remember*)

1. What is the correct pronunciation of *pyrexia?*

   a. pie-RECK-si-a   **d.** pie-REK-see-ah

   b. PIE-RECK-ci-a   **e.** py-rek-SEE-ah

   c. PY-rek-sia

2. What is the correct pronunciation of *costovertebral?*

   a. KOSTO-ver-TREE-bral   **d.** COSTO-ver-tree-bral

   b. cost-o-VER-tre-bal   **e.** kosto-ver-tree-BAL

   c. kos-toe-VER-tee-bral

3. What is the correct pronunciation of *radiopaque?*

   a. ray-dee-oh-PAKE   **d.** radio-PAKE

   b. ra-di-o-PAKE   **e.** ray-DI-o-pake

   c. RADIOH-plaque

C. **To help you master plurals, practice changing singular endings to plural and plural endings to singular in the following exercise.** If you are given a singular word, change it to plural. If you are given a plural word, change it back to singular. <u>The first one is done for you</u>. Fill in the chart; then pick any two terms (singular or plural) and write a sentence for each term for questions 16 and 17. (**LO 3.3,** *Remember, Apply*)

Word	Singular	Plural
1. carcinomata	carcinoma	
2. ovary		
3. ganglia		
4. lumen		
5. villi		
6. cortices		
7. calyx		
8. epididymis		
9. axilla		
10. viscus		
11. appendices		
12. corpora		
13. septum		
14. diagnosis		
15. thorax		

16. _____

17. _____

D. **Word elements are the building blocks of medical terminology.** Being able to define word elements will help you use them correctly. Identify the element by placing a checkmark (√) in the correct column; then define the meaning of the element. In the last column, give an example of a medical term containing that element. Fill in the chart. (**LO 3.1, 3.2,** *Remember, Apply*)

Element	Prefix	Root/ Combining Form	Suffix	Meaning of Element	Medical Term
1. cardi				2.	3.
4. entero				5.	6.
7. dermato				8.	9.
10. logy				11.	12.
13. gastro				14.	15.
16. scopy				17.	18.
19. itis				20.	21.
22. gynec				23.	24.
25. logist				26.	27.

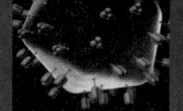

Word Analysis and Communication

E. The answers to all these questions can be found in the WAD on page 39. (**LO 3.1, 3.2,** *Understand*)

1. Which three terms in the WAD refer to tooth repair and maintenance?

    a. _____

    b. _____

    c. _____

2. Which term is a structure? _____

3. Which term means to bleed profusely? _____

4. If you show up in the ER with a temperature of 105, you have _____.

5. What term describes an abnormal heart sound? _____

F. Correct knowledge of medical terms means you can explain them to someone else. Describe the difference between the following terms. (**LO 3.2, 3.6,** *Understand*)

1. hypertension _____

2. hypotension _____

3. ureter _____

4. urethra _____

G. True or false. Circle the correct answer. On the lines below, rewrite any false answer *correctly.* (**LO 3.1, 3.2,** *Understand*)

1. A term never has more than one root.   T   F

2. Some terms will have no combining vowel.   T   F

3. Modification may be necessary to make a word easier to pronounce.   T   F

4. A vowel must always be present in a combining form.   T   F

5. Corrected statements:

    _____

    _____

    _____

    _____

H. **Focus on all the text carefully because some information in the text does not appear in the WAD.** Fill in the blanks with appropriate medical language found in the text. (**LO 3.2,** *Understand*)

1. Explain *splinter hemorrhages.*

_____

2. The root *hem* is the Greek word for _____.

3. Describe the location of the costovertebral angle. _____

_____

4. The costovertebral angle is a surface anatomy marking for what organ? _____

5. Define *surface anatomy.* _____

> **Study Hint**
>
> *Pyrexia* means *fever* or *heat.* Equate that to the glass cookware you bake in to help you remember what the term means.

I. **Precision in documentation means using the correct form of the term, as well as the correct term.** Medical terms can take the forms of noun (thing), verb (action), or adjective (description). Insert the correct term in the appropriate line. (**LO 3.6,** *Understand, Apply*)

diagnosis   diagnose   diagnostic   diagnoses

1. After performing several _____ tests, the physician has confirmed his _____.

2. In addition to her diabetes, the patient has several other _____.

3. The physician was unable to _____ the patient's condition because the patient refused the prescribed tests.

4. Which of the terms used is a verb? _____

5. Which of the terms is an adjective? _____

J. **The suffix in this exercise remains the same, but changing the root will change the specialist.** You are looking for a position as a medical assistant. The following practices have advertised on the County Medical Society's job hotline. What are their specialties? (Use a dictionary or glossary if needed.) (**LO 3.1, 3.2,** *Understand, Apply*)

Type of Physician   Medical Specialty

1. urologist   _____

2. gynecologist   _____

3. gastroenterologist   _____

4. hematologist   _____

5. cardiologist   _____

6. dermatologist   _____

Word Analysis and Communication

K. **Use the appropriate medical language to answer the questions.** Circle the correct answer. (**LO 3.1, 3.2,** *Apply*)

1. Which one of the following terms is an x-ray technician likely to use?

   a. hypertension

   b. radiopaque

   c. hypotension

   d. pyrexia

   e. hemorrhage

2. Which one of the following terms is *not* a symptom?

   a. pyrexia

   b. hypotension

   c. hemorrhage

   d. colic

   e. endocardium

3. Inflammation of the lining of the heart is

   a. cardiology

   b. cardiac

   c. endocarditis

   d. cardiologist

   e. endocardium

4. Which term might be used to describe a baby?

   a. hypertensive

   b. colicky

   c. hypotensive

   d. costovertebral

   e. abdominal

5. Which one of the following terms would a heart specialist use?

   a. colic

   b. urethra

   c. murmur

   d. abdominal

   e. costovertebral

L. Using the elements from the list in the previous exercise, answer the following questions. (LO 3.1, 3.2, *Apply*)

1. Name the specialist for the digestive tract: _____

2. What is study of the heart called? _____

3. What is inflammation of the skin called? _____

4. What specialist would you see for an inflammation of the skin? _____

5. What is inserting a tube into the stomach for a visual examination called? _____

M. Spelling is most important in medical terminology. For example, **ilium** and **ileum** may be similar in appearance and sound, but the difference of one letter makes each a different body part. Choose the correct spelling for the following terms. Fill in the blanks. (**LO 3.6, *Apply***)

1. A Pap smear is part of a _____ exam.

                 gynecologik   gyneckologic   gynecologic

2. After a difficult delivery, the patient started to _____.

                 hemorage   hemmorhage   hemorrhage

3. Inflammation of the heart is _____.

                 carditus   carditis   cardiitis

4. A muscle in the back is the _____.

                 trapeze   trapezium   trapezius

5. A bony protuberance in your ankle is the _____.

                 maleus   malius   malleolus

N. Constructing terms is taking the building blocks of elements and correctly arranging them to form the term you need. Employ your knowledge of prefixes, roots, combining forms, and suffixes to construct the term required. Fill in the chart. (**LO 3.2, *Apply***)

Meaning	Prefix	Root(s)	Combining Form	Suffix	Term
inflammation of the stomach and intestines	1.	2.	3.	4.	5.
pertaining to the rib and spine	6.	7.	8.	9.	10.
inflammation of a joint	11.	12.	13.	14.	15.
visual examination of the stomach	16.	17.	18.	19.	20.
blood bursting forth	21.	22.	23.	24.	25.
pertaining to or on top of the skin	26.	27.	28.	29.	30.
one who studies the heart	31.	32.	33.	34.	35.
visual examination within the body	36.	37.	38.	39.	40.

Word Analysis and Communication

O. Use the word elements to identify the correct medical term. Circle the appropriate medical term. (**LO 3.2,** *Analyze*)

1. Which medical term has an element meaning to flow profusely?

    a. dentistry

    b. endocardium

    c. hemorrhage

    d. pyrexia

    e. diagnosis

2. Which medical term has an element meaning a structure?

    a. endocarditis

    b. cardiologist

    c. endocardium

    d. dental

    e. cardiology

3. Which medical term has an element meaning condition?

    a. pyrexia

    b. murmur

    c. diagnoses

    d. hemostasis

    e. gastroenterology

4. Which medical term has an element meaning inflammation?

    a. gastroenterologist

    b. gastritis

    c. gastrologist

    d. gastric

    e. gastrology

5. Which medical term has an element meaning knowledge of an abnormal condition?

    a. murmur

    b. diagnosis

    c. convulsion

    d. seizure

    e. pyrexia

P. Outline the method of attack on a medical term to deconstruct it. Where do you start, and where do you go from there? (**LO 3.1,** *Analyze*)

1. Start: _____.

2. Next, check the _____.

3. Finally, analyze the _____.

4. Give an example below of a term you have deconstructed:

_____

Q. Speak and spell with precision in medical communication. All terms in the WAD boxes are spelled phonetically to make them easier for you to learn to pronounce. Be sure you can speak them correctly as well as spell them correctly! Practice, practice, practice. You may be called upon to pronounce them in class. Circle the best answer, and then fill in the blanks. (**LO 3.5, 3.6,** *Analyze*)

1. The correct pronunciation for an inflammation of the heart is

   a. **EN**-do-kar-di-tis

   b. en-**DO**-kard-itis

   c. **EN**-doh-kar-**DIE**-tis

   The correct spelling of this term is _____.

2. An abnormally high body temperature is

   a. pie-**REK**-see-ah

   b. **PIE**-rek-seeah

   c. pie-**REK**-see-**AH**

   The correct spelling of this term is _____.

3. Profuse bleeding is termed a

   a. **HEM**-oh-raj

   b. hem-**OH**-raj

   c. **HEM**-oh-**RAJ**

   The correct spelling of this term is _____.

R. Analyze the following medical terms on the basis of your knowledge of elements. Put a slash (/) between each element of the terms listed as follows; then write the definition of each term. (**LO 3.1, 3.2,** *Analyze*)

1. enteric: _____

2. abdominopelvic: _____

3. arthroplasty: _____

4. gastric: _____

5. costovertebral: _____

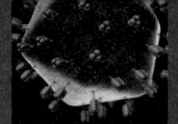

Word Analysis and Communication

S. **Precision is the mark of an educated professional.** Review these statements for accuracy, and correct where necessary. The sentence may contain a spelling or a factual error. Some sentences are correct. Rewrite the incorrect statements on the lines that follow. (**LO 3.6,** *Analyze*)

1. Patient has a bad case of the hives. I referred her to a neurologist.

2. Discharge diagnosis: resolving cardiitis and cardiopathy.

3. Because of a possible bowel obstruction, I have asked a gastroenterologist to see the patient.

4. Patient is suffering from a topical dermatitis.

5. Due to prolonged hemmorrhaging, the patient needed a blood transfusion.

6. Patient will be scheduled for gastrodesis of her knee on Monday.

7. Corrected statements:

_____

_____

_____

_____

_____

T. **Terminology challenge.** Fill in the blanks. (**LO 3.2,** *Analyze*)

1. Which two prefixes in this chapter are opposites, and what do they mean?

_____ means _____, and _____ means _____.

2. Name two suffixes in this chapter that mean *pertaining to.* _____ and _____

3. List two medical specialties that were mentioned in this chapter. _____ and _____

4. What is the medical term for *to bleed profusely?* _____

5. What is the medical term for stopping this bleeding? _____ *(Watch your spelling!)*

U. **Analyze your word choice to be precise.** Errors in medical documentation are a threat to patient safety and a legal liability. Circle the correct answer. (**LO 3.6,** *Analyze*)

1. A visual **examination** of the stomach is a

        gastroscopy   gastropexy   gastrodesis   gastroplasty

2. An **abdominoplasty** would be a surgical

        fusion   fixation   repair   examination

3. **Endogastric** would be

        above the stomach   below the stomach   within the stomach   outside the stomach

4. **Arthropathy** is a disease of

        skin   joints   arteries   blood vessels

5. If you have a painful **skin** rash, what type of specialist do you need?

        cardiologist   urologist   neurologist   dermatologist

6. The root **respir-** means

        to walk   to hear   to breathe   to feel

7. If **rhin/o** means *nose*, what is a surgical repair of a broken nose called?

        rhinodesis   rhinoscopy   rhinoplasty   rhinopexy

V. **Case report questions.** This Case Report is taken from the beginning of Chapter 3. You should feel more comfortable with the medical terminology now. Read the report again, and you will be able to answer the questions. Fill in the blanks. (**LO 3.1, 3.2,** *Analyze, Evaluate*)

Case Report 3.1

You are

. . . an **EMT** employed in the Emergency Department at Fulwood Medical Center.

Your patient is

. . . Barbara Rotelli, a 17-year-old woman, who presents with **pyrexia** and shaking chills. On her medical record, you read that her physical examination reveals splinter **hemorrhages** under her fingernails and a heart **murmur**. There is blood in her urine. She had **dental** surgery four days ago. A provisional **diagnosis** is made of acute **endocarditis**. You are to prepare her for admission to intensive care.

1. *Pyrexia* has an element that means *fever* or *heat*. What is that element? _____

2. What is a *heart murmur?* _____

3. *Endocarditis* has a prefix that means _____

4. What is a *diagnosis?* _____

Chapter 3 Review

Word Analysis and Communication

CHAPTER SUMMARY EXERCISE

A. **Spelling comprehension.** Circle the correct spelling of the term. (**LO 3.6,** *Remember*)

1. pyrexcia	pyrexia	pirixia	pyrixea	pirexia
2. mumur	mermer	murmur	mirmur	mumrur
3. endocardites	endocarditis	endocaritis	endocarites	endacardites
4. hemorrhege	hemorrage	hemmorrhage	hemmorage	hemorrhage
5. dintal	dentel	dental	dendal	denttal
6. diagnosis	deagnossis	diagnnosis	diaggnosis	diagnosiss
7. hypotenssion	hopotension	hypotension	hypotennsion	hipotension
8. costovertebrral	costovertebral	costoverrtibral	castovertebal	costovertebal
9. hemostassis	hemostasis	hemmostassis	hematsasis	hemastasis
10. urethrra	ureathra	urettra	ureathrra	urethra

B. **Match the number of the correct spelling of the term in Exercise A with the brief description of the term below.** (**LO 3.2,** *Apply*)

1. abnormally high fever _____

2. pertaining to the ribs and spine _____

3. stopping bleeding _____

4. abnormal heart sound _____

5. low blood pressure _____

6. canal that leads to the outside _____

7. determination of the cause of a disease _____

8. pertaining to the teeth _____

9. to bleed profusely _____

10. inflammation of the inside of the heart _____

C. Using your knowledge of terms 1–10 in Exercises A and B and their correct spelling, write a brief sentence for each of the terms as it might appear in patient documentation. **(LO 3.6,** *Apply***)**

1. _____

2. _____

3. _____

4. _____

5. _____

6. _____

7. _____

8. _____

9. _____

10. _____

D. Meet the goals of each of the chapter outcomes and provide the correct answers to the questions. **(LO 3.1–3.6,** *Analyze, Apply***)**

1. Deconstruct a medical term into its basic elements. Slash the following medical term into its basic elements. **(LO 3.1)**

costovertebral _____ / _____ / _____

                                          P   R/CF   S

2. Use word elements to identify a medical term. On the basis of the word elements, identify the correct medical term. **(LO 3.2)**

a. hypertension	i. high fever
b. pyrexia	ii. structure within the heart
c. hemorrhage	iii. high blood pressure
d. endocardium	iv. profuse bleeding
e. hypotension	v. low blood pressure

Word Analysis and Communication

3. Use the WADs to describe the phonetic pronunciation, word elements, and definitions of terms used in the book. Refer to the WAD on page 43 to answer the following questions. **(LO 3.3)**

    a. The correct pronunciation of radiopaque is

        i. RAY-de-o-pak

        ii. ray-de-o-PAK

        iii. ray-dee-oh-PAKE

    b. TENS is an element meaning

        i. breathing

        ii. pressure

        iii. flow profusely

        iv. blood

        v. fever, heat

    c. Pertaining to the rib and spine is the definition for

        i. colic

        ii. hemorrhage

        iii. costovertebral

        iv. abdominal

        v. murmur

4. Connect the singular and plural components of medical terms. Select the correct plural for the following singular terms. Circle the appropriate term.

    a. carcinoma

        carcinomae   carcinomum   carcinomata   carcinomus

    b. septum

        septae   septa   septus   septy

    c. corpus

        corporal   corporum   corpora   corporax

    d. appendix

        appendixes   appendixs   appendixes   appendices

    e. thorax

        thoraces   thoraxes   thoraxies   thoracum

5. Employ the phonetic system used to describe pronunciation. Which of the following is the correct pronunciation for the medical term *hemorrhage?* (**LO 3.5**)

   a. **HEM**-oh-raj

   b. hehm-o- **RAJ**

   c. hemmo- **RHAGE**

   d. **HEM**-o-**RAJ**

   e. **HEMO**-rhage

6. Communicate with precision in both written and verbal communication in all health care fields. (**LO 3.6**)

   a. The physician has diagnosed the patient with an abnormal heart sound; the patient has a heart _____.

   b. If a physician tells you the patient has endocarditis, you know the patient has a _____ problem.

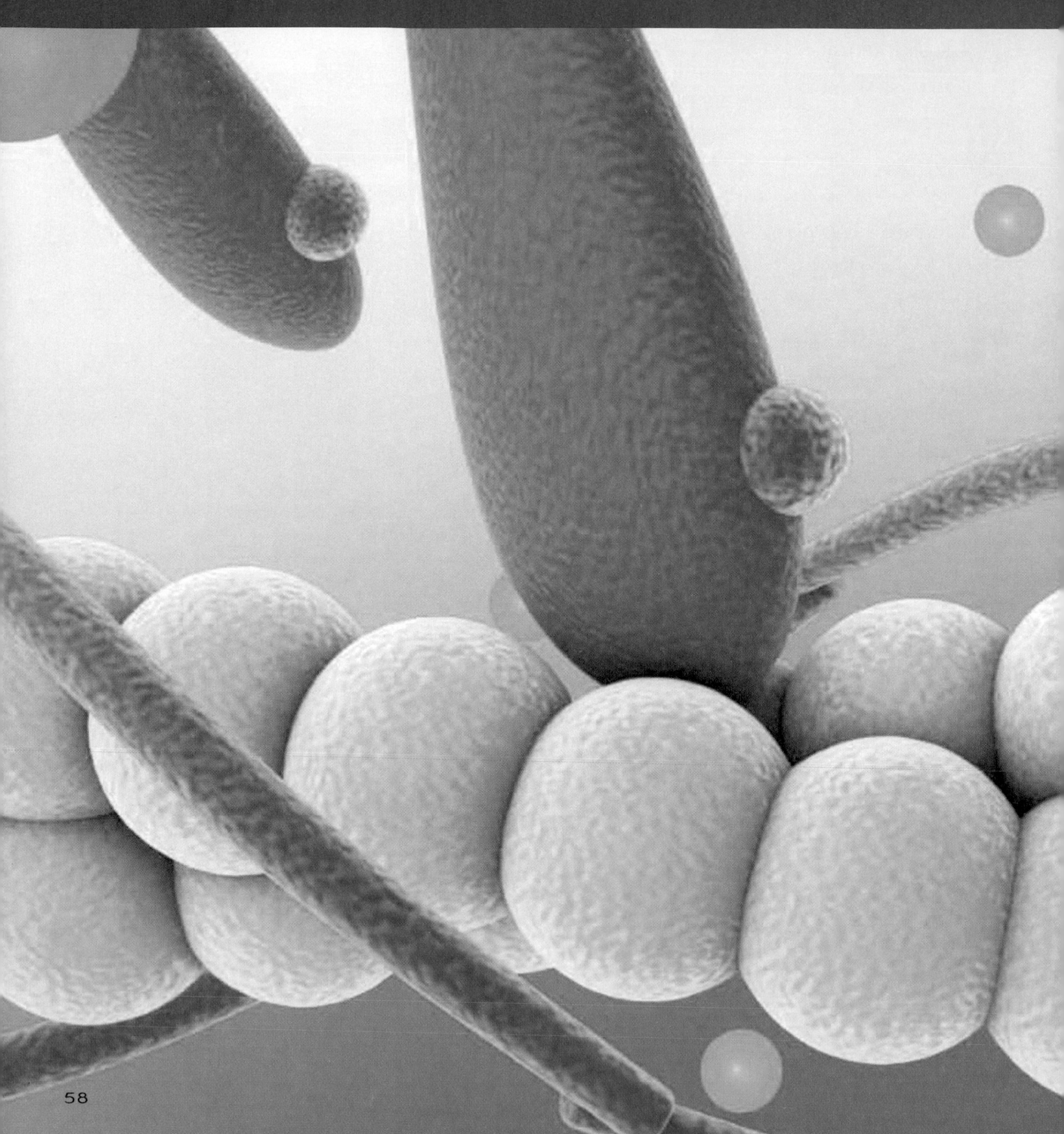

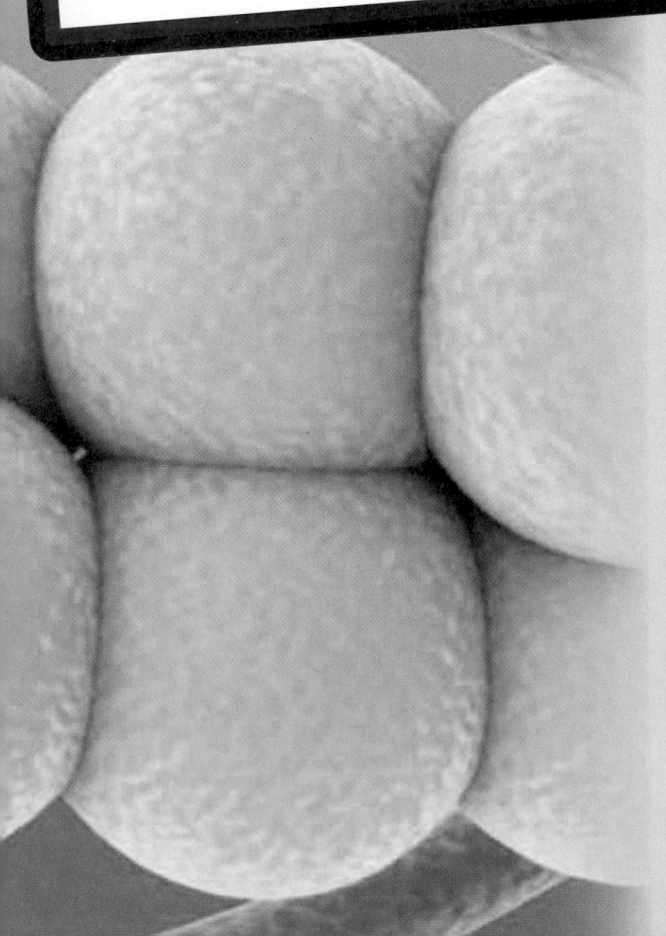

4

Case Report (CR) 4.1

You are

... a certified medical assistant (CMA) employed as an in vitro fertilization coordinator in the Assisted Reproduction Clinic at Fulwood Medical Center.

Your patient is

... Mrs. Mary Arnold, a 35-year-old woman who has been unable to conceive. **In vitro fertilization (IVF)** was recommended. After hormone therapy, several healthy and mature eggs were recovered from her ovary. The eggs were combined with her husband's sperm in a laboratory dish where fertilization occurred to form a single cell, called a **zygote**. The cells were allowed to divide for 5 days to become **blastocysts**, and then four blastocysts were implanted in her uterus.

Your role is to guide, counsel, and support Mrs. Arnold and her husband through the implementation and follow-up for the IVF process.

Chapter Learning Outcomes

Each of us begins as a zygote and becomes a whole person. Effective medical diagnosis and treatment recognizes that each organ, tissue, and cell in your body functions in harmony with and affects every other organ, tissue, and cell. Your whole body also includes your thoughts, emotions, and perceptions that affect your health, disease, and recovery. This concept of treating the body as a whole is called **holistic** and requires you to be able to:

LO 4.1 Apply correct medical terms to the anatomy and physiology of the body as a whole.

LO 4.2 Discuss the medical terms associated with the structures and functions of cells, tissues, and organs.

LO 4.3 Relate individual body systems to the organization and function of the body as a whole.

LO 4.4 Integrate the medical terms of the different anatomic positions, planes, and directions of the body into everyday medical language.

LO 4.5 Map the body cavities.

LO 4.6 Describe the nine regions of the abdomen.

LO 4.7 Use medical terms pertaining to the body as a whole to communicate and document in writing accurately and precisely in any health care setting.

LO 4.8 Use medical terms pertaining to the body as a whole to communicate verbally with accuracy and precision in any health care setting.

Lesson 4.1 Organization of the Body

LESSON OBJECTIVES

All the elements of your body interact with one another to enable your body to be in constant change as it reacts to the environment and to the nourishment you give it.

To understand the structure and function of your body, you need to be able to use correct medical terminology to:

4.1.1 Identify the structure and functions of the components of a cell.

4.1.2 List the four primary groups of tissue and describe their functions.

4.1.3 Identify major organs and list the smaller organs contained within them.

4.1.4 Name the medical terms associated with cells, tissues, and organs.

Composition of the Body

- The whole body or organism is composed of **organ** systems.
  - Organ systems are composed of **organs**.
    - Organs are composed of **tissues**.
      - Tissues are composed of **cells**.
        - Cells are composed in part of **organelles**.
          - Organelles are composed of **molecules**.
            - Molecules are composed of **atoms**.

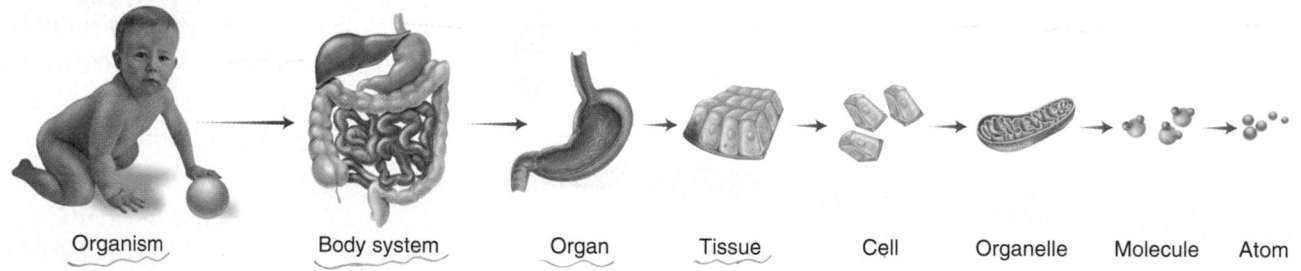

| Organism | Body system | Organ | Tissue | Cell | Organelle | Molecule | Atom |

Abbreviation	
IVF	in vitro fertilization

LO 4.1, 4.2 The Cell

This single fertilized cell, the **zygote**, is the result of the **fertilization** of an egg **(oocyte)** by a sperm and is the origin of every cell in your body (*Figure 4.1*). The oocyte divides and multiplies into millions of cells that are the basic unit of every tissue and organ. The structure and all of the functions of your tissues and organs are due to their cells. The **cell** is the basic unit of life. **Cytology** is the study of this cell structure and function. Your understanding of the cell will form the basis for your knowledge of the anatomy and physiology of every tissue and organ.

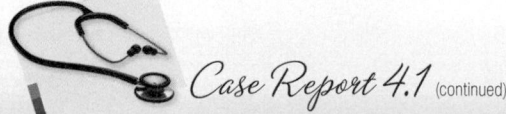

Case Report 4.1 (continued)

Mrs. Arnold achieved pregnancy and delivered a healthy girl at term.

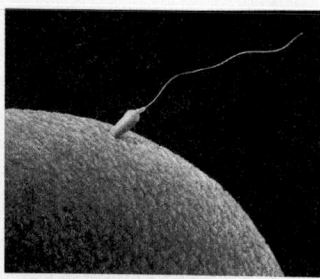

▲ **Figure 4.1** Fertilization of Egg by Single Sperm.

WORD	PRONUNCIATION		ELEMENTS	DEFINITION
atom	AT-om		Greek *indivisible*	A small unit of matter
blastocyst	BLAS-toe-sist	R/CF S/	blast/o *immature cell* -cyst *cyst, sac, bladder*	First 2 weeks of the developing embryo
cell	SELL		Latin *a storeroom*	The smallest unit capable of independent existence
cellular (adj) cytology	SELL-you-lar SIGH-tol-oh-gee	S/ R/ S/ R/CF	-ar *pertaining to* cellul- *small cell* -logy *study of* cyt/o- *cell*	Pertaining to a cell Study of the cell
fertilization fertilize (verb)	FER-til-eye-ZAY-shun FER-til-ize	S/ R/	-ation *process* fertiliz- *to bear*	Union of a male sperm and a female egg
holistic	ho-LIS-tik	S/ R/	-ic *pertaining to* holist- *whole*	Pertaining to the care of the whole person in physical, mental, emotional, and spiritual dimensions
molecule molecular (adj) (**Note:** The two suffixes are joined by two vowels, therefore the *e* in *ule* is not used.)	MOLL-eh-kyul mo-LEK-you-lar	S/ R/ S/	-ule *small* molec- *mass* -ar *pertaining to*	Very small particle consisting of two or more atoms held tightly together
oocyte	OH-oh-site	R/ R/CF	-cyte *cell* o/o- *egg*	Female egg cell
organ organelle	OR-gan OR-gah-nell	S/ R/	Latin *instrument, tool* -elle *small* organ- *organ*	Structure with specific functions in a body system Part of a cell having a specialized function(s)
tissue	TISH-you		Latin *to weave*	Collection of similar cells
vitro in vitro fertilization (IVF)	VEE-troh IN VEE-troh FER-til-eye-ZAY-shun		Latin *glass*	Process of combining a sperm and egg in a laboratory dish and placing resulting embryos inside a uterus
zygote	ZYE-goat		Greek *yolked*	Cell resulting from the union of the sperm and egg

Exercises

A. As you begin your study of *medical language,* it is important to realize the logic of how terms are formed. *Elements are building blocks. You may not see a root in the same position in every term. Not every term requires a prefix and/or a suffix. Build your terms after first reviewing the above WAD box. Fill in the blanks.* **LO 4.1, 4.2**

1. The female egg cell is known as an <u>egg</u> / <u>oocyte</u> / _____. This term is composed of two elements. What are they? <u>o</u> and <u>cyte</u>

> *Study Hint*
> Notice the position of the root in questions 1, 2, and 3. A root can appear at the end of a term or at the beginning of a term, as well as in the middle of a term (its usual place).

2. This term does not start with a prefix; it starts with a combining form and ends with a suffix.

   Study of the cell: <u>cytology</u> /_____/_____

3. This term begins with a combining form, which is a root plus a combining vowel. The term ends with a suffix.

   Pertaining to the cell: _____/_____/_____

B. Elements are building blocks. *You may not see a root in the same position in every term. Not every term requires a prefix and/or a suffix. Build your terms after first reviewing the above WAD box. Fill in the blanks.* **LO 4.1, 4.2**

1. The five elements used to build medical terms are _____, _____, _____, _____, and _____.

2. Which element is missing from all the terms in this WAD?_____

3. Which elements in the WAD means *small*? _____

4. _____ is a (identify the element) _____ and means _____.

LO 4.1, 4.2 Structure and Functions of Cells

As the zygote divides, every cell derived from it becomes a small, complex factory that carries out these **basic functions of life:**

- *Manufacture* of proteins and lipids
- *Production* and use of energy
- *Communication* with other cells
- *Replication* of **deoxyribonucleic acid** (**DNA**)
- *Reproduction*

All your cells contain a fluid called **cytoplasm** (**intracellular** fluid) surrounded by a **cell membrane** *(Figure 4.2)*. A single cell may have 10 billion protein molecules inside it.

The cell membrane is made of proteins and lipids and allows water, oxygen, glucose, **electrolytes**, **steroids**, and alcohol to pass through it. On the outside of the cell membrane are receptors that bind to chemical messengers, such as **hormones** sent by other cells. These are the chemical signals by which your cells communicate with each other. The cytoplasm is a clear, gelatinous substance crowded with different organelles. **Organelles** are small structures that carry out special **metabolic** tasks, the chemical processes that occur in the cell. Examples of organelles are

- Nucleus
- Endoplasmic reticulum
- Golgi complex or apparatus
- **Mitochondria**
- Nucleolus
- Ribosomes
- Lysosomes

These are defined and their functions detailed in the succeeding pages.

Organelles

The **nucleus** is the largest organelle *(Figure 4.2)*. It directs all the activities of the cell. Most of your cells have one nucleus; red blood cells have none, and some liver cells and muscle cells contain many nuclei. The nucleus is surrounded by its own membrane, which has small openings called *pores*. Every minute, hundreds of molecules pass through the pores. These molecules include the raw materials for the DNA and ribonucleic (RNA) synthesis that is ongoing inside the nucleus. Forty-six molecules of DNA and their associated **proteins** are packed into each nucleus as thin strands called **chromatin**. When cells divide, the chromatin condenses to form 46 more densely coiled bodies called **chromosomes**.

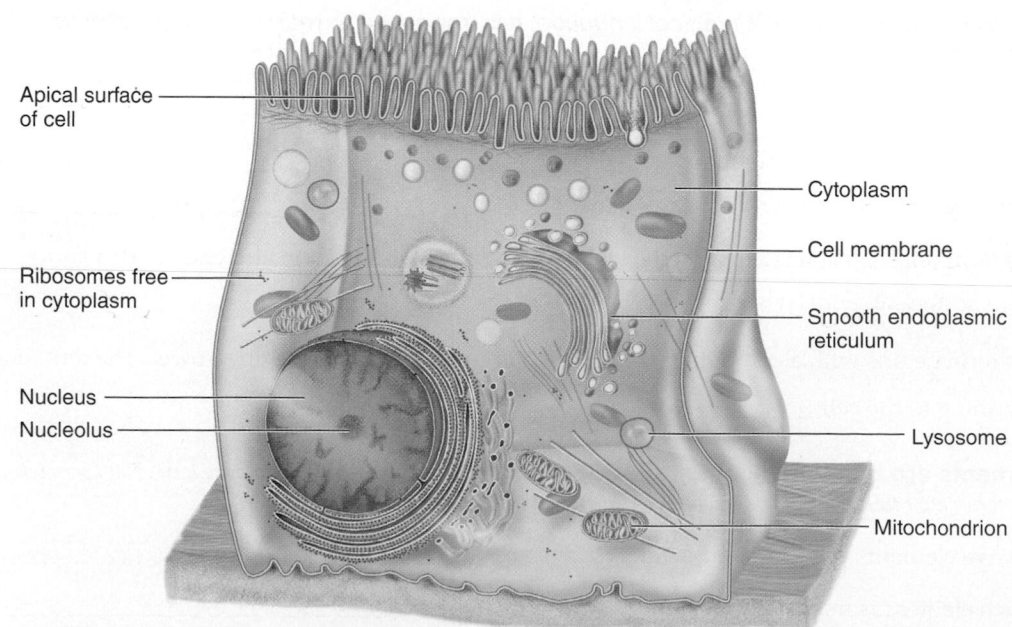

Apical surface of cell

Ribosomes free in cytoplasm

Nucleus

Nucleolus

Cytoplasm

Cell membrane

Smooth endoplasmic reticulum

Lysosome

Mitochondrion

▲ **Figure 4.2**   **Structure of a Representative Cell.**

WORD	PRONUNCIATION	ELEMENTS		DEFINITION
cytoplasm	**SIGH**-toe-plazm	S/ R/CF	-plasm *something formed* cyt/o- *cell*	Clear, gelatinous substance that forms the substance of a cell except for the nucleus
chromatin	**KROH**-ma-tin	S/ R/	-in *substance, chemical compound* chromat- *color*	Substance composed of DNA that forms chromosomes during cell division
chromosome	**KROH**-moh-sohm	S/ R/CF	-some *body* chrom/o- *color*	Body in the nucleus that contains DNA and genes
deoxyribonucleic acid (DNA)	dee-**OCK**-see-**RYE**-boh-noo-**KLEE**-ik **ASS**-id		deoxyribose *sugar* nucleic acid *protein*	Source of hereditary characteristics found in chromosomes
electrolyte	ee-**LEK**-troh-lite	S/ R/CF	-lyte *soluble* electr/o- *electric*	Substance that, when dissolved in a suitable medium, forms electrically charged particles
hormone hormonal (adj)	**HOR**-mohn hor-**MOHN**-al		Greek *set in motion*	Chemical formed in one tissue or organ and carried by the blood to stimulate or inhibit a function of another tissue or organ
intracellular	in-trah-**SELL**-you-lar	S/ P/ R/	-ar *pertaining to* intra- *within* -cellul- *small cell*	Within the cell
membrane membranous (adj)	**MEM**-brain **MEM**-brah-nus		Latin *parchment*	Thin layer of tissue covering a structure or cavity
metabolism metabolic (adj)	meh-**TAB**-oh-lizm met-ah-**BOL**-ik	S/ R/ S/	-ism *condition* metabol- *change* -ic *pertaining to*	The constantly changing physical and chemical processes occurring in the cell Pertaining to metabolism
mitochondrion mitochondria (pl)	my-toe-**KON**-dree-on my-toe-**KON**-dree-ah	S/ R/CF R/CF	-ion *action, condition* mit/o- *thread* chondr/o- *cartilage, rib, granule*	Organelle that generates, stores, and releases energy for cell activities
nucleus nuclear (adj)	**NYU**-klee-us **NYU**-klee-ar	S/ R/	-us *pertaining to* nucle- *nucleus*	Functional center of a cell or structure
nucleolus	nyu-**KLEE**-oh-lus	S/ R/CF	-lus *small* nucle/o- *nucleus*	Small mass within the nucleus
steroid steroidal (adj)	**STER**-oyd **STER**-oy-dal	S/ R/	-oid *resemble* ster- *solid*	Large family of chemical substances found in many drugs, hormones, and body components

Exercises

A. Continue building your knowledge of elements. *Add the elements that will complete this medical term. Write under the line the element(s) you have used (P = prefix, R = root, CF = combining form, and S = suffix). Fill in the blanks.*   **LO 4.1, 4.2**

1. Within the cell   _____/cellul/_____

2. Substance of a cell except for the nucleus   _____/_____/plasm

3. Chemical substance found in drugs   _____/_____/oid

4. What makes the difference between a root and a combining form? _____

B. Seek and find in the above WAD the medical term that is defined as follows.   LO 4.1, 4.2

1. small organ _____

2. thin layer of tissue covering a structure or cavity _____

3. electrically charged particles _____

4. powerhouse of the cell _____

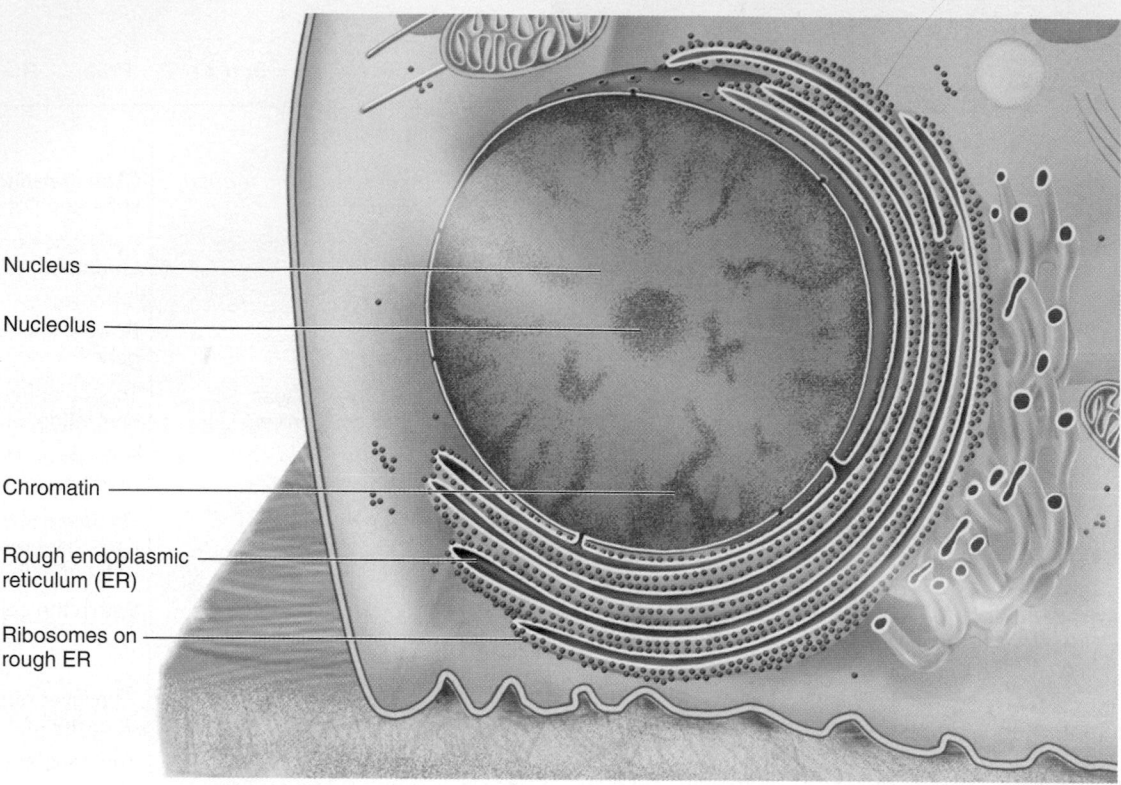

Nucleus

Nucleolus

Chromatin

Rough endoplasmic
reticulum (ER)

Ribosomes on
rough ER

▲ **Figure 4.3**   The Nucleus.

LO 4.1, 4.2 Structure and Functions of Cells (continued)

Ribosomes are organelles involved in the manufacture of protein from simple materials. This process is called **anabolism**.

Organelles (Continued)

Each nucleus (*Figure 4.3*) contains a **nucleolus**, a small dense body composed of RNA and protein. It manufactures ribosomes that migrate through the nuclear membrane pores into the cytoplasm.

The **endoplasmic reticulum** is an organelle that manufactures steroids, cholesterol and other lipids, and proteins. It also detoxifies alcohol and other drugs.

Lysosomes are organelles that are the garbage disposal units of the cell. They digest and dispose of worn-out organelles as part of the process of cell death. They also digest foreign particles and bacteria.

Mitochondria are the powerhouses of the cells. They extract energy by breaking down compounds such as glucose and fat. This process is called **catabolism**. The energy is used to do the work of the cell: for example, to make a muscle contract.

WORD	PRONUNCIATION	ELEMENTS		DEFINITION
anabolism	an-**AB**-oh-lizm	S/ R/	-ism *condition* **anabol-** *build up*	The buildup of complex substances in the cell from simpler ones as a part of metabolism
carbohydrate	kar-boh-**HIGH**-drate	S/ R/CF R/	-ate *composed of, pertaining to* **carb/o-** *carbon* **-hydr-** *water*	Group of organic food compounds that includes sugars, starch, glycogen, and cellulose
catabolism	kah-**TAB**-oh-lizm	S/ R/	-ism *condition* **catabol-** *break down*	Breakdown of complex substances into simpler ones as a part of metabolism
lysosome	**LIE**-soh-sohm	S/ R/CF	-some *body* **lys/o-** *decompose*	Enzyme that digests foreign material and worn-out cell components
protein	**PRO**-teen	S/ R/CF	-in *substance, chemical compound* **prot/e-** *first*	Class of food substances based on amino acids
ribosome	**RYE**-bo-sohm	S/ R/CF	-some *body* **rib/o-** *like a rib*	Structure in the cell that assembles amino acids into protein

Exercises

A. Continue analyzing the logic of *medical language*. *Add the element that will complete this medical term.* <u>Write under the line</u> *the element you have used (P, R, CF, S). Fill in the blanks.*   **LO 4.1, 4.2**

1. Which medical term in the above WAD has an element meaning *color*? _____

2. Which term in the above WAD refers to an enzyme? _____

3. Find a term in the above WAD that contains an element that means *water*. _____

4. Which term in the above WAD refers to breaking substances down? _____

B. Fill in the blanks, or circle the answer with the correct medical terminology.   LO 4.1, 4.2, 4.3

1. What is the small mass within the nucleus called? _____

2. Which of the following terms is associated with metabolism?

   a. nucleus

   b. chromatin

   c. membrane

   d. anabolism

   e. holistic

3. Every one of the following medical terms has a function. Briefly describe what they do.

   a. nucleus   Function: _____

   b. nucleolus   Function: _____

   c. ribosomes   Function: _____

   d. anabolism   Function: _____

   e. catabolism   Function: _____

You are

... a physical therapy assistant employed in the Rehabilitation Unit in Fulwood Medical Center.

Your patient is

... Mr. Richard Josen, a 22-year-old man who injured tissues in his left knee playing football (Figure 4.4).

Case Report 4.2

Using arthroscopy, the orthopedic surgeon removed Mr. Josen's torn **anterior cruciate ligament (ACL)** and replaced it with a **graft** from his patellar ligament. The torn **medial collateral ligament** was sutured together. The tear in his medial **meniscus** was repaired. His rehabilitation, in which you play a key role, focuses on strengthening the **muscles** around his knee joint and helping him regain joint mobility.

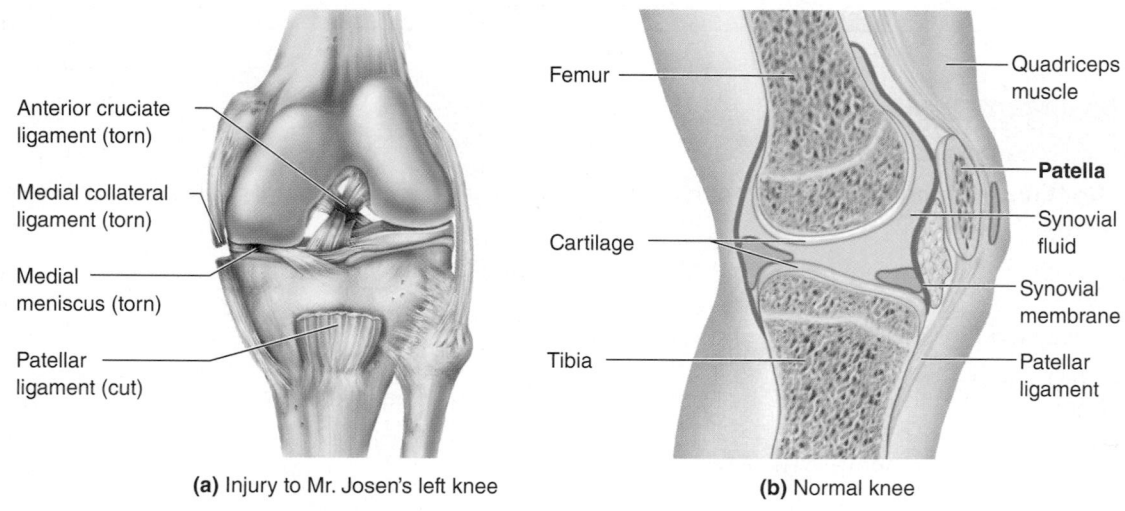

Anterior cruciate ligament (torn)

Medial collateral ligament (torn)

Medial meniscus (torn)

Patellar ligament (cut)

Femur

Cartilage

Tibia

Quadriceps muscle

Patella

Synovial fluid

Synovial membrane

Patellar ligament

(a) Injury to Mr. Josen's left knee

(b) Normal knee

▲ **Figure 4.4**   Knee Anatomy.

Keynote

Different tissues are made of specialized cells with unique materials around them that are manufactured by the cells.

Abbreviation	
ACL	anterior cruciate ligament

LO 4.2 Tissues

The knee contains examples of all the different major groups of tissue and will be used in this lesson to illustrate the relation of structure to function in the different tissues. To understand the condition of the 22-year-old in Case Report 4.2, you need a knowledge of tissue structure and function. Ultimately, this is important for your understanding of the anatomy and physiology of organs, organ systems, and the whole body.

Tissues hold your body together. The many tissues of your body have different structures for specialized functions. The different tissues are made of similar cells with unique materials around them that are manufactured by the cells. **Histology** is the study of the structure and function of tissues. The four primary tissue groups are outlined in *Table 4.1*.

Table 4.1 The Four Primary Tissue Groups

Type	Function	Location
Connective	Bind, support, protect, fill spaces, store fat	Widely distributed throughout the body; for example, in blood, bone, cartilage, and fat
Epithelial	Protect, **secrete**, absorb, **excrete**	Cover body surface, cover and line internal organs, compose glands
Muscle	Movement	Attached to bones, in the walls of hollow internal organs, and in the heart
Nervous	Transmit impulses for **coordination**, sensory reception, motor actions	Brain, spinal cord, nerves

WORD	PRONUNCIATION	ELEMENTS		DEFINITION
anterior (opposite of posterior)	an-**TER**-ee-or	S/ R/	-ior *pertaining to* anter- *before, front part*	Front surface of body; situated in front
collateral	koh-**LAT**-er-al	S/ P/ R/	-al *pertaining to* co- *together* -later- *side*	Situated at the side; having an accessory function
coordinate	ko-**OR**-din-ate	S/ R/CF P/	-ate *composed of, -pertaining to* -ordin- *arrange* co- *together*	To bring together different structures into a harmonious function.
coordination (noun)	ko-**OR**-di-**NAY**-shun	S/	-ation	The harmonious function of interrelated structures
cruciate	**KRU**-she-ate		Latin *cross*	Shaped like a cross
epithelium	ep-ih-**THEE**-lee-um	S/ P/ R/CF	-um *structure* epi- *upon* -thel/i- *nipple*	Tissue that covers surfaces or lines cavities
epithelial (adj)	ep-ih-**THEE**-lee-al	S/	-al *pertaining to*	Pertaining to epithelium
excrete	eks-**KREET**		Latin *separate*	To pass waste products of metabolism out of the body
excretion (noun)	eks-**KREE**-shun			Removal of waste products of metabolism out of the body
graft	GRAFT		French *transplant*	Transplantation of living tissue
histology	his-**TOL**-oh-jee	S/ R/CF	-logy *study of* hist/o- *tissue*	Structure and function of cells, tissues, and organs
histologist	his-**TOL**-oh-jist	S/	-logist *one who studies*	Specialist in the structure and function of cells, tissues, and organs
ligament	**LIG**-ah-ment		Latin *band*	Band of fibrous tissue connecting two structures
medial (opposite of lateral)	**ME**-dee-al		Latin *middle*	Nearer to the middle of the body
meniscus **menisci** (pl)	meh-**NISS**-kuss meh-**NISS**-key		Greek *crescent*	Disc of connective tissue cartilage between the bones of a joint; for example, in the knee joint
muscle	**MUSS**-el		Latin *muscle*	A tissue consisting of contractile cells
patella	pah-**TELL**-ah		Latin *small plate*	Thin, circular bone in front of the knee joint that is embedded in the patellar tendon. Also called the kneecap
secrete **secretion** (noun)	se-**KREET** se-**KREE**-shun		Latin *release*	To produce a chemical substance in a cell and release it from the cell

Exercises

A. Change the elements; change the word. *Find a set of terms in the above WAD for which changing a single element will change the meaning of the term. Fill in the blanks.* **LO 4.2, 4.3**

1. _____/ _____/ _____ means _____.

       P   R/CF   S

   _____/ _____/ _____ means_____.

       P   R/CF   S

The element that changed was the _____.

Examples of opposite terms are given in the above WAD. Write the terms and their opposites below.

2. _____ is the opposite of _____.

3. _____ is the opposite of _____.

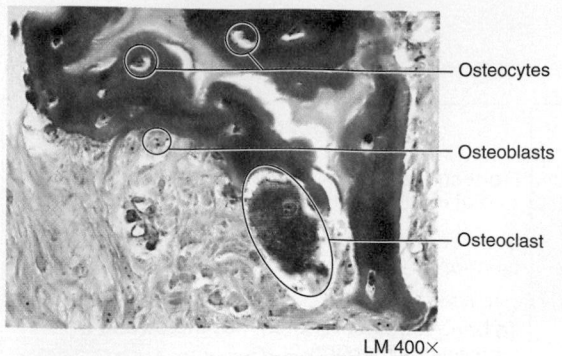

Osteocytes

Osteoblasts

Osteoclast

LM 400×

▲ **Figure 4.5**   **Bone Tissue.**

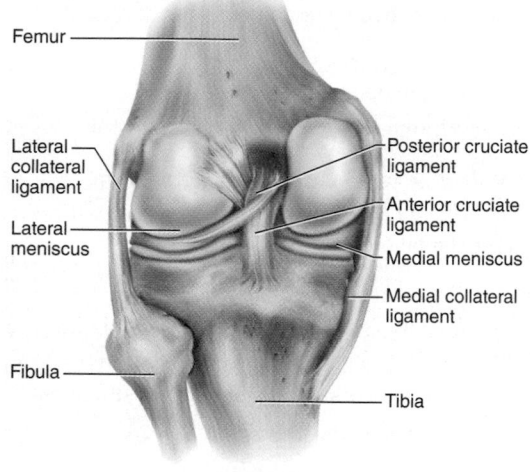

Femur

Lateral collateral ligament

Lateral meniscus

Fibula

Posterior cruciate ligament

Anterior cruciate ligament

Medial meniscus

Medial collateral ligament

Tibia

Anterior view

▲ **Figure 4.6**   **Ligaments of the Knee Joint.**

LO 4.2, 4.3 Connective Tissues in the Knee Joint

- **Bones** of the knee joint are the femur, tibia, and patella. Bone is the hardest connective tissue due to the presence of calcium mineral salts, mostly calcium phosphate. Bone **matrix** is deposited by bone cells, **osteoblasts** (*Figure 4.5*), in concentric patterns around a central canal containing a blood vessel. As a result, every osteoblast is close to a supply of **nutrients** from the blood. This enables bones to heal after being fractured. **Osteocytes** are former osteoblasts that maintain the bone matrix. **Osteoclasts** dissolve the bone matrix to release calcium and phosphate into the blood when these chemicals are needed elsewhere. Bones as a whole are covered with a thick fibrous tissue called the **periosteum**.

- **Cartilage** has a flexible, rubbery matrix that allows it, as a meniscus, to function as a shock absorber and as a gliding surface at **articulations** where two bones meet to form a joint. Cartilage has very few blood vessels and heals poorly or not at all. When it is injured or torn, surgical repair is usually necessary. Sometimes (for example, in osteoarthritis) it cannot be repaired. Cartilage also forms the shape of your ear, the tip of your nose, and your larynx.

- **Ligaments** are strips or bands of fibrous connective tissue (*Figure 4.6*). Cells called **fibroblasts** form a gelatinous (jellylike) matrix and closely packed, parallel **collagen** fibers. These fibers provide the strength the ligament needs. The knee joint has a complex array of 11 ligaments that hold it together, prevent it from rotating when we stand upright, and help prevent dislocations. Their blood supply is poor, so they do not heal well without surgery.

- **Tendons** are thick, strong ligaments that attach muscles to bone.

- The **joint capsule** of the knee joint is attached to the tibia and femur, encloses the joint cavity, and is made of thin, collagenous fibrous connective tissue. It is strengthened by fibers that extend over it from the ligaments and muscles surrounding the knee joint. These features are common to most joints.

- The inner surface of many joint capsules is lined with **synovial membrane**, which secretes **synovial fluid**. This fluid is a slippery lubricant retained in the joint cavity by the capsule. It has a texture similar to raw egg white. It makes joint movement almost friction-free and distributes nutrients to the cartilage on the joint surfaces of bone.

- **Muscle tissue** stabilizes the knee joint. Extensions of the tendons of the *quadriceps femoris*, the large muscle in front of the thigh, and of the *semimembranosus muscle* on the rear of the thigh, are major stabilizers. The muscles themselves respectively extend and flex the joint. The structure and functions of these and other skeletal muscles are described in *chapter 14*.

- **Nervous tissue** extensively supplies all the knee structures, which is why a knee injury is excruciatingly painful. The structure and functions of nervous tissue are described in *chapter 9*.

WORD	PRONUNCIATION	ELEMENTS		DEFINITION
articulate articulation (noun)	ar-**TIK**-you-late ar-tik-you-**LAY**-shun		Latin *jointed*	To form a joint so as to allow movement Joint formed to allow movement
capsule capsular (adj)	**KAP**-syul **KAP**-syu-lar	S/ R/	-ule *little* caps- *box*	Fibrous tissue layer surrounding a joint or some other structure
cartilage	**KAR**-tih-lage		Latin *gristle*	Nonvascular firm, connective tissue found mostly in joints
collagen	**KOL**-ah-jen	S/ R/CF	-gen *produce, form* coll/a- *glue*	Major protein of connective tissue, cartilage, and bone
fibroblast	**FIE**-bro-blast	R/ R/CF	-blast *germ cell* fibr/o- *fiber*	Cell that forms collagen fibers
matrix	**MAY**-triks		Latin "mater" *mother*	Substance that surrounds cells, is manufac- tured by the cells, and holds them together
nutrient	**NYU**-tree-ent	S/ R/	-ent *end result* nutri- *nourish*	A substance in food required for normal physiologic function
osteoblast	**OS**-tee-oh-blast	R/ R/CF	-blast *germ cell* oste/o- *bone*	Bone-forming cell
osteoclast osteocyte	**OS**-tee-oh-klast **OS**-tee-oh-site	S/ S/	-clast *break* -cyte *cell*	Bone-removing cell Bone-maintaining cell
periosteum	**PER**-ee-**OSS**-tee-um	S/ P/ R/	-um *tissue* peri- *around* -oste- *bone*	Fibrous membrane covering a bone
synovial (adj)	si-**NOH**-vee-al	S/ P/ R/CF	-al *pertaining to* syn- *together* -ov/i- *egg*	Pertaining to synovial fluid and synovial membrane
tendon	**TEN**-dun		Latin *sinew*	Fibrous band that connects muscle to bone

Exercises

A. Understanding elements is the key to a large medical vocabulary. *Work with the following exercise to increase your knowledge of medical language. Fill in the blanks.*   **LO 4.2, 4.3**

osteoblast   osteoclast   osteocyte

1. These terms all refer to (circle one)   cartilage   bone   collagen   *with the element*_____.

2. The element that changes in every term is the (circle one):   P   R   CF   S

3. Osteo**blast** means _____.

4. Osteo**clast** means _____.

5. Osteo**cyte** means _____.

B. Match the appropriate medical term in the first column to the descriptions given in the second column.   LO 4.2

_____ 1. synovial   **a.** to form a joint

_____ 2. articulate   **b.** fibrous membrane covering a bone

_____ 3. meniscus   **c.** connects muscle to bone

_____ 4. tendon   **d.** slippery lubricant

_____ 5. periosteum   **e.** shock absorber

An 84-year-old man with advanced **Parkinson disease** was having difficulty breathing because his stooped **posture** was compressing his lungs and his muscle spasticity made respiration more difficult. A bout of influenza increased his breathing difficulty, and a **tracheostomy** tube was inserted to help him breathe. He then became unable to swallow, and a feeding tube was inserted. Because of **hypertrophy** of his prostate, he developed a **urinary** tract infection. This led to **septicemia.** The bloodborne infection attacked his kidneys, heart, and lungs, leading to failure of these organs and their organ systems and, ultimately, death.

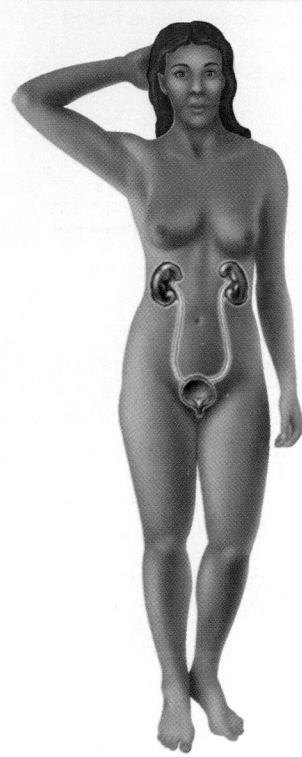

▲ **Figure 4.7**   Urinary
System.

LO 4.2, 4.3 Organs and Organ Systems

As described in Case Report 4.3, when organs and organ systems do not function in an **integrated** way, a person can die.

An **organ** is a structure composed of several tissues that work together to carry out specific functions. For example, the skin is an organ that has different tissues in it such as epithelial cells, hair, nails, and glands.

An **organ system** is a group of organs with a specific collective function, such as digestion, circulation, or respiration. For example, the nose, pharynx, larynx, trachea, and bronchi work together to achieve the total function of respiration.

Organ Systems

The body has 11 organ systems, shown in *Table 4.2*. The muscle and skeleton can be considered one organ system, the musculoskeletal system.

All your organ systems work together to ensure that your body's internal environment remains relatively constant. This process is called **homeostasis**. For example, your digestive, respiratory, and circulatory organ systems work together so that (a) every cell in your body receives adequate nutrients and oxygen and (b) waste products from the breakdown of these nutrients during cell metabolism are removed. Your cells can then function normally. Disease affecting an organ or organ system disrupts this game plan of homeostasis.

Organs

Go to *Table 4.2*, and see that each organ system contains several organs. An organ is composed of two or more tissue types that perform a particular function. Each organ has well-defined anatomic boundaries separating it from adjacent structures. The different organs in an organ system are usually interconnected. For example, in the urinary organ system, the organs are the kidneys, ureters, bladder, and urethra, and they are all connected *(Figure 4.7).*

Table 4.2 Organ Systems

Organ System	Major Organs	Major Functions
Integumentary	Skin, hair, nails, sweat glands, sebaceous glands	Protect tissues, regulate body temperature, support sensory receptors
Skeletal	Bones, ligaments, cartilages, tendons	Provide framework, protect soft tissues, provide attachments for muscles, produce blood cells, store inorganic salts
Muscular	Muscles	Cause movements, maintain posture, produce body heat
Nervous	Brain, spinal cord, nerves, sense organs	Detect changes, receive and interpret sensory information, stimulate muscles and glands
Endocrine	Glands that secrete hormones: pituitary, thyroid, parathyroid, adrenal, pancreas, ovaries, testes, pineal, thymus	Control metabolic activities of organs and structures
Cardiovascular	Heart, blood vessels	Move blood and transport substances throughout body
Lymphatic	Lymph vessels and nodes, thymus, spleen	Return tissue fluid to the blood, carry certain absorbed food molecules, defend body against infection
Digestive	Mouth, tongue, teeth, salivary glands, pharynx, esophagus, stomach, liver, gallbladder, pancreas, small and large intestines	Receive, break down, and absorb food, eliminate unabsorbed material
Respiratory	Nasal cavity, pharynx, larynx, trachea, bronchi, lungs	Control Intake and output of air, exchange gases between air and blood
Urinary	Kidneys, ureters, urinary bladder, urethra	Remove wastes from blood, maintain water and electrolyte balance, store and transport urine
Reproductive	*Male:* scrotum, testes, epididymides, vas deferens, seminal vesicles, prostate, bulbourethral glands, urethra, penis	Produce and maintain sperm cells, transfer sperm cells into female reproductive tract, secrete male hormones
	Female: ovaries, uterine (fallopian) tubes, uterus, vagina, vulva	Produce and maintain egg cells, receive sperm cells, support development of an embryo, function in birth process, secrete female hormones

WORD	PRONUNCIATION	ELEMENTS		DEFINITION
homeostasis (**Note:** Hemostasis is very different.)	ho-mee-oh-**STAY**-sis	S/ R/CF	**-stasis** *stand still, control* **home/o-** *the same*	Stability or equilibrium of a system or the body's internal environment
hypertrophy	high-**PER**-troh-fee	P/ R/	**hyper-** *excessive* **-trophy** *development*	Increase in size, but not in number, of an individual tissue element
integrate	**IN**-teh-grate	S/	**-ate** *composed of, pertaining to*	To bring together into a complete and harmonious whole
integration (noun)	**IN**-teh-**GRAY**-shun	R/	**integr-** *whole*	
organ	**OR**-gan		Greek *instrument*	Structure with specific functions in a body system
Parkinson disease	**PAR**-kin-son diz-**EEZ**		James Parkinson, British physician, 1755–1824	Disease of muscular rigidity, tremors, and a masklike facial expression
posture	**POSS**-chur		Latin *placement*	The carriage of the body as a whole and the position of the limbs
septicemia	sep-tih-**SEE**-mee-ah	S/ R/	**-emia** *blood condition* **septic-** *infected*	Microorganisms circulating in and infecting the blood (blood poisoning)
spastic (adj)	**SPAZ**-tik	S/ R/	**-ic** *pertaining to* **spast-** *tight*	Increased muscle tone on movement with exaggeration of the tendon reflexes
spasticity (noun) (**Note:** This term has 2 suffixes.)	spaz-**TIS**-ih-tee	S/	**-ity** *condition, state*	The condition or state of increased muscle tone on movement
tracheostomy	tray-kee-**OST**-oh-me	S/ R/CF	**-stomy** *new opening* **trache/o-** *windpipe*	Incision into the windpipe, usually so that a tube can be inserted to assist breathing
urinary	**YUR**-in-ary	S/ R/	**-ary** *pertaining to* **urin-** *urine*	Pertaining to urine

Exercises

A. Use your knowledge of the building blocks of terms, and *deconstruct* the following terms into their basic elements.

This will give you a better picture of how the words were formed. Fill in the blanks. **LO 4.2, 4.3, 4.7**

Medical Term	Prefix	Root and/or Combining Form	Suffix	Meaning of Term
homeostasis	1.	2.	3.	4.
hypertrophy	5.	6.	7.	8.
septicemia	9.	10.	11.	12.
tracheostomy	13.	14.	15.	16.
urinary	17.	18.	19.	20.

B. Assign the correct body system to the function. Fill in the blanks. LO 4.3

1. The function is breathing. The correct body system is _____.

2. The function is the birth process. The correct body system is _____.

3. The function is control of metabolic activities. The correct body system is _____.

4. The function is removal of wastes from blood. The correct body system is _____.

5. The function is movement of blood and transport of substances throughout the body. The correct body system is _____.

Anatomical Positions, Planes, and Directions

Terms have been developed over the past several thousand years to enable you to describe clearly where different anatomic structures and lesions are in relation to each other. To communicate effectively with other health professionals, it is critical that you are able to use the terminology to describe these positions and relative positions. To do this, you need to be able to use correct medical terminology to:

4.2.1 Define the fundamental anatomic position on which all descriptions of anatomic locations are based.

4.2.2 Describe the different anatomic planes and directions.

4.2.3 Locate the body cavities.

4.2.4 Identify the four abdominal quadrants and nine abdominal regions.

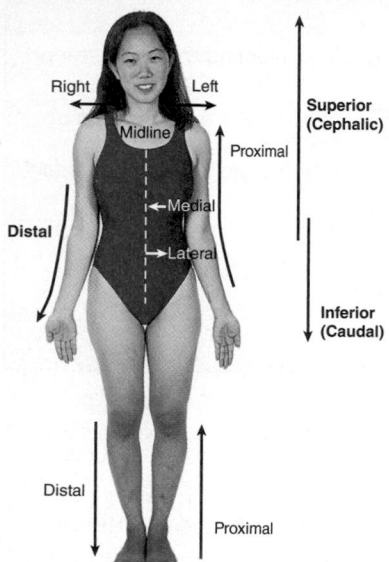

▲ **Figure 4.8** Anatomic Position with Directional Terms.

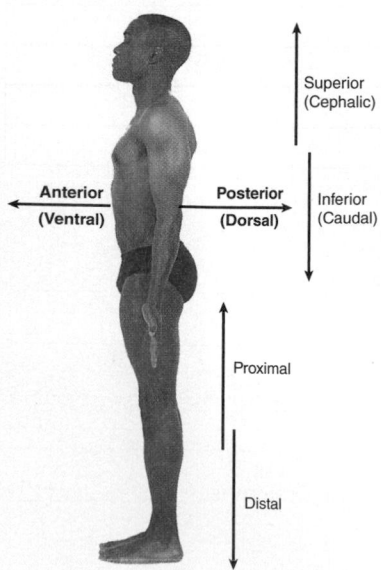

▲ **Figure 4.9** Directional Terms.

LO 4.4 Anatomic Position

When all **anatomic** descriptions are used, it is assumed that the body is in the anatomic position. The body is standing erect with feet flat on the floor, face and eyes facing forward, and arms at the sides with the palms facing forward *(Figure 4.8)*.

When your palms face forward, the forearm is **supine**. When you lie down flat on your back, you are supine. When your palms face backward, the forearm is **prone**. When you lie down flat on your abdomen, you are prone.

LO 4.4 Directional Terms

Directional terms describe the position of one structure or part of the body relative to another. These directional terms are shown in *Figures 4.8* and *4.9*.

LO 4.4 Anatomic Planes

Different views of the body are based on imaginary "slices" producing flat surfaces that pass through the body *(Figure 4.10)*. The three major anatomic planes are

- **Transverse** or **horizontal**—a plane passing across the body parallel to the floor and perpendicular to the body's long axis. It divides the body into an upper (**superior**) portion and a lower (**inferior**) portion.
- **Sagittal**—a vertical plane that divides the body into right and left portions.
- **Frontal** or **coronal**—a vertical plane that divides the body into front (**anterior**) and back (**posterior**) portions.

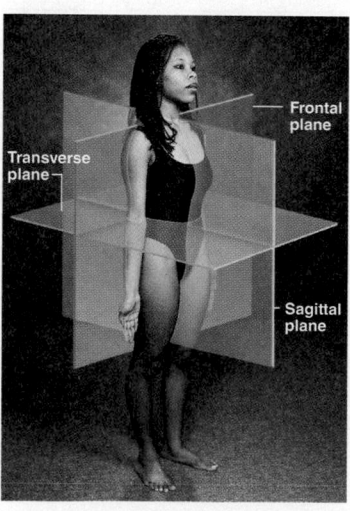

▲ **Figure 4.10** Anatomic Planes.

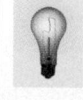 *Study Hint*

Help your memory with little tricks of association for medical terms. *Example:* The medical term *supine* has the word *up* in it. The meaning of supine is *lying with the face and the anterior part of the body UP.* Associate *UP* with s*UP*ine, and you will have no trouble remembering its definition.

Then associate the opposite term, and you will know the meaning of *prone* as well.

WORD	PRONUNCIATION	ELEMENTS		DEFINITION
anatomy	ah-**NAT**-oh-mee	S/ P/ R/ S/	-y *process* ana- *apart from* -tom- *section*	Study of the structures of the human body
anatomic (adj)	an-ah-**TOM**-ik	S/	-ic *pertaining to*	Pertaining to anatomy
anterior (opposite of posterior)	an-**TER**-ee-or	S/ R/	-ior *pertaining to* anter- *coming before*	Front surface of body; situated in front
caudal (opposite of cephalic)	**KAW**-dal	S/ R/	-al *pertaining to* caud- *tail*	Pertaining to or nearer to the tail
cephalic (opposite of caudal)	se-**FAL**-ik	S/ R/	-ic *pertaining to* cephal- *head*	Pertaining to or nearer to the head
coronal (equivalent to frontal)	**KOR**-oh-nal	S/ R/	-al *pertaining to* coron- *crown*	Pertaining to the vertical plane dividing the body into anterior and posterior portions
distal (opposite of proximal)	**DISS**-tal	S/ R/	-al *pertaining to* dist- *away from the center*	Situated away from the center of the body
dorsal (equivalent to posterior)	**DOR**-sal	S/ R/	-al *pertaining to* dors- *back*	Pertaining to the back or situated behind
frontal (equivalent to coronal)	**FRON**-tal	S/ R/	-al *pertaining to* front- *front*	In front; relating to the anterior part of the body
inferior (opposite of superior)	in-**FEE**-ree-or	S/ R/	-ior *pertaining to* infer- *below*	Situated below
posterior (opposite of anterior)	pos-**TER**-ee-or	S/ R/	-ior *pertaining to* poster- *coming behind*	Pertaining to the back surface of the body; situated behind
prone (opposite of supine)	PRONE		Latin *bending forward*	Lying face-down, flat on your abdomen
proximal (opposite of distal)	**PROK**-sih-mal	S/ R/	-al *pertaining to* proxim- *nearest*	Situated nearest the center of the body
sagittal	**SAJ**-ih-tal	S/ R/	-al *pertaining to* sagitt- *arrow*	Pertaining to the vertical plane through the body, dividing it into right and left portions
superior (opposite of inferior)	soo-**PEE**-ree-or	S/ R/	-ior *pertaining to* super- *above*	Situated above
supine (opposite of prone)	soo-**PINE**		Latin *bend backward*	Lying face-up, flat on your spine
transverse	trans-**VERS**		Latin *crosswise*	Pertaining to the horizontal plane dividing the body into upper and lower portions
ventral (equivalent to anterior)	**VEN**-tral	S/ R/	-al *pertaining to* ventr- *belly*	Pertaining to the abdomen or situated nearer the surface of the abdomen

Exercises

A. Each of the following terms from the above WAD box has one element in bold. *You need to identify what type of element it is and define its meaning. Then answer the questions. Fill in the blanks.*   **LO 4.4**

1. Poster**ior**   Type of element: _____   Meaning: _____

2. **caud**al   Type of element: _____   Meaning: _____

3. **cephal**ic   Type of element: _____   Meaning: _____

4. **dist**al   Type of element: _____   Meaning: _____

5. **infer**ior   Type of element: _____   Meaning: _____

6. The three elements with the same meaning are _____, _____, and _____.

7. They all mean _____.

> 💡 *Study Hint*
> Terms will be easier to remember if you study them in *pairs of opposites*.

Figure 4.11 Body Cavities (a) lateral view; (b) frontal view.

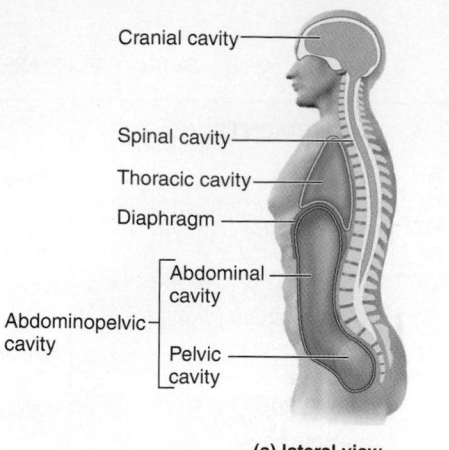

(a) lateral view

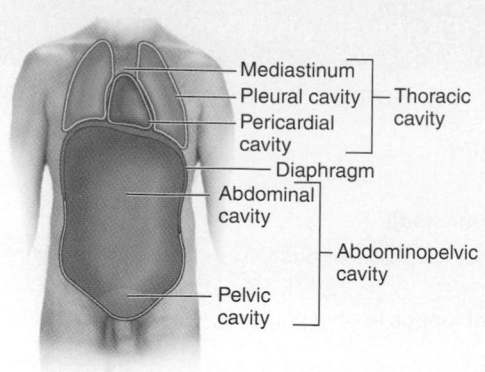

(b) frontal view

LO 4.5 Body Cavities

The body contains many **cavities**. Some, like the nasal cavity, open to the outside. Five cavities do not open to the outside and are shown in *Figure 4.11*.

- **Cranial cavity**—contains the brain within the skull.
- **Thoracic cavity**—contains the heart, lungs, thymus gland, trachea, and esophagus, as well as numerous blood vessels and nerves.
- **Abdominal cavity**—is separated from the thoracic cavity by the **diaphragm** and contains the stomach, intestines, liver, spleen, pancreas, and kidneys.
- **Pelvic cavity**—is surrounded by the pelvic bones and contains the urinary bladder, part of the large intestine, the rectum, the anus, and the internal reproductive organs.
- **Spinal cavity**—contains the spinal cord.

The abdominal cavity and pelvic cavity are collectively referred to as the **abdominopelvic cavity**.

LO 4.6 Abdominal Quadrants and Regions

Abbreviations	
LLQ	left lower quadrant
LUQ	left upper quadrant
RLQ	right lower quadrant
RUQ	right upper quadrant

One way of referring to the locations of abdominal structures and to the site of abdominal pain and other abnormalities is to divide the abdominal region into **quadrants**, as shown in *Figure 4.12a*. The locations are **right upper quadrant (RUQ), left upper quadrant (LUQ), right lower quadrant (RLQ)**, and **left lower quadrant (LLQ)**. Each quadrant has a three letter abbreviation as shown—for example, RUQ.

The abdomen can also be divided into nine **regions** *(Figure 4.12b)*. The central region is called the **umbilical** region, as it is located around the umbilicus. The areas above and below that region are named relative to the stomach—**epigastric**, above the stomach, and **hypogastric**, below the stomach.

The six remaining regions are on the right and left sides of these three central regions. The upper regions on either side of the epigastric region, which sit below the ribs, are named the right and left **hypochondriac** regions. The regions on either side of the umbilical region are named the right and left **lumbar** regions (according to the area of the spine nearby). The regions on either side of the hypogastric region are named the right and left **inguinal** (groin) regions.

▼ **Figure 4.12** Regional Anatomy.

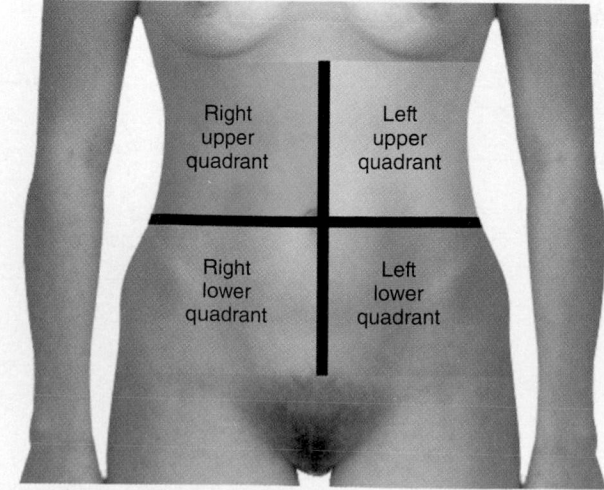

(a) Abdominal quadrants

(b) Abdominal regions

WORD	PRONUNCIATION		ELEMENTS	DEFINITION
abdomen abdominal (adj)	**AB**-doh-men ab-**DOM**-in-al	S/ R/	-al *pertaining to* abdomin- *abdomen*	Part of the trunk between the thorax and pelvis Pertaining to the abdomen
abdominopelvic	ab-**DOM**-ih-no-**PEL**-vik	S/ R/CF R/	-ic *pertaining to* abdomin/o- *abdomen* -pelv- *pelvis*	Pertaining to the abdomen and pelvis
cavity cavities (pl)	**KAV**-ih-tee **KAV**-ih-tees		Latin *hollow place*	Hollow space or body compartment
diaphragm	**DIE**-ah-fram		Greek *diaphragm, fence*	The musculomembranous partition separating the abdominal and thoracic cavities
epigastric	ep-ih-**GAS**-trik	S/ P/ R/CF	-ic *pertaining to* epi- *above* -gastr/i- *stomach*	Pertaining to the abdominal region above the stomach
epigastrium (noun)	ep-ih-**GAS**-tree-um	S/	-um *structure*	Abdominal region above the stomach
hypogastric	high-poh-**GAS**-trik	S/ P/ R/	-ic *pertaining to* hypo- *below* -gastr- *stomach*	Pertaining to the abdominal region below the stomach
quadrant	**KWAD**-rant		Latin *one quarter*	One-quarter of a circle
umbilical umbilicus (noun)	um-**BIL**-ih-kal um-**BIL**-ih-kuss	S/ R/	-al *pertaining to, around* umbilic- *belly button (navel)*	Pertaining to or around the umbilicus or the center of the abdomen

Exercises

A. Take a closer look at the breakdown of medical terms. *The medical term is given to you. Break it down into elements with a slash (/). Below each element, write the meaning of the element. See how the combination of elements will give you the meaning of the entire term.* <u>The first one is done for you</u>. *Fill in the blanks.*   **LO 4.5, 4.6**

1. *epigastrium*

    <u> epi </u> / <u> gastri </u> / <u> um </u>
       above   *stomach*   *structure*

    Meaning of **epigastrium**:   <u>a structure above the stomach   </u>

2. *hypogastric*

    <u>   </u> / <u>   </u> / <u>   </u>

    Meaning of *hypogastric*:   <u>   </u>

> 💡 *Study Hint*
> Remember to start with the suffix and work back to the front of the term.

B. One of the following sentences has misspelled terms in it. *Circle the incorrect spellings and rewrite the correct sentence below.*   **LO 4.5**

1. Abdominal structures and pain can be referred to the *abdominal quadrants*.

2. The abdominal cavity is separated from the thoracic cavity by the diafram.

3. The abdominal cavity and the pelvic cavity are collectively referred to as the *abdominopelvic cavity*.

4. The pelvic cavity contains the urinary bladder.

5. There are four abdominal quadrants.

6. Corrected sentence:

    _____

    _____

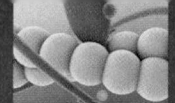

The Body as a Whole

Challenge Your Knowledge

A. Demonstrate your knowledge of directional terms and abbreviations by identifying the correct choice. Circle the correct term. (**LO 4.4, 4.6, 4.7,** *Remember*)

1. The epigastric region is (above/below) the stomach. Therefore, it is (superior/inferior) to the stomach.

2. The umbilical region is so named because it is in the (center/back) of the abdomen and (inferior/superior) to the epigastric region.

3. The hypogastric region is between the (RUQ/LUQ) and the (RLQ/LLQ).

4. In the abbreviation LLQ, the first "L" means (lower/left).

5. The nose is (superior/inferior) to the chin.

6. The spine is (anterior/posterior) to the heart.

7. The umbilicus is (dorsal/ventral) to the spine.

8. The toes are (distal/proximal) to the knee.

B. Functions of the cell. The basic functions of life are all carried on by each and every cell. Fill in the blanks to name all the functions. (**LO 4.2,** *Remember*)

1. _____

2. _____

3. _____

4. _____

5. _____

C. Latin and greek terms. There is no easy way to remember these—you just have to know them so that you can relate to their meanings. Match the terms in 1–10 to the meanings in a-j. Fill in the blanks. (**LO 4.1, 4.2,** *Remember, Understand*)

_____ 1. clot	**a.** a storeroom
_____ 2. graft	**b.** cross
_____ 3. hormone	**c.** yolk
_____ 4. ligament	**d.** crescent
_____ 5. cell	**e.** band
_____ 6. matrix	**f.** to block
_____ 7. cruciate	**g.** mother
_____ 8. membrane	**h.** to set in motion
_____ 9. meniscus	**i.** transplant
_____ 10. zygote	**j.** parchment

D. Knowledge of anatomic locations on the body will make your communications with other health professionals precise. Challenge yourself with the following questions. Circle *T* (true) or *F* (false); then rewrite the false answers correctly below. (**LO 4.4, 4.5, 4.6,** *Remember, Understand*)

1. Standing erect with feet flat on the floor, face and eyes facing forward, and arms at the side with palms facing forward is the anatomical position.   T   F

2. A transverse plane is a horizontal plane.   T   F

3. Frontal and sagittal planes are both vertical planes.   T   F

4. Inferior is situated above another part of the body.   T   F

5. *Dorsal* means the same as *anterior*.   T   F

6. The abdominal cavity contains the urinary bladder.   T   F

7. The thoracic cavity is superior to the pelvic cavity, and the pelvic cavity is inferior to the abdominal cavity.   T   F

8. The diaphragm divides the pelvic cavity and the abdominal cavity.   T   F

9. In RUQ, "Q" means *quadrant*.   T   F

10. The RUQ and the LUQ are divided by a sagittal plane.   T   F

11. Corrected statements:

_____

_____

E. The following terms and abbreviations apply either to a body region, body cavity or body quadrant. Circle the correct choice. (**LO 4.5, 4.6,** *Remember, Apply*)

1. RUQ, RLQ, LUQ, LLQ   body region   body cavity   body quadrant

2. thoracic   body region   body cavity   body quadrant

3. hypogastric   body region   body cavity   body quadrant

4. spinal   body region   body cavity   body quadrant

5. umbilical   body region   body cavity   body quadrant

F. Answer the following true/false questions about the body planes. Circle the correct answer. Any false statement rewrite as correct on the lines provided. (**LO 4.4,** *Remember, Apply*)

1. The transverse plane is a horizontal plane.   T   F

2. The transverse plane divides the body into inferior and superior portions.   T   F

3. The sagittal plane is a horizontal plane.   T   F

4. Frontal plane is the same as coronal plane.   T   F

5. The frontal plane divides the body into anterior and posterior portions.   T   F

6. Corrected statement:

_____

_____

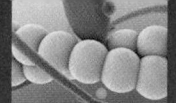

The Body as a Whole

G. **What am I?** Fill in the blanks with the correct answers. (**LO 4.1, 4.2, 4.4,** *Remember, Apply*)

1. Anabolism + catabolism = _____.

2. The largest organelle that directs all the activities of the cell is the _____.

3. This forms the tip of your nose, the shape of your ear, and the larynx: _____.

4. The relatively constant internal environment in the body is _____.

5. Standing erect, with feet flat on the floor, face and eyes facing forward and arms at the side, palms facing

   forward is _____.

H. **Use the language of anatomy to answer the questions.** Circle the correct answer. (**LO 4.4,** *Remember, Apply*)

1. Which of the following medical terms is NOT an anatomic plane?

   a. transverse   **d.** supine

   b. lateral   **e.** coronal

   c. sagittal

2. Which of the following medical terms is NOT a correct pair of opposites?

   a. anterior   posterior

   b. inferior   superior

   c. dorsal   ventral

   d. prone   supine

   e. caudal   cephalic

3. Which of the following medical terms has an element meaning *nearest*?

   a. ventral   **d.** sagittal

   b. proximal   **e.** superior

   c. supine

4. Which of the following terms means the same thing as *coronal*?

   a. frontal   **d.** dorsal

   b. superior   **e.** cephalic

   c. ventral

5. If dorsal is *equivalent to* posterior, it means they are

   a. nouns   **d.** the same

   b. verbs   **e.** the opposite

   c. adjectives

I. **Anatomic positions and planes.** You must know anatomic positions to prepare a patient for any type of procedure or surgery. Anatomic planes can help define radiologic studies. Using this knowledge, complete the following. (**LO 4.4,** *Understand*)

1. The surgeon needs his patient in the _____ position to remove a lesion on his back.

2. To prepare for a knee arthroscopy, the patient will be in the _____ position.

3. The body is standing erect with feet flat on the floor, face and eyes facing forward, and arms at the sides with the palms facing

   forward; this is the _____ position.

4. A plane that divides the body into an upper, or superior, portion and a lower, or inferior, portion is called a _____ plane.

5. A frontal plane can also be called a _____ plane.

J. Directional terms. Along with knowing planes, body cavities, and quadrants, you must know body directional terms in order to be able to document and communicate accurately. (**LO 4.4,** *Understand*)

Proximal and distal: Proximal means _____ ; distal means _____ .

Anterior and posterior: Anterior means _____ ; posterior means _____ .

Dorsal and ventral: Dorsal means _____ ; ventral means _____ .

Superior and inferior: Superior means _____ ; inferior means _____ .

K. Organs and body systems. Knowledge of the body's systems will help you master medical terminology. Assign the following organs to an organ system, and describe one major function of that system. (**LO 4.2, 4.3, 4.7, 4.8,** *Understand*)

Organ	Organ System	System Function
blood vessels	1.	2.
cartilage	3.	4.
testes	5.	6.
fallopian tubes	7.	8.
hair	9.	10.
larynx	11.	12.
liver	13.	14.
muscles	15.	16.
spinal cord	17.	18.
spleen	19.	20.
sweat glands	21.	22.
teeth	23.	24.
thymus	25.	26.
thyroid gland	27.	28.

L. Place the organ in the correct body system. Place a checkmark (√) in the correct system column. (**LO 4.2, 4.3,** *Understand, Apply*)

Organ	Integumentary	Respiratory	Cardiovascular	Digestive	Nervous
1. blood vessels					
2. skin					
3. spinal cord					
4. pharynx					
5. stomach					
6. heart					
7. bronchus					
8. lungs					
9. gallbladder					
10. esophagus					

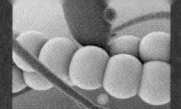
The Body as a Whole

M. **Select from among the following pairs of terms the ones that are opposites.** Circle the correct choices for opposites. **(LO 4.4,** *Understand, Apply*)

1. anterior   posterior

2. caudal   cephalic

3. coronal   frontal

4. distal   proximal

5. dorsal   posterior

6. inferior   superior

7. prone   supine

8. ventral   anterior

9. In the selection above (1–8) which pairs of terms mean the same thing?

_____

10. These medical terms are used to describe _____ of the body.

N. **Use the language of anatomy to answer the following questions about the cell. (LO 4.2,** *Understand, Apply*)

1. Which one of the following medical terms is not an organelle?

   a. lysosomes

   b. nucleolus

   c. endoplasmic reticulum

   d. sulcus

   e. mitochondria

2. The fluid contained inside the cell is

   a. cytoplasm

   b. endoplasm

   c. ectoplasm

   d. synovial fluid

   e. plasma

3. What surrounds and protects the cell?

   a. Golgi complex

   b. endoplasmic reticulum

   c. lysosomes

   d. ribosomes

   e. cell membrane

4. What are the chemical messenger cells called?

   a. lymphocytes

   b. erythrocytes

   c. electrolytes

   d. hormones

   e. minerals

5. What type of tasks do organelles carry out?

   a. excretory

   b. sensory

   c. metabolic

   d. communicative

   e. reproductive

O. Organs, organelles, and tissue types. Through attention and effort, you will learn to recognize the correct spelling of medical terms. Review the pairs of medical terms in the first chart that follows, and circle the correctly spelled word in each pair (read the terms from top to bottom of the chart). Then insert the correct spelling of each term in the first column of the second chart, and place a checkmark (√) in the appropriate column to show whether it is an organ, organelle, or tissue type. (**LO 4.1, 4.2, Understand, Apply**)

1. Circle the correct spelling.

ribosome	galbladder	nevus	mitocondria	conective	nucleolus
ribosomme	gallbladder	nerrvous	mitochondria	connective	nucliolus
muscle	nuceus	lysosones	pancreas	epithelial	reticculum
mussel	nucleus	lysosomes	panncreas	epithellial	reticulum

2. Enter the correctly spelled terms from the above chart in O. into the first column in the following chart; then finish filling in the chart by indicating whether the term is an organ, organelle, or tissue type.

Correctly Spelled Term	Organ	Organelle	Tissue Type
2.	3.		
4.	5.		
6.	7.		
8.	9.		
10.	11.		
12.	13.		
14.	15.		
16.	17.		
18.	19.		
20.	21.		
22.	23.		
24.	25.		

P. Apply this knowledge of organ systems to answer the following questions. Circle your choice, but remember to rewrite any false information *correctly* on the blanks at the end of the exercise. (**LO 4.2, 4.3, Apply**)

1. Organs make basic functions happen in an organ system.   T   F

2. Glands that secrete hormones are in the endocrine system.   T   F

3. There are 13 different body systems.   T   F

4. An organ system has more than one organ.   T   F

5. Organ systems that are not functioning correctly can disrupt homeostasis.   T   F

6. Rewrite any false statement(s) with correct information.

_____

_____

_____

_____

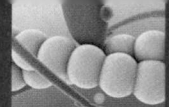
The Body as a Whole

Q. **Build medical terms using your knowledge of elements and their proper position in a medical term.** Fill in the blanks. (**LO 4.1, 4.2, 4.7, 4.8,** *Apply*)

1. Small mass   molec/_____

2. Pertaining to below the stomach   _____/_____ /ic

3. Instrument for viewing a joint   _____/scope

4. Pertaining to urine   urin/_____

5. A change in condition (when the elements are taken literally)   _____/ism

6. Small organ   organ/_____

7. Small nucleus   nucleo/_____

8. Enzyme that digests foreign material   lyso/_____

Note: More than one element can have the same meaning. List the elements in this exercise that have the same meaning.

9. _____ all mean _____.

10. _____ all mean _____.

R. **Abbreviations.** Select any three of these abbreviations, define their meanings, and create a sentence for each one. (**LO 4.1,** *Analyze*)

IVF   ACL   LLQ   LUQ   RLQ   RUQ

1. _____ means _____.

Sentence: _____

_____

2. _____ means _____.

Sentence: _____

_____

3. _____ means _____.

Sentence: _____

_____

S. Knowing the meaning of word elements will help you to deconstruct the following terms to explain the differences in their meaning. First, divide the word into its elements with slashes (/). Circle the suffix, and then fill in the table. (**LO 4.1, 4.2, 4.7, *Analyze***)

Term	Meaning of Root(s)/ Combining Form	Meaning of Suffix	Meaning of Term
homeostasis	1.	2.	3.
anabolism	4.	5.	6.
catabolism	7.	8.	9.
metabolism	10.	11.	12.
nucleus	13.	14.	15.
nucleolus	16.	17.	18.
ribosome	19.	20.	21.
lysosome	22.	23.	24.

T. Body cavities. The organ is given to you in the following chart. Fill in the chart. Organize the terms in the correct body cavity, and then place the organ in the correct body system. *Note:* There are two answers to every question. (**LO 4.3, 4.5, *Analyze***)

Organ	Body Cavity	Body System
brain	1.	2.
gallbladder	3.	4.
heart	5.	6.
kidneys	7.	8.
lungs	9.	10.
pituitary	11.	12.
ribs	13.	14.
spleen	15.	16.
uterus	17.	18.

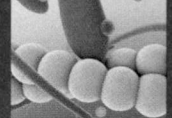

The Body as a Whole

U. **Multiple choice is the format used for most national certification examinations.** Circle the correct answer to the statement or question. (**LO 4.2, 4.3, 4.4,** *Analyze*)

1. The single, fertilized cell is called the

   a. mitochondria

   b. ribosome

   c. organelle

   d. zygote

   e. blastocyst

2. The word *membrane* means

   a. small organ

   b. fluid inside a cell

   c. thin layer of tissue

   d. chemical substance

   e. molecule with electrical charge

3. Patella is the medical term for

   a. ankle

   b. muscle

   c. kneecap

   d. ligament

   e. meniscus

4. Which of the following functions as a shock absorber?

   a. cartilage

   b. muscle

   c. tendon

   d. ligament

   e. blood vessel

5. The prefix *endo-* means

   a. outside

   b. within

   c. around

   d. behind

   e. across

6. The study of the function of tissues is called

   a. cytology

   b. cardiology

   c. dermatology

   d. histology

   e. gastroenterology

7. Two bones that have formed a joint are called

   a. graft

   b. articulation

   c. homeostasis

   d. metabolism

   e. cartilage

8. How many quadrants are in the body?

   a. one

   b. two

   c. three

   d. four

   e. five

9. *Hypogastric* refers to a

   a. body region

   b. body opening

   c. body quadrant

   d. body cavity

   e. body plane

10. What forms the gliding surface at articulations where two bones meet to form a joint?

   a. cartilage

   b. blood vessels

   c. collagen

   d. ligaments

   e. lymph

V. **Short answer and/or class discussion.** Building up to larger components in the body, expand your knowledge of cells and tissues to organs and organ systems. Write a short answer to each question, and be prepared to discuss your answers with the instructor and class. (**LO 4.2, 4.3,** *Analyze*)

1. Describe an *organ*.

_____

_____

_____

_____

2. What is the difference between an organ and an organ system?

_____

_____

_____

_____

3. It is difficult to imagine skin as an "organ" because it is not a compact size like a liver or heart. Basing your answer on the previous answers, why, then, is skin an organ?

_____

_____

_____

_____

4. Which body system has skin as a major organ?

_____

_____

_____

_____

5. There can be smaller organs within a large organ. Name the smaller organs within the skin and some of their functions.

_____

_____

_____

_____

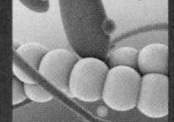

The Body as a Whole

W. **Unscramble the letters to form medical terms that will list all the organ systems in the body.** Use every letter in each scramble to form the correct medical term. (**LO 4.2, 4.3,** *Analyze*)

1. gnmtuaierteyn _____

2. uanriry _____

3. cvraaacsruldio _____

4. ecinrodne _____

5. riaryr eotps _____

6. dseie ivtg _____

7. satklee _____

8. nveosru _____

9. ltayhcpmi _____

10. urcmuals _____

11. roc veteru idp _____

X. **Now that you have had some practice with the new medical terms, you are ready to read again the following Case Report from earlier in this chapter.** Underline all the medical terms, and then answer all the questions. Fill in the blanks. (**LO 4.1, 4.2, 4.3, 4.4,** *Analyze*)

Case Report 4.2

You are

...a physical therapy assistant employed by the Rehabilitation Unit in Fulwood Medical Center.

Your patient is

...Richard Josen, a 22-year-old man who injured tissues in his left knee playing football. Using arthroscopy, the orthopedic surgeon removed his torn anterior cruciate ligament (ACL) and replaced it with a graft from his patellar ligament. The torn medial collateral ligament was sutured together. The tear in his medial meniscus was repaired. Rehabilitation focused on strengthening the muscles around his knee joint and regaining joint mobility.

1. Define *arthroscopy*. _____

2. What type of specialist will use an *arthroscope*? _____

3. *ACL* is the abbreviation for _____.

4. What is a *graft*? _____

5. What does a *meniscus* resemble? _____

6. What is the *patella* also called? _____

7. What is the opposite of *medial*? _____

8. Define *ligament*. _____

9. Describe *anterior*. _____

10. Define *collateral*. _____

CHAPTER SUMMARY EXERCISE

A. Spelling comprehension. Circle the correct spelling of the term. (**LO 4.7,** *Remember*)

1. organale	orgenele	organelle	orgenelle	organel
2. sinovial	sinnovial	synoveal	synevial	synovial
3. rybosome	ribosonme	rhibosome	ribosome	rhybosone
4. diaphram	diaphrame	diaphragm	deaphragm	diafragm
5. traciostomy	trackeostomy	trachiostomy	treckeostomy	tracheostomy
6. nucklii	nucleei	nuclei	neuclei	nucklie
7. zygoat	zigote	zygote	zigotte	zygoate
8. endockrine	endocrine	endoccrine	endockryne	endocrin
9. meniscus	menniscus	menickus	meniskus	meniscuss
10. historyology	histology	hystology	hestology	historology

B. Match the correct spelling of the terms in Exercise A with the brief description of each of the following terms. (**LO 4.1, 4.2, 4.5,** *Apply*)

1. Manufacture protein _____

2. Plural of nucleus _____

3. Opening for tube to assist in breathing _____

4. Contains a sufffix meaning *small* _____

5. Separating two body cavities _____

6. Gland _____

7. Study of function of tissues _____

8. Origin of every cell in body _____

9. Crescent shaped _____

10. Lubricant _____

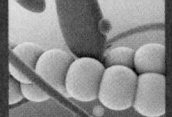
The Body as a Whole

C. Using your knowledge of terms 1–10 in Exercises A and B and their correct spelling, write a brief sentence for each of the terms as it might appear in patient documentation. (LO 4.7, 4.8, *Apply*)

1. _____

2. _____

3. _____

4. _____

5. _____

6. _____

7. _____

8. _____

9. _____

10. _____

D. Meet a learning outcome and begin applying medical terminology to answer the following questions. (LO 4.2, 4.5, 4.6, *Apply*)

1. List the four primary tissue groups and describe their functions.

   a. _____

   b. _____

   c. _____

   d. _____

2. Identify any major organ and list the smaller organs contained in it.

   _____

   _____

3. Identify the structure and functions of the components of a cell.

   Structure: _____

   _____

   Functions: _____

   _____

4. Be able to demonstrate on your own body or on a classroom skeleton the names and locations of the

   a. body cavities   **b.** abdominal quadrants   **c.** abdominal regions

5. Describe the fundamental anatomic position.

   _____

E. **Meet the goals of each of the chapter learning outcomes and insert the correct answers to the questions. (LO 4.1–4.8,** *Analyze*)

1. Apply correct medical terms to the anatomy and physiology of the body as a whole. Circle the correct answers and rewrite the false statement on the lines below. **(LO 4.1)**

   a. Muscles are in the immune system.   T   F

   b. The reproductive system vocabulary is divided into male and female terms.   T   F

   c. Teeth are considered part of the digestive system.   T   F

   d. One of the functions of the urinary system is to remove wastes from the blood.   T   F

   e. The musculoskeletal system provides movement for the body.   T   F

   f. Rewrite the false statement:

   _____

   _____

2. Discuss the medical terms associated with the structures and functions of cells, tissues, and organs. Which term does not belong with medical terms associated with cells, tissues, and organs? Circle the incorrect term. **(LO 4.2)**

   a. cytology

   b. membrane

   c. histology

   d. cytoplasm

   e. cavity

3. Integrate individual body systems into the organization and function of the body as a whole. Next to each body system, list one of its major functions. **(LO 4.3)**

   a. Urinary   Function: _____

   b. Endocrine   Function: _____

   c. Skeletal   Function: _____

   d. Male reproductive   Function: _____

   e. Integumentary   Function: _____

4. Describe the medical terms for the different anatomic positions (AP), planes (P), and directions of the body (D). Identify which of the following terms apply to anatomic positions, planes, or directions of the body. Circle the correct choice. **(LO 4.4)**

   a. caudal   AP   P   D

   b. transverse   AP   P   D

   c. superior   AP   P   D

   d. prone   AP   P   D

   e. distal   AP   P   D

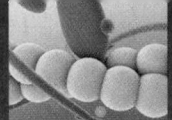

The Body as a Whole

5. Discuss the body cavities. Place each organ in the correct body cavity. Fill in the blanks. (**LO 4.5**)

a. brain   cavity: _____

b. spinal cord   cavity: _____

c. bladder   cavity: _____

d. spleen   cavity: _____

e. thymus gland   cavity: _____

6. Describe the nine regions of the abdomen. (**LO 4.6**)

a. _____

b. _____

c. _____

d. _____

e. _____

f. _____

g. _____

h. _____

i. _____

7. Comprehend, spell, and write medical terms pertaining to the body as a whole so that you communicate and document accurately and precisely in any health care setting. You are given the meaning of the term. Spell it correctly and write it on the line. (**LO 4.1, 4.2, 4.3**)

a. muscle separating the thoracic and abdominal cavities   _____

b. abdominal region above the stomach   _____

c. in the body system building path, what organelles are composed of   _____

d. a group of organic food compounds that includes sugar and starch   _____

e. pertaining to, or nearer, the head   _____

8. Recognize and pronounce medical terms pertaining to the body as a whole so that you communicate verbally with accuracy and precision in any health care setting. (**LO 4.8**)

   a. If a physician tells you to put the patient in the *supine* position, what should you do?

   _____

   b. If the physician tells you she wants x-rays of the abdominopelvic cavity, what parts of the body would you be looking at?

   _____

   c. What is the correct pronunciation of *abdominopelvic*?

     a. ad-domino-PELV-ic

     b. ab-DOM-in-no-PEL-vik

     c. ab-domino-PELV-ik

     d. ab-DOM-ih-no-PEL-vik

Lesson 5.1 The Digestive System

There are basic elements of anatomy, physiology, and medical terminology that apply throughout the different parts of the digestive system. These elements are discussed in this lesson. That information will enable you to:

5.1.1 Select the correct medical terminology to describe the structure and functions of the digestive system.

5.1.2 List the organs and accessory organs of the digestive system.

5.1.3 Discuss the basic processes of digestion.

Abbreviation	
GI	gastrointestinal

Tongue

Esophagus

Stomach

Gallbladder

Duodenum
Pancreas

1.6 feet (.5 m)
(from tongue to duodenum)

3.28 ft.
1.0 m

Jejunum
7.2–7.9 ft.
(2.2–2.4 m)

18–19.7 feet (5.5 – 6.0 m)
(small intestine)

Ileum
10.8–11.8 ft.
(3.3–3.6 m)

Appendix
Cecum

Large
intestine

4.9 feet (1.5 m)
(large intestine)

Anus

▲ **Figure 5.1** **Alimentary Canal.**

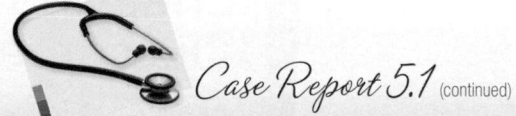

Case Report 5.1 (continued)

In Mrs. Martha Jones's case, the **Roux-en-Y** procedure reduced the size of her available stomach from 2 quarts to 2 ounces. This resulted in her being able to eat less and to absorb less. She had no complications from the **laparoscopic** procedure. In the succeeding 2 months, she lost 15 pounds in weight.

LO 5.1 Alimentary Canal and Accessory Organs

Every cell in your body requires a constant supply of nourishment. The cells cannot travel, so the nourishment has to be brought to them in a form that can be absorbed across their cell membrane. The foods that you **ingest** cannot be used in their existing form by the cells. The digestive system, through its alimentary canal, breaks down the nutrients in the food into elements that can be transported to the cells via the blood and **lymphatics**. These elements can then be transported across the cell membrane into the cell.

The **digestive system** consists of the **alimentary canal** (digestive tract), which extends from the **mouth** to the **anus**, and **accessory organs** connected to the canal to assist in digestion.

The term **gastrointestinal (GI)** technically refers to the stomach and **intestines** but is often used to mean the whole digestive system. **Gastroenterology** is the study of the digestive system. A **gastroenterologist** is a physician who specializes in the digestive system.

The alimentary canal (*Figure 5.1*) includes the

- Mouth
- Pharynx
- **Esophagus**
- Stomach
- Small intestine
- Large intestine

The **accessory organs** of digestion include the

- Teeth
- Tongue
- Salivary glands
- Liver
- Gallbladder
- Pancreas

Word Analysis and Definition

S = Suffix   P = Prefix   R = Root   R/CF = Combining Form

WORD	PRONUNCIATION	ELEMENTS		DEFINITION
alimentary	al-ih-**MEN**-tar-ee	S/ R/	-ary *pertaining to* **aliment-** *nourishment*	Pertaining to the digestive tract
bariatric	bar-ee-**AT**-rik	S/ R/	-atric *treatment* **bari-** *weight*	Treatment of obesity
digestion	die-**JEST**-shun	S/ R/	-ion *action* **digest-** *to break down*	Breakdown of food into elements suitable for cell metabolism
digestive (adj)	die-**JEST**-iv	S/	-ive *nature of*	Pertaining to digestion
esophagus	ee-**SOF**-ah-gus		Greek *gullet*	Tube linking the pharynx and the stomach
gastric	**GAS**-trik	S/ R/	-ic *pertaining to* **gastr-** *stomach*	Pertaining to the stomach
gastroenterology	**GAS**-troh-en-ter-**OL**-oh-gee	S/ R/CF R/CF	-logy *study of* **gastr/o-** *stomach* **-enter/o-** *intestine*	Medical specialty of the stomach and intestines
gastroenterologist	**GAS**-troh-en-ter-**OL**-oh-jist	S/	-logist *one who studies*	Medical specialist in gastroenterology
gastrointestinal (GI)	**GAS**-troh-in-**TESS**-tin-al	S/ R/CF R/	-al *pertaining to* **gastr/o-** *stomach* **-intestin-** *gut, intestine*	Pertaining to the stomach and intestines
intestine intestinal (adj)	in-**TES**-tin in-**TES**-tin-al	S/ R/	-al *pertaining to* **intestin-** *intestine, gut*	The digestive tube from stomach to anus
laparoscopy	lap-ah-**ROS**-koh-pee	S/ R/CF	-scopy *to view* **lapar/o-** *abdomen in general*	Examination of the contents of the abdomen using an endoscope
laparoscope	**LAP**-ah-roh-skope	S/	-scope *instrument for viewing*	Instrument (endoscope) used for viewing the abdominal contents
laparoscopic (adj)	**LAP**-ah-rah-**SKOP**-ik	S/	-ic *pertaining to*	Pertaining to laparoscopy
lymph	LIMF		Latin *spring water*	A clear fluid collected from tissues and trans- ported by vessels to venous circulation
lymphatic (adj)	lim-**FAT**-ik	S/ R/	-atic *pertaining to* **lymph-** *lymph*	Pertaining to lymph
mouth	MOWTH		Old English *mouth*	External opening of a cavity or canal
Roux-en-Y	**ROO**-on-**Y**		César Roux, a Swiss surgeon, 1857–1934	Surgical procedure to reduce the size of the stomach
transcript	**TRAN**-skript	P/ R/	trans- *across, through* **-script** *writing, thing copied*	An exact copy or reproduction
transcription transcriptionist	tran-**SCRIP**-shun tran-**SCRIP**-shun-ist	S/ S/	-ion *action, condition* -ist *a specialist in*	The action of making a copy of dictated material One who makes a copy of dictated material

Exercises

A. Analyzing the elements can tell you a lot about a medical term. *Review the above WAD box before you start the exercise. Fill in the blanks.* **LO 5.1, 5.3**

1. Analyzing the two combining forms shows that the term **gastroenterology** relates to the _____ and the _____.

2. In the term **gastric**, the root _____ has the same meaning as the combining form _____ in the term **gastroenterology**.

3. _____ symptoms pertain to the stomach only. Because Mrs. Jones had stomach and intestinal prob-lems, her symptoms can be described as _____. For this condition, she will need a specialist in the study of the stomach and intestines, a field known as _____. This type of physician is referred to as a _____.

LO 5.2 Functions of the Digestive System

1. **Ingestion**—the selective intake of food into the mouth. Alternatively, food can be inserted directly into the stomach via a **nasogastric** or stomach tube.

2. **Propulsion**—the mechanical movement of food from the mouth to the anus *(Figure 5.2)*. Normally, this takes 24 to 36 hours. **Mastication** (chewing) breaks down the food into smaller particles so that **digestive enzymes** have a larger surface area with which to interact. **Deglutition**, or swallowing, moves the **bolus** of food from the mouth into the esophagus. **Peristalsis**, or waves of contraction and relaxation, moves material through most of the alimentary canal. **Segmental contractions** in the small intestine move food back and forth to mix it with digestive secretions.

3. **Digestion**—the breakdown of foods into forms that can be transported to and absorbed into cells. This process has two components:

   a. Mechanical digestion breaks larger pieces of food into smaller ones without altering their chemical composition. This process exposes a larger surface area of the food to the action of digestive enzymes.

   b. Chemical digestion breaks down large molecules of food into smaller and simpler chemicals. This process is carried out by digestive enzymes produced by the salivary glands, stomach, small intestine, and pancreas.

   The digestive enzymes have three main groups:
   - **Amylases** that digest carbohydrates
   - **Lipases** that digest fats
   - **Proteases** that digest proteins

4. **Secretion**—the addition throughout the digestive tract of secretions that lubricate, liquefy, and digest the food. Mucus lubricates the food and the lining of the tract. Water liquefies the food to make it easier to digest and absorb. Enzymes break down the food.

5. **Absorption**—the movement of nutrient molecules out of the digestive tract and through the epithelial cells lining the tract into the blood or lymph for transportation to body cells.

6. **Elimination**—the process by which the unabsorbed residue of food is removed from the body.

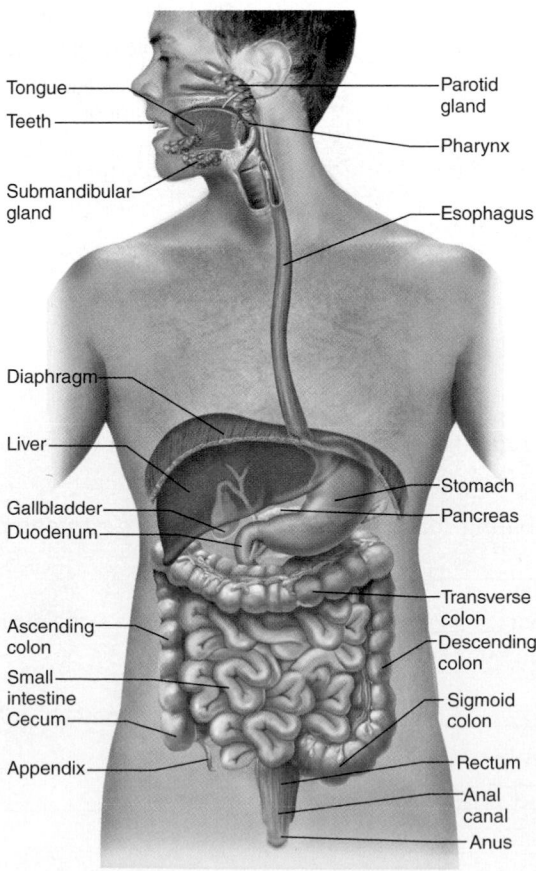

▲ **Figure 5.2**　The Digestive System.

Word Analysis and Definition

S = Suffix   P = Prefix   R = Root   R/CF = Combining Form

WORD	PRONUNCIATION	ELEMENTS		DEFINITION
absorption absorb (verb)	ab-**SORP**-shun ab-**SORB**		Latin *to swallow*	Uptake of nutrients and water by cells in the GI tract
amylase	**AM**-il-aze	S/ R/	-ase *enzyme* **amyl-** *starch*	One of a group of enzymes that break down starch
bolus	**BOH**-lus		Greek *lump*	Single mass of a substance
deglutition	dee-glue-**TISH**-un	S/ R/	-ion *action* **deglutit-** *to swallow*	The act of swallowing
elimination	e-lim-ih-**NAY**-shun	S/ R/	-ation *process* **elimin-** *throw away*	Removal of waste material from the digestive tract
ingestion	in-**JEST**-shun	S/ R/	-ion *action* **ingest-** *carry in*	Intake of food, either by mouth or through a nasogastric tube
lipase	**LIE**-paze	S/ R/	-ase *enzyme* **lip-** *fat*	Enzyme that breaks down fat
nasogastric	**NAY**-zoh-**GAS**-trik	S/ R/CF R/	-ic *pertaining to* **nas/o-** *nose* **-gastr-** *stomach*	Pertaining to the nose and stomach
peristalsis	per-ih-**STAL**-sis	P/ R/	peri- *around* -stalsis *constrict*	Waves of alternate contraction and relaxation of alimentary canal wall to move food along the digestive tract
protease	**PRO**-tee-aze	S/ R/CF	-ase *enzyme* **prot/e-** *protein*	Group of enzymes that break down protein
secrete secretion (noun)	seh-**KREET** seh-**KREE**-shun		Latin *to separate*	To release or give off, as substances produced by cells
segment segmental (adj)	**SEG**-ment **SEG**-ment-al	S/ R/	-al *pertaining to* **segment-** *section*	A section of an organ or structure Pertaining to a segment

Exercises

A. The body process or action has been described for you. *Match the definition in the left column to the correct medical term in the right column.* **LO 5.2, 5.3, 5.4**

_____ 1. Swallowing

_____ 2. Helps lubricate, liquefy, and digest food

_____ 3. Chewing

_____ 4. Removal of waste material

a. mastication

b. elimination

c. deglutition

d. secretion

B. Build the medical terms by filling in their missing elements.   LO 5.2, 5.3, 5.4

1. Enzymes that break down protein   _____/_____/ase

2. Removal of waste material from the digestive tract   _____/_____/ation

3. Enzyme that breaks down fat   _____/lip/_____

4. Enzyme that breaks down starch   _____/_____/ase

5. Pertaining to a section of an organ or structure   _____/_____/al

6. Waves that move food in intestines   peri/_____/_____.

Lesson 5.2 Mouth, Pharynx, and Esophagus

LESSON OBJECTIVES

When you pop a piece of chicken and some vegetables into your mouth, you start a cascade of digestive tract events that occur during the following 24 to 36 hours. In this chapter, you will follow a meal of chicken and vegetables as it goes through the digestive tract. In this lesson, you will review the first stages in the cascade while the food is in the mouth and then is swallowed. The information in this lesson will enable you to:

5.2.1 Select the correct medical terminology to describe the anatomy, physiology, and disorders of the mouth, pharynx, and esophagus.

5.2.2 Identify the structure and functions of the teeth, tongue, and salivary glands.

5.2.3 Describe the composition and functions of saliva.

5.2.4 Describe the process and outcomes of mastication and deglutition.

5.2.5 Discuss some common disorders of the mouth, pharynx, and esophagus.

You are

. . . a Certified Medical Assistant working with Susan Lee, MD, a primary care physician at Fulwood Medical Center.

Your patient is

. . . Mrs. Helen Schreiber, a 45-year-old high school principal. Your task is to document her care.

Case Report 5.2

Documentation.

Mrs. Helen Schreiber, a 45-year-old high school principal, presents with a 6-month history of dry mouth, bleeding gums, and difficulty in chewing and swallowing food.

Questioning by Dr. Susan Lee, her primary care physician, reveals that she also has dry eyes, is having pain in some joints of both hands, and has felt fatigued. Her previous medical history is uneventful. Physical examination shows a dry mouth, mild **gingivitis**, and an **ulcer** on the back of the lower lip. Her salivary glands are not swollen. Her eyes show no **ulceration** or conjunctivitis. The metacarpophalangeal joints of both index fingers are swollen, stiff, and tender. All other systems show no abnormality.

Initial laboratory reports show anemia, decreased **WBC** count, and an elevated **ESR**. Dr. Lee made a provisional diagnosis of **Sjögren syndrome**. The results of blood studies for **SSA** and **SSB** antibodies (Sjögren syndrome antibodies A and B) and for rheumatoid factor titers are pending, as are x-rays of her hands.

Mrs. Schreiber was given advice about symptomatic treatment for her dry mouth and will be seen again in 1 week.

Luisa Guitterez, **CMA** 06/12/12, 1530 hrs.

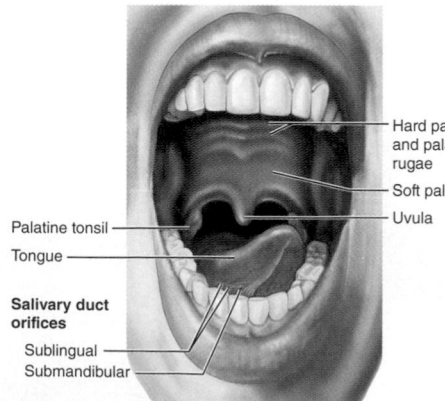

▲ **Figure 5.3** Mouth (Oral Cavity).

Hard palate and palatal rugae
Soft palate
Uvula
Palatine tonsil
Tongue
Salivary duct orifices
Sublingual
Submandibular

▲ **Figure 5.4** Tongue.

Epiglottis
Lingual tonsils
Lingual tonsils
Palatine tonsil

Abbreviations

CMA	Certified Medical Assistant
ESR	erythrocyte sedimentation rate
SSA	Sjögren syndrome antibodies A
SSB	Sjögren syndrome antibodies B
WBC	white blood cell

LO 5.6 The Mouth and Mastication

The mouth, or **oral** cavity *(Figure 5.3)*, is the entrance to your digestive tract and is the first site of mechanical digestion (through **mastication**, or chewing) and of chemical digestion (through an **enzyme** in saliva).

The cheeks contain the **buccinator** muscles. These muscles hold the chicken and vegetable in place while you chew and your teeth crush and tear them.

The roof of the mouth is called the **palate**. The anterior two-thirds is the bony hard palate. The posterior one-third is the muscular soft palate. The hard palate is covered with folds of epithelium called *rugae*, which assist the tongue to manipulate food prior to swallowing. The skeletal muscle of the soft palate has a projection called the **uvula** that closes off the nasopharynx during swallowing.

The **tongue** *(Figure 5.4)* moves food around your mouth and helps the cheeks, lips, and gums hold the food in place while you chew it. Small, rough, raised areas on the tongue, called **papillae**, contain some 4000 **taste buds** that react to the chemical nature of the food to give you the different sensations of taste. A taste bud cell lives for 7 to 10 days and is then replaced.

WORD	PRONUNCIATION	ELEMENTS		DEFINITION
buccinator	**BUCK**-sin-a-tor	S/ R/	-ator *agent* buccin- *the cheek*	Buccinator muscle is the muscle in the cheek
enzyme	**EN**-zime	P/ R/	en- *in* -zyme *fermenting, enzyme*	Protein that induces changes in other substances
gingivitis	jin-jih-**VI**-tis	S/ R/	-itis *inflammation* gingiv- *gums*	Inflammation of the gums
masticate	**MAS**-tih-kate	S/	-ate *composed of, pertaining to*	To chew
mastication (noun)	mas-tih-**KAY**-shun	R/	mastic- *chew*	
oral	**OR**-al	S/ R/	-al *pertaining to* or- *mouth*	Pertaining to the mouth
palate	**PAL**-uht		Latin *palate*	Roof of the mouth
papilla papillae (pl)	pah-**PILL**-ah pah-**PILL**-ee		Latin *small pimple*	Any small projection
Sjögren syndrome	**SHOW**-gren **SIN**-drome		Henrik Sjögren, 1899–1986, Swedish ophthalmologist	Autoimmune disease that attacks the glands that produce saliva and tears
taste	TAYST		Latin *to taste*	Sensation from chemicals on the taste buds
tongue	TUNG		Latin *tongue*	Mobile muscle mass in mouth; bears the taste buds
ulcer ulceration	**ULL**-cer ull-cer-**A**-shun	S/ R/	Latin *sore* -ation *a process* ulcer- *a sore*	Erosion of an area of skin or mucosa Formation of an ulcer
uvula	**YOU**-vyu-lah		Latin *grape*	Fleshy projection of the soft palate

Exercises

A. After reading Case Report 5.2 on the opposite page, answer the following questions. *Be prepared to discuss your answers in class.*
LO 5.3, 5.4

1. What are Mrs. Schreiber's presenting symptoms? _____

_____

2. What other complaints does Dr. Lee discover on further questioning of the patient? _____

_____

3. What does Dr. Lee find on physical examination of the patient? _____

_____

B. Continue using the language of the digestive system to answer the following questions.   LO 5.3

1. What does *symptomatic treatment* mean? _____

_____

2. What symptoms are specific to the patient's mouth? _____

_____

3. Where are the *salivary glands?* _____

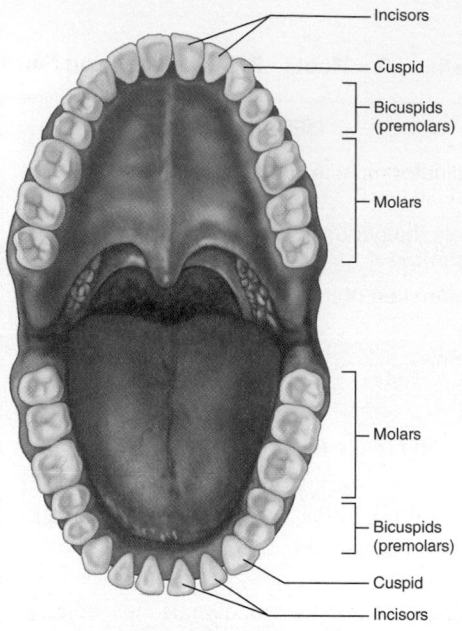

▲ **Figure 5.5** Adult Teeth.

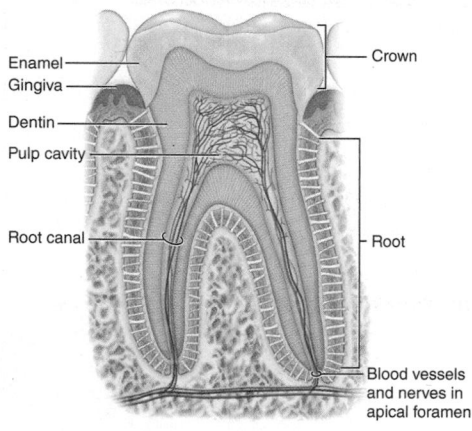

▲ **Figure 5.6** Anatomy of a Molar.

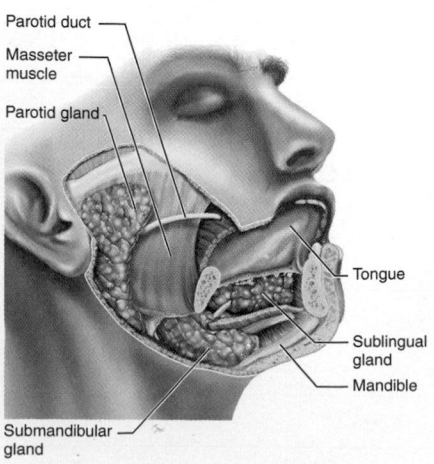

▲ **Figure 5.7** Salivary Glands.

LO 5.6 The Mouth and Mastication (continued)

Adult Teeth

The normal adult has 32 teeth, 16 rooted in the upper jaw (maxilla) and 16 in the lower jaw (mandible). The teeth are the hardest structures in your body, and different teeth *(Figure 5.5)* are designed to handle food in different ways. The eight **incisors** are shaped like a chisel to slice and cut into food. The four **cuspids** have a pointed tip for puncturing and tearing. The eight **bicuspids** and twelve **molars** have flattened surfaces for grinding and crushing food. Your wisdom teeth are molars.

Each tooth has two main parts:

- The **crown**, which projects above the gum and is covered in **enamel**, the hardest substance in the body.

- The **root**, which anchors the tooth to the jaw.

The bulk of the tooth is composed of **dentin**, a substance like bone but harder *(Figure 5.6)*. The dentin surrounds a central **pulp cavity** that contains blood vessels, nerves, and connective tissue. The blood vessels and nerves reach this cavity from the jaw through tubular **root canals**.

Salivary Glands

Salivary glands secrete saliva. The two **parotid** glands, the two **submandibular** glands, the two **sublingual glands** *(Figure 5.7)*, and numerous minor salivary glands scattered in the mucosa of the tongue and cheeks secrete more than a quart of saliva each day.

Saliva is 95% water, and its functions are to

- Begin starch digestion with the enzyme **amylase**.
- Begin fat digestion with the enzyme **lipase**.
- Prevent the growth of bacteria in the mouth with the enzyme **lysozyme** and the protective **immunoglobulin A (IgA)** *(see Chapter 12)*.
- Produce **mucus** to lubricate food to make it easier to swallow.

Imagine that you are eating a piece of chicken with some vegetables. By the end of the mastication process, the chicken has been torn and ground into small pieces by your teeth, and its fat has begun to be digested by the lipase in your saliva. The vegetables have been ground into small pieces as well, and the starch in them has begun to be digested by the amylase in your saliva. The food has been lubricated, mixed together, and formed into a bolus ready to be swallowed.

Case Report 5.2 (continued)

Mrs. Helen Schreiber has Sjögren syndrome, an autoimmune disease *[see Chapter 12]* that affects her salivary glands, stopping production of saliva. This leads to a dry mouth, difficulty in swallowing, and increased bacterial activity in the mouth, causing gingivitis. It is associated with dry eyes and with rheumatoid arthritis, which is beginning in her hands. There is no known cure, and treatment is **symptomatic**.

WORD	PRONUNCIATION	ELEMENTS		DEFINITION
bicuspid (also called premolar)	by-**KUSS**-pid	S/ P/ R/	**-id** *having a particular quality* **bi-** *two* **-cusp-** *point*	Having two points; a bicuspid (premolar) tooth has two points
crown	KROWN		Latin *crown*	Part of the tooth above the gum
cuspid	**KUSS**-pid	S/ R/	**-id** *having a particular quality* **-cusp-** *point*	Tooth with one point
dentin (also spelled dentine)	**DEN**-tin	S/ R/	**-in** *substance, chemical compound* **dent-** *tooth*	Dense, ivory-like substance located under the enamel in a tooth
enamel	ee-**NAM**-el		French *enamel*	Hard substance covering a tooth
incisor	in-**SIGH**-zor		Latin *to cut into*	Chisel-shaped tooth
lysozyme	**LIE**-soh-zime	S/ R/CF	**-zyme** *enzyme* **lys/o-** *dissolve*	Enzyme that dissolves the cell walls of bacteria
molar	**MO**-lar		Latin *millstone*	One of six teeth in each jaw that grind food
parotid	pah-**ROT**-id	S/ P/ R/	**-id** *having a particular quality* **par-** *beside* **-ot-** *ear*	Parotid gland is the salivary gland beside the ear
pulp	PULP		Latin *flesh*	Dental pulp is the connective tissue in the cavity in the center of the tooth
root	ROOT		Old English *beginning*	Fundamental or beginning part of a structure
saliva salivary (adj)	sa-**LIE**-vah **SAL**-ih-var-ee	 S/ R/	Latin *spit* **-ary** *pertaining to* **saliv-** *saliva*	Secretion in mouth from salivary glands
sublingual	sub-**LING**-wal	S/ P/ R/	**-al** *pertaining to* **sub-** *underneath* **-lingu-** *tongue*	Underneath the tongue
submandibular	sub-man-**DIB**-you-lar	S/ P/ R/	**-ar** *pertaining to* **sub-** *underneath* **-mandibul-** *the jaw*	Underneath the mandible
symptom	**SIMP**-tum		Greek *sign*	Departure from the normal experienced by a patient
symptomatic	simp-toe-**MAT**-ik	S/ R/	**-ic** *pertaining to* **symptomat-** *symptom*	Pertaining to the symptoms of a disease

Exercises

A. Analyze and define the following terms, and determine what makes them similar and what makes them different. *Fill in the blanks.* **LO 5.3, 5.4, 5.6**

1. submandibular   Definition: _____

2. sublingual   Definition: _____

3. Now that you have written the definition of each term, it should be obvious what is similar. The similarity is

_____

4. What makes the terms different? _____

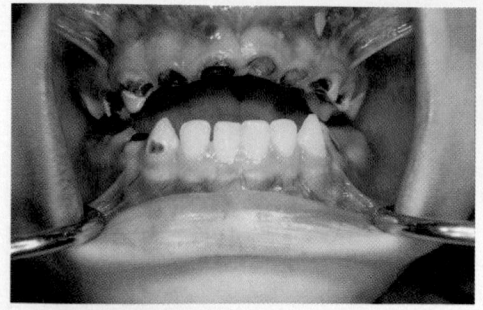

▲ **Figure 5.8** **Dental Caries.** Child with dental caries.

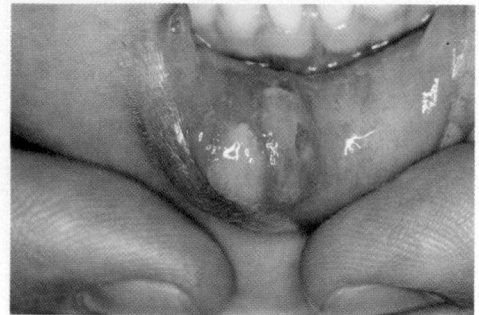

▲ **Figure 5.9** **Cold Sores.** Ulcer inside lower lip.

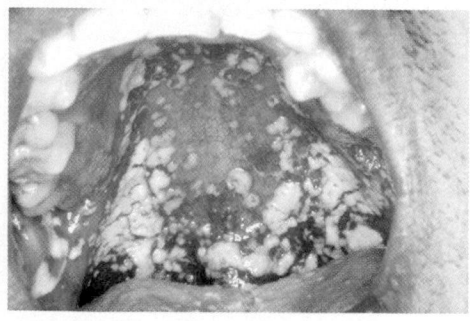

▲ **Figure 5.10** **Oral Thrush.**

LO 5.7 Disorders of the Mouth

An accumulation of dental **plaque** (a collection of oral microorganisms and their products) or **dental calculus (tartar)**, calcified deposits at the gingival margin of the teeth, is a precursor to dental disease.

Dental caries, tooth decay and cavity formation, is an erosion of the tooth surface caused by bacteria *(Figure 5.8)*. If untreated, it can lead to an abscess at the root of the tooth. **Gingivitis** is an infection of the gums. **Periodontal disease** occurs when the gums and the jawbone are involved in a disease process. In **periodontitis**, infection causes the gums to pull away from the teeth, forming pockets that become infected. The infection can spread to the underlying bone. Infection of the gums with a purulent discharge is called **pyorrhea**.

The term **stomatitis** is used for any infection of the mouth. The most common infections are

- **Mouth ulcers**, also called **canker** sores, which are erosions of the mucous membrane lining the mouth. The most common type are **aphthous** ulcers, which occur in clusters of small ulcers and last for 3 or 4 days. They are usually related to stress or illness. Ulcers can also be caused by trauma.

- **Cold sores**, also known as fever blisters *(Figure 5.9)*, which are recurrent ulcers of the lips, lining of the mouth, and gums due to infection with the virus **herpes simplex type 1 (HSV-1)**. Acyclovir (Zovirac) is a treatment used, but the ulcers usually clear spontaneously.

- **Thrush** *(Figure 5.10)*, an infection occurring anywhere in the mouth and caused by the fungus *Candida albicans*. This fungus typically is found in the mouth, but it can multiply out of control as a result of prolonged antibiotic or steroid treatment, cancer chemotherapy, or diabetes. A newborn baby can acquire oral thrush from the mother's vaginal yeast infection during the birth process. Treatment with antifungal agents, such as nystatin (Mycostatin) or clotrimazole (Lotrimin), is usually successful *(see Chapter 19)*.

- **Leukoplakia**, a white plaque seen anywhere in the mouth. It is more common in the elderly, is often associated with smoking or chewing tobacco, and approximately 3% turn into oral cancer. Patients whose immune systems are compromised (for example, with **human immunodeficiency virus [HIV]**) are susceptible to leukoplakia.

- **Oral cancer** *(Figure 5.11)*, which is mostly squamous cell carcinoma, occurring often on the lip. Eighty percent of oral cancers are associated with smoking or chewing tobacco. Metastasis occurs to lymph nodes, bone, lung, and liver. The 5-year-survival rate is only 51%.

- **Halitosis**, the medical term for bad breath, which can be found in association with any of the above mouth disorders.

- **Glossodynia**, a painful burning sensation of the tongue. It occurs in postmenopausal women. Its etiology is unknown, and there is no successful treatment.

- **Cleft palate** is a congenital fissure in the median line of the palate. It is often associated with a cleft lip.

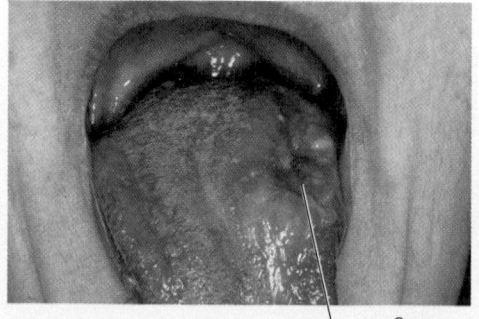

— Cancer

▲ **Figure 5.11** **Oral Cancer.** Cancer of the tongue.

WORD	PRONUNCIATION	ELEMENTS		DEFINITION
aphthous ulcer	**AF**-thus **UL**-ser		Greek *ulcer*	Painful small oral ulcer (canker sore)
canker; canker sore (also called **mouth ulcer**)	**KANG**-ker SOAR		Latin *crab*	Nonmedical term for aphthous ulcer
caries	**KARE**-eez		Latin *dry rot*	Bacterial destruction of teeth
gingiva gingival (adj)	**JIN**-jih-vah **JIN**-jih-vul	S/ R/	Latin *gum* -al *pertaining to* **gingiv-** *gums*	Tissue surrounding teeth and covering the jaw Pertaining to the gums
gingivitis gingivectomy	jin-jih-**VI**-tis jin-jih-**VEC**-toe-me	S/ S/	-itis *inflammation* -ectomy *surgical excision*	Inflammation of the gums Surgical removal of diseased gum tissue
glossodynia	gloss-oh-**DIN**-ee-ah	S/ R/CF	-dynia *pain* **gloss/o-** *tongue*	Painful, burning tongue
halitosis	hal-ih-**TOE**-sis	S/ R/	-osis *condition* **halit-** *breath*	Bad odor of the breath
leukoplakia	loo-koh-**PLAY**-kee-ah	S/ R/CF R/	-ia *condition* **leuk/o-** *white* -plak- *plate, plaque*	White patch on oral mucous membrane, often precancerous
periodontal	**PER**-ee-oh-**DON**-tal	S/ P/ R/	-al *pertaining to* peri- *around* **-odont-** *tooth*	Around a tooth
periodontics	**PER**-ee-oh-**DON**-tiks	S/	-ics *knowledge of*	Branch of dentistry specializing in disorders of tissues around the teeth
periodontist periodontitis	**PER**-ee-oh-**DON**-tist **PER**-ee-oh-don-**TIE**-tis	S/ S/	-ist *specialist* -itis *inflammation*	Specialist in periodontics Inflammation of tissues around a tooth
plaque	PLAK		French *plate*	Patch of abnormal tissue
pyorrhea	pie-oh-**REE**-ah	S/ R/CF	-rrhea *flow* **py/o-** *pus*	Purulent discharge
tartar (also called **dental calculus**)	**TAR**-tar		Latin *crust on wine casks*	Calcified deposit at the gingival margin of the teeth
thrush	THRUSH		Root unknown	Infection with *Candida albicans*

Exercises

A. Find the correct suffix to complete the medical terms. *Use each suffix only one time. Fill in the blanks.*   **LO 5.3, 5.7**

1. Inflammation of the gums   gingiv/ _____

2. Specialized branch of dentistry   periodont/ _____

3. Painful, burning tongue   glosso/ _____

4. Around a tooth   periodont/ _____

5. Bad breath   halit/ _____

6. Surgical removal of diseased gums   gingiv/ _____

7. Precancerous white patches   leukoplak/ _____

B. Find the correct suffix to complete the medical terms. *Use each suffix only one time. Fill in the blanks; then answer the questions.*
   LO 5.3, 5.7

1. One who specializes in periodontics is a periodont/ _____

2. *Aphthous, oral,* and *ulcer* are all terms connected with _____.

3. Dental caries is another name for _____.

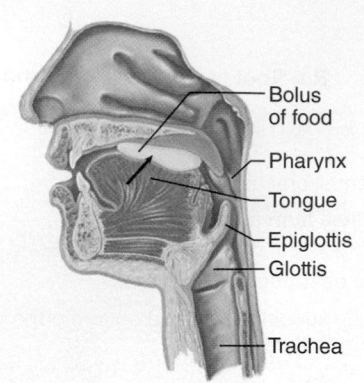

▲ **Figure 5.12** Deglutition (Swallowing): Phase One.

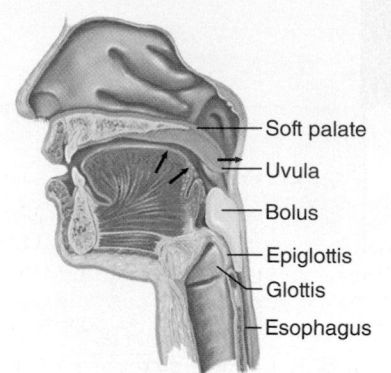

▲ **Figure 5.13** Deglutition (Swallowing): Phase Two.

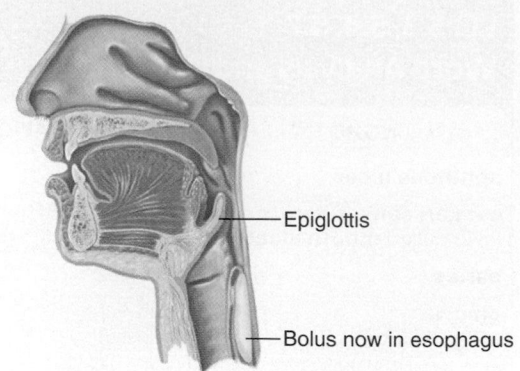

▲ **Figure 5.14** Deglutition (Swallowing): Phase Three.

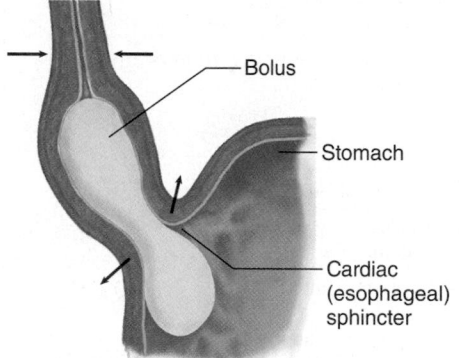

▲ **Figure 5.15** Deglutition (Swallowing): Phase Four.

Abbreviation	
GERD	gastroesophageal reflux disease

LO 5.8 Deglutition (Swallowing)—Pharynx and Esophagus

The pieces of chicken and vegetable that you ingested have now been sliced and ground into small particles by the teeth, partially digested and lubricated by saliva, and rolled into a bolus between the tongue and the hard palate, the bony roof of the mouth *(Figure 5.12)*. The bolus is now ready to be swallowed **(deglutition)**.

- **Phase One.** As you swallow, the bolus of food is pushed backward by your tongue into the **oropharynx**. Once the bolus is in your oropharynx, the tongue contracts against the hard palate and pushes up the soft palate and **uvula** to close off the **nasopharynx** at the back of the nose. This prevents food from going up into your nasopharynx and nose *(see Figure 5.12)*.

- **Phase Two.** Surrounding the oropharynx are circular muscles called **constrictors**. These muscles contract, forcing the bolus down through the laryngopharynx toward the **esophagus** and pushing the **epiglottis** closed so that food cannot enter the **larynx** and **trachea** *(Figure 5.13)*.

- **Phase Three.** When the bolus reaches the lower end of the **pharynx**, the upper **esophageal sphincter** relaxes and the bolus enters the esophagus, where contractions of the muscles in the wall move the bolus toward the stomach *(Figure 5.14)*.

- **Phase Four.** The esophageal sphincter at the lower end of the esophagus **(cardiac sphincter)** relaxes to allow the bolus to enter the stomach *(Figure 5.15)*.

The **esophagus** *(Figure 5.16)* is a tube 9 to 10 inches long; it pierces the diaphragm at the esophageal **hiatus** to go from the thoracic cavity to the abdominal cavity.

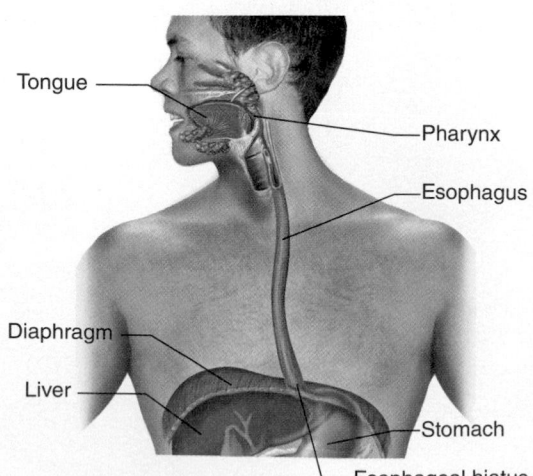

▲ **Figure 5.16** Esophagus.

LO 5.9 Disorders of the Esophagus

Esophagitis is inflammation of the lining of the esophagus that produces a **postprandial** burning chest pain **(heartburn)**, pain on swallowing, and occasional vomiting of blood **(hematemesis)**. The most common cause is **reflux** of the stomach's acid contents into the esophagus, **gastroesophageal reflux disease (GERD)**. **Regurgitation** of stomach contents into the mouth **(water brash)** can occur with resulting hypersalivation.

Hiatal hernia occurs when a portion of the stomach protrudes through the diaphragm alongside the esophagus at the esophageal **hiatus**. Reflux of acid stomach contents into the esophagus causes an esophagitis. Surgical repair sometimes is necessary and is called a **herniorrhaphy**.

Esophageal varices are **varicose** vein of the esophagus. They are **asymptomatic** until they rupture, causing massive bleeding and hematemesis. They are a complication of cirrhosis of the liver *(see Lesson 5.4)*.

Cancer of the esophagus arises from the lining of the tube. Symptoms are difficulty in swallowing **(dysphagia)**, a burning sensation in the chest, and weight loss. Risk factors include cigarettes, alcohol, betel nut chewing, and esophageal reflux. The cancer metastasizes to liver, bone, and lung.

WORD	PRONUNCIATION	ELEMENTS		DEFINITION
deglutition	dee-glue-**TISH**-un		Latin *to swallow*	The act of swallowing
dysphagia	dis-**FAY**-jee-ah	P/ R/	dys- *difficult* -phagia *swallowing*	Difficulty in swallowing
emesis	**EM**-eh-sis	S/ R/	-sis *abnormal condition* eme- *to vomit*	Vomiting
hematemesis	he-mah-**TEM**-eh-sis	R/	hemat- *blood*	Vomiting of red blood
epiglottis	ep-ih-**GLOT**-is	P/ R/	epi- *above* -glottis *windpipe*	Leaf-shaped plate of cartilage that shuts off larynx during swallowing
esophagus esophageal (adj)	ee-**SOF**-ah-gus ee-**SOF**-ah-**JEE**-al	 S/ R/	Greek *gullet* -eal *pertaining to* esophag- *esophagus*	Tube linking the pharynx and stomach Pertaining to the esophagus
esophagitis	ee-**SOF**-ah-**JI**-tis	S/	-itis *inflammation*	Inflammation of the lining of the esophagus
hernia	**HER**-nee-ah		Latin *rupture*	Protrusion of a structure through the tissue that normally contains it
herniorrhaphy	**HER**-nee-**OR**-ah-fee	S/ R/CF	-rrhaphy *suture* herni/o- *hernia*	Repair of a hernia
herniate (verb)	**HER**-nee-ate	S/	-ate *pertaining to*	To protrude
hiatus hiatal (adj)	high-**AY**-tus high-**AY**-tal	 R/ S/	Latin *an aperture* hiat- *aperture* -al *pertaining to*	An opening through a structure Pertaining to an opening through a structure
larynx	**LAIR**-inks		Latin *larynx*	Organ of voice production
nasopharynx	**NAY**-zoh-**FAIR**-inks	R/CF R/	nas/o- *nose* -pharynx *throat*	Region of the pharynx at the back of the nose and above the soft palate
oropharynx	**OR**-oh-**FAIR**-inks	R/CF R/	or/o- *mouth* -pharynx *throat*	Region at the back of the mouth between the soft palate and the tip of the epiglottis
pharynx	**FAIR**-inks		Greek *throat*	Air tube from the back of the nose to the larynx
postprandial	post-**PRAN**-dee-al	S/ P/ R/	-ial *pertaining to* post- *after* -prand- *meal*	Following a meal
reflux	**REE**-fluks	P/ R/	re- *back* -flux *flow*	Backward flow
regurgitation	ree-gur-jih-**TAY**-shun	S/ P/ R/	-ation *process* re- *back* -gurgit- *flood*	Expelling contents of the stomach into the mouth, short of vomiting
trachea	**TRAY**-kee-ah		Greek *windpipe*	Air tube from the larynx to the bronchi
varix varices (pl) varicose (adj)	**VAIR**-iks **VAIR**-ih-seez **VAIR**-ih-kos		Latin *dilated vein*	Dilated, tortuous vein Characterized by or affected with varices

Exercises

A. Some of the terms in this chapter are particularly hard to spell and pronounce. *Read these sentences aloud after you have circled your choice for the correct spelling.* **LO 5.3, 5.8, 5.9**

1. _____ (Hyatus/Hiatus) is the Latin word for *opening* and is the opening through the diaphragm for the (esophagis/esophagus).

2. The (eppiglotis/epiglottis) is a leaf-shaped plate of cartilage that acts to cover the opening of the (larynix/larynx) during deglutition.

3. Medication may be ordered (postprandially/postperandially), meaning *taken after meals.*

4. (Hemotemasis/Hematemesis) is the (vomiting/vomitting) of blood.

5. (Esophagitis/Esophogitis) can be caused by reflux disease.

6. (Varricces/Varices) is the plural of (varix/varex) and means *dilated, tortuous vein.* The adjective is (varicose/varricose).

Lesson 5.3 Digestion—Stomach and Small Intestine

The bolus of food that you swallowed has passed down the esophagus. It now enters the stomach, and the process of digestion begins in earnest. The stomach continues the mechanical breakdown of the food particles and begins the chemical digestion of protein and fats. It is in the small intestine that the greatest amount of digestion and absorption occurs. The information in this lesson will enable you to:

5.3.1 Describe the process of digestion in the small intestine.
5.3.2 Describe the layers of the wall of the small intestine.
5.3.3 Describe the secretions of the stomach and their functions.
5.3.4 Discuss the secretions of the small intestine and their functions.
5.3.5 Explain how food is propelled through the stomach and small intestine.
5.3.6 Describe how the breakdown products of digestion are absorbed from the small intestine.

You are

... an **EMT-1** working in the Emergency Department at Fulwood Medical Center.

Your patient is

... Mrs. Jan Stark, a 36-year-old pottery maker. Your task is to document her visit.

Case Report 5.3

Documentation

Mrs. Jan Stark, a 36-year-old pottery maker, was admitted to the Emergency Department at 2015 hrs.

She stated that she had passed between 20 and 30 watery, gray stools in the previous 24 hours. She had not passed urine for more than 12 hours. She was markedly **dehydrated** and responded well to infusion of lactated Ringer solution and then D5NS (5% dextrose in normal 0.9% saline).

Questioning revealed that, for the past 10 years, she has had spasmodic episodes of diarrhea and flatulence associated with severe headaches and fatigue. During those episodes her stools were greasy and pale. In the past 3 or 4 months, she has had some difficulties with fine movements as she works on her pottery wheel and has had tingling in her fingers and toes.

Dr. Homer Hilinski, emergency physician, believes her **dehydration** is a result of a **malabsorption syndrome**. An appointment has been made for her to see Dr. Cameron Grabowski, gastroenterologist, tomorrow. She was discharged to her husband's care at midnight. She has been advised to stay on fluids only and to return to the Emergency Room (**ER**) if the diarrhea returns.

Sunil Patel, EMT-1. 10/21/12, 0100 hrs.

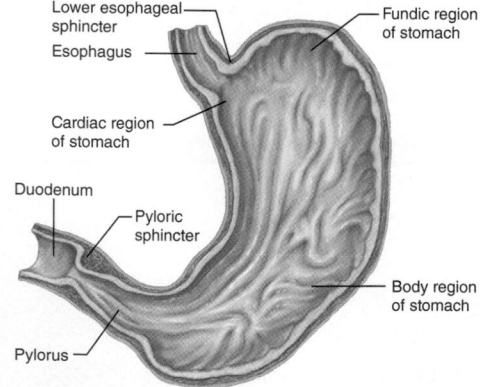

▲ **Figure 5.17** Stomach.

Lower esophageal sphincter
Esophagus
Cardiac region of stomach
Duodenum
Pyloric sphincter
Pylorus
Fundic region of stomach
Body region of stomach

Abbreviations

EMT-1	emergency medical technician–first responder
ER	emergency room
HCl	hydrochloric acid

LO 5.10 Digestion: The Stomach

The stomach's peristaltic contractions mix different boluses of food together and also push the more liquid contents toward the **pylorus** *(Figure 5.17)*. These contractions and the digestive process work on the boluses of food to produce a mixture of semidigested food called **chyme**.

The cells of the lining of the stomach secrete the following:

- **Mucin**—continues to lubricate food and protects the stomach lining.
- **Hydrochloric acid (HCl)**—breaks up the connective tissue of the chicken and the cell walls of the vegetable that you ingested a few seconds ago. It also destroys any pathogens that enter your stomach along with the food you eat.
- **Pepsinogen**—is converted by hydrochloric acid to **pepsin**, an active enzyme that starts to digest the protein in the chicken and vegetable.
- **Intrinsic factor**—is essential for the absorption of vitamin B_{12} in the small intestine. Neither chicken nor vegetables contain this factor.
- **Chemical messengers**—stimulate other cells in the gastric mucosa. One of these messengers, **gastrin**, stimulates both the production of HCl and pepsinogen by the stomach cells and the peristaltic contractions of the stomach.

Liquids exit the stomach within 1½ to 2 hours after ingestion. A typical meal like your chicken and vegetable takes 3 to 4 hours to exit. The resulting chyme is held in the pylorus. Peristaltic waves squirt 2 to 3 mL of the chyme at a time through the **pyloric sphincter** into the **duodenum**.

Anywhere from 40 minutes to 2 hours after consuming that chicken and vegetable dinner mentioned earlier, your food is partially digested by the salivary and stomach enzymes described previously.

Word Analysis and Definition

S = Suffix   P = Prefix   **R = Root**   **R/CF = Combining Form**

WORD	PRONUNCIATION	ELEMENTS		DEFINITION
chyme	KYME		Greek *juice*	Semifluid, partially digested food passed from the stomach into the duodenum
dehydration	dee-high-**DRAY**-shun	S/ P/ R/	-ation *a process* de- *without* -hydr- *water*	Process of losing body water
duodenum	du-oh-**DEE**-num	S/ R/	-um *structure* duoden- Latin for *twelve*	The first part of the small intestine; approximately 12 finger-breadths (9 to 10 inches) in length
duodenal (adj)	du-oh-**DEE**-nal	S/	-al *pertaining to*	Pertaining to the duodenum
fundus	**FUN**-dus	S/ R/	Latin *bottom* -us *pertaining to* fund- *bottom or cul-de-sac*	The portion of the stomach that lies above the entrance of the esophagus
fundic (adj)	**FUN**-dick	S/	-ic *pertaining to*	Pertaining to the fundus
gastrin	**GAS**-trin	S/ R/	-in *substance* gastr- *stomach*	Hormone secreted in the stomach that stimulates secretion of HCl and increases gastric motility
hydrochloric acid (HCl)	high-droh-**KLOR**-ic **ASS**-id	S/ R/CF R/	-ic *pertaining to* hydr/o- *water* -chlor- *green*	The acid of gastric juice
intrinsic factor	in-**TRIN**-sik **FAK**-tor	S/ R/ R/	-ic *pertaining to* intrins- *on the inside* factor *maker*	Substance secreted by the stomach that is necessary for the absorption of vitamin B_{12}
malabsorption	mal-ab-**SORP**-shun	S/ P/ R/	-ion *action, condition* mal- *bad* -absorpt- *to swallow*	Inadequate gastrointestinal absorption of nutrients
mucus	**MYU**-kus	R/	Latin *slime* *muc- mucus*	Sticky secretion of cells in mucous membranes
mucous (adj)	**MYU**-kus	S/	-ous *pertaining to*	Relating to mucus or the mucosa
mucin	**MYU**-sin	S/	-in *chemical compound*	Protein element of mucus
pepsin	**PEP**-sin		Greek *to digest*	Enzyme produced by the stomach that breaks down protein
pepsinogen	pep-**SIN**-oh-jen	S/ R/CF	-gen *produce* pepsin/o- *pepsin*	Enzyme converted by HCl in stomach to pepsin
pylorus	pie-**LOR**-us	S/ R/	-us *pertaining to* pylor- *gate*	Exit area of the stomach proximal to the duodenum
pyloric (adj)	pie-**LOR**-ik	S/	-ic *pertaining to*	Pertaining to the pylorus

Exercises

A. After reading Case Report 5.3 on the opposite page, answer the following questions. *Be prepared to discuss your answers in class.* **LO 5.3, 5.10**

1. What is your body lacking if you are *dehydrated?* _____

2. What is an infusion? _____

3. What are Mrs. Stark's presenting symptoms? _____
_____

4. What symptoms are in Mrs. Stark's past medical history? _____
_____

5. *Malabsorption syndrome* means that Mrs. Stark's body is not absorbing _____.

LO 5.11 Disorders of the Stomach

Gastroesophageal reflux disease (GERD) is the regurgitation of stomach contents back into the esophagus, often when a person is lying down at night. The patient experiences burning sensations in the chest and mouth from the acidity of the regurgitation. The acidity can also irritate and ulcerate the lining of the esophagus, causing it to bleed. Scar tissue can form and cause an esophageal **stricture**, with difficulty in swallowing (dysphagia).

Vomiting can result from distention or irritation of any part of the digestive tract. A message is sent via the **vagus** nerve to the vomiting center in the brain, which, in turn, stimulates the muscles of the diaphragm and abdominal wall to forcefully contract and expel the stomach contents upward into the esophagus and out the mouth.

Gastritis is an inflammation of the lining of the stomach, producing symptoms of epigastric pain, a feeling of fullness, nausea, and occasional bleeding. Gastritis can be caused by common medications such as aspirin and nonsteroidal anti-inflammatory drugs (**NSAIDs**), by radiotherapy and chemotherapy, and by alcohol and smoking. Treatment is directed at removing the factors causing the gastritis by acid neutralization and suppression of gastric acid (see "Pharmacology of Treating Excess Gastric Acid," which follows).

Peptic ulcers occur in the stomach and duodenum when the balance between the acid gastric juices and the protection of the mucosal lining breaks down, causing an **erosion** of the lining by the acid *(Figure 5.18)*. Most peptic ulcers are caused by the bacterium *Helicobacter pylori (H. pylori)*, which produces enzymes that weaken the protective mucus. These ulcers respond to an antibiotic. Use of NSAIDs increases the incidence of peptic ulcers, particularly in the elderly. **Dyspepsia**, epigastric pain with bloating and nausea, is the most common symptom.

Gastric ulcers are peptic ulcers occurring in the stomach. Symptoms are epigastric burning pain after food, nausea, vomiting, and belching. Bleeding can occur from **erosion** of a blood vessel. If untreated, the ulcer can erode through the entire wall, causing a **perforation**.

Gastric cancer can be asymptomatic for a long period and then cause **indigestion**, **anorexia**, abdominal pain, and weight loss. It affects men twice as often as women. It metastasizes to lymph nodes, liver, peritoneum, chest, and brain. It is usually treated with **resection** and chemotherapy.

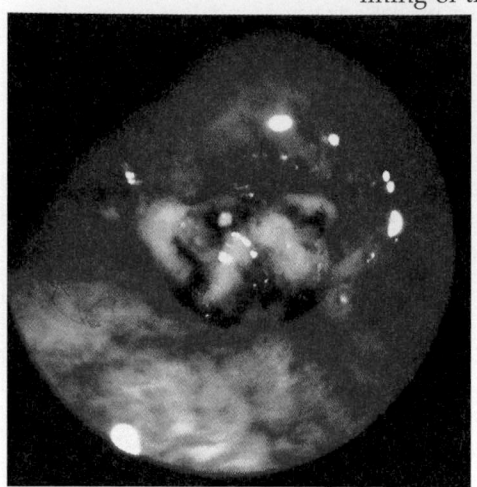

▲ **Figure 5.18** **Bleeding Peptic Ulcer.** The yellow floor of the ulcer shows black blood clots. Fresh blood is around the ulcer margin.

Abbreviations	
GERD	gastroesophageal reflux disease
H₂-blocker	histamine-2 receptor antagonist
NSAIDs	nonsteroidal anti-inflammatory drugs
PPI	proton pump inhibitor

LO 5.12 Pharmacology of Treating Excess Gastric Acid

Antacids are taken orally, neutralize gastric acid, and relieve heartburn and acid indigestion. Examples of antacids include

- Aluminum hydroxide and magnesium hydroxide (Maalox, Mylanta)
- Magnesium hydroxide (Milk of Magnesia)
- Calcium carbonate (Tums, Rolaids)

Histamine-2 receptor antagonists (H₂-blockers) block the production of gastric acid. Examples include

- Cimetidine (Tagamet)
- Famotidine (Pepcid)
- Ranitidine (Zantac)

Proton pump inhibitors (PPIs) suppress gastric acid secretion by blocking in the lining of the stomach the enzyme system that produces gastric acid. Examples include

- Omeprazole (Prilosec)
- Lansoprazole (Prevacid)

Sucralfate coats the site of an ulcer and protects it against gastric acid.

Misoprostol diminishes acid production and protects the mucosa. It is used prophylactically in patients taking NSAIDs.

Anti–*H. pylori* therapy is given with two antibiotics (for example, amoxicillin and clarithromycin) with a proton pump inhibitor.

Word Analysis and Definition

S = Suffix   P = Prefix   R = Root   R/CF = Combining Form

WORD	PRONUNCIATION	ELEMENTS		DEFINITION
anorexia	an-oh-**RECK**-see-ah	S/ P/ R/	**-ia** *condition* **an-** *without* **-orex-** *appetite*	Severe lack of appetite; or an aversion to food
antacid	ant-**ASS**-id	P/ R/	**ant-** *against* **-acid** *acid*	Agent that neutralizes acidity
dyspepsia	dis-**PEP**-see-ah	S/ P/ R/	**-ia** *condition* **dys-** *difficult, bad* **-peps-** *digestion*	"Upset stomach," epigastric pain, nausea, and gas
erosion	ee-**ROE**-shun		Latin *to gnaw away*	A shallow ulcer in the lining of a structure
gastritis	gas-**TRY**-tis	S/ R/	**-itis** *inflammation* **gastr-** *stomach*	Inflammation of the lining of the stomach
gastroesophageal	**GAS**-troh-ee-sof-ah-**JEE**-al	S/ R/CF R/CF	**-al** *pertaining to* **gastr/o-** *stomach* **-esophag/e-** *esophagus*	Pertaining to the stomach and esophagus
gastroscope	**GAS**-troh-skope	S/ R/CF	**-scope** *instrument for viewing* **gastr/o-** *stomach*	Endoscope for examining the inside of the stomach
peptic	**PEP**-tik	S/ R/	**-ic** *pertaining to* **pept-** *digest*	Relating to the stomach and duodenum
perforation	per-foh-**RAY**-shun	S/ R/	**-ion** *action* **perforat-** *bore through*	Erosion that progresses to become a hole through the wall of a structure
proton pump inhibitor (PPI)	**PRO**-ton PUMP in-**HIB**-ih-tor	R/ R/ S/ R/	**proton** *first* **pump** *pump* **-or** *a doer* **inhibit-** *repress*	Agent that blocks production of gastric acid
resection resect (verb)	ree-**SEK**-shun	S/ P/ R/	**-ion** *action, condition* **re-** *back* **-sect-** *cut off*	Removal of a specific part of an organ or structure
vagus	**VAY**-gus		Latin *wandering*	Tenth (X) cranial nerve; supplies many different organs throughout the body

Exercises

A. Deconstruct the following medical terms into basic elements. *The definitions of the elements will help you understand the meaning of the term. Not every type of element will appear in every term. Fill in the chart.* **LO 5.3, 5.11, 5.12**

Medical Term	Meaning of Prefix	Meaning of Root/Combining Form	Meaning of Suffix	Definition of Medical Term
perforation	1.	2.	3.	4.
peptic	5.	6.	7.	8.
gastroesophageal	9.	10.	11.	12.
anorexia	13.	14.	15.	16.
dyspepsia	17.	18.	19.	20.
antacid	21.	22.	23.	24.
gastritis	25.	26.	27.	28.
gastroscope	29.	30.	31.	32.

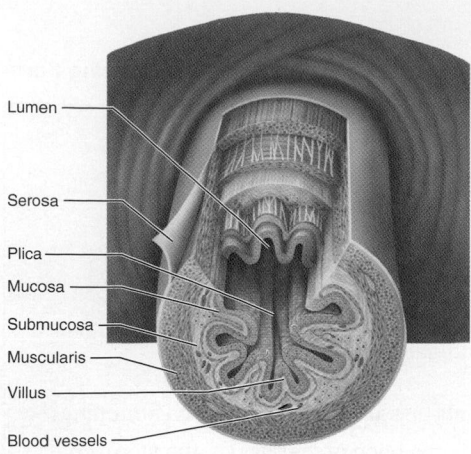

▲ Figure 5.19 **Tissue Layers of Digestive Tract.** An example of the most typical histologic structure of the tract.

Lumen
Serosa
Plica
Mucosa
Submucosa
Muscularis
Villus
Blood vessels

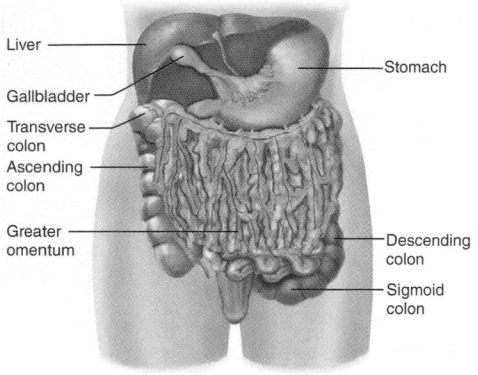

▲ Figure 5.20 **Greater Omentum.**

Liver
Gallbladder
Transverse colon
Ascending colon
Greater omentum
Stomach
Descending colon
Sigmoid colon

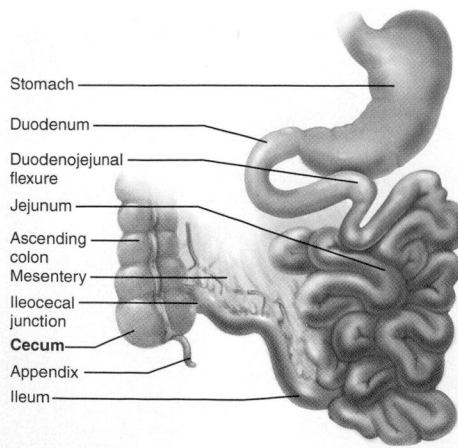

▲ Figure 5.21 **Small Intestine.**

Stomach
Duodenum
Duodenojejunal flexure
Jejunum
Ascending colon
Mesentery
Ileocecal junction
Cecum
Appendix
Ileum

LO 5.10 Small Intestine

The small intestine, called "small" because of its diameter, finishes the process of chemical digestion and is responsible for the absorption of most of the nutrients.

Four major layers are present in the wall of the small intestine and in all areas of the digestive tract (*Figure 5.19*):

1. **Mucosa**, or mucous membrane—the layer containing the epithelial cells that line the tract, intestinal glands that secrete the digestive enzymes, and supportive connective tissue. Fingerlike shapes of mucosa called **villi** project into the lumen of the intestine.

2. **Submucosa**—a thick connective tissue layer containing blood vessels, lymphatic vessels, and nerves.

3. **Muscularis**—an inner, circular layer of **smooth muscle** and an outer longitudinal layer of smooth muscle. When the inner circular layer contracts, it decreases the diameter of the tract. When the outer longitudinal layer contracts, it shortens the tract. These two movements create peristalsis and segmental contractions.

4. **Serosa**—an outermost layer of thin connective tissue and a single layer of epithelial cells.

Most of the digestive organs lie within the abdominal cavity (*see Chapter 4*), which is lined by a moist serous membrane called the **peritoneum**. **Parietal** peritoneum lines the wall of the abdominal cavity. **Visceral** peritoneum (a serosa) covers the external surface of the digestive organs.

The intestines are suspended from the back wall of the abdominal cavity by a **translucent** membrane called the **mesentery**, a continuation of the peritoneum. A fatty portion of the mesentery, called the **greater omentum** (*Figure 5.20*), hangs like an apron in front of all the intestines.

The small intestine (*Figure 5.21*) occupies much of the abdominal cavity, extends from the pylorus of the stomach to the beginning of the large intestine, and has three segments:

1. The **duodenum** is the first 9 to 10 inches of the small intestine. It receives chyme from the stomach, together with pancreatic juices and bile. Here, stomach acid is neutralized, fats are broken up by the bile acids, and pancreatic enzymes take over chemical digestion.

2. The **jejunum** makes up about 40% of the small intestine's length. It is the primary region for chemical digestion and nutrient absorption.

3. The **ileum** makes up about 55% of the small intestine's length. It ends at the **ileocecal** valve, a sphincter that controls entry into the large intestine.

From the duodenum to the middle of the ileum, the lining of the small intestine is folded into circular folds called **plicae**. Along their surface, the plicae have tiny fingerlike villi. The plicae and villi increase the surface area over which secretions can act on the food and through which nutrients can be absorbed. The folds also act as "speed bumps" to slow down the movement of chyme through the small intestine. The cells at the tip of the villi are shed and renewed every 3 or 4 days.

Digestion in the Small Intestine

After leaving the stomach as chyme, the food spends 3 to 5 hours in the small intestine, from which most of the nutrients are absorbed.

Secretion from the small intestine cells is mostly water, mucus, and enzymes. Peristaltic movements of the small intestine have three functions:

1. To mix chyme with intestinal and pancreatic juices and with bile.

2. To churn chyme to make contact with the mucosa for digestion and absorption.

3. To move the residue toward the large intestine.

Anywhere from 4 to 6 hours after consuming that chicken and vegetable dinner mentioned earlier, your food has passed through the small intestine and is ready to be moved into the large intestine. Most of the protein, carbohydrate, and fat of your meal has been broken down by enzymes into basic nutrients and absorbed into your bloodstream.

WORD	PRONUNCIATION	ELEMENTS		DEFINITION
cecum	SEE-kum		Latin *blind*	Blind pouch that is the first part of the large intestine
ileum	ILL-ee-um		Latin *to roll up*	Third portion of the small intestine
ileocecal	ILL-ee-oh-**SEE**-cal	S/ R/CF R/	-al *pertaining to* ile/o- *ileum* -cec- *cecum*	Pertaining to the junction of the ileum and cecum
jejunum	je-**JEW**-num		Latin *empty*	Segment of small intestine between the duodenum and the ileum where most of the nutrients are absorbed
jejunal (adj)	je-**JEW**-nal			
mesentery	**MESS**-en-ter-ree	P/ R/	mes- *middle* -entery *intestine*	A double layer of peritoneum enclosing the abdominal viscera
mesenteric (adj)	**MESS**-en-ter-ik	S/	-ic *pertaining to*	Pertaining to the mesentery
mucosa (another name for **mucous membrane**)	myu-**KOH**-sah		Latin *mucus*	Lining of a tubular structure
mucosal (adj)	myu-**KOH**-sal			Pertaining to the mucosa
muscularis	muss-kyu-**LAR**-is	S/ R/	-aris *pertaining to* muscul- *muscle*	The muscular layer of a hollow organ or tube
omentum	oh-**MEN**-tum		Latin *membrane that drapes over the intestines*	Membrane that drapes over the intestines
omental (adj)	oh-**MEN**-tal			Pertaining to the omentum
pancreas	**PAN**-kree-as		Greek *sweetbread*	Lobulated gland, the head of which is tucked into the curve of the duodenum
peritoneum	per-ih-toe-**NEE**-um		Latin *to stretch over*	Membrane that lines the abdominal cavity
peritoneal (adj)	per-ih-toe-**NEE**-al			Pertaining to the peritoneum
plica	**PLEE**-cah		Latin *fold*	Fold in a mucous membrane
plicae (pl)	**PLEE**-key			
serosa	seh-**ROH**-sa		Latin *serous, watery*	Outermost covering of the alimentary tract
serosal (adj)	seh-**ROH**-sal			Pertaining to serosa
submucosa	sub-mew-**KOH**-sa	P/ R/	sub- *under* -mucosa *lining of a cavity*	Tissue layer underneath the mucosa
villus	**VILL**-us		Latin *shaggy hair*	Thin, hairlike projection, particularly of a mucous membrane lining a cavity
villi (pl)	**VILL**-eye			
viscus (**Note: Viscous** is pronounced the same but means something *sticky*.)	**VISS**-kus		Latin *internal organ*	Hollow, walled, internal organ
viscera (pl)	**VISS**-er-ah		Latin *soft internal organs*	Internal organs, particularly in the abdomen
visceral (adj)	**VISS**-er-al			Pertaining to the internal organs

Exercises

A. Greek and Latin terms do not deconstruct into basic elements, so you must know them for what they are. *Build your knowledge of these terms by matching the phrase in the left column to the correct medical term in the right column.*   **LO 5.3, 5.10**

_____ 1. To roll up

_____ 2. Membrane that drapes over the intestines

_____ 3. Watery

_____ 4. Shaggy hair

_____ 5. Internal organ

_____ 6. Fold

_____ 7. Empty

_____ 8. To stretch over

_____ 9. Lining of a tubular structure

_____ 10. Blind pouch

a. viscus

b. peritoneum

c. mucosa

d. plica

e. cecum

f. omentum

g. ileum

h. serosa

i. villus

j. jejunum

LO 5.11 Disorders of the Small Intestine

The absorption of nutrients occurs primarily through the small intestine. **Impairment of absorption**, including Crohn disease and lactose intolerance, is covered in *Lesson 5.5* of this chapter.

Infections of the small intestine are common and are caused by a variety of agents:

- **Gastroenteritis**, or inflammation of the stomach and small intestine, can result in acute vomiting and diarrhea. It can be caused by a variety of viruses and bacteria (including, occasionally, the parasite *Giardia lamblia*) and is initiated by contact with contaminated food (food poisoning) and water.

- **Bleeding** from the small intestine is usually caused by a duodenal ulcer.

- **Celiac disease** is an allergy to gluten, which is a protein contained in wheat, rye, barley, and other grains. Celiac disease *(Figure 5.22)* damages the lining of the small intestine and can cause abdominal swelling, gas, pain, weight loss, fatigue, and weakness. Treatment is a strict gluten-free diet.

- The symptoms of **irritable bowel syndrome (IBS)** are chronic abdominal pain, bloating, and either diarrhea or constipation or an alternating pattern of the two. X-rays, scans, and endoscopies of patients with IBS show no abnormality. Treatment is difficult and often unsuccessful.

- An **intussusception** *(Figure 5.23)* occurs when a part of the small intestine slides into a neighboring portion of the small intestine—much like the way that parts of a collapsible telescope slide into each other. Eighty percent of intussusceptions can be cured with an enema; the remaining 20% require surgical intervention.

- **Ileus** is a disruption of the normal peristaltic ability of the small intestine. It can be caused by a bowel obstruction or by intestinal paralysis. Risk factors for **paralytic ileus** include GI surgery, diabetic ketoacidosis *(see Chapter 17)*, peritonitis, and medications, such as opiates.

- **Cancer** of the small intestine occurs infrequently compared with tumors in other parts of the GI tract. An **adenocarcinoma** is the most common malignant tumor of the small bowel.

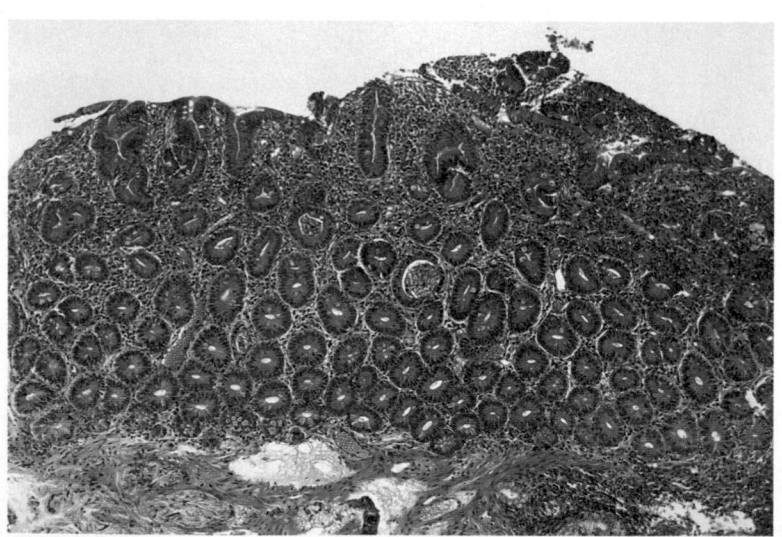

▲ **Figure 5.22** Photomicrograph of Celiac Disease Showing Atrophy of Duodenal Villi.

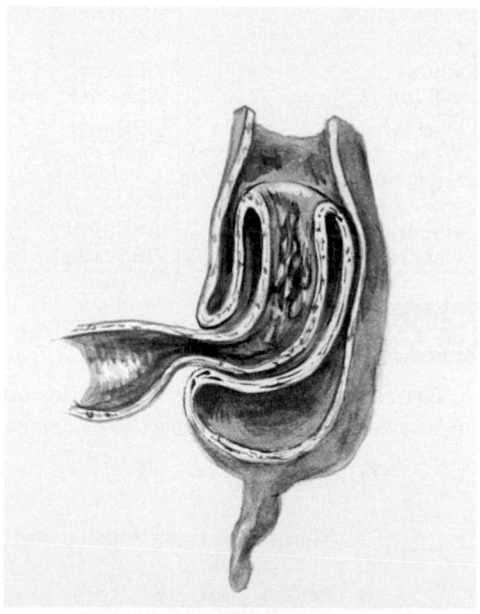

▲ **Figure 5.23** Intussusception.

WORD	PRONUNCIATION		ELEMENTS	DEFINITION
celiac	SEE-lee-ack	S/	Greek belly	Relating to the abdominal cavity
		R/	-ac pertaining to	
			celi- abdomen	
celiac disease	SEE-lee-ack diz-EEZ	P/	dis- apart	Disease caused by a sensitivity to gluten
		R/	-ease normal function	
gastroenteritis	GAS-troh-en-ter-I-tis	S/	-itis inflammation	Inflammation of the stomach and intestines
		R/CF	gastr/o- stomach	
		R/	-enter- intestine	
Giardia	jee-AR-dee-ah	S/	Alfred Giard, 1846–1908	Parasite that can affect the small intestine
		R/CF	French biologist	
ileus	ILL-ee-us		Greek intestinal colic	Dynamic or mechanical obstruction of the small intestine
intussusception	IN-tuss-sus-SEP-shun	S/	-ion action	The slippage of one part of the bowel inside another, causing obstruction
		P/	intus- within	
		R/	-suscept- to take up	

Exercises

A. Match the disorder of the small intestine in column one with the statement describing it in column two.   LO 5.11

_____ 1. ileus

_____ 2. IBS

_____ 3. celiac disease

_____ 4. *Giardia lamblia*

_____ 5. intussusception

a. Parasite that causes gastroenteritis

b. Part of the small intestine slides into a neighboring part

c. Disruption of the normal peristalsis of the small intestine

d. Treatment is difficult and often unsuccessful

e. Allergy to gluten

B. Use your knowledge of the small intestine and answer the questions. *Rewrite the one incorrect statement on the lines below.*   **LO 5.10, 5.11**

1. The absorption of nutrients occurs primarily through the small intestine.	T	F
2. Gastroenteritis can result in acute vomiting and diarrhea.	T	F
3. Bleeding from the small intestine is usually from an infection.	T	F
4. Chronic abdominal pain, bloating, and either diarrhea or constipation can be signs of IBS.	T	F
5. Risk factors for paralytic ileus include GI surgery, diabetic ketoacidosis, and medicines such as opiates.	T	F

6. Corrected statement:

_____

_____

Lesson 5.5 Absorption and Malabsorption

In the previous lessons in this chapter, you have learned the digestive secretions of the different segments of the digestive tract, liver, and pancreas. This information can now be brought together to review the overall process of digestion so that you will be able to:

5.5.1 Describe chemical digestion, absorption, and malabsorption.

5.5.2 Describe disorders of chemical digestion and absorption.

Keynotes

- Proteins are broken down into amino acids.

- Minerals are electrolytes.

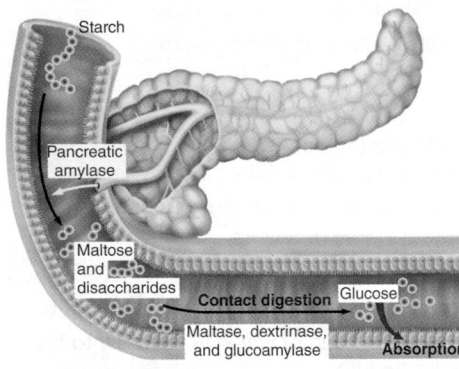

▲ **Figure 5.30** Starch Digestion in the Small Intestine.

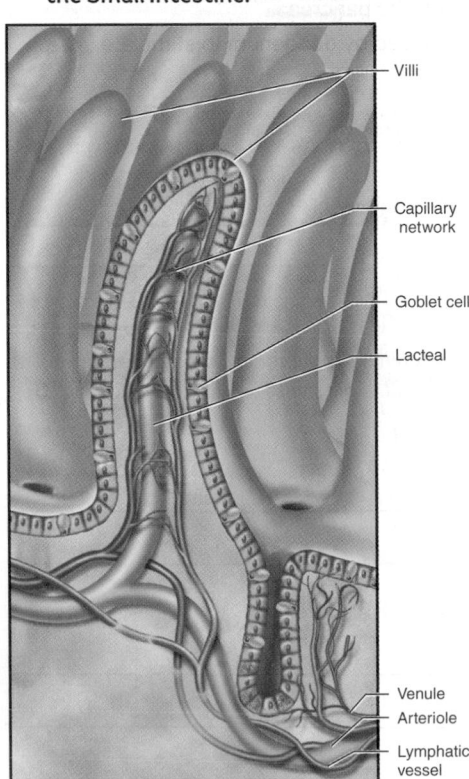

▲ **Figure 5.31** Intestinal Villi.

LO 5.16 Chemical Digestion, Absorption, and Transport

When the remains of the chicken and vegetable arrive in your duodenum, they have been reduced to very small particles by mastication and gastric peristalsis, and they have been mixed with other food to form boluses. Thus far, 10% of their carbohydrates has been partially digested by salivary amylase, operating mostly in the mouth; 10% to 15% of their protein has been partially digested by **proteases** in the stomach; and 10% of their fats has been digested by the salivary lipase operating in the stomach.

Carbohydrates are ingested in three forms:

1. **Polysaccharides**, such as starches.

2. **Disaccharides**, such as sucrose (table sugar) and lactose (milk sugar).

3. **Monosaccharides**, such as glucose (the basic sugar), fructose (found in fruits), and galactose (found in milk).

In the small intestine, polysaccharides are broken down by pancreatic amylase into disaccharides (*Figure 5.30*). Disaccharides are broken down to monosaccharides by maltase and dextrinase, enzymes secreted by the cells lining the villi of the small intestine.

The monosaccharides are taken up by the lining cells and transferred to the capillaries of the villi. They are then carried by the portal vein to the liver, where the nonglucose sugars are converted to glucose.

Proteins arrive in the duodenum and small intestine only 10% to 20% digested by gastric pepsin. Enzymes attached to the villi of the small intestine, together with the pancreatic enzyme trypsin, break down the remaining proteins to **amino acids**.

The amino acids are taken in by the epithelial cells of the small intestine, released into the capillaries of the villi, and carried away in the hepatic portal circulation. They are transported into cells all over the body, to be used as building blocks for new tissue formation.

Lipids (including fats) enter the duodenum and small intestine as large globules that have to be emulsified by bile salts into smaller droplets so that pancreatic lipase can digest the fats into very small droplets of free fatty acids and monoglycerides. There is enough pancreatic lipase in the duodenum to digest average amounts of fat within 1 or 2 minutes.

The very small droplets are absorbed by the intestinal cells and then taken into the lymphatic system by the **lacteals** inside the villi. The white, fatty lymphatic **chyle** eventually reaches the thoracic duct and is transferred into the left subclavian vein of the bloodstream. The chyle is carried by the blood and stored in adipose tissue.

The fat-soluble vitamins (A, D, E, and K) are absorbed with the lipids.

Water that is ingested is 92% absorbed by the small intestine and taken into the bloodstream through the capillaries in the villi (*Figure 5.31*). Water-soluble vitamins (C and the B-complex) are absorbed with water with the exception of vitamin B_{12}. This is a large molecule that has to bind with intrinsic factor from the stomach so that cells in the distant ileum can receive it and pass it through to the bloodstream.

Minerals are absorbed along the whole length of the small intestine. Iron and calcium are absorbed according to the body's needs. The other minerals are absorbed regardless of need, and the kidneys excrete the surplus.

By the time your chicken and vegetable dinner mentioned earlier has reached the end of your small intestine, its carbohydrates have been broken down to monosaccharides and absorbed into the bloodstream through the capillaries in the villi of your small intestine. Its proteins have been broken down into amino acids and also absorbed into the bloodstream via capillaries in the intestinal villi. Its fats have been digested into small droplets of free fatty acids and monoglycerides and taken into the lymphatic system by lacteals inside the intestinal villi.

WORD	PRONUNCIATION	ELEMENTS		DEFINITION
amino acid	ah-**ME**-no **ASS**-id	R/CF	amin/o *nitrogen compound*	The basic building block of protein
carbohydrate	kar-boh-**HIGH**-drate	S/ R/CF R/	-ate *composed of* carb/o- *carbon* -hydr- *water*	Group of organic food compounds that includes sugars, starch, glycogen, and cellulose
chyle (contrast **chyme**, p. 122)	KYLE		Greek *juice*	A milky fluid that results from the digestion and absorption of fats in the small intestine
lacteal	**LAK**-tee-al	S/ R/CF	-al *pertaining to* lact/e- *milk*	A lymphatic vessel carrying chyle away from the intestine
lipid	**LIP**-id		Greek *fat*	General term for all types of fatty compounds; for example, cholesterol, triglycerides, and fatty acids
mineral	**MIN**-er-al	S/ R/	-al *pertaining to* miner- *mines*	Inorganic compound usually found in earth's crust
protein	**PRO**-teen		Greek *first, primary*	Class of food substances based on amino acids

Exercises

A. Apply your medical vocabulary to answer the following questions about digestion. *Circle the best choice.*   **LO 5.3, 5.16**

1. The suffix that is used to form the names of enzymes is

   a. -ic

   b. -al

   c. -ase

   d. -ous

   e. -ion

2. Which of the following terms means *a milky fluid resulting from the digestion and absorption of fats in the small intestine?*

   a. lipid

   b. chyme

   c. protease

   d. chyle

   e. lacteal

3. The group of organic food compounds that includes sugars, starch, glycogen, and cellulose is

   a. proteins

   b. fats

   c. lipids

   d. carbohydrates

   e. calories

4. The root **hydr-** means

   a. blood

   b. juice

   c. water

   d. milk

   e. bile

B. Apply your medical vocabulary to answer the following questions about digestion. *Circle the best choice.*   **LO 5.3, 5.16**

1. The general term for all fatty compounds is

   a. bile

   b. protein

   c. carbohydrate

   d. lipid

   e. protease

2. What is another name for a mineral?

   a. enzyme

   b. electrolyte

   c. lipid

   d. hormone

   e. fatty acid

Mrs. Jan Stark, who presented in the Emergency Department with dehydration, was found to have **celiac disease**, a sensitivity to the protein **gluten** that is found in wheat, rye, barley, and oats. This disease involves the destruction of epithelial cells of the digestive tract lining, so intestinal enzymes are not being produced and absorption is not taking place.

Her difficulties with fine motor movement were the result of a **neuropathy** caused by vitamin B_{12} deficiency because of the lack of intrinsic factor to enable B_{12} to be absorbed. The diagnosis was made by an intestinal biopsy through oral endoscopy. A diet free of such gluten-containing foods as breads, cereals, cookies, and beer relieved her symptoms.

Keynotes

- In malnutrition, the body breaks down its own tissues to meet its nutritional and metabolic needs.

- Milk sugar is lactose. The enzyme lactase breaks down lactose to glucose.

- Diarrhea is caused by irritation of the intestinal lining so that feces pass through the intestine too quickly for adequate amounts of water to be reabsorbed.

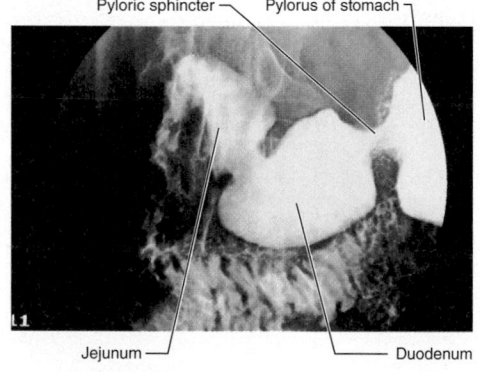

Pyloric sphincter — Pylorus of stomach

Jejunum — Duodenum

▲ **Figure 5.32** **Barium Meal.** Barium meal showing pylorus and duodenum.

LO 5.17 Disorders of Absorption

Malabsorption syndromes refer to a group of diseases in which intestinal absorption of nutrients is impaired.

Malnutrition can arise from malabsorption or from insufficient food intake as a result of famine, poverty, loss of appetite due to cancer, or terminal illness. Many of the poor and elderly in this country suffer from malnutrition. When the body experiences prolonged deprivation of calories and nutrients, it breaks down its own tissues to meet these needs.

Lactose intolerance occurs when the small intestine is not producing sufficient **lactase** to break down the milk sugar lactose. The result is **diarrhea** and cramps. Lactase can be taken in pill form before eating dairy products, and/or lactose can be avoided by using soy products rather than milk products.

Crohn disease (or **regional enteritis**) is an inflammation of the small intestine (frequently in the ileum) and occasionally also in the large intestine. The symptoms are abdominal pain, diarrhea, fatigue, and weight loss. Malabsorption is common, and children with Crohn disease may have delayed development and stunted growth.

Constipation occurs when fecal movement through the large intestine is slow, causing too much water to be reabsorbed by the large intestine. The feces become hardened. Factors causing constipation are lack of dietary fiber, lack of exercise, and emotional upset.

Gastroenteritis (stomach "flu") is an infection of the stomach and intestine that can be caused by a large variety of bacteria and viruses. It causes vomiting, diarrhea, and fever. An outbreak of gastroenteritis can sometimes be traced to contaminated food or water. The Norwalk virus and rotaviruses are major causes of diarrhea in infants and children.

Dysentery is a severe form of bacterial gastroenteritis with blood and mucus in frequent, watery stools. It can lead to dehydration.

Diagnostic Procedures for the Upper Digestive Tract

- **Barium swallow.** The patient ingests barium sulfate, a contrast material, to show details of the pharynx and esophagus on x-ray.

- **Barium meal.** This procedure uses barium sulfate to study the distal esophagus, stomach, and duodenum on x-ray *[Figure 5.32]*.

- **Enteroscopy.** An oral endoscope is used to visualize and biopsy tumors and ulcers and to control bleeding from the esophagus, stomach, and duodenum. This procedure is also called **esophagogastroduodenoscopy.**

- **Angiography.** This procedure uses dye to highlight blood vessels. It can be used to define the site of bleeding in the intestinal tract.

WORD	PRONUNCIATION		ELEMENTS	DEFINITION
celiac celiac disease	SEE-lee-ack SEE-lee-ack diz-EEZ	S/ R/ P/ R/	Greek *belly* -ac *pertaining to* celi- *abdomen* dis- *apart* -ease *normal function*	Relating to the abdominal cavity Disease caused by sensitivity to gluten
constipation	kon-stih-PAY-shun	S/ R/	-ation *process* constip- *press together*	Hard, infrequent bowel movements
Crohn disease (also called **regional enteritis**)	KRONE diz-EEZ RE-jun-al en-ter-I-tis		Burrill Crohn, New York gastroenterologist, 1884–1993	Inflammatory bowel disease with narrowing and thickening of the terminal small bowel
diarrhea	die-ah-REE-ah	P/ R/	dia- *complete, through* -rrhea *flow, discharge*	Abnormally frequent and loose stools
dysentery	DIS-en-tare-ee	P/ R/	dys- *bad, difficult* -entery *intestine*	Disease with diarrhea, bowel spasms, fever, and dehydration
enteroscope	EN-ter-oh-SKOPE	S/ R/CF S/	-scope *instrument for viewing* enter/o- *intestine* -scopy *to examine, to view*	Slender, tubular instrument with light source and camera to visualize the digestive tract
enteroscopy	en-ter-OSS-koh-pee			The examination of the lining of the digestive tract
gastroenteritis	GAS-troh-en-ter-I-tis	S/ R/CF R/	-itis *inflammation* gastr/o- *stomach* -enter- *intestine*	Inflammation of the stomach and intestines
gluten	GLU-ten		Latin *glue*	Insoluble protein found in wheat, barley, and oats
intolerance	in-TOL-er-ance		Latin *unable to cope with*	Inability of the small intestine to digest and dispose of a particular dietary constituent
lactose lactase	LAK-toes LAK-tase	 S/ R/	Latin *milk sugar* -ase *enzyme* lact- *milk*	The disaccharide found in cow's milk Enzyme that breaks down lactose to glucose and galactose
neuropathy	nyu-ROP-ah-thee	S/ R/CF	-pathy *disease* neur/o- *nerve*	Any disease of the nervous system

Exercises

A. Study the terms and elements in the above WAD. *Notice that some terms are formed with only a prefix and a root, while others are formed with a root and a suffix.* **The only element that needs to be present in every term is a root or combining form.** *The definitions for the terms are given, as well as the element placement in the term. Write the correct element on each blank that needs an element.* **LO 5.3, 5.17**

1. Abnormally frequent and loose stools   _____ / _____ / _____
   P   R   S

2. Any disease of the nervous system   _____ / _____ / _____
   P   R   S

3. Instrument for looking in the intestine   _____ / _____ / _____
   P   R   S

4. Infrequent bowel movements   _____ / _____ / _____
   P   R   S

5. Enzyme that breaks down lactose   _____ / _____ / _____
   P   R   S

6. Relating to the abdominal cavity   _____ / _____ / _____
   P   R   S

Lesson 5.6 Elimination and the Large Intestine

After the nutrients have been digested and absorbed in the small intestine, the residual materials have to be prepared in the large intestine for elimination from the body. The information in this lesson will enable you to:

5.6.1 **Describe the anatomy and physiology of the large intestine.**

5.6.2 **Relate the structure of the large intestine to its functions.**

5.6.3 **Discuss common disorders of the large intestine.**

Keynote

A sphincter is a ring of smooth muscle that forms a one-way valve.

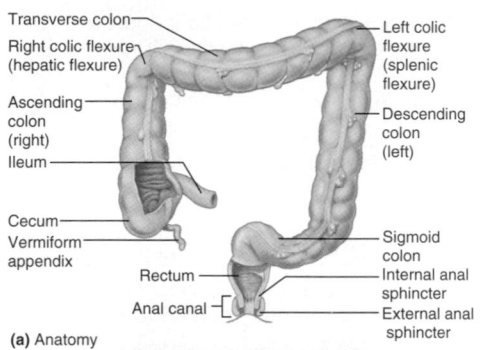

(a) Anatomy

Transverse colon
Right colic flexure (hepatic flexure)
Ascending colon (right)
Ileum
Cecum
Vermiform appendix
Rectum
Anal canal
Left colic flexure (splenic flexure)
Descending colon (left)
Sigmoid colon
Internal anal sphincter
External anal sphincter

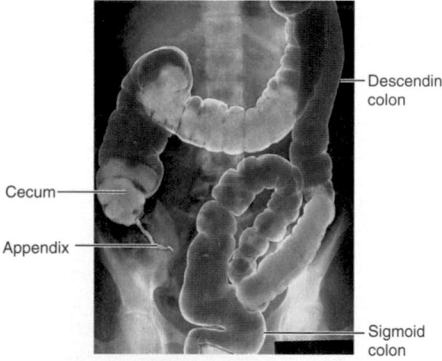

(b) X-ray of large intestine following a barium enema

Descending colon
Cecum
Appendix
Sigmoid colon

▲ **Figure 5.33** **Large Intestine.**
[a] Anatomy. [b] Radiograph of large intestine following barium enema.

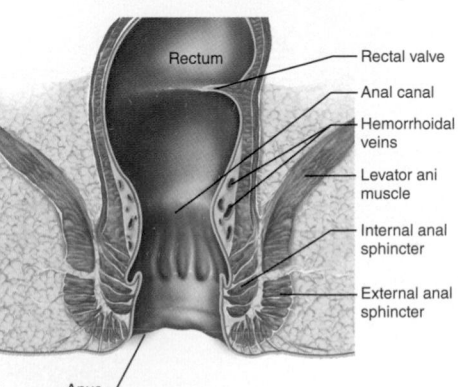

Rectum
Rectal valve
Anal canal
Hemorrhoidal veins
Levator ani muscle
Internal anal sphincter
External anal sphincter
Anus

▲ **Figure 5.34** **Anal Canal.**

LO 5.18 Structure and Functions of the Large Intestine

Structure of the Large Intestine

The **large intestine** is so named because its diameter is much greater than that of the small intestine. It forms a **perimeter** in the abdominal cavity around the central mass of the small intestine (*Figure 5.33a*).

At the junction between the small and large intestines, a ring of smooth muscle called the *ileocecal sphincter* forms a one-way valve. This allows chyme to pass into the large intestine and prevents the contents of the large intestine from backing up into the ileum.

At the beginning of the large intestine, the **cecum** is a pouch in the lower right quadrant of the abdomen (*Figure 5.33b*). A narrow tube with a closed end, the **vermiform appendix**, projects downward from the cecum. The function of the appendix is not known.

The **ascending colon** begins at the cecum, extends upward until, just underneath the liver, it makes a sharp left turn at the hepatic **flexure** and becomes the transverse colon. At the left side of the abdomen, near the spleen at the splenic flexure, the transverse colon turns downward to form the descending colon. At the pelvic brim, the **descending** colon makes an S-shaped curve, the **sigmoid** colon, which descends in the pelvis to become the **rectum** and then the **anal canal**.

The rectum has three transverse folds, rectal valves that enable it to retain feces while passing gas (**flatus**). Intestinal gas is 90% nitrogen and oxygen, ingested while breathing and eating, together with methane, hydrogen, sulfites, and carbon dioxide contributed from bacterial fermentation of undigested food. This yields pungent ammonia and foul-smelling hydrogen sulfide to give gas and feces their characteristic odor.

The anal canal is the last 1 to 2 inches of the large intestine, opening to the outside as the **anus**. The mucous membrane is folded into six to eight longitudinal **anal columns**. **Feces** pressing against the columns causes them to produce more mucus to lubricate the canal during **defecation**. Two sphincter muscles guard the anus (*Figure 5.34*): an internal sphincter, composed of smooth muscle from the intestinal wall, and an external sphincter, composed of skeletal muscle that you can control voluntarily.

Functions of the Large Intestine

- **Absorption** of water and electrolytes. The large intestine receives more than 1 L (1.05 quarts) of chyme each day from the small intestine and reabsorbs water and electrolytes to reduce the volume to 100 to 150 mL of feces to be eliminated by defecation.
- **Secretion** of mucus that protects the intestinal wall and holds particles of fecal matter together.
- **Digestion** by the bacteria that inhabit the large intestine of any food remnants that have escaped the digestive enzymes of the small intestine.
- **Peristalsis**, which, in the large intestine, happens only a few times a day to produce mass movements toward the rectum. Often when you ingest food into your stomach, your **gastrocolic reflex** will generate a mass movement of feces.
- **Elimination** of materials that were not digested or absorbed.

WORD	PRONUNCIATION		ELEMENTS	DEFINITION
anus anal (adj)	**A**-nuss **A**-nal		Latin *ring*	Terminal opening of the digestive tract through which feces are discharged
appendix appendectomy	ah-**PEN**-dicks ah-pen-**DEK**-toe-me	R/ S/	Latin *appendage* **append-** *appendix* **-ectomy** *surgical excision*	Small blind projection from the pouch of the cecum Surgical removal of the appendix
vermiform appendicitis	**VER**-mih-form ah-pen-dih-**SIGH**-tis	S/ S/	Latin *wormlike* **-ic-** *pertaining to* **-itis** *inflammation*	Worm shaped; used as a descriptor for the appendix Inflammation of the appendix
colon	**KOH**-lon		Greek *colon*	The large intestine, extending from the cecum to the rectum
colic	**KOL**-ik	S/ R/	**-ic** *pertaining to* **col-** *colon*	Spasmodic, crampy pains in the abdomen
colitis	koh-**LIE**-tis	S/	**-itis** *inflammation*	Inflammation of the colon
feces fecal (adj)	**FEE**-sees **FEE**-kal	S/ R/	Latin *dregs* **-al** *pertaining to* **-fec-** *feces*	Undigested, waste material discharged from the bowel Pertaining to feces
defecation	def-eh-**KAY**-shun	S/ P/	**-ation** *process* **de-** *from, out of*	Evacuation of feces from the rectum and anus
defecate (verb)	**DEF**-eh-kate	S/	**-ate** *process*	Process of defecation
flatus flatulence flatulent (adj)	**FLAY**-tus **FLAT**-you-lents **FLAT**-you-lent	S/ R/	Latin *blowing* **-ence** *forming* **flatul-** *excessive gas*	Gas or air expelled through the anus Excessive amount of gas in the stomach and intestines
flexure	**FLECK**-shur		Latin *bend*	A bend in a structure
gastrocolic reflex	gas-troh-**KOL**-ik **RE**-fleks	S/ R/CF R/ R/	**-ic** *pertaining to* **gastr/o-** *stomach* **-col-** *colon* **reflex** *bend back*	Mass movement of feces in the colon and the desire to defecate caused by taking food into stomach
ileocecal sphincter	**ILL**-ee-oh-**SEE**-cal **SFINK**-ter	S/ R/CF R/	**-al** *pertaining to* **ile/o-** *ileum* **-cec-** *cecum* **sphincter** Greek *band*	Band of muscle that encircles the junction of the ileum and cecum
perimeter	peh-**RIM**-eh-ter	P/ R/	**peri-** *around* **-meter** *measure*	An edge or border
rectum	**RECK**-tum		Latin *straight*	Terminal part of the colon from the sigmoid to the anal canal
rectal (adj)	**RECK**-tal	S/ R/	**-al** *pertaining to* **rect-** *rectum*	Pertaining to the rectum
sigmoid	**SIG**-moyd	S/ R/	**-oid** *resembling* **sigm-** Greek *letter "S"*	Sigmoid colon is shaped like an "S"

Exercises

A. Attack a medical term with your analytical skills. *Break these terms down into their elements to define the word. Fill in the chart. Deconstruct the medical terms in the first column with a slash so you know what elements you are dealing with. Write the meaning of each element in the appropriate column, then define the term in the last column.* **LO 5.3, 5.18, 5.19**

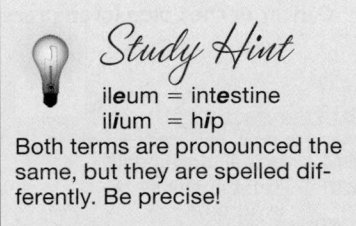

Study Hint

il**e**um = int**e**stine
il**i**um = h**i**p
Both terms are pronounced the same, but they are spelled differently. Be precise!

Medical Term	Meaning of Prefix	Meaning of Root/ Combining Form	Meaning of Suffix	Definition
colitis	1.	2.	3.	4.
defecation	5.	6.	7.	8.
colic	9.	10.	11.	12.
ileocecal	13.	14.	15.	16.

LO 5.19 Disorders of the Large Intestine and Anal Canal

Disorders of the Large Intestine

Appendicitis is the most common cause of acute abdominal pain in the right lower quadrant. On palpation, tenderness over the **McBurney point**, one-third the distance from the anterior superior iliac crest to the umbilicus *(see Chapter 4)*, suggests appendicitis. If neglected, the inflamed appendix can rupture, leading to **peritonitis**. This is strongly suggested by the presence of **rebound tenderness**, in which a stab of severe pain is produced when the abdominal wall, which has been pressed in slowly, is released rapidly. A surgical appendectomy, usually performed through laparoscopy, is the treatment for appendicitis.

Diverticulosis is the presence of small pouches (**diverticula**) bulging outward through weak spots in the lining of the large intestine *(Figure 5.35)*. They are asymptomatic until the pouches become infected and inflamed, a condition called **diverticulitis**. This condition causes abdominal pain, vomiting, constipation, and fever. Complications, such as perforation and abscess formation, can occur. The most likely cause of diverticular disease (diverticulosis and diverticulitis) is a low-fiber diet.

Ulcerative colitis is an extensive inflammation and ulceration of the lining of the large intestine. It produces bouts of bloody diarrhea, crampy pain, and often weight loss and electrolyte imbalance.

Irritable bowel syndrome (IBS) is an increasingly common large-bowel disorder, presenting with crampy pains, gas, and changes in bowel habits to either constipation or diarrhea. There are no anatomic changes seen in the bowel, and the cause is unknown.

Polyps are masses of tissue arising from the wall of the large intestine that protrude into the bowel **lumen**. They vary in size and shape. Most are benign. Endoscopic biopsy can determine if they are **precancerous** or cancerous.

Colon and **rectal cancers** *(Figure 5.36)* are the second leading cause of cancer deaths after lung cancer. The majority occur in the rectum and sigmoid colon. These cancers spread by

1. Direct extension through the bowel wall.
2. **Metastasis** to regional lymph nodes.
3. Moving down the lumen of the bowel.
4. Bloodborne **metastases** to liver, lung, bone, and brain.

Obstruction of the large bowel can be caused by cancers, large polyps, or diverticulitis.

Intussusception is a form of obstruction whereby a tumor in the lumen of the bowel, together with its segment of bowel, is telescoped into the immediately distal segment of bowel.

Proctitis is inflammation of the lining of the rectum, often associated with ulcerative colitis, Crohn disease, or radiation therapy. Symptoms are **anorectal** pain, rectal bleeding, and excess mucus in the **stool**.

Disorders of the Anal Canal

Hemorrhoids are dilated veins in the submucosa of the anal canal, often associated with pregnancy, chronic **constipation**, diarrhea, or aging. They protrude into the anal canal (internal hemorrhoid) or bulge out along the edge of the anus (external hemorrhoid) producing pain and bright red blood from the anus. A **thrombosed** hemorrhoid, in which blood has clotted, is very painful.

Anal fissures are tears in the lining of the anal canal, such as may occur with difficult bowel movements (**BMs**).

Anal fistulas occur following abscesses in the anal glands. The anal canal has six or seven glands in the posterior canal that secrete mucus to lubricate the canal. If the glands become infected, abscesses form that, when they heal, can form a passage (fistula) between the anal canal and the skin outside the anus.

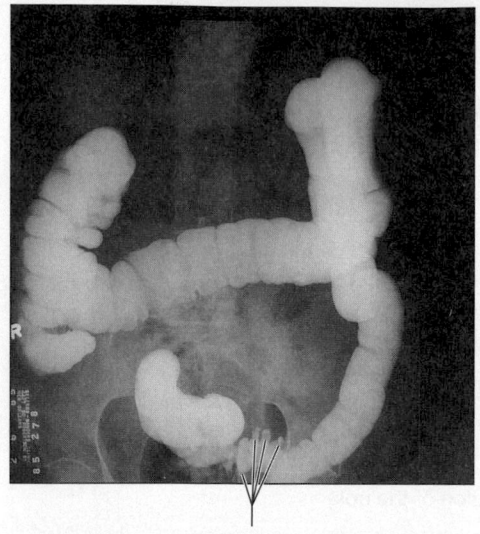

Diverticula

▲ **Figure 5.35**   Barium Enema Showing Diverticulosis.

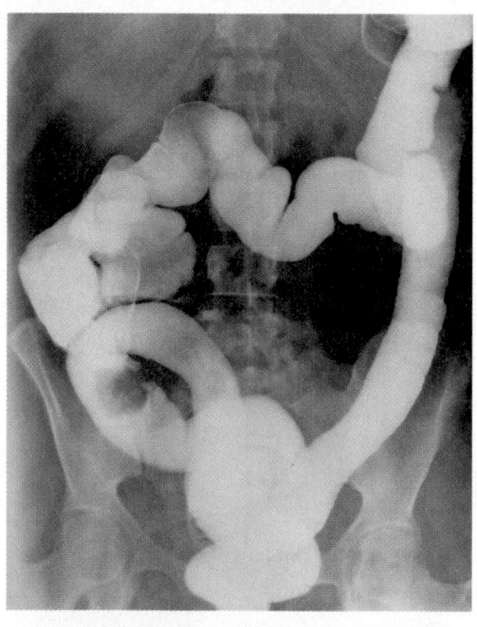

▲ **Figure 5.36**   Barium Enema Showing Cancer of the Colon (orange area).

Abbreviations	
BM	bowel movement
IBS	irritable bowel syndrome

Word Analysis and Definition

S = Suffix   P = Prefix   **R** = Root   **R/CF** = Combining Form

WORD	PRONUNCIATION	ELEMENTS		DEFINITION
bowel	**BOUGH**-el		Latin *sausage*	Another name for intestine
diverticulum	die-ver-**TICK**-you-lum	S/	-um *tissue*	A pouchlike opening or sac from a tubular
diverticula (pl)	die-ver-**TICK**-you-lah	R/	**diverticul-** *byroad*	structure (e.g., gut)
diverticulosis	**DIE**-ver-tick-you-**LOW**-sis	S/	-osis *condition*	Presence of a number of small pouches in the wall of the large intestine
diverticulitis	**DIE**-ver-tick-you-**LIE**-tis	S/	-itis *inflammation*	Inflammation of the diverticula
fissure	**FISH**-ur		Latin *slit*	Deep furrow or cleft
fistula	**FIS**-tyu-lah		Latin *pipe, tube*	Abnormal passage
hemorrhoid	**HEM**-oh-royd	S/	-rrhoid *flow*	Dilated rectal vein producing painful anal swelling
hemorrhoids (pl)		R/CF	**hem/o-** *blood*	
hemorrhoidectomy	**HEM**-oh-roy-**DEK**-toh-me	S/	-ectomy *excision*	Surgical removal of hemorrhoids
intussusception	**IN**-tuss-sus-**SEP**-shun	S/	-ion *action*	The slipping of one part of bowel inside another to cause obstruction
		P/	**intus-** *within*	
		R/	**-suscept-** *to take up*	
lumen	**LOO**-men		Latin *light, window*	The interior space of a tubelike structure
McBurney point	mack-**BUR**-nee POYNT		Charles McBurney, New York surgeon, 1845–1913	One-third the distance from the anterior superior iliac spine to the umbilicus
metastasis	meh-**TAS**-tah-sis	P/	**meta-** *beyond*	Spread of a disease from one part of the body to another
metastases (pl)	meh-**TAS**-tah-seez	R/	**-stasis** *placement*	
peritoneum	per-ih-toe-**NEE**-um	S/	-um *tissue*	Membrane that lines the abdominal cavity
		R/CF	**periton/e-** *stretch over*	
peritoneal (adj)	**PER**-ih-toe-**NEE**-al	S/	-al *pertaining to*	Pertaining to the peritoneum
peritonitis	**PER**-ih-toe-**NIE**-tis	S/	-itis *inflammation*	Inflammation of the peritoneum
polyp	**POL**-ip		Latin *foot, stalk*	Mass of tissue that projects into the lumen of the bowel
		R/	**polyp-** *polyp*	
polyposis	pol-ih-**POH**-sis	S/	-osis *condition*	Presence of several polyps
polypectomy	pol-ip-**ECK**-toh-mee	S/	-ectomy *excision*	Excision or removal of a polyp
precancerous	pree-**KAN**-sir-us	S/	-ous *pertaining to*	Lesion from which a cancer can develop
		P/	**pre-** *before*	
		R/	**-cancer-** *cancer*	
proctitis	prok-**TIE**-tis	S/	-itis *inflammation*	Inflammation of the lining of the rectum
		R/	**proct-** *anus and rectum*	
ulcerative	**UL**-sir-ah-tiv	S/	-ative *quality of*	Marked by an ulcer or ulcers
		R/	**ulcer-** *a sore*	

Exercises

A. This exercise focuses on the suffixes in the above WAD. *The suffix is your first clue to the meaning of a medical term. Challenge your knowledge of suffixes by filling in the blanks. Some answers you will use twice because more than one suffix can have the same meaning. One answer will not be used at all.*
LO 5.3, 5.19

_____ 1. -um

_____ 2. -ous

_____ 3. -osis

_____ 4. -ion

_____ 5. -itis

_____ 6. -rrhoid

_____ 7. -ative

_____ 8. -al

_____ 9. -ectomy

a. flow

b. action

c. inflammation

d. tissue

e. pertaining to

f. condition

g. excision

h. quality of

i. study of

Keynote

Risk factors that can cause GI bleeding include alcohol, smoking, and a low-fiber diet.

LO 5.20 Gastrointestinal Bleeding

Bleeding can occur anywhere in the gastrointestinal (GI) tract from a variety of causes, as described in the preceding sections. The bleeding can be internal and painless. It can present in different ways to provide a clue to the site of bleeding:

- **Hematemesis**—the vomiting of bright red blood, which indicates an upper GI source of ongoing bleeding (esophagus, stomach, duodenum).
- **Vomiting of "coffee grounds"**—occurs when bleeding from an upper GI source has slowed or stopped; red hemoglobin has been converted to brown hematin by gastric acids.
- **Hematochezia**—the passage of bright red bloody stools, which usually indicates lower GI bowel bleeding from the sigmoid colon, rectum, or anus.
- **Melena**—the passage of black tarry stools, which usually indicates upper GI bleeding. The blood is digested and hemoglobin is oxidized as it passes through the intestine to produce the black color. Melena can continue for several days after a severe hemorrhage.
- **Occult blood**—no bleeding seen in the stool, but a chemical fecal occult blood test (**Hemoccult test**) is positive. The chronic source of the bleeding can be anywhere in the GI tract.

Consuming black licorice, Pepto-Bismol, or blueberries can produce black stools.

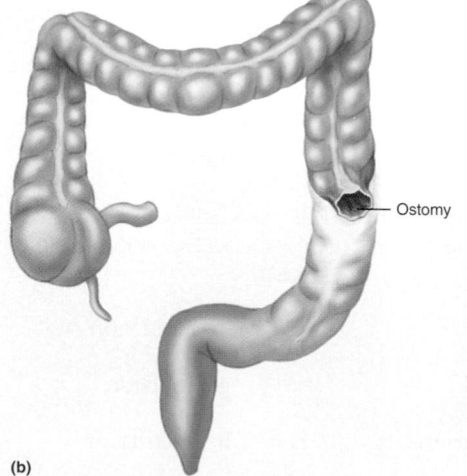

(a)

(b)

Sutures to make anastomosis

Ostomy

▲ **Figure 5.37**   **Intestinal Resections.** (*a*) Anastomosis. (*b*) Ostomy.

LO 5.20 Common Gastrointestinal Diagnostic and Therapeutic Procedures

- **Fecal occult blood test** (Hemoccult) is used to detect the presence of blood not visible to the naked eye.
- **Nasogastric aspiration and lavage**—the presence of bright red blood in the aspiration material indicates active upper GI bleeding; "coffee grounds" indicate the bleeding has slowed or stopped.
- **Upper GI barium x-rays** are less accurate than endoscopy at identifying the bleeding lesion.
- **Barium enema**—a radiographic contrast material is injected into the large intestine as an enema and x-ray films are taken (*see Figures 5.33b, 5.35, and 5.36*).
- **Endoscopy** enables direct visual examination of the intestine with a flexible tube containing light-transmitting glass fibers or a video transmitter that sends back an enlarged image. **Panendoscopy** examines the esophagus, stomach, and duodenum and provides the highest yield of information to establish the source of upper GI bleeding. Endoscopy can also be used to perform a biopsy, remove polyps (**polypectomy**), and **coagulate** bleeding lesions.
- **Anoscopy** examines the anus and lower rectum with a rigid instrument.
- **Flexible sigmoidoscopy** examines the rectum and sigmoid colon.
- **Flexible colonoscopy** examines the whole length of the colon.
- **Gastroscopy** examines the stomach.
- **Intestinal resections** are used to surgically remove diseased portions of the intestine. The remaining portions of the intestine can be joined together through an **anastomosis** (*Figure 5.37a*). If there is insufficient bowel remaining, an **ostomy** (*Figure 5.37b*) can be performed, where the end of the bowel opens onto the skin at a **stoma**. **Ileostomy** and **colostomy** are two common procedures.
- **Digital rectal exam**—the physician palpates the rectum and prostate gland with a gloved index finger.

Word Analysis and Definition

S = Suffix   P = Prefix   R = Root   R/CF = Combining Form

WORD	PRONUNCIATION	ELEMENTS		DEFINITION
anastomosis anastomoses (pl)	ah-**NAS**-to-**MO**-sis ah-**NAS**-to-**MO**-sez	S/ R/	-osis *condition* **anastom-** *join together*	A surgically made union between two tubular structures
coagulate	koh-**AG**-you-late	S/ R/	-ate *composed of,* *-pertaining to* **coagul-** *clotting*	Form a clot
endoscope	**EN**-doh-skope	P/	endo- *within, inside*	Instrument for examining the inside of a tubular or hollow organ
endoscopic (adj)	**EN**-doh-**SKOP**-ik	S/ S/	-ic *pertaining to* -scope *instrument for viewing*	Pertaining to the use of an endoscope

endoscopy
  anoscopy
  colonoscopy
	en-**DOS**-koh-pee
	A-nos-koh-pee
	koh-lon-**OSS**-koh-pee
		S/
		R/CF
		R/CF
			-scopy *to examine*
			an/o- *anus*
			colon/o- *colon*
				The use of an endoscope
				Endoscopic examination of the anus
				Examination of the inside of the colon by endoscopy

gastroscopy
  ileoscopy
  panendoscopy
    (*Note:* two prefixes)
 	
  proctoscopy
 	
  sigmoidoscopy
	gas-**TROS**-koh-pee
	ill-ee-**OS**-koh-pee
	pan-en-**DOS**-koh-pee
	
	prok-**TOSS**-koh-pee
	
	sig-moi-**DOS**-koh-pee
		R/CF
		R/CF
		P/
		P/
		S/
		R/CF
		
		R/CF
			gastr/o- *stomach*
			ile/o- *ileum*
			pan- *all*
			endo *within, inside*
			-scopy *to examine*
			proct/o- *anus and rectum*
			
			sigmoid/o- *sigmoid colon*
				Endoscopic examination of the stomach
				Endoscopic examination of the ileum
				Examination of the inside of the esophagus, stomach, and upper duodenum using a flexible fiberoptic endoscope
				Examination of the inside of the anus and the rectum by endoscopy
				Endoscopic examination of the sigmoid colon

enema	**EN**-eh-mah		Greek *injection*	An injection of fluid into the rectum
hematochezia	he-mat-oh-**KEY**-zee-ah	S/ R/CF	-chezia *pass a stool* **hemat/o-** *blood*	The passage of red, bloody stools
melena	mel-**EN**-ah		Greek *black*	The passage of black, tarry stools
occult Hemoccult test	oh-**KULT** **HEEM**-oh-kult TEST		Latin *to hide*	Not visible on the surface *Hemoccult* (trade name for a fecal occult blood test)

ostomy
 	
  colostomy
 	
  ileostomy
	OS-toe-me
	
	ko-**LOSS**-toe-me
	
	ill-ee-**OS**-toe-me
		S/
		R/
		R/
		
		R/
			-stomy *new opening*
			os- *mouth*
			col- *colon*
			
			ile- *ileum*
				Surgery to create an artificial opening into a tubular structure
				Artificial opening from the colon to the outside of the body
				Artificial opening from the ileum to the outside of the body

stoma	**STOW**-mah		Greek *mouth*	Artificial opening

Exercises

A. *Scope* and *scopy* are two suffixes you will see attached to many medical terms you will meet in later chapters. Scope *is the actual instrument used in the procedure. The procedure itself is the* **scopy**. *Utilize your medical vocabulary to fill in the blanks for this exercise.*   **LO 5.3, 5.19**

Instrument	Procedure Term	Definition of Procedure
endoscope	1.	2.
colonoscope	3.	4.
proctoscope	5.	6.
anoscope	7.	8.
gastroscope	9.	10.
sigmoidoscope	11.	12.

Note: **Endoscope** *is a generic (general) term that means any instrument used to examine the inside of a tubular or hollow organ. The instrument obtains its specific name from the organ it is used to examine. Thus, an instrument used to view a bronchus is a bronchoscope specifically, but it is also an endoscope in general.*

Digestive System

Challenge Your Knowledge

A. **A dental assistant, or anyone working in an Oral Surgery Department, needs to have a thorough knowledge of the mouth and the mastication process.** Your knowledge of medical terms will help you communicate with the dentist or oral surgeon and the patients. Match the correct answer to the statements below. (**LO 5.6**, *Remember, Understand, Apply*)

_____ 1. Grind and crush food

_____ 2. Projects above the gum/covered with enamel

_____ 3. Cheek muscles

_____ 4. Destroys tooth enamel and dentin

_____ 5. Contains blood vessels, nerves, tissue

_____ 6. Harder than bone

_____ 7. Oral cavity

_____ 8. Dental decay

_____ 9. Anchors tooth to jaw

_____ 10. Inflammation of the gum

_____ 11. Nerves reach the tooth through this

_____ 12. Contain the taste buds

a. mouth

b. pulp cavity

c. root canal

d. caries

e. root

f. gingivitis

g. papillae

h. crown

i. tartar

j. buccinator

k. bicuspids and molars

l. dentin

B. **Deconstruct and define.** The following medical terms can all designate a diagnosis. Use your knowledge of basic elements to deconstruct these terms and determine their meanings. First, slash (/) the terms into elements; then fill in the chart. (**LO 5.6**, *Remember, Understand, Apply*)

Medical Term	Prefix	Root/ Combining Form	Suffix	Meaning of Medical Term
dysphagia	1.	2.	3.	4.
esophagitis	5.	6.	7.	8.
hematemesis	9.	10.	11.	12.
pyrosis	13.	14.	15.	16.
reflux	17.	18.	19.	20.
regurgitation	21.	22.	23.	24.

C. Element. The following elements are a mixture of the prefixes, roots, combining forms, and suffixes contained in this chapter. In your study of medical terminology, it is important for you to be able to identify the types of elements and their definitions. This will aid you in determining the meaning of the medical term. Fill in the chart. Identify each element with a checkmark (✓) in the proper column. Then provide a meaning for the element. <u>The first one is done for you.</u> (**LO 5.3**, *Remember, Apply*)

Element	Prefix	Root/ Combining Form	Suffix	Meaning of Element
1. al			✓	2. *pertaining to*
3. atric				4.
5. bari				6.
7. cusp				8.
9. dynia				10.
11. glosso				12.
13. id				14.
15. lingu				16.
17. peri				18.
19. stalsis				20.
21. sub				22.

Now take any combination of elements from this table and form a complete medical term. Define the term using the meaning of the elements given in the chart.

23. Medical term: _____ / _____ / _____

                          P   R/CF   S

24. Meaning of medical term: _____

D. Discussion questions. Draw on your knowledge of the *language of gastroenterology* to discuss the following questions. Prepare a short answer. Be certain you can define every term you are using. (**LO 5.6**, *Remember, Apply*)

1. What is the bony roof of the mouth called? _____

2. What birth defect is associated with this part of the body? _____

3. Why do teeth have to be the hardest structures in the body?

_____

_____

_____

Digestive System

E. Deconstruct. No matter how long or how short the medical term, reducing it to elements will provide the meaning. Deconstruct with slashes the following two medical terms into their elemental meanings. Fill in the blanks. Divide and conquer your terms! (**LO 5.1, 5.3,** *Remember, Apply*)

esophagogastroduodenoscopy

Prefix	Meaning of Prefix	Root(s)/Combining Form	Meaning of Root(s)/Combining Form	Suffix	Meaning of Suffix
1.	2.	3.	4.	5.	6.

7. The meaning of *esophagogastroduodenoscopy* is

_____

_____

_____

oral

Prefix	Meaning of Prefix	Root(s)/Combining Form	Meaning of Root(s)/Combining Form	Suffix	Meaning of Suffix
8.	9.	10.	11.	12.	13.

14. The meaning of *oral* is

_____

F. A medical term that is a noun can also have an adjective form. Each statement has the noun form in parentheses; you must fill in the correct form of the adjective on the blank. Fill in the blanks. (**LO 5.3,** *Remember, Apply*)

1. The patient's (digestion) _____ symptoms were resolved with the new medication.

2. Due to an obstruction, the (pylorus) _____ sphincter was necrotic.

3. The (lymph) _____ tissues were sent to the pathologist for examination.

4. The patient is suffering from (pancreas) _____ cancer.

5. The (saliva) _____ gland was removed and sent to pathology.

6. Due to infection, the patient's (intestine) _____ surgery has been postponed until next week.

7. (Hemolysis) _____ jaundice results from RBC destruction and excess bilirubin.

8. The patient's (esophagus) _____ varices were bleeding.

9. The (laparoscope) _____ surgery poses less risk to the patient.

10. The (segment) _____ resection of the intestine is scheduled for later today.

G. **As a body system, the digestive system has a lot of different disorders.** Can you pair the correct organ with its disease or condition and write a brief definition of the term? Fill in the chart. (**LO 5.7, 5.9, 5.11, 5.15,** *Remember, Analyze*)

Term	Organ	Definition
1. aphthous ulcers	_____	_____
2. cholecystitis	_____	_____
3. choledocholithiasis	_____	_____
4. cirrhosis	_____	_____
5. Crohn disease	_____	_____
6. diverticulitis	_____	_____
7. dysphagia	_____	_____
8. GERD	_____	_____
9. IBS	_____	_____
10. intussusception	_____	_____
11. pancreatitis	_____	_____
12. proctitis	_____	_____

H. **Group recall.** The following colors all have a Latin or Greek term associated with them. Fill in the blanks with the element, and provide a medical term where it is used. (**LO 5.3,** *Understand*)

1. White: _____   Term: _____

2. Yellow: _____   Term: _____

3. Rust: _____   Term: _____

I. **Patient education—in your own words.** If you had to explain each of the specific functions of the digestive system to a patient, what would you say? Translate the medical terms into language the patient can understand. Fill in the blanks. (**LO 5.2, 5.3,** *Understand*)

1. ingestion: _____

2. propulsion: _____

3. digestion: _____

4. secretion: _____

5. absorption: _____

6. elimination: _____

J. **Using all the terms in Exercise I, trace the process of digestion in a single paragraph.** The exercise has been started for you. Underline all the terms in your writing to make sure you have used every one. (**LO 5.2, 5.3,** *Understand*)

The process of digestion begins in the mouth where . . .

_____

_____

_____

Digestive System

K. Abbreviations. Choose the abbreviation that is best described in the statement, and fill it in on the blank provided. On the line below the statement, write out the meaning of the abbreviation you have chosen. *There are more answers than questions.* <u>The first one is done for you.</u> Fill in the blanks. (**LO 5.4,** *Understand, Apply*)

GI   SSA   GERD   BMI   HAV   SGOT   CF   BM

1. Final act of elimination   Abbreviation ___*BM*___

Meaning: <u>Removal of waste matter from the body.</u> _____

2. Backing up into the esophagus   Abbreviation: _____

Meaning: _____

3. Digestive system component   Abbreviation: _____

Meaning: _____

4. Liver disease indicator   Abbreviation: _____

Meaning: _____

5. Inherited disease that affects exocrine glands   Abbreviation: _____

Meaning: _____

L. Be aware of singular and plural terms. Insert the correct medical terms in the blanks; watch for spelling. You will not use all the terms. (**LO 5.3,** *Understand, Apply*)

    diverticulitis   **diverticulum**   **diverticulosis**   **diverticula**

1. What starts out as a single _____ can be followed by many other _____.

    The condition of having a number of these small pouches in the wall intestine is known as _____.

    Should these pouches become inflamed, _____ will result.

    metastasses   **metastases**   **metastize**   **metastasis**

2. What was originally thought to be a single _____ to the patient's lung was proved to be multiple _____ to lung, kidney, and bone.

    polypectomy   **polyposis**   **polyp (singular)**

3. The first polyp was found on sigmoidoscopy. A follow-up colonoscopy 6 months later found several more (plural) _____ in the large intestine. Diagnosis is _____. Proposed treatment is _____.

    peritoneum   **peritonitis**   **peritoneal**

4. The _____ laceration sliced completely through the _____. Because of an infection in the wound, the patient developed _____.

M. Patient education—in your own words. Your knowledge of medical terminology must be translated into layman's terms if you are going to explain things in a way the patient can comprehend. Prepare a short answer that will help your patient understand the *difference* between the following terms. (**LO 5.3,** *Understand, Apply*)

1. A *polypectomy* and an *enteroscopy*:

_____

_____

_____

2. *Sublingual* and *subcutaneous* medication:

_____

_____

_____

N. Word elements are the keys to unlocking medical terms. Assess your knowledge of elements with this exercise. (**LO 5.3,** *Understand, Apply*)

1. Where is the inflammation in **hepatitis**?

   a. the belly

   b. the liver

   c. the pancreas

   d. the mouth

   e. the intestine

2. In the term **submucosa**, the prefix means

   a. over

   b. under

   c. around

   d. inside

   e. across

3. The color denoted in the term **leukoplakia** is

   a. green

   b. black

   c. white

   d. yellow

   e. red

4. The element **os** means

   a. stomach

   b. mouth

   c. eye

   d. liver

   e. ear

5. If the root **cyst** means *bladder*, what is a **cystectomy**?

   a. bladder irrigation

   b. bladder removal

   c. bladder examination

   d. bladder laceration

   e. bladder hemorrhage

6. If a medication is given **postprandially**, you will take it after

   a. exercise

   b. drinking water

   c. a meal

   d. a vitamin

   e. waking up

Digestive System

7. **Gingivitis** has a root that means

   a. opening

   b. teeth

   c. gum

   d. decay

   e. enzyme

8. A **cholecystectomy** is

   a. a procedure

   b. a diagnosis

   c. an inflammation

   d. a discharge

   e. an instrument

9. What is the adjective used to describe a dilated, tortuous vein?

   a. adipose

   b. varicose

   c. edematous

   d. pyloric

   e. segmental

10. On the basis of the suffix, you know that the **peritoneum** will be

   a. an opening

   b. an incision

   c. a structure

   d. a tumor

   e. a matrix

O. **Terminology challenge.** Dr. Lee made a **provisional diagnosis** for Mrs. Schreiber of Sjögren syndrome. Use your glossary or online medical dictionary to learn the meaning of the term *provisional diagnosis*. Write your notes here. (**LO 5.3, *Apply***)

_____

_____

_____

P. **Check the accuracy of your chart documentation.** The following patients have presented to the gastroenterology clinic today. Can you correctly complete their documentation? (**LO 5.3, *Apply, Analyze***)

  1. Caroline Mason presents today with severe _____ (vomiting of blood), which has been getting progressively worse. _____ (looking within by a scope) reveals _____-atous (swollen) _____ (pertaining to the esophagus) _____ (dilated veins).

  2. Andrew Baker reported to the Fulwood Emergency Room yesterday with symptoms of _____ (following a meal) burning chest pain and _____ (vomiting of blood). Dr. Lee admitted him to the GI service for further diagnostic tests and possible surgery.

Q. Medical abbreviations must be interpreted correctly to ensure precision in communication and patient safety. Match the correct abbreviation in the first column to the defined meanings in the second column. (**LO 5.4,** *Apply, Analyze*)

_____ 1. CF   **a.** use increases incidence of peptic ulcers

_____ 2. IBS   **b.** blocks production of gastric acid

_____ 3. GI   **c.** an intestinal diagnosis

_____ 4. PPI   **d.** an inherited disease

_____ 5. NSAIDs   **e.** refers to two specific organs

R. Can you interpret the following colonoscopy report for this patient? First, read the report out loud. Underline the medical terminology. If you need to, consult a dictionary or your glossary for additional help. Fill in the blanks. (**LO 5.3, 5.5,** *Analyze*)

Preoperative Diagnosis: History of (H/O) multiple colonic polyps.

Postoperative Diagnosis: Normal colon.

In the left lateral position, the colonoscope was advanced into the rectum without difficulty. Examination of the rectum was normal. The sigmoid and descending colon revealed extensive diverticular disease but no evidence of colonic polyp disease. The transverse colon was examined to the hepatic flexure. There were no abnormalities of the transverse colon. The ascending colon was examined to the ileocecal valve. This was confirmed by abdominal wall transillumination. There were no abnormalities of the ascending colon. The patient tolerated the procedure well and was discharged from the endoscopy suite in good condition. In view of his age and a clean colonoscopy, I have recommended no further surveillance.

1. Analyze the prefixes. What is the difference between the pre- and postoperative diagnoses?

   pre- = _____ post- = _____

   Why are the diagnoses sometimes different?

   _____

2. Describe the left lateral position. _____

3. What instrument was used for this procedure? _____

4. Give another adjective meaning *extensive*. _____

5. Deconstruct **diverticulosis**, and write its meaning. _____

   _____

6. Define **polyp**. _____

7. On the basis of your understanding of the prefix trans-, in which position does the transverse colon lie? _____

   _____

8. Again, using the prefix *trans*-, what does **transillumination** mean? _____

9. What does a "clean colonoscopy" mean? _____

10. Is it good or bad that the physician is recommending "no further surveillance." Explain your answer.

   _____

Digestive System

S. Precision in documentation. Get the stone in the right place: **cholelithiasis** or **choledocholithiasis**? Make the correct choice of medical terminology for the digestive system. Fill in the blanks. (**LO 5.3, 5.15, *Analyze***)

1. The patient's films revealed a stone in the common bile duct.

   Diagnosis: _____

2. The presence of a stone in the patient's gallbladder was confirmed by the radiologist.

   Diagnosis: _____

T. Supply the missing element that will complete the medical term. Fill in the blanks. <u>The first one is done for you.</u> (**LO 5.18, 5.19, *Analyze***)

1. Inflammation of the appendix   appendic/ <u> itis </u>_____

2. Part of the colon shaped like an "S"   sigm /_____

3. Pertaining to the anus   an /_____

4. Excessive amount of gas   flatul/_____

5. To bend back   re/_____

6. Inflammation of the colon   col /_____

7. Pertaining to the anus   an/_____

8. Evacuation of feces from the rectum and anus   de/ fec/_____

9. An edge or a border   peri/_____

10. Pertaining to the colon   colon/_____

U. Prefixes make the difference in precision. Analyze the two pairs of medical terms. Write a brief description of how they differ, especially after a prefix has been added. (**LO 5.3, 5.11, *Analyze***)

1. *emesis* and *hematemesis*

   _____

   _____

   _____

2. *symptomatic* and *asymptomatic*

   _____

   _____

   _____

V. Documentation. Helen Schreiber's medical record of her visit to Dr. Susan Lee contains terms from this and previous chapters. Reinforce your knowledge of the language of medicine by answering the following questions that are based on this scenario. Fill in the blanks. (**LO 5.3,** *Analyze*)

Case Report 5.2

Mrs. Helen Schreiber, a 45-year-old high school principal, presents with a 6-month history of dry mouth, bleeding gums, and difficulty in chewing and swallowing food.

Questioning by Dr. Susan Lee, her primary care physician, reveals that she also has dry eyes, is having pain in some joints of both hands, and has felt fatigued. Her previous medical history is uneventful. Physical examination shows a dry mouth, mild gingivitis, and an ulcer on the back of the lower lip. Her salivary glands are not swollen. Her eyes show no ulceration or conjunctivitis. The metacarpophalangeal joints of both index fingers are swollen, stiff, and tender. All other systems show no abnormality.

Initial laboratory reports show anemia, decreased WBC count, and an elevated ESR. Dr. Lee makes a provisional diagnosis of Sjögren syndrome. The results of blood studies for SSA and SSB antibodies and for rheumatoid factor titers are pending, as are x-rays of her hands.

Mrs. Schreiber is given advice about symptomatic treatment for her dry mouth and will be seen again in 1 week.

Luisa Guitterez, CMA. 10/12/12, 1530 hrs.

1. List all of Mrs. Schreiber's signs and symptoms. _____

_____

2. Which symptoms pertain to the digestive system? _____

3. Which other body systems are presenting symptoms? _____

4. What procedures are performed to aid in Mrs. Schreiber's diagnosis?

_____

W. Precision in documentation. You may someday find yourself doing medical transcription in a hospital or physician's office. Proofread the letter Dr. Walsh has sent to the patient's insurance company asking for preauthorization for her surgery. Underline or highlight all the errors; then rewrite the correct terms on the lines below the dictation. Then add a brief definition of each term. (**LO 5.3,** *Analyze*)

Request for Authorization of Surgery

Re: Mrs. Martha Jones

Subscriber ID # 056437

Dear Doctor Leavenworth,

Mrs. Jones is a 52-year-old former waitress, recently divorced. She is 5 feet 4 inches tall and weighs 275 pounds. She has type 2 diabeetes with frequent episodes of hyperglycemia and also ketoacidoses, requiring three different hospitalizations. She now has diabetick retinnopathy and peripheral vascullitis. Complicating this is hypertension (185/110), coronery artery disease, and pulmonary edema. Exercise is out of the question because she has marked osteoarrthritis of her knees and hips. Mrs. Jones is now housebound, dependent on her daughter for transportation to our medical center. In spite of monthly meetings with our nutritionist, she has gained 25 pounds in the past 6 months.

Write the correct form of the misspelled words with a brief definition for each term here.

Corrections

_____

_____

_____

Definitions

_____

_____

_____

Digestive System

X. **Your knowledge of medical terminology will increase if you focus on similarities and differences in medical terms.** Adding or changing a suffix or prefix can change the meaning of a term or create a new term. Fill in the blanks. (**LO 5.3, 5.16, 5.19,** *Analyze*)

1. One word element makes lactose different from lactase.

   The word element is a _____.

   Lactose means _____.

   Lactase means _____.

2. *Cuspid* is a medical term. The addition of *bi* to *cuspid* makes two different medical terms.

   What type of element is *bi*? _____

   Cuspid means: _____

   Bicuspid means: _____

Y. **Many medical terms that are nouns also have an adjectival form.** Correctly apply these six medical terms to the following sentences. Fill in the blanks. (**LO 5.3,** *Analyze*)

mucous   mucin   mucus   mucosal   mucosa   submucosa

1. The lining of a tubular structure is referred to as the _____.

2. A sticky film containing mucin is _____.

3. The term for *pertaining to* the mucosa is _____.

4. The tissue layer beneath the mucosa is the _____.

5. _____ is a secretion from the mucosal glands.

6. _____ means *relating to mucus or the mucosa.*

7. Which two terms are differentiated by the addition of a prefix? _____

   and _____

8. Which two terms are pronounced the same but spelled differently? _____

   and _____

CHAPTER SUMMARY EXERCISE

A. Spelling comprehension. Circle the correct spelling of the term. (**LO 5.3, 5.6, 5.7, 5.9, 5.16, 5.20,** *Remember*)

1. laperoscopie   laparoscopy   leperoscopie   leporoscopy   laporoscopie

2. hematemesis   hemmatemisis   hematimisis   hematemis   hematimisus

3. parrotid   paratid   poratid   parotid   parritid

4. jegjunum   jejuunum   jedgejunum   jeghjunem   jejunum

5. mesentery   mesantery   mesenterie   mesanterie   messantery

6. hematochezia   hemetocizia   hemmatocizia   hemocizia   hematocizia

7. leukoplakkia   leukopakia   leukopiccia   leukoplakia   leukkophakia

8. degluetition   deglutition   deeglutition   degglutation   deglutation

9. varices   varixes   verixces   vericces   varicces

10. aphous   aphtous   appthous   aphthous   affthous

B. Match the number of the correct spelling of the term in Exercise A with the brief description of the term below. (**LO 5.3, 5.6, 5.7, 5.9, 5.16, 5.20,** *Apply*)

1. Act of swallowing _____

2. Double layer of peritoneum enclosing viscera _____

3. Small ulcer in the mouth _____

4. Vomiting of blood _____

5. Examining the abdomen with an endoscope _____

6. Dilated, tortuous veins _____

7. Where most nutrients are absorbed _____

8. White plaque in the mouth _____

9. Red, bloody stools _____

10. Salivary gland beside the ear _____

Digestive System

C. Using your knowledge of terms 1–10 in Exercises A and B and their correct spelling, write a brief sentence for each of the terms as it might appear in patient documentation. (LO 5.3, 5.6, 5.7, 5.9, 5.16, 5.20, *Apply*)

1. _____

2. _____

3. _____

4. _____

5. _____

6. _____

7. _____

8. _____

9. _____

10. _____

D. After reading Case Report 5.4, answer the following questions. Be prepared to discuss your answers in class. (LO 5.3, 5.13, 5.15, *Analyze*)

Case Report 5.4

You are

... a Certified Medical Assistant working with Susan Lee, MD, a primary care physician at Fulwood Medical Center.

Your patient is

... Mrs. Sandra Jacobs, a 46-year-old mother of four. Your task is to document her care.

Documentation

Mrs. Sandra Jacobs, a 46-year-old mother of four, presents in Dr. Susan Lee's primary care clinic with episodes of crampy pain in her right upper quadrant associated with nausea and vomiting. The pain often occurs after eating fast food. She has not noticed fever or jaundice. Physical examination reveals an obese white woman with a positive **Murphy sign**. Her BP is 170/90, and she has slight pedal edema. A provisional diagnosis of **gallstones** has been made. She has been referred for an ultrasound examination, and an appointment has been made to see Dr. Stewart Walsh in the Surgery Department.

I explained to her the etiology of her gallstones and the need for surgical removal of the stones, and I discussed with her a low-fat, 1500-calorie diet sheet.

Luisa Guitterez, CMA. 10/12/12, 1430 hrs.

1. Demonstrate to the class the location of your *right upper quadrant*. _____

2. Define *jaundice*. _____

3. What is a *positive Murphy's sign*? _____

4. What makes a diagnosis *provisional*? _____

5. What are the patient's presenting symptoms? _____

_____

6. What additional diagnostic test is Mrs. Jacobs scheduled for? _____

7. In a medical or online dictionary, look up the meaning of the word *etiology*. _____

E. **Meet the goals of each of the chapter outcomes** by using the correct language of the digestive system for the answers. (LO 5.1–5.20, *Analyze*)

1. Describe the alimentary canal and its accessory organs. What are the organ components of the alimentary canal? (**LO 5.1**)

   a. _____

   b. _____

   c. _____

   d. _____

   e. _____

   f. _____

2. Discuss the functions of the digestive system. What is the difference between ingestion and digestion? (**LO 5.2**)

   a. ingestion: _____

   b. digestion: _____

3. Use the medical terms of gastroenterology to communicate and document in writing accurately and precisely in any health care setting. What is the correct spelling of the term that refers to a medical specialist in the disorders and diseases of the stomach and intestines? (**LO 5.3**)

   a. enterogastrologist

   b. gastroenterologist

   c. gastrainterologist

   d. gastrointerologist

   e. endogastrologist

4. Use the medical terms of gastroenterology to communicate verbally with accuracy and precision in any health care setting. What is the correct pronunciation of deglutition? (**LO 5.4**)

   a. de-glue-TIS-ion

   b. dee-GLUE-tis-tion

   c. dee-glue-TISH-un

   d. DI-glu-TISH-tion

   e. DE-glu-tish-ion

5. Match the abbreviation to the medical term. Which of the following abbreviations is a diagnosis/disease? (**LO 5.5**)

   a. NSAIDs

   b. PT

   c. HIV

   d. ESR

   e. RBC

6. Relate the anatomy of the mouth to the function of mastication. What makes the mouth the first site of mechanical and chemical digestion? (**LO 5.6**)

   a. mechanical digestion: _____

   b. chemical digestion: _____

7. Describe disorders of the mouth. An infection occurring anywhere in the mouth that is caused by a fungus describes (**LO 5.7**)

   a. canker sores

   b. leukoplakia

   c. oral cancer

   d. thrush

   e. glossodynia

Digestive System

8. Relate the anatomy of the pharynx and esophagus to the function of swallowing. Describe the four phases of deglutition: (**LO 5.8**)

   a. _____

   b. _____

   c. _____

   d. _____

9. Describe disorders of the esophagus: (**LO 5.9**)

   a. A postprandial burning chest pain is commonly called _____.

   b. Vomiting of blood is termed _____.

   c. The medical term for varicose veins of the esophagus is _____.

   d. What occurs when a portion of the stomach protrudes through the diaphragm? _____

   e. Difficulty in swallowing is called _____.

10. Relate the anatomy of the stomach and small intestine to the process of digestion. (**LO 5.10**)

   a. Food exits the stomach and goes into the small intestine through the _____.

   b. What is the medical term for the circular folds in the lining of the small intestine? _____

   c. What is the sphincter called that controls entry from the small intestine into the large intestine? _____

11. Discuss disorders of the stomach and small intestine. What is the difference between a peptic ulcer and a gastric ulcer? (**LO 5.11**)

   a. peptic ulcer: _____

   b. gastric ulcer: _____

12. Describe the pharmacology of treating excess gastric acid. What is the function of PPIs, and how do they achieve treating excess gastric acid? (**LO 5.12**)

   a. function: _____

   b. treatment: _____

   c. drug examples of a PPI: _____

13. Relate the anatomy of the liver, gallbladder, and pancreas to their functions in digestion. Which three pancreatic secretions aid in digestion? (**LO 5.13**)

   a. _____

   b. _____

   c. _____

14. Explain the function of the different liver function tests. What are the different categories of liver function tests and what do they measure? (**LO 5.14**)

   a. _____

   b. _____

   c. _____

   d. _____

15. Discuss disorders of the liver, gallbladder, and pancreas that affect digestion. Viral hepatitis is related to three major types of virus. Name them, and how they are transmitted. (**LO 5.15**)

   a. Virus (abbreviation)_____ Transmitted by:_____

   b. Virus (abbreviation)_____ Transmitted by:_____

   c. Virus (abbreviation)_____ Transmitted by:_____

16. Explain the digestion and absorption of proteins, carbohydrates, and fats. How does gluconeogenesis function in digestion? (**LO 5.16**)

   a. _____

   b. _____

   c. _____

17. Discuss malabsorption syndromes and their diagnosis. What symptoms may lead to a diagnosis of regional enteritis? (**LO 5.17**)

   a. _____

   b. _____

   c. _____

18. Relate the anatomy of the large intestine to its functions. Which of the following is NOT a function of the large intestine? (**LO 5.18**)

   a. absorption   **d.** elimination

   b. sensation   **e.** secretion

   c. peristalsis

19. Discuss disorders of the large intestine. Small pouches bulging outward through weak spots in the lining of the large intestine describes. (**LO 5.19**)

   a. diverticulitis   **d.** colon cancer

   b. diverticulosis   **e.** intussusception

   c. ulcerative colitis

20. Explain the different forms of gastrointestinal bleeding and their diagnosis and treatment. Listed below are four types of GI bleeding. Define each term and indicate whether it comes from the upper or lower GI tract. (**LO 5.20**)

   a. melena

   Definition: _____ U/L GI Tract: _____

   b. hematemesis

   Definition: _____ U/L GI Tract: _____

   c. vomiting of "coffee grounds"

   Definition: _____ U/L GI Tract: _____

   d. hematochezia

   Definition: _____ U/L GI Tract: _____

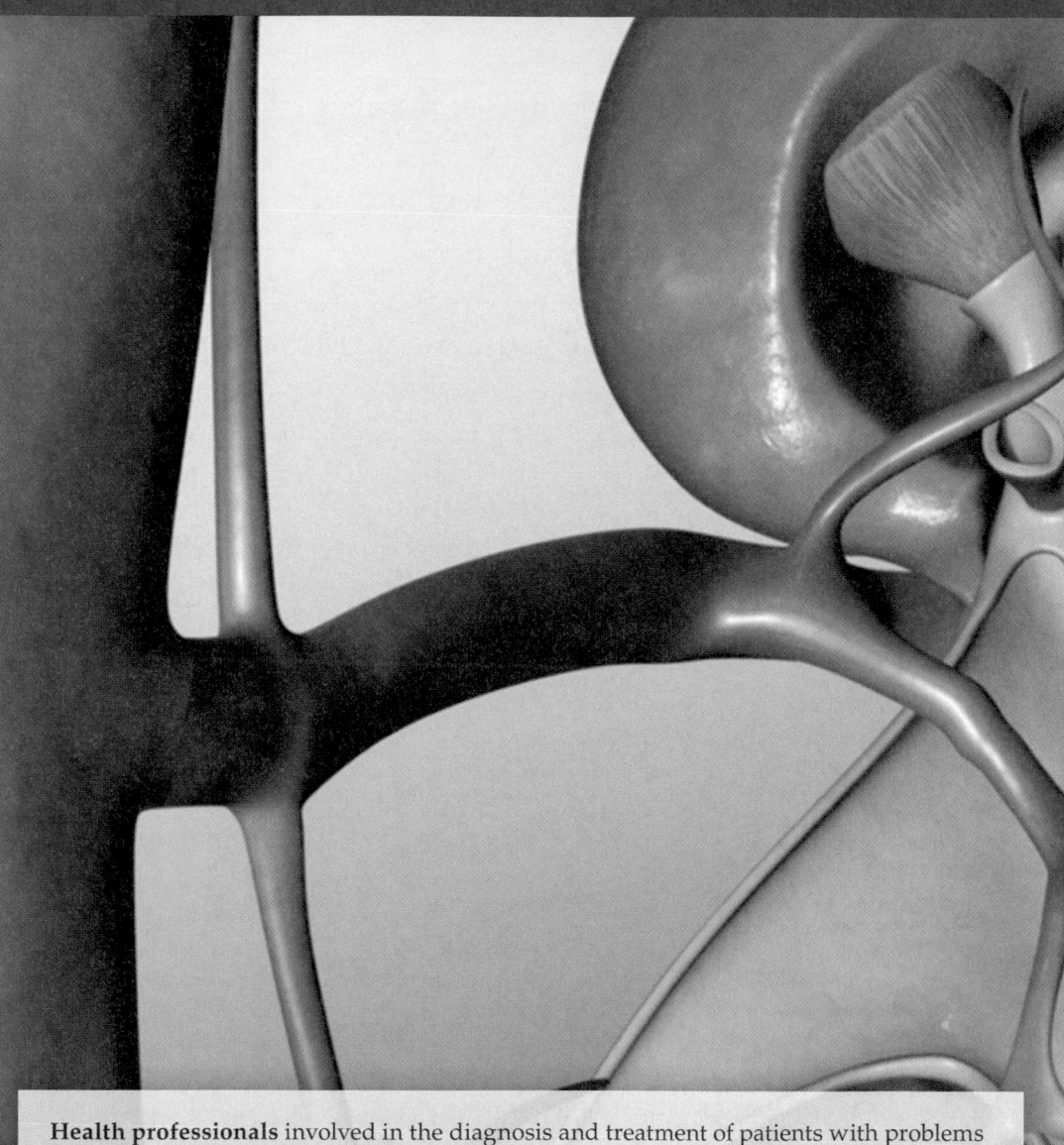

Urinary System
The Language of Urology

Health professionals involved in the diagnosis and treatment of patients with problems with the urologic system include:

- **Urologists**, who are specialists in the diagnosis and treatment of patients with diseases of the urinary system.

- **Nephrologists**, who are specialists in the diagnosis and treatment of diseases of the kidney.

- **Urologic nurses and nurse practitioners**, who are registered nurses with advanced academic and clinical experience in urology.

6

Case Report (CR) 6.1

You are

... a surgical physician assistant working with **urologist** Phillip Johnson, MD, at Fulwood Medical Center.

Your patient is

... Mr. Nelson Hughes, a 58-year-old school principal. You are making your afternoon hospital visits to Dr. Johnson's patients. Earlier today you assisted at Mr. Hughes's surgery. A **laparoscopic radical nephrectomy** for a **tumor node metastasis (TNM) stage II renal cell carcinoma** (cancer) with no evidence of local invasion or lymph node involvement (**metastasis**) was performed.

Your job is to assess Mr. Hughes's postoperative state and determine whether postoperative complications exist.

Chapter Learning Outcomes

To define and understand these areas of concern, communicate with Dr. Johnson and the patient, and document Mr. Hughes's progress, you need to be able to:

LO 6.1 Apply the language of **urology** to the anatomy and the structure of the urinary system.

LO 6.2 Explain the physiology and functions of the urinary system.

LO 6.3 Use the medical terms of urology to communicate in writing and document the terms of urology accurately and precisely in any health care setting.

LO 6.4 Use the medical terms of urology to communicate verbally with accuracy and precision in any health care setting.

LO 6.5 Define abbreviations that relate to the urinary system.

LO 6.6 Explain the effects of common urinary disorders on health.

LO 6.7 Describe the response of common disorders of the urinary system to treatment.

LO 6.8 Describe diagnostic procedures that pertain to the urinary system.

LO 6.9 Explain the use of urinalysis as a diagnostic tool.

LO 6.10 List the abnormal constituents of urine.

LO 6.11 Differentiate the methods of urine collection.

Lesson 6.1 Urinary System, Kidneys, and Ureters

LESSON OBJECTIVES

Although the respiratory system *(see Chapter 13)* excretes carbon dioxide and water, the integumentary system *(see Chapter 15)* excretes water, inorganic salts, and lactic acid in sweat, and the digestive tract *(see Chapter 5)* excretes water, salts, lipids, bile pigments, and other wastes, the urinary system carries the major burden of excretion.

Within the urinary system, the kidneys are the agents that eliminate the waste products. If the kidneys fail to function, the other three systems of excretion are not able to replace them. Therefore, the kidney is a vital organ, and it brings with it a whole new set of terminology.

In this lesson, the information will enable you to:

6.1.1 Identify the location and anatomic features of the kidney.

6.1.2 Describe the functions of the kidney.

6.1.3 Map the flow of fluid through the renal filtration process.

6.1.4 Describe the functional anatomy of the ureters and urinary bladder.

6.1.5 Explain how common disorders of the kidneys and ureters affect health.

6.1.6 Apply correct medical terminology to disorders of the kidneys, ureters, and urinary bladder.

Abbreviation

IVP	intravenous pyelogram
TNM	tumor, node, metastasis (tumor staging method)

LO 6.1, 6.2 Urinary System

The urinary system *(Figure 6.1)* consists of six (6) organs:

- Two **kidneys (2)**
- A single **urinary bladder (1)**
- Two **ureters (2)**
- A single **urethra (1)**

The process of removing metabolic waste is called **excretion.** It is an essential process in maintaining homeostasis *(see Chapter 4)*. The metabolic wastes include carbon dioxide from cellular respiration, excess water and electrolytes, **nitrogenous** compounds from the breakdown of proteins, and **urea**. If these wastes are not eliminated, they poison the whole body.

In the body's cells, protein is broken down *(see Chapter 4)* into **amino acids**. When an amino acid is broken down, **ammonia** is produced. Ammonia is extremely toxic to cells. The liver quickly converts it to the less toxic urea, which is excreted by the kidneys.

Keynotes

- **Urology** is the medical specialty of the diagnosis and treatment of diseases of the urinary system.
- The kidney is the major organ that eliminates the waste products of cellular metabolism.

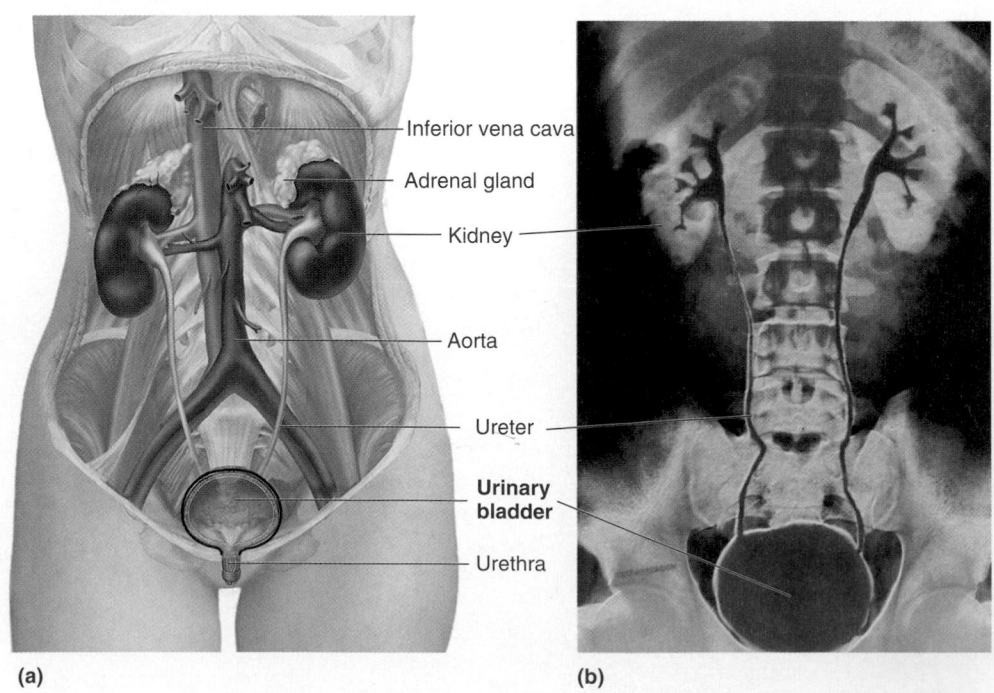

Inferior vena cava

Adrenal gland

Kidney

Aorta

Ureter

Urinary bladder

Urethra

(a)

(b)

▲ **Figure 6.1** **The Urinary System.** *(a)* Major organs. *(b)* Structures of the urinary system are visible in this colored **intravenous pyelogram** (IVP).

WORD	PRONUNCIATION	ELEMENTS		DEFINITION
amino acid	ah-**ME**-no **ASS**-id	R/CF	amin/o *nitrogen containing* acid, Latin *sour*	The basic building block for protein
ammonia	ah-**MOAN**-ih-ah	S/ R/	-ia *condition* ammon- *ammonia*	Toxic breakdown product of amino acids
bladder	**BLAD**-er		Old English *bladder*	Hollow sac that holds fluid; for example, urine or bile
excretion excrete (verb)	eks-**KREE**-shun eks-**KREET**		Latin *remove*	Removal of waste products of metabolism out of the body To pass out of the body the waste products of metabolism
kidney	**KID**-nee		Greek *kidney*	Organ of excretion
nephrectomy	neh-**FREK**-toe-me	S/ R/CF	-ectomy *surgical excision* nephr/o- *kidney*	Surgical removal of a kidney
nephrology nephrologist	neh-**FROL**-oh-jee neh-**FROL**-oh-jist	S/ S/	-logy *study of* -logist *one who studies, specialist*	Medical specialty of diseases of the kidney Medical specialist in diseases of the kidney
nitrogenous	ni-**TROJ**-en-us	S/ R/CF R/	-ous *pertaining to* nitr/o- *nitrogen* -gen- *create*	Containing or generating nitrogen
renal	**REE**-nal	S/ R/	-al *pertaining to* ren- *kidney*	Pertaining to the kidney
urea	you-**REE**-ah		Greek *urine*	End product of nitrogen metabolism
urethra (*Note:* One "e"=one tube.) urethral (adj)	you-**REE**-thra you-**REE**-thral	S/ R/	-al *pertaining to* urethr- *urethra*	Canal leading from the bladder to outside (*Note:* The roots for **urethra** and **ureter** are different.) Pertaining to the urethra
urethritis	you-ree-**THRI**-tis	S/	-itis *inflammation*	Inflammation of the urethra
ureter (*Note:* Two "e's"=two tubes.) ureteral (adj)	you-**RET**-er you-ree-**TER**-al	S/ R/	Greek *urinary canal* -al *pertaining to* ureter- *ureter*	Tube that connects the kidney to the urinary bladder (*Note:* The roots for **urethra** and **ureter** are different.) Pertaining to the ureter
urine urinary (adj)	**YUR**-in **YUR**-in-ary	S/ R/	Latin *urine* -ary *pertaining to* urin- *urine*	Fluid and dissolved substances excreted by kidney Pertaining to urine
urinate (verb)	**YUR**-in-ate	S/	-ate *composed of, pertaining to*	To pass urine
urination	yur-ih-**NAY**-shun	S/	-ation *process*	The act of passing urine
urology	you-**ROL**-oh-jee	S/ R/CF	-logy *study of* ur/o- *urinary system*	Medical specialty of disorders of the urinary system
urologist urological (adj)	you-**ROL**-oh-jist yur-roh-**LOJ**-ik-al	S/ S/	-logist *one who studies* -ical *pertaining to*	Medical specialist in disorders of the urinary system Pertaining to urology

Exercises

A. The same but different. *More than one word element can have the same meaning. In this body system, **nephr/o** and **ren-** both mean kidney. The elements are not interchangeable—one particular element will be used for a specific term. You need to know them individually. Fill in the blanks. Read carefully!* **LO 6.1, 6.2, 6.3**

1. Surgical removal of a kidney   _____/_____/_____

2. Medical specialist in kidney treatment   _____/_____/_____

3. Medical specialty in kidney diseases   _____/_____/_____

4. Pertaining to the kidney   _____/_____/_____

B. Employ the *language of urology* to correctly match the medical term to the brief description. LO 6.1, 6.2

_____ 1. hollow sac that holds fluids

_____ 2. organ of excretion

_____ 3. connects kidney to bladder

_____ 4. canal leading from bladder to outside the body

a. kidney

b. ureter

c. urethra

d. bladder

> 💡 *Study Hint*
> You are keeping a list in the back of your text for all the suffixes meaning *pertaining to*. You should also keep a separate list of various elements like *ren* and *nephr/o* that have the same meaning but generate their own medical terms.

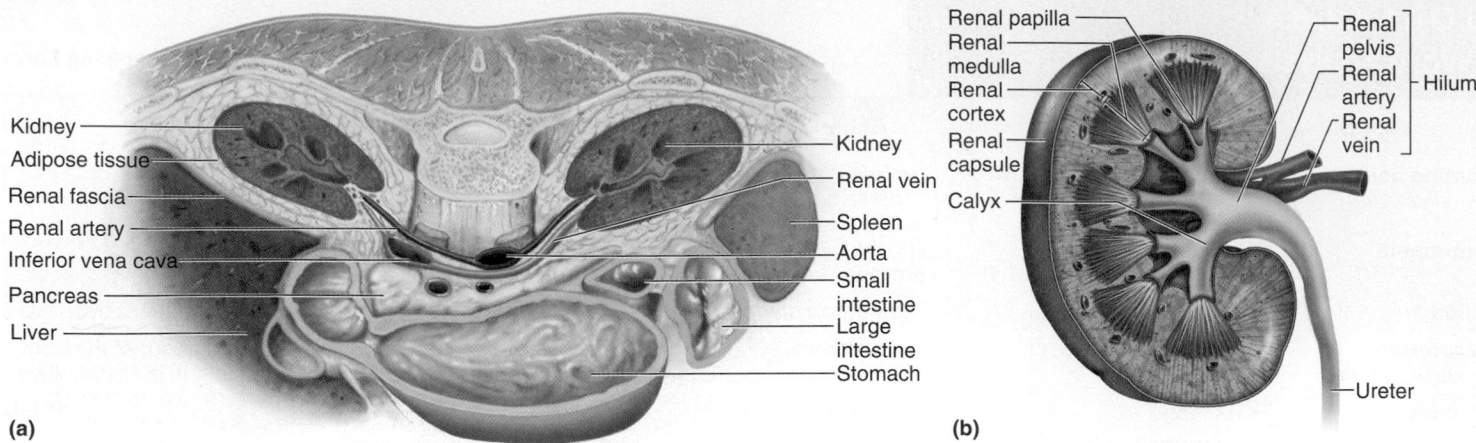

▲ **Figure 6.2** **Kidney.** (*a*) Transverse section of abdomen showing position of kidneys. (*b*) Longitudinal section of a kidney.

Keynote

The functions of the kidneys are to

- **Filter** blood to eliminate wastes.
- **Regulate** blood volume and pressure by eliminating or conserving water as necessary.
- **Maintain homeostasis** by controlling the quantities of water and electrolytes that are eliminated.
- **Secrete** the enzyme **renin**, which raises arterial blood pressure.
- **Secrete** the hormone **erythropoietin**, which acts on the bone to release red blood cells.
- **Synthesize vitamin D** to contribute to maintaining normal blood calcium levels.

LO 6.1, 6.2 Anatomy and Physiology of the Kidneys

Each kidney is a bean-shaped organ about the size of a clenched fist. It is located on either side of the vertebral column behind the peritoneum and lies against the deep muscles of the back. The left kidney is behind the spleen, and the right kidney behind and below the liver *(Figure 6.2a)*.

Waste-laden blood enters the kidney at its **hilum** *(Figure 6.2b)* through the renal artery. Excess water, urea, and other waste products are **filtered** from the blood by the kidney, collected in the ureter, and carried off to the bladder through the renal pelvis at the hilum. The filtered blood exits through the renal vein at the hilum.

Each kidney has three regions *(see Figure 6.2b):*

- An outer renal **cortex**—contains about 1 million **nephrons**, the basic filtration unit of the kidney.
- An inner renal **medulla**—containing the collecting ducts, which merge together to form about 30 papillary ducts, that enter into a **calyx**.
- A central renal **pelvis**—a funnel-shaped structure into which the calyces open, and which forms the ureter.

In the cortex, the renal artery divides into smaller and smaller arterioles, each of which enters a nephron and divides into a network of approximately 50 capillaries, known as a **glomerulus**. Each glomerulus is encased in the **glomerular capsule (Bowman capsule)**. Because the blood is under pressure and the capillaries and glomerular capsule are **permeable**, much of the fluid from the blood filters through the capillary wall and glomerular capsule into the renal tubule, which includes the **loop of Henle**, sometimes called the *nephron loop* *(Figure 6.3)*.

▲ **Figure 6.3** **Glomerulus and Renal Tubule.**

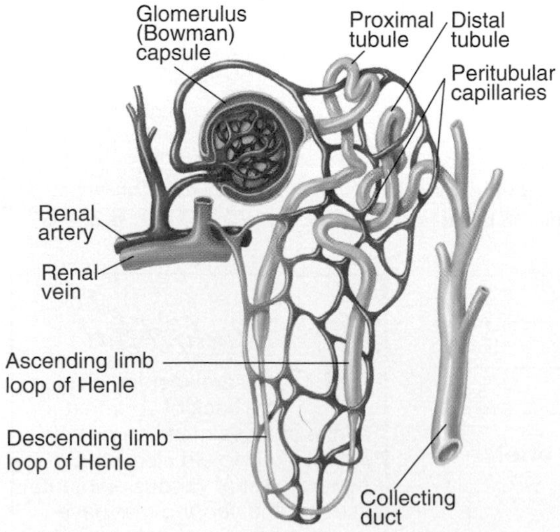

This **filtrate** entering the renal tubule contains water, urea, glucose, electrolytes, amino acids, and vitamins. Red blood cells, platelets, and plasma proteins are too large to pass through the capillary membrane, and they remain in the blood.

Approximately 180 liters (45 gallons) of filtrate are formed each day. As the filtrate passes down the renal tubule, over 90% of the water is returned to the blood by **reabsorption**. Glucose and minerals are also returned to the blood. Some residual wastes in the blood are secreted from the blood into the tubule. These interchanges between the filtrate in the tubule and the blood are made possible by a mesh of capillaries that surrounds the renal tubule *(Figure 6.3)*. The material that remains in the tubule is urine. It consists of excess water, electrolytes, and urea.

The renal tubules merge to form collecting ducts *(Figure 6.3)* that merge into the calyces and then form the **renal pelvis** and become the **ureter**.

Purified blood is returned from the **peritubular** mesh of capillaries to the circulatory system through the renal vein.

S = Suffix   P = Prefix   R = Root   R/CF = Combining Form

WORD	PRONUNCIATION	ELEMENTS		DEFINITION
calyx calyces (pl)	**KAY**-licks **KAY**-lih-sees		Greek *cup of a flower*	Funnel-shaped structure
cortex cortices (pl) cortical (adj)	**KOR**-teks **KOR**-tih-sees **KOR**-tih-kal	 S/ R/	Latin *tree bark* -ical *pertaining to* cort- *cortex*	Outer portion of an organ Pertaining to the cortex
filtrate filter filtration	**FIL**-trate **FIL**-ter fil-**TRAY**-shun	S/ R/ S/	-ate *composed of, pertaining to* filtr- *strain through* Latin *to filter through the* *material felt* -ation *process*	That which has passed through a filter A porous substance through which a liquid or gas is passed to separate out contained particles; or to use a filter Process of passing liquid through a filter
glomerulus glomeruli (pl) glomerular (adj)	glo-**MER**-you-lus glo-**MER**-you-lee glo-**MER**-you-lar		Latin *small ball of yarn*	Plexus of capillaries; part of a nephron Pertaining to or affecting a glomerulus or glomeruli
hilum hila (pl)	**HIGH**-lum **HIGH**-lah		Latin *small bit*	The part where the nerves and blood vessels enter and leave an organ
loop of Henle	**LOOP** of **HEN**-lee		Friedrich Henle, 1809–1885, German anatomist, pathologist, and histologist	Part of the renal tubule where reabsorption occurs
medulla nephron	meh-**DULL-ah** **NEF**-ron		French *middle* Greek *kidney*	Central portion of a structure surrounded by cortex Filtration unit of the kidney; glomerulus+ renal tubule
pelvis	**PEL**-vis		Latin *basin*	A cup-shaped cavity, as in the pelvis of the kidney
peritubular	**PER**-ih-too-**BYU**-lar	S/ P/ R/	-ar *pertaining to* peri- *around* -tubul- *small tube*	Surrounding the small renal tubules
permeable semipermeable impermeable	**PER**-me-ah-bull sem-ee-**PER**-me-ah-bull im-**PER**-me-ah-bull	S/ R/CF P/ P/	-able *capable of* perm/e- *pass through* semi- *half* im- *not, in*	Allowing passage of substances through a membrane Freely permeable to water but not to solutes When nothing is allowed passage
reabsorption (**Note:** This term has two prefixes.)	ree-ab-**SORP**-shun	S/ P/ P/ R/	-ion *process* re- *back* ab- *away from* -sorpt- *swallow*	The taking back into the blood of substances that had previously been filtered out from it
renin	**REE**-nin	S/ R/	-in *substance* ren- *kidney*	Enzyme secreted by the kidney that causes vasoconstriction

Exercises

A. Define and deconstruct the following medical terms into their basic elements. *Write the name of the element on the line below the slash. Fill in the blanks.* **LO 6.1, 6.2, 6.3**

1. Passage of a substance through a membrane   _____ / _____ / _____

2. Enzyme that causes vasoconstriction   _____ / _____ / _____

3. Surrounding the small renal tubules   _____ / _____ / _____

4. Blood that reclaims previously filtered substances   _____ / _____ / _____

B. Three of these terms refer to the regions of the kidney. *Choose the correct three terms and match them to the region.* **LO 6.1, 6.2, 6.3**

peritubular   cortex   Bowman's capsule   pelvis   loop of Henle   medulla

1. outer region   _____

2. inner region   _____

3. central region   _____

Case Report 6.2

Emergency Department, Fulwood Medical Center.
9/12/12 1500hrs

Justin Leandro, a 37-year-old construction worker, presented at 1520 hrs. He complained of a sudden onset of excruciating pain in his right abdomen and back an hour previously while at work. The pain is spasmodic and radiates down into his groin. He has vomited once and keeps having the urge to urinate but cannot. He has no previous medical history of significance.

Vital signs (**VS**): T 99.4°F, P 92, R 20, BP 130/86. Abdomen slightly distended, with tenderness in the right upper and lower quadrants and flank. A dipstick test showed blood in his urine.

Provisional diagnosis: stone in right ureter. An **IV line** was inserted, 2 mg morphine sulfate given by IV push at 1540. He is going to x-ray stat for **KUB** and **IVP**.

Andrea Facundo, **EMT-P**. 1555 hrs.

LO 6.1, 6.2 Ureters

Each ureter is a muscular tube, about 10 inches long (25.5 cm) and ¼ inch (0.6 cm) wide, that carries urine from the renal pelvis to the urinary bladder. It lies on the posterior abdominal wall, which is why Mr. Leandro had pain in his back. It passes behind the bladder and enters it on its posterior inferior surface, which is why the pain radiated into his groin.

Each ureter passes obliquely through the muscle wall of the bladder. As pressure builds in a filling bladder, the muscle wall compresses the ureter and prevents urine from being forced back up the ureter to the kidneys (**reflux**).

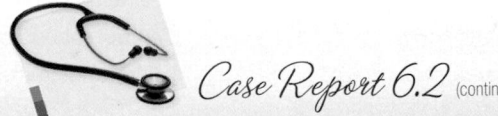

Case Report 6.2 (continued)

Mr. Leandro's x-ray of **k**idney, **u**reter, and **b**ladder (KUB) showed a suspicious lesion halfway down his right ureter. An **IVP** confirmed that this was a stone (renal **calculus**) blocking the ureter and showed the pelvis of the right kidney to be slightly dilated.

In addition to gravity, muscular peristaltic waves, originating in the renal pelvis, squeeze urine down the ureter and squirt it into the bladder. The peristaltic waves are intermittent, which is why Mr. Leandro's pain was **spasmodic**.

Mr. Leandro's stone was large enough to be lodged in the ureter, blocking the flow of urine and, because of the back flow pressure, leading to **hydronephrosis** of his kidney. Mr. Leandro was kept in the hospital overnight with intravenous (IV) pain medication but did not pass the stone. **Extracorporeal shock wave lithotripsy (ESWL)** was successful in crumbling the stone from outside the body. He urinated through a strainer so that the stone fragments could be recovered and chemically analyzed.

LO 6.6, 6.7 Kidney and Ureteral Stones (Nephrolithiasis)

Stones (**calculi**) begin in the pelvis of the kidney as a tiny grain of undissolved material, usually a mineral called calcium oxalate *(Figure 6.4)*. When the urine flows out of the kidney, the grain of material is left behind. Over time, more material is deposited and a stone is formed. The presence of stones is called **nephrolithiasis**.

Most stones enter the ureter while they are still small enough to pass down the ureter into the bladder and out of the body in urine. The passage of urine can be described as **urination**, **micturition**, or **voiding**. Treatment options for renal calculi are

- **Watchful waiting**. With pain medication to relieve symptoms, the hope is that the stone can be passed.
- **ESWL**. A machine called a **lithotripter** produces shock waves that crumble the stone into small pieces that can pass down the ureter.
- **Ureteroscopy**. A small, flexible **ureteroscope** is passed through the urethra and bladder into the ureter. Devices can be passed through the endoscope to remove or fragment the stone.
- **Percutaneous nephrolithotomy**. A **nephroscope** is inserted through the skin and into the kidney to locate and remove the stone.
- **Open surgery**. A surgical incision is made to expose the ureter and remove the stone; this is rarely done.

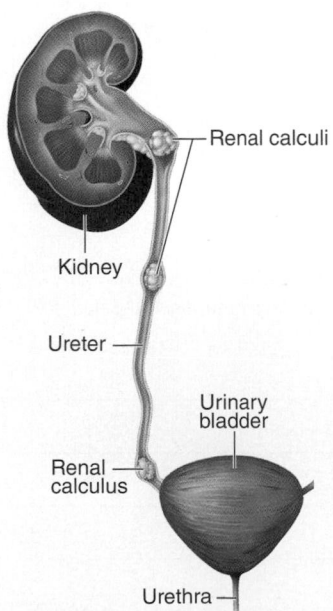

Renal calculi

Kidney

Ureter

Urinary bladder

Renal calculus

Urethra

▲ **Figure 6.4** **Renal Calculi.** Calculi can become lodged at different sites in the ureters.

WORD	PRONUNCIATION	ELEMENTS		DEFINITION
calculus calculi (pl)	**KAL**-kyu-lus **KAL**-kyu-lie		Latin *pebble*	Small stone
extracorporeal	**EKS**-trah-kor-**POH**-ree-al	S/ P/ R/CF	-al *pertaining to* extra- *outside, out of* -corpor/e- *body*	Outside the body
hydronephrosis	**HIGH**-droh-neh-**FRO**-sis	S/ P/ R/CF	-osis *condition* hydro- *water* -nephr/o- *kidney*	Dilation of pelvis and calyces of a kidney
hydronephrotic (adj)	**HIGH**-droh-neh-**FROT**-ik	S/	-tic *pertaining to*	Pertaining to or suffering from the dilation of the pelvis and calyces of the kidney
lithotripsy	**LITH**-oh-trip-see	S/ R/CF	-tripsy *to crush* lith/o- *stone*	Crushing stones by sound waves
lithotripter	**LITH**-oh-trip-ter	S/	-tripter *crusher*	Instrument that generates sound waves
nephrolithiasis	**NEF**-roe-lih-**THIGH**-ah-sis	S/ R/CF R/	-iasis *condition* nephr/o- *kidney* -lith- *stone*	Presence of a kidney stone
nephrolithotomy	**NEF**-roe-lih-**THOT**-oh-me	S/ R/CF R/CF	-tomy *surgical incision* nephr/o- *kidney* -lith/o- *stone*	Incision for removal of a renal stone
nephroscope	**NEF**-roe-skope	S/ R/CF	-scope *instrument for viewing* nephr/o- *kidney*	Endoscope to view the inside of the kidney
nephroscopy	neh-**FROS**-koh-pee	S/	-scopy *to view, examine*	Visual examination of the kidney
peristalsis	per-ih-**STAL**-sis	P/ R/	peri- *around* -stalsis *constrict*	Waves of alternate contraction and relaxation along a tube to move its contents onward.
peristaltic (adj) pyelogram	per-ih-**STAL**-tik **PIE**-el-oh gram	S/ S/ R/CF	-tic *pertaining to* -gram *a record, recording* pyel/o- *renal pelvis*	Relating to peristalsis X-ray image of renal pelvis and ureters
reflux	**REE**-fluks	P/ R/	re- *back* -flux *flow*	Backward flow
spasmodic (**Note:** One "m" is taken out.)	spaz-**MOD**-ik	S/ R/ R/	-ic *pertaining to* spasm- *spasm* -mod- *nature, form*	Having intermittent spasms or contractions
ureteroscope	you-**REE**-ter-oh-scope	S/ R/CF	-scope *instrument for viewing* ureter/o- *ureter*	Endoscope to view the inside of the ureter
ureteroscopy	you-**REE**-ter-os-koh-pee	S/	-scopy *to view, examine*	Examination of the ureter

Exercises

A. After reading both parts of Case Report 6.2, answer the following questions. *Be prepared to discuss your answers in class.*   **LO 6.3, 6.6, 6.7, 6.8**

1. If Mr. Leandro's pain had a "sudden onset," is it acute or chronic? _____

2. What were Mr. Leandro's presenting symptoms?

_____

_____

3. What was the IV for? _____

4. What diagnostic tests did Mr. Leandro have? _____

5. What element in *hydronephrosis* indicates fluid is involved? _____

6. Is ESWL an invasive procedure? _____

> *Study Hint*
>
> Review the WAD again. Find the suffixes *ic* and *tic* which both mean *pertaining to*. Add these to your list.

Abbreviations

AIDS	acquired immunodeficiency syndrome
HIV	human immunodeficiency virus
UTI	urinary tract infection

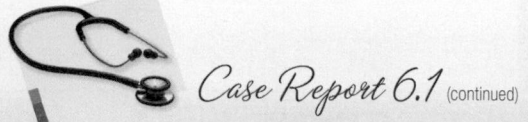

Case Report 6.1 (continued)

Mr. Nelson Hughes had been well until a few months before his surgery, when he noticed a vague, aching pain in his left loin. One week before surgery, he suddenly passed bright red urine. Urinalysis showed red blood cells (RBCs) (**hematuria**). Physical examination revealed an enlarged left kidney. IVP and other imaging tests showed a tumor 3 inches in diameter in the center of the left kidney. Bone scan was normal, indicating no metastases to bone.

Keynotes

- Of all renal cancers, 25% to 30% relate directly to smoking.
- As little as 1mL of blood will turn the urine red.
- Hematuria can be caused by a lesion anywhere in the urinary system.
- The acute form of glomerulonephritis has a 100% recovery rate.
- Acute interstitial nephritis causes 15% of cases of acute renal failure.

LO 6.6, 6.7, 6.8 Disorders of the Kidneys

Renal cell carcinoma is the most common form of kidney cancer and occurs twice as often in men as in women. The cancer develops in the lining cells of the renal tubules, which is why Mr. Hughes had hematuria. Radical **nephrectomy** is the most common treatment for renal cell carcinoma.

Wilms tumor, or **nephroblastoma**, is a malignant kidney tumor of childhood, usually appearing between ages 3 and 8 years, that is treated effectively with a combination of surgery and chemotherapy.

Benign kidney tumors, such as **renal adenoma**, are usually asymptomatic, are discovered incidentally, and are not life-threatening.

Hematuria, blood in the urine, can be caused by lesions anywhere in the urinary system; this includes trauma (including long-distance running), infections, medications (such as quinine and phenytoin), and congenital diseases (such as sickle cell anemia). In **microscopic hematuria**, the urine is not red, and red blood cells can be seen only under a microscope or identified by a urine dipstick. Normal urine contains no blood. Excessive consumption of beets, rhubarb, and red food coloring can cause urine to be colored red. This is not hematuria. Also, in the collection of urine from a woman during menstruation, the urine can be contaminated with blood, giving the impression of hematuria.

Acute glomerulonephritis is an inflammation of the glomerulus. It damages the glomerular capillaries, allows protein and red blood cells to leak into the urine, and interferes with the clearance of waste products. In its acute form, it can develop rapidly after an episode of strep throat infection, most often in children. The *Streptococcus* bacteria do not invade the kidney but stimulate the immune system to overproduce antibodies that damage the glomeruli.

Chronic glomerulonephritis can occur with no history of kidney disease and present as kidney failure. It also occurs in **diabetic nephropathy** and can be associated with autoimmune diseases such as lupus erythematosus; HIV can cause glomerular disease even before developing into AIDS.

Nephrotic syndrome involves large amounts of protein leaking out into the urine so that the level of protein in the blood falls. In children it nearly always responds to treatment with steroids. The causes of nephrotic syndrome are described in *Table 6.1*. The most obvious symptom is fluid retention with edema of the ankles and legs. This is treated with **diuretics**, restriction of salt in the diet, and reduction of fluid intake.

Interstitial nephritis is an inflammation of the spaces between the renal tubules. Most often it is acute and temporary. It can be an allergic reaction to or a side effect of drugs such as penicillin or ampicillin, NSAIDs, and diuretics. Treatment is directed to the underlying disease. Temporary **dialysis** may be necessary.

Pyelonephritis is an infection of the renal pelvis. Most often it occurs as part of a total **urinary tract infection (UTI)**, commencing in the urinary bladder. It has a high mortality rate in the elderly and in people with a compromised immune system (*see Chapter 15*). It requires aggressive antibiotic therapy.

Table 6.1 Types of Nephrotic Syndrome

Disease (as Seen on Biopsy)	Description
Minimal change disease	Most common in children; responds to steroids
Focal segmental glomerulosclerosis (FSGS)	Cause unknown; little response to treatment
Membranous nephropathy	Cause unknown; may respond to immunosuppressive treatment
Diabetes	Occurs if blood sugar has been poorly controlled

WORD	PRONUNCIATION	ELEMENTS		DEFINITION
dialysis	die-**AL**-ih-sis	R/ P/	**-lysis** *to separate* **dia-** *complete*	An artificial method of filtration to remove excess waste materials and water from the body
diuretic (adj)	die-you-**RET**-ik	S/ P/ R/	**-etic** *pertaining to* **di-** *complete (from dia)* **-ur-** *urinary system*	Agent that increases urine output
diuresis (noun)	die-you-**REE**-sis	S/	**-esis** *abnormal condition*	Excretion of large volumes of urine
glomerulonephritis	glo-**MER**-you-low-nef-**RYE**-tis	S/ R/CF R/	**-itis** *inflammation* **glomerul/o-** *glomerulus* **-nephr-** *kidney*	Infection of the glomeruli of the kidney
hematuria	he-mah-**TYU**-ree-ah	S/ R/	**-uria** *urine* **hemat-** *blood*	Blood in the urine
interstitial	in-ter-**STISH**-al	S/ P/ R/	**-ial** *pertaining to* **inter-** *between* **-stit-** *space*	Pertaining to the spaces between cells in a tissue or organ
nephritis	neh-**FRY**-tis	S/ R/	**-itis** *inflammation* **nephr-** *kidney*	Inflammation of the kidney
nephropathy	neh-**FROP**-ah-thee	S/ R/CF	**-pathy** *disease* **nephr/o-** *kidney*	Any disease of the kidney
nephrotic syndrome	neh-**FROT**-ik **SIN**-drome	S/ R/CF	**-tic** *pertaining to* **nephr/o-** *kidney*	Glomerular disease with marked loss of protein
nephrosis (syn)	neh-**FRO**-sis	S/	**-osis** *condition*	
pyelonephritis	**PIE**-eh-loh-neh-**FRY**-tis	S/ R/CF R/	**-itis** *inflammation* **pyel/o-** *renal pelvis* **-nephr-** *kidney*	Inflammation of the kidney and renal pelvis
Wilms tumor	**WILMZ TOO**-mor		Max Wilms, 1867–1918, German surgeon	Cancerous kidney tumor of childhood
nephroblastoma (syn)	**NEF**-roh-blas-**TOE**-mah	S/ R/CF R/	**-oma** *tumor, mass* **nephr/o-** *kidney* **-blast-** *embryonic, immature cell*	

Exercises

A. After reading Case Report 6.1, answer the following questions. *Be prepared to discuss your answers in class.*   **LO 6.3, 6.6, 6.7, 6.8**

1. Define the term *loin*. Use a dictionary if you are not sure of the meaning.

_____

2. "Bright red urine" would indicate the presence of _____ in the urine.

3. What were Mr. Hughes' symptoms?

_____

4. What diagnostic tests has Mr. Hughes had so far?

_____

5. What is the good news for Mr. Hughes?

_____

B. Hematuria is a common urinary disorder. *Normal urine contains no blood. What can cause the presence of blood in the urine?*   **LO 6.8, 6.9**

1. _____

2. _____

3. _____

4. _____

5. _____

LO 6.6, 6.7, 6.8 Disorders of the Kidneys (continued)

Hypertension, with its high blood pressure, can damage the renal arterioles and glomeruli, causing them to thicken and narrow. This reduces their capability to remove wastes and excess water, which can cause the blood pressure (BP) to rise even more. If the cause of hypertension is not known, it is called **primary (or essential) hypertension** *(see Chapter 10)*.

Polycystic kidney disease (PKD) is an inherited disease. Large, fluid-filled cysts grow within the kidneys and press against the kidney tissue. Finally, the kidneys cannot function effectively.

Acute renal failure (ARF) makes the kidneys suddenly stop filtering waste products from the blood. The signs and symptoms can include **oliguria** (reduction of urine output), **anuria** (cessation of urine output), confusion, seizures, and coma.

The causes of acute renal failure include

- **Severe burns**, **trauma**, or **complicated surgery**—with a drastic drop in blood pressure and the release of myoglobin from injured muscles *(see Chapter 14)*. Myoglobin lodges in the renal tubules and blocks the flow of urine.

- **Drugs**—including pain medications such as aspirin and ibuprofen, antibiotics such as streptomycin and gentamicin, and contrast dyes used in angiography.

- **Toxins**—such as heavy metals (mercury is one) and excessive alcohol.

- **Systemic infections**—septicemia.

- **Blood disorders**—such as **idiopathic thrombocytopenic purpura (ITP)** or **disseminated intravascular coagulation (DIC)** *(see Chapter 11)*.

In treatment of ARF, the goal is to treat the underlying disease. Dialysis may be necessary while the kidneys are healing.

Chronic renal failure (CRF), or **chronic kidney disease (CKD)**, is a gradual loss of renal function. Symptoms and signs may not appear until kidney function is less than 25% of normal.

The causes of chronic renal failure include

- **Diabetes**—type 1 and type 2 *(see Chapter 17)*; **hypertension**; **kidney diseases**; **lead poisoning**.

Azotemia is the buildup of nitrogenous waste products in the blood. **Uremia** is the complex of symptoms resulting from excess nitrogenous waste products in the blood, as seen in renal failure.

End-stage renal disease (ESRD) means the kidneys are functioning at less than 10% of their normal capacity. At this point, life cannot be sustained, and either dialysis or kidney **transplant** is needed.

Dialysis is an artificial method of removing waste materials and excess fluid from the blood. It is not a cure but can prolong life. There are several types of kidney dialysis:

- **Hemodialysis** *(Figure 6.5)* filters the blood through an artificial kidney machine (**dialyzer**). Most patients require 12 hours of hemodialysis a week, usually in three sessions.

- **Peritoneal dialysis** uses a dialysis solution that is infused into and drained out of your abdominal cavity through a small, flexible, **implanted** catheter. The dialysis solution extracts wastes and excess fluid from the network of capillaries in the peritoneal lining of the abdominal cavity.

- **Continuous ambulatory peritoneal dialysis (CAPD)** is performed by the patient at home through an implanted abdominal catheter *(Figure 6.6)*, usually four times a day, 7 days a week.

- **Continuous cycling peritoneal dialysis** uses a machine to automatically infuse dialysis solution into and out of the abdominal cavity during sleep.

A **kidney transplant** provides a better quality of life than dialysis—if a suitable donor can be found. The donor has to match the recipient's blood type, cell surface proteins, and antibodies *(see Chapter 12)*. A **sibling** or a blood relative can often qualify as a donor. If not, tissue banks across the country can search for a kidney from an accident victim or a donor who has died.

Keynotes

- Acute renal failure is usually reversible.

- Chronic renal failure has no cure.

Abbreviations

ARF	acute renal failure
CAPD	continuous ambulatory peritoneal dialysis
CKD	chronic kidney disease; also known as chronic renal failure
CRF	chronic renal failure; also known as chronic kidney disease
DIC	disseminated intravascular coagulation
ESRD	end-stage renal disease
ITP	idiopathic thrombocytopenic purpura
PKD	polycystic kidney disease

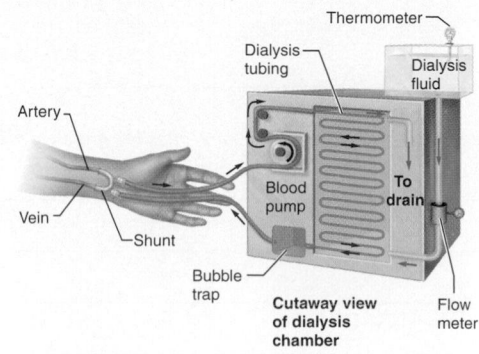

▲ **Figure 6.5** Hemodialysis.

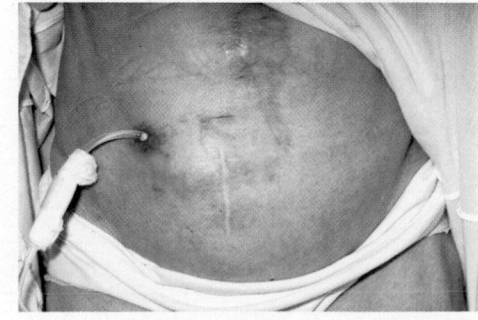

▲ **Figure 6.6** Continuous Ambulatory Peritoneal Dialysis.

WORD	PRONUNCIATION	ELEMENTS		DEFINITION
anuria	an-**YOU**-ree-ah	P/ R/	an- *lack of, without* -uria *urine*	Absence of urine production
azotemia	azo-**TEE**-me-ah	S/ R/	-emia *blood condition* azot- *nitrogen*	Excess nitrogenous waste products in the blood
hemodialysis	**HE**-moh-die-**AL**-ih-sis	P/ R/CF R/	-dia- *complete* hem/o- *blood* -lysis *to separate*	An artificial method of filtration to remove excess waste materials and water directly from the blood
implant	im-**PLANT**	P/ R/	im- *in* -plant *insert or plant*	To insert material into tissues, or the material inserted into tissues
oliguria	ol-ih-**GYUR**-ee-ah	P/ R/	olig- *scanty* -uria *urine*	Scanty production of urine
polycystic	pol-ee-**SIS**-tik	S/ P/ R/	-ic *pertaining to* poly- *many* -cyst- *bladder, cyst*	Composed of many cysts
sibling	**SIB**-ling	S/ R/	-ling *small* sib- *relative*	Brother or sister
transplant	**TRANZ**-plant	P/ R/	trans- *across* -plant *insert, plant*	The act of transferring tissue from one person to another
uremia	you-**REE**-me-ah	S/ R/	-emia *blood condition* ur- *urinary system*	The complex of symptoms arising from renal failure

Exercises

A. Build your knowledge of the elements contained in the *language of urology*. *Specific elements in each term are underlined. Identify the type of element, and provide a meaning for the element. Fill in the blanks.* **LO 6.3, 6.6, 6.7**

Term	Type of Element (P, R, CF, S)	Meaning of Element	Meaning of Term
anuria	1. _____	2. _____	3. _____
hemodialysis	4. _____	5. _____	6. _____
azot**emia**	7. _____	8. _____	9. _____
trans**plant**	10. _____	11. _____	12. _____
oliguria	13. _____	14. _____	15. _____
polycystic	16. _____	17. _____	18. _____
ur**emia**	19. _____	20. _____	21. _____

Remember: Every element at the beginning of a medical term is not necessarily a prefix!

22. Give an example from this exercise: _____

B. Employ the *language of urology* to answer the following questions. **LO 6.7**

1. Hemodialysis is used as a treatment for a major problem in the urinary system. Exactly what does hemodialysis do?

_____

_____

2. Name the other types of kidney dialysis. _____

The urinary bladder is a temporary storage place for urine before it is voided through the urethra. A moderately full bladder contains about 500 mL (1 pint) of urine. The maximum capacity of the bladder is around 750 to 800 mL (1.5 pints). Urination, or emptying of the bladder, is also called *micturition* or *voiding*. The information in this lesson will enable you to use correct medical terminology to:

6.2.1 Describe the structure and functions of the urinary bladder.

6.2.2 Contrast the differences in structure of the male and female urethras.

6.2.3 Explain the greater incidence of urinary tract infections in the female.

6.2.4 Discuss common disorders of the bladder and urethra.

You are

. . . a medical assistant working in the office of Dr. Susan Lee, a primary care physician at Fulwood Medical Center.

Your patient is

. . . Mrs. Caroline Dobson, a 32-year-old housewife. You have asked her to describe the reason for her visit to the office today.

Case Report 6.3

Patient Interview

Mrs. Dobson:

"Since yesterday afternoon I've had a lot of pain low down in my belly and in my lower back. I keep having to go to the bathroom every hour or so to pee. It's often difficult to start, and it burns as it comes out. I've had this problem twice before when I was pregnant with my two kids, so I've started drinking cranberry juice. I've been shivering since I woke up this morning, and the last urine I passed was pink. Was that due to the cranberry juice?"

At the end of this chapter you will be asked to document (using medical terminology) Mrs. Dobson's **history of her present illness (HPI)** and to detail any further questions you have for her.

Abbreviation	
HPI	history of present illness

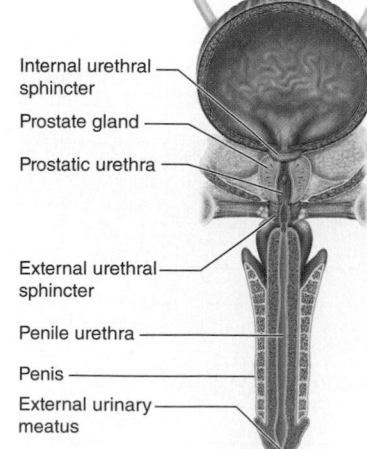

▲ **Figure 6.7** Male Urinary Bladder and Urethra.

Labels:
- Internal urethral sphincter
- Prostate gland
- Prostatic urethra
- External urethral sphincter
- Penile urethra
- Penis
- External urinary meatus

LO 6.1, 6.2 Urinary Bladder and Urethra

The **urinary bladder** is a hollow, muscular organ on the floor of the pelvic cavity, posterior to the pubic symphysis *(Figure 6.7)*. When the bladder is distended, it rises upward and can be palpated above the symphysis pubis.

Urethra

The final passageway for the urine to escape to the outside is the urethra, a thin-walled tube that takes urine from the floor of the bladder to the outside. At the base of the bladder, the muscular wall is thickened to form the **internal urethral sphincter**. As the urethra passes through the skeletal muscles of the pelvic floor, the **external urethral sphincter** provides voluntary control of micturition.

In the female *(see Figure 6.9)*, the urethra is only about 1.5 inches long, and it opens to the outside anterior to the vagina. In the male *(Figure 6.7)*, the urethra is 7 to 8 inches in length and passes through the penis. In both the male and the female, the opening of the urethra to the outside is called the **external urinary meatus**.

Micturition

When the bladder contains about 200 mL of urine, stretch receptors in its wall trigger the **micturition reflex**. However, voluntary control of the external sphincter can keep that sphincter contracted and can hold urine in the bladder until you decide to urinate. Involuntary micturition during sleep in older children or adults is called **enuresis**.

WORD	PRONUNCIATION	ELEMENTS		DEFINITION
enuresis	en-you-**REE**-sis	S/ R/	-esis *abnormal condition* enur- *urinate*	Bed-wetting; urinary incontinence
meatus	me-**AY**-tus		Latin *a passage*	The external opening of a passage
micturition	mik-choo-**RISH**-un	S/ R/	-ition *process* mictur- *pass urine*	Act of passing urine
micturate	**MIK**-choo-rate	S/	-ate *composed of, pertaining to*	Pass urine
reflex	**REE**-fleks		Latin *to bend back*	An involuntary response to a stimulus
sphincter	**SFINK**-ter		Greek *band*	Band of muscle that encircles an opening; when the muscle contracts, the opening squeezes closed
void	VOYD		Latin *to empty*	To evacuate urine or feces

Exercises

A. After reading Case Report 6.3 on the opposite page, answer the following questions. *Be prepared to discuss your answers in class.*   **LO 6.3, 6.6**

1. List all of Mrs. Dobson's "presenting" symptoms. (What symptoms does she have when she comes to the doctor?)

   _____

   _____

2. Has she ever had this condition before? If so, when? _____

3. Insert medical terms for the following phrases from CR 6.3:

   "in my **belly**" _____

   "every hour or so to **pee**" _____

   "I've been **shivering**" _____

4. If the last urine Mrs. Dobson passed was pink, what might be present in her urine now? _____

5. What is the medical term for that condition? _____

6. Right now, is this an acute or chronic condition for Mrs. Dobson? _____

7. How long has Mrs. Dobson had this pain? _____

8. What remedy did Mrs. Dobson try at home? _____

9. What is the difference between micturation and urination? _____

10. To void means to _____

B. Fill out the meanings of these abbreviations and *identify the one abbreviation* that does NOT pertain to the urinary system.   LO 6.5

1. TNM means _____ Applies _____ Does Not Apply _____

2. IVP means _____ Applies _____ Does Not Apply _____

3. ESWL means _____ Applies _____ Does Not Apply _____

4. CV means _____ Applies _____ Does Not Apply _____

5. KUB means _____ Applies _____ Does Not Apply _____

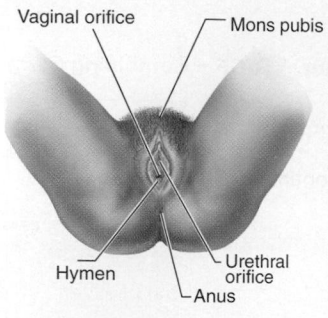

Vaginal orifice — Mons pubis

Hymen — Urethral orifice

Anus

▲ **Figure 6.8** Female External Genitalia.

Ureter

Ureteral openings

Internal urethral sphincter

External urethral sphincter

External urethral orifice

▲ **Figure 6.9** Female Urinary Bladder and Urethra.

Keynotes

- Ten million doctor visits each year are for UTIs.

- Aging itself is not a cause of urinary incontinence.

- Incontinence is not a way of life. It can be helped.

- Cigarette smoking contributes to more than 50% of bladder cancers.

- Bladder cancer is more common in men than women. It is the fourth most common cancer in men and the eighth in women (see Chapter 20).

LO 6.6, 6.7 Disorders of the Urinary Bladder and Urethra

Urinary Tract Infection

A **urinary tract infection (UTI)** occurs when bacteria invade and multiply in the urinary tract. The **portal** of entry for the bacteria is through the urethra. Because the female urethra is shorter than the male urethra and opens to the surface near the anus *(Figure 6.8)*, bacteria from the **gastrointestinal (GI)** tract can more easily invade the female urethra. This is why women are more prone than men to UTIs. Once UTIs have occurred, they often recur.

Infection of the urethra is called **urethritis**; infection of the urinary bladder is cystitis. If **cystitis** is untreated, infection can spread up the ureters to the renal pelvis, causing **pyelitis**, and carry on to reach the renal cortex and nephrons, causing **pyelonephritis**.

The diagnosis can be made through urinalysis. Culture of the organism and testing of its sensitivity to different antibiotics enables appropriate antibiotic therapy to be prescribed. Cranberry juice makes the urine more acid so that bacteria have difficulty multiplying, and chemicals in the juice make the bladder more slippery so that bacteria can't stick to it.

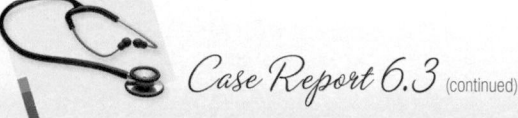

Case Report 6.3 (continued)

Mrs. Dobson described many of the symptoms of cystitis. She had **suprapubic** and low-back pain. She had increased **frequency** of micturition with **dysuria** and had difficulty in and burning on micturition. Her pink urine is probably hematuria.

Urinary Incontinence

Loss of control of your bladder is called **urinary incontinence**. The result is wet clothes. About 12 million adults in America have urinary incontinence. It is most common in women over the age of 50 years.

There are four types of urinary incontinence:

- **Stress incontinence.** Urine leaks because of sudden pressure on the lower stomach muscles when you cough, laugh, sneeze, lift something heavy, or exercise. It is most common in women, with previous pregnancy and childbirth being risk factors.

- **Urge incontinence.** The need to urinate comes on too fast for you to get to the toilet. It is often **idiopathic** but can be associated with UTI, diabetes, stroke, Alzheimer and Parkinson disease, or bladder cancer.

- **Overflow incontinence.** Small amounts of urine leak from a bladder that is always full because you cannot empty it. This occurs when an enlarged prostate gland or tumor blocks the outflow of urine from the bladder. It also occurs in spinal cord injuries and as a side effect of some medications.

- **Functional incontinence.** You cannot get to the toilet in time because of arthritis or any other disease that makes moving quickly difficult.

Treatment depends on the cause. If a medical or surgical problem is present, then the incontinence can go away when the problem is treated. **Bladder training** and **biofeedback** lengthen the time between the urges to go to the toilet. **Kegel exercises** strengthen the muscles of the pelvic floor. Medications, for example oxybutynin, are used for urge incontinence. Surgery can pull up the bladder and secure it if pelvic floor muscles are weak **(cystopexy)**. Absorbent underclothing is available.

Urinary retention is the abnormal, involuntary holding of urine in the bladder. **Acute retention** can be caused by an obstruction in the urinary system; for example, an enlarged prostate in the male *(see Chapter 7)* or neurologic problems such as multiple sclerosis. It can be a side effect of anticholinergic drugs that include tricyclic antidepressants *(see Chapter 18)*. **Chronic retention** can be caused by untreated obstructions in the urinary tract such as an enlarged prostate.

Transitional cell carcinoma is the most common type of bladder cancer, arising in the transitional cells of the lining of the bladder.

A primary symptom of bladder cancer is hematuria. Bladder cancer is diagnosed by

- **Urinalysis** to detect microscopic hematuria.

- **NMP22® BladderChek®**, which detects elevated levels of a specific protein in the urine even in the early stages of cancer.

- **Imaging tests**, such as IVP, CT scan, MRI scan, and ultrasound.

- **Cystoscopy with biopsy**, which is the definitive test.

The cancer is **staged** using the **tumor, node, metastasis (TNM) system** *(see Chapter 20)*.

Word Analysis and Definition

S = Suffix   P = Prefix   R = Root   R/CF = Combining Form

WORD	PRONUNCIATION	ELEMENTS		DEFINITION
cystitis	sis-**TIE**-tis	S/ R/	-itis *inflammation* cyst- *bladder*	Inflammation of the urinary bladder
cystopexy	**SIS**-toh-pek-see	S/ R/CF	-pexy *surgical fixation* cyst/o- *bladder*	Surgical procedure to support the urinary bladder
cystoscope	**SIS**-toh-skope	S/ R/CF	-scope *instrument for viewing* cyst/o- *bladder*	An endoscope inserted to view the inside of the bladder
cystoscopy	sis-**TOS**-koh-pee	S/	-scopy *to examine*	The process of using a cystoscope
dysuria	dis-**YOU**-ree-ah	S/ P/ R/	-ia *condition* dys- *bad, difficult* -ur- *urinary system*	Difficulty or pain with urination
frequency	**FREE**-kwen-see	S/ R/	-ency *state of, quality of* frequ- *repeated, often*	The number of times something happens in a given time (e.g., passing urine)
idiopathic	**ID**-ih-oh-**PATH**-ik	S/ R/CF R/	-ic *pertaining to* idi/o- *personal, distinct* -path- *disease*	Pertaining to a disease of unknown etiology
incontinence	in-**KON**-tin-ence	S/ P/ R/	-ence *state of, quality of* in- *in* -contin- *hold together*	Inability to prevent discharge of urine or feces
incontinent	in-**KON**-tin-ent	S/	-ent *pertaining to, end result*	Denoting incontinence
Kegel exercises	**KEG**-al **EKS**-er-size-ez		Arnold Kegel, 1894–1981, American gynecologist	Contraction and relaxation of the pelvic floor muscles to improve urethral and rectal sphincter function
portal	**POR**-tal		Latin *gate*	The vein that brings blood from the intestines to the liver
pyelitis	pie-eh-**LYE**-tis	S/ R/	-itis *inflammation* pyel- *renal pelvis*	Inflammation of renal pelvis
retention	ree-**TEN**-shun		Latin *hold back*	A holding in of what should normally be discharged (e.g., urine)
stage	**STAJ**		Latin *status, to stand*	A description of the distribution and extent of dissemination of a cancer disease process
suprapubic	**SOO**-prah-pyu-bik	S/ P/ R/	-ic *pertaining to* supra- *above* -pub- *pubis*	Above the symphysis pubis

Exercises

A. After reading Case Report 6.3 on the opposite page, answer the following questions. *Be prepared to discuss your answers in class.*
LO 6.3, 6.6, 6.7

1. What organ in Mrs. Dobson's urinary system has become infected?

_____

2. What is the difference between a UTI and a URI?

UTI: _____   Body system: _____

URI: _____   Body system: _____

3. *Micturition* can also be termed _____ and _____.

4. Name two terms ending in *uria* that are Mrs. Dobson's symptoms.   _____/uria   and   _____/uria

B. Identify in each of the following medical terms exactly which body organ is infected.   LO 6.3, 6.6

1. nephritis   _____
2. cystitis   _____
3. glomerulonephritis   _____

4. pyelonephritis   _____
5. pyelitis   _____
6. urethritis   _____

7. (True or false) The terms in 1-6 above all relate to a diagnosis.   T   F   Circle the correct answer.

LO 6.8, 6.9, 6.10 Diagnostic Procedures

Urinalysis

A **dipstick** (a plastic strip bearing paper squares of reagent) is the most cost-effective method of screening urine *(Figure 6.10)*. After the stick is dipped in the urine specimen, the color change in each segment of the dipstick is compared to a color chart on the container. Dipsticks can screen for pH, specific gravity, protein, blood, glucose, ketones, bilirubin, **nitrite**, and leukocyte esterase (see the following).

Routine urinalysis (UA) in the laboratory can include the following tests:

- **Visual observation** examines **color** and **clarity**. Normal urine is pale yellow or amber in color and clear. Cloudiness indicates excess cells or cellular material. Red and cloudy indicates red blood cells.
- **Odor** of normal urine has a slight "nutty" scent. Infected urine has a foul odor. **Ketosis** gives urine a fruity odor.

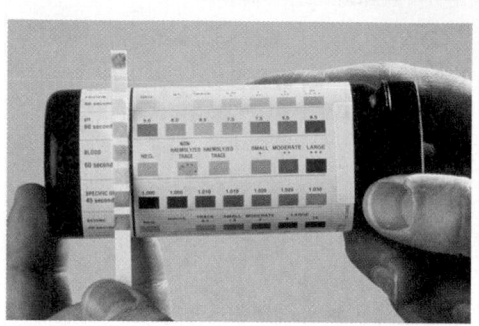

▲ **Figure 6.10** Urinalysis Dipstick Being Compared Against Color Chart on Container.

- **pH** measures how acidic or alkaline urine is *(see Chapter 4)*.
- **Specific gravity (SG)** measures how dilute or concentrated the urine is.
- **Protein** is not detected normally in urine. Its presence **(proteinuria)** indicates infection or urinary tract disease.
- **Glucose** in the urine **(glycosuria)** is a spillover into the urine when the nephrons are damaged or diseased or blood sugar is high in uncontrolled diabetes.
- **Ketones** are present in the urine in **diabetic ketoacidosis** *(see Chapter 17)* or in starvation.
- **Leukocyte esterase** indicates the presence of white blood cells (WBCs) in the urine, which in turn can indicate a UTI.
- **Urine culture** from a clean-catch specimen is the definitive test for a UTI.

Microscopic urinalysis is performed on the solids deposited by centrifuging a specimen of urine. It can reveal

- **Red blood cells (RBCs)**, **WBCs**, renal tubular epithelial cells stuck together to form **casts**, WBCs stuck together to form casts, and bacteria.

Other Diagnostic Procedures

- **KUB**. An x-ray of the abdomen shows the kidneys, ureters, and bladder.
- **IVP**. A contrast material containing iodine is injected intravenously, and its progress through the urinary tract is then recorded on a series of rapid x-ray images.
- **Retrograde pyelogram**. Contrast material is injected through a urinary catheter into the ureters to locate stones and other obstructions.
- **Voiding cystourethrogram (VCUG)**. Contrast material is inserted into the bladder through a catheter and x-rays are taken as the patient voids.
- **Computed tomography (CT) scan**. X-ray images show cross-sectional views of the kidneys and bladder.
- **Magnetic Resonance Imaging (MRI)**. Magnetic fields are used to generate cross-sectional images of the urinary tract.
- **Ultrasound imaging**. High-frequency sound waves and a computer generate noninvasive images of kidneys.
- **Renal angiogram**. X-rays with contrast material are used to assess blood flow to the kidneys.
- **Cystoscopy**. A pencil-thin, flexible, tubelike optical instrument is inserted through the urethra into the bladder to examine directly the lining of the bladder and to take a biopsy if needed.

Abbreviations	
CT	computed tomography
MRI	magnetic resonance imaging
SG	specific gravity
UA	urinalysis
VCUG	voiding cystourethrogram

LO 6.11 Methods of Urine Collection

- **Random collection** is taken with no precautions regarding contamination. It is often used for collecting samples for drug testing.
- **Early morning collection** is used to determine the ability of the kidneys to concentrate urine following overnight dehydration.
- **Clean-catch, midstream specimen** is collected after the external urethral meatus is cleaned. The first part of the urine is passed, and a sterile collecting vessel is introduced into the urinary stream to collect the last part.
- **Twenty-four-hour collection** is used to determine the amount of protein being excreted and to estimate the kidneys' filtration ability.
- **Suprapubic transabdominal needle aspiration** of the bladder is used in newborns and small infants to obtain a pure sample of urine.
- **Catheterization of the bladder** can be used as a last resort to obtain a urine specimen. A soft plastic or rubber tube (catheter) is inserted through the urethra into the bladder to drain and collect urine.

WORD	PRONUNCIATION	ELEMENTS		DEFINITION
cast	KAST		Latin *pure*	A cylindrical mold formed by materials in kidney tubules
cystourethrogram	sis-toh-you-**REETH**-roe-gram	S/ R/CF R/CF	-gram *a record* cyst/o- *bladder* -urethr/o- *urethra*	X-ray image during voiding to show structure and function of bladder and urethra
glycosuria (*Note:* The "s" is added to make the word flow.)	GLYE-koh-**SYU**-ree-ah	S/ R/CF R/	-ia *condition* glyc/o- *glucose* -ur- *urinary system*	Presence of glucose in urine
ketone **ketosis**	**KEY**-tone key-**TOE**-sis	S/ R/CF R/CF	Greek *acetone* -sis *condition* ket/o- *ketones* -acid/o- *acid, low pH*	Chemical formed in uncontrolled diabetes or in starvation Excess production of ketones
ketoacidosis	**KEY**-toe-as-ih-**DOE**-sis			Excessive production of ketones, making the blood acidic
nitrite	**NI**-trite		Greek *niter, saltpeter*	Chemical formed in urine by *Escherichia coli (E.Coli)* and other microorganisms
proteinuria	pro-tee-**NYU**-ree-ah	R/ R/	-uria *urine* protein- *protein*	Presence of protein in urine
retrograde	**RET**-roh-grade	P/ R/	retro- *backward* -grade *going*	Reversal of a normal flow; for example, back from the bladder into the ureters
urinalysis	you-rih-**NAL**-ih-sis	S/ R/CF	-lysis *to separate* urin/a- *urine*	Examination of urine to separate it into its elements and define their kind and/or quantity

Exercises

A. Apply your knowledge of medical language to this exercise. *All the questions can be answered using terms from this spread. Circle the best answer.* **LO 6.8, 6.9, 6.10, 6.11**

1. An x-ray image taken during voiding:

   retrograde   pyelogram   KUB   cystourethrogram

2. Presence of sugar in urine:

   hematuria   polyuria   glycosuria

3. Reversal of normal flow:

   reflex   retrograde   regenerate

4. Excessive ketones in the blood, making it acidic:

   ketosis   ketoacidosis   ketone

5. Separating urine into its elements:

   urinalysis   cystourethrogram   retrograde   pyelogram

Urinary System

Challenge Your Knowledge

A. Brain teaser. Taken directly from your text: "The peristaltic waves are intermittent, which is why Justin's pain was spasmodic." (**LO 6.3,** *Remember*)

1. Define **peristaltic.** _____

2. Which previous body system that you have already studied in this textbook also mentions peristalsis? _____

   Is it the same type of process? _____

B. System review. Understanding the structure and function of the urinary system will give you a better grasp of the terminology. Circle the correct answers to the following questions. (**LO 6.1, 6.2, 6.3,** *Remember*)

1. Where does waste-laden blood enter the kidney?

   a. the fascia   **d.** the renal vein

   b. the glomerulus   **e.** the portal vein

   c. the hilum

2. The medical term to describe urine being forced back up the ureter to the kidneys is

   a. reflux   **d.** absorption

   b. filtration   **e.** micturition

   c. excretion

3. What results if the kidney produces too much renin?

   a. hematuria   **d.** anuria

   b. oliguria   **e.** secondary hypertension

   c. primary hypertension

4. What is the end product of nitrogen metabolism?

   a. ammonia   **d.** nitrates

   b. nitrogen   **e.** renin

   c. urea

5. What do urethritis, cystitis, pyelitis, and pyelonephritis all have in common?

   a. infection   **d.** the same root

   b. skin rash   **e.** the same diagnosis

   c. the same prefix

6. Each kidney is the size of a(n)

   a. orange   **d.** bean

   b. golf ball   **e.** ping-pong ball

   c. clenched fist

7. What protects the kidney?

   a. adipose tissue   **d.** cortex

   b. renal fascia   **e.** hilum

   c. renal capsule

8. The external opening of a passage is called a

   a. meatus   **d.** bladder

   b. urethra   **e.** trigone

   c. ureter

9. The glomerulus is encased in

   a. a blood vessel   **d.** the Bowman capsule

   b. a muscle   **e.** the urethra

   c. renal fascia

10. Nephrotic syndrome involves large amounts of _____ leaking out into the urine.

   a. protein   **d.** blood

   b. sugar   **e.** WBCs

   c. RBCs

C. Plurals. Precision in communication requires the correct use of the singular and/or plural form of the medical term. If the singular form is given in the left column, write in the plural form in the appropriate column. If the plural form is given in the first column, write the singular form in the second column. Be sure to define the term. Fill in the chart. (**LO 6.3**, *Remember*)

Medical Term	Singular	Plural	Meaning of Term
calculus	1.	2.	3.
calices	4.	5.	6.
cortex	7.	8.	9.
glomeruli	10.	11.	12.
hila	13.	14.	15.

To finish this exercise, use any two terms from the table in sentences of documentation that are not definitions.

Sentence 1: _____

_____

Sentence 2: _____

_____

Precision in communication is the mark of a professional.

D. Seek and find. How many medical terms ending in *-itis* have you found in this chapter? List them here, and give a brief definition for each term. Fill in the blanks. (**LO 6.3**, *Remember*)

1. _____itis

   Definition: _____

2. _____itis

   Definition: _____

3. _____itis

   Definition: _____

4. _____itis

   Definition: _____

5. _____ itis

   Definition: _____

6. _____ itis

   Definition: _____

Urinary System

E. System review. Understanding the structure and function of the urinary system will give you a better grasp of the terminology. Circle the correct answers to the following questions. (**LO 6.1, 6.2, 6.3, 6.6,** *Remember, Understand*)

1. *Muscular tube, about 10 inches long, that carries urine to bladder.* This describes

   a. the ureter

   b. the urethra

   c. the portal vein

   d. the renal vein

   e. the aorta

2. Another name for a kidney stone is

   a. UTI

   b. calculus

   c. tumor

   d. hematuria

   e. lithotripsy

3. Water is returned to the blood by

   a. excretion

   b. filtration

   c. resorption

   d. elimination

   e. respiration

4. **Peritoneal** and **continuous cycling** are terms that apply to

   a. incontinence

   b. azotemia

   c. dialysis

   d. nephrectomy

   e. transplants

F. Abbreviations are not helpful if you do not understand their meaning and cannot use them to communicate safely and effectively. The following abbreviations are from this chapter and earlier chapters. Demonstrate that you can put the appropriate abbreviation in the correct context. You will not use every abbreviation listed to fill in the blanks. (**LO 6.5,** *Remember, Apply*)

ARF	**ESWL**	**KUB**	**TNM**
BUN	**GRF**	**PKD**	**UA**
CRF	**IV**	**SG**	**UTI**
ESRD	**IVP**	**SPA**	**MRI**

1. Dr. Lee ordered the _____ medication stat.

2. The patient informed me that there is a history of _____ in his family.

3. The patient with the kidney stone is scheduled for _____ early tomorrow morning.

4. The patient's renal carcinoma was staged using the _____ method.

5. The patient returns with her second _____ this month. Medication is prescribed.

6. Dr. Johnson ordered the following radiologic diagnostic tests for the patient: _____, _____,

   and _____.

7. The patient's _____ progressed to _____,

   and _____ resulted.

G. Review. One or more roots or combining forms can have the same meaning. Demonstrate that you can use these elements correctly. *Remember: They are not interchangeable.* One particular root or combining form goes with a specific suffix. Fill in the blanks. (**LO 6.3,** *Remember, Apply*)

1. Urinary system: These two elements both mean *kidney:* _____ and _____.

Apply the following suffixes to the correct roots or root/combining forms for the urinary system to form the exact medical terms. Fill in the blanks.

-al	-in	-ary	-logist	-ectomy	-itis	-tomy	-logy

2. Incision into the kidney   / nephro/_____

3. Pertaining to the kidney   / ren/_____

4. Removal of the kidney   / nephr/_____

5. Kidney enzyme that causes vasoconstriction   / ren /_____

6. Inflammation of the kidney   / nephr /_____

7. Study of the kidney   / nephro/_____

8. Specialist in kidney diseases   / nephro/_____

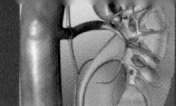

Urinary System

H. Word elements remain your key for understanding a medical term. Deconstruct the following medical terms into their basic elements by putting a slash (/) between each element in every term before you start filling in the chart. Write the elements in the appropriate columns and then write the meaning of the term in the last column. (**LO 6.3,** *Understand*)

Medical Term	Prefix	Root/ Combing Form	Suffix	Meaning of Term
hydronephrosis	1.	2.	3.	4.
incontinence	5.	6.	7.	8.
nephrectomy	9.	10.	11.	12.
nephrolithiasis	13.	14.	15.	16.
nephrolithotomy	17.	18.	19.	20.
peritubular	21.	22.	23.	24.
uremia	25.	26.	27.	28.
nephropathy	29.	30.	31.	32.
nephroblastoma	33.	34.	35.	36.

I. Short answer. You will often be called upon to express yourself in writing documentation. Practice writing clear, concise answers to the following questions. Always be sure to check your spelling! (**LO 6.3,** *Understand*)

1. Explain the difference to the patient's family between a *nephrotomy* and a *nephrectomy.*

   a. nephrotomy: _____

   _____

   b. nephrectomy: _____

   _____

2. The kidneys secrete both an enzyme and a hormone. What are they called, and what are the functions of each?

   a. enzyme: _____

   b. function: _____

   _____

   c. hormone: _____

   d. function: _____

   _____

J. Differences. Being able to explain how terms are different means you understand exactly what they mean. These terms all have the same suffix, but their other elements define them. Fill in the blanks. (**LO 6.3, 6.8,** *Understand, Apply*)

1. The suffix in each term is _____ and means _____.

2. A *nephroscopy* is _____.

3. A *ureteroscopy* is _____.

4. A *cystoscopy* is _____.

K. Matching. Confirm that your knowledge of the language of the urinary system and its functions is accurate. Match the statements in the left column to the correct answers in the right column. (**LO 6.1, 6.2, Apply**)

_____ 1. Chemical formed in uncontrolled diabetes   **a.** uremia

_____ 2. Outside the body   **b.** permeable

_____ 3. Donor organ to recipient   **c.** azotemia

_____ 4. Reversal of normal flow   **d.** flank

_____ 5. Identified by dipstick   **e.** extracorporeal

_____ 6. Loss of bladder control   **f.** dialyzer

_____ 7. Disease state resulting from renal failure   **g.** radical

_____ 8. Extensive removal of diseased part   **h.** incontinence

_____ 9. Side of body between ribs and pelvis   **i.** ketone

_____ 10. Artificial kidney machine   **j.** transplant

_____ 11. Allowing substance to pass through membrane   **k.** retrograde

_____ 12. Excess waste products in blood   **l.** microscopic hematuria

L. Elements. Roots and combining forms may stay the same in similar terms, but you will notice that the suffix can change the entire meaning of the medical term. Insert the correct suffix on the line to provide the precise meaning. Pick the correct ending from among the following choices; you have more choices than you will need. Fill in the blanks. (**LO 6.3, Apply**)

-al	-iasis	-lysis	-scopy
-ectomy	-ion	-osis	-tomy
-emia	-logist	-pexy	-tripsy
-gen	-logy	-scope	-uria

1. Study of the kidney   nephro/_____

2. Dilation of pelvis and calyces of a kidney   hydronephr/_____

3. Instrument for viewing inside a kidney   nephro/_____

4. Presence of a kidney stone   nephrolith/_____

5. Process of eliminating waste products of metabolism   excret/_____

6. Surgical removal of a kidney   nephr/_____

7. Incision for removal of a kidney stone   nephrolitho/ _____

8. Separating urine for examination of elements   urina/_____

9. Medical specialist in disorders of the urinary system   uro/_____

10. Crushing a renal stone with sound waves   litho/_____

11. Blood in the urine   hemat/_____

12. Excess nitrogenous waste products in the blood   azot/_____

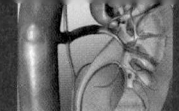

Urinary System

M. Discussion questions. Discussions with patients require effort to get your thoughts organized about what you want to say. Prepare for these discussions by doing one of the following. (**LO 6.1, 6.2, 6.3, 6.7, *Apply***)

- Making a mini-outline of what you want to say.

- Making a list of keywords that will help your memory.

- Making a list of short notes to keep your thoughts on track—try to confine your list/outline to a large index card.

Use any of these methods to prepare a short discussion on one of the following topics:

1. The functions of the kidney: Pick any two functions of the kidney, and be prepared to explain what each function is, how important it is, what other systems may be involved with the function or impacted by it, what urinary structures are involved with the function, and so on. *Be sure that you can define/explain to your classmates any terms you use in your discussion.*

2. Trace the flow of fluid through the renal filtration process. This particular discussion may benefit from a simple illustration you might want to prepare.

   Research this on the Internet.

   Notes (outline, keywords, short notes): _____

   _____

   _____

   _____

   _____

   _____

   _____

   _____

   _____

   _____

   _____

N. Each of these diagnoses relates to a specific organ in the urinary system. Fill in the chart. (**LO 6.1, 6.3, *Apply***)

Diagnosis	Organ in the Urinary System
1. urethritis	
2. cystitis	
3. nephritis	
4. ureteritis	

5. *-itis* means _____

Describe what part(s) of the urinary system are affected by

6. glomerulonephritis: _____

7. pyelonephritis: _____

8. pyelitis: _____

O. Documentation. Case Report 6.3 presents all the information you need to fill out the HPI (History of Present Illness) form for the patient's medical record. *You are translating the patient's own words into medical terminology.* First read Case Report 6.3 about Mrs. Dobson; then read the questions you need to answer. This will help you to fill in the blanks in the HPI form. The last part of the exercise involves asking Mrs. Dobson additional questions you think will provide helpful information for the doctor. Use the correct medical term whenever possible, and be prepared to define each term you use. (**LO 6.3, *Apply, Analyze***)

You are

... a medical assistant working in the office of Dr. Susan Lee, a primary care physician at Fulwood Medical Center.

Your patient is

... Mrs. Caroline Dobson, a 32-year-old housewife. You have asked her to describe the reason for her visit to the office today, 06/09/13.

Case Report 6.3

Patient Interview

Mrs. Dobson:

"Since yesterday afternoon I've had a lot of pain low down in my belly and in my lower back. I keep having to go to the bathroom every hour or so to pee. It's often difficult to start, and it burns as it comes out. I've had this problem twice before when I was pregnant with my two kids, so I've started drinking cranberry juice. I've been shivering since I woke up this morning, and the last urine I passed was pink. Was that due to the cranberry juice?"

What additional questions could you ask Mrs. Dobson that would provide helpful information for Dr. Lee?

1. _____

2. _____

P. Terminology challenge. Medical terminology is full of words that sound and look similar but have very different meanings. Think about the following terms, and explain in plain language how they are different. Notice that these two terms differ by only one letter—this is where precision comes in! Fill in the blanks. (**LO 6.3, *Analyze***)

1. Refl*e*x: _____

2. Refl*u*x: _____

Q. Common denominator. Each of the following groups of terms has something in common. Your knowledge of the terminology and functional anatomy of the urinary system will help you determine the common denominator for each group. Fill in the blanks. (**LO 6.1, 6.2, 6.3, 6.11, *Analyze***)

1. urination, micturition, voiding

   All are _____.

2. ESWL, ureteroscopy, percutaneous nephrolithotomy

   All are _____.

3. stress, urge, overflow, functional

   All are _____.

Chapter 6 Review

Urinary System

R. **Roots and combining forms.** Form the foundation of a medical term. All these terms have the same suffix. Differentiate their meanings by analyzing the rest of the term. On the basis of the word part specify what each term means. Every one of these terms could be a diagnosis for your next patient. Fill in the blanks. (**LO 6.3, 6.7,** *Analyze*)

Medical Term	Meaning of Prefix	Meaning of Root/ Combining Form	Meaning of Suffix	Meaning of Term
anuria	1.	2.	3.	4.
dysuria	5.	6.	7.	8.
glycosuria	9.	10.	11.	12.
hematuria	13.	14.	15.	16.
oliguria	17.	18.	19.	20.
proteinuria	21.	22.	23.	24.

Determine the meaning of these two terms after analyzing the rest of their elements.

25. If **py** means *pus*, then **pyuria** means _____.

26. If **noct** means *night,* then **nocturia** means _____.

S. **Tests and procedures.** Patients with urinary problems will be sent for various renal function tests and diagnostic procedures that may result in a surgical procedure. Any of the following procedures might be ordered for your patient. Do you know their purpose? Be prepared to discuss which terms are tests and which are procedures. (**LO 6.8, 6.11,** *Analyze*)

_____ 1. Contrast material injected to locate stones

_____ 2. Collection of bladder sample in newborns

_____ 3. Incision for removal of kidney stone

_____ 4. Crushing renal stone by sound waves

_____ 5. Assess blood flow to the kidneys

_____ 6. Tissue bank matching of donor to recipient

_____ 7. Treatment for renal cell carcinoma

_____ 8. X-ray of the abdominal urinary organs

_____ 9. Viewing the bladder through a scope

_____ 10. Filtering blood through an artificial kidney machine

a. dialysis

b. transplant

c. KUB

d. retrograde pyelogram

e. cystoscopy

f. nephrolithotomy

g. nephrectomy

h. needle aspiration

i. renal angiogram

j. lithotripsy

Study Hint
Create a study hint for yourself that will make it easy to remember exactly what an IVP is.

Write your hint here: _____
_____
_____

T. Patient documentation. Read the following case history aloud. Then go through the paragraph and underline all the medical terms. Finally, answer the questions. **(LO 6.3, 6.8, *Analyze*)**

Documentation

A 68-year-old female presents with hematuria, dysuria, and left-flank pain. I ordered a KUB and an IVP to ascertain the possibility or extent of obstruction. Test results indicate one large and several small calculi impacted in her left ureter just below the renal hilum. Patient would prefer ESWL, but surgical laparoscopy, I think, will offer better and quicker results to alleviate her pain. Patient will proceed with surgery tomorrow.

1. What are the patient's symptoms?

   _____

2. What diagnostic tests were performed?

   _____

3. What organs were checked in these tests?

   _____

4. What is the singular of *calculi*? _____

5. What does *impacted* mean?

   _____

6. What is meant by *obstructing the ureter*?

   _____

7. Define *ESWL*.

   _____

8. What is a *laparoscopy*? (use the glossary or a medical dictionary if you need to)

   _____

9. What type of doctor performs laparoscopy for renal calculi?

   _____

10. What is a preoperative diagnosis for this patient?

   _____

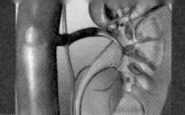

Chapter 6 Review

Urinary System

CHAPTER SUMMARY EXERCISE

A. Spelling comprehension. Circle the correct spelling of the term in the first ten questions, and then in the next ten use the correctly spelled word in a sentence. (**LO 6.3**, *Analyze*)

1. micktutrition	mictrition	mickterition	micterition	micturition
2. incontenince	incontenance	incontinence	incontinance	inccontinance
3. pilitis	pylitis	pyelitis	phylitis	pulitis
4. ureea	uria	urea	urrea	uremia
5. voyd	void	voyid	vuyde	voyde
6. kalyx	calyxx	calyx	kalyxx	calix
7. adventitia	adventishia	adventusa	adventechia	adventia
8. reninne	renine	renin	rynine	rinine
9. Kegelle	Kegele	Keggle	Kegel	Kegale
10. groin	groun	groan	grunne	grune

11. _____

12. _____

13. _____

14. _____

15. _____

16. _____

17. _____

18. _____

19. _____

20. _____

B. Use the appropriate terms to answer the questions. Both questions relate to urine. (**LO 6.10, 6.11**, *Remember*)

1. List some of the abnormal contents of urine:

_____

2. Which of the following is not a urine collection method?

a. catheterization

b. intravenous

c. 24 hour

d. clean catch

e. early morning collection

C. Three for three. Each of these three questions have three answers. Use the language of urology to answer them. (**LO 6.1, 6.2, 6.10,** *Remember*)

1. List three components of normal urine:

   a. _____

   b. _____

   c. _____

2. Name three secretions of the kidney:

   a. _____

   b. _____

   c. _____

3. What three structures form the hilum?

   a. _____

   b. _____

   c. _____

D. Write the correct term for a brief description of each of the following. (**LO 6.1, 6.2, 6.3,** *Remember*)

1. Crease where thigh joins abdomen _____

2. Funnel-shaped structure _____

3. Causes vasoconstriction _____

4. End product of nitrogen metabolism _____

5. Inflammation of the renal pelvis _____

6. Act of passing urine _____

7. Outermost connective tissue layer of any structure _____

8. Exercises to strengthen muscles of pelvic floor _____

9. To evacuate urine or feces _____

10. Loss of control of the bladder _____

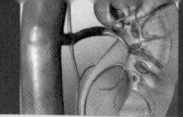

Urinary System

E.   After reading Case Report 6.1 below, answer the following questions. Be prepared to discuss your answers in class. (**LO 6.3,** *Remember*)

You are

...a surgical physician assistant working with **urologist** Phillip Johnson, MD, at Fulwood Medical Center.

Your patient is

...Mr. Nelson Hughes, a 58-year-old school principal. You are making your afternoon hospital visits to Dr. Johnson's patients. Earlier today you assisted at Mr. Hughes's surgery. A **laparoscopic radical nephrectomy** for a **TNM stage II renal cell carcinoma** (cancer) with no evidence of local invasion or lymph node involvement (metastasis) was performed.

Your job is to assess Mr. Hughes's postoperative state and determine whether postoperative complications exist.

1. A *urologist* treats which organs in the urinary system? _____

2. Define

laparoscopic: _____

radical: _____

nephrectomy: _____

3. What does the abbreviation TNM stand for? _____

4. When does *postoperative* occur? _____

5. Why is "no evidence of metastasis" a good thing? _____

Note to student: A *urologist* can operate on any part of the urinary system. A *nephrologist* is not a surgeon, much like a *cardiologist* is not a surgeon. Both specialists **can diagnose the diseases but cannot provide surgical treatment** for them. The *nephrologist* will refer patients who need surgery to a *urologist* for the surgery, and a *cardiologist* will refer patients to a cardiovascular surgeon.

F.   Brain teasers. Employ the language of urology to answer the following questions. (**LO 6.1, 6.3,** *Understand*)

1. What is a catheter, and what is its purpose? _____

2. Ketones are associated with what illnesses? _____

3. Which of the following is *not* a VS?

   a. respiration

   b. voiding

   c. pulse

   d. blood pressure

   e. temperature

G. Meet the goals of each of the chapter outcomes and insert the correct answers to the questions. (LO 6.1–6.11, *Analyze*)

1. Describe the location of the kidneys. (**LO 6.1**) _____

2. What is the main function of the urinary system? (**LO 6.2**) _____

3. Choose the correct medical term to complete the following sentence. (**LO 6.3**)

   "The kidneys maintain _____ by controlling the quantities of water and electrolytes that are eliminated."

4. If a patient's urinalysis comes back with a diagnosis of hematuria, what does that mean? (**LO 6.4**)

   _____

   _____

5. Which of the following abbreviations has no relation to the urinary system? (**LO 6.5**)

   a. LOC

   b. CKD

   c. GI

   d. CAPD

   e. IVP

6. What is a common symptom of urinary calculi? (**LO 6.6**)

   _____

7. What are some of the treatment options for removal of renal calculi? (**LO 6.7**)

   _____

8. Describe how cystoscopy with biopsy can be a diagnostic tool. (**LO 6.8**)

   _____

9. How might a UA function as a diagnostic tool? (**LO 6.9**)

   _____

10. Leukocyte esterase predicts _____. (**LO 6.10**)

11. What two fluids collected from the body can be diagnostic tools? (**LO 6.11**)

    a. Fluid from the urinary system: _____

    b. Fluid from the cardiovascular system: _____

H. Evaluation. Check the following statements and determine the *false* answer. Circle the letter of the false answer. (**LO 6.3**)

1. "A laparoscopic radical nephrectomy for a TNM stage II renal cell carcinoma with no evidence of local invasion or lymph node involvement was performed."

   a. A nephrectomy is a surgery on the urinary system

   b. Carcinoma is the same as cancer

   c. "Local invasion and lymph node involvement" equate to metastasis

   d. "Radical" means they took only a portion of the kidney

   e. Renal cells are located in the kidney

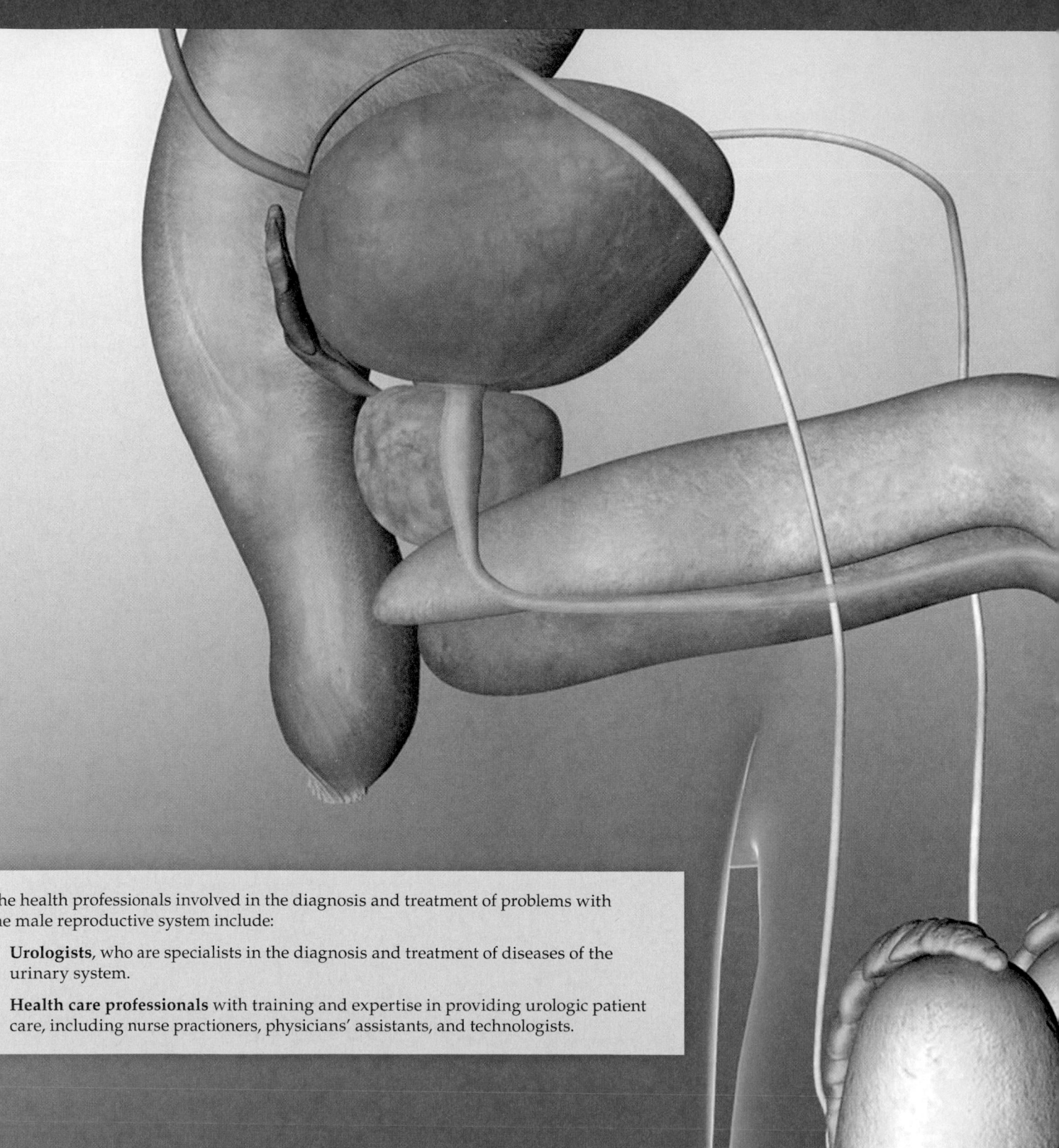

Male Reproductive System
The Language of Reproduction

The health professionals involved in the diagnosis and treatment of problems with the male reproductive system include:

- **Urologists**, who are specialists in the diagnosis and treatment of diseases of the urinary system.

- **Health care professionals** with training and expertise in providing urologic patient care, including nurse practioners, physicians' assistants, and technologists.

7

Case Report (CR) 7.1

You are

. . . an EMT-P working in the Emergency Department at Fulwood Medical Center.

Your patient is

. . . Joseph Davis, a 17-year-old high school senior. He is brought in by his mother at 0400 hrs. He complains of **(c/o)** sudden onset of pain in his left **testicle** 3 hours earlier that woke him up. The pain is intense and has made him vomit. VS: T 99.2°F, P 88, R 15, BP 130/70. Examination reveals his left testicle to be enlarged, warm, and tender. His abdomen is normal to palpation.

At your request, Dr. Helinski, the emergency physician on duty, examines him immediately. He diagnoses a **torsion** of the patient's left testicle.

Chapter Learning Outcomes

As you set up the next stage of Joseph's treatment, there are immediate clinical decisions to be made. You will have to communicate clearly with Dr. Helinski and other health professionals and with Joseph and his mother. You must also document his care.

To participate effectively in all this, you must be able to:

LO 7.1 Apply the language of urology as it relates to the anatomy and physiology of the male reproductive system.

LO 7.2 Use the medical terms of urology as they relate to the male reproductive system to communicate and document in writing accurately and precisely in any health care setting.

LO 7.3 Use the medical terms of urology as they relate to the male reproductive system to communicate verbally with accuracy and precision in any health care setting.

LO 7.4 Describe the anatomy and physiology of the male reproductive organs and the accessory glands.

LO 7.5 Discuss the disorders of the individual reproductive glands and their treatment.

Unlike every other organ system, the reproductive system is not essential for an *individual human* to survive. However, without the reproductive system, the *human species* could not survive. The male reproductive system ensures the sexual maturation of each male, influences male behavior, and produces, maintains, and transports the male sex cells (sperm cells) to the female reproductive tract.

The information in this lesson will enable you to use correct medical terminology to:

7.1.1 Describe the anatomy and physiology of the primary and secondary male sex organs and their accessory glands.

7.1.2 Document the process of spermatogenesis.

7.1.3 List the functions of testosterone.

7.1.4 Discuss disorders of the testes.

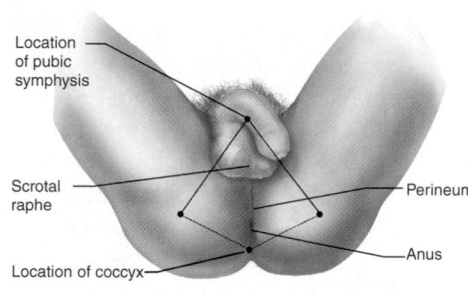

▲ Figure 7.1 Male Perineum.

Abbreviation	
VS	vital signs, which include T (temperature), P (pulse rate), R (respiration rate), and BP (blood pressure).

LO 7.4 Male Reproductive System

The male reproductive organ system *(Figure 7.2)* consists of

1. **Primary sex organs** or **gonads**: the **testes**

2. **Secondary sex organs**:

   a. **Penis**

   b. **Scrotum**

   c. **System of ducts,** including the **epididymis, ductus (vas) deferens,** and **urethra**

3. **Accessory glands**:

   a. **Prostate**

   b. **Seminal vesicles**

   c. **Bulbourethral (Cowper) glands**

Perineum

The **external genitalia** (the penis, scrotum, and testes) occupy the **perineum**, a diamond-shaped region between the thighs. Its border is at the pubic symphysis anteriorly and the coccyx posteriorly *(Figure 7.1).* The anus is also in the perineum.

Scrotum

The **scrotum** is a skin-covered sac between the thighs. Its midline shows a distinct ridge called the **raphe**. It marks the position of the internal **median septum** that divides the scrotum into two compartments. Each compartment contains a testis.

The scrotum's function is to provide a cooler environment for the testes than that inside the body. This is because sperm are best produced and stored at a few degrees cooler than the internal body temperature.

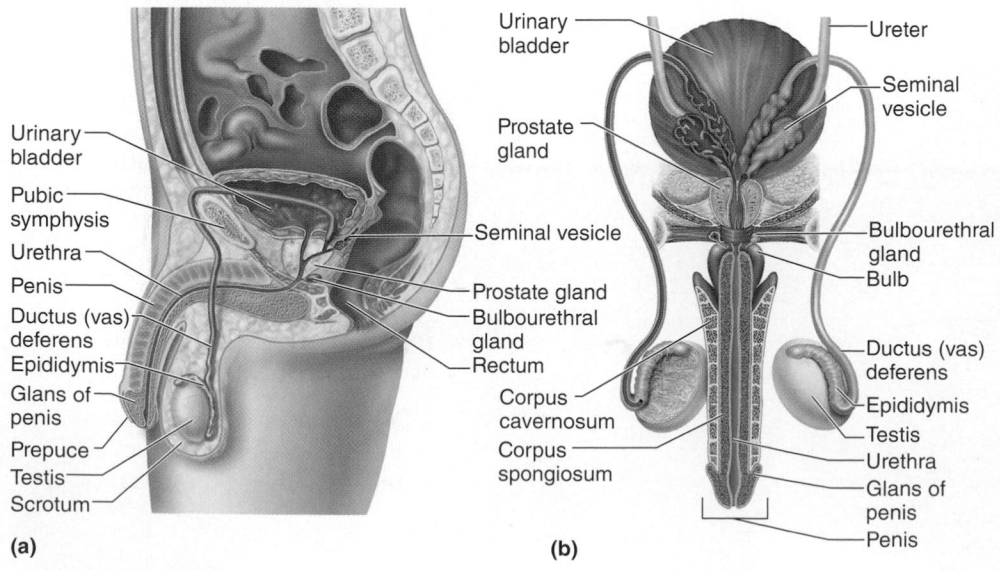

(a)

(b)

▲ Figure 7.2 **Male Reproductive System.** (*a*) Male pelvic cavity: midsagittal section. (*b*) Male reproductive organs.

WORD	PRONUNCIATION	ELEMENTS		DEFINITION
bulbourethral	BUL-boh-you-REE-thral	S/ R/CF R/	-al *pertaining to* bulb/o- *bulb* -urethr- *urethra*	Pertaining to the bulbous penis and urethra
ductus deferens vas deferens (syn)	DUK-tus DEH-fuh-renz VAS DEH-fuh-renz		ductus *Latin to lead* deferens *Latin carry away* vas *Latin blood vessel, duct*	Tube that receives sperm from the epididymis
epididymis	EP-ih-DID-ih-miss	S/ P/ R/	-is *belonging to* epi- *above* -didym- *testis*	Coiled tube attached, to the testis
genitalia	JEN-ih-TAY-lee-ah	S/ R/	-ia *condition* genit- *primary male or female sex organs*	External and internal organs of reproduction
genital	JEN-ih-tal	S/	-al *pertaining to*	Relating to reproduction or to the male or female sex organs
gonad gonads (pl)	GO-nad GO-nads		Greek *seed*	Testis or ovary
maturation	mat-you-RAY-shun	S/ R/	-ation *process* matur- *ripe, ready*	Process to achieve full development
penis penile	PEE-nis PEE-nile	S/ R/	Latin *tail* -ile *pertaining to* pen- *penis*	Conveys urine and semen to the outside Pertaining to the penis
perineum perineal	PER-ih-NEE-um PER-ih-NEE-al	S/ R/CF	Greek *perineum* -al *pertaining to* perin/e- *perineum*	Area between thighs, extending from the coccyx to the pubis Pertaining to the perineum
raphe	RAY-fee		Greek *seam*	Line separating two symmetrical structures
scrotum scrotal (adj)	SKRO-tum SKRO-tal	S/ R/	Latin *scrotum* -al *pertaining to* scrot- *scrotum*	Sac containing the testes Pertaining to the scrotum
semen seminal vesicle seminiferous	SEE-men SEM-in-al VES-ih-kull sem-ih-NIF-er-us	S/ R/ S/ R/ S/ R/CF R/	Latin *seed* -al *pertaining to* semin- *semen* -le *small* vesic- *sac containing fluid* -ous *pertaining to* semin/i- *semen* -fer- *to bear*	Penile ejaculate containing sperm and seminal fluid Sac of ductus deferens that produces seminal fluid Pertaining to carrying semen
testicle (also called testis) testicular testis testes (pl)	TES-tih-kul tes-TICK-you-lar TES-tis TES-tez	S/ R/	Latin *small testis* -ar *pertaining to* testicul- *testicle* Latin *testis*	One of the male reproductive glands Pertaining to the testicle A synonym for testicle
torsion	TOR-shun		Latin *to twist*	The act or result of twisting

Exercises

A. In your own words. *You could be working in the Emergency Department when this patient comes in. Using the information presented in Case Report 7.1, document the case in the patient's record. Use the following terms to fill in the blanks and answer the question.* **LO 7.4**

testicular	testes	testis	testicle

This patient presented to the ED because of pain in his left **1.** _____. Both **2.** _____ were

examined, but the left **3.** _____ was enlarged, warm, and tender. The emergency physician on duty

diagnosed **4.** _____ torsion. Patient will be scheduled for surgery immediately.

5. Is a primary or secondary sex organ involved? _____

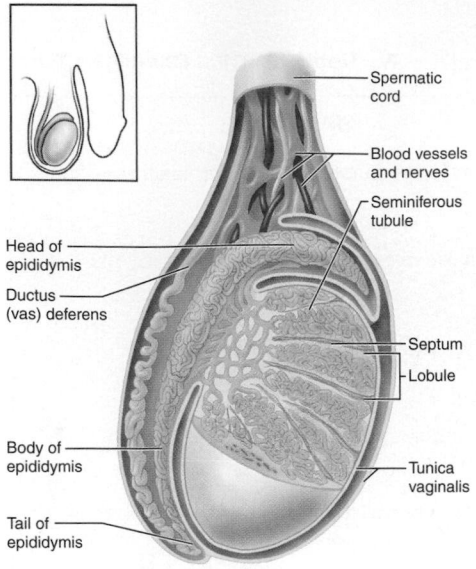

▲ **Figure 7.3** The Testis and Associated Structures.

LO 7.1, 7.4 Testes and Spermatic Cord

In the adult male, each testis is a small, oval organ about 2 inches (5 cm) long and ¾ inch (2 cm) wide *(Figure 7.3)*. Each testis is covered by a serous membrane, the **tunica vaginalis**, which has an outer parietal layer and an inner visceral layer separated by serous fluid.

Inside the testis, thin septa subdivide the testis into some 250 lobules *(Figure 7.3)*.

Each lobule contains three or four **seminiferous tubules** in which several layers of germ cells are in the process of becoming sperm.

Between the seminiferous tubules are the interstitial cells. They produce hormones called **androgens**.

Testosterone is the major androgen produced by the interstitial cells of the testes. It has the following effects:

- **Sustains** the male reproductive tract throughout adulthood.
- **Stimulates** spermatogenesis; testosterone levels peak at age 20, and then decline steadily to one-third of that level at age 65.
- **Inhibits** the secretion of female hormones at age 65, and continue declining after that age.
- **Stimulates** the development of male secondary sex characteristics at puberty.
- **Enlarges** the spermatic ducts and accessory glands of the male reproductive system.
- **Stimulates** a burst of growth at puberty—including increased muscle mass, higher **basal metabolic rate (BMR)**, and larger larynx (this effect deepens the voice).
- **Stimulates** erythropoiesis, giving men a higher red blood cell (RBC) count than women.
- **Stimulates** the brain to increase **libido** (sex drive) in the male.

Spermatic Cord

The blood vessels and nerves to the testis arise in the abdominal cavity. They pass through the inguinal canal, where they join with connective tissue to form a spermatic cord that suspends each testis in the scrotum *(see Figure 7.3)*. The left testis is suspended lower than the right. Within the cord are an artery, a plexus of veins, nerves, a thin muscle, and the ductus (vas) deferens (the passage into which sperm go when they leave the testis).

Keynote

The mature, adult male testes produce up to 100,000,000 sperm per day.

Abbreviation	
BMR	basal metabolic rate

Spermatogenesis

Spermatogenesis is the process in which the germ cells of the seminiferous tubules mature and divide **(mitosis)** and then undergo two divisions called **meiosis**. The four daughter cells differentiate into **spermatids** and then **spermatozoa (sperm)** *(Figure 7.4)*. The germ cells have 23 pairs of chromosomes (a total of 46). Because of meiosis, each sperm has only 23 chromosomes that can combine at fertilization with the 23 chromosomes in a female **oocyte** (egg).

The mature sperm has a pear-shaped head and a long tail *(Figure 7.5)*. The nucleus of the head contains 23 chromosomes.

The tail **(flagellum)** provides the movement as the sperm swims up the female reproductive tract.

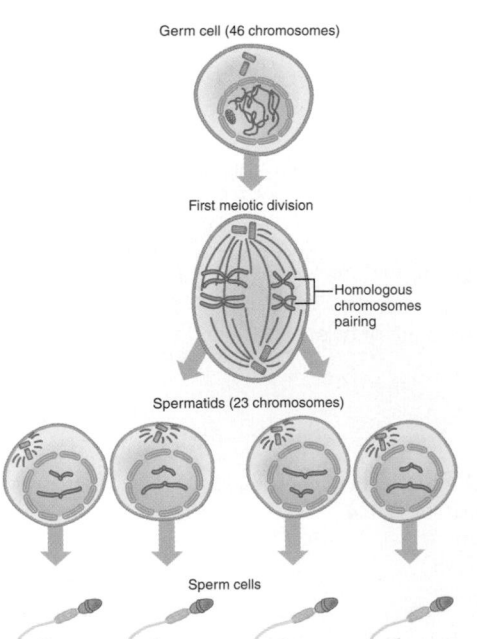

▲ **Figure 7.4** Spermatogenesis.

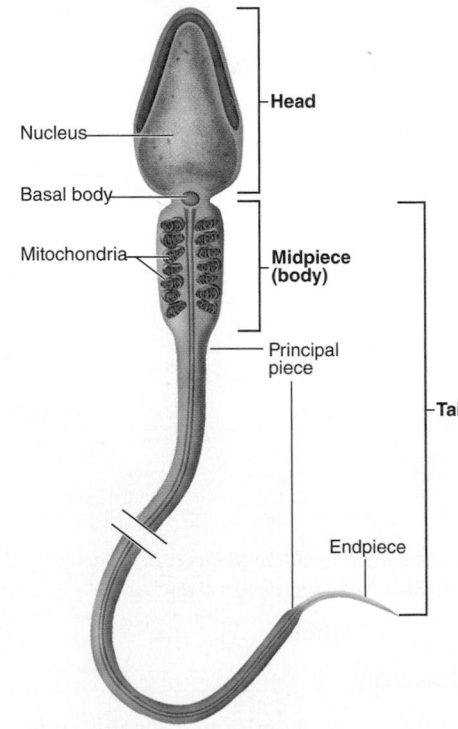

▲ **Figure 7.5** Mature Sperm.

WORD	PRONUNCIATION		ELEMENTS	DEFINITION
androgen	**AN**-droh-jen	S/ R/CF	**-gen** *form, create* **andr/o-** *masculine*	Hormone that promotes masculine characteristics
flagellum **flagella (pl)**	fla-**JELL**-um fla-**JELL**-ah		Latin *small whip*	Tail of a sperm
libido	li-**BEE**-doh		Latin *lust*	Sexual desire
meiosis	my-**OH**-sis	S/ R/	**-osis** *condition* **mei-** *lessening*	Two rapid cell divisions, resulting in half the number of chromosomes
mitosis	my-**TOE**-sis	S/ R/	**-osis** *condition* **mit-** *threadlike structure*	Cell division to create two identical cells, each with 46 chromosomes
oocyte	**OH**-oh-site	S/ R/CF	**-cyte** *cell* **o/o-** *egg*	Female egg cell
oogenesis	oh-oh-**JEN**-eh-sis	R/ S/	**-gen-** *origin, create* **-esis** *abnormal condition*	Development of female egg cell
puberty	**PYU**-ber-tee		Latin *grown up*	Process of maturing from child to young adult
seminiferous tubule	sem-ih-**NIF**-er-us **TU**-byul	S/ R/CF R/	**-ous** *pertaining to* **semin/i-** *semen* **-fer-** *to bear*	Coiled tubes in the testes that produce sperm
sperm (also called **spermatozoon**)	SPERM		Greek *seed*	Mature male sex cell
spermatozoa (pl)	**SPER**-mat-oh-**ZOH**-ah	S/ R/CF	**-zoa** *animals* **spermat/o-** *sperm*	Sperm (plural of spermatozoon)
spermatic (adj)	**SPER**-mat-ik	S/	**-ic** *pertaining to*	Pertaining to sperm
spermatid **spermatogenesis** (**Note:** This term has no prefix or suffix.)	**SPER**-mah-tid **SPER**-mat-oh-**JEN**-eh-sis	S/ R/ R/ R/CF	**-id** *having a particular quality* **spermat-** *sperm* **-genesis** *origin, creation* **spermat/o-** *sperm*	A cell late in the development process of sperm The process by which male germ cells differentiate into sperm
testosterone	tes-**TOSS**-ter-own	S/ R/CF	**-sterone** *steroid* **test/o-** *testis*	Powerful androgen produced by the testes
tunica vaginalis	**TYU**-nih-kah vaj-ih-**NAHL**-iss	S/ R/	*tunica* Latin *coat* **-alis** *pertaining to* **vagin-** *sheath, vagina*	Covering, particularly of a tubular structure. The tunica vaginalis is the sheath of the testis and epididymis

Exercises

A. Deconstruction of medical terms is a tool for analyzing the meaning. *In the following chart, you are given a medical term. Deconstruct the term into its root (or combining form) and suffix. Note that none of these terms have prefixes, and not all of the terms have a suffix. Write the element and its meaning in the appropriate column and the meaning of the term in the last column. <u>The first one is done for you.</u> Then answer the question at the end of the exercise.* **LO 7.1, 7.2, 7.4**

Term	Root/ Combining Form	Suffix	Meaning of Elements	Meaning of Term
vaginalis	**vagin**	**alis**	**sheath,** *pertaining to*	1. *pertaining to the vagina*
testosterone	2.	3.	4.	5.
androgen	6.	7.	8.	9.
spermatid	11.	12.	13.	14.
spermatogenesis	15.	16.	17.	18.

1. In your opinion, which term is the most unusual in the above WAD box, and why? (*Hint: Think of the elements.*)

_____

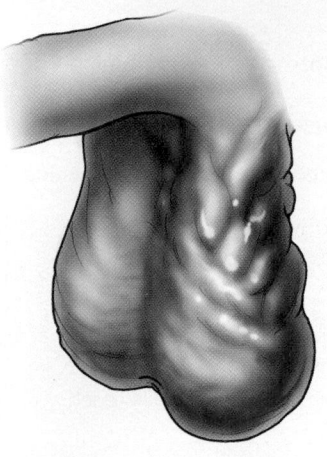

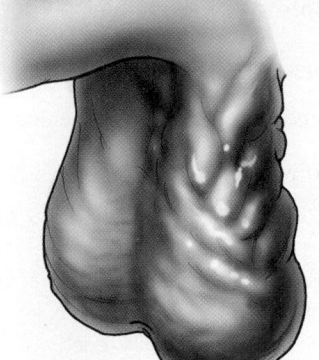

Case Report 7.1 (continued)

In the opening scenario to this chapter, Joseph Davis presented with typical symptoms and signs of testicular torsion. The affected testis rapidly became painful, tender, swollen, and inflamed. Emergency surgery was performed, and the testis and cord were manually untwisted through an incision in the scrotum. The testis was stitched to surrounding tissues to prevent a recurrence.

▲ **Figure 7.6** Illustration of Varicocele, Showing Varicose (Dliated) Veins of the Spermatic Cord in the Scrotum.

LO 7.5 Disorders of the Testes

Testicular torsion is the twisting of a testis on its spermatic cord. As the testis twists, the spermatic cord has to twist because it is fixed in the abdomen. The testicular artery in the twisted cord becomes blocked, and the blood supply to the testis is cut off. The condition occurs in men between puberty and age 25. In half the cases, it starts in bed at night.

Varicocele *(Figure 7.6)* is a condition in which the veins in the spermatic cord become dilated and tortuous as varicose veins. If it is uncomfortable, it can be treated by surgically tying off the affected veins.

Hydrocele is a collection of excess fluid in the space between the visceral and parietal layers of the tunica vaginalis of the testis. It is most common after age 40. The diagnosis can be confirmed by transillumination, shining a bright light on the swelling to see the shape of the testis through the translucent excess fluid *(Figure 7.7)*. Surgical removal is performed for large hydroceles.

Spermatocele is a collection of sperm in a sac formed in the epididymis. It occurs in about 30% of men, is benign, and rarely causes symptoms. It does not require treatment unless it becomes bothersome.

Cryptorchism occurs when a testis fails to descend from the abdomen into the scrotum before the boy is 12 months old. In the **embryo**, the testes develop inside the abdomen at the level of the kidney. They must then migrate down the abdomen into the scrotum. As undescended testicles have a higher risk of infertility and cancer, **orchiopexy** is performed to bring the testis into the scrotum.

Epididymitis and **epididymoorchitis (orchitis)** are both inflammatory diseases. Epididymitis is inflammation of the epididymis; epididymoorchitis is inflammation of the epididymis and testis. Orchitis is usually a consequence of epididymitis. They are most commonly caused by a bacterial infection spreading from a urinary tract infection or infection of the prostate. They can also be caused by **sexually transmitted diseases (STDs)**, such as gonorrhea or chlamydia *(see Chapter 8)*.

A viral cause of orchitis is mumps. In males past puberty who develop mumps, 30% will develop orchitis, and 30% of those will develop resulting testicular atrophy. If the testicular infection is bilateral, **infertility** can result. Mumps is avoidable by immunization during childhood.

Testicular cancer usually develops in men younger than 40.

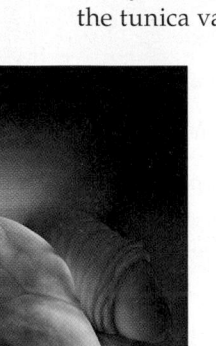

Spermatic cord

Testis

▲ **Figure 7.7** Transillumination of Hydrocele Showing Testis and Spermatic Cord.

Abbreviations

SET	self-examination of the testes
STD	sexually transmitted disease

Keynotes

- The testis in testicular torsion will die in some 6 hours unless the blood supply is restored.
- Self-examination of the testes (SET) for swelling or tenderness should be performed monthly by all men.

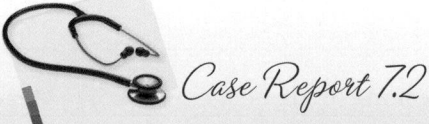

Case Report 7.2

Lance Armstrong, the world-renowned cyclist, presented with hemoptysis (coughing up blood). He had ignored a slight swelling of one testis, and the cancer in that testis had already metastasized to his lungs and brain. He required extensive chemotherapy, with brain surgery to remove several metastases.

Forty percent of testicular cancers are **seminomas**, made up of immature germ cells. Nonseminomas occur in different combinations of **choriocarcinoma**, **embryonal cell**, and **teratoma**. Lance Armstrong's cancer was 60% choriocarcinoma and 40% embryonal cell. The initial treatment for testicular cancer is surgical removal of the affected testis **(orchiectomy)**, followed by chemotherapy and sometimes radiation therapy.

WORD	PRONUNCIATION	ELEMENTS		DEFINITION
choriocarcinoma	**KOH**-ree-oh-kar-sih-**NOH**-mah	S/ R/CF	-oma *tumor* chori/o- *membrane, chorion*	Highly malignant cancer in a testis or ovary
		R/	-carcin- *cancer*	
cryptorchism	krip-**TOR**-kizm	S/ P/ R/	-ism *condition* crypt- *hidden* -orch- *testicle*	Failure of one or both testes to descend into the scrotum
epididymis	ep-ih-**DID**-ih-mis	S/ P/ R/	-is *belonging to* epi- *above* -didym- *testis*	Coiled tube attached to the testis
epididymitis	**EP**-ih-did-ih-**MY**-tis	S/	-itis *inflammation*	Inflammation of the epididymis
epididymoorchitis (syn: orchitis)	ep-ih-**DID**-ih-moh-or-**KIE**-tis	S/ P/ R/ R/	-itis *inflammation* epi- *above* -didym- *testis* -orch- *testicle*	Inflammation of the epididymis and testicle
hydrocele	**HIGH**-droh-seal	S/ R/CF	-cele *cave, swelling* hydr/o- *water*	Collection of fluid in the space of the tunica vaginalis
infertility	in-fer-**TIL**-ih-tee	S/ P/ R/	-ity *condition* in- *not* -fertil- *able to conceive*	Failure to conceive
orchiectomy	or-key-**ECK**-toe-me	S/ R/CF	-ectomy *surgical excision* orch- *testicle*	Removal of one testis or both testes
orchitis epididymoorchitis(syn)	or-**KIE**-tis	S/ R/	-itis *inflammation* orch/i- *testicle*	Inflammation of the testis
orchiopexy (*Note:* The letter "o" is added to make the word flow.)	**OR**-key-oh-**PEK**-see	S/ R/CF	-pexy *surgical fixation* orch/i- *testicle*	Surgical fixation of a testis in the scrotum
seminoma	sem-ih-**NO**-mah	S/ R/	-oma *tumor, mass* semin- *scatter seed*	Neoplasm of germ cells of a testis
spermatocele	**SPER**-mat-oh-seal	S/ R/CF	-cele *cave, swelling* spermat/o- *sperm*	Cyst of the epididymis that contains sperm
teratoma	ter-ah-**TOE**-mah	S/ R/	-oma *tumor, mass* terat- *monster, malformed fetus*	Neoplasm of a testis or ovary containing multiple tissues from other sites in the body
varicocele	**VAIR**-ih-koh-seal	S/ R/CF	-cele *cave, swelling* varic/o- *varicosity*	Varicose veins of the spermatic cord

Exercises

A. After reading Case Report 7.2, answer the following questions. *Be prepared to discuss your answers in class.*   **LO 7.1, 7.2**

1. What element in the word *hemoptysis* confirms that the patient is coughing up blood?

_____

2. You learned in a previous chapter the medical term for *swelling*. Write it here:

_____

3. What does "already metastasized to his lungs and brain" mean for the patient?

_____

4. What is another medical term for *testis?* _____

5. What did the patient's follow-up treatment plan include? _____

_____

Spermatic Ducts and Accessory Glands

The information provided in this lesson will enable you to:

7.2.1 **Trace the pathway taken by a sperm cell from a testis to its ejaculation.**
7.2.2 **Identify the structure and functions of the prostate and other male accessory glands.**
7.2.3 **Describe the origins, composition, and functions of semen.**
7.2.4 **Discuss disorders of the prostate gland.**
7.2.5 **Identify the causes of male infertility.**

You are

. . . a surgical technologist **(LCC-ST)** working with **urologist** Phillip Johnson, MD, in the **Urology** Clinic at Fulwood Medical Center.

Your patient is

. . . Mr. Ronald Detrick, a 60-year-old man who has been referred to the Urology Clinic c/o having to get out of bed to urinate four or five times at night.

Case Report 7.3

Mr. Detrick has difficulty starting urination, has a weak stream, and feels he is not emptying his bladder completely. His symptoms have been gradually worsening over the past year. He has lost interest in sex. His physical examination is unremarkable except that **digital rectal examination (DRE)** reveals a diffusely enlarged prostate with no nodules.

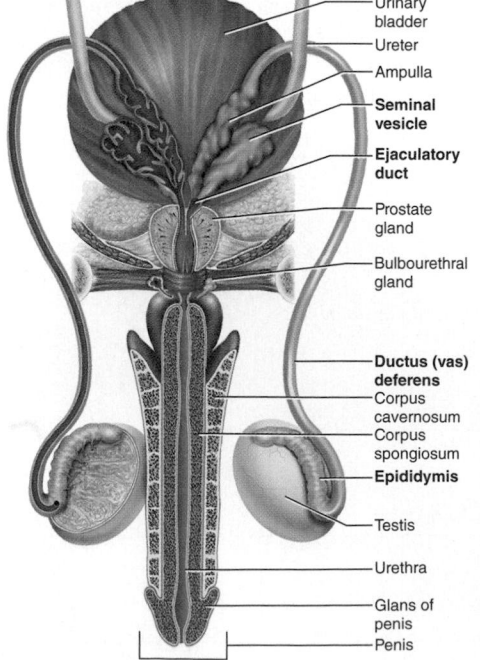

▲ **Figure 7.8** **Components of Male Reproductive Ducts.**

- Urinary bladder
- Ureter
- Ampulla
- **Seminal vesicle**
- **Ejaculatory duct**
- Prostate gland
- Bulbourethral gland
- **Ductus (vas) deferens**
- Corpus cavernosum
- Corpus spongiosum
- **Epididymis**
- Testis
- Urethra
- Glans of penis
- Penis

Abbreviations

DRE	digital rectal examination
LCC-ST	Liaison Council on Certification for the Surgical Technologist

LO 7.4 Spermatic Ducts

The male prostate and urethra have both **urologic** and **reproductive** functions, as the flow of urine and semen goes through both organs. Disorders of the prostate and urethra produce symptoms and signs that arise in both areas. This makes it essential to have knowledge of their anatomy, physiology, and terminology to be able to understand both functions.

Spermatic Ducts

As the sperm cells mature in the testes over a 60-day period, they move down the seminiferous tubules and pass into a network of tubules called the **rete testis**. From here, they move into the epididymis, the ductus (vas) deferens, the ejaculatory duct, and finally the urethra to reach the outside of the body *(Figure 7.8)*.

The epididymis adheres to the posterior side of the testis. It is a single coiled duct in which the sperm are stored for 12 to 20 days until they mature and become **motile**. Stored sperm remain fertile for 40 to 60 days. If they become too old without being **ejaculated**, they disintegrate and are reabsorbed in the epididymis.

The ductus (vas) deferens is a muscular duct that travels up from the epididymis in the scrotum and through the inguinal canal *(see Chapter 5)* into the pelvic cavity *(see Figure 7.8)*. Here the ductus turns medially and passes behind the urinary bladder and widens into a terminal **ampulla**, which joins with the duct of the seminal **vesicle**.

The **ejaculatory duct**, formed by the ductus deferens and seminal **vesicle**, is a short (¾-inch or 2 cm) duct that passes through the prostate gland and empties its contents of sperm and seminal fluid (semen) into the urethra.

WORD	PRONUNCIATION		ELEMENTS	DEFINITION
ampulla	am-**PULL**-ah		Latin *two-handled bottle*	Dilated portion of a canal or duct
ejaculate (*Note:* This term can be a verb or noun.)	ee-**JACK**-you-late	S/ R/	-ate *composed of, pertaining to* ejacul- *shoot out*	To expel suddenly, or the semen expelled in ejaculation
ejaculation	ee-**JACK**-you-**LAY**-shun	S/	-ation *process*	Process of expelling semen
motile	**MOH**-til	S/ R/	-ile *capable* mot- *to move*	Capable of spontaneous movement
motility (noun)	moh-**TILL**-ih-tee	S/	-ility *condition, state of*	The ability for spontaneous movement
reproductive	ree-pro-**DUC**-tiv	S/ P/ R/	-ive *nature of, pertaining to* re- *again* -product- *lead forth*	Relating to the process by which organisms produce offspring
reproduction (noun)	ree-pro-**DUC**-shun	S/	-ion *action, process*	The process by which organisms produce offspring
rete testis	**REE**-teh **TES**-tis		rete Latin *net* testis Latin *testis*	Network of tubules between the seminiferous tubules and the epididymis
urology	you-**ROL**-oh-jee	S/ R/CF	-logy *study of* ur/o- *urinary system*	Medical specialty of disorders of the urinary system
urologist	you-**ROL**-oh-jist	S/	-logist *one who studies, specialist*	Medical specialist in disorders of the urinary system
urologic (adj)	yur-oh-**LOJ**-ih-k	S/ S/	-log- *study of* -ic *pertaining to*	Pertaining to urology
vesicle	**VES**-ih-kull		Latin *a blister*	Small sac containing liquid; for example, a blister or, in this case, semen

Exercises

A. Recall and review. *Certain medical terms can appear in more than one body system. You need to know both applications of the same term. An example is given below as a series of questions that should help you learn to make various connections across the study material when you meet one of these terms.* **LO 7.1, 7.2, 7.4**

1. In the above WAD, the Latin definition of *vesicle* is _____.

2. In what other *body system* would you see this term? _____

3. The specialist treating the body system in question 2 would be a _____.

4. In what type of condition in the other body system might a *vesicle* appear? _____

5. What is the role or function of a *vesicle* in this chapter's body system?

_____

_____

6. How are the uses of the term *vesicle* in these two body systems similar? Dissimilar?

_____

_____

_____

_____

Study Hint

"SEVEN UP" is used to remember the pathway of sperm.
S = seminiferous tubules
E = epididymis
V = vas deferens (now called ductus deferens)
E = ejaculatory duct
(N = nothing)
U = urethra
P = penis

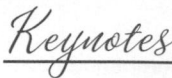
- Combined with sperm, the seminal fluid becomes semen.

- The male testes produce up to 100 million sperm per day.

- A normal sperm count is in the range of 75 to 150 million sperm per mL of semen.

- A normal ejaculation consists of 2 to 5 mL of semen.

Abbreviations

mL	milliliter
PSA	prostate-specific antigen
UTI	urinary tract infection

LO 7.4 Accessory Glands

Seminal fluid contains components produced by all three accessory glands (*Figure 7.9*). The functions of seminal fluid are to

- **Provide nutrients** to the sperm as they are in the urethra and female reproductive tract.
- **Neutralize acid secretions** of the vagina (in which sperm cannot survive).
- **Provide hormones** (**prostaglandins**) that widen the opening of the cervix to enable sperm to enter more easily.
- **Provide the fluid vehicle** in which sperm can swim.

The two seminal vesicles are located on the posterior surface of the urinary bladder. The wall of each vesicle contains mucosal folds. They produce a viscous, yellowish, alkaline fluid that contains fructose and prostaglandins. Fructose is a sugar that provides energy for the sperm.

The single **prostate gland** is located immediately below the bladder and anterior to the rectum and surrounds the urethra and the **ejaculatory** duct. It is composed of 30 to 50 glands that open directly into the urethra. The glands secrete a slightly milky fluid that contains

- **Citric acid**, a nutrient for sperm.
- **An antibiotic** that combats **urinary tract infections (UTIs)** in the male.
- **Clotting factors** that hold the sperm together in a sticky mass until **ejaculation**.
- **Prostate-specific antigen (PSA)**, an enzyme that helps liquefy the sticky mass following ejaculation.

The two bulbourethral glands are located one on each side of the membranous urethra. Each gland has a short duct leading into the spongy (penile) urethra. The glands secrete a clear, slippery, alkaline mucus that protects the sperm as they pass through the urethra by neutralizing any residual acid urine. It also acts as a lubricant during sexual intercourse.

Semen is derived from the secretions of several glands:

- 5% comes from the testicles and epididymis.
- 50% to 80% comes from the seminal vesicles.
- 15% to 33% comes from the prostate gland.
- 2% to 5% comes from the bulbourethral glands.

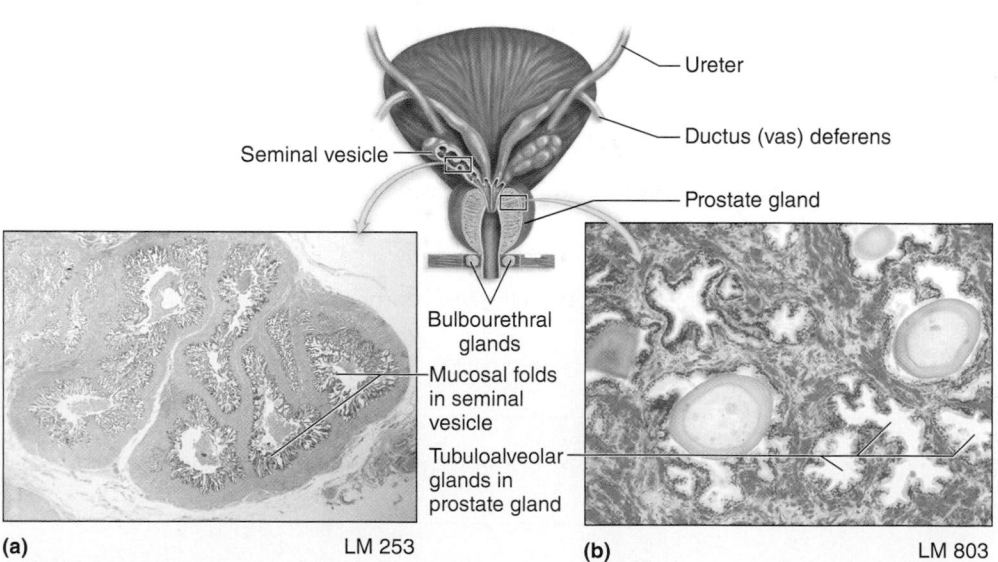

(a) LM 253 (b) LM 803

▲ **Figure 7.9** **Accessory Glands of the Male Reproductive System.** (*a*) Seminal vesicle. (*b*) Prostate gland.

WORD	PRONUNCIATION	ELEMENTS		DEFINITION
prostate	**PROS**-tate (*Note: not* **PROS**-trate.)		Greek *one standing before*	Organ surrounding the beginning of the urethra
prostatic (adj)	pros-**TAT**-ik	S/ R/	-**tic** *pertaining to* **prosta-** *prostate*	Pertaining to the prostate
prostaglandin	**PROS**-tah-**GLAN**-din	S/ R/ R/	-**in** *chemical* **prosta-** *prostate* -**gland-** *gland*	Hormone present in many tissues, but first isolated from the prostate gland

Exercises

A. Elements. *Test your knowledge of the* language of male reproduction. *Circle the best answer.*   **LO 7.1, 7.2, 7.3, 7.4**

1. PSA and prostaglandin are
   a. an enzyme and a hormone
   b. a hormone and an enzyme
   c. a hormone and an antibiotic
   d. a diagnostic test and an antibiotic
   e. none of the above

2. The two bulbourethral glands are located
   a. near the ureters
   b. on each side of the membranous urethra
   c. behind the seminal vesicles
   d. on top of the prostate gland
   e. under the vas deferens

3. The suffix in the term **prostaglandin** tells you it is a
   a. hormone
   b. enzyme
   c. protein
   d. chemical
   e. blood cell

4. In the abbreviation **UTI**, the "T" stands for
   a. torsion
   b. testicle
   c. tract
   d. testosterone
   e. tunica

5. **Semen** is derived from the secretions of several glands:
   a. testicles, epididymis
   b. accessory glands
   c. thymus gland
   d. a, b, and c
   e. a and b only

6. The **prostate gland** is located
   a. below the bladder and posterior to the rectum
   b. beside the bladder and anterior to the rectum
   c. below the bladder and anterior to the rectum
   d. beside the bladder and posterior to the rectum
   e. between the bladder and the kidney

7. The root for **prostatic** is
   a. adeno-
   b. prosta-
   c. gland-
   d. ren-
   e. nephro-

8. Every term in this WAD is composed of
   a. two roots
   b. a root and a combining form
   c. a root and a prefix
   d. at least one root and a suffix
   e. two prefixes and a root

9. What provides energy for sperm?
   a. citric acid
   b. prostaglandins
   c. fructose
   d. a and c
   e. none of these

10. What is a nutrient for sperm?
    a. alkaline mucus
    b. acid urine
    c. citric acid
    d. normal flora
    e. acid secretions of the vagina

11. In the abbreviation **PSA**, the "A" stands for
    a. antidiuretic
    b. antibiotic
    c. antigen
    d. antibody
    e. allergen

12. What is the fluid vehicle for sperm?
    a. bloodstream
    b. lymph system
    c. plasma
    d. aqueous humor
    e. seminal fluid

BPH	benign prostatic hyperplasia
DRE	digital rectal examination
NIH	National Institutes of Health
PSA	prostate specific antigen
TURP	transurethral resection of the prostate

Keynotes

- Survival from prostate cancer is up to 80% if it is detected before it spreads outside the gland.

- Male infertility is involved in 40% of the 2.6 million infertile married couples in the United States (data from the **National Institutes of Health [NIH]**).

- Vasectomy is almost 100% successful in producing male sterility.

- **Vasovasostomy** is a microsurgical procedure to suture back together (anastomosis) the cut ends of the ductus deferens if requested sometime after vasectomy.

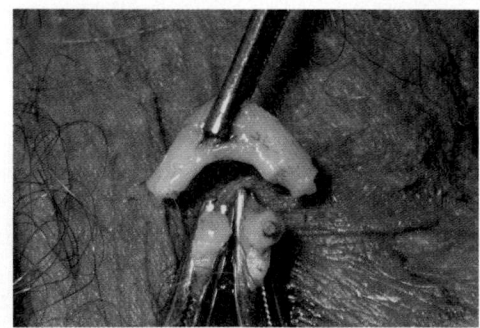

▲ **Figure 7.10** Vasectomy Being Performed.

LO 7.5 Disorders of the Prostate Gland

By the age of 20, the prostate weighs about 20 grams. It remains at that weight until age 45 to 50, when it begins to grow again. By age 80, some 90% of men have **benign prostatic hyperplasia (BPH)**. This is a noncancerous enlargement that compresses the prostatic urethra to produce symptoms of

- Difficulty starting and stopping the urine stream.
- **Nocturia**, **polyuria**, and dysuria.

In some patients, surgical treatment by **transurethral resection of the prostate (TURP)** relieves the symptoms. An endoscope called a **resectoscope** is inserted into the urethra and used to remove the tissue surrounding and compressing the urethra.

Prostatic cancer affects more than 10% of men over the age of 50, and its incidence is increasing. It forms hard nodules in the periphery of the gland and is often asymptomatic in its early stages because it does not compress the urethra.

Screening for prostatic cancer is performed by

- **Digital rectal exam (DRE)**. The size and texture of the prostate is palpated by a finger inserted into the rectum.
- **Prostate-specific antigen (PSA)** levels in the blood. Even though cancer can be present when the level is zero, the benefit of the test is to see if levels rise rapidly over time. The value of this test is a matter of debate at this time.

Several treatment options involving radiotherapy are available *(see Chapter 20)*. Sometimes, a **radical prostatectomy**, with complete surgical removal of the prostate and surrounding tissues, is performed.

Prostatitis is inflammation of the prostate gland. It occurs in three main types:

Type I—an acute bacterial infection with fever, chills, frequency, dysuria, and hematuria.

Type II—a chronic bacterial infection with less severe symptoms.

Type III—a chronic nonbacterial prostatitis in which the urinary symptoms are present but no bacteria can be detected. This is the most common type. Its etiology is unknown, and treatment is difficult.

Male Infertility

Male infertility is the inability to conceive after at least 1 year of unprotected intercourse. The primary causes of infertility are

1. Impaired sperm production:
   a. Cryptorchism
   b. **Anorchism** (absence of one or both testes)
   c. Testicular trauma
   d. Testicular cancer
   e. Orchitis after puberty
2. Impaired sperm delivery:
   a. Infections and blockage of spermatic ducts.
3. Testosterone deficiency **(hypogonadism)**:
   a. Medications to treat hypertension and/or high cholesterol.
   b. Environmental endocrine disrupters that adversely affect the endocrine system; examples are phthalates in plastics and dioxins in paper production.

In the United States each year, 500,000 men choose to be made infertile **(sterile)** by having a **vasectomy** *(Figure 7.10)*. Under local anesthesia, the ductus deferens is pulled through a small incision in the scrotum and cut in two places, a 1-centimeter segment is removed, and the ends are cauterized and tied. The site of the surgery makes the man infertile (still able to produce but not ejaculate sperm) but still able to produce and ejaculate seminal fluid.

WORD	PRONUNCIATION	ELEMENTS		DEFINITION
anastomosis anastomoses (pl)	ah-**NAS**-to-**MO**-sis	S/ R/	-osis *condition* **anastom-** *join together*	A surgically made union between two tubular structures
anorchism	an-**OR**-kizm	S/ P/ R/	-ism *condition* **an-** *without, lack of* **-orch-** *testicle*	Absence of testes
hyperplasia	high-per-**PLAY**-zee-ah	S/ P/ R/	-ia *condition* **hyper-** *excessive* **-plas-** *molding, formation*	Increase in the number of the cells in a tissue or organ
hypogonadism	**HIGH**-poh-**GOH**-nad-izm	S/ P/ R/	-ism *condition* **hypo-** *deficient* **-gonad-** *testes or ovaries*	Deficient gonad production of sperm or eggs or hormones
nocturia	nok-**TYU**-ree-ah	P/ R/	**noct-** *night* **-uria** *urine*	Excessive urination at night
polyuria	pol-ee-**YOU**-ree-ah	P/ R/	**poly-** *excessive* **-uria** *urine*	Excessive production of urine
prostatectomy	pross-tah-**TEK**-toe-me	S/ R/	-ectomy *surgical excision* **prostat-** *prostate*	Surgical removal of the prostate
prostatitis	pross-tah-**TIE**-tis	S/ R/	-itis *inflammation* **prostat-** *prostate*	Inflammation of the prostate
resectoscope	ree-**SEK**-toe-skope	S/ R/CF	-scope *instrument* **resect/o-** *cut off*	Endoscope for transurethral removal of lesions
sterile sterility	**STER**-isle steh-**RIL**-ih-tee	 S/ R/	Latin *barren* -ity *state, condition* **steril-** *barren*	Unable to fertilize or reproduce Inability to reproduce
vasectomy	vah-**SEK**-toe-me	S/ R/	-ectomy *surgical excision* **vas-** *duct*	Excision of a segment of the ductus deferens
vasovasostomy (also called **vasectomy reversal**)	**VAY**-soh-vay-**SOS**-toe-me	S/ R/CF R/ S/	stomy *new opening* **vas/o-** *duct* **-vas-** *duct* -stomy	Reanastomosis of the ductus deferens to restore the flow of sperm

Exercises

A. Recognition. *As you become more familiar with elements (especially suffixes), you will be able to recognize medical terms that are procedures and diagnoses. Practice with the terms in the above WAD. Fill in the blanks.* **LO 7.1, 7.2, 7.5**

1. List all the terms in the above WAD that could be a possible diagnosis for a patient.

_____

_____

2. List all the terms in the above WAD that are a procedure.

_____

3. Which term in the above WAD is an instrument?

_____

4. Which term or terms involve a surgical reconnection?

_____

5. What is another meaning for the word *sterile*?

_____

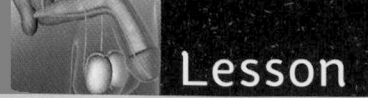

Lesson 7.3 The Penis and Its Disorders

MALE REPRODUCTIVE SYSTEM

The structure of the penis is specifically designed to meet its two main functions:
- Deposit semen in the female vagina around the cervix.
- Enable urine to flow to the outside.

It is essential that the anatomy, physiology, and terminology of the penis as related to performing these two functions be understood. The information in this lesson will enable you to:

7.3.1 Describe the structure and functions of the penis.

7.3.2 Summarize the processes and functions of erection and ejaculation.

7.3.3 Describe common disorders of the penis, prepuce, and urethra.

Abbreviations

ED	erectile dysfunction
STD	sexually transmitted disease

Keynote

Erectile dysfunction (ED) occurs in some 20 million American men.

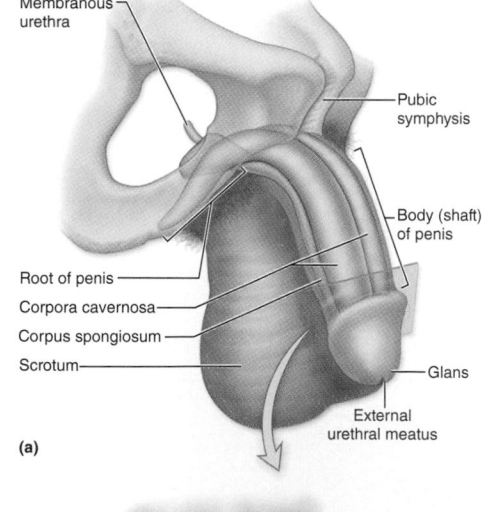

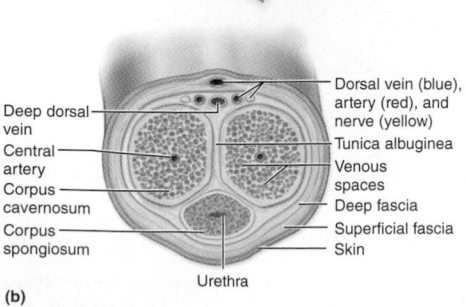

Membranous urethra

Pubic symphysis

Body (shaft) of penis

Root of penis

Corpora cavernosa

Corpus spongiosum

Scrotum

Glans

External urethral meatus

(a)

Deep dorsal vein

Central artery

Corpus cavernosum

Corpus spongiosum

Dorsal vein (blue), artery (red), and nerve (yellow)

Tunica albuginea

Venous spaces

Deep fascia

Superficial fascia

Skin

Urethra

(b)

▲ **Figure 7.11** **Anatomy of Penis.**
(a) External anatomy. (b) Cross-sectional view.

LO 7.1, 7.4, 7.5 Penis

The external, visible part of the penis comprises the **shaft** and the **glans** (*Figure 7.11a*), at the tip of which the external urethral meatus is located. The skin of the penis is very loosely attached to the shaft to permit expansion during erection. The skin continues over the glans as the **prepuce** (foreskin). A ventral fold of tissue, the **frenulum**, attaches the skin to the glans. The glans and facing prepuce contain sebaceous glands that produce a waxy secretion called **smegma**.

The shaft of the penis contains three **erectile** vascular bodies (*Figure 7.11b*):

- Paired **corpora cavernosa** are located dorsolaterally.
- A single **corpus spongiosum** is located inferiorly. It contains the urethra and goes on to form the glans.

The corpora cavernosa are composed of a network of venous sinuses surrounding a central artery. **Erection** occurs when the sinuses fill with blood, causing the erectile bodies to distend and become rigid. It is a parasympathetic nervous system response to stimulation.

Ejaculation occurs when the sympathetic nervous system stimulates the smooth muscle of the ductus deferens, ejaculatory ducts, and the prostate gland to contract. The seminal vesicles contract so that their fluids join to form semen. The internal urethral sphincter also contracts so that urine cannot enter the urethra and semen cannot enter the bladder.

Disorders of the Penis

Trauma to the penis can vary from being caught in a pants zipper to a fracture of an erect penis during vigorous sexual intercourse.

Peyronie disease is a marked curvature of the erect penis caused by fibrous tissue. Its etiology is unknown, and there is no successful treatment.

Priapism is a persistent, painful erection when blood cannot escape from the erectile tissue. It can be caused by drugs (such as epinephrine), blood clots, or spinal cord injury.

Cancer of the penis occurs most commonly on the glans and is rare in circumcised men. Circumcision also offers some protection against HIV infection.

Syphilis can cause flat pink or gray growths called **condylomata** or a sore called a **chancre**.

Other **sexually transmitted diseases (STDs)** can produce small, firm genital warts called **condylomata acuminata** or firm, dimpled growths called **molluscum contagiosum**. The STDs are discussed in detail in *Chapter 13*.

Erectile dysfunction (ED), or **impotence**, is the inability to have a satisfactory erection. **Premature ejaculation** occurs when a man ejaculates so quickly during intercourse that it causes embarrassment.

WORD	PRONUNCIATION	ELEMENTS		DEFINITION
acuminata	a-**KYU**-min-ah-ta	S/	-ata *action, place*	Tapering to a point
		R/	**acumin-** *to sharpen*	
cavernosa	kav-er-**NOH**-sah	S/	-osa *like*	Resembling a cave
		R/	**cavern-** *cave*	
chancre	**SHAN**-ker		Latin *cancer*	Primary lesion of syphilis
condyloma condylomata (pl)	kon-dih-**LOW**-ma kon-dih-**LOW**-ma-tah		Greek *a knob*	Warty growth on external genitalia
contagiosum contagious (adj)	kon-**TAY**-jee-oh-sum kon-**TAY**-jus		Latin *to touch closely*	Infection spread from one person to another by direct contact. Able to be transmitted, as infections transmitted from person to person or from person to air or surface to person
corpus corpora (pl)	**KOR**-pus kor-**POR**-ah		Latin *body*	Major part of a structure
erection	ee-**REK**-shun	S/	-ion *process, condition*	Distended and rigid state of an organ
		R/	**erect-** *straight, to set up*	
erectile	ee-**REK**-tile	S/	-ile *capable of*	Capable of erection or being distended with blood
frenulum	**FREN**-you-lum		Latin *small bridle*	Fold of mucous membrane between the glans and prepuce
glans	GLANZ		Latin *acorn*	Head of the penis or clitoris
impotence	**IM**-poh-tence		Latin *inability*	Inability to achieve an erection
molluscum	moh-**LUS**-kum		Latin *soft*	Soft, round tumor of skin caused by a virus
Peyronie disease	pay-**ROH**-nee **DIZ**-eez		François de la Peyronie, 1678–1747, French surgeon	Penile bending and pain on erection
prepuce	**PREE**-puce		Latin *foreskin*	Fold of skin that covers the glans penis
priapism	**PRY**-ah-pizm		Priapus, mythical Roman god of procreation	Persistent erection of the penis
smegma	**SMEG**-mah		Greek *ointment*	Oily material produced by the glans and prepuce
spongiosum	spun-jee-**OH**-sum	S/	-um *tissue*	Spongelike tissue
		R/	**spongios-** *sponge*	
syphilis	**SIF**-ih-lis		Possibly from the Latin poem "Syphilis sive Morbus Gallicus" by Fracastorius	Sexually transmitted disease caused by a spirochete
trauma traumatic	**TRAW**-mah traw-**MAT**-ik	S/ R/	-tic *pertaining to* **trauma-** *injury*	A physical or mental injury Pertaining to or caused by trauma

Exercises

A. Latin and Greek terms stand alone and do not deconstruct into several elements the way other terms do. *Match the medical term in the left column to its meaning in the right column. Fill in the blanks.*   **LO 7.1, 7.2**

_____ 1. corpus

_____ 2. chancre

_____ 3. molluscum

_____ 4. condyloma

_____ 5. impotence

_____ 6. contagious

a. warty growth on external genitalia

b. Transmitted, as an infection spread from one person to another by direct contact

c. inability to achieve an erection

d. primary lesion of syphilis

e. soft, round tumor of skin caused by a virus

f. major part of a structure

B. What types of body injuries could be considered trauma? *Be prepared to discuss your answers in class.*   **LO 7.1, 7.2, 7.3**

1. _____

2. _____

3. _____

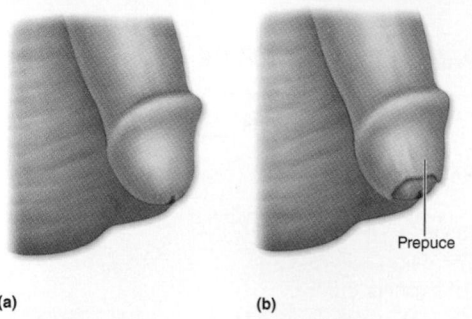

(a)   **(b)**

▲ **Figure 7.12**   Prepuce.
(a) Circumcised penis. (b) Uncircumcised penis.

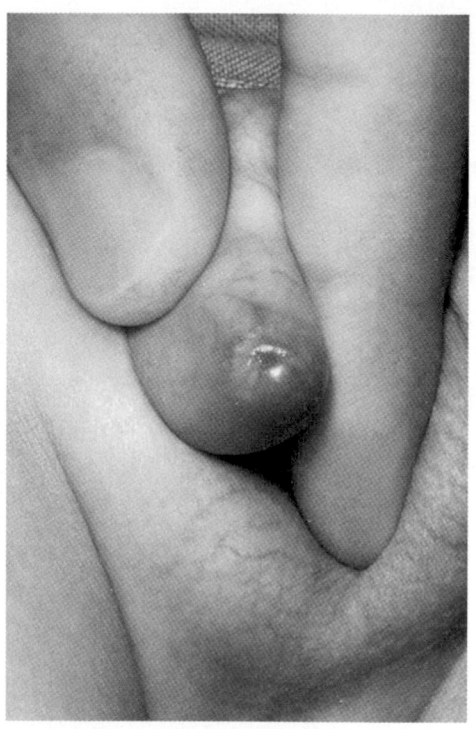

▲ **Figure 7.13**   Phimosis.

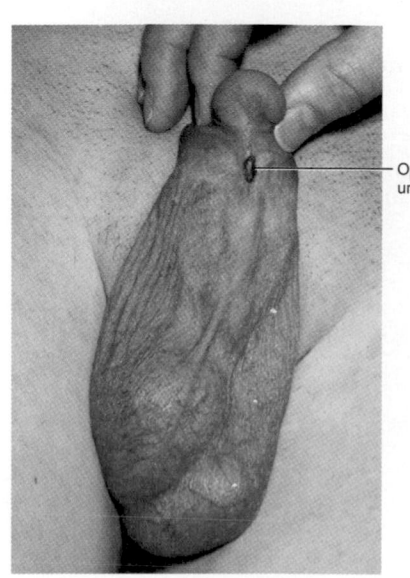

Opening of urethra

▲ **Figure 7.14**   Hypospadias.

LO 7.4, 7.5 Prepuce (Foreskin) and Urethra

Prepuce (Foreskin)

The functions of the **prepuce (foreskin)** are to cover and protect the glans and produce smegma, a lubricant containing lipids, cell debris, and some natural antibiotics.

Removal of the foreskin is called **circumcision** (*Figure 7.12*). In many religions, circumcision is a ritual in the neonatal period or at varying ages before puberty. In the United States, 85% of all males are circumcised in the neonatal period. In Europe, less than 20% are circumcised. Circumcision is painful at any age and may be complicated by bleeding or infection.

Studies suggest that circumcision provides a degree of protection against acquiring HIV infection and also a decreased risk of acquiring penile cancer later in life.

Disorders of the Prepuce

Disorders of the prepuce include

- **Balanitis**—infection of the glans and foreskin with bacteria or yeast.
- **Phimosis**—a condition in which the foreskin is tight because of a small opening and cannot be retracted over the glans for cleaning (*Figure 7.13*). It can lead to balanitis.
- **Paraphimosis**—a condition in which the retracted foreskin cannot be pulled forward to cover the glans.

In all of these conditions, particularly if they are recurrent, circumcision as an adult may be necessary.

Penile Urethra

The **penile urethra** passes through the single erectile body, the corpus spongiosum, to the external urethral meatus.

Disorders of the Penile Urethra

Urethritis is an inflammation of the urethra. It can be caused by

- The same bacteria that cause UTIs (*see Chapter 6*).
- STDs such as chlamydia and gonorrhea (*see Chapter 8*).
- Herpes simplex virus and cytomegalovirus (*see Chapter 8*).
- Chemical irritants such as **spermicides** and **contraceptive** gels.

Urethritis presents with dysuria, increased frequency of urination, and discharge from the penis. After urine culture to identify the organism, antibiotics will clear a bacterial infection, usually without complications.

Urethral stricture is scarring that narrows the urethra. It results from infection or injury. It produces a less forceful stream of urine and can be a cause of UTI. A urologist uses a cystoscope to examine the urethra and to cut the stricture **(urethrotomy)**.

Hypospadias is a congenital defect in which the opening of the urethra is on the undersurface of the penis instead of at the head of the glans (*Figure 7.14*). It can be corrected surgically.

Epispadias is a congenital defect in which the opening of the urethra is on the **dorsum** of the penis. It can be corrected surgically.

WORD	PRONUNCIATION	ELEMENTS		DEFINITION
balanitis	bal-ah-**NIE**-tis	S/ R/	-itis *inflammation* **balan-** *glans penis*	Inflammation of the glans and prepuce of the penis
circumcision	ser-kum-**SIZH**-un	S/ P/ R/	-ion *process, action* **circum-** *around* **-cis-** *to cut*	To remove part or all of the prepuce
contraception	kon-trah-**SEP**-shun	S/ P/ R/	-ion *process, action* **contra-** *against* **-cept-** *to receive*	Prevention of conception
dorsum	**DOR**-sum		Latin *back*	Upper, posterior, or back surface
epispadias	ep-ih-**SPAY**-dee-as	S/ P/ R/	-ias *condition* **epi-** *above* **-spad-** *tear or cut*	Condition in which the urethral opening is on the dorsum of the penis
foreskin	**FOR**-skin	P/ R/	fore- *in front* **-skin** *skin*	Skin that covers the glans penis
hypospadias	high-poh-**SPAY**-dee-as	S/ P/ R/	-ias *condition* **hypo-** *below* **-spad-** *tear or cut*	Urethral opening more proximal than normal on the ventral surface of the penis
paraphimosis	**PAR**-ah-fi-**MOH**-sis	S/ P/ R/	-osis *condition* **para-** *abnormal* **-phim-** *muzzle*	Condition in which a retracted prepuce cannot be pulled forward to cover the glans
phimosis	fi-**MOH**-sis	S/ R/	-osis *condition* **phim-** *muzzle*	Condition in which the prepuce cannot be retracted
spermicide	**SPER**-mih-side	S/ R/CF	-cide *to kill* **sperm/i-** *sperm*	Agent that destroys sperm
spermicidal (adj)	**SPER**-mih-side-al	S/	-al *pertaining to*	Pertaining to the destruction of sperm
stricture	**STRICK**-shur		Latin *to draw tight*	Narrowing of a tube
urethrotomy	you-ree-**THROT**-oh-me	S/ R/CF	-tomy *surgical incision* **urethr/o-** *urethra*	Incision of a stricture of the urethra

Exercises

A. Refine your knowledge of the *language of urology* by choosing the correct term to complete the statement. *Circle the best choice. Be precise and watch the spelling!* **LO 7.1, 7.2, 7.3, 7.4, 7.5**

1. Inflammation of the glans and prepuce is

   urethritis   cystitis   balanitis   hypospadias

2. Condition in which a retracted prepuce cannot be pulled forward to cover the glans is

   hypospadias   phimosis   spongiosum   paraphimosis

3. Incision of a stricture of the urethra is

   Urethrectomy   urethroplasty   urethropexy   urethrotomy

4. To remove all or part of the prepuce is

   circumcision   circumscion   circummcision   circumsion

5. Skin that covers the glans penis is

   forskin   fourskin   forksin   foreskin

6. Narrowing of a tube is

   dilation   anastomosis   stricture   retraction

Male Reproductive System

Challenge Your Knowledge

A. **Language of urology.** Every day on the job in the Urology Clinic you will be asked to apply the language of urology to the anatomy and physiology of the male reproductive system. Circle the correct choice. (**LO 7.1, 7.2, 7.4,** *Remember, Understand*)

1. The prostate, seminal vesicles, and bulbourethral glands are

   a. gonads

   b. primary sex organs

   c. accessory glands

   d. secondary sex organs

   e. accessory vessels

2. A surgical procedure that makes a male sterile is

   a. nephrectomy

   b. vasovasostomy

   c. orchiopexy

   d. vasectomy

   e. lithotripsy

3. Shining a bright light on a swelling to see the shape of the testes is

   a. maturation

   b. micturition

   c. vasoepididymostomy

   d. orchiopexy

   e. transillumination

4. Scarring that narrows the urethra is called

   a. UTI

   b. urethral stricture

   c. ureteroscope

   d. urethrotomy

   e. urethropexy

5. The diamond-shaped region between the thighs is called

   a. rete testis

   b. perineum

   c. median septum

   d. ductus deferens

   e. anal triangle

B. Apply the language of urology to the anatomy and physiology of the male reproductive system. Circle the correct choice. **(LO 7.1, 7.2, 7.4,** *Remember, Understand*)

1. Androgens are

   a. enzymes

   b. vitamins

   c. hormones

   d. special nerve cells

   e. flagellum

2. The penis, scrotum, and testes collectively are known as

   a. primary sex organs

   b. accessory glands

   c. secondary sex organs

   d. external genitalia

   e. the perineum

3. Measured in a blood test to check for prostate cancer is

   a. BPH

   b. TURP

   c. BMR

   d. PSA

   e. ED

4. A female egg cell is called

   a. flagellum

   b. spermatozoa

   c. spermatid

   d. oocyte

   e. varicocele

5. The distinct ridge in the scrotum is called the

   a. dartos

   b. raphe

   c. hydrocele

   d. epididymis

   e. cavernosa

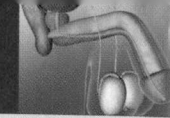

Chapter 7 Review

Male Reproductive System

F. Terminology challenge. Briefly answer the following question. Why does "cryptorchism" mean "hidden"? **(LO 7.1, 7.2, 7.5,** *Remember, Understand, Apply***)**

_____

_____

G. Patient education. Patients will always have questions that you must be able to answer professionally. How well could you explain to your patient the difference between the following terms. **(LO 7.2, 7.4, 7.5,** *Remember, Understand, Apply***)**

1. The surgical procedures of *vasectomy* and *vasovasostomy:*

_____

_____

_____

2. A *radical prostatectomy* and a *TURP:*

_____

_____

_____

H. Circle the incorrect answer and then rewrite it correctly on the lines below. (LO 7.1, 7.2, *Remember, Understand, Apply***)**

1. Which of the following statements is incorrect about the perineum?

   a. The perineum is occupied by the external genitalia.

   b. The perineum is the oval-shaped region between the thighs.

   c. The penis, scrotum, and testes occupy the perineum.

   d. The border of the perineum is located at the pubic symphysis anteriorly.

   e. The anus is also in the perineum.

2. Correction:

   _____

   _____

I. Abbreviations are another form of precise communication. Demonstrate that you know the meanings of the abbreviations in this exercise. Circle the best answer. **(LO 7.1, 7.2,** *Remember, Understand, Apply***)**

1. The following is a diagnosis for a type of prostate disease:

   a. BPH

   b. TURP

   c. PSA

2. The following can produce *condylomata acuminata:*

   a. STD

   b. UTI

   c. ED

3. The abbreviation *BMR* relates to

   a. metabolism

   b. bowel movement

   c. bulbourethral glands

J. Disorder or disease. Complete the diagnosis documentation for the following patients. Fill in the blanks with the correct medical term for the disorder or disease mentioned in each statement. (**LO 7.1, 7.5,** *Remember, Understand, Apply*)

1. Excess fluid has collected in the space between the visceral and parietal layers of the tunica vaginalis of the patient's right

    testis: hydro_____.

2. Noncancerous enlargement compressing the prostatic urethra is: benign _____ plasia.

3. Marked curvature of the erect penis caused by fibrous tissue is _____ disease.

4. Undescended testicles in a 10-month-old male is _____ism.

5. Veins in the spermatic cord become tortuous and dilated: varico _____.

6. Opening of the urethra is on the undersurface of the penis instead of at the head of the glans:

    hypo_____.

7. Yeast infection of the glans and foreskin is _____itis.

8. Foreskin is tight and cannot be retracted over the glans for cleaning: _____sis.

9. Inflammation of the epididymis is _____itis.

K. Trace the pathway taken by a sperm cell from the testes to its ejaculation. Number the following terms in the correct order. Fill in the blanks. *Remember your study hint!* (**LO 7.1, 7.2, 7.4,** *Understand*)

_____ a. epididymis

_____ b. urethra

_____ c. testis

_____ d. seminiferous tubules

_____ e. ejaculatory duct

_____ f. ductus deferens

_____ g. penis

L. Brain teaser. The following brain teaser is taken directly from this chapter: "If it (a varicose vein in the spermatic cord) is uncomfortable, it can be treated by surgically tying off the affected veins." Rewrite this information in more precise medical language. (**LO 7.1, 7.2, 7.5,** *Understand*)

_____

_____

_____

_____

_____

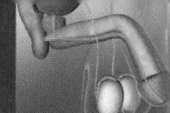

Chapter 7 Review

Male Reproductive System

CHAPTER SUMMARY EXERCISE

A. **Spelling comprehension.** Circle the correct spelling of the term. (**LO 7.1,** *Remember*)

1. gonad	gonnad	gonade	gunad	gunade
2. perikneal	perikneeal	perineal	perrineal	peraneal
3. coriocarcinoma	corriocarcinoma	choriacarcinoma	choriocarcinoma	corheacarcinoma
4. insemination	insemmination	insimination	insimmination	insimation
5. tortion	torsion	tortsion	tortcion	tostion
6. epidydimis	epidydimus	epididymis	epididymus	epodidymis
7. frinulum	frenullum	frenulum	frennulum	frenulumn
8. tistosterune	testosterine	testosterone	tistosterone	testosteron
9. priaprism	piaprism	priapism	prapism	piapresm
10. flagilla	flaggila	flagella	flaggela	flaggilla

B. **Match the number of the correct spelling of the term in Exercise A with the brief description of the term below.** (**LO 7.2,** *Apply*)

1. Androgen produced by testis: _____

2. Highly malignant cancer in testis or ovary: _____

3. Tail of a sperm (plural): _____

4. The act or result of twisting: _____

5. Deposition of semen in female reproductive tract: _____

6. Pertaining to the area between the thighs: _____

7. Testis or ovary: _____

8. Structure on posterior surface of testis: _____

9. Persistent, painful erection: _____

10. Fold of mucous membrane: _____

C. Using your knowledge of terms 1–10 in Exercises A and B and their correct spelling, write a brief sentence for each of the terms as it might appear in patient documentation. (LO 7.2, *Apply*)

1. _____

2. _____

3. _____

4. _____

5. _____

6. _____

7. _____

8. _____

9. _____

10. _____

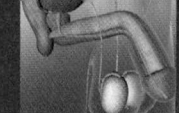

Male Reproductive System

D. **After rereading Case Report 7.1, answer the following questions.** Be prepared to discuss your answers in class. (**LO 7.1, 7.2, 7.5,** *Apply, Analyze*)

Case Report 7.1

You are

...an EMT-P working in the Emergency Department at Fulwood Medical Center.

Your patient is

...Joseph Davis, a 17-year-old high school senior. He is brought in by his mother at 0400 hrs. He complains of (c/o) sudden onset of pain in his left testicle 3 hours earlier that woke him up. The pain is intense and has made him vomit. VS: T 99.2°F, P 88, R 15, BP 130/70. Examination reveals his left testicle to be enlarged, warm, and tender. His abdomen is normal to palpation.

At your request, Dr. Helinski, the emergency physician on duty, examines him immediately. He diagnoses a torsion of the patient's left testicle.

Joseph Davis presented with typical symptoms and signs of testicular torsion. The affected testis rapidly became painful, tender, swollen, and inflamed. Emergency surgery was performed, and the testis and cord were manually untwisted through an incision in the scrotum. The testis was stitched to surrounding tissues to prevent a recurrence.

1. In nonmilitary time, when is 0400 hrs? _____

2. Joseph has "sudden onset of pain." Is that acute or chronic? _____

3. Interpret (spell out) each of the VS:

   T = _____

   P = _____

   R = _____

   BP = _____

4. What action is performed in *palpation?* _____

5. What is the difference between a *symptom* and a *sign?* _____

   Symptom: _____

   Sign: _____

6. In testicular tortion, what gets twisted? _____

7. What is the medical term for "stitched to surrounding tissues"? _____

E. Meet the goals of each of the chapter outcomes by using the correct language of the male reproductive system for the answers. (LO 7.1–7.5, *Analyze*)

1. Apply the language of urology as it relates to the anatomy and physiology of the male reproductive system. What is the purpose of having the scrotum outside the body? (**LO 7.1**)

   _____

   _____

2. Use the medical terms of urology as they relate to the male reproductive system to communicate and document in writing accurately and precisely in any health care setting. What is another term for the bulbourethral glands? (**LO 7.2**)

   a. vas deferens

   b. fallopian

   c. flagellum

   d. Cowper

   e. Peyronie

3. Use the medical terms of urology as they relate to the male reproductive system to communicate verbally with accuracy and precision in any health care setting. You tell the doctor the patient has been experiencing *nocturia, polyuria,* and *dysuria.* What do those terms mean? (**LO 7.3**)

   a. nocturia: _____

   b. polyuria: _____

   c. dysuria: _____

4. Which medical term in this group involves movement? Circle the correct answer. (**LO 7.4**)

   a. testosterone

   b. flagellum

   c. torsion

   d. varicocele

   e. teratoma

5. Discuss the disorders of the individual reproductive glands and their treatment. *Orchitis* can have either a bacterial or viral cause. Give an example of each. (**LO 7.5**)

   a. Bacterial:_____

   b. Viral: _____

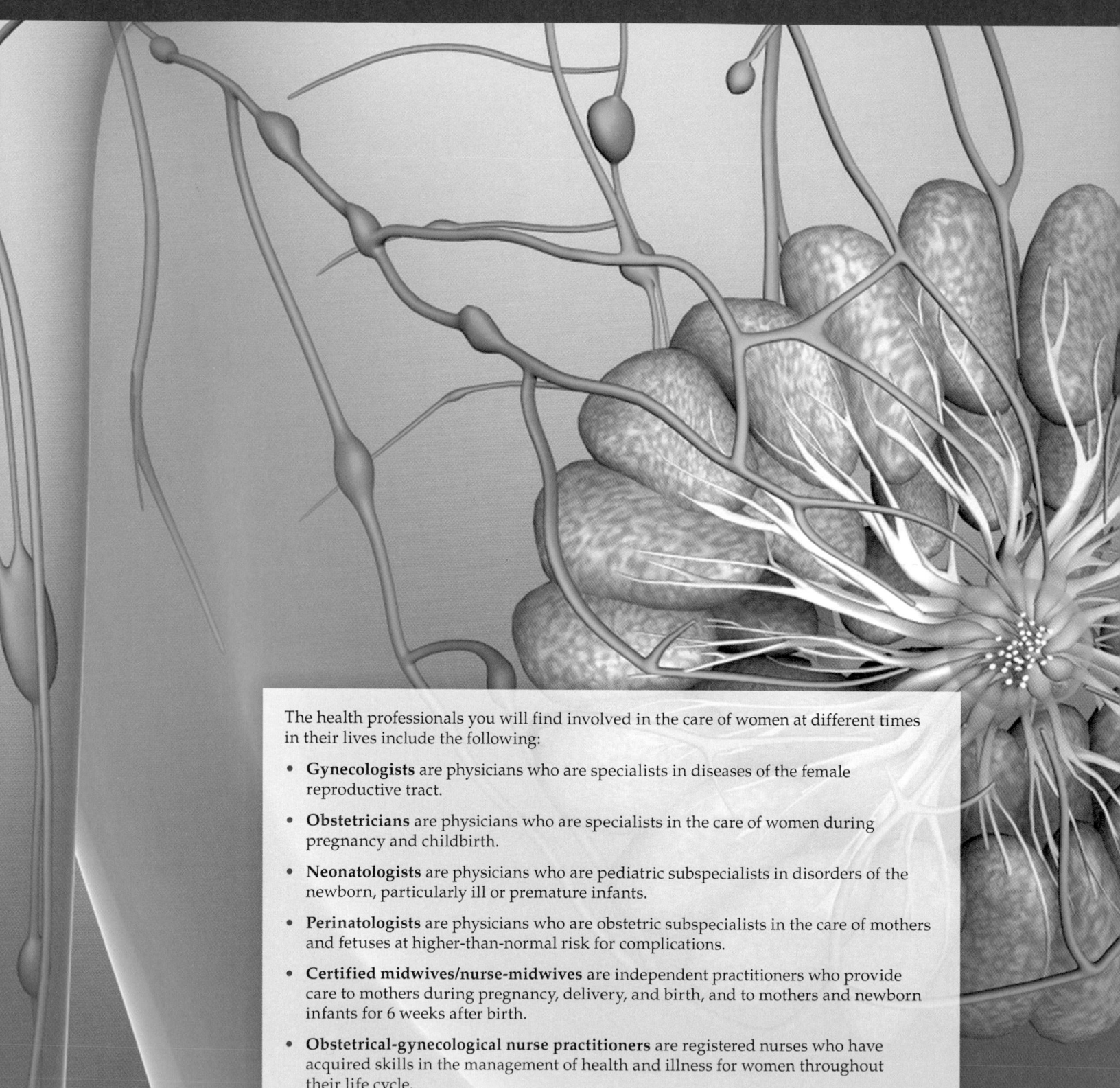

Female Reproductive System
The Languages of Gynecology and Obstetrics

The health professionals you will find involved in the care of women at different times in their lives include the following:

- **Gynecologists** are physicians who are specialists in diseases of the female reproductive tract.

- **Obstetricians** are physicians who are specialists in the care of women during pregnancy and childbirth.

- **Neonatologists** are physicians who are pediatric subspecialists in disorders of the newborn, particularly ill or premature infants.

- **Perinatologists** are physicians who are obstetric subspecialists in the care of mothers and fetuses at higher-than-normal risk for complications.

- **Certified midwives/nurse-midwives** are independent practitioners who provide care to mothers during pregnancy, delivery, and birth, and to mothers and newborn infants for 6 weeks after birth.

- **Obstetrical-gynecological nurse practitioners** are registered nurses who have acquired skills in the management of health and illness for women throughout their life cycle.

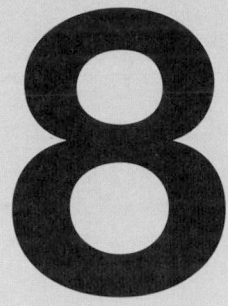

Case Report (CR) 8.1

You are

. . . a **registered nurse (RN)** working in the Emergency Department at Fulwood Medical Center.

Your patient is

. . . Ms. Lara Baker, a 32-year-old single mother who works in the billing department of the medical center. You have been asked to take her vital signs (VS). For the past couple of days she has had muscle aches and a feeling of general uneasiness that she had thought were due to her heavy menstrual period. In the past 3 hours, she has developed a severe headache with nausea and vomiting. A diffuse rash over her trunk that looks like sunburn is now spreading to her upper arms and thighs.

VS: T 104.2°F, P 120 and irregular, R 20, BP 86/50. As you took her VS, you noted that she did not seem to understand where she was. She was unable to pass a urine specimen.

For this patient, the treatment she receives in the next few minutes is vital for her survival. You have your supervising nurse and the emergency physician come to see her immediately. As you participate in this patient's care, clear communication among the team members is essential.

CHAPTER

8

Chapter Learning Outcomes

The information in this chapter will enable you to:

LO 8.1 Use the medical terms of gynecology and obstetrics to communicate and document in writing accurately and precisely in any health care setting.

LO 8.2 Use the medical terms of gynecology and obstetrics to communicate verbally with accuracy and precision in any health care setting.

LO 8.3 Describe the anatomy and physiology of the female reproductive system.

LO 8.4 Describe the effects and treatments of sexually transmitted diseases.

LO 8.5 Identify the hormones of the female sexual cycle.

LO 8.6 Discuss disorders of the female reproductive tract.

LO 8.7 Explain the causes of and the investigation of female infertility.

LO 8.8 Identify methods of contraception for the female and male.

LO 8.9 Describe conception, implantation, and development of the embryo and fetus.

LO 8.10 Discuss the changes that occur in the female reproductive system during pregnancy and childbirth.

LO 8.11 Understand the effects of common disorders of pregnancy and childbirth on the mother and **fetus**.

LO 8.12 Describe the structure and functions of the female breast.

LO 8.13 Discuss disorders of the breast and their treatment.

LESSON OBJECTIVES

Both the female and male reproductive systems are dormant until **puberty**, when the gonads (**ovaries** in the female and testes in the male) begin to secrete significant quantities of sex hormones (**estrogen** and **progesterone** in the female, androgens in the male). In the female, the external **genitalia** become more prominent, pubic hair develops, the **vagina** becomes lubricated, and breast enlargement occurs. Understanding the anatomy and physiology of the mature external genitalia and vagina is an important introduction to the female **reproductive** system.

The information in this lesson will enable you to:

8.1.1 Identify the female external genitalia.

8.1.2 Detail the anatomy and physiology of the vagina.

8.1.3 Discuss the disorders of the vagina.

8.1.4 Describe common sexually transmitted diseases.

LO 8.3 External Genitalia

Abbreviations

RN	registered nurse
GYN	gynecology
OB	obstetrics

Keynotes

• Obstetrics (OB) is the medical specialty for the care of women during pregnancy and the **postpartum** period.

• Gynecology (GYN) is the medical specialty for the care of the female reproductive system.

The female external genitalia occupy most of the **perineum** and are collectively called the **vulva** *(Figure 8.1)*. The structures of the vulva include the

- **Mons pubis**—a mound of skin and adipose tissue overlying the symphysis pubis. In **postpubescent** females it is covered with **pubic** hair.
- **Labia majora**—a pair of thick folds of skin, connective tissue, and adipose tissue. In postpubescent females, their outer surface is covered with coarse hair, and the inner surface has numerous sweat and sebaceous glands.
- **Labia minora**—a pair of thin folds of hairless skin immediately internal to the labia majora. Sebaceous glands are present on these folds, together with melanocytes *(see Chapter 15)* that give the folds a dark melanin pigmentation. Anteriorly, the labia minora join together to form the prepuce (hood) of the clitoris. Posteriorly they merge with the labia majora.
- **Clitoris**—a small erectile body capped with a glans. It has two corpora cavernosa surrounded by connective tissue. The clitoris contains many sensory nerve receptors.

Deep to the labia majora on either side of the vaginal orifice is an erectile body called the **vestibular bulb** *(Figure 8.1b)*. The two bulbs become congested with blood and more sensitive during sexual arousal. Posterior to the vestibular bulbs on each side of the vaginal orifice is a pea-size **Bartholin gland**. These glands secrete mucin, which lubricates the vagina. Secretion is increased during sexual arousal and intercourse.

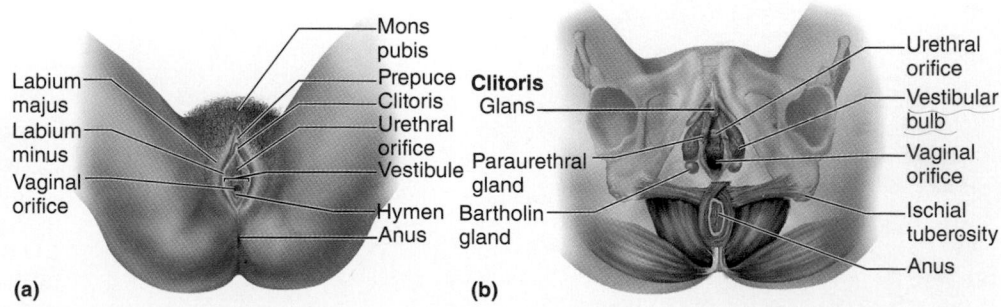

Labium majus · Labium minus · Vaginal orifice · Mons pubis · Prepuce · Clitoris · Urethral orifice · Vestibule · Hymen · Anus · **Clitoris** Glans · Paraurethral gland · Bartholin gland · Urethral orifice · Vestibular bulb · Vaginal orifice · Ischial tuberosity · Anus

(a)   (b)

▲ **Figure 8.1** **Female Perineum and Vulva.** *(a)* Surface anatomy. *(b)* Subcutaneous structures.

WORD	PRONUNCIATION	ELEMENTS		DEFINITION
clitoris	**KLIT**-oh-ris		Greek *clitoris*	Erectile organ of the vulva
estrogen	**ES**-troh-jen	S/ R/CF	-gen *produce, create* **estr/o-** *woman*	Generic term for hormones that stimulate female secondary sex characteristics
gynecology	guy-nih-**KOL**-oh-jee	S/ R/CF	-logy *study of* **gynec/o-** *female*	Medical specialty for the care of the female reproductive system
gynecologist	guy-nih-**KOL**-oh-jist	S/	-logist *specialist*	Specialist in gynecology
labium labia (pl)	**LAY**-bee-um **LAY**-bee-ah		Greek *lip*	Fold of the vulva
majus majora (pl)	**MAY**-jus **MAY**-jora		Latin *greater*	Bigger or greater; for example, labia majora
minus minora (pl)	**MY**-nus **MY**-nora		Latin *smaller*	Smaller or lesser; for example, labia minora
mons pubis	MONZ **PYU**-bis		**mons** Latin *mountain* **pubis** Latin *pubic bone*	Fleshy pad with pubic hair, overlying the pubic bone
obstetrics (OB)	ob-**STET**-ricks		Latin *a midwife*	Medical specialty for the care of women during pregnancy and the postpartum period
obstetrician	ob-steh-**TRISH**-un	S/ R/	-ician *expert, specialist* **obstetr-** *midwifery*	Medical specialist in obstetrics
perineum	**PER**-ih-**NEE**-um		Latin *perineum*	Area between the thighs, extending from the coccyx to the pubis
perineal (adj)	**PER**-ih-**NEE**-al			Pertaining to the perineum
postpartum	post-**PAR**-tum	P/ R/	post- *after* -partum *childbirth*	After childbirth
postpubescent	post-pyu-**BESS**-ent	S/ P/ R/	-ent *pertaining to, end result* post- *after* -pubesc- *to reach puberty*	After the period of puberty
progesterone (*Note:* Two suffixes.)	pro-**JESS**-ter-own	S/ S/ P/ R/	-one *chemical substance, hormone* -er- *agent* pro- *before* -gest- *pregnancy*	Hormone that prepares uterus for pregnancy
puberty	**PYU**-ber-tee	S/ R/	-ty *quality, state* **puber-** *growing up*	Process of maturing from child to young adult capable of reproducing
pubis	**PYU**-bis		Latin *pubic bone*	Bony front arch of the pelvis of the hip; also called pubic bone
pubic (adj)	**PYU**-bik	S/ R/	-ic *pertaining to* **pub-** *pubis*	Pertaining to the pubis
vulva vulvar (adj)	**VUL**-vah		Latin *a wrapper or covering*	Female external genitalia

Exercises

A. Latin and Greek terms cannot be further deconstructed into prefix, root, or suffix. *You must know them for what they are. Match the meaning in the left column with the correct medical term in the right column.*   **LO 8.3**

_____ 1. A covering or wrapper   **a.** labia

_____ 2. Pubic bone   **b.** pubis

_____ 3. Mountain   **c.** majora

_____ 4. Lesser   **d.** vulva

_____ 5. Lip   **e.** minora

_____ 6. Greater   **f.** mons

LO 8.3, 8.6 Vagina and Disorders

The **vagina**, or birth canal, is a fibromuscular tube, 4 to 5 inches (10 to 13 cm) in length (*Figure 8.2*). It connects the vulva with the uterus. It has three main functions:

- Discharge of menstrual fluid
- Receipt of the penis and semen
- Birth of a baby

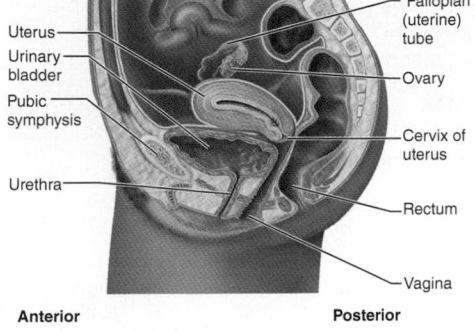

Uterus
Urinary bladder
Pubic symphysis
Urethra

Fallopian (uterine) tube
Ovary
Cervix of uterus
Rectum
Vagina

Anterior   Posterior

▲ **Figure 8.2**   **Female Reproductive Organs.**

It is located between the rectum and the urethra. The urethra is embedded in its anterior wall. In the wall of the vagina around the urethra are several small **paraurethral (Skene) glands** that open into the urethra.

At its posterior end, the vagina extends beyond the cervix of the uterus to form blind spaces called the anterior and posterior **fornices**. The lower end of the vagina contains numerous transverse folds, or **rugae**. The rugae project into the vaginal orifice to form the **hymen**, which stretches across the orifice. The intact hymen contains one or two openings to allow the escape of menstrual fluid.

Bacterial vaginosis is the most common cause of vaginitis in women of childbearing age. Different types of invading bacteria outnumber the normal bacteria of the vagina. The main symptom is an abnormal vaginal discharge with a fishlike odor. Diagnosis is made by laboratory examination of a specimen taken by vaginal swab. Treatment is with antibiotics such as clindamycin or metronidazole.

Toxic shock syndrome is a life-threatening illness caused by toxins circulating in the bloodstream. Certain rare strains of bacteria produce these toxins. In the most common form of toxic shock syndrome, the bacteria are in the vagina of women, and their growth is encouraged by the presence of a superabsorbent **tampon** that is not changed frequently (*see Case Report 8.1*).

Vulvovaginal candidiasis is a common cause of genital itching or burning, with a "cottage-cheese" **vaginal** discharge. It is caused by an overgrowth of the yeast fungus called *Candida* and can occur after taking antibiotics. Recent research has found that it is associated with vitamin D deficiency. Diagnosis is made by microscopic examination of a specimen taken by a vaginal swab. Treatment is with antifungal drugs that can be applied topically and used vaginally (miconazole or clotrimazole). If necessary, oral medications can be used (ketoconazole or fluconazole).

Allergic and irritative causes of **vulvovaginitis** can be found in vaginal hygiene products, spermicides, detergents, and synthetic underwear.

Vulvodynia is a chronic, lasting, severe pain around the vaginal orifice, which feels raw. Painful intercourse **(dyspareunia)** is common. The vulva may look normal or be slightly swollen. The etiology is unknown. Treatment varies from local anesthetics and creams to biofeedback therapy with exercises to the muscles of the pelvic floor. Surgical removal of the affected area **(vestibulectomy)** has been tried with variable results.

Keynotes

- Bacterial vaginosis is associated with increased risk of gonorrhea and **human immunodeficiency virus (HIV) infection.**
- Seventy-five percent of adult women have at least one genital yeast infection in their lifetime.
- Ten million office visits annually are for vulvodynia.
- **Vaginal cancers** are uncommon, comprising 1% to 2% of gynecologic malignancies. They can be effectively treated with surgery and radiation therapy.

Case Report 8.1 (continued)

In the opening Case Report to this chapter, Ms. Lara Baker presented to the Emergency Department with toxic shock syndrome. Because of her heavy period, she was using a superabsorbent tampon. She was admitted to intensive care. The **tampon** was removed and cultured, IV fluids and antibiotics were administered, and her kidney and liver functions were monitored. The causative organism was *Staphylococcus aureus.* She recovered well but had a second episode 6 months later.

S = Suffix   P = Prefix   **R = Root   R/CF = Combining Form**

WORD	PRONUNCIATION		ELEMENTS	DEFINITION
Candida candidiasis (also called **thrush**)	**KAN**-did-ah kan-dih-**DIE**-ah-sis	S/ R/	Latin *dazzling white* -iasis *state of, condition* candid- *Candida, a yeast*	A yeastlike fungus Infection with the yeastlike fungus *Candida*
dyspareunia	dis-pah-**RUE**-nee-ah	S/ P/ R/	-ia *condition* dys- *painful* -pareun- *lying beside, sexual intercourse*	Pain during sexual intercourse
fornix fornices (pl)	**FOR**-niks **FOR**-nih-seez		Latin *arch, vault*	Arch-shaped, blind-ended part of the vagina behind and around the cervix
hymen	**HIGH**-men		Greek *membrane*	Thin membrane partly occluding the vaginal orifice
paraurethral	**PAR**-ah-you-**REE**-thral	S/ P/ R/	-al *pertaining to* para- *alongside* -urethr- *urethra*	Situated around the urethra
ruga rugae (pl)	**ROO**-gah **ROO**-jee		Latin *a wrinkle*	A fold, ridge, or crease
Skene glands paraurethral glands (syn)	SKEEN GLANZ		Alexander Skene, 1838–1900, New York gynecologist	Paraurethral glands in the anterior wall of the vagina
tampon	**TAM**-pon		French *plug*	Plug or pack in a cavity to absorb or stop bleeding
vagina	vah-**JIE**-nah		Latin *a sheath*	Female genital canal extending from the uterus to the vulva
vaginal (adj)	**VAJ**-in-al	S/ R/	-al *pertaining to* vagin- *vagina*	Pertaining to the vagina
vaginosis vaginitis	vah-jih-**NOH**-sis vah-jih-**NIE**-tis	S/ S/	-osis *condition* -itis *inflammation*	Any disease of the vagina Inflammation of the vagina
vestibulectomy	ves-tib-you-**LEK**-toe-me	S/ R/	-ectomy *surgical excision* vestibul- *entrance*	Surgical excision of the vulva
vulvodynia	vul-voh-**DIN**-ee-uh	S/ R/CF	-dynia *pain* vulv/o- *vulva*	Chronic vulvar pain
vulvovaginitis	**VUL**-voh-vaj-ih-**NIE**-tis	S/ R/CF R/	-itis *inflammation* vulv/o- *vulva* -vagin- *vagina*	Inflammation of the vagina and vulva
vulvovaginal (adj)	**VUL**-voh-**VAJ**-ih-nal	S/	-al *pertaining to*	Pertaining to the vulva and vagina

Exercises

A. After reading Case Report 8.1, answer the following questions. *Be prepared to discuss your answers in class.*   **LO 8.6**

1. What makes *toxic shock syndrome* life-threatening?

_____

2. Is the causative agent for the patient's condition a bacterium or a virus?

_____

3. How do you know the correct answer in question 2 above?

_____

4. Why does the patient require intensive care?

_____

5. What was the treatment plan for the patient?

_____

Abbreviations

CDC	Centers for Disease Control and Prevention
DNA	deoxyribonucleic acid
HIV	human immunodeficiency virus
PID	pelvic inflammatory disease
STD	sexually transmitted disease

Keynotes

- Three million cases of chlamydia are recognized annually in the United States and could be prevented by using a **condom**.

- Infection with gonorrhea can be prevented by using a condom.

- Three million cases of trichomoniasis occur annually in the United States and could be prevented by using a condom.

LO 8.4 Sexually Transmitted Diseases

According to the **Centers for Disease Control and Prevention (CDC)**, 15 million cases of sexually transmitted diseases **(STDs)** are reported annually in the United States, with adolescents and young adults being at the greatest risk. Some of the common STDs are described as follows:

Chlamydia is known as the "silent" disease because up to 75% of infected women and men have no symptoms. When there are signs, a vaginal or penile discharge and irritation with dysuria are common. The diagnosis is made by laboratory testing of a **swab** from the cervix or male urethra. Highly accurate urine tests and DNA probes are now available.

Treatment is with oral antibiotics such as doxycycline, erythromycin, or azithromycin. Untreated, chlamydia can spread higher into the female reproductive tract and cause **pelvic inflammatory disease (PID)**. It can be passed on to a newborn during childbirth, causing eye infections or pneumonia. It is a reason why antibiotic eyedrops are given to newborns.

Gonorrhea is spread by unprotected sex and can be passed on to a baby in childbirth, causing a serious eye infection. This is another reason why newborns are given eyedrops. Symptoms in both male and female adults may not be present. In the female, they can include a vaginal discharge, bleeding, and dysuria. Gonorrhea is also a cause of PID. Laboratory testing on a swab taken from the surface of the infected area can confirm the diagnosis; **DNA** probes are also available.

Gonorrhea can be treated with a single dose of an antibiotic such as cefixime, but its causative agent, *Neisseria gonorrhoeae*, is developing resistance to antibiotics.

Syphilis, caused by a **spirochete**, is transmitted sexually and can then spread through the bloodstream to every organ in the body. It is also transmitted among intravenous drug users who share needles. **Primary syphilis** begins 10 to 90 days after infection as an ulcer, a **chancre**, at the place of infection *(Figure 8.3)*. Four to ten weeks later, if the primary syphilis is not treated, **secondary syphilis** appears as a rash on the hands and soles of the feet, with swollen glands and muscle and joint pain. **Tertiary syphilis** can occur years after the primary infection and can cause permanent damage to the brain with dementia. Because primary syphilis is curable with penicillin or other antibiotics, tertiary syphilis is rarely seen today. A pregnant woman with untreated syphilis can transmit the infection to her fetus before birth.

Chancroid is an ulcerative disease (not caused by a spirochete) and is without system-wide effects, unlike syphilis. It develops as a chancre with swollen, tender lymph nodes in the groin. Antibiotics such as azithromycin and ceftriaxone are effective.

Trichomoniasis ("trich") is caused by the parasite *Trichomonas vaginalis*. Men can carry the infection in their urethra and almost never have symptoms. The vagina is the common site of infection in women. It can produce a frothy yellow-green discharge with irritation and itching of the vulva. Because it is a "ping-pong" infection that goes back and forth between partners, both individuals should be treated with metronidazole.

Molluscum contagiosum is caused by a virus that can be sexually transmitted; the resulting tumors are small, shiny bumps that have a milky-white fluid inside *(Figure 8.4)*. They can disappear and reappear anywhere on the body. Molluscum contagiosum is often seen in children and is not sexually transmitted in such cases. The lesions can be treated with podophyllin ointment, or liquid nitrogen and laser surgery can be used.

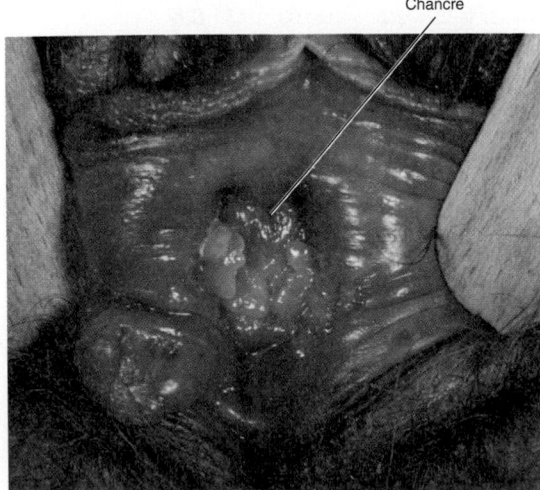

▲ **Figure 8.3** Chancre of Primary Syphilis in Female.

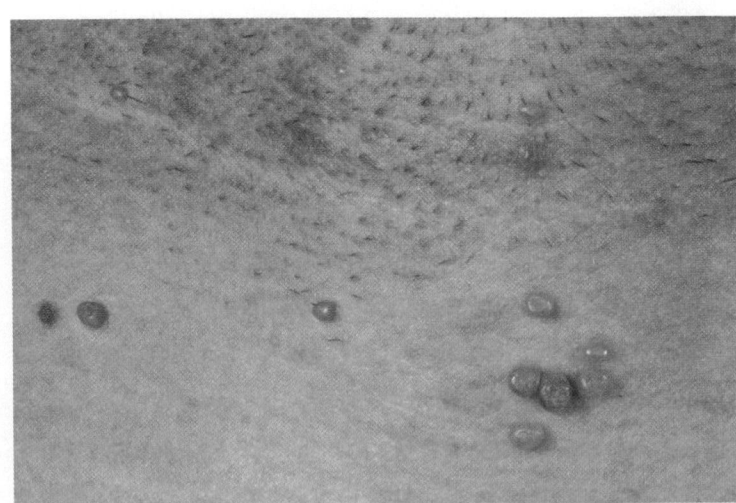

▲ **Figure 8.4** Molluscum Contagiosum.

WORD	PRONUNCIATION		ELEMENTS	DEFINITION
chancre	**SHAN**-ker		Latin *cancer*	Primary lesion of syphilis
chancroid	**SHAN**-kroyd	S/ R	-oid *resembling* chancr- *chancre*	Infectious, painful, ulcerative STD not related to syphilis
chlamydia	klah-**MID**-ee-ah		Latin *cloak*	A species of bacteria causing an STD
condom	**KON**-dom		Old English *sheath or cover*	A sheath or cover for the penis or vagina to prevent conception and infection
gonorrhea	gon-oh-**REE**-ah	S/ R/CF	-rrhea *flow or discharge* gon/o- *seed*	Specific contagious sexually transmitted infection
molluscum contagiosum (**Note:** The "s" in contagiosum is added to make the word flow.)	moh-**LUS**-kum kon-**TAY**-jee-oh-sum	S/ R/ R/CF	-um *structure* mollusc- *soft* contagi/o- *transmissible by contact*	STD caused by a virus
spirochete	**SPY**-roh-keet	S/ R/CF	-chete *hair* spir/o- *spiral*	Spiral-shaped bacterium causing an STD (syphilis)
swab	SWOB		Old English *to sweep*	Wad of cotton used to remove or apply something from/to a surface
syphilis	**SIF**-ih-lis		Possibly from Latin poem, "Syphilis Sive Morbus Gallicus," by Fracastorius Alteration	Sexually transmitted disease caused by a spirochete
Trichomonas trichomoniasis	trik-oh-**MOH**-nas **TRIK**-oh-moh-**NIE**-ah-sis	S/ R/CF R/	-iasis *condition* trich/o- *hair, flagellum* -mon- *single*	A parasite causing an STD Infection with *Trichomonas vaginalis*

Exercises

A. Disease. *Test your knowledge of diseases. Anyone working in a gynecology clinic or internal medicine practice will have patients diagnosed with sexually transmitted diseases. Make the correct association between the name of the STD and its description by matching the statement in the left column with the medical term in the right column.*   **LO 8.4**

_____ 1. "Silent disease"

_____ 2. Curable with penicillin

_____ 3. Can be treated with single dose of antibiotic

_____ 4. Chlamydia or gonorrhea can cause this

_____ 5. Can cause dementia if untreated

_____ 6. Appears as a rash with joint pain

_____ 7. "Ping-pong" infection

_____ 8. Ulcerative disease

a. secondary syphilis

b. trichomoniasis

c. chlamydia

d. primary syphilis

e. PID

f. tertiary syphilis

g. chancroid

h. gonorrhea

Note: These diseases can be particularly difficult to spell. Work with a fellow student. Ask your partner to spell these terms; then have your partner ask you to spell them. Master these terms now—they will surely be in a test question.

9. Spelling: _____

_____

_____

_____

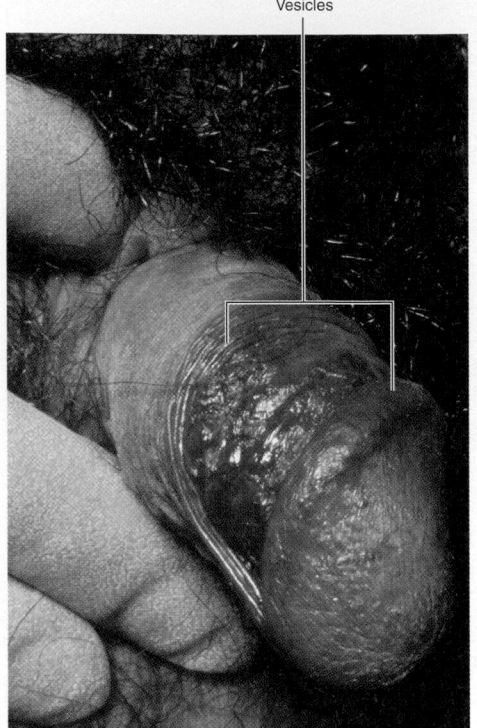

Vesicles

▲ **Figure 8.5** **Genital Herpes Simplex in Male.**

LO 8.4 Sexually Transmitted Diseases (continued)

Genital herpes simplex is a disease caused by the virus **herpes simplex type 2 (HSV-2)** *(Figure 8.5)*. The sores are painful, and the disease can present with fever, joint pains, and enlarged, tender lymph nodes. The genital sores can recur throughout life. After the initial infection, the virus remains dormant in the dorsal root ganglia of nerves. Blisters around the mouth ("cold sores") are caused by a related virus, **herpes simplex type 1 (HSV-1)**.

There is no cure for genital herpes. Three antiviral medications can provide clinical benefit by limiting the **replication** of the virus. These are acyclovir (Zovirax), valacyclovir (Valtrex), and famcyclovir (Famvir). In people who have recurrent outbreaks, medication taken every day can reduce the recurrences by 70% to 80%.

Herpes of the newborn occurs when a pregnant woman with genital herpes sores delivers her baby vaginally and transmits the virus to the baby *(Figure 8.6)*. Because the baby's immune system is not well developed, the infection is destructive and can be fatal. If there is evidence of genital herpes lesions in the mother, the fetus should be delivered by **cesarean section (C-section)**.

Human papilloma virus (HPV) causes genital warts in both men and women *(Figure 8.7)* and can also cause changes to the cells in the **cervix**. Some strains of the virus can increase a woman's risk for **cervical** cancer. More than 90% of abnormal Papanicolaou **(Pap)** smears are caused by HPV infections. A vaccine is now available that can prevent lasting infections from the two HPV strains that cause 70% of cervical cancers and another two strains that cause 90% of genital warts. The vaccine will be offered to girls and women aged 9 to 26 and may be given to boys and men of the same age group.

Medications such as podophyllin, trichloracetic acid, and Aldara cream can be applied to the warts, and cryotherapy or laser therapy can also be used. Because of the sites of the warts around the genitalia, condoms cannot provide complete protection.

HIV is a virus that attacks the immune system and usually leads to **acquired immunodeficiency syndrome (AIDS)**. Because HIV is carried in body fluids, it is transmitted during unprotected sex. Sharing needles can spread the virus. The virus can also pass from an infected pregnant woman to her unborn child, and she must take medications to protect the baby.

Symptoms often do not appear until years after the initial infection. The initial symptoms of HIV are similar to the flu. A person is diagnosed HIV-positive using a blood test that identifies antibodies to the virus **(ELISA)**, with a confirmatory western blot that identifies the specific antibody proteins. The CDC considers an HIV-infected person with a CD4 count below 200 to have AIDS, whether the person is sick or well; CD4 cells, also known as helper T cells, play key roles in the body's defense mechanisms.

There is no cure for HIV or AIDS, but combinations of anti-HIV medications are taken to stop the replication of the virus in the cells of the body and stop the progression of the disease. Development of resistance to the drugs is a problem.

Human immunodeficiency virus damages the immune system, so infections will develop that the body would normally cope with easily. These are **opportunistic infections** and include herpes simplex, candidiasis, syphilis, and tuberculosis.

Abbreviations

AIDS	acquired immunodeficiency syndrome
C-section	cesarean section
ELISA	enzyme-linked immunosorbent assay
HPV	human papilloma virus
HSV	herpes simplex virus
Pap	papanicolaou

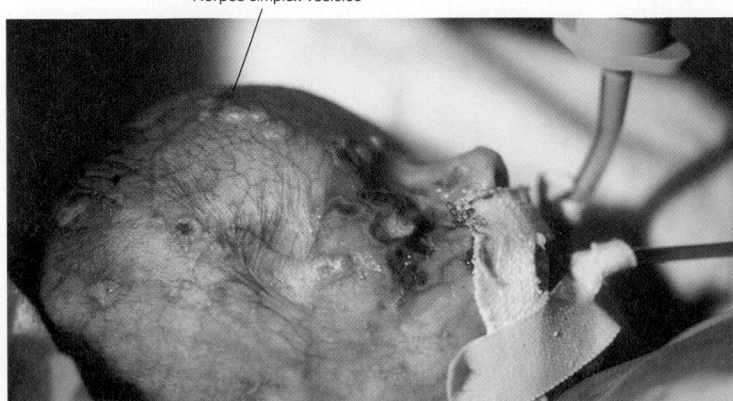

Herpes simplex vesicles

▲ **Figure 8.6** **Premature Baby Born with Herpes Simplex Infection.**

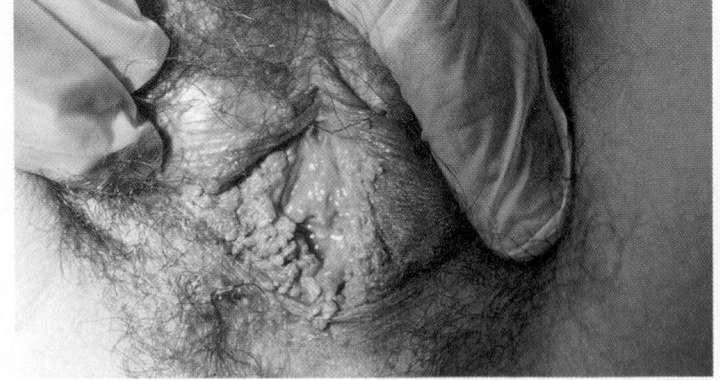

▲ **Figure 8.7** **HPV in the Female Vulva.**

WORD	PRONUNCIATION	ELEMENTS		DEFINITION
acquired immunodeficiency syndrome (AIDS)	ah-**KWIRED** **IM**-you-noh-de-**FISH**-en-see **SIN**-drome	S/ R/CF R/ P/ R/	**acquired** Latin *obtain* -**ency** *condition* **immun/o-** *immune response* -**defici-** *lacking, inadequate* **syn-** *together* -**drome** *running*	Infection with the HIV virus
cervix cervical (**Note:** This term also means *pertaining to the neck region.*)	**SER**-viks **SER**-vih-kal	S/ R/	Latin *neck* -**al** *pertaining to* **cervic-** *cervix*	Lower part of the uterus Pertaining to the cervix
cesarean section (C-section) (syn)	seh-**ZAH**-ree-an **SEK**-shun		Roman law under the Caesars required that pregnant women who died be cut open and the fetus extracted	Extraction of the fetus through an incision in the abdomen and uterine wall
herpes simplex virus (HSV)	**HER**-peez **SIM**-pleks **VIE**-rus		**herpes** Greek *spreading skin eruption*	An infection that manifests with painful, watery blisters on the skin and mucous membranes
human immunodeficiency virus (HIV)	**HYU**-man **IM**-you-noh-dee-**FISH**-en-see **VIE**-rus	S/ R/CF R/ R/	**human** Latin *human being* -**ency** *condition* **immun/o-** *immune response* -**defici-** *lacking, inadequate* **virus** *poison*	Etiologic agent of AIDS
human papilloma virus (HPV)	**HYU**-man pap-ih-**LOW**-mah **VIE**-rus	S/ R/	-**oma** *tumor* **papill-** *pimple*	An infection that causes warts on the skin and genitalia and can increase the risk for cervical cancer
opportunistic infection (**Note:** This term contains two suffixes.)	**OP**-or-tyu-**NIS**-tik in-**FEK**-shun	S/ S/ R/	-**ic** *pertaining to* -**ist-** *specialist in* **opportun-** *take advantage of*	An infection that causes disease when the immune system is compromised for other reasons
replication	rep-lih-**KAY**-shun	S/ R/	-**ation** *process* **replic-** *reply*	Reproduction to produce an exact copy

Exercises

A. Disease. *Continue working with the medical terminology for sexually transmitted diseases. Make the correct association between the description of the disease in the left column and its medical term listed in the right column.* **LO 8.1, 8.4, 8.6**

_____ 1. Causes cold sores around the mouth

_____ 2. Virus remains dormant

_____ 3. Virus attacks the immune system

_____ 4. This disease has no cure

_____ 5. Infections that would not normally develop

_____ 6. Not an inherited syndrome

_____ 7. Transmitted during vaginal delivery

_____ 8. Can be treated with laser or cryotherapy

    a. herpes simplex type 2

    b. AIDS

    c. herpes of the newborn

    d. HIV and AIDS

    e. HPV

    f. herpes simplex type 1

    g. opportunistic

    h. HIV

9. *Abbreviations: Take this opportunity to write out the meaning of any one of the abbreviations in this exercise.*

Ovaries, Fallopian (Uterine) Tubes, and Uterus

The female gonads, the primary sex organs, are the ovaries. The female internal accessory organs include a pair of **fallopian (uterine) tubes**, a **uterus**, and a vagina. Women are born with all the eggs **(ova)** that they will release, but it is not until puberty that the eggs mature and start to leave the ovary. The ovarian hormones, estrogen and progesterone, are involved in **menstruation** and **pregnancy (PGY)**. The pituitary gland at the base of the brain produces other hormones that control the functions of the ovaries, uterus, and breast *(see Chapter 17)*.

These complex interactions are the core of the human reproductive system and an essential part of understanding the human body. The information in this lesson will enable you to:

8.2.1 Describe the anatomy of an ovary, the fallopian tubes, and the uterus.

8.2.2 Identify the major events of oogenesis.

8.2.3 List the functions of estrogen and progesterone.

8.2.4 Explain the control of the pituitary gland over the female reproductive system.

8.2.5 Discuss the female sexual cycle.

Case Report 8.2

You are
. . . a certified health education specialist **(CHES)** employed by Fulwood Medical Center.

Your patient is
. . . Ms. Claire Marcos, a 21-year-old student referred to you by Anna Rusack, MD, a gynecologist.

Ms. Marcos has been diagnosed with **polycystic ovarian syndrome (PCOS)**, and your task is to develop a program of self care as part of her overall plan of therapy.

From her medical record, you see that she has presented with irregular, often missed menstrual periods since the beginning of puberty, persistent acne, patches of dark skin on the back of her neck and under her arms, loss of hair from the front of her scalp, and inability to control her weight. She is 5 feet 4 inches and weighs 150 pounds.

Her self-care program is to include exercise, diet, and regular use of birth control medication and metformin to lower insulin levels and help reduce her weight.

She has written out a list of questions that she hands to you. These include

- Why are my periods so irregular?
- Why doesn't my acne respond to all the treatment I've had?
- Am I going bald?
- Will I be able to have children some day?
- Why am I taking birth control pills when I'm not sexually active?
- What are all these other health problems they say I'm at risk for?

At the end of this chapter you will be asked to answer these questions.

Abbreviations

CHES	certified health education specialist
PCOS	polycystic ovarian syndrome
PGY	pregnancy

WORD	PRONUNCIATION	ELEMENTS		DEFINITION
fallopian tubes (also called uterine tubes)	fah-**LOW**-pee-an		Gabriello Fallopio, 1523–1562, Italian anatomist	Uterine tubes connected to the fundus of the uterus
menses menstruation (syn)	**MEN**-seez men-stru-**A**-shun	S/ R/CF	Latin *month* -ation *action* menstr/u- *menses*	Monthly uterine bleeding
menstruate (verb)	**MEN**-stru-ate	S/	-ate *composed of, pertaining to*	The act of menstruation
menstrual (adj)	**MEN**-stru-al	S/	-al *pertaining to*	Pertaining to menstruation
ovary ovaries (pl) ovarian (adj)	**OH**-va-ree **OH**-vah-rees oh-**VAIR**-ee-an	S/ R/	Latin *egg* -an *pertaining to* ovari- *ovary*	One of the paired female egg-producing glands Pertaining to the ovary
ovum (syn) ova (pl)	**OH**-vum **OH**-va		Latin *egg*	Egg
polycystic	pol-ee-**SIS**-tik	S/ P/ R/	-ic *pertaining to* poly- *many* -cyst- *cyst*	Composed of many cysts
pregnant	**PREG**-nant	S R/	-ant *forming, pertaining to* pregn- *with child, pregnant*	Having conceived
pregnancy gestation	**PREG**-nan-see jes-**TAY**-shun	S/ S/ R/	-ancy *state of* -ion *condition, process* gestat- *gestation, pregnancy*	State of being pregnant Period from conception to birth
uterus uterine (adj)	**YOU**-ter-us **YOU**-ter-ine		Latin *womb*	Organ in which an egg develops into a fetus

Exercises

A. Elements. *Knowing the meaning of word elements is your best tool for building and analyzing medical terms. Choose from among the following word elements, and insert the correct element in the blank to complete the medical term. Then use any term from the above WAD box in a sentence of patient documentation.* **LO 8.3, 8.9**

1. Pertaining to many cysts: _____cystic

   mono   poly   cyano   endo

2. Pertaining to the ovary: _____an

   gestat   ovari   menstru   pregn

3. This term is synonymous with *menstruation*: _____

   gynecology   gynecologic   menses   menstrual

4. Having conceived: _____ant

   pregn   gyneco   gestat   estra

5. From conception to birth: _____ion

   ovari   gestat   gyneco   menstru

6. Sentence: _____

   _____

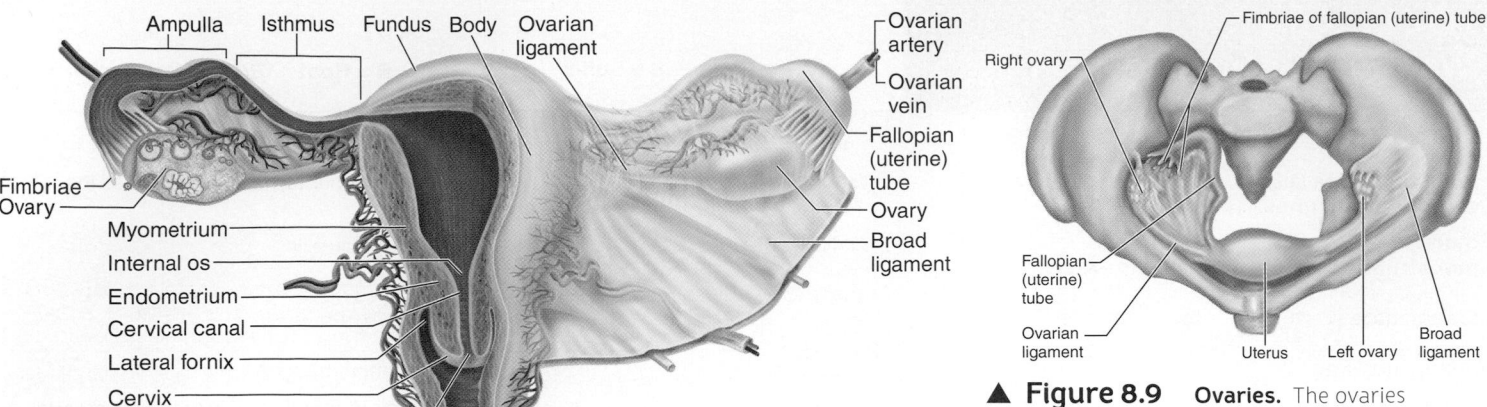

▲ Figure 8.8   Female Reproductive Tract.

▲ Figure 8.9   **Ovaries.** The ovaries are located on each side against the lateral walls of the pelvic cavity. The right fallopian (uterine) tube is retracted to reveal the ovarian ligament.

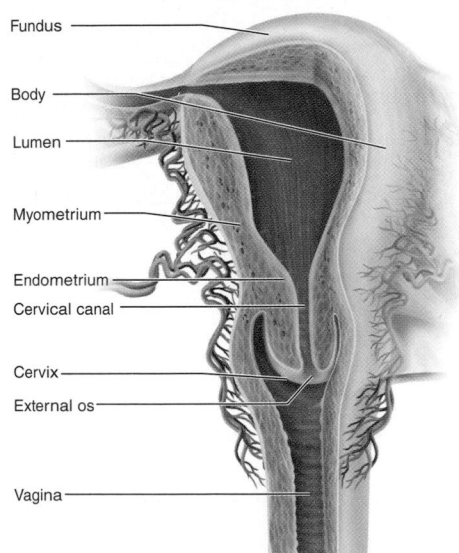

▲ Figure 8.10   Uterus.

Keynotes

The wall of the uterus has three layers. From the outside, these are

- The **perimetrium**—a continuation of the broad ligament.
- The **myometrium**—a thick layer of smooth muscle.
- The **endometrium**—the lining that sheds in menstruation.

LO 8.3 Anatomy of the Female Reproductive Tract

Ovaries

Each ovary is an almond-shaped organ located in a shallow depression (ovarian fossa) in the lateral wall of the pelvic cavity *(Figure 8.8)*. The ovary is about 1 inch (2.5 cm) long and ½ inch (1.3 cm) in diameter. It is enclosed in a capsule called the *tunica albuginea*. Each ovary is held in place by ligaments that attach it to the pelvic wall and uterus *(Figure 8.9)*.

Fallopian (Uterine) Tubes

Each fallopian (uterine) tube is a canal about 4 inches (10 cm) long, extending from the uterus and opening to the abdominal cavity near the ovary. At the ovarian end, the outer one-third flares out into a funnel-shaped **infundibulum**, with fingerlike folds called **fimbria**. At ovulation, the **fimbriae** enclose the ovary *(see Figure 8.8)*. The inner one-third of each tube approaching the uterus is called the **isthmus**. The tubes are supported by the broad ligament.

The wall of the tube has an inner layer of mucosal cells that secrete mucus. Some are ciliated. The cilia beat toward the uterus and transport the egg down the uterine tube with peristaltic contractions, a journey that takes 3 or 4 days.

The ovaries and uterine tubes are called the **adnexa** of the uterus.

Uterus

The uterus *(Figure 8.10)* is a thick-walled, muscular organ in the pelvic cavity. It normally tilts forward **(anteverted)** over the urinary bladder. If it were to be tilted backward toward the rectum, its position would be **retroverted**, a condition found in 20% of women. Anatomically, it is divided into three regions:

- **Fundus**—the broad, curved upper region between the lateral attachments of the fallopian (uterine) tubes.
- **Body**—the midportion.
- **Cervix**—the cylindrical inferior portion that projects into the vagina.

The cavity of the uterus is triangular, with its upper two corners receiving the openings of the fallopian (uterine) tubes. Its lower end communicates with the vagina through the **cervical canal**, which has an **internal os** from the lumen and an **external os** into the vagina *(see Figure 8.8)*.

The cervical canal contains mucous glands; secretions of mucus help prevent the spread of infection from the vagina. The uterus is supported by the muscular floor of the pelvic outlet and by ligaments that extend to the pelvic wall from the uterus and cervix.

WORD	PRONUNCIATION	ELEMENTS		DEFINITION
adnexa (pl) adnexum (sing)	ad-**NEK**-sa ad-**NEK**-sum	S/ R/	Latin *connected parts* -**um** *mass* -**adnex-** *connected parts*	Parts accessory to an organ or structure
adnexal (adj)	ad-**NEK**-sal	S/	-**al** *pertaining to*	Pertaining to accessory structures; for example, structures alongside the uterus, fallopian tubes, and ovaries
anteverted	an-teh-**VERT**-ed	S/ P/ R/	-**ed** *pertaining to* **ante-** *before, forward* -**vert** *to turn*	Tilted forward
anteversion	an-teh-**VER**-shun	S/	-**ion** *condition, process*	Forward tilting of the uterus
endometrium	en-doh-**ME**-tree-um	S/ P/ R/CF	-**um** *tissue* **endo-** *within, inside* -**metr/i-** *uterus*	Inner lining of the uterus
endometrial (adj)	en-doh-**ME**-tree-al	S/	-**al** *pertaining to*	Pertaining to the inner lining of the uterus
fimbria fimbriae (pl)	**FIM**-bree-ah **FIM**-bree-ee		Latin *fringe*	A fringe-like structure on the surface of a cell or a microorganism
fundus	**FUN**-dus		Latin *bottom*	Part farthest from the opening of a hollow organ
infundibulum infundibula (pl)	**IN**-fun-**DIB**-you-lum **IN**-fun-**DIB**-you-lah		Latin *funnel*	Funnel-shaped structure
isthmus	**IS**-mus		Greek *isthmus*	Part connecting two larger parts; in this case, the uterus to the uterine tube
myometrium	my-oh-**ME**-tree-um	S/ R/CF R/CF	-**um** *tissue* **my/o-** *muscle* -**metr/i-** *uterus*	Muscle wall of the uterus
os	OS		Latin *mouth*	Opening into a canal; for example, the cervix
perimetrium	per-ih-**ME**-tree-um	S/ P/ R/CF	-**um** *tissue* **peri-** *around* -**metr/i-** *uterus*	The covering of the uterus; part of the peritoneum
retroversion	reh-troh-**VER**-shun	S/ P/ R/	-**ion** *process, condition* **retro-** *backward* -**vers-** *turned*	The tipping backward of the uterus
retroverted	reh-troh-**VERT**-ed	S/ R/	-**ed** *pertaining to* -**vert** *to turn*	Tilted backward

Exercises

A. Demonstrate your understanding of the *language of gynecology* employed on this and the opposite page.   LO 8.1, 8.3

1. Which two terms in the above WAD are opposites, and what do they mean?

   _____ means _____, and

   _____ means _____.

2. What is the "collective" (as a group) medical term for the ovaries and uterine tubes? _____

3. What is another name for the *uterine tube*? _____

4. Describe *peristaltic contractions*.

   _____

5. Where else in the body does this action occur?

   _____

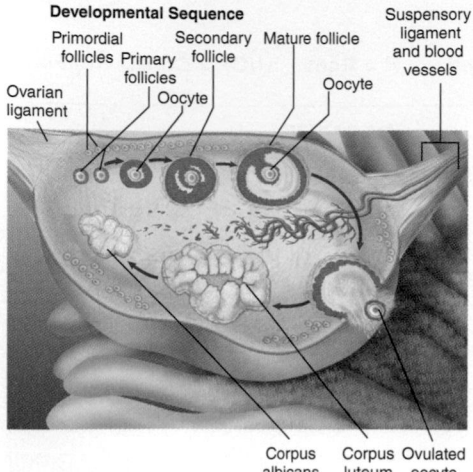

Developmental Sequence

Primordial follicles
Primary follicles
Secondary follicle
Mature follicle
Oocyte
Oocyte
Ovarian ligament
Suspensory ligament and blood vessels
Corpus albicans
Corpus luteum
Ovulated oocyte

▲ **Figure 8.11** **Oogenesis.**
The development of the oocyte begins with the primordial follicles.

Abbreviations

FSH follicle-stimulating hormone
GnRH gonadotropin-releasing hormone
LH luteinizing hormone

Keynotes

• Menarche cannot occur until at least 17% of a girl's weight is body fat.

• High levels of estrogen and progesterone inhibit the secretion of GnRH. This is the basis for most forms of contraceptive medications.

LO 8.5 Oogenesis (Egg Formation)

During **prenatal** development, small groups of cells in the ovarian cortex form some 2 million **follicles**. In each group there is a single large cell, the primary oocyte, surrounded by a layer of **follicular cells**. Many of these degenerate, a process called *atresia*.

At puberty, some 400,000 primary oocytes remain, each containing 23 pairs of chromosomes. They undergo meiosis to produce secondary oocytes, each containing 23 single chromosomes. As they mature, the follicular cells form a fluid-filled **primary follicle**, in which the egg is located *(Figure 8.11)*. Surrounding the oocyte (egg) and lining the fluid-filled **antrum** of the follicle are **granulosa cells** that secrete estrogen.

At the beginning of the menstrual cycle, as many as 20 primary follicles can start the maturing process, but only one develops fully. The remainder degenerate. By the midpoint of the menstrual cycle, the mature follicle bulges out on the surface of the ovary and ruptures **(ovulation)**. The oocyte and lining cells from the follicle can either be taken into the fallopian (uterine) tube or fall into the pelvic cavity and degenerate.

Ovarian Hormones

The ovaries of the sexually mature female secrete estrogens and progesterone.

Estrogens are produced in the ovarian follicles. Their sexual functions are to

1. Convert girls into sexually mature women through the onset of breast development, the growth of pubic hair, and the establishment of menstruation.
2. Participate in the menstrual cycle *(see Figure 8.12)*.
3. Participate in pregnancy when that occurs.

Progesterone is produced by the corpus luteum of the ovary and by the adrenal glands *(see Chapter 17)*. Its sexual functions are to

1. Prepare the lining of the uterus for implantation of the egg *(see Figure 8.12)*.
2. Inhibit lactation during pregnancy.
3. Produce menstrual bleeding if pregnancy does not occur.

The synthesis and secretion of estrogen is stimulated by **follicle-stimulating hormone (FSH)** from the pituitary gland. FSH is controlled by the hypothalamic **gonadotropin-releasing hormone (GnRH)**. Progesterone production is stimulated by **luteinizing hormone (LH)** from the pituitary gland, which is also stimulated by GnRH.

The ovaries also secrete small amounts of androgens, male hormones.

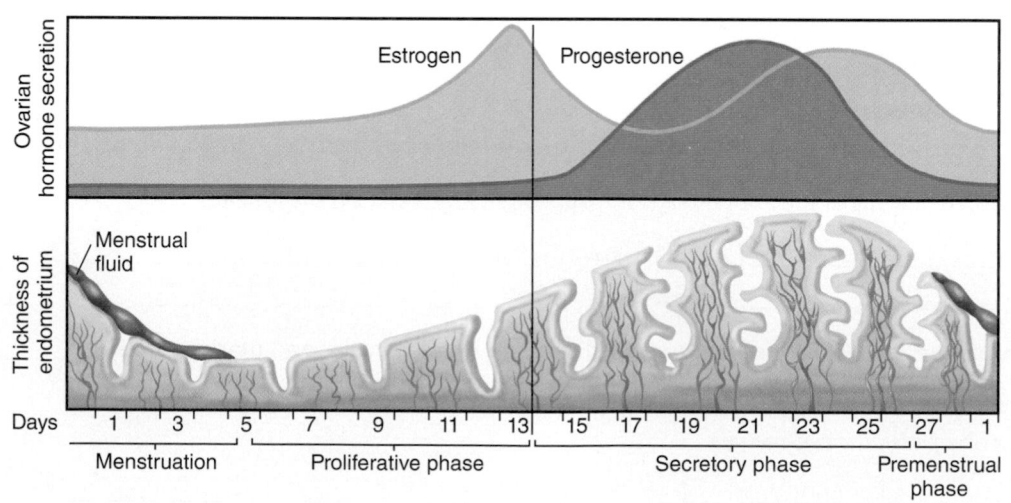

▲ **Figure 8.12** **Menstrual Cycle.**

WORD	PRONUNCIATION	ELEMENTS		DEFINITION
antrum	**AN**-trum		Greek *cave*	A nearly closed cavity or chamber
follicle	**FOLL**-ih-kull		Latin *small sac*	Spherical mass of cells containing a cavity or a small cul-de-sac, such as a hair follicle
follicular (adj)	fo-**LIK**-you-lar	S/ R/	-ar *pertaining to* follicul- *follicle*	Pertaining to a follicle
gonadotropin	**GO**-nad-oh-**TROH**-pin	S/ R/CF	-tropin *nourishing* gonad/o- *gonad*	Hormone capable of promoting gonad function
granulosa cell	gran-you-**LOW**-sah SELL	S/ R/	-osa *like* granul- *small grain*	Cell lining the ovarian follicle
ovulation	**OV**-you-**LAY**-shun	S/ R/	-ation *process* ovul- *egg*	Release of an oocyte from a follicle
ovulate (verb)	ov-you-**LATE**	S/	-ate *composed of, pertaining to*	To release an oocyte from a follicle
prenatal	pree-**NAY**-tal	S/ P/ R/	-al *pertaining to* pre- *before* -nat- *born*	Before birth

Exercises

A. Deconstruct these medical terms into the meanings of their basic elements. *This will help you learn the meaning of the term. Fill in the table, and answer the questions.* **LO 8.1, 8.5**

Medical Term	Meaning of Prefix	Meaning of Root/Combining Form	Meaning of Suffix	Meaning of Medical Term
follicular	1.	2.	3.	4.
ovulation	5.	6.	7.	8.
prenatal	9.	10.	11.	12.
granulosa	13.	14.	15.	16.
gonadotropin	17.	18.	19.	20.

Review the above WAD before you fill in the blanks.

21. Release of an *oocyte* from a follicle is known as _____.

22. Which term in the above WAD is the name of a *hormone*? _____.

23. The meaning of *prenatal* is _____.

LO 8.5 The Sexual Cycle

The sexual cycle averages 28 days in length and includes the menstrual cycle. It begins with a 2-week follicular phase *(Figure 8.13)*. The beginning of the cycle is recognized by physiologists as menstruation, which occurs during the first 3 to 5 days.

After menstruation ends, the uterus starts to replace the endometrial tissue lost during menstruation. The developing ovarian follicles mature, and one of them ovulates around day 14 *(Figure 8.14)*. Around this time, the fimbriae of the uterine tube envelope and caress the ovary in time with the mother's heartbeat.

After ovulation, in the postovulatory phase, the endometrial lining continues to grow. The residual ovarian follicle becomes a **corpus luteum** containing **lutein** cells that are involved in progesterone production. Around day 24, the corpus luteum **involutes**. By day 26, it is an inactive scar called a **corpus albicans**. At this time, the arteries supplying the endometrium of the uterus contract. This leads to ischemia, tissue necrosis, and the start of menstruation.

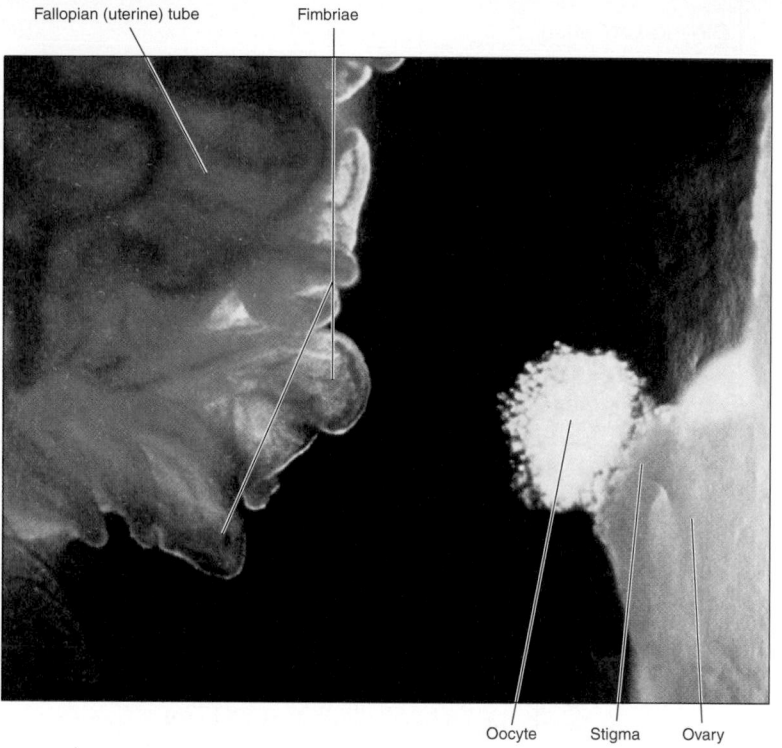

▲ Figure 8.13   Ovarian Cycle.

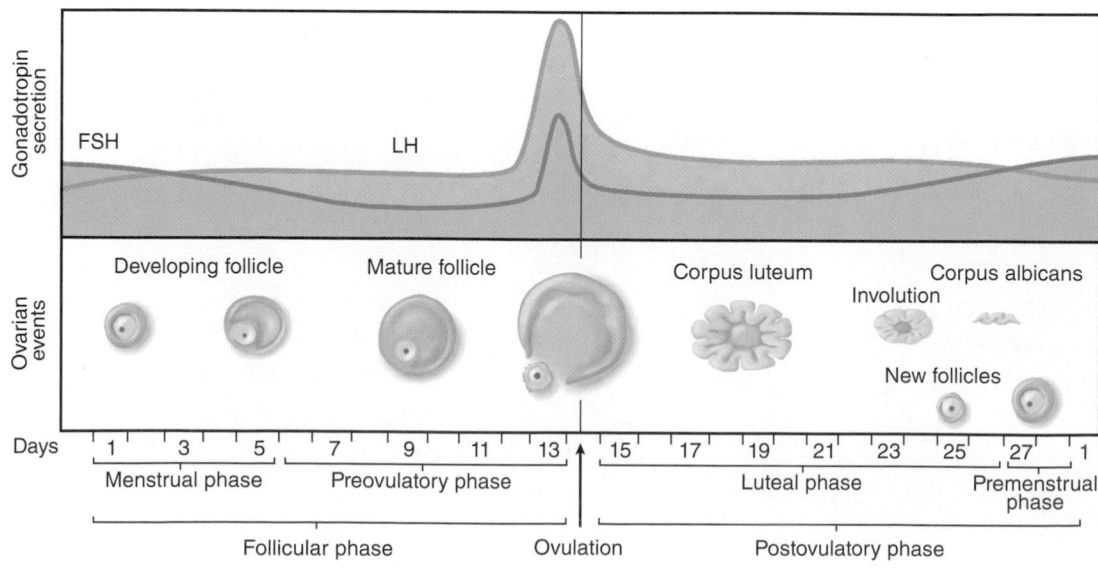

▲ Figure 8.14   Ovulation.

WORD	PRONUNCIATION	ELEMENTS		DEFINITION
corpus albicans corpus luteum	**KOR**-pus **AL**-bih-kanz **KOR**-pus **LOO**-teh-um		**albicans** Latin *white* **luteum** Latin *yellow*	An atrophied corpus luteum Yellow structure formed at the site of a ruptured ovarian follicle
involution involute (verb)	in-voh-**LOO**-shun	S/ P/ R/	**-ion** *process, condition* **in-** *in* **-volut-** *roll up, shrink*	A decrease in size or vigor
lutein	**LOO**-tee-in	R/	Latin *saffron yellow* **lute-** *yellow*	Yellow pigment
luteal (adj)	**LOO**-tee-al	S/	**-al** *pertaining to*	Pertaining to a corpus luteum

Exercises

A. Employ the *language of gynecology* and your understanding of the female sexual cycle to match the phrases in the left column with the correct medical terminology in the right column.   LO 8.5

_____ 1. After menses ends, uterus replaces this

_____ 2. Formed where ovarian follicle ruptures

_____ 3. Envelope the ovary

_____ 4. Decreases in size

_____ 5. Averages 28 days in length

_____ 6. Inactive scar

_____ 7. Mature ovarian follicle does this

_____ 8. Cells involved in progesterone production

_____ 9. After ovulation

_____ 10. Menses occurs during first 3 to 5 days

a. sexual cycle

b. ovulates

c. lutein

d. corpus albicans

e. follicular phase

f. postovulatory phase

g. corpus luteum

h. endometrial tissue

i. involutes

j. fimbriae

A clear understanding of the medical terms used to explain the sexual cycle will help you answer the following questions:

11. Where is the *endometrial lining*? _____

12. What do *lutein cells* produce? _____

13. Is the answer in question 12 above a hormone or an enzyme? _____

14. When the corpus luteum *involutes*, what happens? _____

15. "When the arteries supplying the uterus contract, this leads to ischemia, tissue necrosis, and the start of menses."

    Explain this in layman's language to your patient.

    _____

Disorders of the Female Reproductive Tract

Use correct medical terminology to:

8.3.1 Describe disorders of the ovaries, uterus, and fallopian (uterine) tubes, and their effects on a woman's health.

8.3.2 Discuss the etiologies of infertility and modern treatments for the condition.

8.3.3 Identify modern methods of contraception and their rates of success.

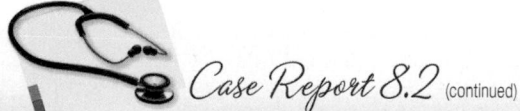

Case Report 8.2 (continued)

When Ms. Claire Marcos first presented in the Gynecology Clinic, Dr. Rusack examined her abdomen and pelvis. Dr. Rusack was able to **palpate** both enlarged ovaries on vaginal examination. A vaginal ultrasound scan showed multiple small cysts in each ovary. Blood tests showed high levels of testosterone and luteinizing hormone. Dr. Rusack prescribed birth control pills because they contain estrogen and progesterone. These can correct the hormonal imbalance, regulate menses, and lower the level of testosterone to diminish acne and hair problems. Metformin was also prescribed.

Abbreviations

PCOS polycystic ovarian syndrome
PMS premenstrual syndrome

LO 8.6 Disorders of the Ovaries

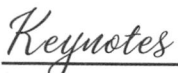

- The peak incidence of ovarian cancer is in women in their fifties and sixties.
- More than 20,000 new cases of ovarian cancer are diagnosed in the United States each year.
- More than 15,000 deaths from ovarian cancer occur in the United States each year.
- Screening tests for ovarian cancer are in research trials.

Ovarian Cysts

An ovarian cyst is a fluid-filled sac in the ovary. Most cysts are normal and are called *functional cysts*. They follow ovulation and disappear within 3 months.

Polycystic ovarian syndrome (PCOS), in which multiple follicular cysts form in both ovaries *(Figure 8.15)*, is the disorder diagnosed in Ms. Marcos. Because of the repeated cyst formation, no egg matures and is released, ovulation does not occur, and progesterone is not produced. Without progesterone, her menstrual cycle is irregular or absent.

The cysts produce androgens, which prevent ovulation and produce acne, the male-pattern hair loss from the front of the scalp, and weight gain. In addition, women with PCOS make too much insulin, which interferes with normal fat metabolism and prevents it being used for energy. This leads to difficulty in losing weight and causes patches of dark skin. Metformin, a medication that affects glucose and insulin metabolism, can help with the weight problems associated with PCOS.

Women with PCOS are also at increased risk for endometrial cancer, type 2 diabetes, high blood cholesterol, hypertension, and heart disease.

Ovarian cancer is the second most common gynecologic cancer after endometrial cancer, but it accounts for more deaths than any other gynecologic malignancy. Symptoms develop late and are usually vague, making early diagnosis difficult. A mass in the abdomen may be detected during routine pelvic examination.

Treatment is to surgically remove the tumor and give chemotherapy. A majority of patients experience a recurrence. The 5-year survival rate is below 20%.

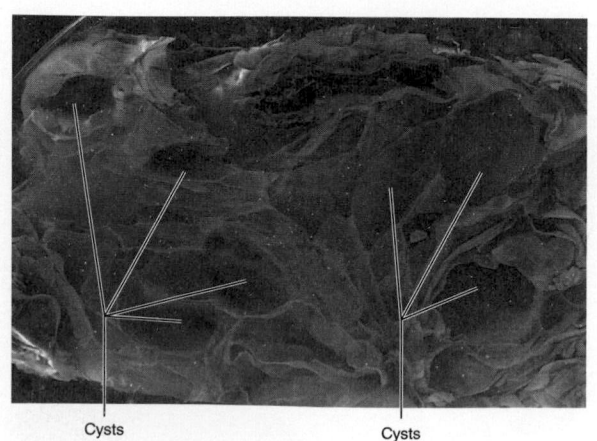

Cysts   Cysts

▲ **Figure 8.15** Polycystic Ovary.

WORD	PRONUNCIATION	ELEMENTS		DEFINITION
menopause (*Note:* This term has no suffix, only a combining form and a root.)	MEN-oh-paws	R/ R/CF	-pause men/o- *month, menses*	Permanent ending of menstrual periods
menopausal (adj)	MEN-oh-paws-al	S/	-al *pertaining to*	Pertaining to menopause
palpate (verb) palpation (noun)	PAL-pate pal-PAY-shun	S/ R/	Latin *to touch* -ion *process, action* palpat- *touch, stroke*	To examine with the fingers and hands Examination using the fingers and hands
premenstrual	pree-MEN-stru-al	S/ P/ R/	-al *pertaining to* pre- *before* -menstru- *menses*	Pertaining to the time immediately before the menses

Exercises

A. Apply your knowledge of the *language of gynecology* by choosing the correct answer to the following questions. *Circle the best choice.*   **LO 8.5, 8.6**

1. The term *palpate* means to

   excise   touch   incise

2. In the medical term *menopause*, the combining form means

   menses   monthly   cycle

3. The *gynecologic malignancy* that accounts for the most deaths is

   cervical cancer   breast cancer   ovarian cancer

4. If this *hormone* is not present, the menstrual cycle is irregular or absent:

   estrogen   testosterone   lutein

B. Critical thinking. Use the *language of gynecology* to complete this exercise.   **LO 8.6**

1. PCOS is an abbreviation used in the female reproductive system. Write out this abbreviation in words,

   _____

2. In PCOS, what process does *not* occur in the woman's body?

   _____

3. Women with PCOS are at increased risk for which other diseases?

   _____

4. As a result of PCOS, a woman's body will produce too much _____

5. Name some of the symptoms of PCOS.

   _____

LO 8.6 Disorders of the Uterus and Fallopian (Uterine) Tubes

Primary amenorrhea occurs when a girl has not menstruated by age 16. This can occur with or without other signs of puberty. There are numerous possible causes: drastic weight loss from malnutrition; dieting; bulimia, or anorexia nervosa *(see Chapter 18)*; extreme exercise, as in some young gymnasts; extreme obesity; chronic illness; congenital abnormalities of the uterus or vagina; and congenital hormonal disorders. Treatment is directed to the basic cause.

Secondary amenorrhea occurs when a woman who has menstruated normally then misses three or more periods in a row and is not in her **menopause**. The causes include pregnancy (by far the most common cause); ovarian disorders such as PCOS; excessive weight loss; low body fat percentage; excessive exercise (e.g., in marathon runners); certain drugs, including antidepressants; and stress.

Primary dysmenorrhea, or **premenstrual syndrome (PMS)**, refers to pain or discomfort associated with menstruation. The pain can begin 1 or 2 days before menses, peak on the first day of flow, and then slowly subside. The pain can be cramping or aching and be associated with headache, diarrhea or constipation, and urinary frequency. Treatment is with **nonsteroidal anti-inflammatory drugs (NSAIDs)**. If these are ineffective, oral contraceptives are 80% to 90% effective.

Secondary dysmenorrhea is pain associated with disorders such as infection in the genital tract or endometriosis.

Endometriosis is said to affect 1 in 10 American women of childbearing age. The endometrium becomes implanted outside the uterus on the fallopian (uterine) tubes, the ovaries, and the pelvic peritoneum. The displaced endometrium continues to go through its monthly cycle. It thickens and bleeds; but because there is nowhere for the blood to go, it leads to cysts and scar tissue and produces pain. The etiology of endometriosis is unknown.

Salpingitis is an inflammation of the fallopian (uterine) tubes and is part of pelvic inflammatory disease. A bacterial infection, often from an STD, spreads from the vagina through the cervix and uterus. Symptoms are lower abdominal pain, fever, and a vaginal discharge. Treatment is with appropriate antibiotics. If a pelvic abscess has developed, it may be necessary to remove the damaged tube **(salpingectomy)**.

Uterine Prolapse

The uterus is normally supported by the muscles, ligaments, and connective tissue of the pelvic floor. Difficult childbirth can weaken these tissues, so the uterus can descend into the vaginal canal. Aging, obesity, lack of exercise, chronic coughing, and chronic constipation are also thought to play a role in the development of the **prolapse** *(Figure 8.16)*.

Uterine prolapse can be accompanied by prolapse of the bladder and anterior vaginal wall, called a **cystocele**, or the rectum and posterior wall of the vagina, called a **rectocele**.

Treatment can be an individually fitted vaginal **pessary** inserted into the vagina to support the uterus. Surgical procedures such as **sacral colpopexy**, in which a mesh is inserted into the pelvic floor, or a **vaginal hysterectomy**, in which the uterus is removed through the vagina, achieve good results.

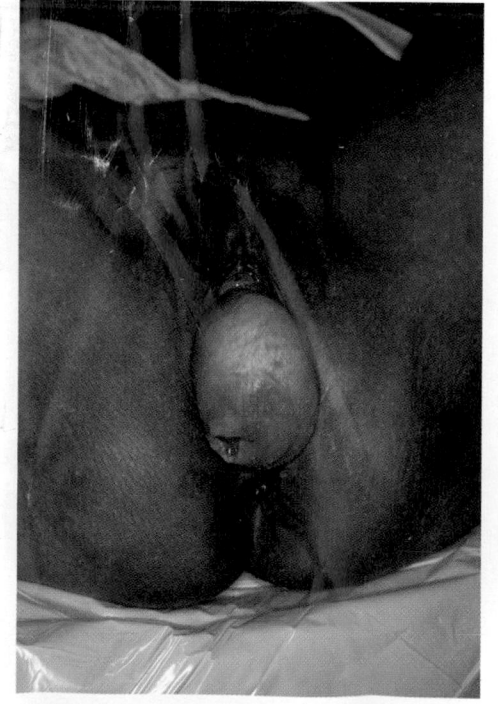

▲ **Figure 8.16** Complete Prolapse of the Uterus which Protrudes Outside the Vaginal Canal.

WORD	PRONUNCIATION	ELEMENTS		DEFINITION
amenorrhea	a-men-oh-**REE**-ah	S/ P/ R/CF	-rrhea *flow or discharge* a- *without* -men/o- *month, menses*	Absence or abnormal cessation of menstrual flow
dysmenorrhea	dis-men-oh-**REE**-ah	S/ P/ R/CF	-rrhea *flow or discharge* dys- *painful or difficult* -men/o- *month, menses*	Painful and difficult menstruation
colpopexy	**KOL**-poh-peck-see	S/ R/CF	-pexy *surgical fixation* colp/o- *vagina*	Surgical fixation of the vagina
cystocele	**SIS**-toh-seal	S/ R/CF	-cele *swelling, hernia* cyst/o- *bladder*	Hernia of the bladder into the vagina
endometriosis	**EN**-doh-me-tree-**OH**-sis	S/ P/ R/CF	-osis *condition* endo- *within, inside* -metr/i- *uterus*	Endometrial tissue in the abdomen outside the uterus
hysterectomy	his-ter-**EK**-toe-me	S/ R/	-ectomy *surgical excision* hyster- *uterus*	Surgical removal of the uterus
pessary	**PES**-ah-ree		Greek *an oval stone*	Appliance inserted into the vagina to support the uterus
prolapse	pro-**LAPS**		Latin *a falling*	The falling or slipping of a body part from its normal position
rectocele	**REK**-toe-seal	S/ R/CF	-cele *swelling, hernia* rect/o- *rectum*	Hernia of the rectum into the vagina
salpingitis	sal-pin-**JIE**-tis	S/ R/	-itis *inflammation* salping- *fallopian tube*	Inflammation of the uterine tube
salpingectomy	sal-pin-**JECT**-oh-me	S/	-ectomy *surgical excision*	Surgical removal of fallopian tube(s)

Exercises

A. Refer to the above WAD for the answers to the following questions. *Circle the best choice.*   **LO 8.6**

1. Which of the following statements is true about the term *salpingectomy*?

   a. it refers to the uterus

   b. it is only performed on a male

   c. it refers to the fallopian tube

   d. it is not a surgery

   e. it is a diagnostic test

2. The term *colpopexy* refers to

   a. surgical excision of the uterus

   b. surgical fixation of the uterus

   c. surgical incision into the fallopian tubes

   d. surgical fixation of the vagina

   e. surgical incision into the uterus

3. A hysterectomy is a surgical procedure

   a. that removes the vagina

   b. that removes the uterus

   c. that removes the fallopian tubes

   d. that removes the ovaries

   e. that removes the ureters

4. Which of the following suffixes means *hernia*?

   a. pexy

   b. cele

   c. ectomy

   d. osis

   e. ary

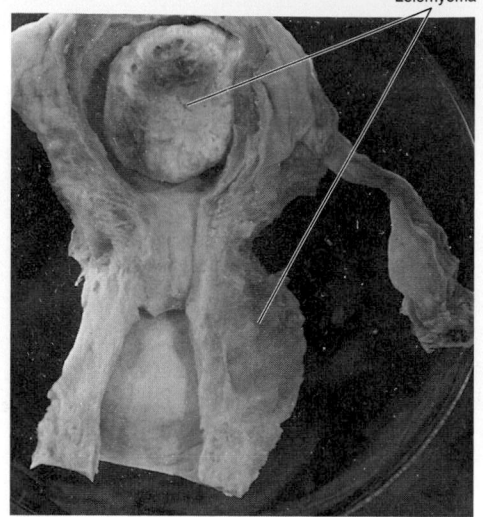

Leiomyoma

▲ Figure 8.17 **Leiomyomas (Fibroids).** In this sectioned uterus a smaller rounded leiomyoma is present, causing a small, rounded bulge in the uterine wall. The larger mass at the top is another leiomyoma projecting from the surface into the uterine cavity.

Keynotes

- In postmenopausal women, the risk of heart disease becomes almost the same as it is in men.
- Menopause affects every woman differently: 50% never suffer any symptoms.

Abbreviations

CT	computed tomography
D&C	dilation and curettage
DUB	dysfunctional uterine bleeding
HRT	hormone replacement therapy
MRI	magnetic resonance imaging

LO 8.6 Disorders of the Uterus and Fallopian (Uterine) Tubes (continued)

Uterine Fibroids

Fibroids are noncancerous growths of the uterus that appear during childbearing years. Three out of four women have them, but only one out of four women has symptoms from them.

The symptoms they can produce include

- **Menorrhagia**—abnormally long, heavy menstrual bleeding.
- **Metrorrhagia**—irregular bleeding between menstrual periods.
- **Polymenorrhea**—too frequent periods (occur more often than every 21 days) and no ovulation in the cycle.
- **Pelvic pressure**—low-back pain, urinary incontinence, and frequency.

Uterine fibroids are also called **fibromyomas**, **leiomyomas**, or **myomas** (*Figure 8.17*). They arise in the myometrium, producing a pale, firm, rubbery mass separate from the surrounding tissue. They vary in size from seedlings to large masses that distort the uterus. They can protrude into the uterine cavity, causing menorrhagia, or project outside the uterus and press on the bladder or rectum to produce symptoms.

Diagnostic studies include endometrial biopsy, transabdominal ultrasound, transvaginal ultrasound, hysterosonography, hysterosalpingography, hysteroscopy, computed tomography (CT), and magnetic resonance imaging (MRI).

Treatment options are numerous and include

- **Expectant management**, or watchful waiting.
- **Myomectomy**, removal of the fibroids surgically leaving the uterus in place.
- **Hormone therapy**, which uses **GnRH agonists** to cause estrogen and progesterone levels to fall so that menstruation stops and fibroids shrink.
- **Hysterectomy**, major surgery that is performed by many gynecologists as a last resort.

Other Causes of Uterine Bleeding

Dysfunctional uterine bleeding (DUB) is a term applied when no cause can be found for a patient's menorrhagia. Treatment is with oral contraceptives. If that fails, **dilation and curettage (D&C)** may be effective. This procedure involves dilating the entrance to the uterus through the cervix so that a thin instrument can be inserted to scrape or suction away the lining of the uterus and take tissue samples. An alternative treatment is **endometrial ablation**, in which a heat-generating tool or a laser removes or destroys the lining of the uterus and prevents or reduces menstruation. Endometrial ablation and hysterectomy are used in women who have finished childbearing.

Endometrial polyps are benign extensions of the endometrium that can cause irregular and heavy bleeding. They can be removed by hysteroscopy or D&C.

Menopause

Menopause is diagnosed when a woman has not menstruated for a year and is not pregnant; she is in the "change of life." In this normal, natural, biological process of reproductive aging, levels of estrogen and progesterone start to decline around the age of 40. For most women, menstruation ceases between the ages of 45 and 55. Significant quantities of estrogen and progesterone are no longer secreted, so the endometrial lining of the uterus cannot grow and be shed as in a normal menstrual period.

Without estrogen and progesterone, the uterus, vagina, and breasts atrophy, and more bone is lost than is replaced. Blood vessels constrict and dilate in response to changing hormone levels and can cause hot flashes.

The risks, types, and benefits of **hormone replacement therapy** (HRT) as a treatment for menopausal symptoms are a source of ongoing debate.

WORD	PRONUNCIATION	ELEMENTS		DEFINITION
ablation	ab-**LAY**-shun	S/ P/ R/	-ion *action, condition* ab- *away from* -lat- *to take*	Removal of tissue to destroy its function
agonist	**AG**-on-ist		Greek *contest*	Agent that combines with receptors on cells to initiate drug actions
curettage	kyu-reh-**TAHZH**	S/ R/	-age *related to* curett- *to cleanse*	Scraping of the interior of a cavity
dysfunctional	dis-**FUNK**-shun-al	S/ P/ R/	-al *pertaining to* dys- *painful, difficult* -function- *perform*	Having difficulty in performing
fibroid	**FIE**-broyd	S/ R/	-oid *resembling* fibr- *fiber*	Uterine tumor resembling fibrous tissue
Fibromyoma (also called **fibroid**)	**FIE**-bro-my-**OH**-mah	S/ R/CF R/	-oma *tumor, mass* fibr/o- *fiber* -my- *muscle*	Benign neoplasm derived from smooth muscle containing fibrous tissue
leiomyoma (also called **fibroid**)	**LIE**-oh-my-**OH**-mah	S/ R/ R/CF	-oma *tumor, mass* -my- *muscle* lei/o- *smooth*	Benign neoplasm derived from smooth muscle
menorrhagia	men-oh-**RAY**-jee-ah	S/ R/CF	-rrhagia *excessive flow, discharge* men/o- *menses*	Excessive menstrual bleeding
metrorrhagia	**MEH**-troh-**RAY**-jee-ah	S/ R/CF	-rrhagia *excessive flow, discharge* metr/o- *uterus*	Irregular uterine bleeding between menses
myoma	my-**OH**-mah	S/ R/	-oma *tumor, mass* my- *muscle*	Benign tumor of muscle
myomectomy	my-oh-**MEK**-toe-me	S/ R/	-ectomy *surgical excision* -om- *tumor, body*	Surgical removal of a myoma (fibroid)
polymenorrhea	**POL**-ee-men-oh-**REE**-ah	S/ P/ R/CF	-rrhea *flow* poly- *many* men/o- *menses*	More than normal frequency of menses

Exercises

A. Build the *language of gynecology* by completing the medical term with the correct element. *Fill in the blanks.* **LO 8.1, 8.6**

1. benign neoplasm derived from smooth muscle   leio/_____ /_____

2. irregular bleeding between menses   metro/_____

3. removal of tissue to destroy its function   _____ /_____ /ion

4. uterine tumor resembling fibrous tissue   _____ /oid

5. benign tumor of muscle   _____ /oma

6. more than normal frequency of menses   _____ /meno/_____

7. surgical removal of a fibroid   _____ /ectomy

8. excessive menstrual bleeding   meno/_____

9. having difficulty in performing   _____ /_____ /al

10. scraping of the interior of a cavity   _____ /age

Note: Although the suffix -oma *means tumor (or mass), it is not necessarily a malignancy. Fibromyomas, leiomyomas, and myomas are all benign neoplasms or tumors. This is an important distinction for coders especially to note.*

• More than 600,000 hysterectomies are performed each year in the United States.

• Cervical cancer is extremely rare in women under 25 years.

Abbreviation	
LEEP	loop electrosurgical excision procedure
LMP	last menstrual period

LO 8.6 Disorders of the Uterus and Fallopian (Uterine) Tubes (continued)

Endometrial Cancer

Endometrial cancer is the fourth most common cancer in women (after lung, breast, and colon cancer). Forty thousand new cases are diagnosed each year, mostly in women between ages 60 and 70. The most common symptom is vaginal bleeding after the menopause. It can also cause a vaginal discharge, pelvic pain, and dyspareunia. Higher levels than normal of estrogen are thought to be a risk factor for endometrial cancer.

Endometrial cancer is staged at the time of any surgical procedure into four groups, depending on its localization to the uterus or its spread outside. Surgery is the most common treatment. It can be a total hysterectomy, in which the uterus and cervix are removed, or a radical hysterectomy, in which the uterine tubes and ovaries are removed and a pelvic lymph node dissection is also done. If the cancer has spread to other parts of the body, progesterone therapy, radiation therapy, and chemotherapy are used.

Cervical Cancer

Cervical cancer is less common than endometrial cancer, but 50% of cases occur between ages 35 and 55. Some 10,000 new cases are diagnosed in the United States each year.

Early cervical cancer produces no symptoms or signs and may be found on a routine Pap test (see below). In the precancerous stage, abnormal cells **(dysplasia)** are found only in the outer layer of the cervix.

Thirteen types of human papilloma virus can convert these **dysplastic** cells to cancer cells *(Figure 8.18)*. A vaccine has been developed that makes people immune to two of the most common types of HPV.

Treatment depends on the stage of the cancer. In preinvasive cancer, when it is only in the outer layer of the lining of the cervix, treatment can include

- **Conization.** A cone-shaped piece of tissue from around the abnormality is removed with a scalpel.
- **Loop electrosurgical excision procedure (LEEP).** A wire loop carries an electrical current to slice off cells from the mouth of the cervix.
- **Laser surgery.** A laser beam is used to kill precancerous and cancerous cells.
- **Cryosurgery.** Freezing is used to kill the precancerous and cancerous cells.

In an invasive stage when cancer has invaded the cervix and beyond, treatment can include total or radical hysterectomy, chemotherapy, and radiation therapy.

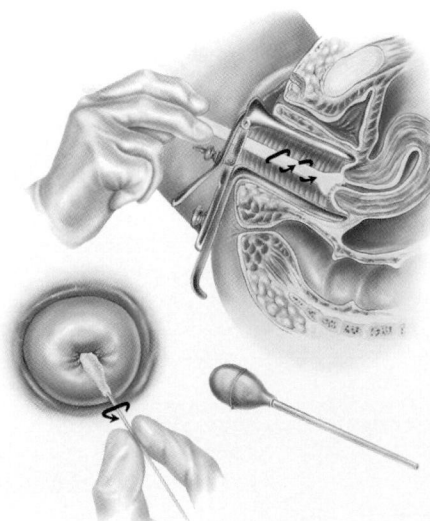

Normal cells   Dysplastic cells

▲ **Figure 8.18** Abnormal Pap Smear with Dysplastic Cells.

Pap Test

In a Pap test, the doctor brushes cells from the cervix *(Figure 8.19)*. The cells are smeared onto a slide or rinsed into a special liquid and sent to the laboratory for examination. The test enables abnormal cells, precancerous or cancerous, to be detected. It is the most successful and accurate test for early detection of abnormalities and should be scheduled according to current guidelines issued in 2012 by the National Cancer Institute, the American Cancer Society, and other national organizations:

- **Initial Pap test**—at age 21.
- **Age 21 to 29**—every 3 years.
- **Age 30–65**—Pap and HPV cotesting every 5 years or Pap alone every 3 years.
- **Age 65 onward**—continue screening if risk factors are present including HIV infection, immunosuppression, previous treatment for precancerous cervical lesion or cervical cancer. Schedule individually with your doctor.
- **Any abnormal result** at any age mandates working out the best schedule for follow-up testing with your doctor.

A Pap test is best performed 10 to 20 days after the first day of the **last menstrual period (LMP)**.

▲ **Figure 8.19** Pap Smear Being Performed.

WORD	PRONUNCIATION	ELEMENTS		DEFINITION
conization	koh-nih-**ZAY**-shun	S/ R/	**-ation** *process* **coniz-** *cone*	Surgical excision of a cone-shaped piece of tissue
cryosurgery	cry-oh-**SUR**-jer-ee	S/ **R/CF** R/	**-ery** *process of* **cry/o-** *icy cold* **-surg-** *operate*	Use of liquid nitrogen or argon gas in surgery to freeze and kill abnormal tissue
dysplasia	dis-**PLAY**-zee-ah	S/ P/ R/	**-ia** *condition* **dys-** *painful, difficult* **-plas-** *molding*	Abnormal tissue formation
dysplastic (adj)	dis-**PLAS**-tic	S/	**-tic** *pertaining to*	Pertaining to abnormal tissue function
Pap test	PAP TEST		George Papanicolaou, 1883–1962, Greek-U.S. physician, anatomist, and cytologist	Examination of cells taken from the cervix

Exercises

A. Proofread the following sentences for errors in documentation. *It may be an error of fact and/or spelling. Rewrite the correct form of the entire sentence on the lines below.*   **LO 8.1, 8.6**

1. Cervixal cancer is more common than endometrial cancer.

   _____

   _____

2. The most common symptom of endometrial cancer is vaginal bleeding after mennopause.

   _____

   _____

3. Displasia is abnormal tissue formation.

   _____

   _____

4. Surgical excision of a wedge-shaped piece of tissue is colonization.

   _____

   _____

5. The Pap test should be examined by a citologist.

   _____

   _____

6. A total hysterectomy removes the uteris and the cervix.

   _____

   _____

Precision is everything!

- Approximately 20% of women now have their first child when they are aged 35 or older.

- In 20% to 30% of female infertility problems, no identifiable cause is found.

- The success rate for IVF is approximately 30% for each egg retrieval.

Abbreviation

IVF	in vitro fertilization

LO 8.7 Female Infertility

Infertility is the inability to become pregnant after 1 year of unprotected intercourse. It affects 10% to 15% of all couples. The causes of infertility are due to

- The female factor alone in 35%

- The male factor alone in 30%

- Male and female factors in 20%

- Unknown factors in 15%

In women, fertility begins to decrease as early as age 30, and pregnancy rates are very low after age 44.

Causes of Infertility in the Female

- **Infrequent ovulation** is responsible in 20% of female infertility problems when both ovulation and menses occur at intervals of longer than 1 month. Bulimia, anorexia nervosa, rapid weight loss, excessive exercise training, low body weight, obesity, and polycystic ovarian syndrome are among the causes.

- **Scarring of the fallopian (uterine) tubes** is responsible for 30% of female infertility problems. Scarring can result from previous surgery, previous tubal pregnancy, pelvic inflammatory disease, or endometriosis. The scarring blocks the sperm from reaching the egg.

- **Structural abnormalities of the uterus** are responsible for 20% of female infertility problems. Fibroid tumors, uterine polyps, and scarring from infections, abortions, and miscarriages can all produce abnormalities of the uterus. These abnormalities also block the sperm from reaching the egg.

After a complete history and physical examination, including vagina and pelvic organs, other diagnostic tools include

- **Hormone blood levels** of progesterone, estrogens, and FSH.

- **Hysterosalpingogram**, in which x-rays of the uterus and fallopian (uterine) tubes are taken after dye is injected into the uterus through a slender catheter (*Figure 8.20*).

- **Ultrasound** of the abdomen, which can show the shape and size of the uterus, and vaginal ultrasound, which can show the shape and size of the ovaries.

- **Hysteroscopy**, which can visualize the inside of the uterus and be used to take an endometrial biopsy and remove polyps or fibroids.

- **Laparoscopy**, which allows inspection of the outside of the uterus and ovaries and removal of any scar tissue blocking tubes.

- **Postcoital testing**, in which the cervix is examined soon after unprotected intercourse to see if sperm can travel through into the uterus.

Treatment is of any underlying cause arising from the results of the infertility evaluation. Infrequent ovulation can be treated with hormones to stimulate release of the egg. These include clomiphene citrate and injectable forms of FSH, LH, and GnRH.

Surgical procedures to initiate pregnancy include

- **Intrauterine insemination**. Sperm are inserted directly into the uterus via a special catheter.

- **In vitro fertilization (IVF)**. Eggs and sperm are combined in a laboratory dish, and two resulting embryos are placed inside the uterus. This can result in twins.

Figure 8.20 **Hysterosalpingogram of a Normal Uterus, Fallopian Tubes, and Ovaries.** ▶

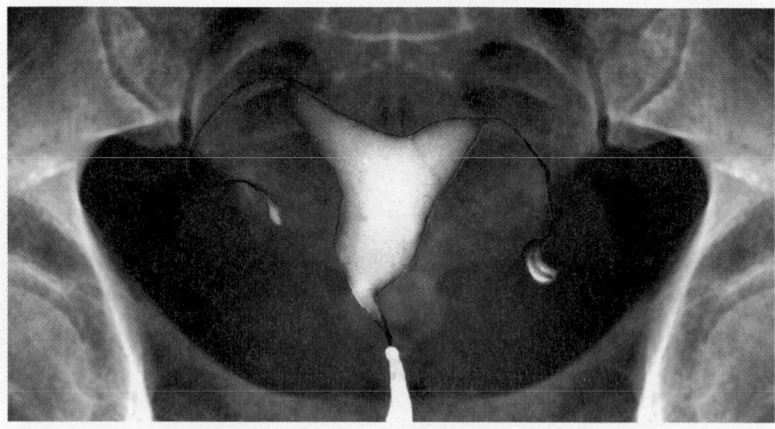

WORD	PRONUNCIATION	ELEMENTS		DEFINITION
hysterosalpingogram	HIS-ter-oh-sal-PING-oh-gram	S/ R/CF R/CF	-gram *a record* hyster/o- *uterus* -salping/o- *fallopian tube*	Radiograph of uterus and uterine tubes after injection of contrast material
hysteroscopy	his-ter-OS-koh-pee	S/ R/CF	-scopy *view or examine* hyster/o- *uterus*	Visual inspection of the uterine cavity using an endoscope
infertility infertile (adj)	in-fer-TIL-ih-tee in-FER-tile	S/ P/ R/	-ity *condition* in- *not* -fertil- *able to conceive*	Inability to conceive over a long period of time
insemination inseminate (verb)	in-sem-ih-NAY-shun in-SEM-ih-nate	S/ P/ R/	-ation *process* in- *in* -semin- *scatter seed*	Introduction of semen into the vagina
intrauterine	IN-trah-YOU-ter-ine	S/ P/ R/	-ine *pertaining to* intra- *inside* -uter- *uterus*	Inside the uterine cavity
in vitro fertilization (IVF)	IN VEE-troh FER-til-eye-ZAY-shun	S/ R/	in vitro Latin *in glass* -ization *process of creating* fertil- *able to conceive*	Process of combining sperm and egg in a laboratory dish and placing the resulting embryos inside the uterus
postcoital	post-KOH-ih-tal	S/ P/ R/	-al *pertaining to* post- *after* -coit- *sexual intercourse*	After sexual intercourse

Exercises

A. Build your knowledge of the meaning of elements. *Write the correct element or term on the line to complete the term.*   **LO 8.1, 8.3, 8.7**

1. If it occurs after intercourse, it is _____coital.

    (pre   post)

2. Visual inspection of the uterine cavity using an endoscope is a _____scopy.

    (cysto   hystero)

3. The patient is unable to conceive and suffers from _____.

    (infertility   insemination)

4. Inside the uterine cavity is referred to as _____uterine.

    (intra   inter)

5. The process of combining sperm and egg in a laboratory dish is _____ fertilization.

    (intrauterine   in vitro)

6. Introduction of semen into the vagina is _____.

    (infertility   insemination)

7. A radiograph of the uterus and uterine tubes is a _____.

    (hysterogram   hysterosalpingogram)

8. Sperm can be _____ directly into the uterus via a catheter.

    (inseminated   insemination)

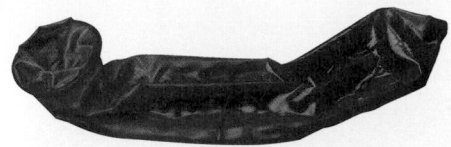

▲ **Figure 8.21** Female Condom.

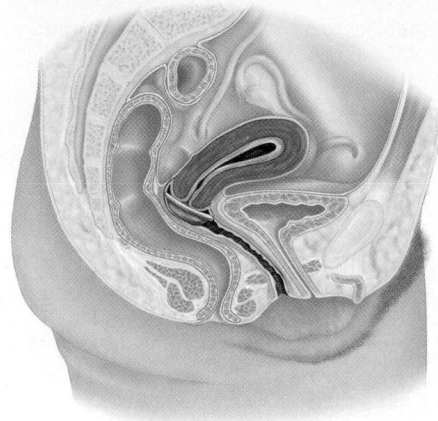

▲ **Figure 8.22** Diaphragm.

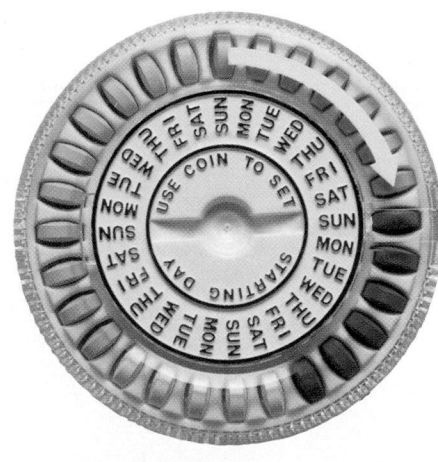

▲ **Figure 8.23** Oral Contraceptives.

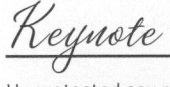

Keynote

Unprotected sex results in pregnancy 85% of the time.

Abbreviations	
IUD	intrauterine device
RU-486	mifepristone

LO 8.8 Contraception

Contraception is the prevention of pregnancy. Common methods of contraception include the following.

Behavioral Methods

- **Abstinence** is reliable if followed consistently.
- **Rhythm method** avoids intercourse near the time of expected ovulation, which is difficult to determine. It has a 25% failure rate.
- **Coitus interruptus** involves the male withdrawing his penis before ejaculation. There is a 20% failure rate.

Barrier Methods

- **Male condom**—a sheath of latex or rubber rolled on over the erect penis. There is a 14% to 15% failure rate for pregnancy.
- **Female condom**—a polyurethane sheath that fits into the vagina with a ring at one end to go over the cervix and a larger ring at the other end to go over the vulva *(Figure 8.21)*. Both male and female condoms help protect against STDs. They have a 5% to 10% failure rate for pregnancy.
- **Diaphragm** *(Figure 8.22)* **and cervical cap**—a latex or rubber dome inserted into the vagina and placed over the cervix. When used with a spermicide, they have a 5% to 10% failure rate for pregnancy.
- **Spermicidal foam and gel**—inserted into the vagina. Used on their own, they have a 25% failure rate.
- **Sponge**—a spermicidal-coated polyurethane barrier placed in the vagina to inhibit sperm. It has a 10% failure rate.

Intrauterine Devices

Intrauterine devices (IUDs) are T-shaped flexible plastic or copper devices inserted into the uterus and left in place for 1 to 4 years. Failure rate is less than 3%.

Hormonal Methods

- **Oral contraceptives** (birth control pills) utilize a mixture of estrogen and progesterone to prevent follicular development and ovulation *(Figure 8.23)*. They are taken orally and have a 5% failure rate, usually due to inconsistent pill taking.
- **Estrogen/progestin patches** deliver the hormones transdermally. Some are applied monthly, some weekly. Their failure rate is less than 1% when reapplied at the correct time.
- **Injected progestins**, such as Depo-Provera, are given by injection every 3 months. Their failure rate is less than 1%.
- **Implanted progestins**, such as Implanon, are contained in porous silicone tubes that are inserted under the skin and slowly release the progestin for up to 5 years. Their failure rate is less than 1%.
- **Morning-after pills**, such as Plan B, contain large doses of progestins to inhibit or delay ovulation. They are a backup when taken within 72 hours of unprotected intercourse. Their failure rate is around 10%.
- **Mifepristone (RU-486)**, when taken with a prostaglandin, induces a miscarriage. It has an 8% failure rate.

Surgical Methods

- **Tubal ligation** ("getting your tubes tied") is performed with laparoscopy. Both fallopian (uterine) tubes are cut, a segment is removed, and the ends are tied off and cauterized shut. Failure rate is less than 1%. A **tubal anastomosis** is the procedure of rejoining the tubes if there is a subsequent change of mind.
- **Vasectomy** in the male is discussed in *Chapter 7*.

Word Analysis and Definition

S = Suffix   P = Prefix   R = Root   R/CF = Combining Form

WORD	PRONUNCIATION	ELEMENTS		DEFINITION
anastomosis anastomoses (pl)	ah-**NAS**-to-**MO**-sis	S/ R/	-osis *condition* anastom- *join together*	A surgically made union between two tubular structures
coitus	**KOH**-it-us		Latin *come together*	Sexual intercourse
condom	**KON**-dom		Old English *sheath or cover*	A sheath or cover for the penis or vagina to prevent conception and infection
contraception	kon-trah-**SEP**-shun	S/ P/ R/	-ion *process* contra- *against* -cept- *receive*	Prevention of pregnancy
contraceptive	kon-trah-**SEP**-tiv	S/	-ive *quality of*	An agent that prevents conception
diaphragm (***Note:** Diaphragm also is the term for the muscle that separates the thoracic and abdominal cavities.*)	**DIE**-ah-fram		Greek *partition or wall*	A ring and dome-shaped material inserted in the vagina to prevent pregnancy
ligature	**LIG**-ah-chur		Latin *band*, *tie*	Thread or wire tied around a tubal structure to close it
ligation	lie-**GAY**-shun	S/ R/	-ion *process* ligat- *tie up*	Use of a tie to close a tube
progestin	pro-**JESS**-tin	S/ P/ R/	-in *chemical compound* pro- *before* -gest- *produce, pregnancy*	A synthetic form of progesterone

Exercises

A. Review all the terms in the above WAD. *With critical thinking, you will be able to answer the following questions using these terms. Fill in the blanks.* **LO 8.8**

1. What is the Latin term for *sexual intercourse*? _____

2. If a patient has a *tubal ligation* and later changes her mind, what procedure is necessary to repair this? _____

   _____

   Briefly describe what this term means. _____

   _____

3. Write the two definitions of the word *diaphragm* and one sentence for each meaning.

   a. Definition 1: _____

   b. Sentence: _____

   _____

   c. Definition 2: _____

   d. Sentence: _____

   _____

4. A *contraceptive* works against something—what does it work against? _____

   _____

5. What is the medical term for a thread or wire that is used to close a tube? _____

Obstetrics: Pregnancy and Childbirth

The nuclei of the male and female cells unite; their chromosomes mingle. Fertilization (**conception**) is complete, and a **zygote** is formed. So begins the incredible, dramatic, and wondrous development of an embryo and a new human being. This process will be described in this lesson to enable you to:

8.4.1 Specify the stages of embryonic development.

8.4.2 Describe the implantation of the embryo in the uterus.

8.4.3 List the functions of the placenta.

8.4.4 Identify the major events of fetal development.

8.4.5 Explain the process of childbirth.

8.4.6 Discuss some of the most common problems of fetal development and childbirth.

8.4.7 Recognize and use appropriately the medical terminology for embryonic and fetal development, pregnancy, and childbirth.

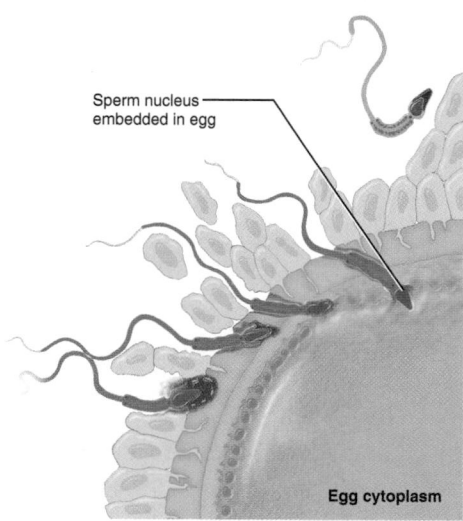

Sperm nucleus embedded in egg

Egg cytoplasm

▲ **Figure 8.24**   Fertilization.

LO 8.9 Conception

When released from the ovary, an egg takes 72 hours to reach the uterus, but it must be **fertilized** *(Figure 8.24)* within 12 to 24 hours to survive. Therefore, **fertilization** must normally take place in the distal third of the fallopian (uterine) tube.

Between 200 million and 600 million sperm are deposited in the vagina near the cervix. Many are destroyed by the acidity in the vagina or just drain out. Others fail to get through the cervical mucus. Approximately half the survivors will go up the wrong fallopian (uterine) tube. The journey through the uterus into the fallopian (uterine) tube takes about an hour. Some 2000 to 3000 sperm reach the egg. Several of these penetrate the outer layers of the egg and clear the path for the one sperm that will penetrate all the way into the egg cytoplasm to fertilize it *(see Figure 8.24).*

Implantation

While still in the fallopian (uterine) tube, the zygote divides, producing a ball of cells called a **morula**. Within the morula, a fluid-filled cavity develops, and the morula becomes a **blastocyst**. A week after fertilization, the blastocyst enters the uterine cavity and burrows into the endometrium (**implantation**). A group of cells in the blastocyst, the inner cell mass, differentiate into the germ layers and form the embryo. Other cells from the blastocyst, together with endometrial cells, form the **placenta**.

Twins (and other multiple births) can be produced in two ways:

- **Dizygotic** twins are produced when two eggs are released by the ovary and fertilized by two separate sperm. They can be of different sexes and are only as genetically similar as other siblings would be.

- **Monozygotic** twins are produced when a single egg is fertilized and later two inner cell masses form within a single blastocyst, each producing an embryo. These twins share a single placenta, are genetically identical, are the same sex, and look alike.

Word Analysis and Definition

S = Suffix   P = Prefix   R = Root   R/CF = Combining Form

WORD	PRONUNCIATION	ELEMENTS		DEFINITION
blastocyst	BLAS-toe-sist	S/ R/CF	-cyst *bladder* blast/o- *germ cell*	The developing embryo during the first 2 weeks
conception	kon-SEP-shun		Latin *something received*	Fertilization of the egg by sperm to form a zygote
dizygotic	die-zye-GOT-ik	S/ P/ R/	-ic *pertaining to* di- *two* -zygot- *yoked together*	Twins from two separate zygotes
fertilize	FER-til-ize		Latin *make fruitful*	To penetrate an oocyte with a sperm so as to impregnate
fertilization	FER-til-eye-ZAY-shun	S/ R/	-ation *process* fertiliz- *make fruitful*	Union of a male sperm and a female egg
implantation	im-plan-TAY-shun	S/ P/ R/	-ation *process* im- *in* -plant- *to plant*	Attachment of a fertilized egg to the endometrium
monozygotic	MON-oh-zye-GOT-ik	S/ P/ R/	-ic *pertaining to* mono- *one* -zygot- *yoked together*	Twins from a single zygote
morula	MOR-you-lah		Latin *mulberry*	Ball of cells formed from divisions of a zygote
placenta placental (adj)	plah-SEN-tah plah-SEN-tal		Latin *a cake*	Organ that allows metabolic interchange between the mother and fetus
zygote	ZYE-goat		Greek *joined together*	Cell resulting from the union of the sperm and egg

Exercises

A. Meet a learning outcome by tracing the pathway of embryo implantation. *You are given the terminology—put it in the correct order of the implantation process.* **LO 8.1, 8.9**

placenta   morula   sperm   embryo

blastocyst   uterine tube   implantation   zygote

fertilization   egg   endometrium

1. _____   7. _____

2. _____   8. _____

3. _____   9. _____

4. _____   10. _____

5. _____   11. _____

6. _____

B. Terminology challenge. *Use the medical language you have learned in this chapter to construct your answers to the following question.* **LO 8.1, 8.9**

1. Describe the difference between dizygotic and monozygotic twins.

  a. dizygotic twins:

  _____

  _____

  b. monozygotic twins:

  _____

  _____

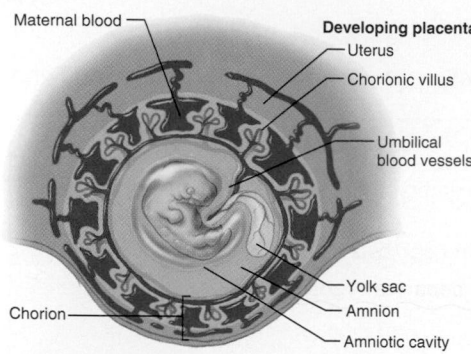

▲ Figure 8.25   Embryo at 4.5 Weeks.

LO 8.9, 8.10 Embryo and Fetus

Embryo

From week 2 until week 8 is the **embryonic period**, in which most of the external structures and internal organs of the **embryo** are formed, together with the placenta, **umbilical** cord, **amnion**, **yolk sac**, and **chorion** *(Figure 8.25)*. The **amnion** is a fluid-filled sac that protects the embryo. The yolk sac is a small sac arising from the ventral surface of the embryo. It contributes to the formation of the digestive tract and produces blood cells and future sex germ cells. The **chorion** forms the placenta by penetrating deeply into the endometrium. At the eighth week, all the organ systems are present; the embryo is just over 1 inch long and is now called a **fetus**.

The **placenta** is a disc of tissue that increases in size as pregnancy proceeds *(Figure 8.26)*. The surface facing the fetus is smooth and gives rise to the **umbilical cord**, which contains two arteries and one vein. The surface attached to the uterine wall consists of treelike structures called **chorionic villi**. The cells of the villi keep the maternal and fetal circulations largely separate, but they are very thin and allow an exchange of gases, nutrients, and waste products to occur.

The functions of the placenta are to

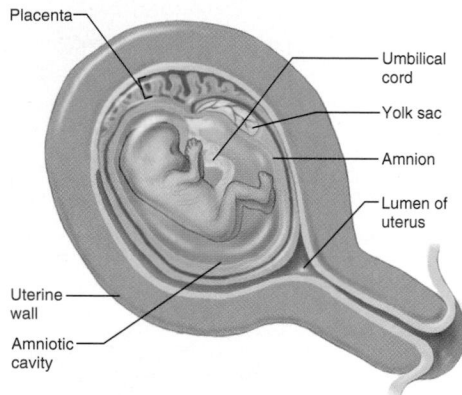

▲ Figure 8.26   Embryo and Placenta at 13.5 Weeks.

- **Transport nutrients** (such as glucose, amino acids, fatty acids, minerals) from mother to fetus.
- **Transport nitrogenous wastes** (such as ammonia, urea, creatinine) from fetus to mother, who can excrete them.
- **Transport oxygen** from mother to fetus and carbon dioxide from fetus to mother, who can excrete it.
- **Transport maternal antibodies** to the fetus.
- **Secrete hormones** (such as estrogen and progesterone) and allow maternal hormones to pass to the fetus.

Unfortunately, some undesirable items and many medications can also cross the placenta. These include the HIV and rubella viruses and the bacteria that cause syphilis. Alcohol, nicotine, carbon monoxide from smoking, and drugs (for example, heroin and cocaine), all have bad effects on the fetus.

Amniocentesis and **chorionic** villus sampling are performed to test for chromosomal abnormalities and genetic birth defects.

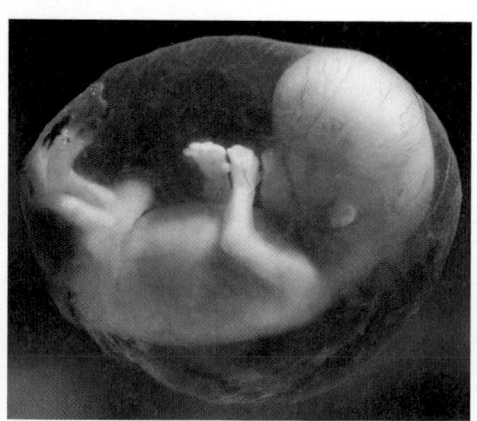

▲ Figure 8.27   Developing Fetus at 20 Weeks.

Fetus

The **fetal period** lasts from the eighth week until birth. At the eighth week, the heart is beating. By the twelfth week, the bones have begun to calcify, and the external genitalia can be differentiated as male or female. In the fourth month, downy hair called **lanugo** appears over the body. In the fifth month, skeletal muscles become active, and the baby's movements are felt between 16 and 22 weeks of gestation *(Figure 8.27)*. A protective substance called **vernix caseosa** covers the skin. In the sixth and seventh months, weight gain is increased, and body fat is deposited.

At 38 weeks, the baby is at full term and ready for birth.

The length of pregnancy, the gestation, is often considered to be 40 weeks, which is the time from a woman's last menstrual period to birth. However, the woman does not become pregnant until she ovulates 2 weeks after her last period, so gestation is really 38 weeks. Gestation is also divided into **trimesters**. The first trimester is up to week 12, the second from week 13 to 24, and the third from week 25 to birth.

A pregnant woman is described as a **gravida**. A woman in her first pregnancy is a **primigravida**. A woman in her second pregnancy is a gravida 2. **Parity** relates to outcome of the pregnancy: Deliveries after the twentieth week are numbered successively as para 1, 2, 3, and so on. **Abortus** refers to losses of pregnancy before the twentieth week. The total of abortus and paras equals a woman's gravidity.

WORD	PRONUNCIATION		ELEMENTS	DEFINITION
abortion	ah-**BOR**-shun	S/ R/	**-ion** *action, process* **abort-** *fail at onset*	Spontaneous or induced expulsion of an embryo or fetus from the uterus
abortus	ah-**BOR**-tus	S/	**-us** *pertaining to*	Product of abortion
amnion	**AM**-nee-on		Greek *membrane around fetus*	Membrane around the fetus that contains amniotic fluid
amniotic (adj)	am-nee-**OT**-ic	S/ R/CF	**-tic** *pertaining to* **amni/o-** *amnion*	Pertaining to the amnion
amniocentesis	**AM**-nee-oh-sen-tee-sis	S/	**-centesis** *puncture*	Removal of amniotic fluid for diagnostic purposes
chorion	**KOH**-ree-on		Greek *membrane*	The fetal membrane that forms the placenta
chorionic (adj)	koh-ree-**ON**-ick	S/ R/	**-ic** *pertaining to* **chorion-** *chorion*	Pertaining to the chorion
embryo	**EM**-bree-oh		Greek *a young one*	Developing organism from conception until the end of the second month
embryonic (adj)	em-bree-**ON**-ic	S/ R/CF	**-nic** *pertaining to* **embry/o-** *embryo*	Pertaining to the embryo
fetus	**FEE**-tus		Latin *offspring*	Human organism from the end of the eighth week after conception to birth
fetal (adj)	**FEE**-tal	S/ R/	**-al** *pertaining to* **fet-** *fetus*	Pertaining to the fetus
gravid (adj)	**GRAV**-id		Latin *pregnant*	Pregnant
gravida	**GRAV**-ih-dah		Latin *pregnant woman*	A pregnant woman
primigravida	pree-mih-**GRAV**-ih-dah	P/ R/	**primi-** *first* **-gravida** *pregnant woman*	First pregnancy
lanugo	la-**NYU**-go		Latin *wool*	Fine, soft hair on the fetal body
parity	**PAIR**-ih-tee		Latin *to bear*	Number of deliveries
para	**PAH**-rah		Latin *bring forth*	Abbreviation for number of deliveries
trimester	**TRY**-mes-ter		Latin *of 3 months' duration*	One-third of the length of a full-term pregnancy
umbilicus	um-**BIL**-ih-kus		Latin *navel*	Pit in the abdomen where the umbilical cord entered the fetus
umbilical (adj)	um-**BIL**-ih-kal	S/ R/	**-al** *pertaining to* **umbilic-** *umbilicus*	Pertaining to the umbilicus or the center of the abdomen
vernix caseosa	**VER**-nicks kay-see-**OH**-sah		**vernix** Latin *varnish* **caseosa** Latin *cheese*	Cheesy substance covering skin of the fetus
yolk sac	YOKE SACK		**yolk** Latin *yellow* **sac** Latin *pouch or bag*	Source of blood cells and future sex cells for the fetus

Exercises

A. Precision in documentation includes using the correct form (noun, verb, adjective) of the medical term. *Practice precision in this written* **language of obstetrics***. Fill in the blanks.*   **LO 8.1, 8.9, 8.10**

amniocentesis   amnion   amniotic

1. The _____ will be punctured in the procedure _____ in order to withdraw the _____ fluid.

embryo   embryonic

2. The _____ stage of gestation means the _____ has formed in the first 8 weeks of human development.

umbilical   umbilicus

3. The medical term for navel is _____. The _____ cord enters the fetus in the abdomen.

Practice your precision in spelling, please!

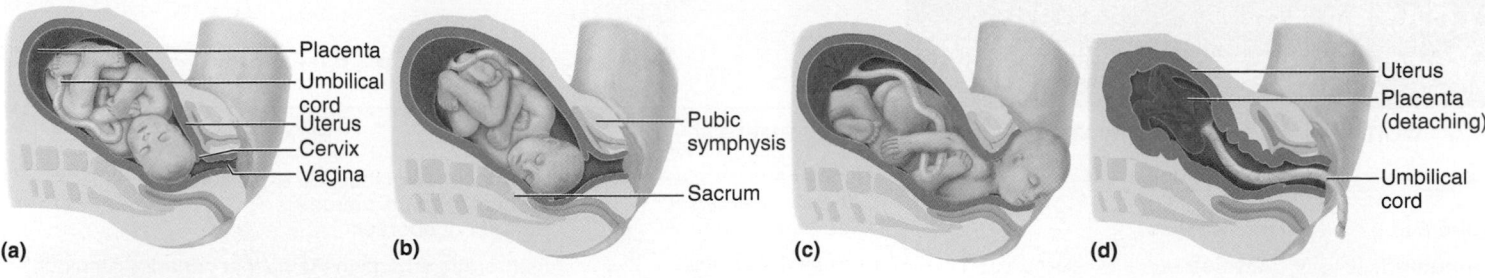

▲ **Figure 8.28** **The Stages of Childbirth.** (*a*) First stage: Early dilation of cervix. (*b*) First stage: Late dilation of cervix. (*c*) Second stage: Expulsion of the fetus. (*d*) Third stage: Expulsion of the placenta.

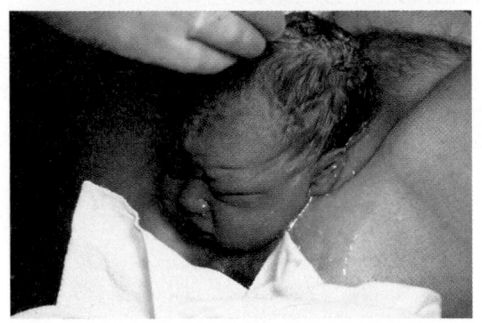

▲ **Figure 8.29** Delivery of Head.

Keynote

The 6 weeks **postpartum** (after the birth) are called the **puerperium**. The uterus shrinks (**involution**) through self-digestion (**autolysis**) of uterine cells by their own lysosomal enzymes. This generates a vaginal discharge called **lochia** that lasts about 10 days.

Abbreviations	
FSH	follicle-stimulating hormone
HCG	human chorionic gonadotropin
LH	luteinizing hormone

LO 8.10 Pregnancy and Childbirth

Hormones of Pregnancy

Human chorionic gonadotropin (HCG) is secreted by the blastocyst and the placenta. Its presence in the mother's blood and urine is the basis for laboratory and home pregnancy tests. It can be detected as early as 9 or 10 days after conception. Human chorionic gonadotropin stimulates the growth of the corpus luteum and its production of estrogen and progesterone.

Estrogen stimulates the mother's uterus to enlarge and her breasts to increase to twice their normal size. It makes the pelvic joints and ligaments more flexible so that the pelvic outlet widens for childbirth.

Progesterone is secreted by the corpus luteum and the placenta. It suppresses further ovulation, prevents menstruation, stimulates the proliferation of the endometrium to support the implantation, and inhibits contractions of the uterine muscle.

Follicle-stimulating hormone (FSH) and **luteinizing hormone (LH)** from the pituitary gland stimulate the maintenance of the corpus luteum and its estrogen and progesterone production.

Childbirth

Labor contractions begin about 30 minutes apart. They have to be intermittent because each contraction shuts down the maternal blood supply to the placenta and therefore shuts down the blood supply to the fetus. Labor pains are due to ischemia of the myometrium.

Labor is divided into three stages, each of which is usually longer in a **primipara** (first-time birth) than in a **multipara** (two or more births).

First Stage—Dilation of the Cervix This is the longest stage. It can be a few minutes in a multipara to more than 1 day in a primipara. **Dilation** is widening of the cervical canal to the same diameter as the baby's head (*Figure 8.28 a and b*). At the same time the wall of the cervix becomes thinner, a process called **effacement**. During dilation, the fetal membranes rupture, and the "waters break" as amniotic fluid is released.

Second Stage—Expulsion of the Fetus As the uterus continues to contract, additional pain is generated by the stretching of the cervix and vagina by the baby's head. When the head reaches the vaginal opening and stretches the vulva, the head is said to be **crowning** (*Figure 8.29*). This process is sometimes helped by performing an **episiotomy**, an incision in the perineum to prevent tearing.

After the baby is delivered, the umbilical cord is clamped in two places and cut between the two clamps.

Third Stage—Expulsion of the Placenta After the baby is delivered, the uterus continues to contract. It pushes the placenta off the uterine wall and expels it out of the vagina. This usually takes 5 to 15 minutes; after 30 minutes the placenta is said to be **retained** and may have to be removed manually by the obstetrician. The use of the hormone **oxytocin**, either IM or IV, can reduce the incidence of retained placenta.

WORD	PRONUNCIATION		ELEMENTS	DEFINITION
autolysis	awe-**TOL**-ih-sis	P/ R/	auto- *self* -**lysis** *destruction*	Self-destruction of cells by enzymes within the cells
crowning	**KROWN**-ing	S/ R/	-ing *doing, quality of* **crown-** *crown*	During childbirth, when the maximum diameter of the baby's head comes through the vulvar ring
dilation	die-**LAY**-shun	S/ R/	-ion *process* **dilat-** *open out*	Stretching or enlarging of an opening
effacement	ee-**FACE**-ment	S/ R/	-ment *resulting state* **efface-** *wipe out*	Thinning of the cervix during labor
episiotomy	eh-piz-ee-**OT**-oh-me	S/ R/CF	-tomy *surgical incision* **episi/o-** *vulva*	Surgical incision of the vulva
labor	**LAY**-bore		Latin *toil, suffering*	Process of expulsion of the fetus
lochia	**LOW**-kee-uh		Greek *relating to childbirth*	Vaginal discharge following childbirth
multipara	mul-**TIP**-ah-ruh	P/ R/	multi- *many* -**para** *to bring forth*	Woman who has given birth to two or more children
oxytocin	**OCK**-see-toe-sin	S/ R/CF R/	-in *chemical compound* **ox/y-** *oxygen* -**toc-** *labor, birth*	Pituitary hormone that stimulates the uterus to contract and causes breast milk to be ejected from the alveoli into the duct system
postpartum	post-**PAR**-tum	P/ R/	post- *after* -**partum** *childbirth*	After childbirth
primipara	pree-**MIP**-ah-ruh	P/ R/	primi- *first* -**para** *to bring forth*	Woman who has given birth for the first time
puerperium (**Note:** This term is composed only of roots.)	pyu-er-**PEE**-ree-um	R/ R/	**puer-** *child* -**perium** *bringing forth*	Six-week period after birth in which the uterus involutes

Exercises

A. Several of these elements you have seen before, and you will certainly see them again in other terms. *Learn each once, and recognize it all the time. Circle the best answer to the questions.*   **LO 8.1, 8.10**

1. The term that contains the prefix meaning *many* is

   primipara   lochia   multipara

2. The term that contains the suffix meaning *incision* is

   episiotomy   effacement   dilation

3. The term that contains the root meaning *to bring forth* is

   primipara   involution   effacement

4. The term that contains the root meaning *child* is

   lochia   multipara   puerperium

5. The term that contains the suffix meaning *process* is

   effacement   episiotomy   involution

6. The term that contains the prefix meaning *first* is

   multipara   puerperium   primipara

7. The term that contains the prefix meaning *self* is

   multipara   autolysis   lochia

8. The term that contains the prefix meaning *after* is

   primipara   postpartum   multipara

B. Review the text on the opposite page and then circle the best answer for the following questions.   LO 8.5, 8.10

1. The hormones involved in pregnancy and childbirth are

   a. FSH, LH, progesterone, BMT, MRI

   b. HCG, estrogen, FSH, LH, BMT

   c. HCG, FSH, LH, estrogen, progesterone

   d. LH, insulin, BMT, FSH, estrogen

   e. progesterone, insulin, FSH, BMT, estrogen

2. Which of the following statements is not true about the first stage of labor?

   a. the first stage is dilation of the cervix

   b. the first stage is the shortest stage of labor

   c. the first stage includes the process of effacement

   d. the first stage includes the rupture of the fetal membranes

   e. the first stage can be shorter in multipara and longer in primipara

You are

. . . an obstetric assistant working with Garry Joiner, MD, an obstetrician at Fulwood Medical Center.

Your patient is

. . . Mrs. Gloria Maggay, a 29-year-old housekeeper.

Case Report 8.3

Mrs. Maggay's last menstrual period was 8 weeks ago, and she has a positive home pregnancy test. This is her first pregnancy. She has breast tenderness and mild nausea. For the past 2 days, she has had some cramping and right-sided, lower abdominal pain, and this morning she had vaginal spotting. Her VS are T 99°F, P 80, R 14, BP 130/70.

While you are waiting for Dr. Joiner to come and examine Mrs. Maggay, she complains of feeling faint and has a sharp, severe pain in her lower abdomen on the right side. Her pulse rate has increased to 92. You need to recognize what is happening. Mrs. Maggay's symptoms are those of an ectopic pregnancy. The sudden increase in the pain and the rise in pulse rate can indicate that the tube has ruptured and is hemorrhaging into the abdominal cavity. The gynecologist should see her immediately and, if necessary, take her to the **operating room (OR)** for laparoscopic surgery to stop the bleeding and evacuate the products of conception.

LO 8.11 Disorders of Pregnancy

Ectopic Pregnancy

If the fallopian (uterine) tube is obstructed, the fertilized egg will be prevented from moving into the uterus and will continue its development in the fallopian (uterine) tube. This is called an **ectopic pregnancy**. Tubal disorders that cause ectopic pregnancy include previous salpingitis, pelvic inflammatory disease (PID), and endometriosis.

Preeclampsia and Eclampsia

Preeclampsia is a sudden, abnormal increase in blood pressure after the twentieth week of pregnancy, with proteinuria and edema.

Eclampsia is a life-threatening condition, characterized by the signs and symptoms of preeclampsia and with the addition of convulsions. Management involves immediate admission to the hospital with control of the mother's blood pressure. The baby is delivered as soon as the mother is stabilized, regardless of maturity.

Amniotic Fluid Abnormalities

Amniotic fluid abnormalities occur in the second trimester. Normally, the fetus breathes in and swallows amniotic fluid to promote development of the gastrointestinal tract and lungs.

- **Oligohydramnios** is too little amniotic fluid. It is associated with an increase in the risk of birth defects and poor fetal growth. Its etiology is unknown.
- **Polyhydramnios** is too much amniotic fluid. It causes abdominal discomfort and breathing difficulties for the mother. It also is associated with **preterm delivery**, placental problems, and fetal growth problems.

Gestational Diabetes Mellitus

In some pregnant women, the amount of insulin they can produce decreases. This leads to **gestational diabetes mellitus (GDM)** and increased risk of preeclampsia. For the neonate, it increases the risk of **perinatal mortality**. Later in life, both mother and child are at increased risk for developing type 2 diabetes and obesity.

Hyperemesis Gravidarum

Eighty percent of pregnant women experience some degree of "morning sickness." It is at its worst between 2 and 12 weeks and resolves in the second trimester. For a few women, nausea and vomiting persist. This is **hyperemesis gravidarum**. Severe cases may have to be admitted to the hospital for intravenous (IV) fluids.

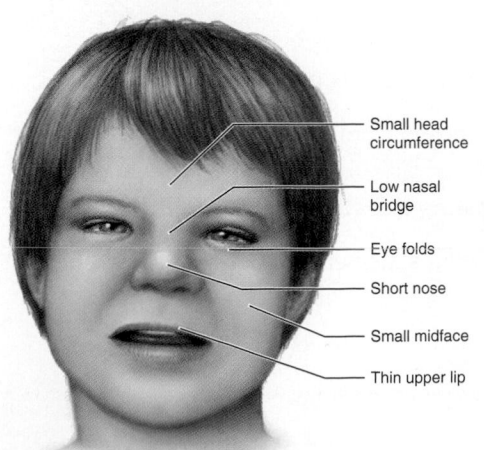

Small head circumference

Low nasal bridge

Eye folds

Short nose

Small midface

Thin upper lip

▲ **Figure 8.30** Fetal Alcohol Syndrome.

WORD	PRONUNCIATION		ELEMENTS	DEFINITION
eclampsia	ek-**LAMP**-see-uh		Greek *a shining forth*	Convulsions in a patient with preeclampsia
ectopic	ek-**TOP**-ik	S/ R/	**-ic** *pertaining to* **ectop-** *on the outside, displaced*	Out of place, not in a normal position
hyperemesis	high-per-**EM**-ee-sis	P/ R/	**hyper-** *excessive* **-emesis** *vomiting*	Excessive vomiting
mortality	mor-**TAL**-ih-tee	S/ S/ R/	**-al-** *pertaining to* **-ity** *condition, state* **mort-** *death*	Fatal outcome or death rate
oligohydramnios	**OL**-ih-goh-high-**DRAM**-nee-os	P/ R/ R/	**oligo-** *too little, scanty* **-hydr-** *water* **-amnios** *amnion*	Too little amniotic fluid
polyhydramnios	**POL**-ee-high-**DRAM**-nee-os	P/	**poly-** *many*	Too much amniotic fluid
perinatal	per-ih-**NAY**-tal	S/ P/ R/	**-al** *pertaining to* **peri-** *around* **-nat-** *birth*	Around the time of birth
preeclampsia	pree-eh-**KLAMP**-see-uh	S/ P/ R/	**-ia** *condition* **pre-** *before* **-eclamps-** *shining forth*	Hypertension, edema, and proteinuria during pregnancy
preterm premature (syn)	**PREE**-term pree-mah-**TYUR**	P/ R/	**pre-** *before* **-term** *normal gestation*	Baby delivered before 37 weeks of gestation Occurring before the expected time; for example, an infant born before 37 weeks of gestation
teratogen	**TER**-ah-toe-jen	S/ R/CF	**-gen** *produce, create* **terat/o-** *monster, malformed fetus*	Agent that produces fetal deformities
teratogenesis teratogenic (adj)	**TER**-ah-toe-**JEN**-eh-sis **TER**-ah-toe-**JEN**-ik	S/ S/	**-esis** *condition* **-ic** *pertaining to*	Process involved in producing fetal deformities Capable of producing fetal deformities

Exercises

A. After reading both parts of Case Report 8.4 on the opposite page, answer the following questions. *Be prepared to discuss your answers in class.*   **LO 8.1, 8.10, 8.11**

1. What symptoms did Mrs. Maggay have when she came into the office?

   _____

   _____

2. What symptoms did she develop while she was there?

   _____

   _____

3. What does the phrase "the tube had ruptured" mean? _____

4. What is occurring if Mrs. Maggay is "hemorrhaging into the abdominal cavity"?

   _____

   _____

5. Why is this an emergency? _____

   _____

6. What is the function of the laparoscope? _____

   _____

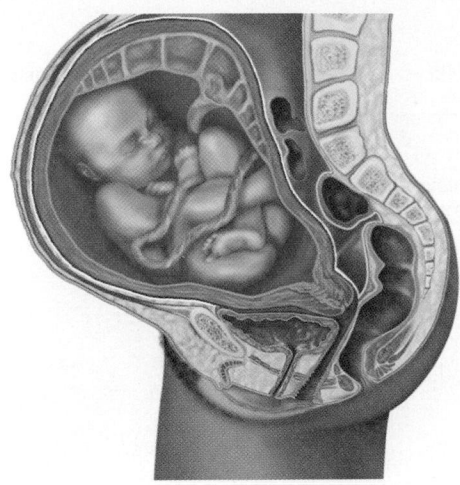

▲ **Figure 8.31**   Breech Presentation.

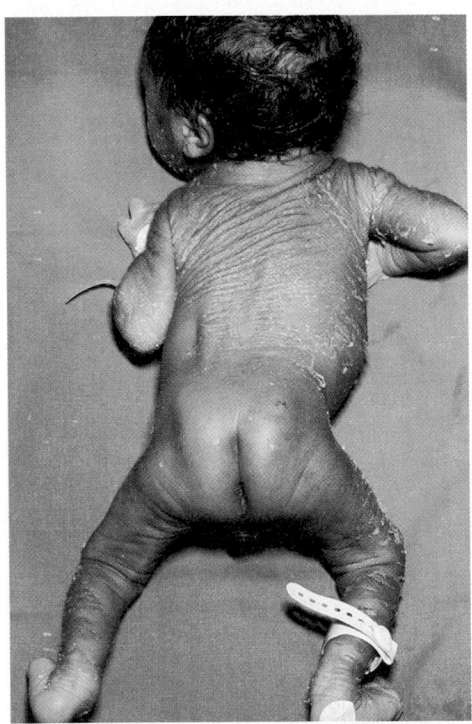

▲ **Figure 8.32**   Postmature Infant.

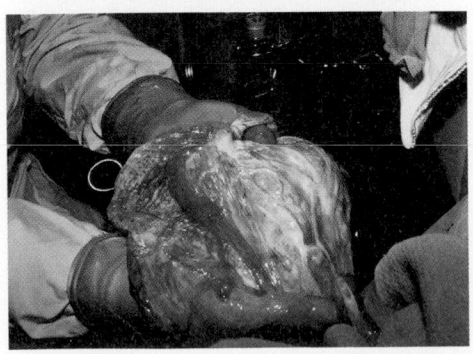

▲ **Figure 8.33**   Placenta (Afterbirth).

LO 8.11 Disorders of Childbirth

Fetal distress due to lack of oxygen is an uncommon complication of labor but is detrimental if not recognized. During labor, there is electronic fetal heart monitoring to determine whether the baby is in distress. Treatment is to give the mother oxygen or increase IV fluids. If distress persists, the baby is delivered as quickly as possible by **forceps extraction**, vacuum extractor, or C-section.

Abnormal position of fetus occurs when the baby at the beginning of labor is not in a head-first **(vertex)** presentation facing rearward. Abnormal positions include

- **Breech.** The buttocks present *(Figure 8.31)*.
- **Face.** The face instead of the top of the head presents.
- **Shoulder.** The shoulder and upper back are trying to exit the uterus first.

If the baby cannot be turned into a vertex presentation, a C-section is usually performed.

Prolapsed umbilical cord occurs when the cord precedes the baby down the birth canal. Pressure on the cord can cut off the baby's blood supply, which is still being provided through the umbilical arteries.

Nuchal cord is the condition of having the cord wrapped around the baby's neck during delivery. This occurs in 20% of deliveries.

Premature rupture of the membranes occurs in 10% of normal pregnancies and increases the risk of infection of the uterus and fetus.

Gestational Classification

Every newborn **(neonate)** is either:

- **Premature**—less than 37 weeks gestation.
- **Full-term**—between 37 to 42 weeks gestation.
- **Postmature**—longer than 42 weeks gestation *(Figure 8.32)*.

Prematurity occurs in about 8% of newborns. The earlier the baby is born, the more life-threatening problems occur.

Because their lungs are underdeveloped, premature babies can develop **respiratory distress syndrome (RDS)**, also called **hyaline membrane disease**. The premature baby's lungs are not mature enough to produce **surfactant**, a mixture of lipids and proteins that keeps the alveoli from collapsing.

If their brains are underdeveloped, premature newborns can have inconsistent breathing with **apnea**. They are susceptible to bleeding into the brain. Their immune systems have low levels of antibodies to provide protection from infection.

An immature liver can impair the excretion of bilirubin *(see Chapter 5)*, and premature babies become jaundiced. High levels of bilirubin can produce **kernicterus**, in which deposits of bilirubin in the brain cause brain damage.

Postmaturity is much less common than prematurity. Its etiology is unknown, but the placenta begins to shrink and is less able to supply sufficient nutrients to the baby. This leads to hypoglycemia; loss of subcutaneous fat; dry, peeling skin; and, if oxygen is lacking, fetal distress. The baby can pass stools **(meconium)** into the amniotic fluid. In its distress, the baby can take deep gasping breaths and inhale the meconium fluid. This leads to **meconium aspiration syndrome** and respiratory difficulty at birth.

Placental Disorders

Placenta abruptio is separation of the placenta from the uterine wall before delivery of the baby. The baby's oxygen supply is cut off, and fetal distress appears quickly. It is an obstetric (OB) emergency, and usually a C-section is indicated.

Placenta previa is a low-lying placenta between the baby's head and the internal os of the cervix. It can cause severe bleeding during labor, and a C-section may be necessary.

Retained placenta means that all or part of the placenta and/or membranes remain behind in the uterus 30 minutes to an hour after the baby has been delivered. The expulsion of the placenta *(Figure 8.33)* can happen naturally. The result of retained placenta is heavy uterine bleeding called **postpartum hemorrhage (PPH)**. Manual removal of the retained product may be necessary under spinal, epidural, or general anesthesia.

Abbreviations	
OB	obstetrics
PPH	postpartum hemorrhage
RDS	respiratory distress syndrome

Word Analysis and Definition

S = Suffix   P = Prefix   R = Root   R/CF = Combining Form

WORD	PRONUNCIATION		ELEMENTS	DEFINITION
abruptio	ab-**RUP**-she-oh		Latin *to break off*	Placenta abruptio is the premature detachment of the placenta
apnea	**AP**-nee-ah		Greek *lack of breath*	Absence of spontaneous respiration
breech	BREECH		Old English *trousers*	Buttocks-first presentation of fetus at delivery
forceps extraction	**FOR**-seps ek-**STRAK**-shun		Latin *a pair of tongs* Latin *to draw out*	Assisted delivery of the baby by an instrument that grasps the head of the baby
kernicterus	ker-**NICK**-ter-us	R/ R/	**kern-** *nucleus* **-icterus** *jaundice*	Bilirubin staining of basal nuclei of the brain
meconium	meh-**KOH**-nee-um		Greek *a little poppy*	The first bowel movement of the newborn
neonate	**NEE**-oh-nate	P/ S/	**neo-** *new* **-al** *pertaining to*	A newborn infant
neonatal (adj)	**NEE**-oh-**NAY**-tal	R/	**-nat-** *born*	Pertaining to the newborn infant or the newborn period
nuchal cord	**NYU**-kul KORD		**nuchal** French *the back (nape) of the neck*	Loop of umbilical cord around the fetal neck
postmature (adj)	post-mah-**TYUR**	P/ R/	**post-** *after* **-mature** *ripe, ready*	Pertaining to an infant born after 42 weeks of gestation
postmaturity (noun)	post-mah-**TYUR**-ih-tee	S/	**-ity** *condition*	Condition of being postmature
premature (adj)	pree-mah-**TYUR**	P/ R/	**pre-** *before, in front of* **-mature** *ripe*	Occurring before the expected time; for example, when an infant is born before 37 weeks of gestation
prematurity (noun) **preemie (informal)**	pree-mah-**TYUR**-ih-tee **PREE**-me	S/	**-ity** *condition, state*	Condition of being premature Premature baby
previa	**PREE**-vee-ah	P/ R/	**pre-** *before, in front of* **-via** *the way*	Anything blocking the fetus during its birth; for example, am abnormally situated placenta, *placenta previa*
surfactant	ser-**FAK**-tant		surface active agent	A protein and fat compound that creates surface tension to hold lung alveolar walls apart
vertex	**VER**-teks		Latin *whorl*	Topmost point of the vault of the skull

Exercises

A. Elements. *Real familiarity with obstetrical and reproductive terms means you can look at an element and identify it as either a prefix, root or combining form, or suffix. Identify each element by writing its type and meaning in the appropriate columns. The first one is done for you. Fill in the blanks.* **LO 8.1, 8.10, 8.11**

Element	Type	Meaning		Element	Type	Meaning
1. post	P	after		6. pre		
2. obstetr				7. ician		
3. kern				8. icterus		
4. via				9. ity		
5. mature						

B. Employ the *language of obstetrics* and create two sentences of clinical documentation using any two terms in the above WAD. The sentences cannot be definitions or come directly from the text. **LO 8.1, 8.10, 8.11**

1. Sentence:

_____

_____

_____

2. Sentence:

_____

_____

_____

It is important to complete your understanding of reproduction by being able to use correct medical terminology to:

8.5.1 Describe the anatomy of the breast.

8.5.2 Differentiate the breast from the mammary gland.

8.5.3 Explain the physiology and mechanisms of lactation.

8.5.4 Discuss common disorders of the breast.

Keynotes

- There is no relationship between breast size and the ability to breastfeed.

- Breastfeeding is not a reliable means of contraception. It has a failure rate of around 10%.

LO 8.12 The Breast

Until the relatively recent introduction of bottles filled with liquid supplied by cows or soybeans, the milk produced by the female breast was essential for the survival of the human species. Nourishment of the infant remains the breast's major function, even though our culture has made the breast a visible, tangible, and beautiful symbol of femininity.

Anatomy of the Breast

The breasts of males and females are identical until puberty, when ovarian hormones stimulate the development of the breast in females. Adult males still have main milk ducts in their breasts.

Each adult female breast has a **body** located over the pectoralis major muscle and an **axillary tail** extending toward the armpit. The **nipple** projects from the breast and contains multiple openings of the main milk ducts. The reddish-brown **areola** surrounds the nipple. The small bumps on its surface are **areolar glands**. These are sebaceous glands, the secretions of which prevent chapping and cracking during breastfeeding.

Internally, the breasts are supported by **suspensory ligaments** that extend from the skin to the fascia overlying the pectoralis major muscle (*Figure 8.34*).

The **nonlactating breast** consists mostly of adipose and connective tissues. It has a system of ducts that branch through the connective tissue and converge on the nipple.

Mammary Gland

When the **mammary gland** develops during pregnancy, it is divided into 15 to 20 lobes that contain the secretory **alveoli** that produce milk. Each lobe is drained by the main milk ducts, called **lactiferous ducts** (*see Figure 8.34*). Immediately before opening onto the nipple, each lactiferous duct dilates to form a **lactiferous sinus** in which milk is stored before being released from the nipple.

Lactation

When the mammary gland develops during pregnancy, high estrogen levels cause the lactiferous ducts to grow and branch, and progesterone stimulates the budding of alveoli at the ends of the ducts. The alveoli are formed in grapelike clusters. The percentage of adipose and connective tissue diminishes.

In late pregnancy, the alveoli and ducts contain **colostrum**. This secretion contains more protein but less fat than human milk, but it also contains high levels of **immunoglobulins** (*see Chapter 12*) to give the newborn infant protection from infections. Colostrum is replaced by milk 2 or 3 days after the baby's birth, and this replacement is complete by day 5.

Milk production is mainly controlled by **prolactin**, a hormone from the pituitary gland. The other essential stimulus to milk production is the baby's sucking (*Figure 8.35*), which stimulates prolactin production. In addition, the **sucking reflex** stimulates the pituitary gland to produce **oxytocin** (*see Chapter 17*), which causes milk to be ejected from the alveoli into the duct system.

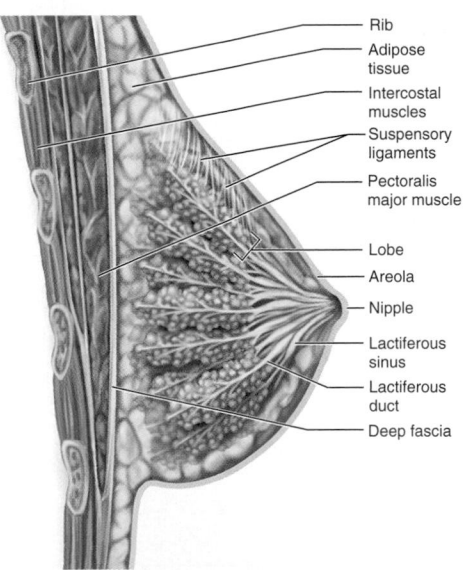

Rib
Adipose tissue
Intercostal muscles
Suspensory ligaments
Pectoralis major muscle
Lobe
Areola
Nipple
Lactiferous sinus
Lactiferous duct
Deep fascia

▲ **Figure 8.34** Anatomy of Lactating Breast.

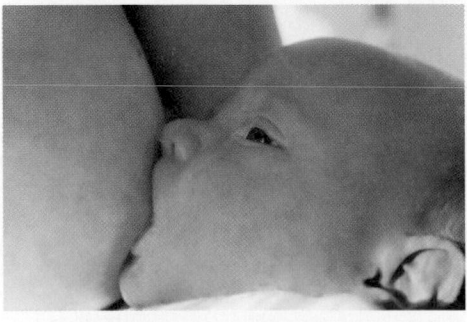

▲ **Figure 8.35** Breastfeeding.

WORD	PRONUNCIATION	ELEMENTS		DEFINITION
areola areolar (adj)	ah-**REE**-oh-luh		Latin *small area*	Circular reddish area surrounding the nipple
colostrum	koh-**LOSS**-trum		Latin *foremilk*	The first breast secretion at the end of pregnancy
lactation	lak-**TAY**-shun	S/ R/CF	-ation *process* lact/i- *milk*	Production of milk
lactiferous (adj) lactate (verb)	lak-**TIF**-er-us	S/ R/	-ous *pertaining to* -fer- *to bear, carry*	Pertaining to or yielding milk
mammary	**MAM**-ah-ree	S/ R/	-ary *pertaining to* mamm- *breast*	Relating to the lactating breast
nipple	**NIP**-el		Old English *small nose*	Projection from the breast into which the lactiferous ducts open
prolactin	pro-**LAK**-tin	S/ P/ R/	-in *chemical compound* pro- *before* -lact- *milk*	Pituitary hormone that stimulates production of milk

Exercises

A. Spelling your documentation correctly is a mark of an educated professional. *Read the following statements, and insert the correctly spelled term in the blanks.*   **LO 8.12**

1. (Prolectin/Prolactin) _____ is the pituitary hormone that stimulates production of milk.

2. The circular, reddish area surrounding the nipple is the (aireola/areola) _____.

3. (Oxitocin/Oxytocin) _____ is the pituitary hormone that stimulates the uterus to contract.

4. The first breast secretion at the end of pregnancy is known as (colestrium/colostrum) _____.

5. The projection from the breast into which the milk ducts open is the (nippel/nipple) _____.

6. (Laktiferous/Lactiferous) _____ means *pertaining to or yielding milk.*

7. The areolar glands are (cebaceous/sebaceous) _____ glands.

B. Find the one false statement in the following choices. *Circle the correct choices and then rewrite the false statement to be true.*   **LO 8.12**

1. The secretory alveoli produce milk.   T   F

2. In late pregnancy, the alveoli and ducts contain colostrum.   T   F

3. High levels of immunoglobulins are in breast milk.   T   F

4. Milk production is mainly controlled by prolactin.   T   F

5. The sucking reflex produces estrogen.   T   F

6. Corrected statement:

_____

_____

Abbreviations	
BRCA1, BRCA2	breast cancer genes
BSE	breast self-examination

LO 8.13 Disorders of the Breast

Mastitis, inflammation of the breast, can occur in association with breastfeeding if the nipple or areola is cracked or traumatized. It is usually segmental in one of the lobes of the breast and responds well to antibiotics. It is not an indication for stopping breastfeeding.

Mastalgia (breast pain) is the most common benign breast disorder. The pain can be associated with breast tenderness and be part of PMS. If the pain is not relieved by acetaminophen or NSAIDs, danazol or tamoxifen can be used for a short time.

Paget disease of the nipple presents as a scaling, crusting lesion of the nipple, sometimes with a discharge from the nipple (*Figure 8.36*). It is indicative of an underlying cancer that has to be the focus of diagnosis and treatment.

Nipple discharge, particularly if it is from one breast and bloody, is an indication of an underlying disorder such as breast cancer and warrants investigation.

Fibroadenomas are circumscribed, small, benign tumors that can be either cystic or solid and can be multiple. They can be excised surgically.

Fibrocystic disease of the breast presents as a dense, irregular cobblestone consistency of the breast, often with intermittent breast discomfort (*Figure 8.37*). It occurs in over 60% of all women and is considered by many doctors as a normal variant.

Breast cancer affects one in eight women in their lifetime. Risk factors include a family history, particularly if a woman carries either of the breast cancer **genes**, *BRCA1* or *BRCA2*; the use of postmenopausal estrogen therapy; and an early menarche and late menopause.

Most breast cancers are discovered as a lump by the patient, which is why **monthly breast self-examinations (BSEs)** are so important. Another 40% are discovered on routine **mammogram** (*Figure 8.37*). Routine **mammography** reduces breast cancer mortality by 25% to 30% (*Figure 8.38*).

Most breast cancers occur in the upper and outer quadrant of the breast. If cancer is suspected, biopsy should be planned. This is being performed more and more often as a **stereotactic biopsy**, a needle biopsy performed during mammography.

The surgical treatments for breast cancer include

- **Excisional biopsy** to remove the breast tumor with a surrounding margin of normal breast tissue.
- **Lumpectomy** or **quadrantectomy**, which are breast-conserving surgeries.
- **Simple mastectomy** to remove the breast with skin and nipple.
- **Modified radical mastectomy**, which is a simple mastectomy plus lymph node dissection.
- **Radical mastectomy**, with complete removal of breast tissue, pectoralis major muscle, and all associated lymph nodes.

Additional radiotherapy, combination chemotherapy, and Herceptin and Tamoxifen therapy are also used. Two new research drugs, pertuzumab (Omnitag) and everolimus (Afenitor), have been shown to hold cancer at bay for several months. Both can cost up to $10,000 per month.

Breast cancer can metastasize to lymph nodes, lungs, liver, bone, brain, and skin.

Galactorrhea is the production of milk when a woman is not breastfeeding. Sometimes the cause cannot be found, but it can occur in association with hormone therapy, antidepressants, tumor of the pituitary gland (*see Chapter 17*), and use of street drugs such as opiates and marijuana. In most cases, the milk production ceases with time.

Gynecomastia, enlargement of the breast, can be unilateral or bilateral and occur in both sexes. It is usually associated with either liver disease, marijuana, or drug therapy such as estrogens, calcium channel blockers, and antineoplastic drugs. It remits or disappears after the drug is withdrawn. Occasionally **suction lipectomy** and/or cosmetic surgery is needed.

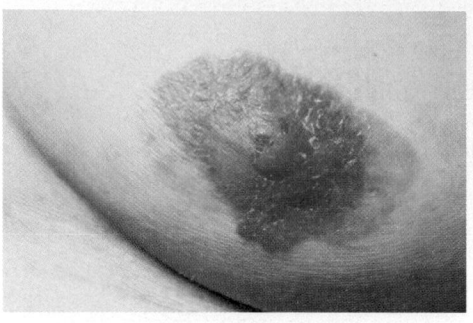

▲ **Figure 8.36** Paget Disease of the Nipple Is Associated with Breast Cancer.

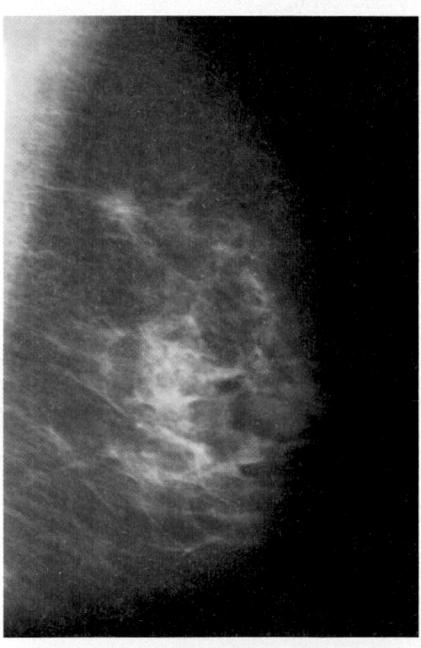

▲ **Figure 8.37** Mammogram showing Fibrocystic Disease of the Breast.

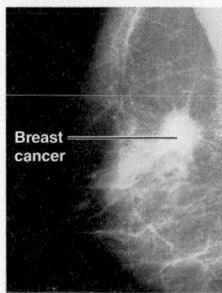

Breast cancer

▲ **Figure 8.38** Mammogram Showing Breast Cancer.

WORD	PRONUNCIATION	ELEMENTS		DEFINITION
fibroadenoma	FIE-broh-ad-en-OH-mah	S/ R/ R/CF	-oma *tumor* -aden- *gland* fibr/o- *fiber*	Benign tumor containing much fibrous tissue
fibrocystic disease	fie-broh-SIS-tik DIZ-eez	S/ R/CF R/	-ic *pertaining to* fibr/o- *fiber* -cyst- *cyst*	Benign breast disease with multiple tiny lumps and cysts
galactorrhea	gah-LAK-toe-REE-ah	S/ R/CF	-rrhea *flow* galact/o- *milk*	Abnormal flow of milk from the breasts
gynecomastia	GUY-nih-koh-MAS-tee-ah	S/ R/CF R/	-ia *condition* gynec/o- *female* -mast- *breast*	Enlargement of the breast
lipectomy	lip-ECK-toe-me	S/ R/	-ectomy *surgical excision* lip- *fatty tissue*	Surgical removal of adipose tissue
lumpectomy	lump-ECK-toe-me	S/ R/CF	-ectomy *surgical excision* lump- *piece*	Removal of a lesion with preservation of surrounding tissue
mammogram	MAM-oh-gram	S/ R/CF	-gram *a record* mamm/o- *breast*	The record produced by x-ray imaging of the breast
mammography	mah-MOG-rah-fee	S/	-graphy *process of recording*	Process of x-ray examination of the breast
mastalgia	mass-TAL-jee-uh	S/ R/	-algia *pain* mast- *breast*	Pain in the breast
mastectomy	mass-TECK-toe-me	S/ R/	-ectomy *surgical excision* mast- *breast*	Surgical excision of the breast
mastitis	mass-TIE-tis	S/ R/	-itis *inflammation* mast- *breast*	Inflammation of the breast
quadrant quadrantectomy	KWAD-rant kwad-ran-TEK-toe-me	 S/ R/	Latin *quarter* -ectomy *surgical excision* quadrant- *quarter*	One-quarter of a circle Surgical excision of a quadrant of the breast
stereotactic	STER-ee-oh-TAK-tic	S/ R/ R/CF	-ic *pertaining to* -tact- *orderly arrangement* stere/o- *three-dimensional*	Pertaining to a precise three-dimensional method to locate a lesion

Exercises

A. Build your knowledge of suffixes, which always provide a big clue to the meaning of a medical term. *Review all the terms in the above WAD; then answer the following questions. All of these questions can be answered by analyzing the elements in each term. Which of the terms in the above WAD mean the following terms?*   **LO 8.13**

1. *surgical excision?* List them here. _____

2. *a glandular tumor?* _____

3. *condition of enlarged breasts?* _____

4. *precise, three-dimensional method to locate a lesion?* _____

5. *an inflammation of the breast?* _____

6. *breast pain?* _____

7. *an abnormal flow of milk?* _____

B. Use the medical terminology you have learned in this chapter to answer the following question.   LO 8.13

1. Explain to a fellow student the difference between *mastitis* and *mastalgia*.

   1. mastitis: **2. mastalgia:**

   _____   _____

   _____   _____

   _____   _____

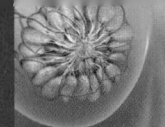

Female Reproductive System

Challenge Your Knowledge

A. **Prefixes.** The following medical terms all have the same prefix, but the rest of their elements make them entirely different terms. Analyze each medical term into its basic elements and meaning; then use the terms in sentences of your own making. Fill in the chart, and then write your sentences. (**LO 8.1, 8.6,** *Remember*)

Medical Term	Prefix	Root/ Combining Form	Suffix	Meaning of Term
dysplasia	1.	2.	3.	4.
dysmenorrhea	5.	6.	7.	8.
dysplastic	9.	10.	11.	12.
dysfunctional	13.	14.	15.	16.
dyspareunia	17.	18.	19.	20.

Sentences:

21. _____

22. _____

23. _____

24. _____

25. _____

B. **Precise communication in medical language includes correct spelling of medical terms. (LO 8.1, 8.6,** *Remember, Understand*)

    1. Circle the pair of terms that are incorrectly spelled.

        a. lumpectomy   mastectomy

        b. gynecomastea   galactorhea

        c. fibrocystic   fibroadenoma

        d. mastitis   mastalgia

        e. modified   excisional

C. Abbreviations. There are many abbreviations in this chapter, and they are of no use to you if you cannot interpret them correctly. Practice using abbreviations in this exercise. Everything in the sentence is spelled out—rewrite the sentence on the following lines, inserting abbreviations where appropriate. (**LO 8.1, 8.3, 8.6, 8.8,** *Remember, Understand, Apply*)

1. Patient was advised to take naproxen sodium to relieve the symptoms of her premenstrual syndrome; she wishes to discontinue the birth control pills, and try an intrauterine device for contraception instead.

_____

_____

_____

2. The patient's untreated sexually transmitted disease, chlamydia, has progressed to pelvic inflammatory disease and needs immediate treatment.

_____

_____

_____

3. Following a difficult labor and cesarean delivery, the patient suffered postpartum hemorrhage, and the infant is suffering from respiratory distress syndrome.

_____

_____

_____

4. Patient has been referred to the Gynecology Clinic for a consultation regarding the need for a dilation and curettage.

_____

_____

_____

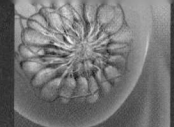

Female Reproductive System

H. **Latin and Greek terms cannot be further deconstructed into prefix, root, combining form, or suffix.** You must know them for what they are. Test your knowledge of these terms with this exercise. Match the medical term in the left column with the correct meaning in the right column. (**LO 8.1, 8.3,** *Remember, Understand, Apply*)

_____	1. fornix	**a.** plug
_____	2. menses	**b.** membrane
_____	3. ruga	**c.** egg
_____	4. ulcer	**d.** month
_____	5. os	**e.** sheath
_____	6. hymen	**f.** neck
_____	7. ovary	**g.** arch, vault
_____	8. vagina	**h.** mouth
_____	9. cervix	**i.** ridge or crease
_____	10. tampon	**j.** cancer

I. **Plurals of some medical terms can be difficult to convert from the singular because there are so many different rules for plurals.** Practice makes perfect in your ability to form the correct plural of the term. Fill in the plural column; then choose any one term, and write a sentence of clinical documentation using that term. (**LO 8.1, 8.3,** *Remember, Understand, Apply*)

Singular Term	Plural Term
cilium	1.
fimbria	2.
fornix	3.
infundibulum	4.
labium	5.
majus	6.
minus	7.
ovary	8.
ovum	9.
ruga	10.

11. Sentence: _____

_____

J. Terminology challenge. Autolysis is a new term you learned in this chapter. It is composed of two elements you have encountered in previous chapters. Recall other terms you have already learned that have those elements. (**LO 8.1, 8.10,** *Remember, Apply*)

Autolysis means _____.

Other terms with the same elements and their meanings:

auto-: _____

-lysis: _____

K. Dictionary. **Tertiary** is a term used in connection with the disease syphilis. Using your dictionary or an online medical dictionary, look up its meaning. (**LO 8.1, 8.4,** *Understand*)

1. tertiary: _____

2. Discuss. Prepare a brief discussion on the different stages of syphilis and its various signs, symptoms, and treatments. Write your discussion notes on the following lines.

_____

_____

_____

_____

L. Trace the pathway of conception. The following phrases describe the process of fertilization. Number the items A to H to indicate the correct order of their occurrence. (**LO 8.1, 8.3, 8.9,** *Understand*)

_____ 1. Nuclei of male and female cells unite.

_____ 2. Morula becomes a blastocyst.

_____ 3. Inner cell mass differentiates and forms embryo.

_____ 4. Zygote produces morula.

_____ 5. Ovary releases egg.

_____ 6. All organ systems are present; embryo becomes fetus.

_____ 7. Blastocyst implants in the endometrium.

_____ 8. Zygote is formed.

Note: Notice how the various terms change, as what starts out as the "egg" progresses through different stages and terms to become the "fetus."

List the terms in the descriptions here: _____

_____

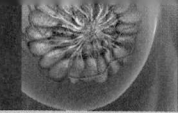

Female Reproductive System

M. **Translation please.** How well do you understand what you read? Use your knowledge of OB/GYN terminology to translate the following sentences taken directly from this chapter into layman's terms. Fill in the blanks. (**LO 8.1, 8.2, 8.10,** *Understand, Apply*)

1. "Gestation is divided into trimesters."

_____

_____

_____

2. "Tubal ligation is performed with laparoscopy."

_____

_____

_____

N. **Roots/combining forms are the core foundation of every term.** Underline just the roots or combining forms in the following terms, and give their meanings. (**LO 8.1,** *Understand, Apply*)

Term	Meaning
1. amenorrhea	_____
2. progesterone	_____
3. leiomyoma	_____
4. menstruation	_____
5. antevert	_____
6. endometrial	_____
7. paraurethral	_____
8. amniocentesis	_____
9. perimetrium	_____
10. hysterosalpingogram	_____

O. Language of obstetrics. Pregnancy has its own associated set of obstetric terms. Apply your knowledge of obstetric terms to answering the following questions. Circle the correct answer. (**LO 8.1, 8.9, 8.10, *Apply, Analyze***)

1. The *nuchal cord* is

   a. only present in ectopic pregnancy

   b. wrapped around the baby's neck during delivery

   c. a congenital malformation

   d. only present in breech births

   e. present in 50% of births

2. What keeps the maternal and fetal blood circulations separated?

   a. umbilical cord

   b. amnion

   c. yolk sac

   d. cells of the villi

   e. placenta

3. A test for chromosomal abnormalities and genetic birth defects is

   a. teratogenesis

   b. hyperemesis

   c. dilation

   d. labor

   e. amniocentesis

4. When the head is just starting to push out of the vaginal opening, it is said to be

   a. effacing

   b. crowning

   c. dilating

   d. ovulating

   e. none of these

5. Which undesirable item can cross the placenta into the fetus?

   a. rubella virus

   b. oxygen

   c. maternal antibodies

   d. glucose

   e. hormones

6. The pit in the abdomen where the umbilical cord enters the fetus is the

   a. meatus

   b. navel

   c. yolk sac

   d. a and b

   e. none of these

7. Postpartum vaginal discharge is called

   a. puerperium

   b. lochia

   c. polyhydramnios

   d. amniocentesis

   e. oligohydramnios

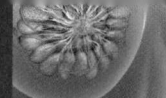

Female Reproductive System

P. Short answer. If you understand the terminology in these questions, you can explain it to someone else, as you will often have to do on the job. Fill in the blanks. (**LO 8.2, Apply, Analyze**)

1. Explain how the difference of one word element changes the meanings of these words: conception   contraception

_____

_____

2. Explain what is meant by "an STD develops *resistance* to antibiotics."

_____

_____

3. A new patient's chart says she is "gravida 4, para 3." What does that mean?

_____

_____

_____

Q. Patient Claire Marcos. Go back and reread the scenario in Case Report 8.2. Now that you have completed this chapter, you should be able to answer her questions in language she will understand. Fill in the blanks. (**LO 8.1, 8.2, 8.6, Apply, Analyze**)

1. Why are my periods so irregular?

_____

_____

2. Why doesn't my acne respond to all the treatment I've had?

_____

_____

3. Am I going bald?

_____

_____

4. Will I be able to have children some day?

_____

_____

5. Why am I taking birth control pills when I'm not sexually active?

_____

_____

6. What are all these other health problems they say I'm at risk for?

_____

_____

R. Language of obstetrics. Pregnancy has its own associated set of obstetric terms. Apply your knowledge of obstetric terms to answering the following questions. Circle the correct answer. (**LO 8.1, 8.2, 8.9, 8.10,** *Apply, Analyze*)

1. Where does fertilization actually take place?

   a. left ovary

   b. distal third of the fallopian (uterine) tube

   c. right ovary

   d. proximal third of the fallopian (uterine) tube

   e. uterus

2. During the first stage of labor, what is the process in which the wall of the cervix becomes thinner?

   a. crowning

   b. effacement

   c. delivery

   d. autolysis

   e. involution

3. What is the term for a fertilized egg's development in the fallopian (uterine) tube instead of the uterus?

   a. preeclampsia

   b. postpartum

   c. eclampsia

   d. ectopic

   e. endometriosis

4. The protective covering of the skin of fetus is the

   a. estrogen

   b. lanugo

   c. vernix caseosa

   d. chorion

   e. morula

5. A woman who has given birth for the first time is

   a. multipara

   b. gravidarum

   c. primipara

   d. postpartum

   e. puerperium

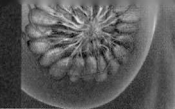

Female Reproductive System

S. **Patient education.** Breast cancer affects one in eight women in their lifetime. If a patient were to ask, could you give a brief description of each of the following surgical treatments for breast cancer? (**LO 8.12, 8.13,** *Apply, Analyze*)

1. excisional biopsy:

_____

_____

2. lumpectomy:

_____

_____

3. quadrantectomy:

_____

_____

4. simple mastectomy:

_____

_____

5. modified radical mastectomy:

_____

_____

6. radical mastectomy:

_____

_____

T. Patient documentation. The following mammogram report for a patient contains terminology you should understand after reading this chapter. Answer the questions about the report by filling in the blanks. (**LO 8.12, 8.13,** *Analyze*)

Exam: Diagnostic bilateral mammogram

Reason for exam: Discomfort in both breasts

The glandular tissue is heterogeneously dense. There are scattered fibroglandular densities bilaterally. There is a benign-appearing curvilinear area of glandular tissue in the right lower inner breast. There are a few faint calcifications in the lower inner left breast and in the central left breast. Magnification views were performed of the left breast calcifications in two positions, and they have an appearance most consistent with benign process. There is no associated mass or distortion.

Impression: Heterogeneously dense glandular tissue with focal glandular density in the medial aspect of the right breast and faint calcifications in the left breast. Probably benign.

Recommendation: Comparison with prior films. If prior films are not available, recommend follow-up mammogram in 6 months. Findings were submitted to the patient in writing.

1. Define *bilateral*. _____

2. Deconstruct the term *fibroglandular* by putting slashes between each element.

   _____

3. Define *calcification*. Use a dictionary if needed.

   _____

4. Define *benign process*. Use a dictionary if needed.

   _____

5. Define *heterogeneously*. Use a dictionary if needed.

   _____

Discussion questions on this report and the breast:

6. Why does the radiologist recommend follow-up in 6 months if no previous films are available?

   _____

7. What is the difference between *mastitis* and *mastalgia*?

   _____

8. With what is *gynecomastia* usually associated?

   _____

9. Define *fibroadenoma*.

   _____

10. Does this patient's report show any *malignancies*? _____

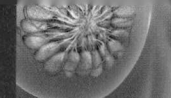
Female Reproductive System

CHAPTER SUMMARY EXERCISE

A. **Spelling comprehension.** *Circle the correct spelling of the term.* (**LO 8.1,** *Remember*)

1. mensstuation	menstruation	menstuation	mensstruation	menstrruation
2. falopian	fallopian	faloppian	fallopean	falopean
3. anteverted	antiverted	anteverrted	antiverrted	antevertted
4. postpubescent	postpubiscient	postpubescient	postpubisent	postpubessient
5. cotus	cottus	coitus	coituss	cutois
6. fimbeia	fimmbria	fembria	fimbria	fembrea
7. dyspareeunia	dispareunia	dyspareunia	disspariunia	despariunia
8. liomioma	lyomyoma	leiomyoma	liomyoma	leomyoma
9. gonorhea	gonorrhea	gonnorhea	gonorhea	gonorheea
10. epesiotomy	episiotomy	eppesiotomy	epessiotomy	epeziotomy

B. **Match the number of the correct spelling of the term in Exercise A with the brief description of the term below.** (**LO 8.1, 8.3,** *Apply*)

1. Pain during sexual intercourse _____

2. Synonym for menses _____

3. Uterine tubes _____

4. Fringelike structure _____

5. Contagious infection of genital mucosa _____

6. After the age of puberty _____

7. Tilted forward _____

8. Sexual intercourse _____

9. Benign neoplasm derived from smooth muscle _____

10. Surgical incision of the vulva _____

C. Using your knowledge of terms 1–10 in Exercises A and B and their correct spelling, write a brief sentence for each of the terms as it might appear in patient documentation. (LO 8.1, *Apply*)

1. _____

   _____

2. _____

   _____

   _____

3. _____

   _____

4. _____

   _____

5. _____

   _____

6. _____

   _____

7. _____

   _____

8. _____

   _____

9. _____

   _____

10. _____

   _____

Female Reproductive System

8. Identify methods of contraception for the female and male. Place a checkmark (✓) beside the term to indicate whether it is used for male or female contraception. **(LO 8.8)**

Method	Male	Female
a. tubal ligation		
b. spermicidal foam & gel		
c. diaphragm		
d. oral contraceptives		
e. sponge		
f. vasectomy		
g. IUD		
h. cervical cap		
i. condom (usual user)		

9. Describe conception, implantation, and development of the embryo and fetus. Which of the following terms is *not* involved in conception, implantation, and development of the embryo and fetus? **(LO 8.9)**

a. fertilization

b. zygote

c. ovary

d. coitus

e. anastomosis

10. Discuss the changes that occur in the female reproductive system during pregnancy and childbirth. List the changes the female's body undergoes during pregnancy. **(LO 8.10)**

a. What enlarges? _____ and the _____

b. Which body parts become more flexible? _____ and _____

c. What body part widens? _____

d. What gets suppressed? _____

e. What gets stimulated? _____

f. What is prevented? _____

11. Understand the effects of common disorders of pregnancy and childbirth on the mother and fetus. Discuss how eclampsia affects the mother and the fetus. (**LO 8.11**)

    a. Define eclampsia:

      _____

      _____

    b. Describe eclampsia's effect on the mother:

      _____

      _____

    c. Describe eclampsia's effect on the fetus:

      _____

      _____

    d. Why is eclampsia a life-threatening condition?

      _____

      _____

12. Describe the structure and functions of the female breast. Only one of the following statements about the breast is false. Rewrite the false statement correctly. (**LO 8.12**)

    a. The breasts of males and females are identical until puberty.

    b. Ovarian hormones stimulate the growth of breasts in females.

    c. Adult males still have main milk ducts in their breasts.

    d. The reddish-brown areola surrounds the nipple.

    e. The nonlactating breast consists mostly of adipose and muscular tissue.

    f. Correction:

      _____

      _____

      _____

13. Discuss disorders of the breast. Explain the difference between *mastitis* and *mastalgia*. (**LO 8.13**)

    a. mastitis:

      _____

      _____

    b. mastalgia:

      _____

      _____

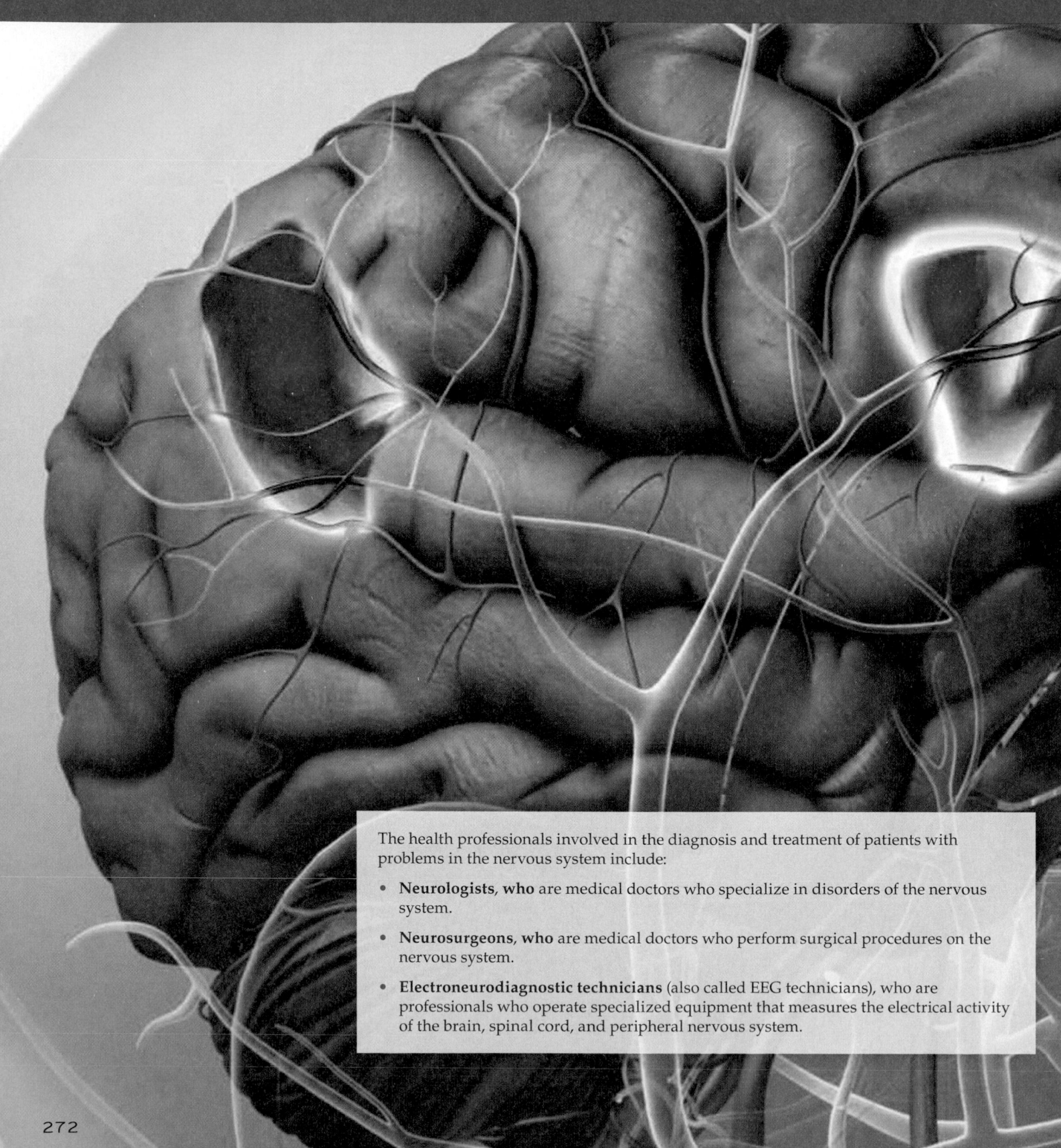

Nervous System
The Language of Neurology

The health professionals involved in the diagnosis and treatment of patients with problems in the nervous system include:

- **Neurologists, who** are medical doctors who specialize in disorders of the nervous system.

- **Neurosurgeons, who** are medical doctors who perform surgical procedures on the nervous system.

- **Electroneurodiagnostic technicians** (also called EEG technicians), who are professionals who operate specialized equipment that measures the electrical activity of the brain, spinal cord, and peripheral nervous system.

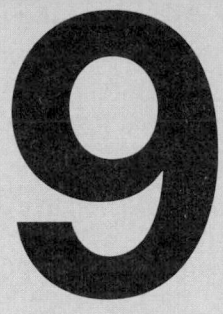

9

Case Report (CR) 9.1

You are

. . . an **electroneurodiagnostic technologist** working with Gregory Solis, MD, a **neurosurgeon** at Fulwood Medical Center.

Your patient is

. . . Ms. Roberta Gaston, a 39-year-old woman, who has been referred by Raul Cardenas, MD, a **neurologist**, for evaluation for possible **neurosurgery**.

Ms. Gaston has had **epileptic seizures** since the age of 16. She has **generalized tonic-clonic seizures** occurring once a week. She also has daily minor spells when she stops interacting with her surroundings and blinks rhythmically for about 20 seconds, after which she returns to normal. Numerous **antiepileptic** drugs, including phenobarbital, valproic acid, and phenytoin, have been tried with no relief. She is not able to work and is cared for by her parents.

Her neurologic examination is normal. Her **EEG** (electroencephalogram) shows diffuse spike-and-wave discharges with a left-sided frontal predominance. Her **CT** (computed tomography) is normal. An **MRI** (magnetic resonance imaging) shows a 20-mm diameter mass adjacent to the anterior horn of her left **ventricle**. Continuous EEG/video monitoring shows **ictal** activity in the left frontal lobe.

Chapter Learning Outcomes

Your roles are to communicate with Ms. Gaston and her parents; communicate with other health professionals involved in her care; and maintain, review, and document her history. Also, you are to assist Dr. Solis with studies to identify the site and cause of her epilepsy and determine if surgery is needed.

To perform these roles you must be able to:

LO 9.1 Recognize the health professionals involved in the care of patients with neurologic problems.

LO 9.2 Apply the language of neurology to the anatomy, structures, and cells of the nervous system.

LO 9.3 Use the language of neurology to describe the physiology and functions of the nervous system.

LO 9.4 Write the medical terms of neurology to communicate and document accurately and precisely in any health care setting.

LO 9.5 Use the medical terms of neurology to communicate verbally with accuracy and precision in any health care setting.

LO 9.6 Define abbreviations that pertain to the nervous system.

LO 9.7 Describe the major regions of the brain, cranial nerves, and their functions.

LO 9.8 Define the structure and functions of the spinal cord, spinal nerves, and the meninges.

LO 9.9 Explain the effects of common disorders of the brain and cranial nerves on health.

LO 9.10 Explain the effects of common disorders of the spinal cord, spinal and peripheral nerves, and meninges on health.

LO 9.11 Recognize diagnostic procedures that pertain to the nervous system.

LO 9.12 Discuss the pharmacology of the drugs that affect the nervous system.

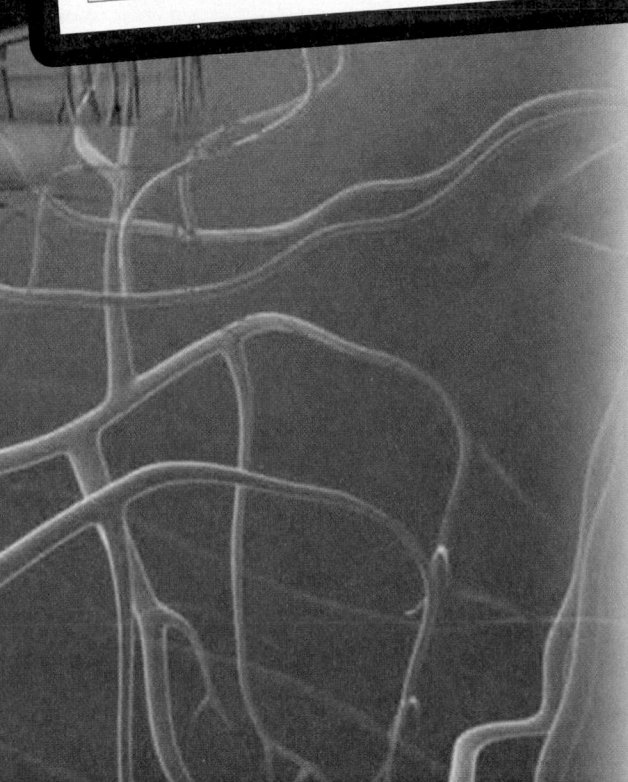

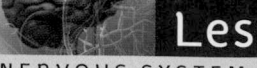
Functions and Structure of the Nervous System

Every time you stop to smell the roses, touch a petal, bend down, cut a stem, carry it indoors, place it in a vase, and admire its color, a wide range of sensations and actions are interpreted and controlled by your nervous system.

The trillions of cells in your body must communicate and work together for you to function effectively. This is done through your nervous system, and it is essential that you understand how this system operates. You can then understand how your body functions and maintains its homeostasis to respond to changes in your internal and external environments.

In this lesson, you will learn to use correct medical terminology to:

9.1.1   **Describe the specific functions of the nervous system.**

9.1.2   **Relate the specific functions of the nervous system to the structures of its components.**

9.1.3   **List the subdivisions of the nervous system.**

9.1.4   **Define the basic cells of the nervous system.**

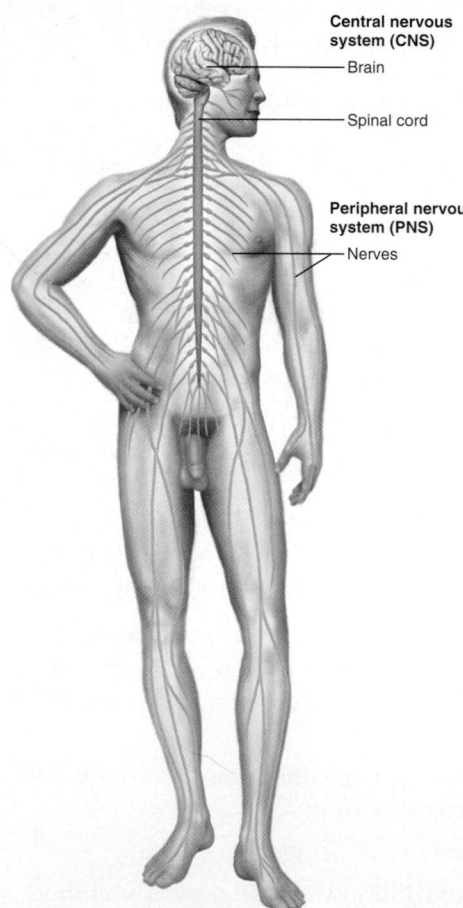

Central nervous system (CNS)
- Brain
- Spinal cord

Peripheral nervous system (PNS)
- Nerves

▲ **Figure 9.1   The Nervous System.**

Abbreviations

EEG	electroencephalogram
CNS	central nervous system
CT	computed tomography
MRI	magnetic resonance imaging
PNS	peripheral nervous system

LO 9.3 Functions of the Nervous System

1. **Sensory input** to the brain comes from receptors all over the body at both the conscious and subconscious levels. Seeing the rose, touching it, smelling it, and noting your body position as you bend are external stimuli of which you are aware. Inside your body, internal stimuli about the amount of oxygen and carbon dioxide in your blood and other homeostatic variables are being continually processed at the subconscious level.

2. **Motor output** from the brain stimulates the skeletal muscles to contract and enables you to bend down, cut a stem, or move in any way. Smooth muscle in the walls of blood vessels contracts when stimulated by the nervous system. The production of sweat, saliva, and digestive enzymes is controlled by the nervous system.

3. **Evaluation and integration** occur in the brain to process the sensory input, initiate a motor response, and store the event in memory.

4. **Homeostasis** is maintained by the nervous system taking in internal sensory input and, for example, responding by stimulating the heart to deliver the correct volume of blood for oxygenation and removal of waste products.

5. **Mental activity** occurs in the brain so that you can think, feel, understand, respond, and remember.

   - The brain and spinal cord are called the **central nervous system (CNS)** *(Figure 9.1)*.
   - Nerves all over the body outside the CNS are called the **peripheral nervous system (PNS)** *(Figure 9.1)*.
   - The medical specialty of disorders of the nervous system is called **neurology**.
   - A specialist in neurology is called a **neurologist**, and a specialist who operates on the nervous system is a **neurosurgeon**.

Word Analysis and Definition

S = Suffix   P = Prefix   R = Root   R/CF = Combining Form

WORD	PRONUNCIATION	ELEMENTS		DEFINITION
antiepileptic	**AN**-tee-epih-**LEP**-tik	S/ P/ R/	**-tic** *pertaining to* **anti-** *against* **-epilep-** *seizure*	A pharmacologic agent capable of preventing or arresting epilepsy
convulsion	kon-**VUL**-shun	S/ P/ R/	**-ion** *process* **con-** *with, together* **-vuls-** *tear, pull*	Alternative name for seizure
electroencephalogram (EEG)	ee-**LEK**-troh-en-**SEF**-ah-low-gram	S/ R/CF R/CF	**-gram** *a record* **electr/o-** *electricity* **-encephal/o-** *brain*	Record of the electrical activity of the brain
electroencephalograph	ee-**LEK**-troh-en-**SEF**-ah-low-graf	S/	**-graph** *to record*	Device used to record the electrical activity of the brain
electroencephalography	ee-**LEK**-troh-en-**SEF**-ah-**LOG**-raf-ee	S/	**-graphy** *process of recording*	The process of recording the electrical activity of the brain
electroneurodiagnostic	ee-**LEK**-troh-**NYUR**-oh-die-ag-**NOS**-tik	S/ R/CF R/CF R/	**-ic** *pertaining to* **electr/o-** *electricity* **-neur/o-** *nerve* **-diagnost-** *decision*	Pertaining to the use of electricity in the diagnosis of a neurologic disorder
epilepsy	**EP**-ih-**LEP**-see		Greek *seizure*	Chronic brain disorder due to paroxysmal excessive neuronal discharges
epileptic (adj)	**EP**-ih-**LEP**-tik	S/ R/	**-tic** *pertaining to* **epilep-** *seizure*	Pertaining to or suffering from seizures
ictal	**ICK**-tal	S/ R/	**-al** *pertaining to* **ict-** *seizure*	Pertaining to, or condition caused by, a stroke or epilepsy
motor	**MOH**-tor		Latin *to move*	Pertaining to nerves that send impulses out to cause muscles to contract or glands to secrete
neurology	nyu-**ROL**-oh-jee	S/ R/CF	**-logy** *study of* **neur/o-** *nerve*	Medical specialty of disorders of the nervous system
neurologist	nyu-**ROL**-oh-jist	S/	**-logist** *one who studies, specialist*	Medical specialist in disorders of the nervous system
neurologic (adj) neurosurgeon neurosurgery	**NYUR**-oh-**LOJ**-ik **NYU**-roh-**SUR**-jun **NYU**-roh-**SUR**-jer-ee	S/ S/ R/CF R/ S/	**-ic** *pertaining to* **-eon** *one who does* **neur/o-** *nerve* **-surg-** *operate* **-ery** *process of*	Pertaining to the nervous system Specialist in operating on the nervous system Medical specialty in surgery of the nervous system
psychoactive	sigh-co-**AK**-tiv	R/CF S/	**psych/o** *soul, mind* **active** *agent of change*	An agent with the ability to alter mood, anxiety, behavior, cognitive processes, or mental tension
seizure	**SEE**-zhur	S/ R/	**-ure** *process* **seiz-** *to grab, convulse*	Event due to excessive electrical activity in the brain
sensory	**SEN**-soh-ree	S/ R/	**-ory** *having the function of* **sens-** *feel*	Having the function of sensation; relating to structures of the nervous system that carry impulses to the brain
tonic	**TON**-ik	S/ R/	**-ic** *pertaining to* **ton-** *pressure, tension*	In a state of muscular contraction
tonic–clonic seizure	**TON**-ik-**KLON**-ik **SEE**-zhur	R/	**clon-** *violent action*	Generalized seizure due to epileptic activity in all or most of the brain

Exercises

A. Documentation. *Fill in the following paragraph with the appropriate language of neurology. There is one extra term you will not need.*   **LO 9.4**

electroencephalography
epilepsy
neurologist
antiepileptic

electroneurodiagnostic
electroencephalograph
electroencephalogram

Ms. Roberta Gaston and her parents were sent to this office by her _____. Dr. Solis has ordered some _____ tests because of her _____. The particular type of test is a(n) _____, which will produce an EEG on the (machine) _____. The process of doing this test is _____.

LO 9.2, 9.3, 9.4 Components of the Nervous System

The nervous system has two major anatomical subdivisions *(Figure 9.2)*:

1. The **central nervous system** (CNS), consisting of the brain and spinal cord.
2. The **peripheral nervous system** (PNS) consisting of all the **neurons**, **nerves**, **ganglia**, and **plexuses** outside the central nervous system. It includes 12 pairs of cranial nerves originating from the brain and 31 pairs of spinal nerves originating from the spinal cord.

The PNS in turn, is further subdivided into

   i. **Sensory division**, in which sensory nerves (**afferent nerves**) carry messages toward the spinal cord and brain from sense organs *(Figure 9.3)*. **Visceral nerves** carry signals from the viscera in the thoracic and abdominal cavities; for example, the heart and lungs and the stomach and intestines. **Somatic nerves** carry signals from the skin, muscles, bones, and joints.

   ii. **Motor division**, in which motor nerves (**efferent nerves**) carry messages away from the brain and spinal cord to muscles and organs.

      a. The visceral motor division is called the **autonomic nervous system (ANS)**. It carries signals to glands and to cardiac and smooth muscle. It operates at a subconscious level outside your voluntary control. It has two subdivisions:

         i. The **sympathetic division** arouses the body for action; for example, by increasing the heart and respiratory rates to increase oxygen supply to brain and muscles. At the same time, it slows digestion, so less blood flow is needed to the digestive system. Blood can be directed where it is needed more.

         ii. The **parasympathetic division** calms the body, slowing down the heartbeat but stimulating digestion.

      b. The **somatic motor division** carries signals to the skeletal muscles and is under voluntary control.

Study Hint

Remember the acronym **SAME**: The **S**ensory nerves are **A**fferent (toward the brain) and the **M**otor nerves are **E**fferent (away from the brain or spinal cord).

Motor—**E**fferent SA**ME** (opposite of **afferent**)

Sensory—**A**fferent **SA**ME (opposite of efferent)

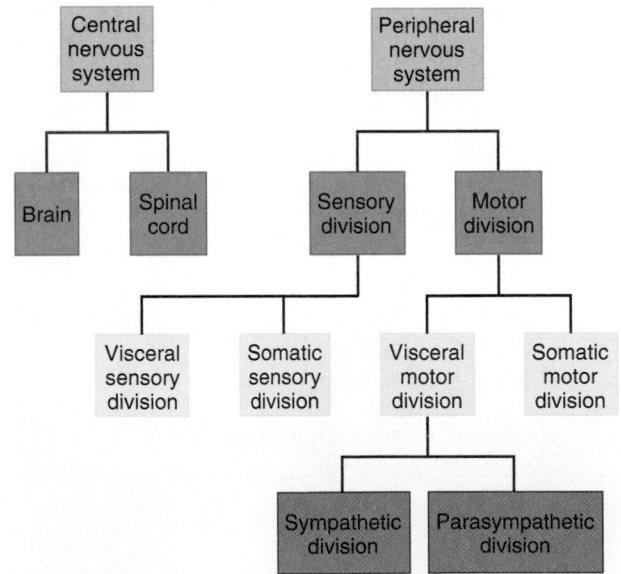

▲ **Figure 9.2** Components of the Nervous System.

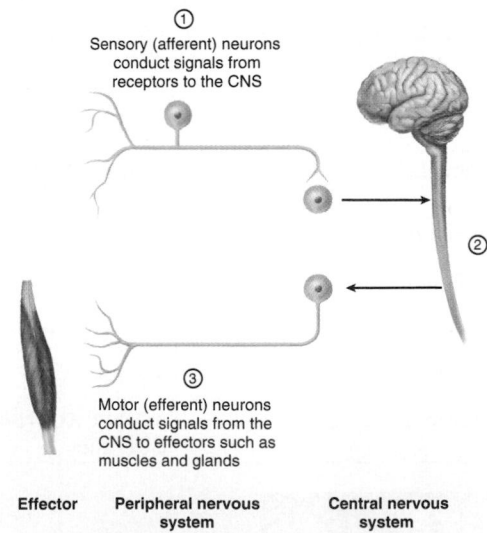

▲ **Figure 9.3** Afferent and Efferent Neurons.

WORD	PRONUNCIATION	ELEMENTS		DEFINITION
afferent	**AF**-eh-rent		Latin *to bring to*	Conducting impulses inward *toward* the spinal cord or brain
autonomic	awe-toh-**NOM**-ik	S/ P/ R/	-ic *pertaining to* auto- *self* -nom- *law*	Not voluntary; pertaining to the self—governing visceral motor division of the peripheral nervous system
efferent	**EF**-eh-rent		Latin *to bring away from*	Conducting impulses outward *away from* the brain or spinal cord
ganglion ganglia (pl)	**GANG**-lee-on **GANG**-lee-ah		Greek *swelling*	Collection of nerve cell bodies outside the CNS
nerve nervous (adj)	NERV **NER**-vus		Latin *nerve*	A cord of fibers in connective tissue conduct impulses
neuron	**NYUR**-on		Greek *nerve*	Technical term for a nerve cell; consists of the cell body with its dendrites and axons
parasympathetic (**Note:** This term has two prefixes.)	par-ah-sim-pah-**THET**-ik	S/ P/ P/ R/	-ic *pertaining to* para- *beside* -sym- *together* -pathet- *suffering*	Pertaining to division of autonomic nervous system; has opposite effects of the sympathetic division
peripheral	peh-**RIF**-er-al	S/ R/	-al *pertaining to* peripher- *outer part*	Pertaining to the periphery or external boundary
plexus plexuses (pl)	**PLEK**-sus **PLEK**-sus-ez		Latin *braid*	A weblike network of joined nerves
somatic	soh-**MAT**-ik	S/ R/	-ic *pertaining to* somat- *body*	Pertaining to a division of peripheral nervous system serving the skeletal muscles
sympathetic	sim-pah-**THET**-ik	S/ P/ R/	-ic *pertaining to* sym- *together* -pathet- *suffering*	Pertaining to the part of the autonomic nervous system operating at the unconscious level
visceral	**VISS**-er-al	S/ R/	-al *pertaining to* viscer- *internal organs*	Pertaining to the internal organs

Exercises

A. The nervous system has two major anatomical subdivisions, each with specialized functions. *Keep in mind that there are systems and divisions of systems. Use the precise* **language of neurology** *to answer the following questions.*   **LO 9.2, 9.3, 9.4**

1. This division carries signals to the skeletal muscles and is under voluntary control: _____

2. This system consists of the brain and spinal cord: _____

3. This division carries messages to the brain from the sensory organs: _____

4. The visceral motor division is also called the _____ system.

5. This division arouses the body for action: _____

6. This system consists of neurons, nerves, ganglia, and plexuses: _____

7. This division calms the body and slows the heartbeat: _____

8. Motor and sensory are further subdivisions of which system? _____

9. This division has efferent nerves to carry messages from the brain to muscles and organs: _____

10. Somatic nerves are in the _____ division of the _____ system.

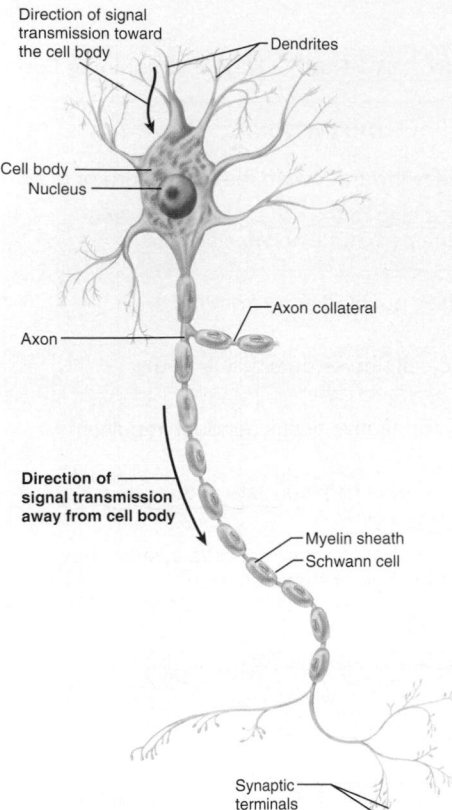

Figure 9.4 Neuron.

Abbreviations	
C5	fifth cervical vertebra or nerve
T1	first thoracic vertebra or nerve

LO 9.2, 9.3 Cells of the Nervous System

Neurons (nerve cells) receive stimuli and transmit impulses to other neurons or to receptors in other organs. Each neuron consists of a **cell body** and two types of processes or extensions, called **axons** and **dendrites** (Figure 9.4).

Dendrites are short, highly branched extensions of the neuron's cell body. They conduct impulses toward the cell body. The more dendrites a neuron has, the more impulses it can receive from other neurons.

A single axon, or nerve fiber, arises from the cell body and carries impulses away from the cell body. Each axon has a constant diameter but can range in length from a few millimeters to a meter. The axon is covered in a fatty **myelin** sheath that is covered by a membrane called the **neurilemma**. The myelin sheath, like the plastic covering of electrical wire, enables the nerve impulse to travel faster.

The axon terminates in a network of small branches. Each branch ends in a **synaptic terminal** that forms a **synapse** (junction) with a dendrite from another neuron or with a receptor on a muscle cell or gland cell (Figure 9.5). The synaptic terminals contain vesicles full of **neurotransmitters** that cross the synapse to stimulate or inhibit the receptor on a dendrite of another neuron or the cell of a muscle or gland. Examples of neurotransmitters are

- **Acetylcholine**—stimulates muscle cells to contract.
- **Norepinephrine**—found in many areas of the brain and spinal cord; has a stimulatory effect that is increased by cocaine and amphetamines.
- **Serotonin**—found in many areas of the brain and spinal cord; is involved with mood, anxiety, and sleep.
- **Dopamine**—confined to small areas of the brain; its absence is associated with **Parkinson disease**.
- **Endorphins**—found in areas around the brainstem; are the body's natural pain relievers.

Groups of cell bodies cluster together to form ganglia, and axons collect together to form nerves. Groups of nerves collect together to form a **plexus**, in which nerve fibers from different spinal nerves are sorted and recombined so that all the fibers (motor and sensory) going to a specific body part are located in a single nerve. The three plexuses are the **cervical plexus** to the neck, the **brachial plexus** to the arm, and the **lumbosacral plexus** to the pelvis and legs. Figure 9.6 shows an example of a plexus, the brachial plexus, in which spinal nerves **C5** to **T1** unite to form three **roots** that go on to supply the motor and sensory functions of the arm. The labeling of nerves is addressed in a later lesson in this chapter.

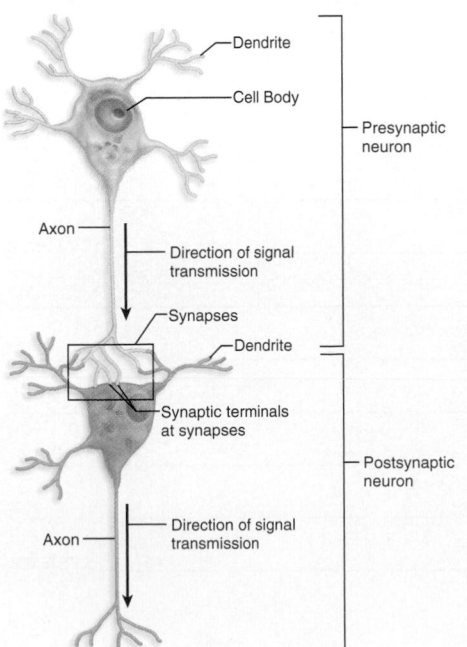

Figure 9.5 Synapse.

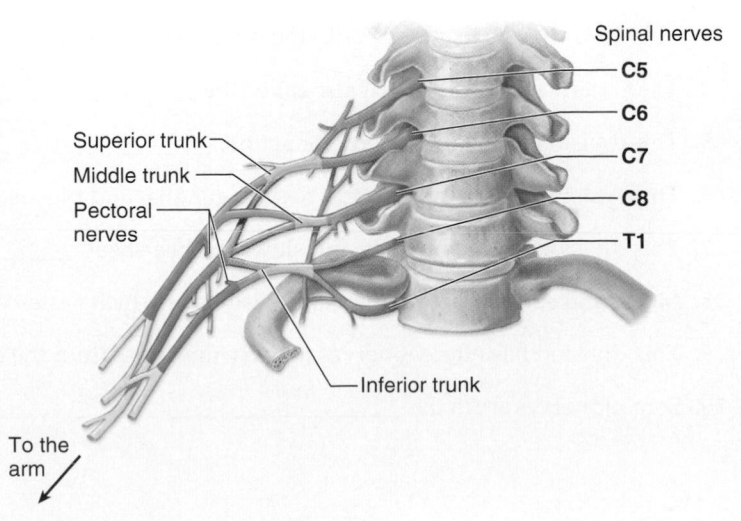

Figure 9.6 Brachial Plexus.

WORD	PRONUNCIATION	ELEMENTS		DEFINITION
acetylcholine	AS-eh-til-KOH-leen	R/ R/	acetyl- *acetyl* -choline *choline*	Parasympathetic neurotransmitter
axon	ACK-son		Greek *axis*	Single process of a nerve cell carrying nervous impulses away from the cell body
dendrite	DEN-dright		Greek *looking like a tree*	Branched extension of the nerve cell body that receives nervous stimuli
dopamine	DOH-pah-meen		Precursor of norepinephrine	Neurotransmitter in some specific small areas of the brain
endorphin (*Note:* The "m" of morphine is not used.)	en-DOR-fin	P/ R/	end- *within* -morphin *morphine*	Natural substance in the brain that has the same effect as opium
myelin	MY-eh-lin	S/ R/	-in *substance, chemical compound* myel- *spinal cord*	Material of the sheath around the axon of a nerve
neurilemma	nyu-ri-LEM-ah	S/ R/CF	-lemma *covering* neur/i- *nerve*	Covering of a nerve around the myelin sheath
neurotransmitter	NYUR-oh-trans-MIT-er	S/ R/CF P/ R/	-er *agent* neur/o- *nerve* -trans- *across* -mitt- *to send*	Chemical agent that relays messages from one nerve cell to the next
norepinephrine (*Note:* Two prefixes)	NOR-ep-ih-NEFF-rin	P/ P/ R/ S/	nor- *normal* -epi- *upon, above* -nephr- *kidney* -ine *pertaining to*	Parasympathetic neurotransmitter
Parkinson disease	PAR-kin-son DIZ-eez		James Parkinson, British physician, 1755–1824	Disease of muscular rigidity, tremors, and a masklike facial expression
serotonin	ser-oh-TOE-nin	S/ R/CF R/	-in *chemical compound* ser/o- *serum, serous* -ton- *tension*	Neurotransmitter in the central and peripheral nervous systems
synapse synaptic (adj)	SIN-aps sih-NAP-tik	P/ R/	syn- *together* -apse *clasp*	Junction between two nerve cells, or a nerve fiber and its target cell; where electrical impulses are transmitted between the cells

Exercises

A. Spelling is very important for every medical term. *Choose the correct spelling in the* **language of neurology.** *Circle the best choice; then fill in the blanks.* **LO 9.2, 9.3, 9.4**

1. Junction between two nerve cells: synapses   sinapse   synapse

2. The material of the sheath around a nerve axon: myelin   myalin   myeline

3. Branched extension of the nerve cell body that
   receives an impulse: denderite   dendrite   dendryte

4. Chemical agent that relays messages: neutrontransmitter   neurontransmitter   neurotransmitter

5. Covering of a nerve around the sheath: neurelemma   neurilemmia   neurilemma

B. Using the terms in the above WAD, fill in the blanks in the following questions.   LO 9.2

1. Which terms contain a prefix? _____

2. Which term contains a combining form and a suffix? _____

3. Which root means *the spinal cord*? _____

4. Which term contains two prefixes? _____

LO 9.2, 9.3 Neuroglia

The trillion neurons in the nervous system are outnumbered 50 to 1 by the supportive **glial** cells (**neuroglia**). There are six types of neuroglia. Four are found in the CNS (*Figure 9.7*):

1. **Astrocytes** are the most abundant glial cells. They are involved in the transportation of water and salts from capillaries to the neurons.

2. **Oligodendrocytes** form the myelin sheaths around axons in the brain and spinal cord. Axons that have myelin sheaths are called *myelinated axons.* Bundles of these axons appear white and create the **white matter** of the brain and spinal cord. Neuron cell bodies, dendrites, and synapses appear gray and create the **gray matter**.

3. **Microglia** phagocytose bacteria and cell debris.

4. **Ependymal cells** line the central canal of the spinal cord and the ventricles of the brain. They help regulate the composition of the **cerebrospinal fluid (CSF)**.

Two types of neuroglial cells are found in the PNS:

1. **Schwann cells** form the myelin sheaths of the peripheral nerves that speed up signal conduction in the nerve fiber.

2. **Satellite cells** are found around the neuron cell bodies. Their function is unknown.

Abbreviations

BBB	blood-brain barrier
CSF	cerebrospinal fluid

The **blood-brain barrier (BBB)** is a physical barrier between the capillaries that supply the CNS and most parts of the CNS. Astrocytes and the tight junctions between endothelial cells of the capillaries work together to prevent foreign substances, toxins, and infection from reaching the brain. Many medications are unable to pass this barrier, but alcohol gets through, producing its buzz and problems with coordination and **cognition**.

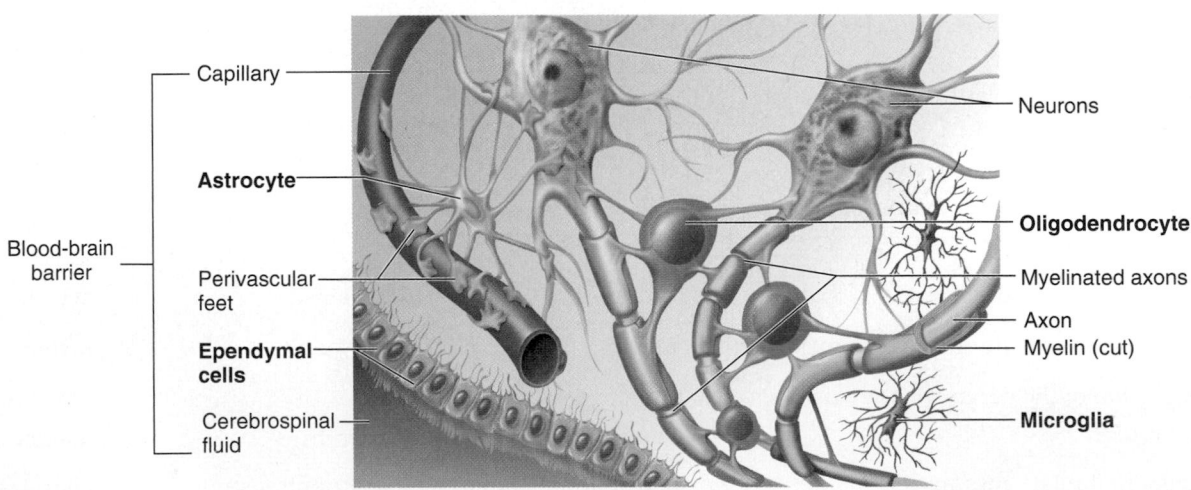

▲ **Figure 9.7**   Neuroglial Cells in the CNS.

WORD	PRONUNCIATION	ELEMENTS		DEFINITION
astrocyte	**ASS**-troh-site	S/ R/CF	-cyte *cell* astr/o- *star*	Star-shaped connective tissue cell in the nervous system
blood-brain barrier (BBB)	BLUD BRAYN **BAIR**-ee-er			A selective mechanism that protects the brain from toxins and infections
cerebrospinal cerebrospinal fluid (CSF)	**SER**-eh-broh-**SPY**-nal	S/ R/CF R/	-al *pertaining to* cerebr/o- *brain* -spin- *spinal cord*	Pertaining to the brain and spinal cord Fluid formed in the ventricles of the brain; surrounds the brain and spinal cord
cognition cognitive (adj)	kog-**NIH**-shun **KOG**-nih-tiv		Latin *knowledge*	Process of acquiring knowledge through thinking, learning, and memory Pertaining to the mental activities of thinking and learning
ependyma ependymal (adj)	ep-**EN**-dih-mah ep-**EN**-dih-mal		Greek *garment*	Membrane lining the central canal of the spinal cord and the ventricles of the brain
glia glial (adj) microglia neuroglia	**GLEE**-ah **GLEE**-al my-**KROH**-glee-ah nyu-roh-**GLEE**-ah	 P/ R/ R/CF	Greek *glue* micro- *small* -glia *glue, supportive tissue of the nervous system* neur/o- *nerve*	Connective tissue that holds a structure together Small nervous tissue cells that are phagocytes Connective tissue holding nervous tissue together
gray matter	GRAY **MATT**-er			Regions of the brain and spinal cord occupied by cell bodies and dendrites
oligodendrocyte	**OL**-ih-goh-**DEN**-droh-site	S/ P/ R/CF	-cyte *cell* oligo- *scanty* -dendr/o- *treelike*	Connective tissue cell of the central nervous system that forms a myelin sheath
Schwann cell	SHWANN SELL		Theodor Schwann, German anatomist, 1810–1882	Connective tissue cell of the peripheral nervous system that forms a myelin sheath
white matter	WITE **MATT**-er			Regions of the brain and spinal cord occupied by bundles of axons

Exercises

A. Identify the correct meaning for each element. *Knowing the definitions of elements is your key to unlocking the meaning of medical terms. Match the element in the left column with its correct meaning in the right column.* **LO 9.2, 9.3, 9.4**

_____ 1. oligo

_____ 2. glia

_____ 3. cerebro

_____ 4. astro

_____ 5. spin

_____ 6. cyte

_____ 7. dendro

_____ 8. al

_____ 9. neuro

_____ 10. micro

a. cell

b. nerve

c. small

d. spinal cord

e. treelike

f. scanty

g. brain

h. glue

i. star

j. pertaining to

B. Precision in documentation is key to patient safety. *Use the appropriate abbreviation to convey correct information about the patient.* **LO 9.6**

EEG   CNS   MRI   CT   ANS   BBB   CSF   PNS   UTI

1. The doctor has ordered the following diagnostic tests for the patient. (*Hint:* Which of the above abbreviations represent diagnostic tests?) _____

2. The patient's excess _____ will require a shunt to relieve the pressure.

3. The patient's problems with coordination and cognition result from alcohol penetrating the _____.

Lesson 9.2 The Brain and Cranial Nerves

Smelling the roses, seeing them, and touching them are recognized and interpreted in the brain, as are all sensations. The actions of bending down, cutting the rose stem, walking into the house, and placing it in a vase originate in the brain, as do all our voluntary actions. The integration of a sensory stimulus with a motor response occurs in the brain. The brain is the control center for many of the body's functions. The brain carries out the higher mental functions, such as reasoning, planning, forming ideas, and all aspects of memory.

The information in this lesson will enable you to:

9.2.1   Use correct medical terminology to describe the anatomy and physiology of the brain.
9.2.2   Identify the 12 pairs of cranial nerves and their functions.
9.2.3   Locate the major sensory and motor areas of the brain.
9.2.4   Describe how the brain is protected and supported.
9.2.5   Explain how common disorders of the brain and spinal cord affect health.

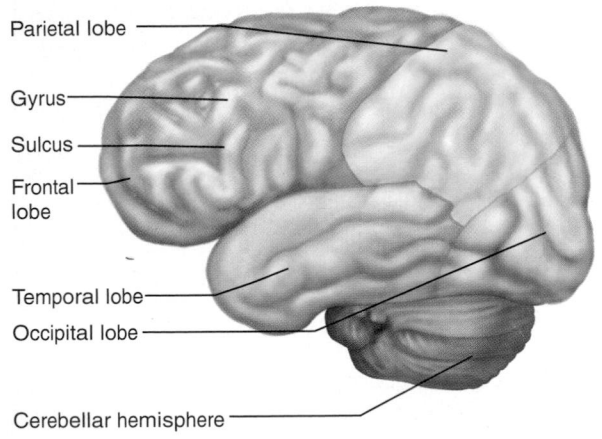

(a) View from left side

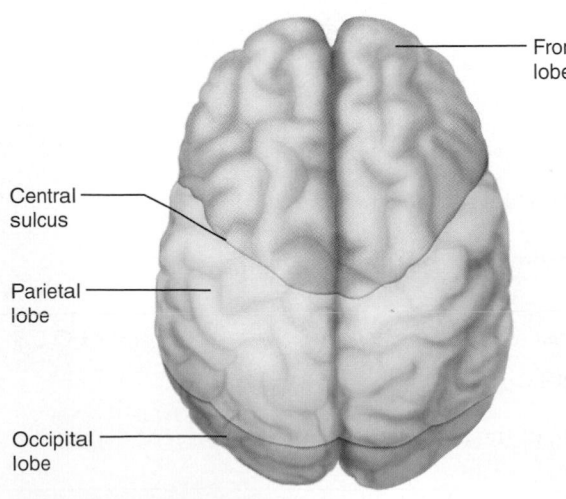

(b) View from above

▲ **Figure 9.8**   Brain.

LO 9.2, 9.3 Brain

The adult brain weighs about 3 pounds. Its size and weight are proportional to body size, not intelligence.

The brain is divided into three major regions, the **cerebrum**, the **brainstem**, and the **cerebellum**.

The cerebrum is about 80% of the brain and consists of two **cerebral hemispheres** that are anatomically mirror images of each other *(Figure 9.8)*. They are separated by a deep longitudinal fissure, at the bottom of which they are connected by a bridge of nerve fibers called the **corpus callosum**.

On the surface of the cerebrum, numerous ridges **(gyri)** are separated by fissures called **sulci**.

Each cerebral hemisphere is divided into four lobes *(see Figure 9.8a)*:

1. The **frontal lobe** is located behind the forehead. It forms the anterior part of the hemisphere. It is responsible for memory, intellect, concentration, problem solving, emotion, and the planning and execution of behavior, including voluntary motor control of muscles.
2. The **parietal lobe** located above the ear, is posterior to the frontal lobe. The parietal lobe receives and interprets sensations of pain, pressure, touch, temperature, and body part awareness.
3. The **temporal lobe** located behind the ear, is below the frontal and parietal lobes. The temporal lobe is involved in interpreting sensory experiences, sounds, and spoken words.
4. The **occipital lobe** located at the back of the head, forms the posterior part of the hemisphere. The occipital lobe interprets visual images and the written word.

The cerebral hemispheres are covered by a thin layer of gray matter (unmyelinated nerve fibers) called the **cerebral cortex**. It is folded into the gyri, sulci, and fissures and contains 70% of all the neurons in the nervous system. Below the cerebral cortex is a mass of white matter, in which bundles of myelinated nerve fibers connect the neurons of the cortex to the rest of the nervous system.

S = Suffix   P = Prefix   **R = Root   R/CF = Combining Form**

WORD	PRONUNCIATION		ELEMENTS	DEFINITION
brainstem	BRAYN-STEM		Old English *brain* **stem** *support*	Region of the brain that includes the thalamus, pineal gland, pons, fourth ventricle, and medulla oblongata
cerebellum	ser-eh-**BELL**-um	S/ R/	-um *structure* **cerebell-** *little brain*	The most posterior area of the brain
cerebrum cerebral (adj)	**SER**-ee-brum **SER**-ee-bral		Latin *brain*	The major portion of the brain divided into two hemispheres (cerebral hemispheres) separated by a fissure
corpus callosum	**KOR**-pus kah-**LOW**-sum	R/ S/ R/	**corpus** *body* -um *structure* **callos-** *thickening*	Bridge of nerve fibers connecting the two cerebral hemispheres
cortex cortical (adj)	**KOR**-teks **KOR**-ti-kal		Latin *shell*	Gray covering of cerebral hemispheres
frontal lobe	**FRON**-tal LOBE	S/ R/	-al *pertaining to* **front-** *forehead* **lobe** Greek *lobe*	Area of brain behind the frontal bone
gyrus gyri (pl)	**JI**-rus **JI**-ree		Greek *circle*	Rounded elevation on the surface of the cerebral hemispheres
occipital lobe	ock-**SIP**-it-al LOBE	S/ R/	-al *pertaining to* **occipit-** *back of head* **lobe** Greek *lobe*	Posterior area of cerebral hemispheres
parietal lobe	pah-**RYE**-eh-tal LOBE	S/ R/	-al *pertaining to* **pariet-** *wall* **lobe** Greek *lobe*	Area of brain under the parietal bone
sulcus sulci (pl)	**SUL**-cuss **SUL**-sigh		Latin *furrow, ditch*	Groove on the surface of the cerebral hemispheres that separates gyri
temporal lobe	**TEM**-por-al LOBE	S/ R/	-al *pertaining to* **tempor-** *temple, side of head* **lobe** Greek *lobe*	Posterior two-thirds of cerebral hemispheres

Exercises

A. Roots. *The lobes of the cerebral hemispheres share a common suffix -al, meaning pertaining to. It is the root that describes the exact location of the lobe in the cerebral hemispheres. Use your knowledge of roots to understand the anatomical location of the lobes. Fill in the blanks.*   **LO 9.2, 9.3, 9.4**

1. _____/al   Root means _____.

   Lobe is located _____.

   Lobe is responsible for _____.

2. _____/al   Root means _____.

   Lobe is located _____.

   Lobe is responsible for _____.

3. _____/al   Root means _____.

   Lobe is located _____.

   Lobe is responsible for _____.

4. _____/al   Root means _____.

   Lobe is located _____.

   Lobe is responsible for _____.

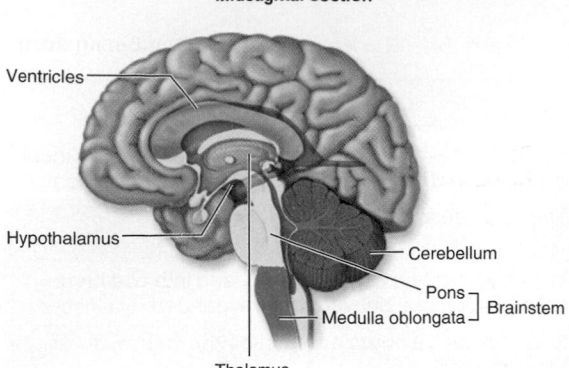

Midsagittal section

Ventricles

Hypothalamus

Cerebellum

Pons ⎤
Medulla oblongata ⎦ Brainstem

Thalamus

▲ **Figure 9.9** Lateral View of Functional Regions of Brain.

LO 9.2, 9.3, 9.7 Functional Brain Regions

Deep inside each cerebral hemisphere are spaces called **ventricles**. They contain the watery **cerebrospinal fluid (CSF),** which circulates through the ventricles and around the brain and spinal cord. The CSF helps protect, cushion, and provide nutrition for the brain and spinal cord.

Underneath the cerebral hemispheres and the ventricles are important regions of the brain *(Figures 9.9 and 9.10):*

1. **Thalamus**—receives all sensory impulses and channels them to the appropriate region of the cortex for interpretation. As the sensory fibers carrying impulses pass through the thalamus, they **decussate** (cross over) so that the impulses from the left side of the body go to the right brain, and impulses coming from the right side of the body go to the left brain. Similarly, motor impulses coming from the right brain decussate and supply the left side of the body, and motor impulses coming from the left brain decussate and supply the right side of the body. If a lesion caused by a stroke is in the right brain, the left side of the body will be affected, and vice versa.

2. The **hypothalamus** regulates:
   a. Blood pressure
   b. Body temperature
   c. Water and electrolyte balance
   d. Hunger and body weight
   e. Sleep and wakefulness
   f. Movements and secretions of the digestive tract

3. The **basal nuclei** are collections of gray matter lateral to the thalamus that aid in controlling the amplitude of our voluntary muscular movements and posture, as well as playing a part in emotion and cognition.

4. The **limbic system** controls emotional experience, fear, anger, pleasure, and sadness. If your limbic system is destroyed, you go into a **comatose** state.

5. The **brainstem** *(Figure 9.9)* contains two major areas:

a. The **pons** *(Figure 9.9),* which relays sensory impulses from peripheral nerves to higher brain centers.

b. The **medulla oblongata** *(Figure 9.9),* within which nuclei of gray matter form centers to control vital visceral activities, such as

   i. **Cardiac center**—regulates heart rate.
   ii. **Respiratory center**—regulates breathing.
   iii. **Vasomotor center**—regulates vasoconstriction and vasodilation of blood vessels.
   iv. **Reticular formation**—responds to sensory impulses by arousing the cerebral cortex into wakefulness.

The most posterior area of the brain, the cerebellum *(Figures 9.9 and 9.10),* coordinates skeletal muscle activity to maintain posture and balance.

Abbreviation	
CSF	cerebrospinal fluid

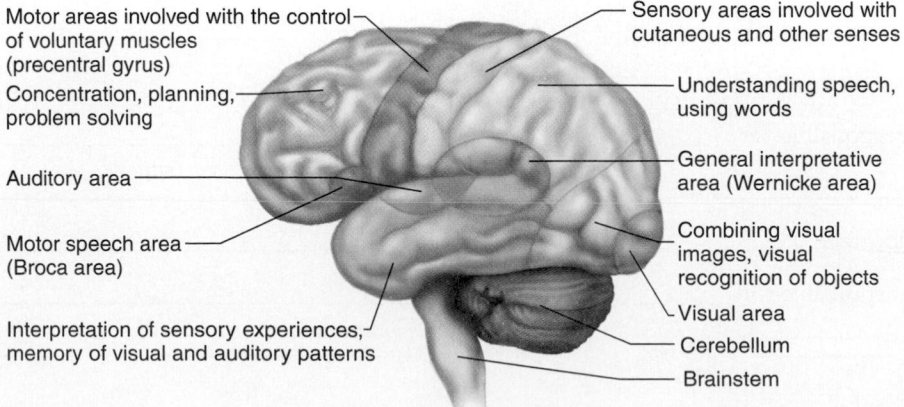

Motor areas involved with the control of voluntary muscles (precentral gyrus)

Concentration, planning, problem solving

Auditory area

Motor speech area (Broca area)

Interpretation of sensory experiences, memory of visual and auditory patterns

Sensory areas involved with cutaneous and other senses

Understanding speech, using words

General interpretative area (Wernicke area)

Combining visual images, visual recognition of objects

Visual area

Cerebellum

Brainstem

▲ **Figure 9.10** Cerebral Cortex, Functional Regions.

WORD	PRONUNCIATION	ELEMENTS		DEFINITION
coma comatose	KOH-mah KOH-mah-toes		Greek *deep sleep, trance*	State of deep unconsciousness Being in a coma
decussate	DEE-kuss-ate		Latin *to make in the form of a cross*	Cross over like the arms of an "X"
hypothalamus hypothalamic	high-poh-**THAL**-ah-muss high-poh-tha-**LAM**-ik	S/ P/ R/ S/	-us *pertaining to* hypo- *below* -thalam- *thalamus* -ic *pertaining to*	Area of gray matter forming part of the walls and floor of the third ventricle Pertaining to the hypothalamus
limbic	LIM-bic		Latin *border*	Pertaining to the limbic system, an array of nerve fibers surrounding the thalamus
medulla oblongata	meh-**DULL**-ah ob-lon-**GAH**-tah	R/ S/ R/	medulla *middle* -ata *place* oblong- *elongated*	Most posterior subdivision of the brainstem, continuation of the spinal cord
pons	PONZ		Latin *bridge*	Part of the brainstem
reticulum reticular (adj)	reh-**TIK**-you-lum reh-**TIK**-you-lar	S/ R/ S/	-um *structure* reticul- *fine net* -ar *pertaining to*	Fine network of cells in the medulla oblongata Pertaining to the reticulum
thalamus	**THAL**-ah-mus		Greek *inner room*	Mass of gray matter underneath the ventricle in each cerebral hemisphere
ventricle ventricular	**VEN**-trih-kel ven-**TRIK**-you-lar	 S/ R/	 -ar *pertaining to* ventricul- *ventricle*	A cavity of the heart or brain Pertaining to a ventricle

Exercises

A. Latin and Greek terms cannot be deconstructed into prefix, root, and suffix. *You must know them for what they are. Test your knowledge of these terms with the following exercise. Match the terms in the left column to their correct meaning in the right column.* **LO 9.2, 9.3, 9.7**

_____ 1. thalamus   a. deep sleep

_____ 2. decussate   b. bridge

_____ 3. limbic   c. inner room

_____ 4. coma   d. border

_____ 5. pons   e. cross over

B. Recall from the lesson the correct medical terms that identify the appropriate answers to the questions.   **LO 9.2, 9.3**

1. What is the center of the brain that controls vital and visceral activity?

_____

2. What part of the brain regulates heartbeat?

_____

3. What responds to sensory impulses by arousing the cerebral cortex into wakefulness?

_____

4. Where in the brain is breathing regulated?

_____

5. What regulates vasoconstriction and vasodilation of blood vessels?

_____

6. All this terminology relates to which area of the brain?

_____

Table 9.1 Mnemonic for the Cranial Nerves

Oh	(olfactory-I)
once	(optic-II)
one	(oculomotor-III)
takes	(trochlear-IV)
the	(trigeminal-V)
anatomy	(abducens-VI)
final	(facial-VII)
very	(vestibulocochlear-VIII)
good	(glossopharyngeal-IX)
vacations	(vagus-X)
are	(accessory-XI)
heavenly!	(hypoglossal-XII)

Figure 9.11   Cranial ▶ Nerves. Base of brain showing origins of the 12 cranial nerves.

LO 9.2, 9.7 Cranial Nerves

To function, the brain must communicate with the rest of the body, and it does this through the spinal cord and the **cranial nerves**. Twelve pairs of cranial nerves arise from the base of the brain (*Figure 9.11*). A mnemonic to help you remember their names is in *Table 9.1*.

The two pairs of nerves for smell and vision contain only sensory fibers. The other 10 pairs are mixed nerves containing sensory, motor, and parasympathetic fibers. The cranial nerves have, from front to back, both names and numbers. The latter are always written in Roman numerals (*Table 9.2*).

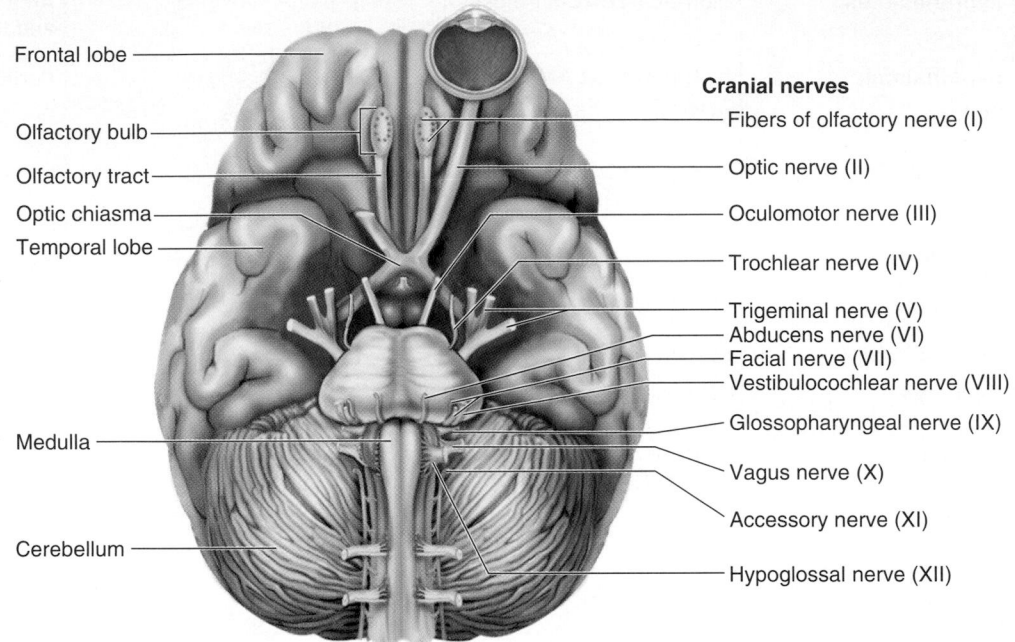

Frontal lobe
Olfactory bulb
Olfactory tract
Optic chiasma
Temporal lobe
Medulla
Cerebellum

Cranial nerves
Fibers of olfactory nerve (I)
Optic nerve (II)
Oculomotor nerve (III)
Trochlear nerve (IV)
Trigeminal nerve (V)
Abducens nerve (VI)
Facial nerve (VII)
Vestibulocochlear nerve (VIII)
Glossopharyngeal nerve (IX)
Vagus nerve (X)
Accessory nerve (XI)
Hypoglossal nerve (XII)

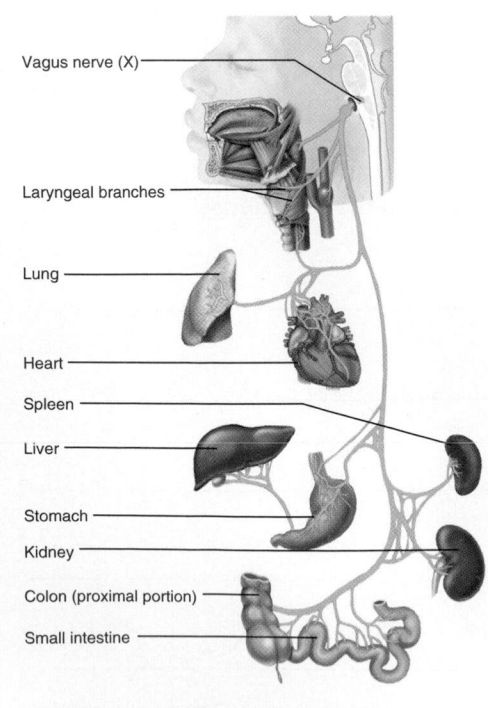

Vagus nerve (X)
Laryngeal branches
Lung
Heart
Spleen
Liver
Stomach
Kidney
Colon (proximal portion)
Small intestine

▲ **Figure 9.12**   **Left Vagus Nerve.**

Table 9.2 Cranial Nerves

Roman Numeral	Name	Description
I	**Olfactory** nerves	Sensory nerves for smell
II	**Optic** nerves	Sensory nerves for vision
III	**Oculomotor** nerves	Predominantly motor nerves for eye movement and pupil size
IV	**Trochlear** nerves	Predominantly motor nerves for eye movement
V	**Trigeminal** nerves	Sensory and motor nerves responsible for face, nose, and mouth sensations and for chewing
VI	**Abducens** nerves	Predominantly motor nerves responsible for eye movement
VII	**Facial** nerves	Mixed nerves associated with taste (sensory), facial expression (motor), and production of tears and saliva (parasympathetic fibers of motor nerves)
VIII	**Vestibulocochlear (auditory)** nerves	Predominantly sensory nerves associated with hearing and balance
IX	**Glossopharyngeal** nerves	Mixed nerves for sensation and swallowing in the pharynx
X	**Vagus** nerves	Mixed sensory and parasympathetic nerves supplying the pharynx, larynx (speech), and the viscera of the thorax and abdomen (*Figure 9.12*)
XI	**Accessory** nerves	Predominantly motor nerves supplying neck muscles, pharynx, and larynx
XII	**Hypoglossal** nerves	Predominantly motor nerves that move the tongue in speaking, chewing, and swallowing

WORD	PRONUNCIATION	ELEMENTS		DEFINITION
abducens	ab-**DYU**-senz		Latin *abduct, draw away from*	Sixth (VI) cranial nerve; responsible for eye movement
accessory	ack-**SESS**-oh-ree		Latin *move toward*	Eleventh (XI) cranial nerve; supplying neck muscles, pharynx, and larynx
auditory	**AW**-dih-tor-ee	S/ R/	-ory *having the function of* **audit-** *hearing*	Pertaining to the sense of or the organs of hearing
cranial	**KRAY**-nee-al	S/ R/	-al *pertaining to* **crani-** *skull, cranium*	Pertaining to the skull
facial	**FAY**-shal		Latin *face*	Seventh (VII) cranial nerve; supplying the forehead, nose, eyes, mouth, and jaws
glossopharyngeal	**GLOSS**-oh-fah-**RIN**-jee-al	S/ R/CF R/	-eal *pertaining to* **gloss/o-** *tongue* **-pharyng-** *pharynx*	Ninth (IX) cranial nerve; supplying the tongue and pharynx
hypoglossal	high-poh-**GLOSS**-al	S/ P/ R/	-al *pertaining to* **hypo-** *below, under* **-gloss-** *tongue*	Twelfth (XII) cranial nerve; supplying muscles of the tongue
oculomotor	**OCK**-you-loh-**MOH**-tor	S/ R/CF R/	-or *doer* **ocul/o-** *eye* **-mot-** *move*	Third (III) cranial nerve; moves the eye
olfactory	ol-**FAK**-toh-ree	S/ R/	-ory *having the function of* **olfact-** *smell*	First (I) cranial nerve; carries information related to the sense of smell
optic	**OP**-tick		Greek *eye*	Second (II) cranial nerve; carries visual information
trigeminal	try-**GEM**-in-al	S/ P/ R/	-al *pertaining to* **tri-** *three* **-gemin-** *double, twin*	Fifth (V) cranial nerve, with its three different branches supplying the face
trochlear	**TROHK**-lee-are	S/ R/	-ar *pertaining to* **trochle-** *pulley*	Fourth (IV) cranial nerve; supplies one muscle of the eye
vagus	**VAY**-gus		Latin *to wander*	Tenth (X) cranial nerve; supplies many different organs throughout the body
vestibulocochlear (**Note:** This term starts with a combining form, not a prefix.)	ves-**TIB**-you-loh-**KOK**-lee-ar	S/ R/CF R/	-ar *pertaining to* **vestibul/o-** *vestibule of inner ear* **-cochle-** *cochlea*	Eighth (VIII) cranial nerve; carrying information for the senses of hearing and balance

Exercises

A. Elements. *Continue your work with elements to help build your knowledge of the language of neurology. One element in each of the following medical terms is set in bold. Identify the type of element (prefix, root, root/combining form, suffix) in the middle column; then write the meaning of the element in the right column. Fill in the chart.* **LO 9.4, 9.7**

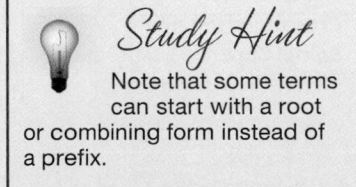

Study Hint
Note that some terms can start with a root or combining form instead of a prefix.

Medical Term	Type of Element	Meaning of Element	Meaning of Term
glosso*pharyngeal*	1.	2.	3.
tri*geminal*	4.	5.	6.
audit*ory*	7.	8.	9.
olfact*ory*	10.	11.	12.

B. Fill in the blanks with the appropriate language of neurology.   LO 9.3, 9.4, 9.7

The thalamus is a functional region of the brain. What does it regulate?

1. _____

_____

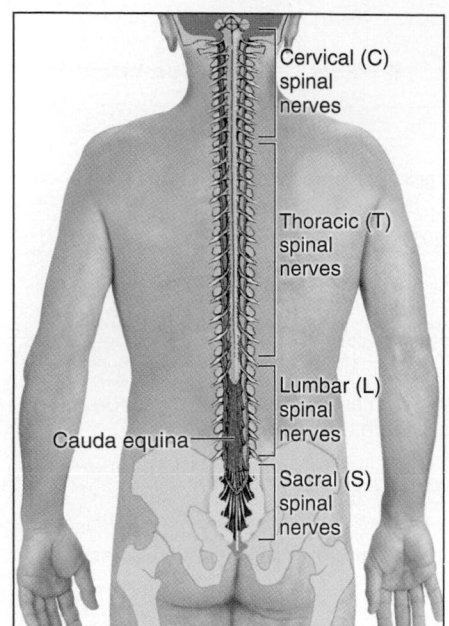

▲ **Figure 9.13** Spinal Cord Regions.

(Labels on figure: Cervical (C) spinal nerves; Thoracic (T) spinal nerves; Lumbar (L) spinal nerves; Cauda equina; Sacral (S) spinal nerves)

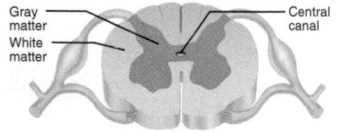

(Labels on figure: Gray matter; White matter; Central canal)

▲ **Figure 9.14**
Cross-Section of Spinal Cord.

LO 9.8 Spinal Cord and Meninges

Spinal Cord

This part of the central nervous system consists of 31 segments, each of which gives rise to a pair of spinal nerves. These are the major link between the brain and the peripheral nervous system and are a pathway for sensory and motor impulses.

The spinal cord occupies the upper two-thirds of the vertebral canal, extending from the base of the skull to the first lumbar vertebra. From here, a group of nerve fibers continues down the vertebral canal and is called the **cauda equina**.

The spinal cord is divided into four regions *(Figure 9.13):*

1. The **cervical region** is continuous with the medulla oblongata. It contains the motor neurons that supply the neck, shoulders, and upper limbs through eight pairs of cervical spinal nerves **(C1–C8)**.

2. The **thoracic region** contains the motor neurons that supply the thoracic cage, rib movement, vertebral column movement, and postural back muscles through 12 pairs of thoracic spinal nerves **(T1–T12)**.

3. The **lumbar region** supplies the hips and front of the lower limbs through five pairs of lumbar nerves **(L1–L5)**.

4. The **sacral region** supplies the buttocks, genitalia, and backs of the legs through five sacral nerves **(S1–S5)** and one coccygeal nerve.

A cross-section of the spinal cord *(Figure 9.14)* reveals that it has a core of gray matter shaped like a butterfly surrounded by white matter. In the center of the gray matter is the central canal that contains CSF. The gray matter contains the axons of sensory neurons bringing impulses into the cord and the neurons of motor nerves that send impulses out to skeletal muscles.

The white matter contains myelinated nerve fibers organized into **tracts** that conduct either sensory impulses up the cord to the brain or motor impulses down the cord from the brain.

All individual spinal nerves except C1 supply a specific segment of skin called a **dermatome**.

Meninges

The brain and spinal cord are protected by the cranium and the vertebrae, cushioned by the CSF, and covered by the **meninges** *(Figure 9.15)*. The meninges have three layers:

1. **Dura mater**—the outermost layer, composed of tough connective tissue attached to the inner surface of the cranium but separated from the vertebral canal by the **epidural space**, into which **epidural injections** are introduced.

2. **Arachnoid mater**—a thin web over the brain and spinal cord. The CSF is contained in the subarachnoid space between the arachnoid and pia mater.

3. **Pia mater**—the innermost layer of the meninges, attached to the surface of the brain and spinal cord. It supplies nerves and blood vessels that nourish the outer cells of the brain and spinal cord.

To obtain a specimen of CSF, a **lumbar puncture (spinal tap,** *Figure 9.16)* is performed. A needle is inserted through the skin, back muscles, spinal ligaments of an **intervertebral space**, epidural space, dura mater, and arachnoid mater into the **subarachnoid space**. The CSF can then be aspirated.

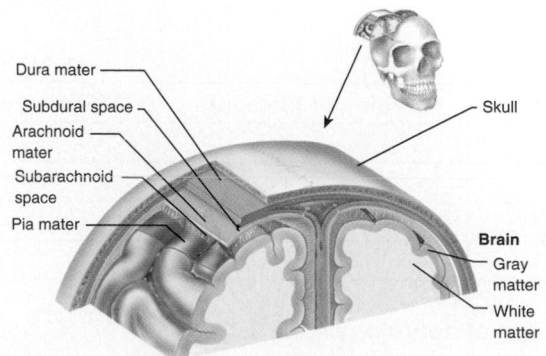

(Labels on figure: Dura mater; Subdural space; Arachnoid mater; Subarachnoid space; Pia mater; Skull; Brain; Gray matter; White matter)

▲ **Figure 9.15** Meninges of Brain.

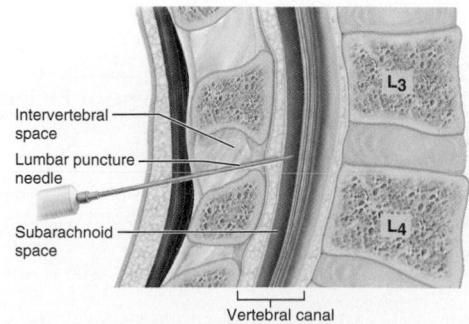

(Labels on figure: Intervertebral space; Lumbar puncture needle; Subarachnoid space; L3; L4; Vertebral canal)

▲ **Figure 9.16** Lumbar Puncture (Spinal Tap).

WORD	PRONUNCIATION	ELEMENTS		DEFINITION
arachnoid mater	ah-**RACK**-noyd **MAY**-ter	S/ R/ R/	**-oid** *resembling* **arachn-** *cobweb, spider* **mater** *mother*	Weblike middle layer of the three meninges
cauda equina (***Note:*** Both these terms are stand-alone roots.)	**KAW**-dah eh-**KWY**-nah	R/CF R/CF	**caud/a** *tail* **equin/a** *horse*	Bundle of spinal nerves in the vertebral canal below the ending of the spinal cord
cervical (***Note:*** Cervical also is used to refer to a region of the uterus.)	**SER**-vih-kal	S/ R/	**-al** *pertaining to* **cervic-** *neck*	Pertaining to the neck region
dermatome	**DER**-mah-tome	S/ R/CF	**-tome** *instrument to cut* **derm/a-** *skin*	The area of skin supplied by a single spinal nerve; alternatively, an instrument used for cutting thin slices
dura mater (***Note:*** Both terms are stand-alone roots.)	**DYU**-rah **MAY**-ter	R/CF R/	**dur/a** *dura mater* **mater** *mother*	Hard, fibrous outer layer of the meninges
epidural **epidural space**	ep-ih-**DYU**-ral ep-ih-**DYU**-ral SPASE	S/ P/ R/	**-al** *pertaining to* **epi-** *above* **-dur-** *dura mater*	Above the dura Space between the dura mater and the wall of the vertebral canal or skull
intervertebral	in-ter-**VER**-teh-bral	S/ P/ R/	**-al** *pertaining to* **inter-** *between* **-vertebr-** *vertebra*	The space between two vertebrae
lumbar	**LUM**-bar		Latin *loin*	Pertaining to the region in the back and sides between the ribs and pelvis
meninges	meh-**NIN**-jeez		Greek *membrane*	Three-layered covering of the brain and spinal cord
pia mater (***Note:*** Both terms are stand-alone roots.)	**PEE**-ah **MAY**-ter	R/ R/	**pia** *delicate* **mater** *mother*	Delicate inner layer of the meninges
sacral	**SAY**-kral	S/ R/	**-al** *pertaining to* **sacr-** *sacrum*	In the neighborhood of the sacrum
spinal tap	**SPY**-nal TAP	S/ R/	**-al** *pertaining to* **spin-** *spine* **tap** Old English *to open*	Placement of a needle through an intervertebral space into the subarachnoid space to withdraw CSF
subarachnoid space	sub-ah-**RACK**-noyd SPASE	S/ P/ R/	**-oid** *resembling* **sub-** *under* **-arachn-** *cobweb, spider*	Space between the pia mater and the arachnoid membrane
thoracic	**THOR**-ass-ik	S/ R/	**-ic** *pertaining to* **thorac-** *chest*	Pertaining to the chest (thorax)
tract	TRAKT		Latin *draw out*	Bundle of nerve fibers with common origin and destination

Exercises

A. Describe the location of the following spinal nerves and what they affect in that body region. *Do this in language your patient can understand.* **LO 9.8**

1. Cervical: location _____   affect _____

2. Thoracic: location _____   affect _____

3. Lumbar: location _____   affect _____

4. Sacral: location _____   affect _____

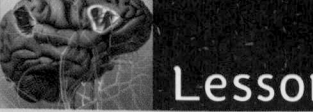

Lesson 9.3 Disorders of the Brain and Cranial Nerves

LESSON OBJECTIVES

When patients communicate with you as a health professional, they will often enhance your continual, ongoing learning by informing you of and reinforcing your knowledge about a specific disorder.

Information in this lesson will enable you to:

9.3.1 Describe common disorders of the brain and cranial nerves.

9.3.2 Match common disorders of the brain and cranial nerves to normal and abnormal anatomy and physiology.

9.3.3 Use correct terminology to communicate about the brain and cranial nerves and their disorders with patients and other health professionals.

You are

. . . a medical assistant working with Dr. Raoul Cardenas, a neurologist at Fulwood Medical Center.

Your patient is

. . . Mr. Lester Rood, a 75-year-old man who was diagnosed a year ago as having dementia.

Case Report 9.2

Mr. Rood lives with his daughter, Judy, and she is with him today.

Patient Interview:

Mr. Lester Rood: "How am I feeling? Scared stiff. Sometimes I don't know where I am. I get so messed up. I can't cook anymore. I forget what I'm doing. I find myself in the street and don't know how I got there. Judy has to help me shower and remind me to go to the bathroom. And it's only going to get worse. I don't want to be a burden. I used to have 100 people work for me. Now, it's frustrating, so frightening. And the future . . ."

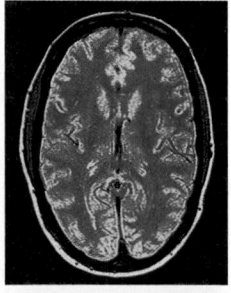

(a)

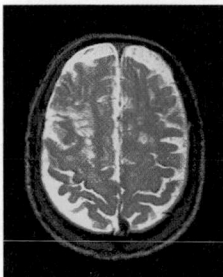

(b)

▲ **Figure 9.17**

Brain Sections.
(*a*) MRI scan of normal brain. (*b*) MRI scan of Alzheimer disease showing cerebral atrophy (*yellow*).

LO 9.9 Disorders of the Brain

Dementia

Your **empathy** allowed Mr. Rood to talk without interruption. He reminded you that the symptoms of **dementia** include short-term memory loss, inability to solve problems, confusion, inappropriate behavior (such as wandering away), and impaired intellectual function that interferes with normal activities and relationships. In its early stages it is a very frightening and frustrating situation for the patient. It requires a lot of **sympathy** and understanding from family and caregivers.

Dementia is *not* a normal part of aging and is *not* a specific disease. It is a term used for a collection of symptoms that can be caused by a number of disorders affecting the brain.

Alzheimer disease is the most common form of dementia. It affects 10% of the population over 65 and 50% of the population over 85. Nerve cells in the areas of the brain associated with memory and cognition are replaced by abnormal clumps and tangles of a protein (*Figure 9.17*).

Vascular dementia is the second most common form of dementia. It can come on gradually when arteries supplying the brain become arteriosclerotic (narrowed or blocked), depriving the brain of oxygen, or can occur suddenly after a **stroke** (*see Chapter 7*).

Confusion is used to describe people who cannot process information normally. For example, they cannot answer questions appropriately, understand where they are, or remember important facts. Confusion is often part of dementia or delirium.

Delirium is the sudden onset of disorientation, an inability to think clearly or pay attention. There is a change in the level of **consciousness**, varying from increased wakefulness to drowsiness. It is a mental state, not a disease. It can be part of dementia or a stroke.

Other conditions causing dementia are often treatable. They include

- **Reactions to medications** (e.g., sedatives, antiarthritics). Remove or lower the dose of the medication.
- **Metabolic abnormalities** (e.g., hypoglycemia). Correct the metabolic abnormality.
- **Nutritional deficiencies** (e.g., vitamins B_1 and B_6). Remedy the nutritional deficiency.
- **Emotional problems** (e.g., depression in the elderly). Use behavioral therapy or antidepressives.
- **Infections** (e.g., AIDS, encephalitis). Treat the underlying infection.

WORD	PRONUNCIATION	ELEMENTS		DEFINITION
Alzheimer disease	**AWLZ**-high-mer **DIZ**-eez		Alois Alzheimer, German neurologist, 1864–1915	Common form of dementia
confusion	kon-**FEW**-zhun	S/ R/	-ion *action, condition* confus- *bewildered*	Mental state in which environmental stimuli are not processed appropriately
conscious	**KON**-shus		Latin *to be aware*	Having present knowledge of oneself and one's surroundings
consciousness	**KON**-shus-ness	S/ R/	-ness *quality, state* conscious- *aware*	The state of being aware of and responsive to the environment
unconscious	un-**KON**-shus	P/	un- *not*	Not conscious, lacking awareness
delirium	de-**LIR**-ee-um	S/ R/	-um *structure* deliri- *confusion, disorientation*	Acute altered state of consciousness with agitation and disorientation; condition is reversible
dementia	dee-**MEN**-she-ah	S/ P/ R/	-ia *condition* de- *without* -ment- *mind*	Chronic, progressive, irreversible loss of the mind's cognitive and intellectual functions
empathy	**EM**-pah-thee	P/ R/	em- *into* -pathy *disease*	Ability to place yourself into the feelings, emotions, and reactions of another person
sympathy	**SIM**-pa-thee	P/ R/	sym- *together* -pathy *disease*	Appreciation and concern for another person's mental and emotional state
stroke	STROHK		Old English *to strike*	Acute clinical event caused by an impaired cerebral circulation

Exercises

A. Identify the elements in each medical term, and unlock the meaning of the word. *Fill in the chart; then use one of the terms in a sentence of your choice that is not a definition.* **LO 9.4, 9.9**

Medical Term	Meaning of Prefix	Meaning of Root/ Combining Form	Meaning of Suffix	Meaning of the Term
dementia	1.	2.	3.	4.
sympathy	5.	6.	7.	8.
unconscious	9.	10.	11.	12.
delirium	13.	14.	15.	16.
confusion	17.	18.	19.	20.
empathy	21.	22.	23.	24.

25. Sentence:

_____

_____

B. Identify the one incorrect statement in the following group. *Circle your answers.*   **LO 9.9**

1. Alzheimer disease is the most common form of dementia.   T   F

2. Delirium is a mental state and not a disease.   T   F

3. Reaction to medication can cause dementia.   T   F

4. Metabolic abnormalities have no effect on the brain.   T   F

5. Confusion is used to describe people who cannot process information normally.   T   F

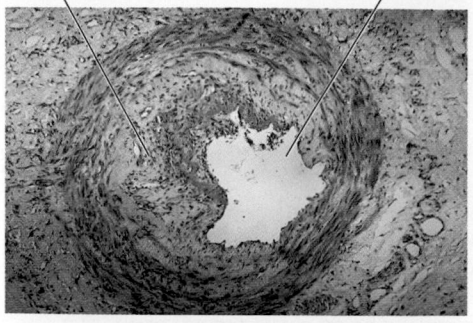

Atherosclerosis   Residual lumen of artery

(a)

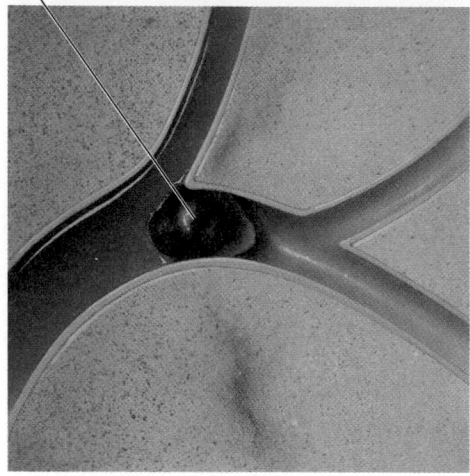

Embolus

(b)

▲ **Figure 9.18**   **Causes of Ischemic Strokes.** (*a*) Atherosclerosis in a cerebral artery leaving a small, residual lumen. (*b*) Embolus blocking an artery. Healthy tissue is on the left (*pink*); blood-starved tissue is on the right (*blue*).

Keynotes

- Risk factors for ischemic strokes are hypertension, diabetes mellitus, high cholesterol levels, cigarettes, and obesity.

- Risk factors for hemorrhagic strokes are hypertension, cerebral arteriovenous malformations, and cerebral aneurysms.

- One-third of people who have had a TIA will have more TIAs, and one-third will have a full-blown stroke later.

- One in twenty people who suffer a TIA will have a stroke within 2 days.

LO 9.9 Cerebrovascular Accidents (CVAs) or Strokes

A **stroke** (also known as a *cerebrovascular accident*, or *CVA*) occurs when the blood supply to a part of the brain is suddenly interrupted and thus brain cells are deprived of oxygen (*see Chapter 10*). Some cells die; others are left badly damaged. With timely treatment, the damaged cells can be saved. There are two types of stroke:

1. **Ischemic strokes** account for 90% of all strokes and are caused by
   a. **Atherosclerosis**—plaque in the wall of a cerebral artery (*Figure 9.18a*).
   b. **Embolism**—blood clot in a cerebral artery originating from elsewhere in the body (*Figure 9.18b*).
   c. **Microangiopathy**—occlusion of small cerebral arteries.

   Treatment of many acute ischemic strokes is by **thrombolysis** using clotbusters such as **tissue plasminogen activator (tPA)** within 4½ hours of the stroke, with supportive measures followed by rehabilitation.

2. **Hemorrhagic strokes (intracranial hemorrhage)** occur when a blood vessel in the brain bursts or when a cerebral **aneurysm** or **arteriovenous malformation (AVM)** ruptures.

   Cerebral arteriography can determine the site of bleeding in hemorrhagic strokes, enabling surgery to be performed to stop the bleeding or to clip off the aneurysm or AVM.

Symptoms of Strokes

The symptoms of a stroke can include the sudden onset of numbness or weakness, especially on one side of the body; difficulty in walking, balance, or coordination; trouble speaking or understanding speech; trouble seeing in one or both eyes; dizziness; confusion; and severe headache. A method to remember common warning signs of stroke is to use the acronym FAST:

Face—Ask the person to smile. Does one side of the face droop?

Arms—Ask the person to raise both arms. Does one arm drift downward?

Speech—Ask the person to repeat a simple phrase. Is his or her speech slurred or strange?

Time—If any of the previous signs is present, call 911 immediately.

Disability after Strokes

Although stroke is a disease of the brain, it can affect the whole body. A common residual disability is complete paralysis of one side of the body, called **hemiplegia**. If one side of the body is weak rather than paralyzed, the disability is called **hemiparesis**. Problems with forming and understanding speech and problems with awareness, attention, learning, judgment, and memory can remain after a stroke. Stroke patients may have difficulty controlling their emotions and may experience depression. All of these disabilities require well-planned rehabilitation.

Transient Ischemic Attack

Transient ischemic attacks **(TIAs)** are short-term, small strokes with symptoms lasting for less than 24 hours. If neurologic symptoms persist for more than 24 hours, then it is a full-blown stroke with brain cell damage and death.

The most frequent cause is a small **embolus** that occludes a small artery in the brain. Often, the embolus arises from a clot in the atrium in atrial fibrillation or from an atherosclerotic plaque in a carotid artery. If the impairment of blood supply lasts more than a few minutes, the affected nerve cells can die and cause permanent neurologic deficit.

Treatment is directed at the underlying cause. **Carotid endarterectomy** may be necessary if a carotid artery is significantly occluded with plaque.

Abbreviations	
AVM	arteriovenous malformation
CVA	cerebrovascular accident
TIA	transient ischemic attack
tPA	tissue plasminogen activator

WORD	PRONUNCIATION	ELEMENTS		DEFINITION
aneurysm aneurysmal (adj)	**AN**-yur-izm an-yur-**RIZ**-mal		Greek *dilation*	Circumscribed dilation of an artery or cardiac chamber
arteriography	ar-teer-ee-**OG**-rah-fee	S/ R/CF	-graphy *process of recording* **arteri/o-** *artery*	X-ray visualization of an artery after injection of contrast material
arteriovenous malformation	ar-**TEER**-e-o-**VE**-nus mal-for-**MAY**-shun	S/ R/ S/ P/ R/	-ous *pertaining to* **-ven-** *vein* -ion *process* mal- *bad* **-format-** *to form*	An abnormal communication between an artery and a vein
carotid endarterectomy	kah-**ROT**-id **END**-ar-ter-**EK**-toe-me	R/ S/ P/ R/	**carotid** *large neck artery* -ectomy *surgical excision* end- *inside* **-arter-** *artery*	Surgical removal of diseased lining from the carotid artery to leave a smooth lining
hemiparesis	**HEM**-ee-pah-**REE**-sis	P/ R/	hemi- *half* **-paresis-** *weakness*	Weakness of one side of the body
hemiplegia hemiplegic (adj)	hem-ee-**PLEE**-jee-ah hem-ee-**PLEE**-jik	S/ P/ R/ S/	-ia *condition* hemi- *half* **-pleg-** *paralysis* -ic *pertaining to*	Paralysis of one side of the body Pertaining to or suffering from hemiplegia
microangiopathy	**MY**-kroh-an-jee-**OP**-ah-thee	S/ P/ R/CF	-pathy *disease* micro- *small* **-angi/o-** *blood vessel*	Disease of the very small blood vessels (capillaries)
thrombolysis thrombolytic (adj)	throm-**BOL**-ih-sis **THROM**-boh-**LIT**-ik	S/ R/CF S/	-lysis *dissolve* **thromb/o-** *clot* -lytic *relating to dissolving or destroying*	Dissolving a thrombus (clot) Capable of breaking up or dissolving a thrombus

Exercises

A. Prefixes are applicable to terms from various body systems and will appear repeatedly. *Define the terms below; then define a term with the same prefix from a different body system or chapter. Fill in the blanks.* **LO 9.4, 9.9**

1. **malformation** Prefix is _____ and means _____.

   Definition of malformation: _____

   Term from a different body system/chapter with the same prefix: _____

   This term means _____.

2. **endarterectomy** Prefix is _____ and means _____.

   Definition of endarterectomy: _____

   Term from a different body system/chapter with the same prefix: _____

   This term means _____.

3. **hemiparesis** Prefix is _____ and means _____.

   Definition of hemiparesis: _____

   Term from a different body system/chapter with the same prefix: _____

   This term means _____.

4. **microangiopathy** Prefix is _____ and means _____.

   Definition of microangiopathy: _____

   Term from a different body system/chapter with the same prefix: _____

   This term means _____.

Keynotes

- CP is caused by damage to the developing brain. Of all CP cases, 75% occur during pregnancy; 5%, during childbirth; and 15% during infancy up to age 3.

- Spastic CP is the most common type, occurring in 70% to 80% of all cases.

- Spastic CP can occur as spastic hemiplegia, spastic diplegia, and spastic quadriplegia.

- Babies with very low birth weights are more likely to have CP.

LO 9.9 Cerebral Palsy

Definition

Cerebral palsy (CP) is the term used to describe the motor **impairment** resulting from brain damage in an infant or young child, regardless of the cause or the effect on the child. It is not hereditary. In congenital CP, the cause is often unknown but can be brain malformations or maternal use of cocaine; CP developed at birth or in the neonatal period is usually related to an incident causing hypoxia of the brain.

Cerebral palsy causes delay in the development of normal milestones in infancy and childhood.

The medical terminology of the classification and effects of CP is important, and it is used in many other conditions, including the aftereffects of strokes. The technical terms that follow are labels used to describe the type and extent of a problem. They do not describe the individual.

Classification by Number of Limbs Impaired

- **Quadriplegia.** All four limbs are involved (*Figure 9.19*).
- **Diplegia.** All four limbs are involved, but the legs are affected more than the arms.
- **Hemiplegia.** The arm and leg of one side of the body are affected (*Figure 9.20*).
- **Monoplegia.** Only one limb is affected, usually an arm (*Figure 9.21*).
- **Paraplegia.** Both lower extremities are involved (*Figure 9.22*).
- **Triplegia.** Three limbs are involved.

Classification by Movement Disorder

- **Spastic**—pertaining to tight muscles that are resistant to being stretched. They can become overactive when used and produce clonic movements.
- **Athetoid**—pertaining to difficulty in controlling and coordinating movements, leading to involuntary writhing movements in constant motion.
- **Ataxic**—pertaining to a poor sense of balance and depth perception, leading to a staggering walk and unsteady hands.

Combined Classifications

- The classifications of movement disorder and number of limbs involved are combined, for example, **spastic diplegia**.

Treatment of Cerebral Palsy

A multidisciplinary team of health professionals is required to develop an individualized treatment plan and to involve the patients, families, teachers, and caregivers in decision making and planning.

Physical therapy is designed to prevent muscles from becoming weak or rigidly fixed with **contractures**, to improve motor development, and to facilitate independence. Speech therapy and psychotherapy complement physical therapy.

Muscle relaxants, such as diazepam, can reduce **spasticity** for short periods of time, and a variety of devices and mechanical aids ranging from muscle braces to motorized wheelchairs help overcome physical limitations.

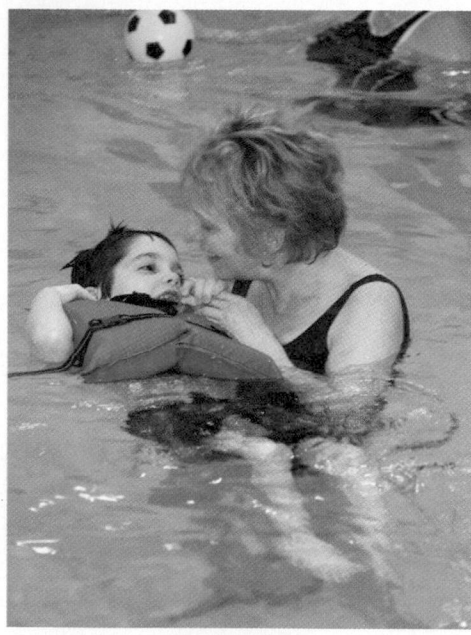

▲ **Figure 9.19** Quadriplegia.

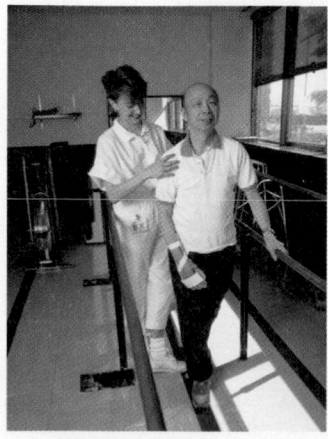

▲ **Figure 9.20** Hemiplegia.

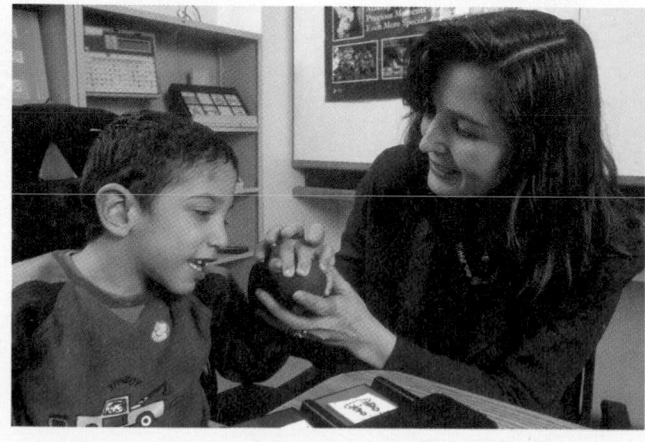

▲ **Figure 9.21** Monoplegia.

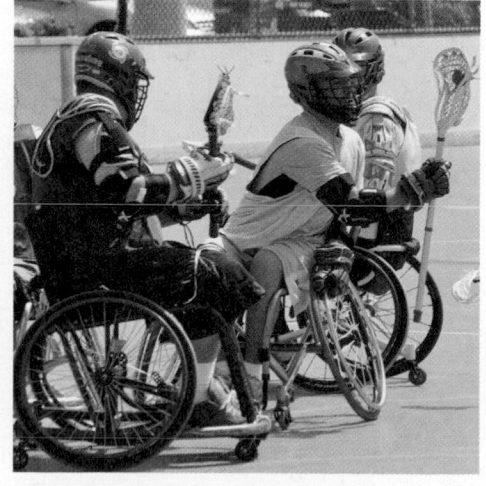

▲ **Figure 9.22** Paraplegia.

WORD	PRONUNCIATION	ELEMENTS		DEFINITION
ataxia ataxic (adj)	a-**TAK**-see-ah a-**TAK**-sik	S/ P/ R/	-ia *condition* a- *without* -tax- *coordination*	Inability to coordinate muscle activity, leading to jerky movements
athetosis	ath-eh-**TOE**-sis	S/ R/	-osis *condition* **athet-** *uncontrolled, without position*	Slow, writhing involuntary movements
athetoid (adj)	**ATH**-eh-toyd	S/	-oid *resembling*	Resembling athetosis
contracture	kon-**TRAK**-chur	S/ R/	-ure *result of, process* **contract-** *draw together*	Muscle shortening due to spasm or fibrosis
diplegia diplegic (adj)	die-**PLEE**-jee-ah die-**PLEE**-jik	S/ P/ R/	-ia *condition* di- *two* -pleg- *paralysis*	Paralysis of all four limbs, with the two legs affected most severely
impairment	im-**PAIR**-ment	S/ R/	-ment *action, state* **impair-** *worsen*	Diminishing of normal function
monoplegia monoplegic (adj)	**MON**-oh-**PLEE**-jee-ah **MON**-oh-**PLEE**-jik	S/ P/ R/	-ia *condition* mono- *one* -pleg- *paralysis*	Paralysis of one limb
palsy	**PAWL**-zee		Latin *paralysis*	Paralysis or paresis from brain damage
paraplegia	par-ah-**PLEE**-jee-ah par-ah-**PLEE**-jik	S/ P/ R/	-ia *condition* para- *abnormal, beside* -pleg- *paralysis*	Paralysis of both lower extremities
paraplegic (adj)		S/	-ic *pertaining to*	Pertaining to or suffering from paraplegia
quadriplegia	kwad-rih-**PLEE**-jee-ah	S/ P/ R/	-ia *condition* quadri- *four* -pleg- *paralysis*	Paralysis of all four limbs
quadriplegic (adj)	kwad-rih-**PLEE**-jik	S/	-ic *pertaining to*	Pertaining to or suffering from quadriplegia
spasm	SPASM		Greek *spasm*	Sudden involuntary contraction of a muscle group Increased muscle tone on movement
spastic (adj)	**SPAZ**-tik	S/ R/	-ic *pertaining to* **spast-** *tight*	Pertaining to or suffering from increased muscle tone on movement
triplegia triplegic (adj)	tri-**PLEE**-jee-ah tri-**PLEE**-jik	S/ P/ R/	-ia *condition* tri- *three* -pleg- *paralysis*	Paralysis of three limbs

Exercises

A. Prefixes. *Continue your work with prefixes of number. The following prefixes signify a number from 1 to 4. List an English and a medical term that uses the same number as a prefix. Try to think of terms from another chapter with that prefix. Fill in the blanks.* **LO 9.4, 9.5, 9.9**

1. **monoplegia** Prefix is _____ and means _____.

   English word: _____

   Medical term: _____

2. **diplegic** Prefix is _____ and means _____.

   English word: _____

   Medical term: _____

3. **triplegia** Prefix is _____ and means _____.

   English word: _____

   Medical term: _____

4. **quadriplegia** Prefix is _____ and means _____.

   English word: _____

   Medical term: _____

- Between 1% and 3% of the population will develop some form of epilepsy.
- Up to 50,000 Americans die each year from seizures and related causes, including drownings.
- Two-thirds of epileptic patients are manageable with medication and surgery; one-third are not.
- Status epilepticus is a medical emergency.
- First-aid treatment of a seizure is to place the person in a reclining position and cushion the head.
- A common tic disorder is *transient tic disorder*, occurring in 10% of children during the early school years. It goes away within 1 year.

Abbreviation	
IV	intravenous
LOC	loss of consciousness

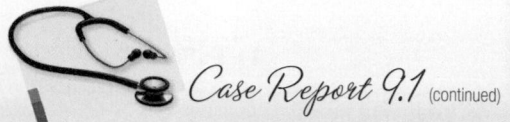

Case Report 9.1 (continued)

For Ms. Roberta Gaston, who was seen in Dr. Solis' neurosurgery clinic, the EEG did not localize an epileptic source. Therefore, deep brain electrodes were inserted into the region of the suspicious mass that showed on MRI. Seizures were recorded as arising in the mass itself. Dr. Solis performed a surgical resection of the mass, which was a **glioma**. Ms. Gaston has been seizure-free since the surgery a year ago.

LO 9.9 Epilepsy

Epilepsy is a chronic disorder in which clusters of neurons in the brain discharge their electrical signals in an abnormal rhythm. This disturbed electrical activity (a seizure) can cause strange sensations and behavior, convulsions, and loss of consciousness.

The causes of epilepsy are numerous, from abnormal brain development to brain damage.

An accepted classification of seizures is from the **International League Against Epilepsy**:

1. **Partial seizures** occur when the epileptic activity is in one area of the brain only. For example, in a partial seizure the only symptom of an epileptic attack could be a series of involuntary jerking movements of a single limb.

2. **Generalized seizures**:
   a. **Absence seizures**, previously known as "**petit mal**," begin between ages 5 and 10 years and may cease at puberty or continue through adult life. The child stares vacantly for a few seconds, apparently out of contact with surroundings. Recovery is quick. The child may be accused of daydreaming.
   b. **Tonic-clonic seizures**, previously called "**grand mal**," are dramatic. The person experiences a **loss of consciousness (LOC)**, breathing stops, the eyes roll upward, and the jaw is clenched. This "tonic" phase lasts for 30 to 60 seconds. It is followed by the "clonic" phase, in which the whole body shakes with a series of violent, rhythmic jerkings of the limbs. The seizures last for a couple of minutes, and consciousness returns.
   c. **Febrile seizures** are triggered by a fever in infants age 6 months to 5 years. Very few of these infants go on to develop epilepsy.

Status epilepticus occurs when the brain is in a state of persistent seizure. It is defined as one continuous seizure or recurrent seizures without regaining consciousness for 30 minutes or more. Many physicians believe that 5 minutes in this state is sufficient to damage neurons. Status epilepticus is a medical emergency and requires maintenance of the airway, breathing, and circulation and the **intravenous (IV)** administration of diazepam and anticonvulsant drugs.

Seizures may be followed by a period of diminished function in the area of brain surrounding the seizure focus. This transient neurologic deficit is called a **postictal state**.

Most epileptic disorders respond to **antiepileptic** medication, but occasionally brain surgery is required. The first-aid treatment during a seizure is to place the person in a reclining position on his or her side and to cushion the head. Do not try to keep the limbs from moving.

Tourette syndrome and other **tic disorders** are characterized by episodes of involuntary, rapid, repetitive, fixed movements of individual muscle groups. They occur with varying frequency and are associated with meaningless vocal sounds or meaningful words and phrases. The tics are probably genetic. There is no cure, but they can be treated pharmacologically with haloperidol or clonidine.

Narcolepsy is a chronic disorder caused by the brain's inability to regulate the sleep-wake cycle. Patients fall asleep during the day for a few seconds or up to an hour. It is associated with **cataplexy**, the sudden loss of voluntary muscle tone with brief episodes of total paralysis and vivid hallucinations. There is no cure, but it can be treated pharmacologically with stimulants.

WORD	PRONUNCIATION	ELEMENTS		DEFINITION
antiepileptic	AN-tee-epih-LEP-tik	S/ P/ R/	-tic *pertaining to* anti- *against* -epilep- *seizure*	A pharmacologic agent capable of preventing or arresting epilepsy
cataplexy	KAT-ah-plek-see	P/ R/	cata- *down* -plexy *stroke*	Sudden loss of muscle tone with brief paralysis
glioma	gli-OH-mah	S/ R/	-oma *tumor, mass* gli- *glue*	Tumor arising in a glial cell
grand mal	GRAHN MAL	R/ R/	grand *big* mal *bad*	Old name for a generalized tonic-clonic seizure
narcolepsy	NAR-coh-lep-see	S/ R/CF	-lepsy *seizure* narc/o- *stupor*	Condition with frequent incidents of sudden, involuntary deep sleep
petit mal	peh-TEE MAL	R/ R/	petit *small* mal *bad*	Old name for an absence seizure
postictal	post-IK-tal	S/ P/ R/	-al *pertaining to* post- *after* -ict- *seizure*	Occurring after a seizure
status epilepticus	STAT-us ep-ih-LEP-tik-us	S/ R/ S/ R/	-us *pertaining to* stat- *standing still* -ic *pertaining to* epilept- *seizure*	A recurrent state of seizure activity lasting longer than a specific time frame (usually 30 minutes)
tic	TIK		French *tic*	Sudden, involuntary, repeated contraction of muscles
Tourette syndrome	tur-ET SIN-drome		Georges Gilles de la Tourette, French neurologist, 1857–1904	Disorder of multiple motor and vocal tics

Exercises

A. After reading Case Report 9.1 on the opposite page, answer the following questions. *Be prepared to discuss your answers in class.* **LO 9.4, 9.9**

1. Basically, what is a *seizure?* _____

_____

_____

2. Explain the phrase *"resection of the mass."* _____

_____

3. Define *glioma.* _____

_____

4. These two terms have an element that means *electricity:* _____ and _____

5. What does the abbreviation MRI mean? _____

6. What is a *tic?* _____

_____

Abbreviations

BSE	bovine spongiform encephalopathy
CJD	Creutzfeldt-Jakob disease
NMS	neurally mediated syncope
TB	tuberculosis

LO 9.9 Other Brain Disorders

Parkinson disease is caused by the degeneration of neurons in the basic ganglia that produce a neurotransmitter called **dopamine**. Motor symptoms of abnormal movements, **tremor** of the hands, rigidity, a shuffling or **festinant** (hastening, falling-forward) gait, and weak voice appear. The symptoms gradually increase in severity. The cause is unknown, and there is no cure.

Huntington disease (also known as **Huntington chorea**) is a hereditary disorder starting with mild personality changes between the ages of 30 and 50. Involuntary, irregular, jerky (**choreic**) movements and muscle weakness follow, and dementia occurs in the later stages. A gene defect is on chromosome 4, but there is no known cure.

Creutzfeldt-Jakob disease (CJD) produces a rapid deterioration of mental function with difficulty in coordination of muscle movement. Some cases are linked to the consumption of beef from cattle with **mad cow disease (bovine spongiform encephalopathy, or BSE)**. Damage to the brain is thought to be caused by an abnormal infectious protein called a **prion**.

Syncope (fainting or passing out) is a temporary loss of consciousness and posture. It is usually due to hypotension and the associated deficient oxygen supply (hypoxia) to the brain. This disorder is called **neurally mediated syncope (NMS)**. In adults, it may be associated with cardiac arrhythmias and other diseases. The first-aid treatment is to place the person in a reclining position.

Migraine produces an intense throbbing, pulsating pain in one area of the head, often with nausea and vomiting. It can be preceded by an **aura**, visual disturbances such as flashing lights or temporary loss of vision. It occurs three times as often in women as men. There are multiple drugs used for prevention and treatment, with varying effectiveness. Stress management strategies can also be of value.

Headache, in its chronic, recurrent form, is classified into three types:

1. **Vascular headaches**, of which migraine is the most common, are caused by blood vessels becoming dilated and distended, producing a throbbing type of pain. **Cluster headaches** with intense, episodic pain are associated with hypertension. Strokes can produce severe headache.
2. **Muscular**, in which there is tension of facial and neck muscles.
3. **Inflammatory**, associated with diseases of the meninges, sinuses, teeth, and ears.

Treatment is to eliminate the basic cause.

Cerebral edema is excess accumulation of water in the intra- or extracellular spaces of the brain. It is associated with trauma, tumors, inflammation, toxins (such as aspirin in **Reye syndrome**), ischemia, and malignant hypertension.

Encephalitis is inflammation of the parenchyma of the brain. It is usually caused by a virus such as human immunodeficiency virus (HIV), West Nile virus, herpes simplex, or the childhood diseases of measles, mumps, chickenpox, and rubella. It occurs most often in the elderly, those with compromised immune systems *(see Chapter 15)*, and children.

Brain abscess is most often a direct spread of infection from sinusitis, otitis media, or mastoiditis *(see Chapter 16)*. It can also be a result of bloodborne pathogens from lung or dental infections. Abscesses are also formed by exotic fungal or protozoan organisms in immunosuppressive diseases like acquired immunodeficiency syndrome (AIDS) and **tuberculosis (TB)**. Protozoa are single-celled organisms that like to live in the damp. An example, *Trichomonas*, is sexually transmitted *(see Chapter 8)*.

Brain tumors are most often secondary tumors that have metastasized from cancers in the lung, breast, skin, or kidney. **Primary brain tumors** arise from any of the glial cells and are called **gliomas** *(Figure 9.23)*. The most malignant form of glioma is called **glioblastoma multiforme**.

Treatment of gliomas is a combination of surgery, radiotherapy, and chemotherapy. The combination is necessary because even if you remove 99% of a tumor, there will be up to 1 billion cells remaining. A more recent therapy, **brachytherapy**, implants small radioactive pellets directly into the tumor. The radiation is released over time.

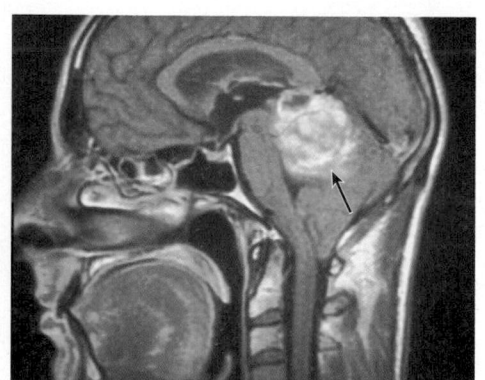

▲ **Figure 9.23** MRI Shows a Glioma *(arrow)*.

WORD	PRONUNCIATION	ELEMENTS		DEFINITION
aura	AWE-rah		Greek *breath of air*	Sensory experience preceding an epileptic seizure or a migraine headache
bovine spongiform encephalopathy (also called **mad cow disease**)	**BO**-vine **SPON**-jee-form en-sef-ah-**LOP**-ah-thee	S/ R/ S/ R/CF S/ P/ R/	-ine *pertaining to* **bov-** *cattle* -form *appearance of* **spong/i-** *sponge* -pathy *disease* en- *in* -cephal/o- *head*	Disease of cattle (mad cow disease) that can be transmitted to humans, causing Creutzfeldt-Jakob disease
brachytherapy	bra-kee-**THAIR**-ah-pee	P/ R/CF	brachy- *short* -therapy *medical treatment*	Radiation therapy in which the source of irradiation is implanted in the tissue to be treated
chorea choreic (adj)	kor-**EE**-ah kor-**EE**-ik		Greek *dance*	Involuntary, irregular spasms of limb and facial muscles
Creutzfeldt-Jakob disease	**KROITS**-felt-**YAK**-op **DIZ**-eez		Hans Creutzfeldt (1885–1964) and Alfons Jakob (1884–1931), German neuropsychiatrists	Progressive incurable neurologic disease caused by infectious prions
festinant	**FES**-tih-nant		Latin *to hasten*	Shuffling, falling-forward gait
glioblastoma	**GLIE**-oh-blas-**TOE**-mah	S/ P/ R/ P/ R/CF	-oma *tumor* glio- *glue* -blast- *germ cell* multi- *many* -form/e *shape, appearance of*	A malignant form of brain cancer
multiforme	**MULL**-tih-**FOR**-meh			
Huntington disease **Huntington chorea (syn)**	**HUN**-ting-ton **DIZ**-eez kor-**EE**-ah		George Huntington, U.S. physician, 1851–1916	Progressive inherited, degenerative, incurable neurologic disease
migraine	**MY**-grain	P/ R/	mi- *derived from hemi; half* -graine *head pain*	Paroxysmal severe headache confined to one side of the head
prion	**PREE**-on		derived from *protein-infectious particle*	Small infectious protein particle
Reye syndrome	RAY **SIN**-drome		R. Douglas Reye, twentieth-century Australian pathologist	Encephalopathy and liver damage in children following an acute viral illness; linked to aspirin use
syncope	**SIN**-koh-peh		Greek *cutting short*	Temporary loss of consciousness and postural tone due to diminished cerebral blood flow
tremor	**TREM**-or		Latin *to shake*	Small, shaking, involuntary, repetitive movements of hands, extremities, neck, or jaw

Exercises

A. Apply the medical terminology you are learning in this chapter, and be prepared to discuss the following information about headaches.   LO 9.4, 9.9

1. What are the three types of headaches that reoccur in chronic form? _____, _____, and

_____

2. What type of headache is associated with hypertension? _____

3. Muscular headaches result from tension in what part of the body? _____

4. What is the most common type of vascular headache? _____

5. Severe headache can be a symptom of impending _____.

LO 9.9 Traumatic Brain Injury

Traumatic brain injury (TBI) causes damage to the brain. Over 1 million people are seen by medical doctors each year following a blow to the head. Of these, 50,000 to 100,000 will have prolonged problems affecting their work and their **activities of daily living (ADLs)**. These injuries can occur during combat situations, but they also occur in sports, such as boxing, ice hockey, and American football, which are all sports that often involve severe contact injuries to the head.

If you are driving your car at 50 miles per hour and are hit head-on, your brain goes from 50 miles per hour to zero instantly. Your soft brain tissue is propelled forward and squished against the front of your hard skull **(coup)**. Then the brain and the rest of your body rebound backward. The soft brain is then squished against the back of your rigid skull **(contrecoup)**. The squished front and back areas are at least bruised. This bruise is called a **contusion** *(Figure 9.24)*.

If the process is more severe, blood vessels tear and blood flows into the brain. In addition, the brain itself can tear and cut brain connections and signals. In any injury, brain swelling can occur. Because the skull is hard and rigid, it cannot expand to cope with this extra volume. So the soft brain tissue is compressed, and some areas can stop working.

A mild head injury is called a **concussion**. You may feel dazed or have a period of confusion during which you do not recall the event that caused the concussion. In more severe cases, you may lose consciousness for a brief period of time and have no memory of the event. Repeated concussions have a cumulative effect, with loss of mental ability and/or traumatically induced Parkinson disease (as happened with professional boxer Muhammad Ali).

In more severe TBIs, the symptoms will depend on the area of the brain damaged. Some symptoms, such as difficulty with memory or concentration, irritability, aggression, **insomnia**, or depression, can be long-term. Traumatic brain injury has become a signature wound of the wars in Iraq and Afghanistan.

Posttraumatic stress disorder (PTSD) arises after significant trauma like a life-threatening incident, loss of a loved one, abuse, or combat in war. Symptoms include re-experiencing the original trauma through flashbacks or nightmares, difficulty in sleeping, anger, and hypervigilance. The symptoms cause significant impairment in social, occupational and family areas of functioning.

The residual effects of brain damage, whether due to trauma or stroke, have a terminology:

- **Impairment** is a deviation from normal function, for example, not being able to control an unwanted muscle movement.

- **Disability** is a restriction in the ability to perform a normal activity of daily living (ADL), for example, a 3-year-old who cannot walk independently.

- **Handicap** is defined as having a disability that prevents a child or adult from achieving a normal role in society commensurate with age and sociocultural setting, for example, a 16-year-old who cannot take care of personal toiletry and hygienic needs.

- **Shaken baby syndrome (SBS)** is a type of TBI produced when a baby is violently shaken. The baby has weak neck muscles and a heavy head. Shaking makes the brain bounce back and forth in the skull, leading to severe brain damage. Other injuries include retinal hemorrhages, damage to the spinal cord, and fractures of the ribs and limb bones. This syndrome usually occurs in children younger than 2 years.

Abbreviations

ADLs	activities of daily living
PTSD	posttraumatic stress disorder
SBS	shaken baby syndrome
TBI	traumatic brain injury

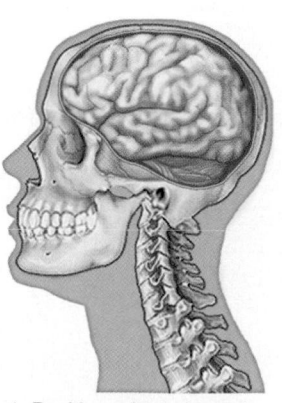

1. Position prior to impact.

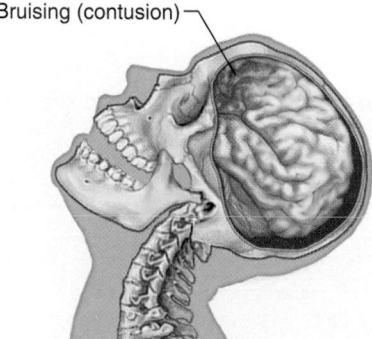

Bruising (contusion)

2. Impact from the front.

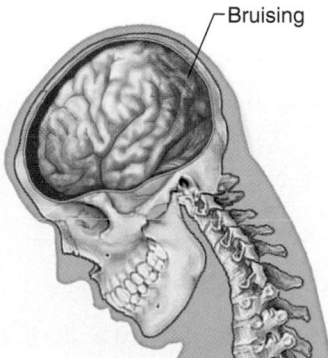

Bruising

3. Contrecoup action.

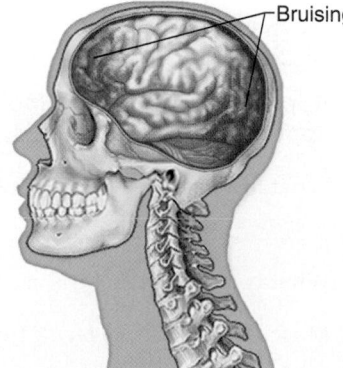

Bruising

4. Subsequent coup-contrecoup injury.

▲ **Figure 9.24** Contusions Caused by Back-and-Forth Movement of Brain in Skull.

S = Suffix   P = Prefix   R = Root   R/CF = Combining Form

WORD	PRONUNCIATION	ELEMENTS		DEFINITION
activities of daily living	ak-**TIV**-ih-tees of **DAY**-lee **LIV**-ing	S/ R/ S/ R/ S/ R/	-ity *condition, state* activ- *movement* -ly *every* dai- *day* -ing *quality of* liv- *life*	Daily routines for mobility and personal care: bathing, dressing, eating, and moving
concussion	kon-**KUSH**-un	S/ R/	-ion *action, condition* concuss- *shake violently*	Mild head injury
contusion	kon-**TOO**-zhun	S/ R/	-ion *action, condition* contus- *bruise*	Bruising of a tissue, including the brain
coup	KOO		French *a blow*	Injury to the brain occurring directly under the skull at the point of impact
contrecoup	**KON**-treh-koo		French *counterblow*	Injury to the brain at a point directly opposite the point of original contact
disability	dis-ah-**BILL**-ih-tee	P/ R/	dis- *away from* -ability *competence*	Diminished capacity to perform certain activities or functions
handicap	**HAND**-ee-cap		French *assess before a race*	Condition that interferes with a person's ability to function normally
insomnia	in-**SOM**-nee-ah	S/ P/ R/	-ia *condition* in- *not* -somn- *sleep*	Inability to sleep

Exercises

A. Apply the correct medical language from the above WAD to the following sentences. *Remember to check your spelling when you are finished. Fill in the blanks.*   **LO 9.4, 9.9**

1. A TBI can cause problems with the (abbreviation) _____.

2. Rewrite sentence 1 without using the abbreviations. (Spell them out.)

   _____

   _____

3. Diminished capacity to perform certain activities or functions is a _____.

4. A condition that interferes with a person's ability to function normally is a _____.

5. A mild head injury can be termed a _____.

6. Bruising of a tissue, including the brain, is a _____.

7. List briefly some activities of daily living (ADLs): _____

B. Use your knowledge of the language of neurology to fill in the correct medical terminology answers.   **LO 9.4, 9.9**

1. Two terms in the above WAD that are diagnoses you might see on an Emergency Room record are _____ and

   _____.

2. What is the difference between a *disability* and a *handicap*?

   Disability _____.

   Handicap _____.

3. What kind of brain injuries are likely to occur in a motor vehicle accident? _____, _____.

4. Can you think of another possible brain injury in an MVA that is not included in the above WAD?

   _____.

LO 9.11 Pain Management

Pain persisting longer than 3 months is said to be **chronic**. It can be caused by cancer, arthritis, fibromyalgia, low-back or neck problems, headache, or injuries that have not healed. Normal activities can be restricted or be impossible.

Among Americans, 6 million to 10 million are affected by fibromyalgia, 5 million are disabled by back problems, 8 million experience chronic neck and facial pain, and 40 million suffer from chronic recurrent headaches. In modern health care, chronic pain management has become essential and often uses a **multidisciplinary** approach. Pain management is now a board-certified subspecialty for **anesthesiologists**.

Medications are the cornerstone of pain management, and the following can be used depending on the severity of the pain:

Abbreviations	
NSAIDs	nonsteroidal anti-inflammatory drugs
RF	radiofrequency

- Mild pain. **Analgesics**, such as acetaminophen, and **nonsteroidal anti-inflammatory drugs (NSAIDs)**, such as ibuprofen, are used.

- Moderate pain. **Opiate** medications in combination with acetaminophen or NSAIDs are used. Some opiates used in combination medications are codeine, hydrocodone, and oxycodone. Examples are hydrocodone/acetaminophen (Vicodin), oxycodone/acetaminophen (Percocet), and oxycodone/aspirin (Percodan). These medications are frequently abused and sold on the street.

- Severe pain. Higher doses of opiates are used, often not as combination products. These include **morphine**, fentanyl, and oxy- and hydromorphone. The opiates can be taken orally, by patch, sublingually, by intravenous (IV) infusion, or by continuous delivery systems.

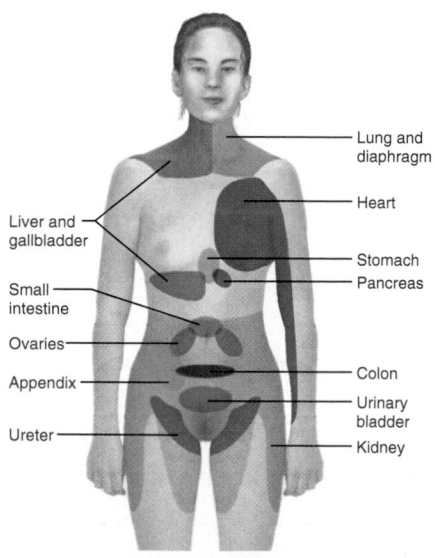

Lung and diaphragm
Heart
Stomach
Pancreas
Liver and gallbladder
Small intestine
Ovaries
Colon
Appendix
Urinary bladder
Ureter
Kidney

▲ **Figure 9.25** Referred Pain.

Central sensitization pain is a new concept describing how neurons in the spinal cord sending messages to the brain become excitable. They exaggerate the pain response in tissues they supply. The input can be somatic from skeletal muscles (as in fibromyalgia) or visceral (as in irritable bowel syndrome).

Interventional pain management, particularly for pain originating in the spine and spinal nerves, is being increasingly used. Examples are

- **Epidural** or **facet nerve blocks**. Anesthetic or anti-inflammatory agents are injected into an area surrounding the pain-generating nerve.

- **Radiofrequency (RF) nerve ablation**. A probe heats the area around a pain-generating spinal nerve and temporarily deactivates it.

- **Spinal infusion pump**. Pain medications such as morphine are delivered through an indwelling catheter into the **intrathecal** CSF surrounding the spinal cord. A pump delivery device is inserted under the skin of the abdomen.

Phantom limb pain occurs following the **amputation** of a limb or part of a limb. Any stimulation of the remaining intact portion of the sensory pathway coming originally from the limb is interpreted by the brain as coming from the original limb. The pain can be severe and debilitating or just an insatiable urge to scratch an itch.

Referred pain occurs when pain in the viscera is felt in the skin or other superficial sites *(Figure 9.25)*. An example is the pain of a heart attack felt along the front of the left shoulder and down the underside of the left arm. This is because spinal cord segments T1 to T5 receive sensory input from the heart, as well as from the skin of the shoulder and arm. This input is transmitted to the brain. The brain cannot distinguish the true source of the pain. It assumes it is coming from the skin, which has more pain receptors than the heart and is injured more often.

WORD	PRONUNCIATION	ELEMENTS		DEFINITION
ablation	ab-**LAY**-shun	S/ P/ R/	-ion *action, condition* ab- *away from* -lat- *to take*	Removal of tissue to destroy its function
amputation	am-pyu-**TAY**-shun	S/ R/	-ation *process* amput- *to prune, lop off*	Process of removing a limb, part of a limb, a breast, or other projecting part
analgesia	an-al-**JEE**-ze-ah	S/ P/ R/	-ia *condition* an- *without* -alges- *sensation of pain*	State in which pain is reduced
analgesic	an-al-**JEE**-zic	S/	-ic *pertaining to*	Substance that produces analgesia
anesthesia	an-es-**THEE**-zee-ah	P/ R/CF	an- *without* -esthesi/a- *sensation, feeling*	Complete loss of sensation
anesthesiologist	**AN**-es-thee-zee-**OL**-oh-jist	S/ P/ R/CF	-logist *one who studies, specialist* an- *without* -esthesi/o- *feeling, sensation*	Medical specialist in anesthesia
anesthesiology	**AN**-es-thee-zee-**OL**-oh-jee	S/	-logy *study of*	Medical specialty related to anesthesia
anesthetic	an-es-**THET**-ic	S/ P/ R/	-ic *pertaining to* an- *without* -esthet- *sensation, perception*	An agent that causes absence of feeling or sensation
facet	**FAS**-et		French *little face*	Small area, in this case around a pain-generating nerve
intrathecal	**IN**-trah-**THEE**-kal	S/ P/ R/	-al *pertaining to* intra- *within* -thec- *sheath*	Within the subarachnoid or subdural space
intravenous	**IN**-trah-**VEE**-nuss	S/ P/ R/	-ous *pertaining to* intra- *within, inside* -ven- *vein*	Inside a vein
morphine	**MOR**-feen		Latin *god of dreams*	Derivative of opium used as an analgesic or sedative
multidisciplinary	mul-tee-**DIS**-ih-plin-**NAR**-ee	S/ P/ R/	-ary *pertaining to* multi- *many* -disciplin- *discipline, instruction*	Involving health care providers from more than one profession
opiate	**OH**-pee-ate		Latin *bringing sleep*	A drug derived from opium

Exercises

A. Deconstruct the following *language of neurology.* *Write the meaning of each element to see how it will aid you in understanding the meaning of the complete term. Fill in the chart.*   **LO 9.4, 9.11**

Medical Term	Meaning of Prefix	Meaning of Root/ Combining Form	Meaning of Suffix	Meaning of Term
intrathecal	1.	2.	3.	4.
ablation	5.	6.	7.	8.
analgesia	9.	10.	11.	12.
anesthesia	13.	14.	15.	16.
amputation	17.	18.	19.	20.

Remember: Every term does not need a prefix!

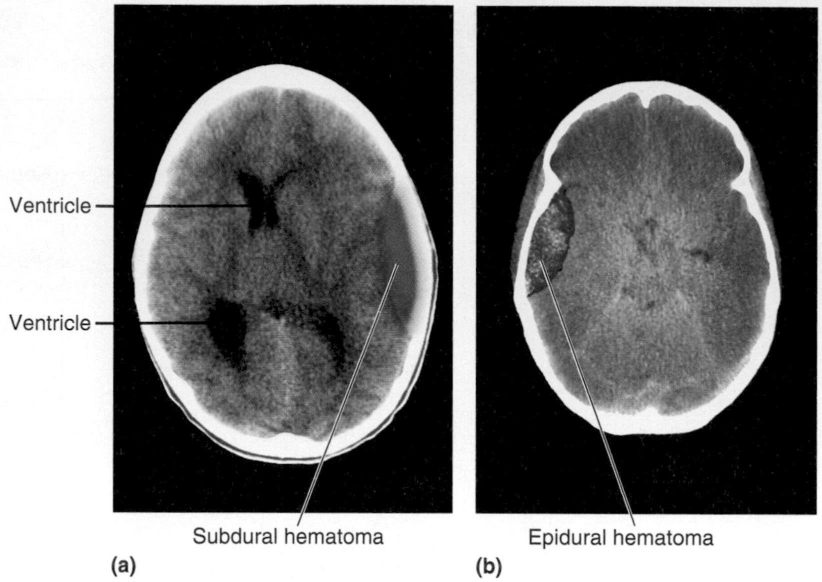

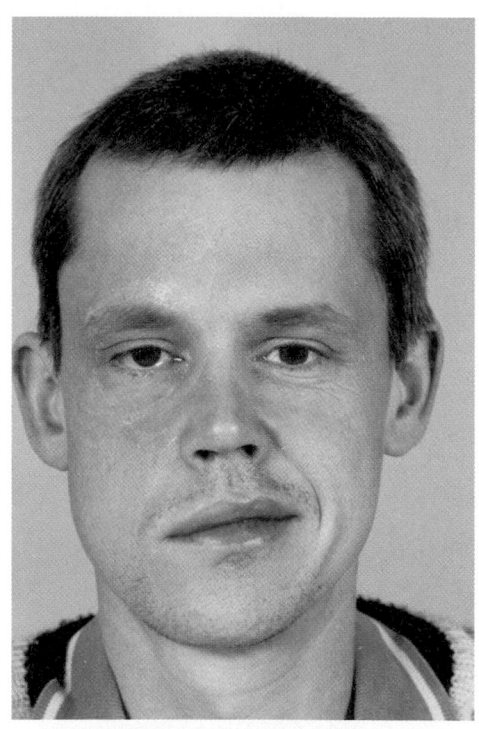

Figure 9.26 Hematomas. ▶
[a] CT scan of subdural hematoma compressing ventricles and pushing them laterally. [b] Epidural hematoma.

Ventricle —

Ventricle —

Subdural hematoma

(a)

Epidural hematoma

(b)

LO 9.10 Disorders of the Meninges

Subdural hematoma is bleeding into the subdural space outside the brain *(Figure 9.26)*. Most subdural hematomas are associated with closed head injuries and bleeding from broken veins caused by violent rotational movement of the head. They have been seen following roller-coaster rides with high-speed turns that jerk and whip the head. Although the blood accumulation is slow, the bleeding must be stopped surgically.

Epidural hematoma is a pooling of blood in the epidural space outside the brain *(Figure 9.26)*. Most are associated with a fractured skull and bleeding from an artery that lies in the meninges. If the bleeding is not stopped surgically by **ligating** (tying off) the blood vessel, brain compression with severe neurologic injury or death can occur.

Meningitis is inflammation of the meninges covering the brain and spinal cord. Viral meningitis is the most common form and occurs at all ages. Bacterial meningitis is more common in the very young or very old. **Meningococcal meningitis** is contagious through droplet infection by coughing and sneezing and through close living conditions, as in college dormitories. Vaccines are available to prevent most causes of meningitis *(see Chapter 12)*.

Meningioma is a tumor originating in the arachnoid cells of the meninges, most commonly overlying the cerebral hemispheres. It is usually benign and produces a slow-growing, focal, spherical tumor. Symptoms can take years to develop. Surgical resection is usually curative.

▲ **Figure 9.27** Bell Palsy of Right Side of Face.

LO 9.10 Disorders of the Cranial Nerves

Bell palsy is a disorder of the seventh cranial nerve (facial nerve), causing a sudden onset of weakness or paralysis of facial muscles on one side of the face *(Figure 9.27)*. Common symptoms are a **hemifacial** inability to smile, whistle, or grimace; drooping of the mouth with drooling of saliva; and inability to close the eye on the affected side. Early treatment with steroids and supportive measures is essential. The facial nerve can also be affected by trauma or tumors.

Trigeminal neuralgia (tic douloureux) is intermittent, shooting pain in the area of the face and head innervated by the fifth cranial nerve. The pain is abrupt (sudden), unilateral, often severe, and can affect any area of the face from the crown of the head to the jaw. Chewing or touching the affected area causes pain. Effective medications are carbamazepine and gabapentin.

Horner syndrome presents with a unilateral droopy eyelid (ptosis), small pupil, and decrease in perspiration on the face. It can occur in lung cancer and injuries to the head, neck, and cervical spinal cord *(Figure 9.28)*.

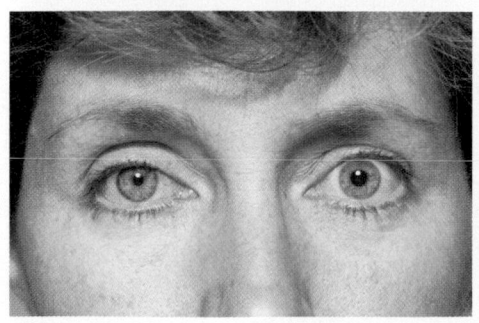

▲ **Figure 9.28** Horner Syndrome Showing Ptosis and Small Pupil of Right Eye.

WORD	PRONUNCIATION	ELEMENTS		DEFINITION
Bell palsy	BELL **PAWL**-zee		Charles Bell, 1774–1842, Scottish surgeon, anatomist, and physiologist	Paresis or paralysis of one side of face
hematoma	he-mah-**TOE**-mah	S/ R/	-oma *tumor, mass* **hemat-** *blood*	Collection of blood that has escaped from the blood vessels into tissue
hemifacial	hem-ee-**FAY**-shal	S/ P/ R/CF	-al *pertaining to* **hemi-** *half* **-fac/i-** *face*	Pertaining to one side of the face
Horner syndrome	**HOR**-ner **SIN**-drome		Johann Friedrich Horner 1831–1886, Swiss ophthalmologist	Disorder of the sympathetic nerves to the face and eye
ligate	**LIE**-gate		Latin *to tie, bind*	Tie off a structure, such as a bleeding blood vessel
meningioma	meh-**NIN**-jee-**OH**-mah	S/ R/CF	-oma *tumor, mass* **mening/i-** *meninges*	Tumor arising from the arachnoid layer of the meninges
meningococcal	meh-nin-goh-**KOK**-al	S/ R/CF R/	-al *pertaining to* **mening/o-** *meninges* **-cocc-** *spherical bacterium*	Pertaining to the *meningococcus* bacterium
meningitis	men-in-**JIE**-tis	S/	-itis *infection*	Inflammation of the membranes surrounding the brain or spinal cord
neuralgia	nyu-**RAL**-jee-ah	S/ R/	-algia *pain* **neur-** *nerve*	Pain in the distribution of a nerve
subdural	sub-**DUR**-al	S/ P/ R/	-al *pertaining to* **sub-** *under* **dur-** *dura mater*	Located in the space between the dura mater and arachnoid membrane
tic douloureux trigeminal neuralgia (syn)	TIK duh-luh-**RUE**		**douloureux** French *painful tic*	Painful, sudden, spasmodic, involuntary contractions of the facial muscles supplied by the trigeminal nerve

Exercises

A. Some suffixes can have more than one meaning, and only one of the meanings will apply to a particular term. *In the following exercise, practice using the suffix* **-oma**. *Fill in the blanks; then fill in the chart.*   **LO 9.4, 9.9**

1. The suffix -oma has two meanings: _____ and/or _____

2. In the term **hematoma**, the meaning of -oma is _____.

3. In the term **meningioma**, the meaning of -oma is _____.

4. Construct the term meaning *a nerve tumor*. _____

B. Now deconstruct the following medical terms into all their basic elements.   LO 9.4

Medical Term	Prefix	Root/ Combining Form	Suffix	Meaning of the Term
hematoma	1.	2.	3.	4.
hemifacial	5.	6.	7.	8.
meningioma	9.	10.	11.	12.
neuralgia	13.	14.	15.	16.

Lesson 9.4 Disorders of the Spinal Cord and Peripheral Nerves

There are many disorders of the nervous system that affect the spinal cord and the peripheral nerves without affecting the brain. In this lesson, the information will enable you to:

9.4.1 Discuss disorders of the spinal cord and peripheral nerves.

9.4.2 Distinguish between different diagnostic tests used for nervous system disorders.

9.4.3 Define methods by which nervous system medications influence disease processes.

9.4.4 Recognize common congenital disorders of the nervous system.

9.4.5 Use the correct terminology to communicate about the nervous system and its disorders with patients and other health professionals.

You are

. . . Tanisha Colis, an electroneurodiagnostic technologist working with Raul Cardenas, MD, a neurologist at Fulwood Medical Center.

Your patient is

. . . Mrs. Suzanne Kalish, a 42-year-old social worker employed by the medical center.

Case Report 9.3

Mrs. Kalish has recently had an exacerbation of her symptoms due to **multiple sclerosis (MS)**. She is going to have a **visual evoked potential (VEP)** test, followed by an MRI of her brain and spinal cord.

Patient Interview:

Tanisha: "Good morning, Mrs. Kalish, I'm Tanisha Colis, the technologist who'll be performing your visual evoked potential test. How are you feeling?"

Mrs. Kalish: "I've been doing OK for the last 4 or 5 years. Then, a few weeks ago, I started dragging my right foot like a wounded witch. I'm tired out, can't come to work. It's a struggle to walk the few yards just to pick up the mail."

Tanisha: "The MRI you are going to have today will give us a lot of information about what's going on."

Mrs. Kalish: "My mind is going 'wheelchair, wheelchair, wheelchair.' Especially since in the last couple of days the vision in my right eye has got all blurred."

Tanisha: "That's the reason you are having the visual evoked potential test."

Mrs. Kalish: "I hate this disease. If I had cancer, I'd have a chance. I'd fight it to the end, whatever that would be."

Tanisha: "Let me help you up, and we'll go get this test done."

Mrs. Kalish: "I can manage on my own, thank you."

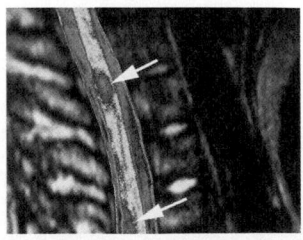

▲ **Figure 9.29**
Multiple sclerosis.
Note areas of spinal cord where myelin sheath has been destroyed (arrows). Normal spinal cord is yellow.

Abbreviations	
MS	multiple sclerosis
VEP	visual evoked potential

LO 9.10 Disorders of the Myelin Sheath of Nerve Fibers

When the myelin sheath surrounding nerve fibers is damaged, nerves do not conduct impulses normally. **Demyelination**, the destruction of an area of the myelin sheath, can occur in the PNS caused by inflammation, vitamin B_{12} deficiency, poisons, and some medications.

Guillain-Barré syndrome is a disorder of the peripheral nerves in which the body makes antibodies against myelin, leading to loss of nerve conduction, muscle weakness, and **paresthesias** (changes in sensation). Treatment is with corticosteroids, and recovery of neurologic function is slow.

Demyelination of nerve fibers in the brain, spinal cord, and optic nerves can also occur. Multiple Sclerosis (MS) is the most common of these demyelination disorders. As you can tell from Mrs. Kalish's story, MS is a chronic, progressive disorder. **Intermittent** myelin damage and scarring slows nerve impulses *(Figure 9.29)*. This leads to muscle weakness, pain, numbness, and vision loss. Because different nerve fibers are affected at different times, MS symptoms often worsen (**exacerbations**) or show partial or complete reduction (**remissions**). Mrs. Kalish is now in an exacerbation.

MS has an average age of onset between 18 and 35 years and is more common in women. Its cause is unknown, but it is thought to be an autoimmune disease.

There is no known cure for MS, but recently developed **disease-modifying** drugs appear to have partial success in slowing down the accumulation of disabilities if started when the diagnosis is first made.

Other causes of demyelination in the CNS are injury, ischemia, toxic agents such as chemotherapy or radiotherapy, and congenital disorders such as **Tay Sachs disease**. After viral infections or vaccinations, **postinfectious encephalomyelitis** is a demyelination process, as is **HIV encephalitis**, which is seen in up to 30% of patients with AIDS.

WORD	PRONUNCIATION	ELEMENTS		DEFINITION
demyelination	dee-**MY**-eh-lin-**A**-shun	S/ P/ R/	-ation *process* de- *away from, without* -myelin- *myelin*	Process of losing the myelin sheath of a nerve fiber
encephalitis	en-**SEF**-ah-**LIE**-tis	S/ R/	-itis *inflammation* **encephal-** *brain*	Inflammation of brain cells and tissues
encephalomyelitis	en-**SEF**-ah-loh-**MY**-eh-lie-tis	R/CF R/	**encephal/o-** *brain* -myel- *spinal cord*	Inflammation of the brain and spinal cord
exacerbation (contrast remission)	ek-zas-er-**BAY**-shun	S/ R/	-ation *process* **exacerbat-** *increase,* *aggravate*	Period when there is an increase in the severity of a disease
Guillain-Barré syndrome	**GEE**-yan-bah-**RAY** **SIN**-drom		Georges Guillain (1876–1961) and Jean-Alexandre Barré (1880–1967), French neurologists	Disorder in which the body makes anti- bodies against myelin, disrupting nerve conduction
intermittent	**IN**-ter-**MIT**-ent	S/ P/ R/	-ent *end result* inter- *between* -mitt- *send*	Alternately ceasing and beginning again
modify	**MOD**-ih-fie		Latin *to limit*	Change the form or qualities of something
paresthesia paresthesias (pl)	par-es-**THEE**-ze-ah	S/ P/ R/	-ia *condition* **par(a)-** *abnormal* -esthes- *sensation, feeling*	Abnormal sensation; for example, tingling, burning, prickling
remission (contrast exacerbation)	ree-**MISH**-un	S/ P/ R/	-ion *action, condition* re- *back* -miss- *send*	Period when there is a lessening or absence of the symptoms of a disease

Exercises

A. Test yourself on the elements and terms in the above WAD. *Practice pronouncing the terms before you start the exercise. Circle the best answer.* **LO 9.4, 9.10**

1. **Guillain-Barré syndrome** disrupts

   nerve conduction   blood flow   metabolism

2. In the term **paresthesia**, the prefix means

   between   abnormal   many

3. **Remission** is the opposite of

   intermittence   exacerbation   demyelination

4. To **modify** something is to

   dispose of it   change it   renew it

5. In the term **demyelination**, the prefix means

   away from   in front of   in between

6. **Encephalomyelitis** is inflammation of

   brain   spinal cord   brain and spinal cord

Abbreviations

ALS	amyotrophic lateral sclerosis
GI	gastrointestinal
polio	poliomyelitis
PPS	postpoliomyelitis syndrome
SCI	spinal cord injury

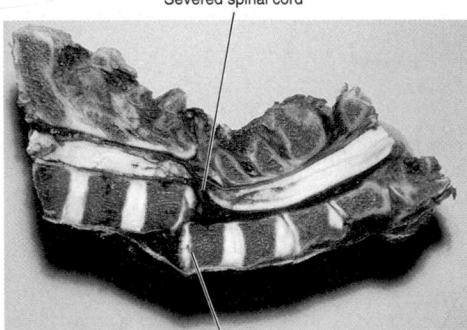

Severed spinal cord

(a) Fracture-dislocation of vertebra

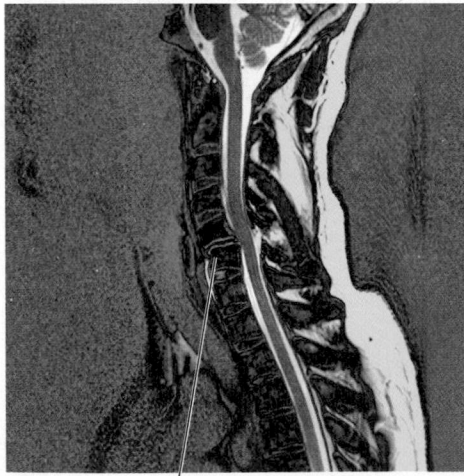

(b) Fractured vertebra

▲ **Figure 9.30** **Spinal Cord Injuries.** (*a*) Severed spinal cord from fracture-dislocation of vertebra. (*b*) Compressed spinal cord with vertebral fracture.

LO 9.10 Disorders of the Spinal Cord

Trauma

The spinal cord is injured in three ways (*Figure 9.30*):

1. **Severed**.

2. **Contused**.

3. **Compressed**, by a broken or dislocated vertebra, bleeding, or swelling.

Because of its anatomy with nerve fibers and tracts going up and down, to and from the brain, injury to the spinal cord results in loss of function *below the injury*. For example, if the cord is injured in the thoracic region, the arms function normally, but the legs can be **paralyzed**. Both muscle control and sensation are lost.

If the spinal cord is severed, the loss is permanent. Contusions can cause temporary loss lasting days, weeks, or months. Compression injuries may require surgical intervention to relieve the pressure. Compression can also be due to a **herniated** disc.

The first goal of treatment is to prevent further damage, which is why you see football players being carried off the field strapped to a board and carefully padded to prevent even slight shifting of the spine.

Approximately half-a-million people in the United States have **spinal cord injuries (SCIs)**. About 8,000 new injuries occur each year; 82% involve males between the ages of 16 and 30. Quadriplegia is slightly more common than paraplegia.

Compression of the cord can also occur slowly from a tumor in the cord or spine. Cancer or osteoporosis can cause a vertebra to collapse and compress the cord.

- **Cervical spondylosis** is a disorder in which the discs and vertebrae in the neck degenerate, narrow the spinal canal, and compress the spinal cord and/or the spinal nerve roots.

- In **syringomyelia**, fluid-filled cavities grow in the spinal cord and compress nerves that detect pain and temperature. There is no specific cure.

Other Disorders

Acute transverse myelitis is a localized disorder of the spinal cord that blocks transmission of impulses up and down the spinal cord. People who have **Lyme disease**, **syphilis**, or **tuberculosis** or those who inject heroin or amphetamines intravenously are at risk of developing this disorder. The disorder causes loss of sensation, muscle paralysis, and loss of bladder and bowel control. There is no specific treatment. Most people recover completely.

Subacute combined degeneration of the spinal cord is due to a deficiency of vitamin B_{12}. The sensory nerve fibers in the spinal cord degenerate, producing weakness, clumsiness, tingling, and loss of the position sense as to where limbs are. Treatment is injections of vitamin B_{12}.

Poliomyelitis (polio) is an acute infectious disease, occurring mostly in children, that is caused by the poliovirus. The virus can be asymptomatic in the nasopharynx and **gastrointestinal (GI)** tract. When it spreads to the nervous system, it replicates in the spinal cord and destroys motor neurons. Symptoms are progressive muscle **paralysis**; paralysis of the respiratory muscles can require mechanical ventilation using the **Drinker respirator** (iron lung). Poliomyelitis is preventable by vaccination and has almost been eradicated in the world.

Postpolio syndrome (PPS), in which people develop tired, painful, and weak muscles many years after recovery from polio, is classified as a motor neuron disorder.

Motor neuron disorders occur when motor nerves in the spinal cord and brain progressively deteriorate. This leads to muscle weakness that can progress to paralysis. **Amyotrophic lateral sclerosis (ALS**, or Lou Gehrig disease) and its variants, **progressive muscular atrophy** and **primary lateral sclerosis**, are examples. There is no cure.

WORD	PRONUNCIATION	ELEMENTS		DEFINITION
amyotrophic	a-my-oh-**TROH**-fik	S/ P/ R/CF R/	**-ic** *pertaining to* **a-** *without* **-my/o-** *muscle* **-troph-** *nourishment,* *development*	Pertaining to muscular atrophy
atrophy	**AT**-roh-fee	P/ R/	**a-** *without* **-trophy** *development,* *nourishment*	Wasting or diminished volume of a tissue or organ
compression	kom-**PRESH**-un	S/ P/ R/	**-ion** *action, condition* **com-** *together* **-press-** *squeeze*	A squeezing together so as to increase density and/or decrease a dimension of a structure
herniation hernia (noun) herniate (verb)	**HER**-nee-ay-shun **HER**-nee-ah **HER**-nee-ate	S/ R/ S/	**-ation** *process* **herni-** *rupture* **-ate** *composed of*	Protrusion of an anatomical structure from its normal location
Lyme disease	LIME **DIZ**-eez		Named in 1977 after a group of children in Lyme, Connecticut	Disease transmitted by the bite of an infected deer tick
myelitis	**MY**-eh-**LIE**-tis	S/ R/	**-itis** *inflammation* **myel-** *spinal cord*	Inflammation of the spinal cord
paralyze paralysis paralytic (adj)	**PAR**-ah-lyze pah-**RAL**-ih-sis par-ah-**LYT**-ik	P/ R/ R/ R/ S/	**para-** *abnormal* **-lyze** *destroy* **-lysis** *destruction* **-ly-** *break down* **-tic** *pertaining to*	To make incapable of movement Loss of voluntary movement Pertaining to or suffering from paralysis
poliomyelitis polio (abbrev) postpolio syndrome	POE-lee-oh-**MY**-eh-lie-tis post-**POE**-lee-oh SIN-drome	S/ R/ R/ P/ P/ R/	**-itis** *inflammation* **polio-** *gray matter* **-myel-** *spinal cord* **post-** *after* **syn-** *together* **-drome** *running*	Inflammation of the gray matter of the spinal cord, leading to paralysis of the limbs and muscles of respiration Progressive muscle weakness in a person previously affected by polio
spondylosis	spon-dih-**LOH**-sis	S/ R/	**-osis** *condition* **spondyl-** *vertebra*	Degenerative osteoarthritis of the spine
syringomyelia	sih-**RING**-oh-my-**EE**-lee-ah	S R R/CF	**-ia** *condition* **myel-** *spinal cord* **syring/o-** *tube, pipe*	Abnormal longitudinal cavities in the spinal cord that cause paresthesias and muscle weakness

Exercises

A. Meet a lesson objective by answering the following questions about the spinal cord. *Fill in the blanks, and be prepared to discuss your answers in class.* **LO 9.10**

1. What has happened to a *severed* spinal cord? _____

_____

2. If the spinal cord is *contused,* what does that mean? _____

_____

3. Briefly define a *compressed* spinal cord injury. _____

_____

B. Recall from the answers in Exercise A the correct answers to the following questions.   LO 9.10

1. Of the three injuries mentioned in Exercise A, which one is permanent? _____

2. Where does loss of *function* occur in a spinal cord injury? _____

3. In the case of paralysis, what is lost? _____

LO 9.10 Disorders of the Peripheral Nerves

The **term neuropathy** is used here as any disorder affecting one or more peripheral nerves.

Mononeuropathy is damage to a single peripheral nerve. Prolonged pressure on a nerve that runs close to the surface over a bony prominence is a common cause. Examples are

- **Carpal tunnel syndrome**. The median nerve at the wrist is compressed between the wrist bones and a strong overlying ligament. Numbness, pain, and tingling of the thumb side of the hand are the symptoms. Incision of the ligament relieves the pressure.

- **Ulnar nerve palsy**. Nerve damage occurs as the ulnar nerve crosses too close to the surface over the humerus at the back of the elbow. Pins-and-needles sensation and weakness in the hand result. Hitting the ulnar nerve is the cause of pain when you hit your "funny bone."

- **Peroneal nerve palsy**. Nerve damage occurs as the peroneal nerve passes too close to the surface near the back of the knee. Compression of the nerve occurs in people who are bedridden or strapped in a wheelchair.

Polyneuropathy is damage to, and the simultaneous malfunction of, many peripheral nerves throughout the body.

Symptoms of acute polyneuropathy include muscle weakness and a pins-and-needles sensation or loss of sensation. The symptoms begin suddenly in the legs and work upward to the arms.

In diabetic chronic polyneuropathy, only sensation is affected, most commonly in the feet. Pins and needles, numbness, and a burning sensation are prominent.

When people with a neuropathy are unable to sense pain, they can injure a joint many times without feeling it. The joint malfunctions and can progress to being permanently destroyed. Joints involved in this **neuropathic joint disease** are called **Charcot joints**.

Herpes zoster (shingles) is an infection of peripheral nerves arising from a reactivation of the primary virus infection in childhood with **chickenpox (varicella)**. During the primary infection of chickenpox, the virus gains entry into sensory dorsal root ganglia. Later in life, for unknown reasons, the virus can produce the painful, unilateral dermatome rash of shingles *(Figure 9.31)*.

Postherpetic neuralgia is acute dermatome pain persisting after the acute rash of shingles has subsided. It is debilitating and very difficult to treat.

Neuromuscular junction disorders occur where nerves connect with muscle fibers and interfere with the **neurotransmitter acetylcholine**. Examples are

- **Myasthenia gravis**, in which the immune system produces antibodies that attack the acetylcholine receptors on the muscle cells. The common symptoms are drooping eyelids; weak eye muscles, causing double vision; difficulty talking and swallowing; and muscle weakness in the limbs. Treatment is with a drug called **pyridostigmine**, which increases the amount of available acetylcholine.

- **Botulism**, a rare, life-threatening food poisoning caused by toxins from the bacterium *Clostridium botulinum*. These **neurotoxins** paralyze the muscles. In certain seasons, shellfish produce a similar neurotoxin.

- Certain **insecticides (organophosphates)** and nerve gases used in chemical warfare that act on neuromuscular junctions.

- Nerve compression occurring when the space around a nerve is constricted. The pinched nerve becomes edematous and later fibrotic and produces pain and paresthesias. Examples are sciatica when the sciatic nerve is compressed in the lower spine and carpal tunnel syndrome when the median nerve is compressed at the wrist.

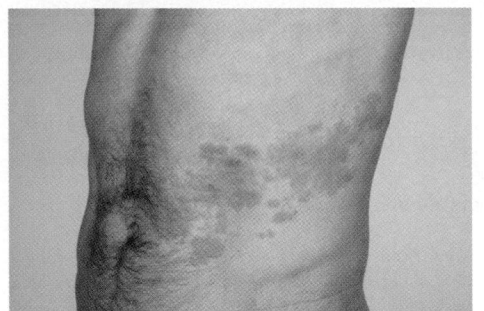

▲ **Figure 9.31** Herpes Zoster (Shingles).

Keynote

Herpes zoster occurs in people with depressed immune responses, HIV infection, or cancer and those on chemotherapy and/or radiation therapy, as well as for no apparent reason.

WORD	PRONUNCIATION		ELEMENTS	DEFINITION
botulism	**BOT**-you-lizm		Latin *sausage*	Food poisoning caused by the neurotoxin produced by *Clostridium botulinum*
Botox	**BO**-tox			Neurotoxin injected into muscles of the face to prevent the muscles from contracting and causing wrinkles
Charcot joint	**SHAR**-koh JOYNT		Jean-Martin Charcot, 1825–1893, French neurologist	Bone and joint destruction secondary to a neuropathy and loss of sensation
chickenpox varicella (syn)	**CHICK**-en-pocks		Disease originally considered a "chicken" (not dangerous) version of smallpox	Acute, contagious viral disease
Clostridium botulinum	klos-**TRID**-ee-um bot-you-**LIE**-num			Bacterium that causes food poisoning
insecticide	in-**SEK**-tih-side	S/ R/CF	–cide *kill* insect/i- *insect*	Agent that destroys insects
myasthenia gravis	my-as-**THEE**-nee-ah **GRA**-vis	S/ R/ P/ R/ R/	-ia *condition* my- *muscle* -a- *without* -sthen- *strength* gravis *serious*	Disorder of fluctuating muscle weakness
neuropathy neuropathic (adj) mononeuropathy polyneuropathy	nyu-**ROP**-ah-thee nyur-oh-**PATH**-ik **MON**-oh-nyu-**ROP**-ah-thee **POL**-ee-nyu-**ROP**-ah-thee	S/ R/CF P/ P/	-pathy *disease* neur/o- *nerve* mono- *one** poly- *many**	Any disease of the nervous system Disorder affecting a single nerve Disorder affecting many nerves
neurotoxin	**NYUR**-oh-tock-sin	R/ R/CF	-toxin *poison* neur/o- *nerve*	Agent that poisons the nervous system
organophosphate	**OR**-ga-no-**FOS**-fate	S/ R/CF R/	-ate *composed of* organ/o- *organic* -phosph- *phosphorus*	Organic phosphorus compound used as an insecticide
sciatica sciatic (adj)	sigh-**AT**-ih-kah sigh-**AT**-ik		Greek *related to the hip joint*	Pain from compression of L5 or S1 nerve roots Pertaining to the sciatic nerve or sciatica

Exercises

A. Complete the definition with the correct medical language. *Review the above WAD for the elements you need to construct the term. Fill in the blanks.*   **LO 9.9, 9.10**

💡 *Study Hint*
Add the terms indicated by asterisks (*) in the above WAD to your list of prefixes designating numbers.

1. Agent to destroy insects   _____/cide

2. Disorder affecting the nervous system   neuro/_____

3. Disorder of fluctuating muscle weakness   my/a/sthen/ _____/_____

4. Disorder affecting many nerves   _____/neuro/_____

B. Complete the definition with the correct medical language. *Review the above WAD for the elements you need to construct the term. Fill in the blanks.*   **LO 9.9, 9.10**

1. Agent that poisons the nervous system   _____/toxin

2. Another term for chickenpox   _____

3. Another term for botulism   _____

4. Used as an insecticide   organo/phosph/_____

5. Prefix meaning *affecting one*   _____

6. Prefix meaning *affecting many*   _____

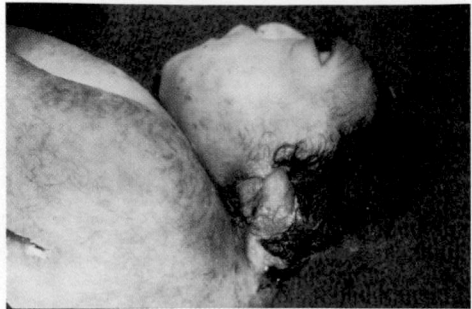

▲ **Figure 9.32**   Newborn with Anencephaly.

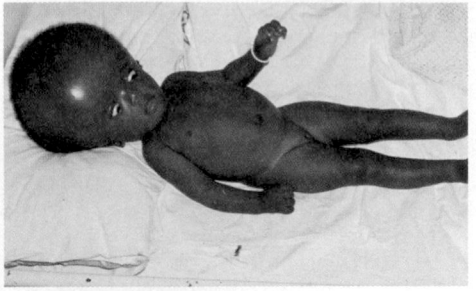

▲ **Figure 9.33**   Infant with Hydrocephalus.

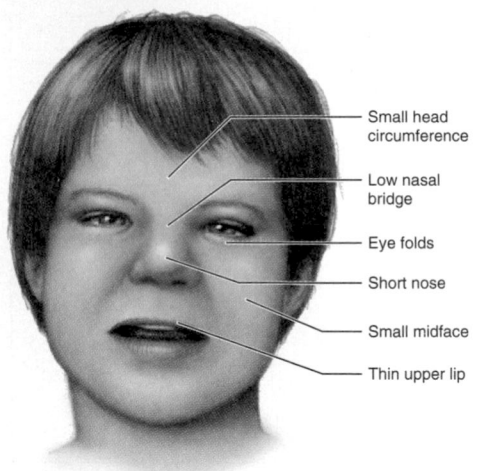

- Small head circumference
- Low nasal bridge
- Eye folds
- Short nose
- Small midface
- Thin upper lip

▲ **Figure 9.34**   Fetal Alcohol Syndrome.

Abbreviation	
FAS	fetal alcohol syndrome

LO 9.9, 9.10 Congenital Anomalies of the Nervous System

Some of the most devastating **congenital neurologic abnormalities** develop in the first 8 to 10 weeks of **gestation**, when the nervous system is in its early stages of formation. These malformations can be detected by using **ultrasonography** and **amniocentesis** *(see Chapter 8)*. Many can be prevented by the mother's taking 4 mg/day of **folic acid** before conception and during early pregnancy.

A **teratogen** is an agent that can cause malformations of an embryo or fetus *(see Chapter 8)*. It can be a chemical, virus, or radiation. Some teratogens are encountered in the workplace and include textile dyes, photographic chemicals, semiconductor materials, lead, mercury, and cadmium. One of the early uses of the drug thalidomide was to control morning sickness in pregnancy, but it caused severe limb and other deformities in the baby.

Anencephaly is absence of the cerebral hemispheres and is always fatal *(Figure 9.32)*.

Microcephaly, decreased head size, is associated with small cerebral hemispheres and with moderate to severe motor and mental retardation.

Hydrocephalus, ventricular enlargement in the cerebral hemispheres with excessive CSF, is usually due to an obstruction that prevents the CSF from exiting the ventricles to circulate around the spinal cord *(Figure 9.33)*. Treatment typically is to place a **shunt** to drain the CSF from the ventricles to either the peritoneal cavity or an atrium of the heart.

Fetal alcohol syndrome (FAS) can occur when a pregnant woman drinks alcohol. The child born with FAS has a small head, narrow eyes, and a flat face and nose *(Figure 9.34)*. Intellect and growth are **impaired.** Fetal alcohol syndrome is a cause of mental retardation.

Spina bifida occurs mostly in the lumbar and sacral regions *(Figure 9.35)*. It is very variable in its presentation and symptoms. **Spina bifida occulta** presents with a small partial defect in the vertebral arch. The spinal cord or meninges does not protrude. Often the only sign is a tuft of hair on the skin overlying the defect. In **spina bifida cystica**, no vertebral arch is formed. The spinal cord and meninges protrude through the opening and may or may not be covered with a thin layer of skin *(see Figure 9.35a and b)*. Protrusion of the meninges only is called a **meningocele**; protrusion of the meninges and spinal cord is called a **meningomyelocele.** Paralysis of the lower limbs may be present. The defect must be closed promptly to preserve spinal cord function and prevent infection. The cause of spina bifida is not known.

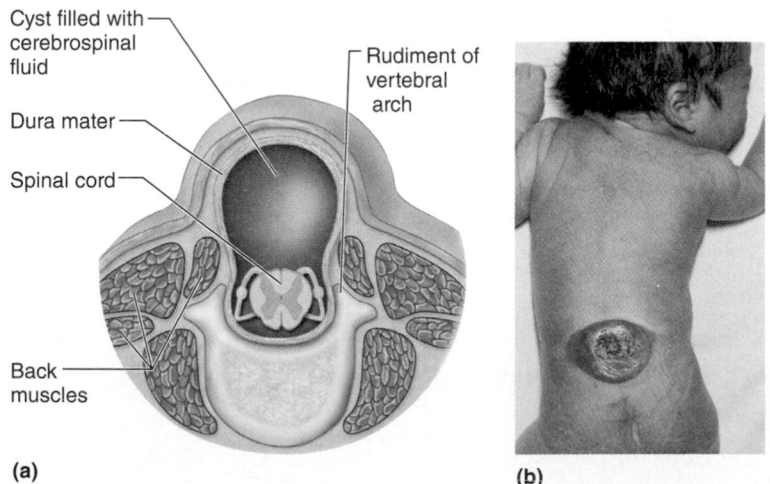

Cyst filled with cerebrospinal fluid

Dura mater

Spinal cord

Rudiment of vertebral arch

Back muscles

(a)

(b)

▲ **Figure 9.35**   **Spina Bifida Cystica.** *(a)* cross section of spinal cord in spina bifida cystica. *(b)* Child with spina bifida cystica.

Word Analysis and Definition

S = Suffix   P = Prefix   R = Root   R/CF = Combining Form

WORD	PRONUNCIATION	ELEMENTS		DEFINITION
anencephaly	**AN**-en-**SEF**-ah-lee	P/ R/	an- *without* -encephaly *condition of the brain*	Born without cerebral hemispheres
anomaly	ah-**NOM**-ah-lee		Greek *abnormality*	A structural abnormality
hydrocephalus	high-droh-**SEF**-ah-lus	S/ R/CF R/	-us *pertaining to* hydr/o- *water* -cephal- *head*	Enlarged head due to excess CSF in the cerebral ventricles
meningocele	meh-**NING**-oh-seal	S/ R/CF	-cele *hernia* mening/o- *meninges*	Protrusion of the meninges from the spinal cord or brain through a defect in the vertebral column or cranium
meningomyelocele	meh-**NIN**-goh-**MY**-el-oh-seal	S/ R/CF R/CF	-cele *hernia* -myel/o- *spinal cord* mening/o- *meninges*	Protrusion of the spinal cord and meninges through a defect in the vertebral arch of one or more vertebrae
microcephaly	**MY**-kroh-**SEF**-ah-lee	P/ R/	micro- *small* -cephaly *condition of the head*	An abnormally small head
spina bifida	**SPY**-nah **BIH**-fi-dah	R/CF P/ R/	spin/a *spine* bi- *two* -fida *split*	Failure of one or more vertebral arches to close during fetal development
spina bifida cystica	**SIS**-tik-ah	S/ R/	-ica *pertaining to* cyst- *cyst*	Meninges and spinal cord protruding through the absent vertebral arch and having the appearance of a cyst
spina bifida occulta	**OH**-kul-tah	R/	occulta *hidden*	The deformity of the vertebral arch is not apparent from the skin surface
teratogen	**TER**-ah-toe-jen	S/ R/CF	-gen *produce, create* terat/o- *monster, malformed fetus*	Agent that produces fetal deformities
teratogenic (adj) (**Note:** Has two suffixes.)	**TER**-ah-toe-jen-ik	S/	-ic *pertaining to*	Capable of producing fetal deformities

Exercises

A. Search and find the correct term for the element you are given. *Circle the best answer.*   **LO 9.4, 9.9, 9.10**

1. Find the term with the prefix meaning *without:*

   hydrocephalus   anencephaly   impairment

2. Find the term with the root meaning *cyst:*

   meningocele   cystica   teratogen

3. Find the term with the root meaning *monster:*

   teratogen   spina   myelomeningocele

4. Find the term with the root meaning *split:*

   bifida   occulta   cystica

5. Find the term with the root meaning *head:*

   anomaly   hydrocephalus   meningocele

6. Find the term with the root meaning *hidden:*

   spina bifida   spina bifida cystica spina bifida occulta

7. Find the term with the combining form meaning *water:*

   teratogenic   hydrocephalus   myelomeningocele

8. Find the term with the suffix meaning *hernia:*

   meningocele   hydrocephalus   anomaly

9. Find the term with the combining form meaning *spinal cord:*

   menigomyelocele cystocele   meningocele

10. Find the term with the prefix meaning *small:*

   anencephaly   teratogenic   microcephaly

LO 9.11 Diagnostic Procedures in Neurology

Lumbar puncture (spinal tap) has been shown earlier. Laboratory examination of the CSF that shows white blood cells suggests meningitis. High protein levels indicate meningitis or damage to the brain or spinal cord. Blood suggests a brain hemorrhage or a traumatic tap.

Electroencephalography records the brain's electrical activity and helps identify seizure disorders, sleep disturbances, degenerative brain disorders, and brain damage *(Figure 9.36)*.

Computed tomography (CT), a computer-enhanced x-ray technique, generates images of slices of the brain and can detect a wide range of brain and spinal cord disorders, including tumors, areas of dead brain tissue due to stroke, and birth defects.

Magnetic resonance imaging (MRI) produces highly detailed anatomical images of most neurologic disorders, including strokes, brain tumors, and myelin sheath damage *(Figure 9.37)*.

Magnetic resonance angiography uses an injection of a radiopaque dye to produce images of blood vessels of the head and neck during MRI.

Cerebral angiography is an invasive procedure in which a radiopaque dye is injected into the blood vessels of the neck and brain. It can detect blood vessels that are partially or completely blocked, aneurysms, or arteriovenous malformations.

Color Doppler ultrasonography uses high-frequency sound (ultrasound) waves to show different rates of blood flow through the arteries of the neck or the base of the brain. This evaluates TIAs and the risk of a full-blown stroke.

Echoencephalography uses ultrasound waves to produce an image of the brain in children under the age of 2 because their skulls are thin enough for the waves to pass through them.

Positron emission tomography (PET) involves attaching radioactive molecules onto a substance necessary for brain function (for example, the sugar glucose). As the molecules circulate in the brain, the radioactive labels give off positively charged signals that can be recorded *(Figure 9.38)*.

Myelography is the use of x-rays of the spinal cord that are taken after a radiopaque dye has been injected into the CSF by spinal tap. It has been replaced by MRI when that is available.

Evoked responses are a procedure in which stimuli for vision, sound, and touch are used to activate specific areas of the brain and their responses are measured with EEG or PET scans. This provides information about how that specific area of the brain is functioning in disorders such as MS.

Electromyography involves placing small needles into a muscle to record its electrical activity at rest and during contraction. It is used to provide information in disorders of muscles, peripheral nerves, and the **neuromuscular** junction.

Nerve conduction studies measure the speed at which motor or sensory nerves conduct impulses. The studies exclude disorders of the brain, spinal cord, and muscles and focus on the peripheral nerves.

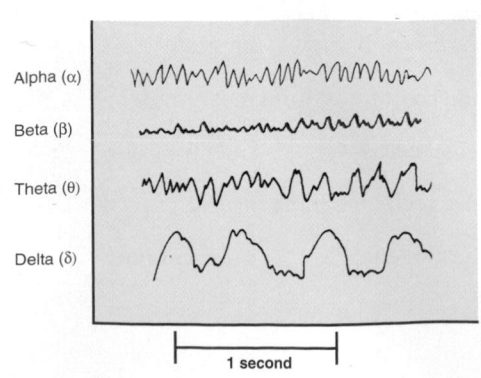

▲ **Figure 9.36** Four Classes of Brain Waves on EEG.

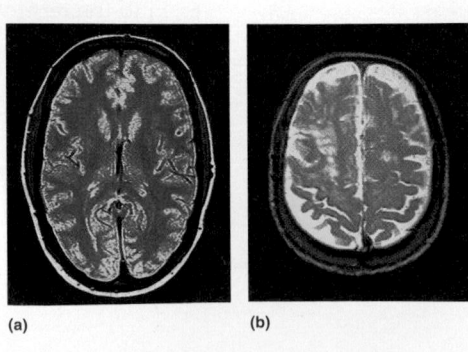

▲ **Figure 9.37** MRI Scans of Brain Sections. *(a)* Scan of normal brain. *(b)* Scan of Alzheimer disease showing cerebral atrophy *(yellow)*.

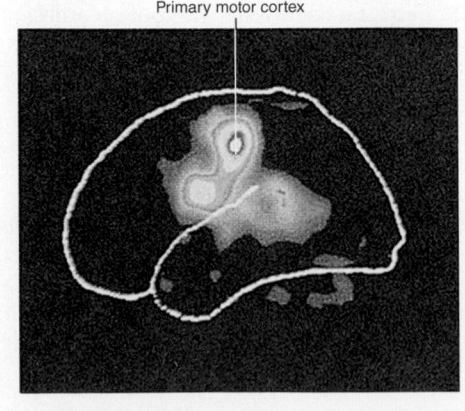

▲ **Figure 9.38** PET Scan of the Brain Showing the Motor Cortex.

S = Suffix   P = Prefix   R = Root   R/CF = Combining Form

WORD	PRONUNCIATION	ELEMENTS		DEFINITION
Doppler	**DOP**-ler		Johann Christian Doppler, 1803–1853, Austrian mathematician and physicist	Diagnostic instrument that sends an ultrasonic beam into the body
Doppler ultrasonography color Doppler ultrasonography	**DOP**-ler **UL**-trah-soh-**NOG**-rah-fee	S/ P/ R/CF	**-graphy** *process of recording* **ultra-** *beyond* **-son/o-** *sound*	Imaging that detects direction, velocity, and turbulence of blood flow; used in workup of stroke patients Computer-generated color image to show directions of blood flow
echoencephalography	**EK**-oh-en-sef-ah-**LOG**-rah-fee	S/ R/CF P/ R/CF	**-graphy** *process of recording* **ech/o-** *sound wave* **-en-** *in* **-cephal/o-** *head*	Use of ultrasound in the diagnosis of intracranial lesions
electroencephalogram (EEG)	ee-**LEK**-troh-en-**SEF**-ah-low-gram	S/ R/CF R/CF	**-gram** *recording* **electr/o-** *electricity* **-encephal/o-** *brain*	Record of the electrical activity of the brain
electroencephalograph	ee-**LEK**-troh-en-**SEF**-ah-low-graf	S/	**-graph** *to write, record*	Device used to record the electrical activity of the brain
electroencephalography	ee-**LEK**-troh-en-**SEF**-ah-**LOG**-rah-fee	S/	**-graphy** *process of recording*	The process of recording the electrical activity of the brain
electromyography	ee-**LEK**-troh-my-**OG**-rah-fee	S/ R/CF R/CF	**-graphy** *process of recording* **electr/o-** *electricity* **-my/o-** *muscle*	Recording of electrical activity in muscle
myelography	my-eh-**LOG**-rah-fee	S/ R/CF	**-graphy** *process of recording* **myel/o-** *spinal cord*	Radiography of the spinal cord and nerve roots after injection of contrast medium into the subarachnoid space
nerve conduction study	NERV kon-**DUK**-shun **STUD**-ee	R/ S/ P/ R/	**nerve** *nerve* **-ion** *action* **con-** *with, together* **-duct-** *lead* **study** *inquiry*	Procedure to measure the speed at which an electrical impulse travels along a nerve
neuromuscular	**NYUR**-oh-**MUSS**-kyu-lar	S/ R/CF R/	**-ar** *pertaining to* **neur/o-** *nerve* **-muscul-** *muscle*	Pertaining to both nerves and muscles

Exercises

A. Meet a learning outcome by demonstrating your knowledge of diagnostic procedures in neurology. *All the answers can be found on the opposite page. Fill in the blanks.*   **LO 9.11**

1. Which procedures can be considered *invasive* procedures? _____

_____

2. What makes a procedure *invasive?* _____

_____

3. Which procedures involve the use of injections of dye or radioactive molecules? _____

_____

4. Which procedures involve high-frequency sound waves? _____

_____

5. Which procedures measure electrical activity? _____

_____

Abbreviations

LSD	lysergic acid diethylamide
MDMA	methylenedioxy-methamphetamine (ecstasy)
PCP	phencyclidine (angel dust)
THC	tetrahydrocannabinol (marijuana)

LO 9.12 Pharmacology of the Nervous System

The transmission of impulses from one neuron to another and from a neuron to a cell is achieved by neurotransmitters at synaptic connections. Drugs that affect the nervous system, called *psychoactive drugs,* target this synaptic mechanism.

Psychoactive drugs are able to change mood, behavior, cognition, and anxiety. They can be classified into several families:

1. Stimulants—caffeine, nicotine, amphetamines, and cocaine—enhance the stimulation provided by the sympathetic nervous system. They cause the level of dopamine to rise in the synapses, leading to the pleasurable effects associated with these drugs.

2. Sedatives—ethanol (beverage alcohol), barbiturates, and meprobamate—decrease the sensitivity of the postsynaptic neurons to quiet the nervous excitement. They also act on the sleep centers to induce sleep.

3. Inhaled anesthetics such as isoflurane act similarly to but are more powerful than sedatives.

4. Opiates—morphine, codeine, heroin, methadone, and oxycodone—-depress nerve transmission in the synapses of sensory pathways of the brain and spinal cord. They also inhibit centers in the brain controlling coughing, breathing, and intestinal motility. Codeine is used in cough medicines. Constipation is a side effect of all these drugs. Opiates are addictive because they produce tolerance and physical dependence.

5. Opiate antagonists, such as naloxone and naltrexone, prevent opiates from acting in the synapses. They can be used in drug overdose and to help recovering heroin addicts stay drug-free.

6. Tranquilizers, such as chlorpromazine, haloperidol, and the benzodiazepines (Librium, Valium, Xanax), act like sedatives but without their sleep-inducing effect.

7. Antidepressants all increase the amount of serotonin at the synapses, where it is a neuro-transmitter. Zoloft and Prozac are examples.

8. Antiepileptics act in different ways on the synaptic junction to keep stimuli from passing across the synapse. Phenytoin and carbamazepine are examples.

9. Psychedelics distort sensory perceptions, particularly sight and sound. They can be natural plant products, such as mescaline, psilocybin, and dimethyltryptamine. They can be synthetic, such as **lysergic acid diethylamide (LSD)**, **methylenedioxymethamphetamine (MDMA** or "ecstasy"), and **phencyclidine (PCP** or "angel dust"). They increase the amount of serotonin in the synaptic junctions, and some have an additional amphetamine stimulation.

10. Marijuana has the active ingredient **tetrahydrocannabinol (THC).** It produces the drowsiness of sedatives like alcohol, the dulling of pain like opiates, and, in high doses, the perception distortions of the psychedelics. Unlike the case with opiates or sedatives, tolerance does not occur.

WORD	PRONUNCIATION	ELEMENTS		DEFINITION
addict	**AD**-ikt	P/ R/	ad- *to* -dict *consent, surrender*	Person with a psychologic or physical dependence on a substance or practice
addiction	ah-**DIK**-shun	S/	-ion *condition, action*	Habitual psychologic and physiologic dependence on a substance or practice
addictive	ah-**DIK**-tiv	S/	-ive *quality of, pertaining to*	Pertaining to or causing addiction
antagonist	an-**TAG**-oh-nist	S/ P/ R/	-ist *agent* ant- *against* -agon- *contest against*	An opposing structure, agent, disease, or process
antagonism	an-**TAG**-oh-nizm	S/	-ism *process, action*	Situation of opposing
marijuana	mar-ih-**HWAN**-ah		Mexican Spanish *María Juana*	Dried, flowering leaves of the plant *Cannabis sativa*
psychedelic	sigh-keh-**DEL**-ik	S/ R/CF R/	-ic *pertaining to* psych/e- *mind, soul* -del- *visible*	Agent that intensifies sensory perception
psychoactive	sigh-koh-**AK**-tiv	S/ R/CF R/	-ive *quality of, pertaining to* psych/o- *mind, soul* -act- *to do*	Able to alter mood, behavior, and/or cognition
sedative	**SED**-ah-tiv	S/	-ive *quality of, pertaining to*	Agent that calms nervous excitement
sedation	seh-**DAY**-shun	R/ S/	sedat- *to calm* -ion *condition, action*	State of being calmed
stimulant	**STIM**-you-lant	S/	-ant *forming*	Agent that excites or strengthens functional activity
stimulate (verb)	**STIM**-you-late	R/	stimul- *excite, strengthen*	
stimulation	stim-you-**LAY**-shun	S/	-ation *process*	Arousal to increased functional activity
synthetic	sin-**THET**-ik	S/ P/	-ic *pertaining to* syn- *together*	Built up or put together from simpler compounds
synthesis (noun)	**SIN**-the-sis	R/ S/	-thet- *place, arrange* -esis *abnormal condition*	The process of building a compound from different elements
tolerance	**TOL**-er-ants	S/ R/	-ance *state of, condition* toler- *endure*	The capacity to become accustomed to a stimulus or drug
tranquilizer	**TRANG**-kwih-lie-zer	S/ R/	-izer *affects in a particular way* tranquil- *calm*	Agent that calms without sedating or depressing

Exercises

A. Deconstruct this *language of neurology* into its basic elements to help understand the meaning of the term. *Write the elements between the slashes. <u>The first one is done for you.</u> Every term does not need every element, so you will have some blanks.*   **LO 9.4, 9.12**

1. antagonist   _____ant_____ / _____agon_____ / _____ist_____

2. addict   _____/_____/_____

3. tranquilizer   _____/_____/_____

4. stimulant   _____/_____/_____

5. synthetic   _____/_____/_____

6. psychedelic   _____/_____/_____

7. tolerance   _____/_____/_____

8. psychoactive   _____/_____/_____

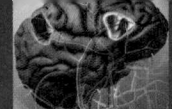

Chapter 9 Review

Nervous System

Challenge Your Knowledge

A. Construct the proper medical terms for the statements. You have an assortment of prefixes, roots, combining forms, and suffixes with which to construct your terms. Fill in the blanks. (**LO 9.4**, *Remember*)

hydro	**lepsy**	**esthesia**
narco	**lysis**	**a**
algia	**occulta**	**para**
neur/o	**itis**	**post**
an	**trophy**	

1. Recurring episodes of falling asleep during the day: _____

2. Complete loss of sensation: _____

3. Pain in the distribution of a nerve: _____

4. Wasting away of tissue: _____

5. Derived from a word meaning *hidden:* _____

B. Terminology challenge. The difference in one or two letters makes for precision in medical language. *Brady-* and *brachy-* have two different meanings. Define them below, and give an example of their use in a term. (**LO 9.3**, *Remember, Understand*)

Brady- means _____. Example: _____.

Brachy- means _____. Example: _____.

C. Similar but different. The following medical terms contain a similar root, but the suffixes change the meaning of the terms. Use the correct form of these terms in the following sentences. Fill in the blanks. (**LO 9.4**, *Remember, Understand*)

neurosurgery	**neurologic**	**neurologist**	**neurosurgeon**	**neurology**

The _____ from the Fulwood _____ Department referred the patient to a _____ for surgical consultation. The patient's _____ condition was deteriorating rapidly, and she would probably need _____.

D. Word building skills. Combine your knowledge of word elements and medical terminology construction, together with the power of your millions of brain cells, to answer the following questions. (**LO 9.2**, *Remember, Apply*)

1. In the term **neuralgia**, the suffix is _____, which means _____. If the element **ceph** means *head*, what does the term **cephalgia** mean? _____

   What does the term **arthralgia** mean? _____. If the element **caus** means *burning*, what is **causalgia**?

   _____

2. Exacerbation and remission are defined by their elements. Using their elements, explain the difference between these two processes.

   Exacerbation means _____.

   Remission means _____.

E. **Diseases and disorders.** The Fulwood Neurology Clinic treats patients with varied diseases and disorders of the nervous system. Are you familiar enough with their terminology and symptoms to match the correct disease or disorder with the appropriate statement for each patient? Circle the correct choice. (**LO 9.9, 9.10,** *Remember, Understand*)

1. Patient has had a hemorrhagic stroke. Another name for this is

   intercranial hemorrhage   intercerebral hemorrhage   intracranial hemorrhage

2. Patient bumped head on low doorway:

   concussion   seizure   convulsion

3. Patient has inflammation of the parenchyma of the brain:

   meningitis   encephalitis   vasculitis

4. Infection of the peripheral nerves arising from a reactivation of the chickenpox (varicella) virus is

   herpes simplex   shingles   post herpetic neuralgia

5. Infant has motor impairment resulting from brain damage at birth:

   Bell palsy   cerebral palsy   palsy

6. Patient had very bad dental infection that resulted in bloodborne pathogens lodging in her brain:

   brain tumor   brain abscess   brain hematoma

7. Patient complains of intermittent, shooting pain in the area of the face and head:

   trigeminal neuralgia   peripheral neuropathy   neuritis

F. **Abbreviations are helpful only if you know what they are meant to communicate.** Rewrite the following sentences without their abbreviations, but communicate the same message. (**LO 9.6,** *Remember, Apply*)

1. The patient's CVA has affected her CNS.

   _____

   _____

2. The BBB exists to protect brain tissue.

   _____

   _____

3. The patient's CSF will be tested today with a LP.

   _____

   _____

G. **Plurals.** Refresh your memory on the rules for plurals. Precision in communication depends on this. The singular form is given; circle the best answer for the plural form. (**LO 9.4, 9.5,** *Understand*)

   1. **ganglion:**   ganglius   ganglia   gangli

   2. **plexus:**   plexuses   plexuia   plexui

   3. **sulcus:**   sulces   sulci   sulcia

   4. **gyrus:**   gyri   gryia   gryuses

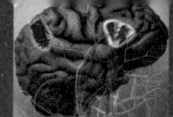

Nervous System

H. Roots and combining forms remain the core of a medical term. Reinforce your knowledge of these elements with this exercise. Match the correct root or combining form in the left column to its meaning in the right column. (**LO 9.4**, *Understand*)

_____ 1. pathy		**a.** hearing
_____ 2. cephalo		**b.** first
_____ 3. algesia		**c.** sleep
_____ 4. syringo		**d.** blood vessel
_____ 5. audit		**e.** tube, pipe
_____ 6. trophy		**f.** disease
_____ 7. proto		**g.** development
_____ 8. pleg		**h.** head
_____ 9. somn		**i.** sensation of pain
_____ 10. angio		**j.** paralysis

I. Prefixes can be a very important part of medical terms. Challenge your knowledge of this chapter's prefixes by correctly filling in the following chart. You are given either the meaning or the prefix—complete the rest of the chart. (**LO 9.4**, *Understand*)

Prefix	Meaning of Prefix	Medical Term Containing This Prefix	Meaning of Medical Term
dis	1.	2.	3.
con	4.	5.	6.
7.	self	8.	9.
re	10.	11.	12.
13.	together	14.	15.
an	16.	17.	18.
de	19.	20.	21.

J. Medical language. The nervous system is a complicated one and has a large range of vocabulary. Assess your knowledge of the nervous system by circling the correct answer in the following questions. (**LO 9.4, 9.5,** *Understand*)

1. Abnormal movements marked by rapid contraction and relaxation of a muscle or muscle groups are called

   a. compression

   b. clonic

   c. coma

   d. contusion

   e. concussion

2. Astrocytes, oligodendrocytes, microglia, ependymal, Schwann, and satellite are all terms relating to

   a. capillaries

   b. tumors

   c. hematomas

   d. neuroglia

   e. ganglia

3. Body temperature is regulated by the

   a. thalamus

   b. hypothalamus

   c. limbic system

   d. pons

   e. cerebellum

4. Centers that control vital visceral activities are located in the

   a. pons

   b. corpus

   c. medulla oblongata

   d. hypothalamus

   e. CSF

K. Latin and Greek terms do not deconstruct like some medical terms. Test your knowledge of these terms with this exercise. Match the terms in the left column to their correct meaning in the right column. (**LO 9.4,** *Understand*)

_____ 1. epilepsy	a.	stroke
_____ 2. sulcus	b.	seizure
_____ 3. efferent	c.	brain
_____ 4. cerebrum	d.	ditch, furrow
_____ 5. ictal	e.	away from

Nervous System

L. Medical language. The nervous system is a complicated one and has a large range of vocabulary. Assess your knowledge of the nervous system by circling the correct answer in the following questions. **(LO 9.4, 9.5, 9.6, *Understand*)**

1. An agent capable of preventing or arresting epilepsy is called an

   a. antidiuretic

   b. antibiotic

   c. antiepileptic

   d. antidepressant

   e. antibody

2. Administration of tPA is for

   a. ALS

   b. thrombolysis

   c. seizures

   d. dementia

   e. meningitis

3. **Hypoglossal** refers to structures that can be found under the

   a. diaphragm

   b. tongue

   c. jawbone

   d. bronchus

   e. alveoli

4. In simple terms, a **synapse** is a

   a. malformation

   b. birth defect

   c. junction

   d. seizure

   e. vesicle

5. Implantation of radioactive pellets directly into a tumor is called

   a. bradytherapy

   b. bradycardia

   c. brachytherapy

   d. brachial plexus

   e. none of the above

6. A state of deep unconsciousness is called

   a. coma

   b. seizure

   c. sulcus

   d. dementia

   e. syncope

7. The groove that separates gyri is called

   a. gyrus

   b. cortex

   c. fissure

   d. sulcus

   e. dermatome

8. The cerebral hemispheres are covered by a thin layer of gray matter called the

   a. basal ganglia

   b. corpus callosum

   c. frontal lobe

   d. cerebral cortex

   e. cerebellum

9. The abbreviation for a short-term, small stroke is

   a. EEG

   b. HACE

   c. TIA

   d. PET

   e. SBS

10. The medical term that means *pertaining to or caused by a seizure* is

    a. clonic

    b. ictal

    c. tonic

    d. visceral

    e. synaptic

M. **In your own words.** Translate into layman's terms these sentences directly from this chapter. How well do you understand what you read? Can you explain these sentences in nonmedical language? Rewrite each sentence in your own words. (**LO 9.4, 9.5, Apply, Analyze**)

1. Brain abscess is most often a direct spread of infection from sinusitis, otitis media, or mastoiditis.

_____

_____

_____

2. Carotid endarterectomy may be necessary if a carotid artery is significantly occluded with plaque.

_____

_____

_____

3. Risk factors for hemorrhagic strokes are hypertension, cerebral arteriovenous malformation, and cerebral aneurysms.

_____

_____

_____

4. Cerebral angiography can detect blood vessels that are occluded, aneurysms, or arteriovenous malformations.

_____

_____

_____

5. Anencephaly is absence of the cerebral hemispheres and is incompatible with life.

_____

_____

_____

Nervous System

N. Test-taking strategy practice. Use your knowledge of medical terminology to insert the correct term in the appropriate statement. Not all answers will be used, and no answer will be used more than once. (**LO 9.4,** *Apply*)

hemiplegia	somatic	afferent
meningitis	meningioma	quadriplegia
festinant	comatose	visceral
neurotransmitters	dendrite	dementia

> **Study Hint**
> Start by answering the questions for which you are sure of the correct answer. Cross off the answer in the column after you insert it in the statement, and then answer the rest of the questions from the choices you have left. You will then be working with a smaller and smaller group of choices, which will make it easier to spot the correct answer.

1. _____ nerves, which carry signals from major organs such as the heart, lungs, stomach, and intestines

2. State of deep unconsciousness: _____

3. A process or extension of a neuron: _____

4. Shuffling gait: _____

5. Loss of the mind's cognitive functions: _____

6. Paralysis of all four limbs: _____

7. Chemicals that cross the synapse to another neuron: _____

8. _____ nerves, which carry signals from the skin, muscles, bones, and joints

O. Proofread your documentation. The radiologist has just dictated the following report for a patient of the Fulwood Neurology Clinic. Before you print a final copy, always proofread the document for errors. Can you find the errors in the report? Circle the incorrect words in the report; then write the corrected words on the lines below, and include a brief definition for each correct word. (**LO 9.1,** *Analyze*)

CT SCAN OF THE HEAD

CT of the head: CT of the head performed without IV contrast demonstrates mild dilutation of the venticular system. The sulcuses are also prominent. These findings are consistent with mild atrophie.

No intracerbral hemorhage, subdaral, or epedural hemetoma is noted. No shift of the midline structures is noted. IMPRESSION: mild cerebral atrohy.

_____

_____

_____

_____

_____

_____

_____

_____

P. **Analyze the following diagnostic procedures on the basis of their elements alone; then answer the questions.** Fill in the blanks. **(LO 9.11, *Analyze*)**

1. **echoencephalography**

   The combining form _____ tells me this is a diagnostic procedure on the _____.

2. **electromyography**

   The combining form _____ tells me this is a diagnostic procedure on the _____.

3. **myelography**

   The combining form _____ tells me this is a diagnostic procedure on the _____.

4. **electroencephalography**

   The combining form _____ tells me this is a diagnostic procedure on the _____.

5. Each of the four procedures listed previously ends with the suffix _____, which means

   _____.

6. Change the suffix in each of these terms to -*gram*, which means the actual record produced by the diagnostic procedure.

   Write the new terms in the following blank. _____

   _____

Use the terms in questions 1 to 6 to identify (define) the statements in questions 7 through 10. (*Hint:* In some cases you are asked for the *record*, and in some cases you are asked for the *recording*.) Be precise! Fill in the blanks.

7. Recording of electrical activity in muscle: _____

8. Use of ultrasound in the diagnosis of intracranial lesions: _____

9. Radiography of the spinal cord and nerve roots after injection of contrast medium into the subarachnoid space:

   _____

10. Record of the electrical activity of the brain: _____

Select any two of the diagnostic procedures in this exercise and describe their function or purpose.

11. Procedure: _____

    Purpose: _____

12. Procedure: _____

    Purpose: _____

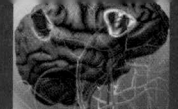

Nervous System

Q. Precision of medical language. Medical language has many terms that look and sound similar. You must use the precise term in spoken and written medical communication and documentation. If a patient were to ask, you should be able to explain to him or her the difference between the following pairs of words a. Write a short explanation for each. (**LO 9.4, 9.5,** *Analyze*)

1. *concussion* and *contusion:*

_____

_____

2. *meningitis* and *meningioma:*

_____

_____

3. *cerebellum* and *cerebrum:*

_____

_____

R. Diagnostic testing. You are responsible for scheduling diagnostic procedures for patients in the Neurology Clinic at Fulwood Medical Center. Practice your *language of neurology* by scheduling these patients appropriately, using the following procedures. (**LO 9.11,** *Analyze*)

CT scan	angiography
myelography	magnetic resonance imaging
evoked responses	nerve conduction studies
electromyography	electroencephalogram
lumbar puncture or spinal tap	magnetic resonance angiography

Patient Needs/Symptoms:	Schedule Patient For:
1. Dr. Solis would like to measure the speed at which a patient's motor nerves conduct impulses.	
2. Doctor has ordered a recording of the electrical activity of the patient's brain.	
3. Dr. Solis suspects a tumor and needs to see a highly detailed anatomical image of the brain.	
4. Patient needs x-rays of the spinal cord taken after dye has been injected into it.	
5. Dr. Solis wants a sample of the patient's CSF.	
6. Patient has to schedule a study with contrast to image the cerebral blood vessels.	
7. Patient has a blocked carotid artery.	
8. Patient has possibly had a stroke; study will be looking for areas of dead brain tissue.	
9. Sensory stimuli will be used to activate specific areas of the brain and measure responses with EEG.	
10. Doctor wants to test and record the electrical activity of a patient's muscle at rest and during contractions	

S. Precision in documentation. One of the five descriptions that follow is clearly the best choice for your answer—circle it, and explain why it is the best choice. (**LO 9.9,** *Analyze*)

What type of tumors arise from glial cells?

tumors   primary tumors   secondary tumors   primary brain tumors   secondary brain tumors

The most precise description is _____ because _____

_____.

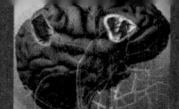
Nervous System

CHAPTER SUMMARY EXERCISE

A. Spelling comprehension. Circle the correct spelling of the term. (**LO 9.4,** *Understand*)

1. synapse	sinapse	synipse	sinipse	synapsse
2. attetosis	athitoses	athitosis	athetosis	atetosis
3. Altheimer	Altzheimer	Alheimer	Alsheimer	Alzheimer
4. poleomielitis	polliomielitis	poliomyelitis	poliomielitis	poleomyelitis
5. serebelum	cerebellum	cerabelum	cerebelum	serabelum
6. perresthesia	paresthesia	peristhesia	parrestetia	peristesia
7. ketaplexy	cataprexie	ketaplexie	cataplexy	cateplexy
8. menninges	minengies	meninges	menningese	minenges
9. fantom	pantom	phantom	pantome	phantum
10. okcipital	ocipital	occipital	ocipitul	occipitule

B. Match the number of the correct spelling of the term in Exercise A with the one of the following brief descriptions of the terms. (**LO 9.4,** *Apply*)

1. Posterior brain between midbrain and cerebral hemispheres _____

2. Three-layered covering of the brain and spinal cord _____

3. Inflammation of the gray matter of the spinal cord _____

4. Junction between two nerve cells _____

5. Abnormal sensation like tingling, burning _____

6. Slow, writhing, involuntary movements _____

7. Sensation of a limb being present after amputation _____

8. Common form of dementia _____

9. Sudden loss of muscle tone with brief paralysis _____

10. Back of the head _____

C. Using your knowledge of terms 1–10 in Exercises A and B and their correct spelling, write a brief sentence for each of the terms as it might appear in patient documentation. (LO 9.4, *Evaluate*)

1. _____

2. _____

3. _____

4. _____

5. _____

6. _____

7. _____

8. _____

9. _____

10. _____

D. Classify each of the lobes of the brain and state their functions. (LO 9.7, *Remember*)

_____

_____

_____

E. Demonstrate your ability to communicate in the language of neurology by answering the following questions. Be prepared to define any of the medical terms in class if asked by the instructor. (**LO 9.4, 9.9,** *Remember, Understand*)

1. Risk factors for ischemic strokes are _____

2. The hypothalamus regulates _____

3. What is a medical term that means the same thing as *hemorrhagic stroke?* _____

4. Name one tic disorder. _____

5. Identify all the prefixes in the following terms and list their common grouping: quadriplegia, monoplegia, triplegia, bilateral.

_____

Prefixes: _____

All can be grouped as prefixes of: _____

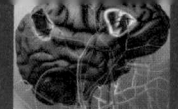

Nervous System

F. **Show your comprehension of the language of neurology by answering the following questions. (LO 9.5, 9.4, 9.6,** *Remember, Understand, Apply*)

1. Interpret (rewrite) this physician's order without using the abbreviations: "Mr. Baker should be scheduled for an MRI and PET scan first thing in the AM." _____

   _____

2. If a patient is suffering from PPS, what previous disease has he recovered from? _____

   _____

3. What is a plexus? _____

   _____

4. What is the logical term to complete this group? axon, dendrite, synapse, _____

   _____

5. Many medications are unable to pass the BBB, but one substance can get through. What is that substance? _____

6. Hypoglossal has the same meaning as _____.

7. TIA and CVA are both abbreviations associated with _____.

8. Quadriplegia, diplegia, hemiplegia, monoplegia, paraplegia, and triplegia *all* refer to _____.

9. Translate into layman's language: "This transient neurologic deficit is called a postictal state." _____

   _____

G. **If you really know it, you can explain it to someone else.** What is the difference among the following choices? (**LO 9.8,** *Remember, Apply*)

1. impairment, handicap, and disability?

   a. impairment

   _____

   b. handicap

   _____

   c. disability

   _____

2. hemiplegia and hemiparesis?

   a. hemiplegia

   _____

   b. hemiparesis

   _____

3. phantom pain and referred pain?

   a. phantom pain

   _____

   b. referred pain

   _____

> ## Study Hint
> The following is an acronym for remembering the functions of the nervous system: MMESH
> M   motor OUTput
> M   mental activity
> E   evaluation and integration
> S   sensory INput
> H   homeostasis

H. Meet the goals of each of the chapter outcomes and insert the correct answers to the following questions. (LO 9.1–9.12, *Analyze*)

1. What does a neurosurgeon do that a neurologist cannot do? _____ **(LO 9.1)**

2. Which of the following vocabulary is not related to cells of the nervous system? **(LO 9.2)**

   a. neurons

   b. axon

   c. dendrite

   d. synapse

   e. sublingual

3. Homeostasis is a **(LO 9.3)**

   a. disease of the nervous system

   b. function of the nervous system

   c. condition of the nervous system

   d. symptom of a nervous condition

   e. structure in the nervous system

4. In the chart of a patient with brain cancer, you would use the term **(LO 9.4)**

   a. Doppler

   b. glioma

   c. angioplasty

   d. EEG

   e. dendrite

5. If you have to tell a patient their cancer has spread, you would use the term **(LO 9.5)**

   a. metastasis

   b. visceral

   c. peripheral

   d. microglia

   e. decussate

6. Which of the following is the only abbreviation that pertains to the nervous system? **(LO 9.6)**

   a. VS

   b. MRI

   c. UTI

   d. URI

   e. C5

7. The thalamus and hypothalamus are major regions of the brain. Describe their functions. **(LO 9.7)**

   Thalamus:

   _____

   Hypothalamus:

   _____

8. Describe the structure and function of the meninges: **(LO 9.8)**

   _____

   _____

9. Choose any three common disorders of the brain and describe their effect on health. **(LO 9.9)**

   _____

   _____

10. What is the difference between an epidural hematoma and a subdural hematoma, and how do their effects differ? **(LO 9.10)**

    _____

    _____

11. What fluid collected from the nervous system can be a diagnostic tool? **(LO 9.11)**

12. Tolerance does not occur in what family of drugs? **(LO 9.12)**

    _____

Cardiovascular System
The Language of Cardiology

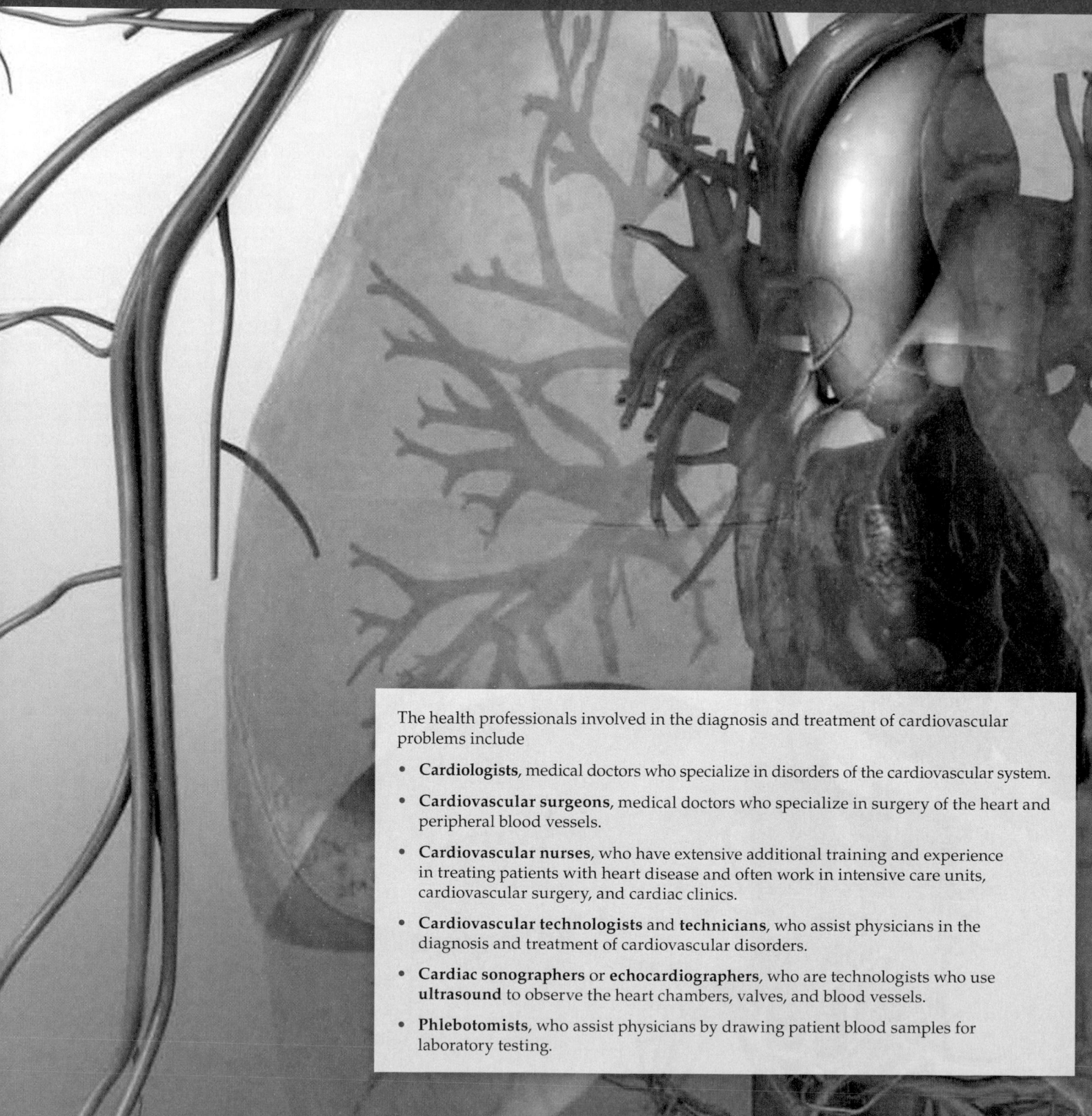

The health professionals involved in the diagnosis and treatment of cardiovascular problems include

- **Cardiologists**, medical doctors who specialize in disorders of the cardiovascular system.

- **Cardiovascular surgeons**, medical doctors who specialize in surgery of the heart and peripheral blood vessels.

- **Cardiovascular nurses**, who have extensive additional training and experience in treating patients with heart disease and often work in intensive care units, cardiovascular surgery, and cardiac clinics.

- **Cardiovascular technologists** and **technicians**, who assist physicians in the diagnosis and treatment of cardiovascular disorders.

- **Cardiac sonographers** or **echocardiographers**, who are technologists who use **ultrasound** to observe the heart chambers, valves, and blood vessels.

- **Phlebotomists**, who assist physicians by drawing patient blood samples for laboratory testing.

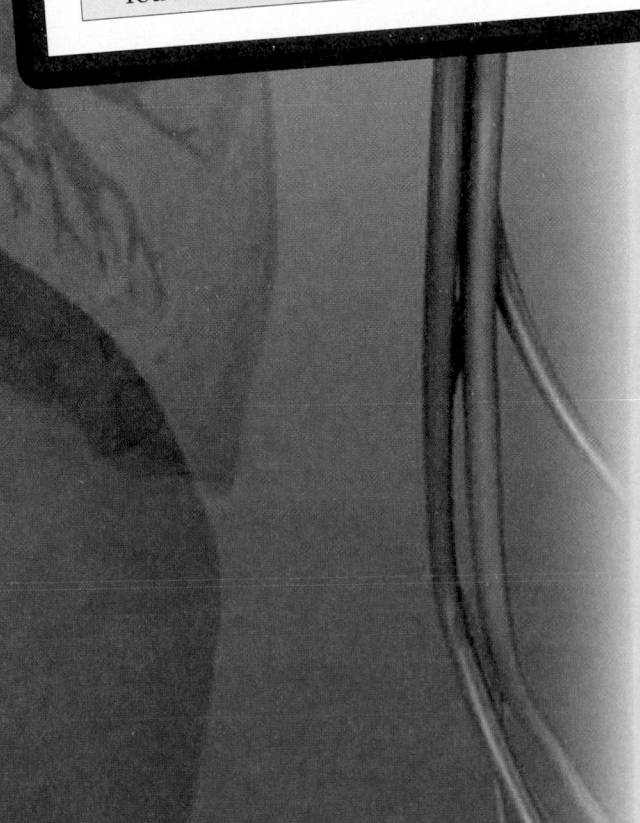

Case Report (CR) 10.1

You are

... a **cardiovascular technologist (CVT)** employed by the **Cardiology** Department at Fulwood Medical Center. You have been called to the Emergency Department immediately **(STAT)** to take an **electrocardiogram (ECG or EKG)**.

Your patient is

... Mr. Hank Johnson. From his medical records, you see that he is the 64-year-old owner of a printing company.

Eight months ago, Mr. Johnson had a left total hip replacement. In the past 3 months, he has returned to his daily workouts. This morning, while riding his exercise bike, he felt tightness in his chest. He kept on cycling and developed pain in the center of his chest radiating down his left arm and up into his jaw. He became **diaphoretic**. His personal trainer called 911.

You perform the ECG, and the automatic report describes abnormalities in the chest leads.

As you remove the electrodes, Mr. Johnson complains that he is feeling faint and has shortness of breath **(SOB)**. You are the only person in the room.

Chapter Learning Outcomes

The **cardiovascular** system includes the heart and blood vessels. In any health care discipline or setting, the condition of a patient's heart will always be a factor during diagnosis, treatment, and communication. In order to understand and communicate that information you need to know the medical terminology involved and be able to:

LO 10.1 Apply the language of cardiology to the anatomy and structure of the cardiovascular system.

LO 10.2 Explain the physiology and functions of the cardiovascular system.

LO 10.3 Describe the blood flow through the heart and the systemic circulations.

LO 10.4 Identify the phases of the cardiac cycle.

LO 10.5 Describe the electrical properties of the heart.

LO 10.6 Use the medical terms of cardiology to communicate and document in writing accurately and precisely in any health care setting.

LO 10.7 Use the medical terms of cardiology to communicate verbally with accuracy and precision in any health care setting.

LO 10.8 Define abbreviations that pertain to the cardiovascular system.

LO 10.9 Explain the effects of common disorders of the heart on health.

LO 10.10 Describe tests used to detect cardiac disorders.

LO 10.11 Define the types of treatment procedures and the effects of cardiac drugs that are in clinical use.

LO 10.12 Match the structure of the different blood vessels in the circulations to their functions.

LO 10.13 Explain the effects of common circulatory disorders on the body as a whole.

Lesson 10.1 Heart

CARDIOVASCULAR SYSTEM

LESSON OBJECTIVES

If you have a healthy heart rate of 60 beats per minute and you live to be 80 years old, your heart will beat (contract and relax) at least 2,522,880,000 times. Your heart pumps approximately 2,000 gallons of blood each day. In 80 years of life, it will have pumped a total of 58,400,000 gallons of blood. If your heart is unable to maintain this ability to pump blood for just a few minutes, your life is in danger.

When your heart fails, there is an inadequate circulation of blood to the body, tissues are deprived of oxygen and nutrients, and metabolic wastes accumulate. Your body cells die.

The information in this lesson will enable you to use correct medical terminology to:

10.1.1 Describe the location of the heart and its relation to other structures.

10.1.2 Discuss the functions of the heart.

10.1.3 Identify the chambers of the heart and the pathway blood takes through them.

10.1.4 Explain the causes of the sounds of the heartbeat heard through a stethoscope.

10.1.5 Identify the blood supply to the heart muscle.

10.1.6 Distinguish between contraction and relaxation during the heart cycle.

10.1.7 Describe the electrical properties of the heart.

Abbreviations

CPR	cardiopulmonary resuscitation
CVT	cardiovascular technician
ECG	electrocardiogram
EKG	electrocardiogram
SOB	shortness of breath
STAT	immediately

LO 10.1 Position of the Heart

Location of the Heart

It is important to know the position of the heart so that you can perform effective **cardiopulmonary resuscitation (CPR)**, position a **stethoscope** to hear heart sounds, or position the **electrodes** correctly for an ECG.

The heart is roughly the size of your fist and weighs around 10 ounces. It is a blunt cone that points down and to the left. The heart lies obliquely between the lungs, with one-third of its mass behind the **sternum** and two-thirds to the left of the sternum *(Figure 10.1a)*. The **apex** can normally be palpated in the fifth **intercostal** space, between the fifth and sixth ribs. The base of the heart lies behind the sternum and the second intercostal space, between the second and third ribs. The region of the thoracic cavity in which the heart lies is called the **mediastinum** *(Figure 10.1b)*.

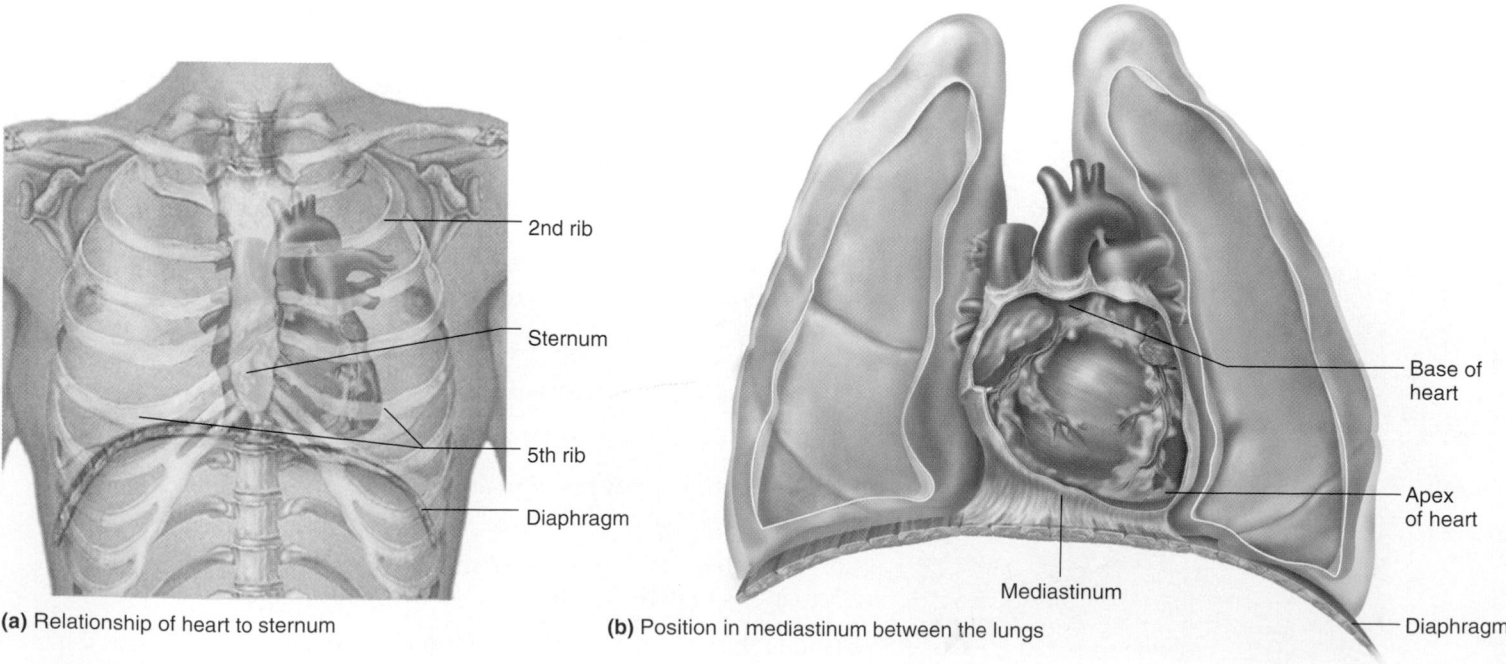

(a) Relationship of heart to sternum

2nd rib
Sternum
5th rib
Diaphragm

(b) Position in mediastinum between the lungs

Base of heart
Apex of heart
Mediastinum
Diaphragm

▲ **Figure 10.1**   **Position of Heart in Thoracic Cavity.**

WORD	PRONUNCIATION		ELEMENTS	DEFINITION
apex	A-peks		Latin *summit or tip*	Tip or end of cone-shaped structure, such as the heart
cardiac	KAR-dee-ak	S/ R/	-ac *pertaining to* **cardi-** *heart*	Pertaining to the heart
cardiogenic	KAR-dee-oh-JEN-ik	S/ R/	-ic *pertaining to* **-gen** *produce, create*	Of cardiac origin
cardiologist	kar-dee-OL-oh-jist	R/CF S/	**cardi/o-** *heart* -logist *specialist*	A medical specialist in diagnosis and treatment of the heart (cardiology)
cardiology	kar-dee-OL-oh-jee	S/	-logy *study of*	Medical specialty of diseases of the heart
cardiopulmonary resuscitation	KAR-dee-oh-PUL-mo-nary ree-sus-ih-TAY-shun	S/ R/CF R/ S/ R/	-ary *pertaining to* **cardi/o-** *heart* **-pulmon-** *lung* -ation *process* **resuscit-** *revival from apparent death*	The attempt to restore cardiac and pulmonary function
cardiovascular	KAR-dee-oh-VAS-kyu-lar	S/ R/CF R/	-ar *pertaining to* **cardi/o-** *heart* **-vascul-** *blood vessel*	Pertaining to the heart and blood vessels
diaphoretic (adj) diaphoresis (noun)	DIE-ah-foh-RET-ic DIE-ah-foh-REE-sis	S/ R/ S/	-etic *pertaining to* **diaphor-** *sweat* -esis *abnormal condition*	Pertaining to sweat or perspiration Sweat or perspiration
electrocardiogram electrocardiograph electrocardiography	ee-lek-troh-KAR-dee-oh-gram ee-lek-troh-KAR-dee-oh-graf ee-LEK-troh-kar-dee-OG-rah-fee	S/ R/CF R/CF S/ S/	-gram *a record* **electr/o-** *electricity* **-cardi/o-** *heart* -graph *to record* -graphy *process of recording*	Record of the electrical signals of the heart Machine that makes the electrocardiogram Interpretation of electrocardiograms
electrode	ee-LEK-trode	S/ R/	-ode *way, road* **electr-** *electricity*	A device for conducting electricity
intercostal	IN-ter-KOS-tal	S/ P/ R/	-al *pertaining to* **inter-** *between* **-cost-** *rib*	The space between two ribs
mediastinum	ME-dee-ass-TIE-num	S/ P/ R/	-um *structure* **media-** *middle* **-stin-** *partition*	Area between the lungs containing the heart, aorta, venae cavae, esophagus, and trachea
sternum	STIR-num		Latin *chest*	Long, flat bone forming the center of the anterior wall of the chest
stethoscope	STETH-oh-skope	S/ R/CF	-scope *instrument* **steth/o-** *chest*	Instrument for listening to cardiac and respiratory sounds

Exercises

A. Build your *language of cardiology* by completing the following documentation. *There is only one best answer for each blank.* **LO 10.6**

1. **cardiology   cardiovascular   cardiologist   cardiac**

   The universal root/combining form in these terms is _____, which means _____.

   The _____ Department sent a specialist to examine the patient in the Emergency Room. The _____ ordered a cardiac catheterization, which showed three obstructed arteries in the patient's heart, so the _____ surgeon was notified immediately to perform _____ surgery.

2. **electrode   electrocardiogram   electrocardiograph   electrocardiography**

   The patient was scheduled for _____ today. The CVT attached the _____ to the patient's chest and proceeded to turn on the _____. Unfortunately, a malfunction of the machine prevented him from obtaining the _____. This study will have to be rescheduled for the patient.

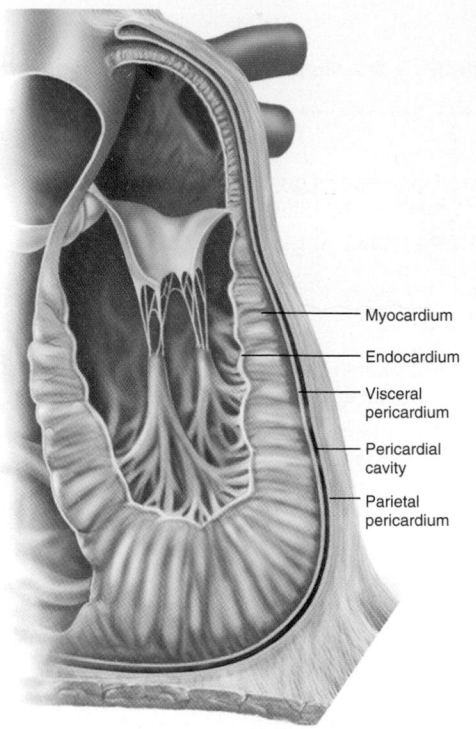

▲ Figure 10.2 **Heart Wall.**

Labels on Figure 10.2:
- Myocardium
- Endocardium
- Visceral pericardium
- Pericardial cavity
- Parietal pericardium

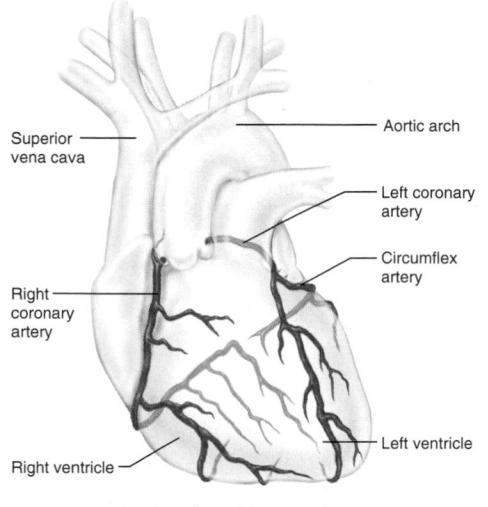

▲ Figure 10.3 **Coronary Arterial Circulation.**

Labels on Figure 10.3:
- Superior vena cava
- Aortic arch
- Left coronary artery
- Circumflex artery
- Right coronary artery
- Left ventricle
- Right ventricle

Abbreviation	
MI	myocardial infarction ("heart attack")

LO 10.1, 10.2 Functions and Structure of the Heart

Functions of the Heart

1. **Pumping blood.** Contractions of the heart generate the pressure to produce movement of blood through the blood vessels.
2. **Routing blood.** The heart can be described as two pumps. A pump on the right side of the heart sends blood through the **pulmonary** circulation of the lungs and back to the pump on the left side, which sends blood through the **systemic** circulation of the body. The valves of the heart ensure this one-way flow of blood.
3. **Regulating blood supply.** The changing metabolic needs of tissues and organs (for example, when you exercise) are met by changes in the rate and force of the heart's contraction.

Structure of the Heart

The heart wall consists of three layers *(Figure 10.2)*:

1. **Endocardium**—a single layer of cells over a thin layer of connective tissue lining the heart.
2. **Myocardium**—cardiac muscle cells that enable the heart to contract.
3. **Epicardium**—a thin serous membrane that is the inner layer of the pericardium.

The **pericardium** is a connective tissue sac that surrounds and protects the heart. It consists of an inner **visceral** layer **(epicardium)** and outer **parietal** layer, between which is the **pericardial** cavity. This cavity contains a **lubricant** fluid that allows the heart to beat with very little friction around it.

Blood Supply to Heart Muscle

Because the heart beats continually and strongly, it requires an abundant supply of oxygen and nutrients. To meet this need, the cardiac muscle has its own blood circulation, the **coronary circulation** *(Figure 10.3)*.

Immediately above the aortic valve in the root of the aorta, the right and left **coronary arteries** exit from the aorta and divide into branches to begin the coronary circulation.

After the blood has flowed through the arteries into the capillaries of the myocardium, 80% drains into veins that flow into the right atrium and 20% flows into the right ventricle. There, the deoxygenated blood mixes with the deoxygenated blood from the rest of the body.

If any of the coronary arteries become blocked, the blood supply to a part of the cardiac muscle is cut off **(ischemia)**, and those cells supplied by that artery die (undergo **necrosis**) within minutes. This is a **myocardial infarction (MI)**, or what many call a "heart attack."

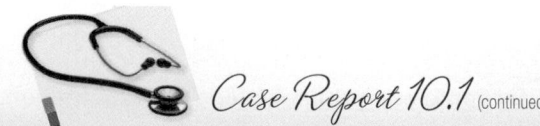

Case Report 10.1 (continued)

Changes on Mr. Johnson's ECG show he was having an MI. Cardiac muscle cells have very limited capability to replicate, and the repair of muscle cell death is mainly by **fibrosis**. This limits cardiac function; Mr. Johnson's heart muscle will have a diminished capacity to contract normally after he recovers from the heart attack.

WORD	PRONUNCIATION	ELEMENTS		DEFINITION
coronary circulation	**KOR**-oh-nair-ee **SER**-kyu-**LAY**-shun	S/ R/	-ary *pertaining to* coron- *crown*	Blood flow through the vessels supplying the heart
endocardium	**EN**-doh-**KAR**-dee-um	S/ P/ R/	-um *structure* endo- *inside* -cardi- *heart*	The inside lining of the heart
endocardial (adj)	**EN**-doh-**KAR**-dee-al	S/	-al	Pertaining to the endocardium
epicardium	**EP**-ih-kar-**DEE**-um	S/ P/ R/	-um *structure* epi- *upon, above* -cardi- *heart*	The outer layer of the heart wall
fibrosis	fie-**BROH**-sis	S/ R/CF	-sis *condition* fibr/o- *fiber*	Repair of dead tissue cells by formation of fibrous tissue
fibrotic (adj)	fie-**BROT**-ik	S/	-tic *pertaining to*	Pertaining to fibrosis
infarct	in-**FARKT**	P/ R/	in- *in* -farct- *stuff*	Area of cell death resulting from an infarction
infarction	in-**FARK**-shun	S/	-ion *process*	Sudden blockage of an artery
ischemia	is-**KEE**-me-ah	R/ R/	-emia *blood* isch- *to keep back*	Lack of blood supply to a tissue
ischemic (adj)	is-**KEE**-mik	S/	-ic *pertaining to*	Pertaining to or affected by ischemia
lubricant	**LOO**-bri-cant	S/ R/	-ant *forming* lubric- *make slippery*	Substance for reducing friction
myocardium	**MY**-oh-**KAR**-dee-um	S/ R/CF R/	-um *structure* my/o- *muscle* -cardi- *heart*	All the heart muscle
myocardial (adj)	**MY**-oh-**KAR**-dee-al	S/	-al *pertaining to*	Pertaining to the myocardium
necrosis	neh-**KROH**-sis	S/ R/	-osis *condition* necr- *death*	Pathologic death of tissue or cells
necrotic (adj)	neh-**KROT**-ik	S/ R/CF	-tic *pertaining to* necr/o- *death*	Affected by necrosis
parietal	pah-**RYE**-eh-tal	S/ R/	-al *pertaining to* pariet- *wall*	Pertaining to the outer layer of the pericardium and other body cavities
pericardium	per-ih-**KAR**-dee-um	S/ P/ R/	-um *structure* peri- *around* -cardi- *heart*	Structure around the heart
pericardial (adj)	per-ih-**KAR**-dee-al	S/	-al *pertaining to*	Pertaining to the pericardium
pulmonary	**PULL**-moh-nar-ee	S/ R/	-ary *pertaining to* pulmon- *lung*	Pertaining to the lungs and their blood supply
systemic	sis-**TEM**-ik	S/ R/	-ic *pertaining to* system- *body as a whole*	Relating to the entire organism
visceral	**VISS**-er-al	S/ R/	-al *pertaining to* viscer- *an organ*	Pertaining to the internal organs

Exercises

A. Deconstruct the following medical terms into their basic elements by filling in the chart. *Knowledge of elements will help increase your medical vocabulary.*   **LO 10.2, 10.6**

Medical Term	Prefix	Root/ Combining Form	Suffix	Meaning of Term
myocardium	1.	2.	3.	4.
infarction	5.	6.	7.	8.
endocardium	9.	10.	11.	12.
visceral	13.	14.	15.	16.
parietal	17.	18.	19.	20.
ischemia	21.	22.	23.	24.
pericardium	25.	26.	27.	28.

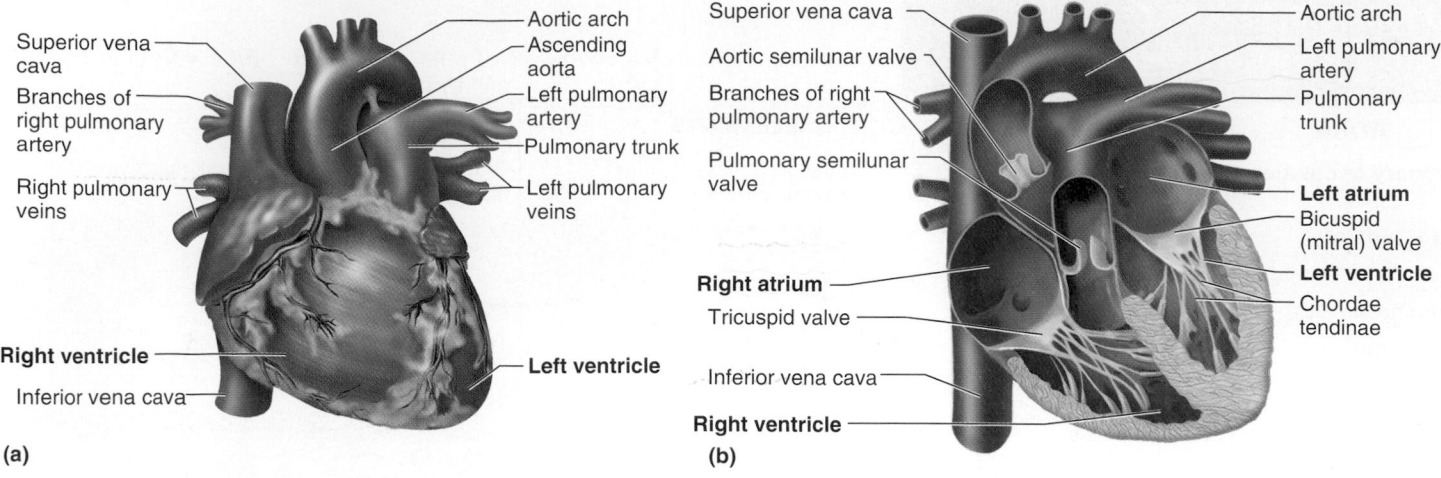

(a)

(b)

▲ **Figure 10.4** External (*a*) and Internal (*b*) Anatomy of the Heart: Frontal View.

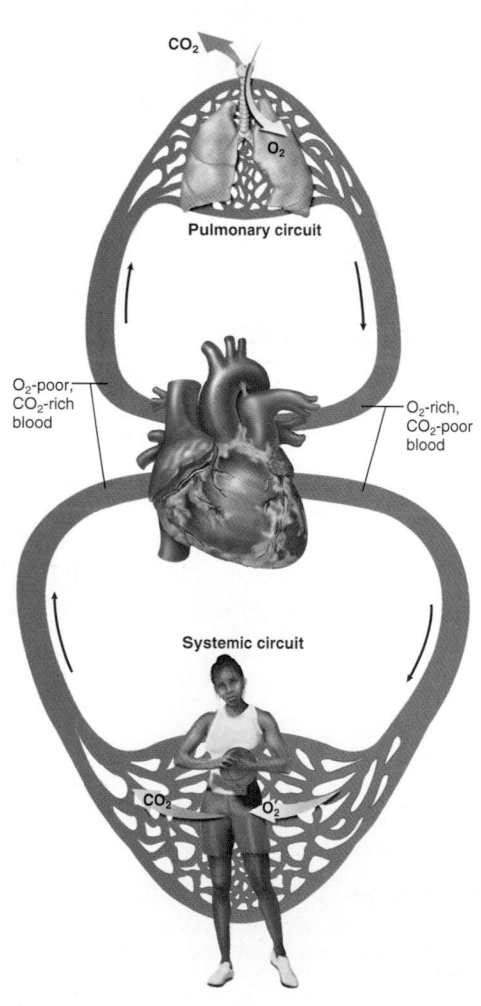

▲ **Figure 10.5** General Schematic of the Cardiovascular Circulation.

Keynote

The pulmonary circulation is the only place in the body where deoxygenated blood is carried in arteries and oxygenated blood is carried in veins.

LO 10.3 Blood Flow through the Heart

The heart has four chambers (*Figure 10.4b*):

1. Right **atrium**

2. Right **ventricle**

3. Left atrium

4. Left ventricle

The right and left sides of the heart are separated by the cardiac **septum**, which can be described in two sections:

- The right and left atria are separated by a thin muscle wall called the **interatrial** septum.

- The right and left ventricles are separated by a thicker muscle wall called the **interventricular** septum.

In addition, the **atrioventricular (AV) septum** is located between and behind the right atrium and left ventricle.

Blood circulates around the body (through the systemic circulation) to unload oxygen and nutrients and pick up carbon dioxide and metabolic waste products. This **deoxygenated** blood returns to the heart via the **superior and inferior venae cavae**. These large veins open into the right atrium. When the right atrium contracts, the blood flows through the **tricuspid valve** into the right ventricle. The tricuspid valve then shuts so when the right ventricle contracts, blood cannot flow back into the atrium.

When the right ventricle contracts, the blood is pushed out through the **semilunar pulmonary valve** into the **pulmonary trunk** (*Figure 10.4a and b*) to begin the pulmonary circulation. The pulmonary valve then shuts to prevent blood flowing back into the ventricle. The pulmonary trunk divides into two arteries; the right pulmonary artery goes to the right lung, and the left pulmonary artery goes to the left lung. In the lungs, carbon dioxide is unloaded, and oxygen is picked up from the air by the blood. The oxygen-rich blood is returned to the heart by the pulmonary veins (*Figure 10.4a and b*).

The blood from the pulmonary veins flows into the left atrium. When the atrium contracts, the blood flows through the **mitral** (or **bicuspid**) valve into the left ventricle. The bicuspid valve then shuts so that blood cannot flow back into the left atrium when the ventricle contracts. The bicuspid and tricuspid valves are anchored to the floor of the ventricles by stringlike **chordae tendineae** (*see Figure 10.4b*).

When the left ventricle contracts, the oxygenated blood is forced out under pressure through the **aortic** semilunar valve into the **aorta**, to return to circulating round the body in the systemic circulation (*Figure 10.5*). The aortic valve then shuts so blood cannot flow back into the left ventricle. The four valves all allow the blood to flow only in one direction.

WORD	PRONUNCIATION	ELEMENTS		DEFINITION
aorta aortic (adj)	a-**OR**-tuh a-**OR**-tic		Greek *lift up*	Main trunk of the systemic arterial system
atrium atria (pl) atrial (adj)	**A**-tree-um **A**-tree-ah **A**-tree-al		Latin *entrance*	Chamber where blood enters the heart on both right and left sides
atrioventricular (AV)	**A**-tree-oh-ven-**TRICK**-you-lar	S/ R/CF R/	-ar *pertaining to* atri/o- *entrance, atrium* -ventricul- *ventricle*	Pertaining to both the atrium and the ventricle
bicuspid	by-**KUSS**-pid	S/ P/ R/	-id *having a particular quality* bi- *two* -cusp- *point*	Having two points; a bicuspid heart valve has two flaps
chordae tendineae	**KOR**-dee ten-**DIN**-ee		Latin *cord* Latin *tendon*	Tendinous cords attaching the bicuspid and tricuspid valves to the heart wall
interatrial	**IN**-ter-**AY**-tree-al	S/ P/ R/	-al *pertaining to* inter- *between* -atri- *atrium, entrance*	Between the atria of the heart
interventricular	**IN**-ter-ven-**TRIK**-you-lar	S/ P/ R/	-ar *pertaining to* inter- *between* -ventricul- *ventricle*	Between the ventricles of the heart
mitral	**MY**-tral		Latin *turban*	Shaped like the headdress of a Catholic bishop
semilunar	sem-ee-**LOO**-nar	S/ P/ R/	-ar *pertaining to* semi- *half* -lun- *moon*	Appears like a half moon
septum septa (pl)	**SEP**-tum **SEP**-tah		Latin *partition*	A wall dividing two cavities
tricuspid	try-**KUSS**-pid	S/ P/ R/	-id *having a particular quality* tri- *three* -cusp- *point*	Having three points; a tricuspid heart valve has three flaps
vena cava venae cavae (pl)	**VEE**-nah **KAY**-vah **VEE**-nee **KAY**-vee	R/CF R/	ven/a *vein* cava *cave*	One of the two largest veins in the body
ventricle	**VEN**-trih-kel		Latin *small belly*	Chamber of the heart or brain

Exercises

A. Plurals of medical terms follow certain established rules. *Apply these rules and change the singular forms into plurals. Then write one sentence for either the singular or plural term.*   **LO 10.1, 10.6**

1. Singular: **atrium**   Plural: _____

   Sentence: _____

2. Singular: **septum**   Plural: _____

   Sentence: _____

3. Singular: **vena cava**   Plural: _____

   Sentence: _____

4. Singular: **ventricle**   Plural: _____

   Sentence: _____

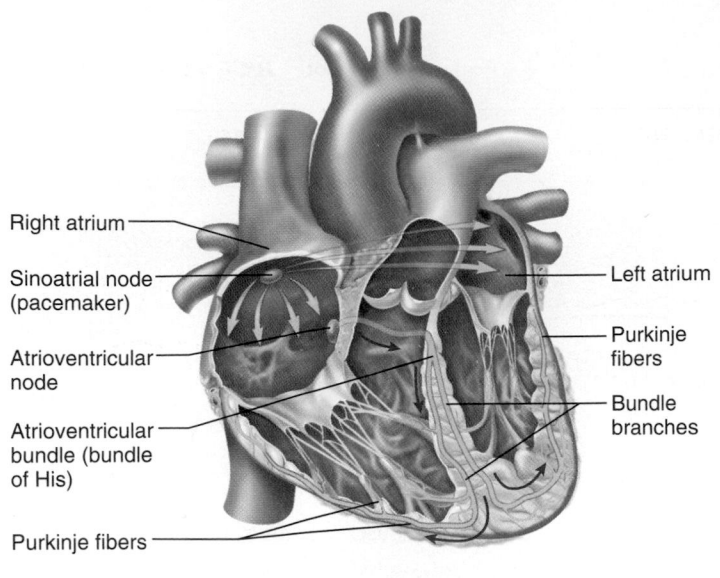

Right atrium

Sinoatrial node (pacemaker)

Atrioventricular node

Atrioventricular bundle (bundle of His)

Purkinje fibers

Left atrium

Purkinje fibers

Bundle branches

▲ **Figure 10.6** **Cardiac Conduction System.**

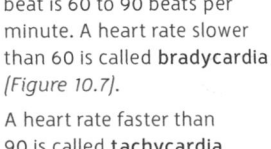

Abbreviations	
AV	atrioventricular
SA	sinoatrial

Keynotes

- The normal rate of heartbeat is 60 to 90 beats per minute. A heart rate slower than 60 is called bradycardia *(Figure 10.7)*.

- A heart rate faster than 90 is called tachycardia *(Figure 10.8)*.

- The normal heartbeat with normal electrical conduction *(Figure 10.9)* through the heart leading to a ventricular rate of around 60 to 90 beats per minute is called sinus rhythm. Any abnormal cardiac rhythm is called an arrythmia or a dysrhythmia.

LO 10.4, 10.5 The Cardiac Cycle

The action of the four heart chambers is coordinated. When the atria contract (atrial **systole**), the ventricles relax (ventricular **diastole**, or ventricular filling). When the atria relax (atrial diastole), the ventricles contract (ventricular systole). Then the atria and ventricles all relax briefly. This series of events is a complete cardiac cycle, or heartbeat.

The "*lub*-dub, *lub*-dub" sounds heard through the stethoscope are made by the snap of the heart valves as they close.

A valve closure abnormality will produce an abnormal sound called a **murmur**. If the abnormal sound is harsh, it can be called a **bruit**.

Electrical Properties of the Heart

As the cardiac muscles contract, they generate a small electrical current. Because the muscle cells are coupled together electrically, they stimulate their neighbor cells so that the myocardium of the atria, and that of the ventricles, each acts as a *single* unit.

To keep the heart beating in a rhythm, a **conduction system** is in place. It consists of five components *(Figure 10.6)*:

1. A small region of specialized muscle cells in the right atrium initiates the electrical current and, therefore, the heartbeat. This area is called the **sinoatrial (SA) node**. It is the **pacemaker** of heart rhythm.

2. Electrical signals from the SA node spread out through the atria and then come back together at the **atrioventricular (AV) node**. This is the electrical gateway to the ventricles, and normally electrical currents cannot get to the ventricles by any other route. The AV node delays impulses to ensure that the atria have injected their blood into the ventricles before the ventricles contract.

3. Electrical signals leave the AV node to reach the ventricles through the AV bundle, called the **bundle of His**.

4. This AV bundle divides into the right and left **bundle branches**, which supply the two ventricles.

5. From the two bundle branches, **Purkinje fibers** spread through the ventricular myocardium and distribute the electrical stimuli to cause contraction of the ventricular myocardium.

An instrument called an *electrocardiograph* picks up the electrical changes in the heart muscle and amplifies them to record an electrocardiogram in the form of five waves *(Figure 10.9)*. The waves are labeled P, Q, R, S, and T.

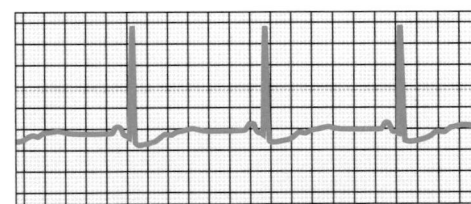

▲ **Figure 10.7** **Bradycardia.**

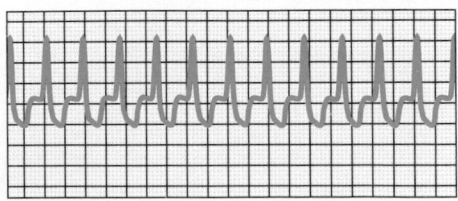

▲ **Figure 10.8** **Tachycardia.**

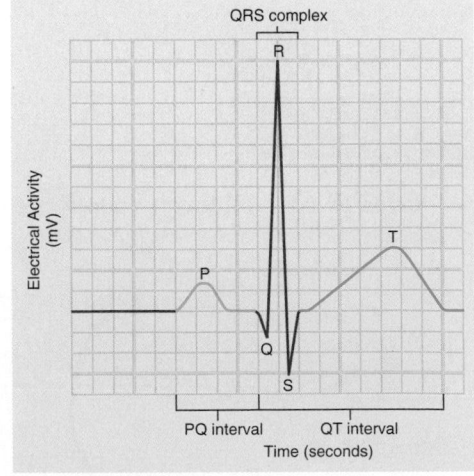

▲ **Figure 10.9** **Normal Electrocardiogram.**

WORD	PRONUNCIATION	ELEMENTS		DEFINITION
arrhythmia (note the double "rr")	a-**RITH**-me-ah	S/ P/ R/	-ia *condition* a- *without* -rrhythm- *rhythm*	An abnormal heart rhythm
atrioventricular	A-tree-oh-ven-**TRICK**-you-lar	S/ R/CF R/	-ar *pertaining to* atri/o- *entrance, atrium* -ventricul- *ventricle*	Pertaining to both the atrium and ventricle
auscultation	aws-kul-**TAY**-shun	S/ R/	-ation *process* auscult- *listen to*	Diagnostic method of listening to body sounds with a stethoscope
bradycardia	brad-ee-**KAR**-dee-ah	S/ P/ R/	-ia *condition* brady- *slow* -card- *heart*	Slow heart rate (below 60 beats per minute)
bruit	brew-**EE**		French *harsh musical sound*	A harsh abnormal sound heard on auscultation of the heart
bundle of His	**BUN**-del of HISS		Wilhelm His, 1831–1904, Swiss anatomist	Pathway for electrical signals to be transmitted to the ventricles
conduction	kon-**DUCK**-shun	S/ P/ R/	-ion *process* con- *together, with* -duct- *lead*	Process of transmitting energy
diastole diastolic (adj)	die-**AS**-toe-lee die-as-**TOL**-ik		Greek *dilation*	Dilation of heart cavities, during which they fill with blood
dysrhythmia (note the single "r")	dis-**RITH**-me-ah	S/ P/ R/	-ia *condition* dys- *bad, difficult* -rhythm- *rhythm*	An abnormal heart rhythm
murmur	**MUR**-mur		Latin *low voice*	Abnormal heart sound heard on auscultation of the heart or blood vessels
pacemaker	**PACE**-may-ker	S/ R/	-maker *one who makes* pace- *step, pace*	Device that regulates cardiac electrical activity
Purkinje fibers	per-**KIN**-jee fi-**BERS**		Johannes von Purkinje, Bohemian anatomist and physiologist, 1787–1869	Network of nerve fibers in the myocardium
sinoatrial node	sigh-noh-**AY**-tree-al NODE	S/ R/CF R/	-al *pertaining to* sin/o- *sinus* -atri- *entrance, atrium*	The center of modified cardiac muscle fibers in the wall of the right atrium that acts as the pacemaker for the heart rhythm
sinus rhythm	**SIGH**-nus **RITH**-um		sinus *channel, cavity* rhythm Greek *to flow*	The normal (optimal) heart rhythm arising from the sinoatrial node
systole systolic (adj)	**SIS**-toe-lee sis-**TOL**-ik		Greek *contraction*	Contraction of the heart muscle
tachycardia	tak-ih-**KAR**-dee-ah	S/ P/ R/	-ia *condition* tachy- *rapid* -card- *heart*	Rapid heart rate (above 100 beats per minute)

Exercises

A. Both of the following terms have similar roots and suffixes, but the prefixes make the difference. *Deconstruct each term using the slashed lines. Then analyze the terms, and explain how they are different.* **LO 10.4, 10.5, 10.6**

1. bradycardia: _____ / _____ / _____
                                           P   R   S

2. tachycardia: _____ / _____ / _____
                                           P   R   S

3. The difference between bradycardia and tachycardia is _____

B. Use the appropriate abbreviations to complete the following documentation. *You have more abbreviations than you will need.* **LO 10.8**

STAT   KUB   CPR   CVT   VS   ECG   SOB   UTI

1. Because the patient was complaining of _____, an _____ was ordered by the doctor. The patient went into cardiac arrest during the test and the _____ had to perform _____ until the doctor arrived.

Every different structure within the heart may not function properly. In this lesson, you will learn the common disorders of the heart and the medical terminology to describe them and their treatment.

10.2.1 Describe common types of cardiac arrhythmias.

10.2.2 Explain common disorders of the heart valves.

10.2.3 Discuss common disorders of the heart wall and its blood supply.

10.2.4 Describe hypertensive heart disease and congestive heart failure.

10.2.5 Discuss congenital heart disease.

10.2.6 Detail cardiologic tests, treatment procedures, and drug treatments.

LO 10.9 Disorders of the Heart

Abnormal Heart Rhythms

There are four common types of **arrhythmias**, abnormal or irregular heartbeats:

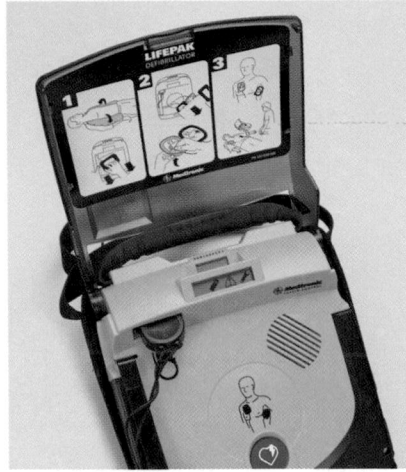

▲ **Figure 10.10** Automatic External Defibrillator.

1. **Premature** beats may originate in either the atrium and the ventricle or both, may occur in individuals of all ages, and may be associated with caffeine and stress.

2. **Atrial fibrillation** occurs when the two atria quiver rather than contract in an organized fashion to pump blood into the ventricle. This causes blood to pool in the atria and sometimes clot. **Paroxysmal atrial tachycardia (PAT)** presents with periods of rapid, regular heartbeats that originate in the atrium. The episodes begin and end abruptly. The heart rate speeds up to 160 to 200 beats per minute.

3. **Ventricular arrhythmias** consist of several types. **Ventricular tachycardia** is a rapid heartbeat arising in the ventricles. **Premature ventricular contractions (PVCs)** occur when extra impulses arise from a ventricle. **Ventricular fibrillation (V-fib)** is characterized by ventricles going out of control, quivering, and beating ineffectively instead of pumping.

4. **Heart block** occurs when interference in cardiac electrical conduction causes the contractions of the atria to fail to coordinate with the contractions of the ventricles.

Palpitations are unpleasant sensations of a rapid or irregular heartbeat that last a few seconds or minutes. They can be brought on by exercise, anxiety, and stimulants like caffeine. Occasionally, they can be caused by an arrhythmia.

Arrhythmias can be treated with medications, but some patients require mechanical **pacemakers.** These artificial pacemakers consist of a battery, electronic circuits, and computer memory to generate electronic signals. The signals are carried along thin, insulated wires to the heart muscle. The most common need for a pacemaker is a very slow heart rate (bradycardia).

People with life-threatening arrhythmias may need an **implantable cardioverter/defibrillator (ICD),** which senses abnormal rhythms and gives the heart a small electrical shock to return the rhythm to normal.

In emergency situations, external **cardioversion** is performed through **automatic external defibrillators (AEDs)** *(Figure 10.10)* that send an electrical shock to the heart to restore a normal contraction rhythm.

Abbreviations	
AED	automatic external defibrillator
ICD	implantable cardiovertor/defibrillator
PAT	paroxysmal atrial tachycardia
PVC	premature ventricular contraction
V-fib	ventricular fibrillation

WORD	PRONUNCIATION	ELEMENTS		DEFINITION
cardioversion (also called defibrillation)	KAR-dee-oh-VER-shun	S/ R/CF R/	-ion *action, process* cardi/o- *heart* -vers- *turn*	Restoration of a normal heart rhythm by electrical shock
cardioverter	KAR-dee-oh-VER-ter	R/	-verter *that which turns*	Device used to generate the electrical shock to the heart
defibrillation	dee-fib-rih-LAY-shun	S/ P/ R/	-ation *process* de- *without, away from* -fibrill- *small fiber*	Restoration of uncontrolled twitching of cardiac muscle fibers to normal rhythm
defibrillator	dee-fib-rih-LAY-tor	S/	-ator *instrument*	Instrument for defibrillation
fibrillation	fi-brih-LAY-shun	S/ R/	-ation *process* fibrill- *small fiber*	Uncontrolled quivering or twitching of the heart muscle
implantable	im-PLAN-tah-bul	S/ P/ R/	-able *capable of* im- *in* -plant- *insert*	Able to be inserted into tissues
pacemaker	PACE-may-ker	S/ R/	-maker *one who makes* pace- *step, pace*	Device that regulates cardiac electrical activity
palpitation	pal-pih-TAY-shun	S/ R/	-ation *process* palpit- *throb*	Forcible, rapid beat of the heart felt by the patient
paroxysmal	par-ock-SIZ-mal	S/ R/	-al *pertaining to* paroxysm- *irritation*	Occurring in sharp, spasmodic episodes

Exercises

A. The definitions for the medical terms in the above WAD box are given to you—break the term down into its basic elements. *Notice in particular which terms do not have prefixes or suffixes. Every term must have a root and/or combining form.*   **LO 10.5, 10.6**

1. Forcible, rapid beat of the heart

_____ / _____ / _____
P   R/CF   S

2. Uncontrolled heart muscle twitching

_____ / _____ / _____
P   R/CF   S

3. Changes abnormal rhythm to normal

_____ / _____ / _____
P   R/CF   S

4. Device inserted into body tissue

_____ / _____ / _____
P   R/CF   S

5. Sharp, spasmodic episode

_____ / _____ / _____
P   R/CF   S

6. Device that regulates cardiac electrical activity

_____ / _____ / _____
P   R/CF   S

7. What is another term for cardioversion? _____

8. What are the only terms in the above WAD that contain all three elements? _____ and _____

Use one of the terms in question #8 in a sentence that is not a definition.

9. Sentence: _____

_____

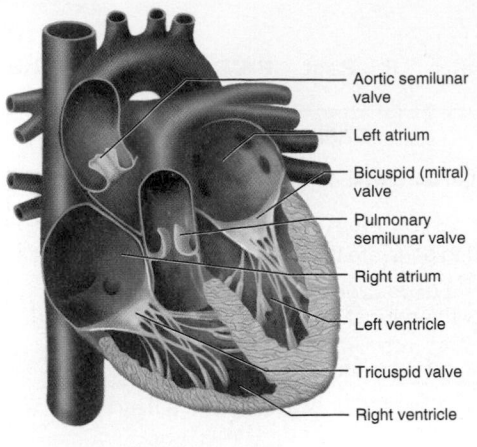

▲ Figure 10.11   Heart Valves.

Labels on figure:
- Aortic semilunar valve
- Left atrium
- Bicuspid (mitral) valve
- Pulmonary semilunar valve
- Right atrium
- Left ventricle
- Tricuspid valve
- Right ventricle

Keynotes

- **Malfunctions** of the valves on the right side of the heart are much less common than those of valves on the left side.

- **Cor pulmonale** is failure of the right ventricle to pump properly. Almost any chronic lung disease causing low blood oxygen (hypoxia) can cause this disorder.

LO 10.9 Disorders of the Heart (continued)

Disorders of the Heart Valves

Heart valves can **malfunction** in two basic ways:

1. **Stenosis** occurs when the valve does not open fully, and its opening is narrowed (constricted). Blood cannot flow freely through the valve and accumulates behind the valve.

2. **Incompetence** or **insufficiency** occurs when the valve cannot close fully, and blood can **regurgitate** (flow back) through the valve to the chamber from which it started.

Mitral valve stenosis can occur following rheumatic fever. Because the blood cannot flow freely through the valve, the left atrium becomes dilated. Eventually, **chronic heart failure** results. (*Figure 10.11* enables you to review the locations of the valves and chambers.)

Mitral valve incompetence occurs when there is leakage back through the valve as the left ventricle contracts. The left atrium becomes dilated. Again, chronic heart failure results.

Mitral valve prolapse occurs when the cusps of the valve bulge back into the left atrium when the left ventricle contracts, thus allowing blood to flow back into the atrium.

A prolapsed or incompetent mitral valve can often be repaired. There are two valve replacement options:

1. **A mechanical (prosthetic) valve.** Various models and designs are made from different metal alloys and plastics.

2. **Tissue valve.** This can come from a pig (porcine) or cow (bovine). Occasionally, a tissue valve can come from a human donor, or a valve can be constructed of tissue from the patient's own pericardium.

Aortic valve stenosis is common in the elderly when the valves become calcified due to **atherosclerosis**. Blood flow into the systemic circuit is diminished, leading to dizziness and fainting. The left ventricle dilates, hypertrophies, and ultimately fails.

Aortic valve incompetence initially produces few symptoms other than a murmur, but eventually the left ventricle fails.

Rheumatic fever is an inflammatory disease. If a sore throat caused by group A beta-hemolytic streptococcus (*see Chapter 13*) is not treated with a complete course of antibiotics, antibodies to the bacteria can develop and attack normal tissue. Multiple joints are inflamed, and endocarditis can affect the function of the heart valves—particularly the mitral and aortic valves.

Disorders of the Heart Wall

Endocarditis is inflammation of the lining of the heart. It is usually secondary to an infection elsewhere. Intravenous drug users and people with damaged heart valves are at high risk for endocarditis.

Myocarditis is inflammation of the heart muscle. It can be bacterial, viral, or fungal in origin or a complication of other diseases, such as influenza.

Pericarditis is inflammation of the covering of the heart. The inflammation causes an **exudate** (pericardial **effusion**) to be released into the pericardial space. This interferes with the heart's ability to contract and expand normally, and cardiac output falls—a condition called **cardiac tamponade**.

Cardiomyopathy is a weakening of the heart muscle that causes it to pump inadequately. The etiology can be viral, idiopathic (when the cause is unknown), or alcoholic. It causes **cardiomegaly** and heart failure.

WORD	PRONUNCIATION	ELEMENTS		DEFINITION
cardiomegaly	KAR-dee-oh-MEG-ah-lee	S/ R/CF	-megaly *enlargement* cardi/o- *heart*	Enlargement of the heart
cardiomyopathy	KAR-dee-oh-my-OP-ah-thee	S/ R/CF R/CF	-pathy *disease* cardi/o- *heart* -my/o- *muscle*	Disease of heart muscle, the myocardium
cor pulmonale	KOR pul-moh-NAH-lee	S/ R/ R/	-ale *pertaining to* cor *heart* pulmon- *lung*	Right-sided heart failure arising from chronic lung disease
effusion	eh-FYU-shun		Latin *pouring out*	Collection of fluid that has escaped from blood vessels into a cavity or tissues
endocarditis	EN-doh-kar-DIE-tis	S/ P/ R/	-itis *inflammation* endo- *within* -card- *heart*	Inflammation of the lining of the heart
exudate	EKS-you-date	S/ P/ R/	-ate *process, composed of* ex- *out of* -ud- *sweat*	Fluid that has come out of a tissue or its capillaries because of inflammation or injury
incompetence	in-KOM-peh-tense	S/ P/ R/	-ence *quality of* in- *not* -compet- *strive together*	Failure of valves to close completely
insufficiency	in-suh-FISH-en-see	S/ P/ R/CF	-ency *quality of* in- *not* -suffic/i- *enough*	Lack of completeness of function; in the heart, failure of a valve to close properly
malfunction	mal-FUNK-shun	S/ P/ R/	-ion *action, condition* mal- *bad, inadequate* -funct- *perform*	Inadequate or abnormal function
myocarditis	MY-oh-kar-DIE-tis	S/ R/CF R/	-itis *inflammation* my/o- *muscle* -card- *heart*	Inflammation of the heart muscle
pericarditis	PER-ih-kar-DIE-tis	S/ P/ R/	-itis *inflammation* peri- *around* -card- *heart*	Inflammation of the pericardium, the covering of the heart
prolapse	pro-LAPS		Latin *a falling*	The falling or slipping of a body part from its normal position
prosthesis prosthetic (adj)	PROS-thee-sis pros-THET-ik		Greek *an addition*	A manufactured substitute for a missing or diseased part of the body
regurgitate	ree-GUR-jih-tate	S/ P/ R/	-ate *pertaining to* re- *back* -gurgit- *flood*	To flow backward; in this case, through a heart valve
stenosis	steh-NOH-sis	S/ R/CF	-sis *abnormal condition* sten/o- *narrow*	Narrowing of a canal or passage, as in the narrowing of a heart valve
tamponade	tam-po-NAID	S/ R/	-ade *process* tampon- *plug*	Pathologic compression of an organ such as the heart

Exercises

A. Use your knowledge of the *language of cardiology* to match the description in the left column with the correct medical term in the right column. *Fill in the blanks.*   **LO 10.9**

_____	1. Weakening of heart muscle	a.	incompetence
_____	2. Inflammation that causes exudates	b.	cardiomegaly
_____	3. Cusps of valve bulge back into atrium	c.	cor pulmonale
_____	4. Constricted valve opening	d.	pericarditis
_____	5. Failure of right ventricle to pump properly	e.	rheumatic fever
_____	6. Cardiomyopathy can be the cause	f.	cardiomyopathy
_____	7. Causes valve regurgitation	g.	prolapse
_____	8. Inflammatory disease that affects the heart	h.	stenosis

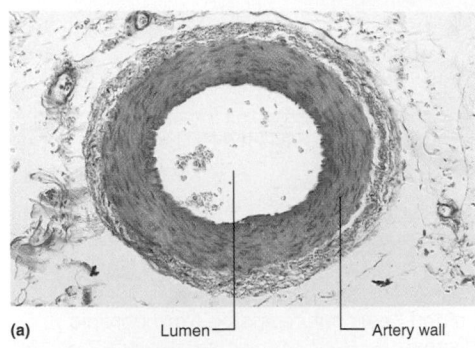

(a) Lumen — Artery wall

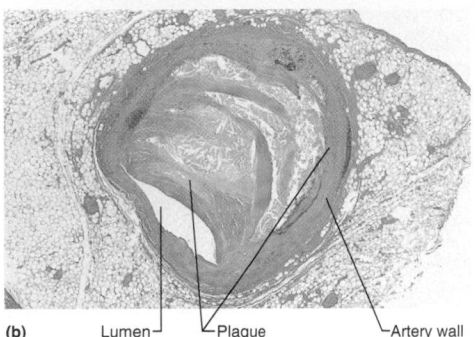

(b) Lumen — Plaque — Artery wall

▲ **Figure 10.12** **Arterial Structure.** (*a*) Normal coronary artery. (*b*) Advanced atherosclerosis.

Keynotes

All of the following risk factors can be reduced by changes in lifestyle.

Risk factors for CAD include

- Obesity
- Lack of exercise (**sedentary**)
- Tobacco
- Diabetes mellitus
- High BP (**hypertension**)
- Elevated serum cholesterol
- Stress

Abbreviations

ASHD	arteriosclerotic heart disease
BP	**blood pressure**
CAD	coronary artery disease
MI	myocardial infarction

Keynote

Cardiac arrest is the sudden cessation of cardiac activity resulting from **anoxia**. The ECG shows a flat line, **asystole** (*Figure 10.13*).

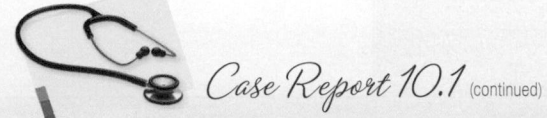

Case Report 10.1 (continued)

In the Emergency Room, the ECG indicated that Mr. Johnson was having a **myocardial infarction (MI)** affecting the anterior wall of his left ventricle. The cardiovascular technician did not want to leave Mr. Johnson, so he used the call system to summon help.

LO 10.9 Disorders of the Heart (continued)

Coronary Artery Disease (CAD)

The arteries supplying the myocardium become narrowed by atherosclerotic **plaques**, called **atheroma**. As the atheroma increases, the lumen of the artery becomes increasingly narrow (*compare Figure 10.12a and b*). The blood supplied to the cardiac muscle by the artery is reduced. Platelet aggregation can occur on the plaque to form a blood clot (**coronary thrombosis**). **Atherosclerosis** is the most common form of **arteriosclerosis** (hardening of the arteries) and can lead to **arteriosclerotic heart disease (ASHD)**.

Angina pectoris, pain in the chest on exertion, is often the first symptom of reduced oxygen supply to the myocardium. The pain goes away if the exertion is stopped or if a **nitroglycerin** tablet is placed under the tongue (**sublingually**).

Myocardial infarction (MI) is the death of myocardial cells caused by the lack of blood supply (ischemia) when an artery eventually becomes blocked (**occluded**). Sudden, severe, crushing **substernal** or left chest pain is experienced. If the ischemia is not reversed within 4 to 6 hours, the muscle cells die (undergo necrosis).

Cardiogenic shock occurs when the heart fails to pump effectively and organs and tissues are **perfused** inadequately. The pulse is weak and rapid, and **blood pressure (BP)** drops. The patient becomes pale, cold, sweaty, and anxious.

The other form of circulatory shock is **hypovolemic shock**, in which there is a loss of blood volume, often from hemorrhage or dehydration.

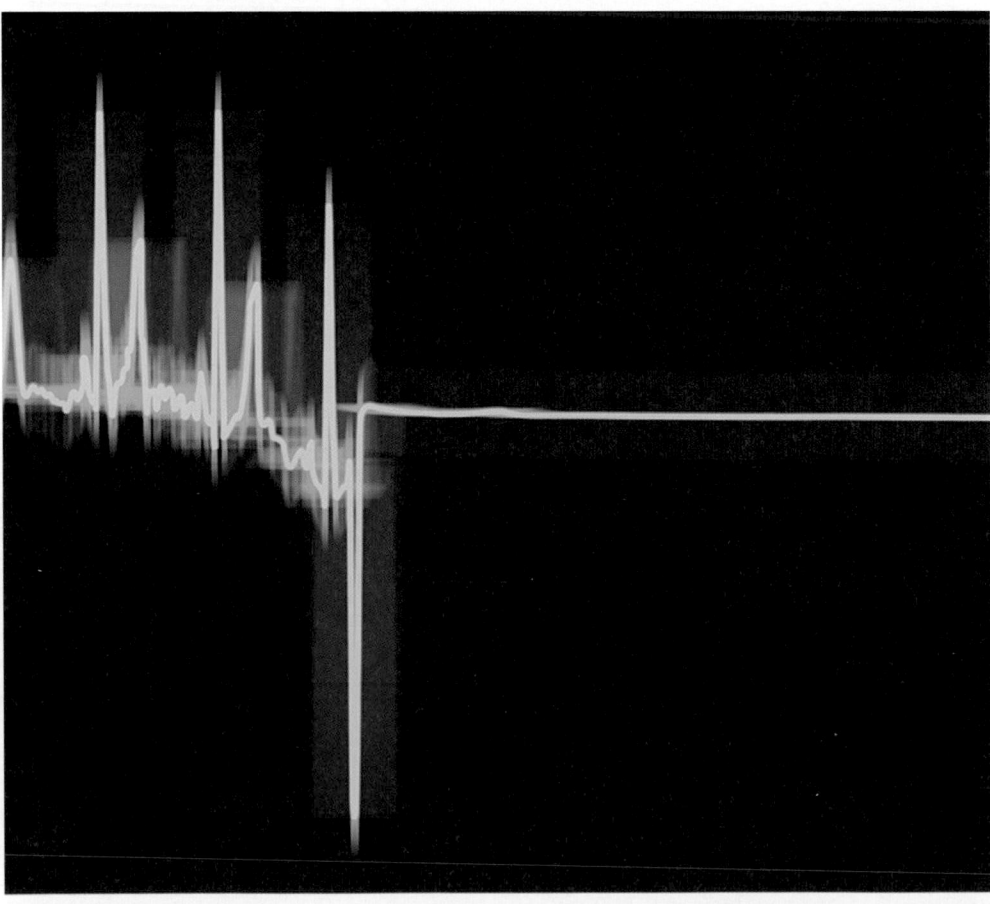

▲ **Figure 10.13** **Electrocardiogram (ECG) Showing Asystole.**

WORD	PRONUNCIATION	ELEMENTS		DEFINITION
anoxia	an-OCK-see-ah	S/ P/ R/	-ia *condition* an- *without* -ox *oxygen*	Without oxygen
anoxic (adj)	an-OCK-sik	S/	-ic *pertaining to*	Pertaining to or suffering from a lack of oxygen
arteriosclerosis	ar-TIER-ee-oh-skler-OH-sis	S/ R/CF R/CF	-sis *abnormal condition* arteri/o- *artery* -scler/o- *hardness*	Hardening of the arteries
arteriosclerotic (adj)	ar-TIER-ee-oh-skler-OT-ik	S/	-tic *pertaining to*	Pertaining to or suffering from arteriosclerosis
asystole	a-SIS-toe-lee	P/ R/CF	a- *without* -systole/e *contraction*	Absence of contractions of the heart
atheroma	ath-er-ROE-mah	S/ R/	-oma *tumor* ather- *porridge, gruel*	Lipid deposit in the lining of an artery
atherectomy	ath-er-EK-toe-me	S/ R/CF	-ectomy *excision* ather/o- *porridge, gruel*	Surgical removal of the atheroma
atherosclerosis	ATH-er-oh-skler-OH-sis	S/ R/CF	-sis *abnormal condition* -scler/o- *hardness*	Atheroma in arteries
hypovolemic	HIGH-poh-vo-LEE-mick	S/ P/ R/	-emic *in the blood* hypo- *below* -vol- *volume*	Having decreased blood volume in the body
occlude (verb) occlusion (noun)	o-KLUDE o-KLU-zhun		Latin *to close*	To close, plug, or completely obstruct A complete obstruction
perfuse	per-FYUSE		Latin *to pour*	To force blood to flow through a lumen or a vascular bed
perfusion (noun)	per-FYU-shun	S/ R/	-ion *action, condition* perfus- *to pour*	The act of perfusing
plaque	PLAK		French *a plate*	Patch of abnormal tissue
sedentary	sed-en-TER-ee	S/ R/	-ary *pertaining to* sedent- *sitting*	Accustomed to little exercise or movement
sublingual	sub-LING-wal	S/ P/ R/	-al *pertaining to* sub- *under* -lingu- *tongue*	Underneath the tongue
substernal	sub-STER-nal	S/ P/ R/	-al *pertaining to* sub- *under* -stern- *breastbone*	Under the sternum, or breastbone

Exercises

A. Consult the above WAD for the best medical terms to complete the following sentences in patient documentation. *Fill in the blanks.* **LO 10.6, 10.9**

1. His _____ (little exercise or movement) lifestyle, coupled with obesity, increases his risk factors for a heart attack.

2. Schedule the patient for a(n) _____ (surgical removal of lipid deposit in artery lining) as soon as possible.

3. _____ (absence of heart contractions) occurred at 2251 hrs, and the patient was pronounced dead.

4. Angioplasty showed a large clot _____ (completely obstructing) her left coronary artery.

5. The bullet entered his left _____ (under the breastbone) area and exited his back.

6. The patient's diagnostic studies show clear evidence of _____ (patch of abnormal tissue) in a coronary heart artery.

7. Cardiogenic shock occurred, and the patient's tissues were not _____ (forcing blood through a vascular bed or lumen) adequately.

LO 10.9 Disorders of the Heart (continued)

Hypertensive Heart Disease

Hypertension is the most common cardiovascular disorder in this country, affecting more than 20% of the adult population. It results from a prolonged elevated blood pressure (BP) throughout the vascular system. The high pressure forces the ventricles to work harder to pump blood. Eventually, the myocardium becomes strained and less efficient. It is the major cause of heart failure, stroke, and kidney failure.

High BP is currently defined as a BP reading at or above 140/90 mm **Hg** (mercury). A normal BP is below 120/80 mm Hg. The first number, or **systolic** reading, reflects the BP when the heart is contracting. The second number, or **diastolic** reading, reflects BP when the heart is relaxed between contractions.

Primary (essential) hypertension is the most common type of hypertension. Its etiology is unknown. Its risk factors are

- Being overweight
- Stress
- Lack of exercise
- Using tobacco
- Using alcohol

Secondary hypertension results from other diseases, such as kidney disease, atherosclerosis, and hyperthyroidism.

Malignant hypertension is a rare, severe, life-threatening form of hypertension in which the BP reading can be greater than 200/120 mm Hg. Aggressive intervention is indicated to reduce the blood pressure.

Prehypertension, with a systolic pressure between 120 and 139 mm Hg and a diastolic pressure between 80 and 90 mm Hg, may indicate an increased risk for cardiovascular disease.

Congestive Heart Failure (CHF)

Congestive heart failure occurs with the inability of the heart to supply enough cardiac output to meet the body's metabolic needs. The patient shows **shortness of breath (SOB)** and **orthopnea**.
The most common conditions leading to CHF are

- Cardiac ischemia
- Cardiomyopathy
- Chronic lung disease
- Valvular regurgitation
- Severe hypertension
- Aortic **stenosis**

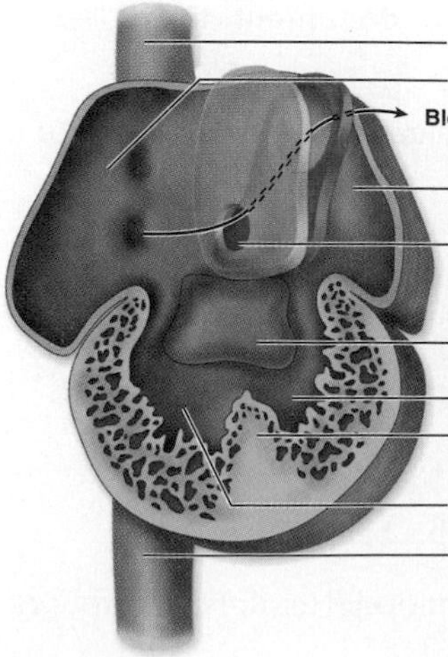

Congenital Heart Disease (CHD)

Congenital heart disease is the result of abnormal development of the heart in the fetus. Common congenital defects include

- **Atrial septal defect (ASD).** A hole in the interatrial septum allows blood to **shunt** from the higher-pressure left atrium to the lower-pressure right atrium *(Figure 10.14)*.
- **Ventricular septal defect (VSD).** A hole in the interventricular septum allows blood to shunt from the higher-pressure left ventricle to the lower-pressure right ventricle *(see Figure 10.14)*.
- **Patent ductus arteriosus (PDA).** The ductus arteriosus is a normal blood vessel in the fetus that usually closes within 24 hours of birth. When the artery remains open (patent), blood can shunt from the aorta to the pulmonary artery, and the higher pressure causes damage to the lungs.
- **Coarctation of the aorta.** This is a narrowing of the aorta shortly after the artery to the left arm branches from the aorta. It causes **hypertension** in the arms behind the narrowing and **hypotension** in the lower limbs and organs like the kidney below the narrowing.
- **Tetralogy of Fallot (TOF).** This is a **syndrome** with four congenital heart defects.
  All these congenital abnormalities can be surgically repaired.

Superior vena cava
Right atrium
Blood flow
Left atrium
Interatrial septal defect
Interventricular septal defect
Left ventricle
Interventricular septum
Right ventricle
Inferior vena cava

▲ **Figure 10.14** **Atrial and Ventricular Septal Defects.**

Abbreviations	
ASD	atrial septal defect
CHD	congenital heart disease
CHF	congestive heart failure
Hg	mercury
PDA	patent ductus arteriosus
SOB	short(ness) of breath
TOF	tetralogy of Fallot
VSD	ventricular septal defect

Word Analysis and Definition

S = Suffix   P = Prefix   **R = Root**   **R/CF** = Combining Form

WORD	PRONUNCIATION	ELEMENTS		DEFINITION
coarctation	koh-ark-**TAY**-shun	S/ R/	-ation *process* **coarct-** *press together*	Constriction stenosis, particularly of the aorta
congenital	kon-**JEN**-ih-tal	S/ P/ R/	-al *pertaining to* con- *together, with* **-genit-** *bring forth*	Present at birth, either inherited or due to an event during gestation up to the moment of birth
defect	**DEE**-fect		Latin *to lack*	An absence, malformation, or imperfection
hypertension	**HIGH**-per-**TEN**-shun	S/ P/ R/	-ion *action, condition* hyper- *excessive* **-tens-** *pressure*	Persistent high arterial blood pressure
hypertensive hypotension prehypertension	**HIGH**-per-**TEN**-siv **HIGH**-poh-**TEN**-shun pree-**HIGH**-per-**TEN**-shun	S/ P/ P/	-ive *quality of* hypo- *low, below* pre- *before*	Suffering from hypertension Persistent low arterial blood pressure Precursor to hypertension
orthopnea orthopneic (adj)	or-**THOP**-nee-ah or-**THOP**-nee-ik	S/ R/CF S/	-pnea *breathe* **orth/o-** *straight* -ic *pertaining to*	Difficulty in breathing when lying flat Pertaining to or affected by orthopnea
patent ductus arteriosus	**PAY**-tent **DUK**-tus ar-**TER**-ee-oh-sus	R/ R/ R/	**patent** *lie open* **ductus** *leading* **arteriosus** *like an artery*	An open, direct channel between the aorta and the pulmonary artery
shunt	SHUNT		Middle English *divert*	A bypass or diversion of fluid; in this case, blood
syndrome	**SIN**-drohm	P/ R/	syn- *together* -drome *running*	Combination of signs and symptoms associated with a particular disease process
tetralogy of Fallot (TOF)	teh-**TRAL**-oh-jee OF fah-**LOW**	 P/ S/	Etienne-Louis Fallot, French physician 1850–1911 tetra- *four* -logy *study of*	Set of four congenital heart defects occurring together

Exercises

A. Abbreviations need to be used carefully so that you communicate exactly what is necessary. *The following sentences contain abbreviations. Translate the abbreviations into their correct medical terms. Rewrite the sentences without the abbreviations, and convey the same message. Check your spelling!* **LO 10.8**

1. ASD, TOF, VSD, and PDA are all examples of CHD.

_____

_____

2. CHF occurs with the inability of the heart to supply enough cardiac output to meet the body's metabolic needs.

_____

_____

3. High BP is a reading at or above 140/90 mm Hg.

_____

_____

LO 10.10 Cardiologic Tests

Blood Tests

Lipid profile helps determine the risk of CAD and comprises

- **Total cholesterol**
- **High-density lipoprotein (HDL)** ("good cholesterol")
- **Low-density lipoprotein (LDL)** ("bad cholesterol")
- **Triglycerides**

The following are chemical indicators used as risk factors in the diagnosis and monitoring of cardiovascular diseases:

- **B-type natriuretic peptide (BNP)**, a brain hormone, is used to diagnose and monitor congestive heart failure and to predict the course of end-stage heart failure.
- **C-reactive protein (CRP)**, produced by the endothelial cells of arteries, when elevated, has been identified as a risk factor for atherosclerosis and CAD.
- **Homocysteine** is an amino acid in the blood. Elevated levels are related to a higher risk of CAD, stroke, and peripheral vascular disease.
- **Creatine kinase (CK)** is an enzyme released into the blood by dead myocardial cells in MI.
- **Troponin I and T** are part of a protein complex in muscle that is released into the blood during myocardial injury. Troponin I is found in heart muscle but not in skeletal muscle. Its presence in blood is therefore a highly sensitive indicator of a recent MI. Both CK and Troponin I and T are used to confirm a suspected MI.

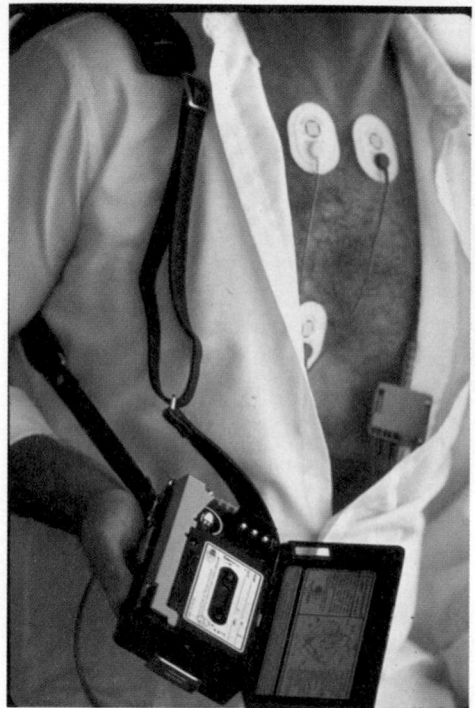

▲ **Figure 10.15**   Holter monitor.

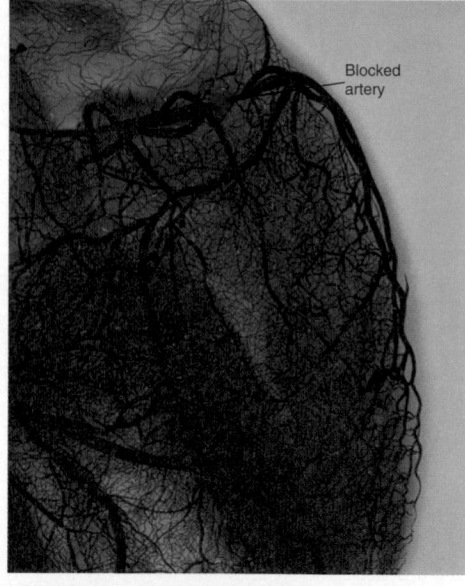

▲ **Figure 10.16**   Coronary angiogram showing blocked artery.

Abbreviations

BNP	B-type natriuretic peptide
CK	creatine kinase
CRP	C-reactive protein
EBT	electron beam tomography
HDL	high-density lipoprotein
LDL	low-density lipoprotein
TEE	transesophageal echocardiography

LO 10.11 Diagnostic Tests

1. An **electrocardiogram** (ECG or EKG) is a paper record of the electrical signals of your heart.

2. **Cardiac stress testing** is an exercise tolerance test to raise your heart rate and monitor the effect on cardiac function. **Nuclear imaging** of the heart, using an injection of a radioactive substance, can be used with the stress test.

3. **Persantine/thallium exercise testing** is used for people unable to engage in physical exercise. It combines nuclear imaging with a drug that increases the demand on the heart.

4. **Echocardiography** uses ultrasound waves to study cardiac function at rest. The test is performed by a **sonographer**, who places a **transducer** on the patient's chest. A stress echocardiogram is performed after the patient has exercised on a treadmill.

5. **Transesophageal echocardiography (TEE)** involves insertion of a small probe into the esophagus to record the anatomy and function of heart valves.

6. A **holter monitor** [Figure 10.15] is a continuous ECG recorded on a tape recorder cassette as you work, play, and rest for 24 to 48 hours. The patient keeps a diary of all symptoms and activities so that the data on the monitor can be correlated with symptoms and activities.

7. An **event monitor** is used for patients whose symptoms occur sporadically. A monitor is held over the chest when an event occurs. The data are stored and transmitted by telephone to a monitoring station.

8. An **ambulatory blood pressure monitor** provides a record of your BP over a 24-hour period as you go about your daily activities.

9. **Electron beam tomography (EBT)** is a scan that identifies calcium deposits in arteries.

10. **Cardiac catheterization** detects patterns of pressures and blood flows in the heart. A thin tube is guided into the heart under x-ray guidance after being inserted into a vein or artery.

11. **Coronary angiogram** [Figure 10.16] uses a contrast dye injected during cardiac catheterization to identify coronary artery blockages.

WORD	PRONUNCIATION	ELEMENTS		DEFINITION
catheter	**KATH**-eh-ter		Greek *to send down*	Hollow tube that allows passage of fluid into or out of a body cavity, organ, or vessel
catheterize (verb)	**KATH**-eh-teh-**RIZE**	S/ S/ R/	-ize *action* -er- *agent* cathet- *catheter*	To introduce a catheter
catheterization (*Note:* Unusual three suffixes.)	**KATH**-eh-ter-ih-**ZAY**-shun	S/	-ation *process*	Introduction of a catheter
creatine kinase	**KREE**-ah-teen **KI**-naze	S/ R/ S/ R/	-ine *pertaining to* creat- *flesh* -ase *enzyme* kin- *motion*	Enzyme elevated in plasma following heart muscle damage in myocardial infarction
echocardiography	**EK**-oh-kar-dee-**OG**-rah-fee	S/ R/CF R/CF	-graphy *process of recording* ech/o- *sound wave* -cardi/o- *heart*	Ultrasound recording of heart function
homocysteine	ho-moh-**SIS**-teen	P/ R	homo- *same* -cysteine *an amino acid*	An amino acid similar to cysteine
lipoprotein	**LIE**-poh-pro-teen	R/CF R/	lip/o- *fat* -protein *protein*	Molecules made of combinations of fat and protein
natriuretic peptide	**NAH**-tree-you-**RET**-ik **PEP**-tide	S/ R/CF R/ S/ R/	-ic *pertaining to* natr/i- *sodium* -uret- *ureter* -ide *having a particular quality* pept- *amino acid*	Protein that increases the excretion of sodium
sonograph	**SON**-oh-graf	S/ R/CF	-graph *to record* son/o- *sound*	Instrument that uses sound waves to create images of structures
sonographer sonogram	so-**NOG**-rah-fer **SON**-oh-gram	S/ S/	-grapher *one who records* -gram *a record*	The technician who performs a sonogram Image obtained by using a sonograph
tomography	toe-**MOG**-rah-fee	S/ R/CF	-graphy *process of recording* tom/o- *section, cut*	Radiographic image of a selected slice of tissue
transducer	trans-**DYU**-sir	P/ R/	trans- *across* -ducer *to lead*	Device that converts energy from one form to another
triglyceride	tri-**GLISS**-eh-ride	S/ P/ R/	-ide *having a particular quality* tri- *three* -glycer- *glycerol*	Any of a group of fats containing three fatty acids

Exercises

A. Identify the type of element and its meaning in the appropriate column. *The first one is done for you.* Fill in the blanks.   **LO 10.6**

Element	Meaning of Prefix	Meaning of Root/Combining Form	Meaning of Suffix
ase			*Enzyme*
1. cardio			
2. creat			
3. echo			
4. graphy			
5. homo			
6. ide			

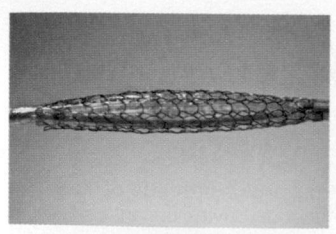

▲ Figure 10.17 Stent.

Abbreviations

ACE	angiotensin-converting enzyme
CABG	coronary artery bypass graft
OR	operating room
PTCA	percutaneous transluminal coronary angioplasty
tPA	tissue plasminogen activator

LO 10.11 Treatment Procedures

The most immediate need in the treatment of MI is to provide perfusion to get blood and oxygen to the affected myocardium. This can be attempted in several ways:

1. **Clot-busting drugs (thrombolysis).** Streptokinase or tissue plasminogen activator (**tPA**) are injected within a few hours of the MI to dissolve the thrombus.

2. **Artery-cleaning angioplasty (percutaneous transluminal coronary angioplasty [PTCA]).** A balloon-tipped catheter is guided to the site of the blockage and inflated to expand the artery from the inside by compressing the plaque against the walls of the artery.

3. **Stent placement.** To reduce the likelihood that the artery will close up again (occlude), a wire mesh tube, or stent (*Figure 10.17*), is placed inside the vessel. Some stents (**drug-eluting** stents) are covered with a special medication to help keep the artery open.

4. **Coronary artery bypass graft (CABG).** In this procedure, mostly used for people with extensive disease in several arteries, healthy blood vessels harvested from the leg, chest, or arm detour blood around blocked coronary arteries. The procedure is performed by using a heart-lung machine that pumps the recipient's blood through the machine to oxygenate it while surgery is performed. More recently, the procedure is being performed "off-pump" with the heart still beating.

5. **Rotational atherectomy.** A high-speed rotational device is used to "sand" away plaque. This procedure has limited acceptance.

Other procedures used in cardiology include the following:

- **Cardioversion**, which uses a therapeutic dose of electrical current to the heart synchronized to a specific moment in the electrical cycle (at the QRS complex) to convert an abnormally fast heart rate or cardiac arrhythmia to a normal rhythm.

- **Defibrillation**, which uses a nonsynchronized electrical shock to terminate ventricular fibrillation or pulseless ventricular tachycardia and revert to a normal rhythm. It is not effective for asystole.

- **Radiofrequency ablation**, which uses a catheter with an electrode in its tip guided into the heart to destroy the cells from which abnormal cardiac rhythms are originating.

- **Heart transplant**, in which the heart of a recently deceased person (donor) is transplanted to the recipient after the recipient's diseased heart has been removed. The immune characteristics of the donor and recipient have to be a close match.

LO 10.11 Cardiac Pharmacology

Clinically, six types of cardiac drugs are in use:

1. **Anticoagulants** are drugs that reduce susceptibility to thrombus formation. These include aspirin, warfarin (Coumadin), heparin, and dabigatran etexilate (Pradaxa).

2. **Chronotropic drugs** alter the heart rate. Epinephrine (adrenaline), norepinephrine, and atropine increase the heart rate. Quinidine, procainamide, lidocaine, and propranolol slow the heart.

3. **Inotropic drugs** alter the contractions of the myocardium. Digitalis and its derivatives, digoxin and digitoxin, increase the strength of contractions of the myocardium, leading to increased cardiac output. **Vasoconstrictor** drugs, such as Vasoxyl (methoxamine) and Aramine (metariminol), cause vasoconstriction. Both classes of drugs work via the autonomic nervous system,. Vasoconstrictors are used in the resuscitation of seriously ill patients and for the treatment of hypotension in the **operating room (OR)**.

4. **Diuretics** indirectly affect the heart by stimulating urinary fluid loss to lessen the fluid volume with which the heart has to cope. Thiazides are an example. Diuril (chlorthiazide) is a thiazide diuretic. Lasix (furosemide) is a loop diuretic; Aldactone (spironolactone) is a potassium-sparing diuretic.

5. **Antiarrhythmics** change the electrical properties of the myocardial cells to restore normal rate and rhythm. Beta-blockers (**beta-adrenergic-blocking agents**) reduce the rate and strength of myocardial contraction and are used in treating arrhythmias.

6. **Vasodilators** relax smooth muscle in arterioles. For example, nitroglycerin dilates both peripheral and coronary blood vessels. **Calcium channel blockers** have the dual effect of reducing contractility and dilating coronary arteries. **Angiotensin-converting enzyme inhibitors** (**ACE** inhibitors) dilate arteries and veins and can be used to treat hypertension.

WORD	PRONUNCIATION	ELEMENTS		DEFINITION
ablation	ab-**LAY**-shun	S/ R/	-ion *process* ablat- *take away*	Removal of a tissue to destroy its function
adrenergic	ad-re-**NER**-jik	S/ R/ R/	-ic *pertaining to* adren- *adrenal gland* -erg- *work*	Relating to the autonomic nervous system
angioplasty	AN-jee-oh-**PLAS**-tee	S/ R/CF	-plasty *formation* angi/o- *blood vessel*	Recanalization of a blood vessel by surgery
angiotensin	an-jee-oh-**TEN**-sin	S/	-tensin *tense, taut*	An agent that constricts blood vessels
beta	**BAY**-tah		Greek	Second letter in the Greek alphabet
chronotropic	**KRONE**-oh-**TROH**-pic	S/ R/CF	-tropic *change* chron/o- *time*	Affecting the rate of rhythmic movements, in this case the heart rate
diuretic	die-you-**RET**-ik	S/ P/ R/	-ic *pertaining to* di- *from dia—throughout* -uret- *urine, urination*	Agent that increases urine output
inotropic	IN-oh-**TROH**-pic	S/ R/	-tropic *change* ino- *sinew*	Affecting the contractility of cardiac muscle
stent	STENT		Charles Stent, English dentist, nineteenth century	Wire mesh tube used to keep arteries open

Exercises

A. Deconstruct the medical terms in this chart to their basic elements. *Fill in the blanks.*   **LO 10.6, 10.11**

Medical Term	Prefix	Root/CF	Suffix
angiotensin	1.	2.	3.
inotropic	4.	5.	6.
ablation	7.	8.	9.
diuretic	10.	11.	12.
adrenergic	13.	14.	15.
chronotropic	16.	17.	18.
angioplasty	19.	20.	21.

B. Choose any two terms from the table in Exercise A above and use each in a sentence that is not a definition.   LO 10.6

1. _____

_____

2. _____

_____

LESSON OBJECTIVES

To understand the etiologies and effects of Mrs. Jones's problems (see CR 10.2) and communicate with her and Dr. Bannerjee about them, you need to have the medical terminology and knowledge to be able to:

10.3.1 Explain the functions of the peripheral circulation.
10.3.2 Identify the major arteries and veins in the body.
10.3.3 Match the structure of the different blood vessels to their functions.
10.3.4 Explain the dynamics and control of blood flow in the circulatory systems.
10.3.5 Describe the effects of common disorders of the circulatory systems on health.

You are

. . . a medical assistant working for Dr. Lokesh Bannerjee, a cardiologist in Fulwood Medical Center.

Your patient is

. . . Mrs. Martha Jones. You are documenting her medical record after Dr. Bannerjee has interviewed, examined, and reported his findings back to Dr. Susan Lee, who referred Mrs. Jones to Dr. Bannerjee.

Keynotes

The peripheral circulation

- Transports oxygen, nutrients, hormones, and enzymes to the cells and carries carbon dioxide and waste products to the lungs, liver, and kidney for excretion

- Maintains homeostasis by enabling cells to meet their metabolic needs and maintains a steady flow of blood and blood presure in the tissues

Case Report 10.2

Documentation.

Fulwood Medical Center
Consultation Request and Report Form

Patient's Name: Jones, MARTHA   Age: 52
To: Dr. LOKESH BANNERJEE   Department: Cardiology
From: Dr. Susan Lee   Department: Primary Care
Patient's Location: FULWOOD MEDICAL CENTER

Type of Consultation Desired:
  ☐ Consultation Only
  ☐ Consulation and follow Jointly
  ☒ Accept in Transfer

Referring Diagnoses: CLAUDICATION, POSSIBLE DVT
Reason for Consultation: Severe pain in both legs on walking

Signature: _____   Date: 12/12/12   Time 1105 hrs
Consultation Report: by Lokesh Bannerjee
Chief complaint: Pt. c/o severe pain in both legs on walking about 100 yards or climbing a flight of stairs. Pain is so severe she must stop and wait 5 mins. before she can go on. For the past two weeks she has noticed soreness and hardness along a vein in her left calf.
Past medical history: Known type 2 diabetic with hypertension, CAD, diabetic retinopathy, and OA of her hips and knees. Several episodes of ketoacidosis and one of pulmonary edema. Bariatric surgery performed 8 months prior at 275 lbs.
Medications: metformin, verapamil, propanolol, Mevacor
Allergies: NKA
Physical examination: Ht: 5'2" WT: 190 lbs. BP: 170/100 sitting. P: 80, regular. Both feet show slight pitting edema and skin is pale, cold, and dry. Small ulcer on lateral margin of each big toe. Varicosities, both legs. Tender cord in superficial vein of left calf. Flexion of left foot produces pain in left calf. Chest clear. Heart sounds unremarkable. No loss of sensation in legs or feet.
Impression: 1. Varicose veins, both legs.
    2. Severe claudication, both legs.
    3. probable deep vein thrombosis, left leg
    4. possible peripheral neuropathy
    5. H/O diabetes type 2, CAD, hypertension, retinopathy, OA
Plan: Admit patient to cardiology unit stat for IV heparin and conversion to oral anticoagulant therapy with Coumadin. Doppler studies, venogram, and angiogram have been ordered.

Signature: _____   Date 12/12/12   Time 1250 hrs

WORD	PRONUNCIATION	ELEMENTS		DEFINITION
angiogram	**AN**-jee-oh-gram	S/ R/CF	**-gram** *a record* **angi/o-** *blood vessel*	Radiograph obtained after injection of radiopaque contrast material into blood vessels
artery	**AR**-ter-ee		Greek *artery*	Thick-walled blood vessel carrying blood away from the heart
circulation	ser-kyu-**LAY**-shun		Latin *to encircle*	Continuous movement of blood through the heart and blood vessels
claudication	klaw-dih-**KAY**-shun	S/ R/	**-ation** *process* **claudic-** *limping*	Intermittent leg pain and limping
Doppler	**DOP**-ler		Johann Doppler, Austrian mathematician and physicist, 1803–1853	Diagnostic instrument that sends an ultrasonic beam into the body
peripheral	peh-**RIF**-er-al	S/ R/	**-al** *pertaining to* **periph-** *outer part*	Pertaining to a part of the body away from a central point. For example, the peripheral circulation is away from the heart
varix varices (pl) varicose (adj) varicosities	**VAIR**-iks **VAIR**-ih-sees **VAIR**-ih-kos vair-ih-**KOS**-ih-tees	 S/ R/ S/	Latin *dilated vein* **-ose** *full of* **varic-** *dilated, tortuous vein* **-ities** *collection of*	Dilated, tortuous vein Characterized by varices Collection of varicose veins
vein venogram venous (adj)	VANE **VEE**-noh-gram **VEE**-nuss	 S/ R/CF S/	Latin *vein* **-gram** *a record* **ven/o-** *vein* **-ous** *pertaining to*	Blood vessel carrying blood toward heart Radiograph of veins after injection of radiopaque contrast material Pertaining to venous blood or the venous circulation

Exercises

A. Terms from the above WAD can all be correctly inserted into the following paragraph of radiology documentation.

Watch your singular and plural forms of terms. Fill in the blanks.   **LO 10.12, 10.13**

veins   varicosities   varix   vein   varicose   varices   venogram

1. The _____ performed on this patient's left saphenous and popliteal _____ shows the following:

   One slightly engorged and dilated _____ at the midpoint of the saphenous _____ and several

   _____ at the terminal end of the popliteal. Diagnosis: _____ veins.

   These _____ need immediate attention by a vascular surgeon.

B. Refer to the consultation form shown above for Mrs. Jones. *Answer the questions regarding her visit to the cardiologist.*   **LO 10.6, 10.9, 10.10, 10.11**

1. Why is Mrs. Jones being transferred to Dr. Bannerjee's care?

   _____

2. What diagnoses did Dr. Lee make prior to Mrs. Jones' visit to the cardiologist?

   _____

3. What diagnostic studies were ordered for Mrs. Jones?

   _____

4. What drugs were immediately ordered for Mrs. Jones?

   _____

5. If this problem is not attended to immediately, what could possibly happen to Mrs. Jones?

   _____

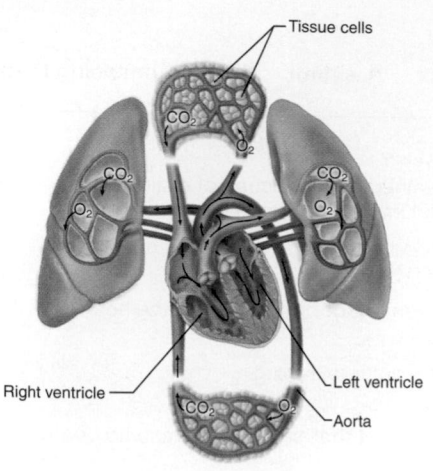

▲ Figure 10.18 Systemic and Pulmonary Circulations.

LO 10.12, 10.13 Blood Circulations

There are two major circulations, the **pulmonary** and the **systemic**.

Pulmonary Circulation

Deoxygenated blood from the body flows into the right atrium of the heart and then into the right ventricle that pumps it out into the pulmonary trunk *(Figure 10.18)*. This trunk branches into the right pulmonary artery to the right lung and the left pulmonary artery to the left lung. Gas exchange occurs between the air in the lungs and blood *(see Chapter 13)*. Carbon dioxide is removed from the blood and excreted into the air. Oxygen is taken into the blood from the air in the lungs.

The blood exits each lung through two pulmonary veins. All four pulmonary veins take blood into the left atrium of the heart.

Systemic Arterial Circulation

The systemic circulation refers to the process wherein oxygenated blood enters the left side of the heart from the pulmonary veins. The blood passes through the left atrium into the left ventricle. The ventricle pumps it out into the **aorta**, which takes the blood to all areas of the body.

The aorta is described in four parts:

1. **Ascending aorta**, which gives rise to the coronary circulation. Right and left coronary arteries branch from it to supply the myocardium.

2. **Aortic arch** *(Figure 10.19)*, which has three main branches:

   a. **Brachiocephalic artery**, a short artery that divides into two arteries:

   i. **Right common carotid artery**, which supplies the right side of the head, brain, and neck.

   ii. **Right subclavian artery**, which supplies the right upper limb.

   b. **Left common carotid artery**, which supplies the left side of the head, brain, and neck. The right and left common carotid arteries divide into two branches:

   i. The **internal carotid** artery, which enters the cranial cavity through a foramen in the base of the skull and supplies the brain.

   ii. The **external carotid** artery, which supplies the neck and face.

   c. **Left subclavian artery**, which supplies the left upper limb.

3. **Thoracic aorta**, which has two major groups of branches:

   a. **Visceral** branches—small **bronchial arteries** that supply the bronchi and bronchioles *(see Chapter 13)*, the esophagus, and the pericardium.

   b. **Parietal** branches—**intercostal arteries** that supply the chest wall and a **phrenic artery** that supplies the diaphragm.

4. **Abdominal aorta**, which has two major groups of branches:

   a. **Visceral branches** that supply the abdominal organs:

   i. **Celiac trunk**, which supplies the stomach, liver, gallbladder, pancreas, and spleen.

   ii. **Superior mesenteric artery**, which supplies the small intestine and part of the large intestine.

   iii. **Inferior mesenteric artery**, which supplies the remainder of the large intestine.

   iv. Paired **renal arteries**, which supply the kidneys and adrenal glands.

   v. Paired **gonadal arteries**, which supply the testes or ovaries.

   b. Four pairs of **lumbar** arteries that supply the abdominal wall.

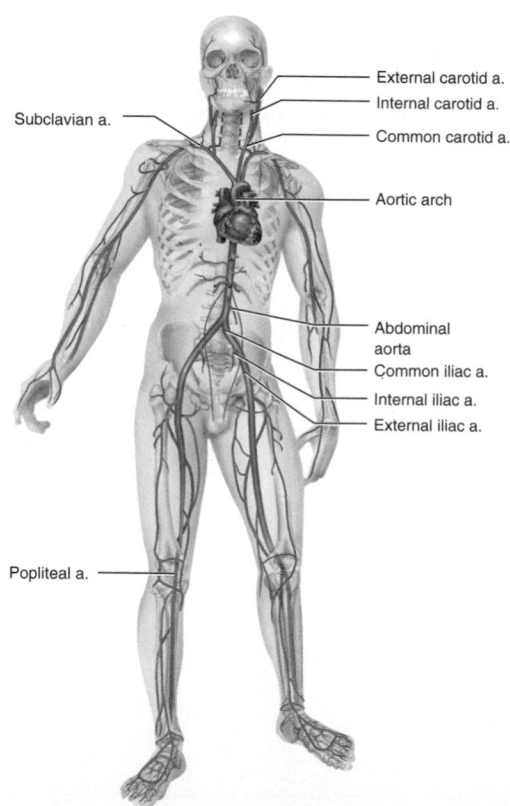

▲ Figure 10.19 The Major Systemic Arteries. *(a. = artery; aa. = arteries)*

At the level of the fifth lumbar vertebra (at the top of the pelvis), the aorta divides into the right and left **common iliac arteries**. Visceral branches from these arteries supply the urinary bladder, uterus, and vagina. The common iliac arteries give off an internal iliac artery to supply the pelvis. The common iliac artery becomes the external iliac artery and then the femoral artery as it goes down the thigh and supplies the lower limb. The pulse that can be felt in the back of the knee is from the **popliteal artery**.

WORD	PRONUNCIATION	ELEMENTS		DEFINITION
brachiocephalic	BRAY-kee-oh-seh-FAL-ik	S/ R/CF R/	-ic *pertaining to* brachi/o- *arm* -cephal- *head*	Pertaining to the head and arm, as an artery supplying blood to both
carotid	kah-ROT-id		Greek *carotid arteries*	Main artery of the neck
gonad gonadal (adj)	GO-nad go-NAD-al		Greek *seed*	Testis or ovary
iliac	ILL-ee-ack		Latin *groin, flank*	Pertaining to or near the ilium (pelvic bone)
popliteal	pop-LIT-ee-al	S/ R/CF	-al *pertaining to* poplit/e- *back of knee*	Pertaining to the back of the knee
subclavian	sub-CLAY-vee-an	S/ P/ R/	-ian *one who does* sub- *under* -clav- *clavicle*	Underneath the clavicle

Exercises

A. Use the medical terminology of the circulatory system and circle the correct answers.   LO 10.12

1. Blood in the systemic circulation is

    oxygenated   viscous   deoxygenated   clotted

2. The blood exits each lung through

    vena cava   pulmonary veins   aorta   pulmonary arteries

3. The *coronary circulation* arises in the

    thoracic aorta   carotid arteries   ascending aorta   subclavian arteries

4. *Carbon dioxide* is removed from the blood and excreted through

    dehydration   inspiration   inhalation   expiration

5. The *gonadal* arteries supply the

    testes   ovaries   kidneys   testes and ovaries

6. *Deoxygenated blood* from the body flows into the

    right atrium   right ventricle   left atrium   left ventricle

7. *Gas exchange* occurs between the air in the lungs and the

    heart   blood   ventricles   windpipe

8. _____ is a term relating to the abdominal cavity.

    thoracic   iliac   celiac   brachiocephalic

9. The pulse that can be felt at the back of the knee is from the

    aorta   popliteal vein   carotid artery   popliteal artery

10. The _____ arteries supply the chest wall.

    phrenic   visceral   intercostal   mesenteric

11. This circulation takes blood to all areas of the body:

    coronary   pulmonary   cardiovascular   systemic

12. The *subclavian* artery is located

    above the heart   below the stomach   above the neck   below the collarbone

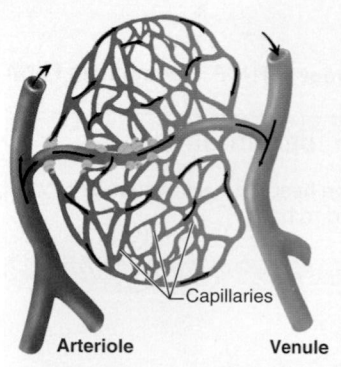

▲ Figure 10.20
Capillary Bed.

LO 10.13 Blood Vessels in the Circulations

Arterioles, Capillaries, and Venules

As the arteries branch farther away from the heart and distribute blood to specific organs, they become smaller, muscular vessels called **arterioles**. By contracting and relaxing, these arterioles are the primary controllers by which the body directs the relative amounts of blood that organs and structures receive.

From there, the blood flows into **capillaries** and **capillary beds** (*Figure 10.20*). There are approximately 10 billion capillaries in the body. Each capillary consists of only a single layer of endothelium supported by a thin connective tissue basement membrane. Between the overlapping endothelial cells are thin slits through which larger water-soluble substances can pass. Red blood cells flow through the small capillaries in single file.

From the capillaries, tiny **venules** accept the blood and merge to form **veins**. The veins form reservoirs for blood; at any moment 60% to 70% of the total blood volume is contained in the venules and veins.

The circulatory system exists to serve the capillaries because capillaries are the only place where water and materials are exchanged between the blood and tissue fluids.

Diffusion is the means by which this capillary exchange occurs. Nutrients and oxygen diffuse from a higher concentration in the capillaries to a lower concentration in the **interstitial** fluid around the cells. Waste products diffuse from a higher concentration in the interstitial fluid to a lower concentration in the capillaries.

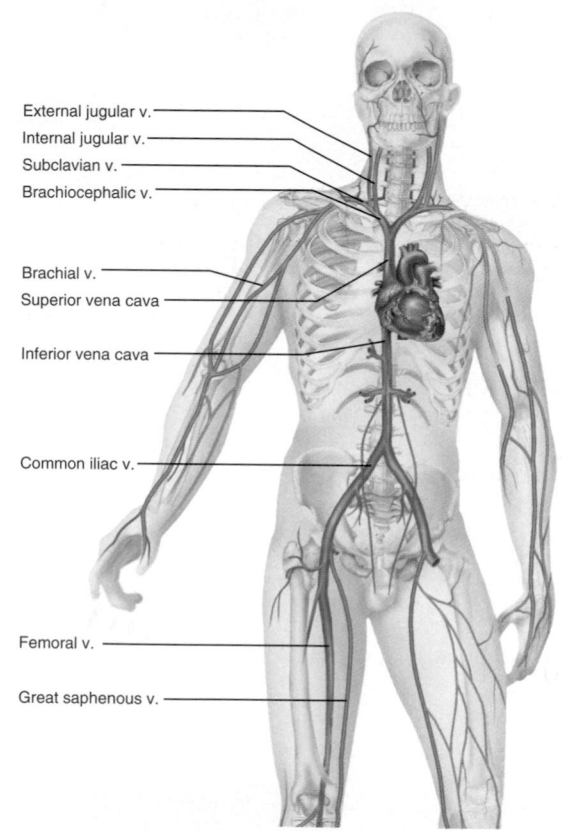

External jugular v.
Internal jugular v.
Subclavian v.
Brachiocephalic v.

Brachial v.
Superior vena cava

Inferior vena cava

Common iliac v.

Femoral v.

Great saphenous v.

▲ Figure 10.21 **The Major Systemic Veins.** (*v.* = vein; *vv.* = veins)

Systemic Venous Circulation

There are three major types of veins (*Figure 10.21*):

1. **Superficial**—such as those you can see under the skin of your arms and hands.

2. **Deep**—running parallel to arteries and draining the same tissues that the arteries supply.

3. **Venous sinuses**—in the head and heart and having specific functions.

In the lower limb, the superficial veins merge to form the **saphenous vein**. The deep veins form the **femoral vein**. They join together with veins from the pelvis to form the **common iliac vein**. The right and left common iliac veins form the **inferior vena cava (IVC)**.

Veins draining the abdominal organs merge into the **hepatic portal vein**, which delivers nutrients from the stomach and intestines to the liver. Within the liver, the nutrients are either stored or converted into chemicals that can be used by other cells in the body. The blood leaves the liver in **hepatic veins** that drain into the IVC.

In the upper limb, the superficial veins merge to form the **axillary vein**. The deep veins alongside the limb arteries empty into the **brachial veins**. These also flow into the axillary vein.

As the axillary vein passes behind the clavicle, its name changes to the **subclavian vein**.

Abbreviations	
IVC	inferior vena cava
SVC	superior vena cava

In the head and neck, the superficial veins outside the skull drain into the right and left **external jugular veins**. Inside the cranial cavity, **venous sinuses** around the brain drain into the right and left **internal jugular veins**.

The external jugular veins empty into the subclavian veins. The internal jugular veins join with the subclavian veins on each side to form the **brachiocephalic veins**. The right and left brachiocephalic veins join together to form the **superior vena cava (SVC)**. The SVC empties into the right atrium.

Word Analysis and Definition

S = Suffix   P = Prefix   R = Root   R/CF = Combining Form

WORD	PRONUNCIATION	ELEMENTS		DEFINITION
arteriole	ar-TER-ee-ole	S/ R/	Latin *small artery* -ole *small* arteri- *artery*	Small terminal artery leading into the capillary network
axilla axillary (adj)	AK-sill-ah AK-sil-air-ee	S/ R/	Latin *armpit* -ary *pertaining to* axill- *armpit*	Medical name for the armpit Pertaining to the axilla
brachial	BRAY-kee-al	S/ R/	-ial *pertaining to* brachi- *arm*	Pertaining to the arm
capillary	KAP-ih-lair-ee	S/ R/	-ary *pertaining to* capill- *hairlike structure*	Minute blood vessel between the arterial and venous systems
femoral	FEM-oh-ral	S/ R/	-al *pertaining to* femor- *femur*	Pertaining to the femur
interstitial	in-ter-STISH-al	S/ R/	-ial *pertaining to* interstit- *spaces within tissues*	Pertaining to spaces between cells in a tissue or organ
jugular	JUG-you-lar	S/ R/	-ar *pertaining to* jugul- *throat*	Pertaining to the throat
saphenous	SAPH-ih-nus		Root unknown	Relating to the saphenous vein in the thigh
vein	VANE		Latin *vein*	Blood vessel carrying blood toward the heart
venule	VEN-yule	S/ R/	Latin *small vein* -ule *small* ven- *vein*	Small vein leading from the capillary network

Exercises

A. Build your knowledge of the elements and terms that make up the *language of the cardiovascular system*. *All your answers can come from the above WAD. Fill in the blanks.*   **LO 10.6, 10.13**

1. The two suffixes in the above WAD that both mean *small* are _____ and _____.

2. A small vein is a _____, and a small artery is an _____.

3. An axillary lymph node is located in the _____.

4. List two terms in the above WAD whose *different* suffixes both mean *pertaining to*.

    Terms are _____ and _____.

    Suffixes are _____ and _____.

5. The brachial pulse can be found in the _____.

6. List the four general terms in the above WAD that are blood vessels: _____, _____, _____, and _____

7. The jugular vein is in the _____ (location).

B. Identify the body location of the following veins. *Fill in the blanks.*   **LO 10.12, 10.13**

1. subclavian vein _____

2. saphenous vein _____

3. femoral vein _____

4. brachial vein _____

5. hepatic vein _____

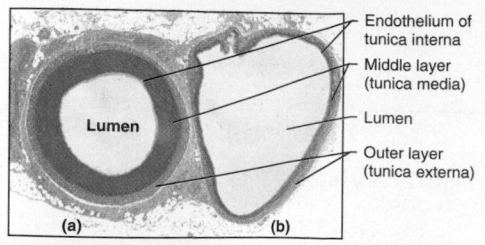

▲ **Figure 10.22** **Anatomy of an Artery and Vein.** (*a*) Artery. (*b*) Vein.

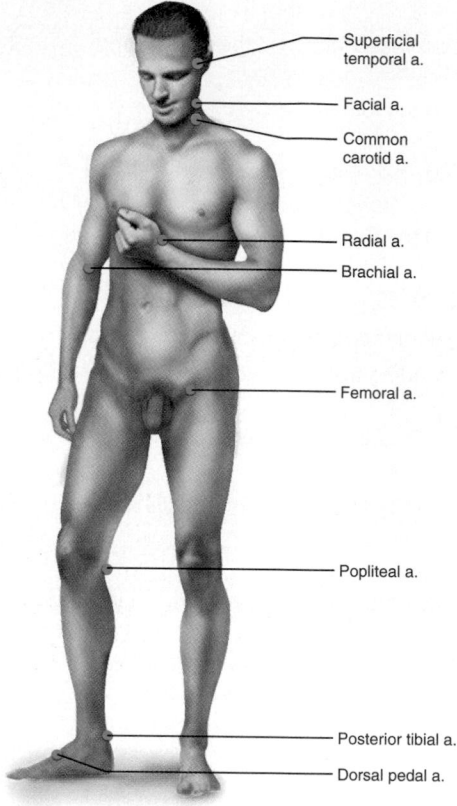

▲ **Figure 10.23** **Arterial Pulses.** (*a.* = artery)

LO 10.13 Blood Vessel Function Related to Structure

Except for the capillaries and venules, all the blood vessel walls show a basic structure of three layers (*Figure 10.22*):

1. **Tunica intima (interna)**—the innermost layer of endothelial cells, with thin layers of fibrous and elastic connective tissue supporting them.

2. **Tunica media**—a middle layer of smooth muscle cells arranged circularly around the blood vessel. A membrane of elastic tissue separates the tunica media from the outer layer of the wall.

3. **Tunica adventitia (externa)**—an outer connective tissue layer of varying density and thickness.

The larger arteries near the heart, the aorta and its major branches, have to cope with large quantities of blood and fluctuating pressures between systole and diastole. Therefore, these arteries have a large number of elastic fibers and a relatively small number of muscle fibers.

The functions of the medium-sized and smaller arteries are to regulate the blood supply to the different regions of the body and to ensure that the blood pressure in the arteries is at an appropriate level. The tunica media of these arteries contains 25 to 40 layers of smooth muscle to enable the muscles to contract (**vasoconstriction**) and to relax (**vasodilation**) to increase flow.

The function of the veins is to return the blood from the periphery to the heart in a low-pressure system. For example, by the time blood reaches the venules, its pressure has dropped from the 120 mm Hg of systole to around 15 mm Hg. By the time the blood is in the venae cavae, the **central venous pressure (CVP)** is down to around 4 to 5 mm Hg.

Veins have a much thinner tunica media than arteries, with few muscle cells and elastic fibers (*Figure 10.22*). They have a larger lumen and a thick tunica adventitia that merges with the connective tissue of surrounding structures. In the limbs, the veins are surrounded and massaged by muscles to squeeze the blood along the veins. One-way valves in the veins allow the blood to flow toward the heart but not away from the heart. They are shaped like and function like the semilunar valves of the heart.

Space Medicine

Normally, gravity helps the blood circulate in the lower limbs. When astronauts are weightless for long periods of time, blood pools in the central and upper areas of the body, and there appears to be an excess blood volume. The kidney compensates by excreting more fluid, leading to a 10% to 20% decrease in blood volume and a low blood pressure. Astronauts compensate for this by wearing lower-body suction suits, which apply a vacuum force to draw blood into the lower limbs.

Arterial Pulses

The pulse is always part of a clinical examination because it can show heart rate, rhythm, and the state of the arterial wall by **palpation**. There are nine locations on each side of the body where large arteries are close to the surface and can be palpated (*Figure 10.23*).

The most easily accessible is the **radial artery** at the wrist, where the pulse is usually taken. The **brachial artery** at the elbow is also used for taking blood pressure readings. All the pulse sites can be used as **pressure points** to temporarily reduce arterial bleeding in an emergency.

The two pulses that can be palpated in the feet are the **pedal** pulses, one in each foot.

Blood Pressure

Blood pressure (BP) is the force the blood exerts on arterial walls as it is pumped around the circulatory system by the left ventricle. The pressure is measured using a **sphygmomanometer** and a stethoscope.

Keynotes

- All blood vessel walls have three layers.

- **Vital signs (VS)** measure temperature (T), pulse rate (P), respiration rate (R), and blood pressure (BP) to assess cardiorespiratory function.

Abbreviations

CVP	central venous pressure
VS	vital signs

S = Suffix   P = Prefix   **R = Root**   **R/CF = Combining Form**

WORD	PRONUNCIATION	ELEMENTS		DEFINITION
adventitia	ad-ven-**TISH**-ah		Latin *from outside*	Outer layer of connective tissue covering blood vessels or organs
intima	**IN**-tih-ma		Latin *inmost*	Inner layer of a structure, particularly a blood vessel
media	**ME**-dee-ah		Latin *middle*	Middle layer of a structure, particularly a blood vessel
palpate palpation (noun)	**PAL**-pate pal-**PAY**-shun	S/ R/	Latin *touch, stroke* -ion *process* **palpat-** *touch, stroke*	To examine with the fingers and hands An examination with the fingers and hands
pedal	**PEED**-al	S/ R/	-al *pertaining to* **ped-** *foot*	Pertaining to the foot
radial	**RAY**-dee-al	S/ R/	-al *pertaining to* **radi-** *radius (forearm bone)*	Pertaining to the forearm
sphygmomanometer	**SFIG**-moh-mah-**NOM**-ih-ter	S/ R/CF R/CF	-meter *instrument to measure* **sphygm/o-** *pulse* -**man/o-** *pressure*	Instrument for measuring arterial blood pressure
tunica	**TYU**-nih-kah		Latin *coat*	A layer in the wall of a blood vessel or other tubular structure
vasoconstriction	**VAY**-soh-con-**STRIK**-shun	S/ R/CF R/	-ion *process* **vas/o-** *blood vessel* -**constrict-** *narrow*	Reduction in diameter of a blood vessel
vasodilation	**VAY**-soh-di-**LAY**-shun	S/ R/CF R/	-ion *process* **vas/o-** *blood vessel* -**dilat-** *open up*	Increase in diameter of a blood vessel
vital signs	**VI**-tal SIGNS		**vital** Latin *life* **signs** Latin *mark*	A procedure during a physical examination in which temperature, pulse rate, respiration rate, and blood pressure are measured to assess general health and cardiorespiratory function

Exercises

A. Match the definition in the left column with the correct medical term in the right column.   LO 10.12

_____ 1. To examine by feeling with fingers and hand

_____ 2. Reduction in diameter of a blood vessel

_____ 3. Inner layer of a structure

_____ 4. Latin for *coat*

_____ 5. Outer tissue covering of an organ

_____ 6. Instrument to measure blood pressure

_____ 7. Pertaining to the foot

_____ 8. Increase in diameter of a blood vessel

_____ 9. Middle layer of a structure

_____ 10. Pertaining to the forearm

a. radial

b. vasodilation

c. adventitia

d. pedal

e. vasoconstriction

f. media

g. intima

h. sphygmomanometer

i. palpate

j. tunica

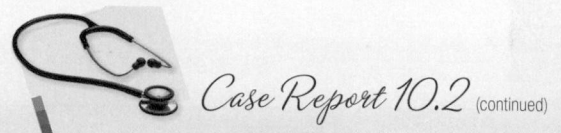

Case Report 10.2 (continued)

Mrs. Martha Jones, who had been referred to Dr. Bannerjee's cardiovascular clinic, has several circulatory problems related to her diabetes and obesity. She was diagnosed previously with hypertension, CAD, and diabetic retinopathy. She now has severe pain in her legs when walking.

Her **ankle/brachial index (ABI)**, which measures the ratio of the blood pressure in her ankle to that in her arm, showed significant blockage of blood flow. Doppler studies confirmed this. This blockage produces the pain when walking (intermittent claudication). It is due to arteriosclerosis of the large arteries in her legs. Angiograms showed several atherosclerotic areas in her popliteal artery.

The ulcers on the edges of her big toes result from thickening of the walls of her capillaries and arterioles and the resulting poor circulation to her feet. Again, this is due to her diabetes.

In the venous system of her legs, the tender cordlike lesion is due to thrombophlebitis of a superficial vein in her left leg.

Pain in the calf on flexion of the ankle (Homans sign) indicates that she may have a **deep vein thrombosis (DVT)**. A venogram confirmed this diagnosis.

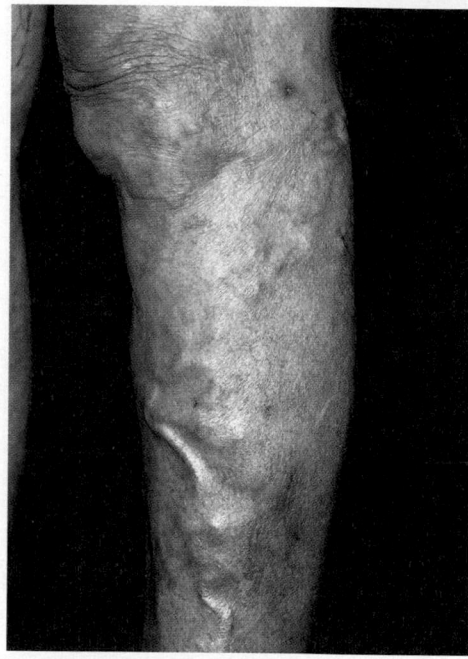

▲ **Figure 10.24**   Varicose Veins of Leg.

Abbreviations

ABI	ankle/brachial index
DVT	deep vein thrombosis
PVD	peripheral vascular disease

LO 10.13 Circulatory Disorders

Disorders of Veins

Thrombophlebitis is an inflammation of the lining of a vein (tunica intima), allowing clots (thrombi) to form.

Deep vein thrombosis (DVT) is thrombus formation in a deep vein, often due to reduced blood flow. Risk factors include immobility, surgery, prolonged travel, and contraception (estrogen). The increased pressure in the capillaries due to back pressure from the blocked blood flow in the veins causes an increase in the flow of fluid from the capillaries to the interstitial spaces. The collection of fluid is called **edema**.

A major complication of thrombus formation is that a piece of the clot can break off and be carried in the bloodstream to lodge in a blood vessel in another organ and block blood flow. The piece that breaks off is called an **embolus**. It often lodges in the lungs, producing a pulmonary embolus *(see Chapter 13)*.

Varicose veins are superficial veins that have lost their elasticity and appear swollen and tortuous *(Figure 10.24)*. Their valves become incompetent, and blood flows backward and pools. Smaller, more superficial varicose veins are called **spider veins**. Varicose veins are associated with a family history, obesity, and prolonged standing. Treatments offered include laser technology and **sclerotherapy**, where solutions that scar **(sclerose)** the veins are injected into them. **Collateral** circulations develop to take the blood through alternative routes.

A **phlebotomist** is a technician who draws blood. The procedure is called **phlebotomy**.

Disorders of Arteries

Peripheral vascular disease (PVD) is a general term describing all the disorders of the systemic arterial and venous systems.

An **aneurysm** is a localized dilation of an artery as a result of a localized weakness of the vessel wall. Common sites occur along the aorta, mostly the abdominal aorta. They can rupture, leading to severe bleeding and hypovolemic shock. Surgical repair consists of excision of the aneurysm and replacement with a synthetic graft.

Intracranial aneurysms, particularly at the base of the brain, are an important cause of bleeds into the cranial cavity *(see Chapter 9)*.

Thromboangiitis obliterans (Buerger disease) is an inflammatory disease of the arteries with clot formation, usually in the legs. The occlusion of arteries and impaired circulation leads to intermittent claudication.

Carotid artery disease affects the two major arteries supplying the brain. They can be involved in arteriosclerosis and the deposition of plaque, which puts the patient at risk for a stroke. If an artery is more than 70% blocked, a carotid **endarterectomy** can be performed to surgically remove the plaque.

WORD	PRONUNCIATION	ELEMENTS		DEFINITION
aneurysm	**AN**-yur-izm		Greek *dilation*	Circumscribed dilation of an artery or cardiac chamber
collateral	koh-**LAT**-er-al	S/ P/ R/	-al *pertaining to* col- *before* -later- *at the side*	Situated at the side, often to bypass an obstruction
edema edematous (adj) pitting edema	ee-**DEE**-mah ee-**DEM**-ah-tus	S/ R/	Greek *swelling* tous *pertaining to* edema- *swelling, edema*	Excessive accumulation of fluid in cells and tissues Pertaining to or marked by edema Edema that maintains for a time indentations made by applying pressure to the area
embolus	**EM**-bo-lus		Greek *plug, stopped*	Detached piece of thrombus, a mass of bacteria, quantity of air, or foreign body that blocks a blood vessel
endarterectomy	**END**-ar-ter-**EK**-toe-me	S/ P/ R/	-ectomy- *surgical excision* end- *within* -arter- *artery*	Surgical removal of plaque from an artery
peripheral phlebitis	peh-**RIF**-er-al fleh-**BIE**-tis	S/ R/ S/ R/	-al *pertaining to* peripher- *outer part* -itis *inflammation* phleb- *vein*	Pertaining to the periphery or an external boundary Inflammation of a vein
phlebotomist phlebotomy	fleh-**BOT**-oh-mist fleh-**BOT**-oh-me	S/ R/CF R/ S/	-ist *specialist* phleb/o- *vein* -tom- *incise* -tomy *surgical incision*	Person skilled in taking blood from veins Taking blood from a vein
sclerotherapy sclerose (verb) sclerosis (noun)	**SKLAIR**-oh-**THAIR**-ah-pee skleh-**ROZE** skleh-**ROH**-sis	S/ R/CF S/ S/	-therapy *treatment* scler/o- *hardness* -ose *full of* -osis *condition*	To collapse a vein by injecting a solution into it to harden it To harden or thicken Thickening or hardening of a tissue
thromboembolism thrombophlebitis	**THROM**-boh-**EM**-boh-lizm **THROM**-boh-fleh-**BY**-tis	S/ R/ R/ S/ R/ R/	-ism *condition* thromb/o- *clot* -embol- *plug* -itis *inflammation* thromb/o- *clot* -phleb- *vein*	A piece of detached blood clot (embolus) blocking a distant blood vessel Inflammation of a vein with clot formation

Exercises

A. Apply the *language of the cardiovascular system,* and circle the best answer.   LO 10.6, 10.13

1. The suffix tells you that **thrombophlebitis** is

   A puncture   an inflammation   an excision

2. **Endarterectomy** means the plaque has been

   incised   excised   repaired

3. **Collateral** means

   at the front   in the middle   at the side

4. **The combining form** *phlebo-* **means**

   artery   vein   capillary

5. The combining form *sclero-* describes a

   softening   clotting   hardening

6. The symptom of **edema** is

   a rash   a swelling   a lesion

7. **Aneurysm** describes a blood vessel that is

   dilated   constricted   collapsed

8. The roots tell you that **thromboembolism** is a(n)

   clot or plug   tear or rupture   swelling or lesion

9. The combining form *thrombo-* means

   clot   lump   plug

10. The prefix *end-* signifies

   within   without   beside

Cardiovascular System

Challenge Your Knowledge

A. Diagnostic tests may yield results that indicate a procedure should be performed. Match up the following cardiac procedures. (**LO 10.11,** *Remember*)

1. to reduce occlusion of an artery, this may be inserted

2. surgical removal of arterial plaque

3. donor to recipient

4. arrhythmia is converted back to normal rhythm

5. clot-busting drug therapy

6. surgical removal of the lipid deposit in an artery

7. catheter with electrode destroys abnormal cells

8. healthy blood vessels are harvested to detour blood around blocked vessels

9. high speed rotational device "sands away" plaque

10. artery-cleaning angioplasty

a. radiofrequency ablation

b. rotational atherectomy

c. atherectomy

d. stent

e. transplant

f. CABG

g. defibrillation

h. PTCA

i. endarterectomy

j. thrombolysis

B. In your own words. Identify one procedure or type of service performed by the following occupations. (**LO 10.6,** *Remember*)

1. CVT: _____

2. phlebotomist: _____

3. cardiologist: _____

4. sonographer: _____

5. cardiovascular surgeon: _____

C. Translate. Rewrite the sentences using medical terms instead of the abbreviations. Make sure you are communicating the same message either way. Check (√) your spelling! Fill in the blanks. (**LO 10.6, 10.8,** *Remember*)

1. The CVT started CPR after checking the patient's ECG. He paged the doctor STAT. Apparently, the patient had had an MI.

_____

_____

2. Because of the patient's PVD, the doctor ordered special stockings to prevent DVT.

_____

_____

3. ASD and VSD are holes in the walls of the chambers of the heart that allow blood to leak through.

_____

_____

4. Risk factors for CAD include hypertension, diabetes, obesity, and stress.

_____

_____

D. Build your knowledge of heart terms by working with the following word elements. Fill in the table. (**LO. 10.6,** *Remember*)

Element	Type of Element (P, R, CF, S)	Meaning of Element
cardio	1.	2.
ar	3.	4.
logy	5.	6.
gram	7.	8.
logist	9.	10.
vascul	11.	12.
electro	13.	14.
graph	15.	16.
pulmon	17.	18.

E. Label. On the lines next to the statements below, write the medical term for the body part the statement refers to. (**LO 10.5,** *Recall*)

1. "Pacemaker of the heart": _____

2. Distribute electrical stimuli, which cause contraction of the ventricular myocardium: _____

3. Electrical gateway to the ventricles: _____

4. Supply both ventricles: _____

5. Superior and inferior venae cavae open into this atrium: _____

6. Electrical signals leaving the AV node reach the ventricles through this: _____

7. Blood from pulmonary veins flows into this atrium: _____

Cardiovascular System

F. Abbreviations are present throughout medical documentation, and you must be absolutely certain you are interpreting them correctly. Fill in the correct abbreviation in the following patient documentation. All of the abbreviations contain some combination of the following letters. You will have to use some letters more than once. (**LO 10.8**, *Remember*)

A   C   D   F   H   I   M   P   S   V   O

1. Studies show that the patient has a hole in the interventricular septum, allowing blood to shunt from the higher-pressure

   left ventricle to the lower-pressure right ventricle. The abbreviation for the diagnosis is _____.

2. The pediatric cardiologist was called to the Neonatal Unit because the baby's fetal blood vessel had not closed normally.

   The baby was diagnosed with _____ .

3. The patient's arterial vessels have become dangerously narrowed due to his _____, and an angioplasty will
   be scheduled.

4. Due to her sedentary lifestyle, obesity, hypertension, and smoking history, the patient is at great risk for _____.

5. This patient's left ventricle is failing because it cannot pump out the blood it receives. He is going into _____.

6. An infant male was born with tetralogy of Fallot (_____). This is a form of _____.

7. This patient's ischemic attack resulted in occlusion of her coronary artery, and a (surgical procedure) _____
   followed.

G. Discussion question. Regurgitation means to *flow backward*. In this chapter, regurgitation through the heart valve is discussed. Employ the language of medical terminology to answer the following questions about regurgitation. Fill in the blanks. (**LO 10.3, 10.7**, *Remember*)

1. Previous chapter that discusses regurgitation: _____

2. Body system in question 1: _____

3. Describe the regurgitation in question 1, as opposed to cardiac regurgitation:

   Regurgitation as discussed in a previous chapter is _____

   _____ .

   Cardiac regurgitation is _____

   _____ .

4. How are they similar? _____

   _____

5. How are they different? _____

   _____

H. Translate from layman's language to medical terminology. Provide a medical term for every underlined word or phrase. Fill in the blanks. (**LO 10.6, 10.7,** *Remember*)

1. If any of the <u>heart</u> (_____) arteries become <u>blocked</u> (_____), the blood supply to a part of the <u>heart muscle</u>

   (_____) is cut off and the cells supplied by that artery are <u>dead</u> (_____) within minutes.

2. Aortic valve <u>narrowing</u> (_____) is common in the elderly when the valves become <u>hardened</u> (_____)

   due to <u>lipid deposits in the lining of an artery</u> (_____).

3. The <u>cause</u> (_____) of weakening of the heart muscle (_____) can be viral, unknown (_____), or

   alcoholic.

4. The other form of circulatory shock presents with <u>loss of blood volume</u> (_____), often from

   <u>excessive bleeding</u> (_____) or <u>water depletion</u> (_____).

5. <u>Inflammation of the lining of a vein</u> (_____) allows <u>clots</u> (_____) to form.

I. You are mentoring a new CVT who has just been hired in the Cardiology Department in Fulwood Medical Center. Because you have been on the job for a while, you should be able to explain briefly the difference between each of the following entries. (**LO 10.7, 10.9,** *Remember*)

1. *Heart valve stenosis* and *heart valve incompetency:* _____

   _____

2. A *thrombus* and an *embolus:* _____

   _____

3. *Essential hypertension, secondary hypertension,* and *malignant hypertension:* _____

   _____

J. The cardiac cycle can be heard through the stethoscope. Apply the correct terms in the appropriate place to describe what happens in the chambers of the heart during the cardiac cycle. One term you will use twice. Three terms you will not use at all. (**LO 10.4,** *Remember, Apply*)

atrial diastole	**relax**	**heartbeat**	**atrial systole**	**ventricular systole**
atria	**ventricular diastole**	**contraction**	**contract**	**murmur**

1. When the atria _____, called _____ (atrial emptying), the ventricles _____,

   called _____ (or ventricular filling).

2. When the atria relax, called _____, the ventricles _____, called _____.

3. Then the atria and ventricles all relax briefly. This series of events is the complete cardiac cycle or _____.

K. Which pair of the following terms is a cardiovascular surgeon likely to use in his/her dictation? Circle the correct terms. (**LO 10.6,** *Remember, Understand*)

1. subcutaneous   subdermal

2. catheter   bypass

3. ureter   urethra

4. transverse   horizontal

5. cervical   lumbar

Cardiovascular System

L. Build your knowledge of the heart's location and function by correctly answering the following questions. (LO 10.2, *Remember, Understand*)

1. Which of the following is *NOT* a function of the heart?

    a. pulmonary circulation

    b. maintaining respiration

    c. systemic circulation

    d. regulating blood supply

    e. pumping blood

2. The heart lies in the thoracic cavity between the lungs in an area called the

    a. sternum

    b. mediastinum

    c. ventricle

    d. atrium

    e. vena cava

3. If the *base* of the heart is the upper end of the heart, what is the tip (or other end) of the heart called?

    a. tricuspid

    b. atrium

    c. aorta

    d. semilunar

    e. apex

4. What is responsible for ensuring the one-way flow of blood in the heart?

    a. blood vessels

    b. pulmonary circulation

    c. coronary circulation

    d. valves

    e. blood pressure

M. **Test your knowledge of the cardiovascular system by circling the correct answer. (LO 10.1, 10.2, 10.3,** *Remember, Understand, Apply*)

1. The long, flat bone forming the center of the anterior wall of the chest is the

   a. mediastinum

   b. sternum

   c. myocardium

   d. apex

   e. pericardium

2. The area of cell death caused by the sudden blockage of a blood vessel is termed

   a. fibrosis

   b. infarct

   c. coronary

   d. sinus

   e. visceral

3. The term **sinus rhythm** refers to

   a. the AV node

   b. normal heartbeat

   c. dysrhythmias

   d. arrthythmias

   e. a pacemaker

4. Pathologic compression of the heart is known as

   a. endocarditis

   b. prolapse

   c. tamponade

   d. regurgitation

   e. effusion

5. The abbreviations that represent cardiac diagnoses are

   a. SOB and EKG

   b. MI and PAT

   c. CPR and CVT

   d. STAT and SA

   e. AED and ID

6. What is the purpose of the four valves in the heart?

   a. Blood flows in only one direction.

   b. Blood gets oxygenated.

   c. The heart muscle can rest between beats.

   d. They prevent infection.

   e. They are the gateway to the heart.

7. In the term **cardioversion**, the suffix *-ion* means

   a. a structure

   b. a process

   c. to pour

   d. pertaining to

   e. small

Cardiovascular System

N. Test your knowledge of the cardiovascular system with the following questions. (LO 10.3, *Remember, Understand, Apply*)

1. Tissue heart valves can come from

   a. rabbits

   b. monkeys

   c. occasionally humans

   d. dogs

   e. horses

2. Abnormality in valve closure produces

   a. exudate

   b. infarct

   c. murmur

   d. necrosis

   e. fibrillation

3. The cordlike tendons that anchor the mitral and tricuspid heart valves to the floor of the ventricles are

   a. semilunar

   b. intraventricular

   c. mesenteric

   d. chordae tendinae

   e. fibrotic

4. The pacemaker of heart rhythm is the

   a. AV node

   b. bundle branch

   c. SA node

   d. coronary sinus

   e. PVC

5. **Marginal, interventricular**, and **circumflex** are all terms applied to heart

   a. veins

   b. capillaries

   c. arteries

   d. tendons

   e. muscles

6. Which of the following terms does NOT apply to blood vessels?

   a. arterioles

   b. venules

   c. hilum

   d. veins

   e. arteries

7. The term **visceral** pertains to

   a. an artery

   b. a vein

   c. a capillary

   d. the aorta

   e. an internal organ

8. Capillary exchange occurs by

   a. infusion

   b. transfusion

   c. perfusion

   d. diffusion

   e. effusion

O. **Challenge your knowledge of medical terminology and provide the correct answers to the following questions. (LO 10.9, *Remember, Apply*)**

1. A *flat line* on an ECG is called _____.

2. *Death of tissue* is _____.

3. *Arrhythmia* is another term for _____.

4. An *abnormal sound* in the closure of a heart valve is a _____.

5. *Cardiomyopathy* can cause _____.

6. *Atherosclerotic plaques* are also called _____.

7. A *bypass* or diversion of fluid is _____

8. *A hollow tube* that allows passage of fluid into or out of a body cavity is _____

9. An agent that *increases* urine output is _____

10. *The main artery* in the neck is _____

P. **Form medical terms to fill in the blanks. (LO 10.6, 10.8, *Remember, Apply*)**

1. A _____ is a specialist in the study of the heart.

2. In the abbreviation CPR, the "C" stands for _____.

3. The abbreviation ECG stands for _____.

4. The study of the heart is the specialty called _____.

5. The term that means *pertaining to the heart and blood vessels* is _____.

6. The instrument used for taking an ECG is _____

7. A specialist in the study of lung diseases is called _____

Cardiovascular System

Q. The following elements are all roots or combining forms. Write the meaning of the root/combining form; then demonstrate its use with a medical term containing that element. Fill in the chart. (**LO 10. 1, 10.6, *Understand***)

Root/Combining Form	Meaning of Root/Combining Form	Medical Term Containing This Element
coron	1.	2.
cost	3.	4.
diaphoret	5.	6.
isch	7.	8.
lun	9.	10.
palpit	11.	12.
resuscitat	13.	14.
stetho	15.	16.
tampon	17.	18.
viscer	19.	20.

Pick any two medical terms from the right column above, and create a sentence of patient documentation for each term.

21. Sentence 1:

_____

_____

22. Sentence 2:

_____

_____

R. The following procedures could all be performed by a cardiovascular surgeon. First, slash the term into its elements. Use the suffix to help you analyze the meaning of the term. Write a brief description of the procedure on the line below. Fill in the blanks. (**LO 10.11, *Understand, Apply***)

1. ablation: _____/_____/_____

　　　　　　　　　　P　　　　　　　R/CF　　　　　　　S

　　Description: _____

2. angioplasty: _____/_____/_____

　　　　　　　　　　P　　　　　　　R/CF　　　　　　　S

　　Description: _____

3. endarterectomy: _____/_____/_____

　　　　　　　　　　P　　　　　　　R/CF　　　　　　　S

　　Description: _____

4. sclerotherapy: _____/_____/_____

　　　　　　　　　　P　　　　　　　R/CF　　　　　　　S

　　Description: _____

5. atherectomy: _____/_____/_____

　　　　　　　　　　P　　　　　　　R/CF　　　　　　　S

　　Description: _____

S. Use your knowledge of cardiac pharmacology and insert the correct medical term for the drugs defined. (LO 10.11, *Understand, Apply*)

1. change the electrical properties of the myocardial cells to restore normal rate and rhythm. _____

2. alter the contractions of the myocardium _____

3. reduce susceptibility to clot formation _____

4. stimulate urinary fluid loss to lesson fluid volume the heart has to cope with _____

5. alter the heart rate _____

6. relax smooth muscles in arterioles _____

7. dilate arteries and veins and can be used to treat hypertension _____

T. Using your knowledge of the terminology in the following report, circle the correct answer for the following questions. (LO 10.1, 10.6, *Understand, Apply*)

CHEST X-RAY REPORT

The left ventricle is slightly enlarged. Right atrium and right ventricle appear to be dilated. There is tortuosity of the thoracic aorta, with arteriosclerosis. The hilar and interstitial structures are somewhat accentuated. There are large pericardial fat pads. Tricuspid and pulmonic valves appear normal but are not well seen. Mitral valve appears grossly normal for age. Aortic valve appears grossly normal for age.

1. Where are the pericardial fat pads?

   a. in the heart

   b. around the heart

   c. below the heart

   d. beside the heart

   e. above the heart

2. Which two heart chambers have a somewhat similar appearance?

   a. right and left ventricle

   b. right and left atrium

   c. left atrium and right ventricle

   d. right atrium and left ventricle

   e. right atrium and right ventricle

3. What is another spelling and pronunciation for *dilation?*

   a. dillation

   b. dilatation

   c. dillatation

   d. diletation

   e. dilletation

4. **Interstitial** means

   a. space between the cells of a structure or organ

   b. cavity between the cells of a structure or organ

   c. fluid between the cells of a structure or organ

   d. membrane between the cells of a structure or organ

   e. wall between the cells of a structure or organ

Cardiovascular System

U. Definitions. Define the following medical terms either by looking them up in a WAD or by breaking them down into elements and defining the elements to get the meaning of the term. (**LO 10.1, *Apply***)

1. ventricle _____

2. atrium _____

3. dilated _____

4. thoracic aorta _____

5. arteriosclerosis _____

6. interstitial _____

7. tricuspid _____

8. pulmonic _____

9. mitral _____

10. aortic _____

V. Knowledge of pharmacology is essential to be certain your patients are receiving the correct drugs for their conditions. The following are six types of cardiac drugs in use. List the main function of each drug; then give an example of that type of drug. (**LO 10.11, *Apply, Analyze***)

Drug Type	Function of the Drug	Example
vasodilators	1.	2.
inotropic drugs	3.	4.
anticoagulants	5.	6.
antiarrhythmic drugs	7.	8.
chronotropic drugs	9.	10.
diuretics	11.	12.

W. **Determine which type of drug would be prescribed for the following conditions. (LO 10.11, *Apply, Analyze*)**

1. The patient has hypertension: _____

2. The patient suffers from atrial fibrillation: _____

3. The patient has excessive platelets: a) _____

   Critical thinking: Based on your knowledge of *Chapter 7*, what then is likely to form, and is that a problem?

   b) _____

   _____

4. On the basis of studies, the patient has poor cardiac output: _____

5. The patient has tachycardia. This drug attempts to alter that rate: _____

6. The patient has CHF and needs a _____ to reduce fluid volume.

X. **Procedures.** You have passed your certification examination and have been hired as the coder for the Cardiology Department at Fulwood Medical Center. You are coding the claims for the following tests performed in the department. How much do you know about cardiology testing? Match the letter to the numbered blank. (**LO 10.11**, *Apply, Analyze*)

_____ 1. Thallium testing	**a.** MRI
_____ 2. EKG, also known as	**b.** through esophagus to record heart valves
_____ 3. Continuous ECG recorded on tape	**c.** echocardiography
_____ 4. Cardiac stress testing	**d.** detects patterns of pressure in the heart
_____ 5. TEE	**e.** people unable to do physical exercise
_____ 6. Helps determine risk of CAD	**f.** coronary angiogram
_____ 7. Event tracker	**g.** exercise tolerance test
_____ 8. Sound waves study heart function	**h.** sporadic symptoms
_____ 9. Electron beam CT	**i.** lipid profile
_____ 10. Cardiac catheterization	**j.** ECG
_____ 11. Radioactive substance injected	**k.** Holter monitor
_____ 12. Can identify ischemic muscle	**l.** identifies calcium in arteries
_____ 13. Dye injected to find heart blockage	**m.** nuclear imaging

Cardiovascular System

Y. **Knowing your word elements will always help you to deconstruct a medical term.** Underline the prefix in each term; then write a brief definition of the term. (**LO 10.11**, *Analyze*)

Prefix: sub means _____

1. subclavian means _____

2. substernal means _____

3. sublingual means _____

4. subaortic means _____

Suffixes: Underline the suffix in each term; then write a brief definition of the term.

5. sonographer means _____

6. sonogram means _____

7. sonography means _____

8. sonograph means _____

Z. **Terminology challenge.** Demonstrate your understanding of cardiac terminology by filling in the blanks. (**LO 10. 2,** *Analyze*)

1. What is the function of a *perfusionist?* _____

2. What is the difference between a *stent* and a *shunt?*

stent: _____

shunt: _____

3. A *dilated,* tortuous *vein* can also be called a _____.

4. What are the two terms for increase and decrease in the diameter of a blood vessel?

increase:_____ decrease:_____

5. Name a function of a *sphygmomanometer* and a function of a *stethoscope:*

sphygmomanometer: _____

stethoscope: _____

CHAPTER SUMMARY EXERCISE

A. Spelling comprehension. Circle the correct spelling of the term. (**LO 10.6,** *Understand*)

1. ishemia	ishima	ischemia	iskemia	ischimia
2. dyuretic	diuretic	dyeretic	dieretic	diyuretic
3. regergitate	reguritate	regersitate	regurgitate	regugitate
4. resuscitation	resucitation	resusitation	risusitation	risusitation
5. thombolisis	thrombolysis	tombolisis	thrombylosis	tombolysis
6. dyastole	diastolye	dyastolie	diastole	diastolee
7. paretial	peretal	parietal	parital	partial
8. adventitia	advintitea	adventia	advinttia	adventetea
9. deaphoresis	diaphoresis	diaporesis	deaporesis	diaporisis
10. thrombopelpitis	thromblitis	thrombophlebitis	thrombuphelitis	thrombopelbitis

B. Match the number of the correct spelling of the terms in Exercise A with the following brief descriptions of the terms below. (**LO 10. 6,** *Understand*)

_____ a. Revival from potential or apparent death

_____ b. Agent that increases urine output

_____ c. Relating to the wall of a cavity

_____ d. Deficiency of blood flow to an organ or tissue

_____ e. To flow backward

_____ f. Profuse sweating

_____ g. Inflammation of a vein with clot formation

_____ h. Destruction of a clot

_____ i. Outer connective tissue covering of a blood vessel or organ

_____ j. Relaxation of the heart chamber as it fills with blood

C. Write a brief definition for each of the following terms, using the language of the cardiovascular system. Then pick any one term and write a brief sentence of patient documentation using that term. (**LO 10.6,** *Remember, Apply, Create*)

1. apex _____

2. systemic _____

3. visceral _____

4. bicuspid _____

5. ventricle _____

6. bruit _____

7. diaphoresis _____

8. ischemia _____

9. sternum _____

10. dysrhythmia _____

11. Sentence:

_____

_____

_____

_____

Cardiovascular System

D. **After rereading Case Report 10.2, answer the following questions.** Be prepared to discuss your answers in class. (**LO 10.14,** *Understand*)

Case Report 10.2 (continued)

Mrs. Martha Jones, who had been referred to Dr. Bannerjee's cardiovascular clinic, has several circulatory problems related to her diabetes and obesity. She was diagnosed previously with hypertension, CAD, and diabetic retinopathy. She now has severe pain in her legs when walking.

Her ankle/brachial index (**ABI**), which measures the ratio of the blood pressure in her ankle to that in her arm, showed significant blockage of blood flow. Doppler studies confirmed this. This blockage produces the pain when walking (intermittent claudication). It is due to arteriosclerosis of the large arteries in her legs. Angiograms showed several atherosclerotic areas in her popliteal artery.

The ulcers on the edges of her big toes result from thickening of the walls of her capillaries and arterioles and the resulting poor circulation to her feet. Again, this is due to her diabetes.

In the venous system of her legs, the tender cordlike lesion is due to thrombophlebitis of a superficial vein in her left leg. Pain in the calf on flexion of the ankle (Homans sign) indicates that she may have a deep vein thrombosis (DVT). A venogram confirmed this diagnosis.

1. What weight problem is a complicating factor to Mrs. Jones's diabetes?

   _____

2. What diagnoses are in Mrs. Jones's past medical history?

   _____

3. What is the medical term for "severe pain in legs on walking"?

   _____

4. What is an angiogram? _____

5. Explain in simple language what a DVT is. _____

   _____

6. What diagnostic tests has Mrs. Jones had so far? _____

7. Where does retinopathy occur? _____

8. Name one circulatory problem Mrs. Jones has as a result of her diabetes.

   _____

E. **Meet the goals of each of the chapter outcomes and insert the correct answers to the questions. (LO 10.1–10.13, *Analyze*)**

1. Describe the coronary circulation of the heart. (**LO 10.1**) _____

_____

2. Explain the functions of the CV system. (**LO 10.2**) _____

_____

3. Map the blood flow through the heart. (**LO 10.3**) _____

_____

4. Summarize the phases of the cardiac cycle. (**LO 10.4**) _____

_____

5. Clarify the electrical phases of the heart. (**LO 10.5**) _____

_____

6. Create one sentence of patient documentation a cardiologist might write in a patient's chart. (**LO 10.6**) _____

_____

7. If a physician tells you his patient needs a "stent," exactly what does that mean? (**LO 10.7**) _____

_____

8. Which of the following abbreviations would not be applicable to the CV system? Circle the correct answer. (**LO 10.8**)

    a. URI   **d.** tPA

    b. CABG   **e.** ACE

    c. PTCA

9. Which of the following statements is not true about arrhythmias? (**LO 10.9**)

    a. arrhythmias are abnormal heartbeats   **d.** arrhythmias can be irregular heartbeats.

    b. ventricular arrhythmias consist of several types   **e.** atrial fibrillation is an arrhythmia

    c. medication is not a treatment for arrhythmias

10. Explain any two diagnostic tests used to determine cardiac disorders. (**LO 10.10**)

    a. _____

    b. _____

11. Define the effects of one cardiac drug that is in current use. (**LO 10.11**)

    Drug: _____

12. Focus on one of the major circulatory systems, and describe its functions. (**LO 10.12**)

_____

_____

13. Select one of the blood vessels and describe how its structure is related to its function in circulation. (**LO 10.13**)

_____

_____

Blood

The Language of Hematology

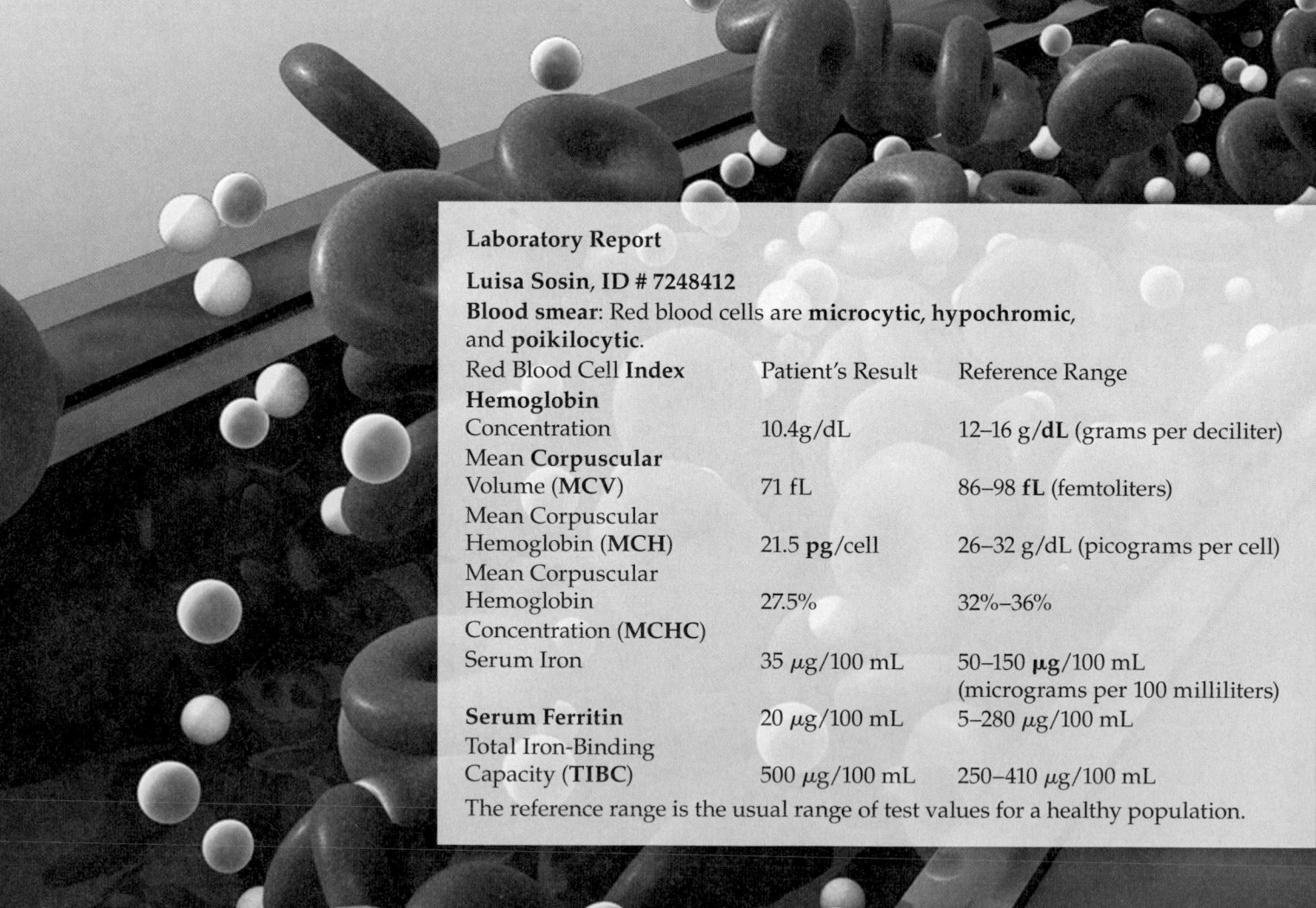

Laboratory Report

Luisa Sosin, ID # 7248412

Blood smear: Red blood cells are **microcytic, hypochromic,** and **poikilocytic.**

Red Blood Cell **Index**	Patient's Result	Reference Range
Hemoglobin Concentration	10.4g/dL	12–16 g/**dL** (grams per deciliter)
Mean **Corpuscular** Volume (**MCV**)	71 fL	86–98 **fL** (femtoliters)
Mean Corpuscular Hemoglobin (**MCH**)	21.5 **pg**/cell	26–32 g/dL (picograms per cell)
Mean Corpuscular Hemoglobin Concentration (**MCHC**)	27.5%	32%–36%
Serum Iron	35 μg/100 mL	50–150 **µg**/100 mL (micrograms per 100 milliliters)
Serum Ferritin	20 μg/100 mL	5–280 μg/100 mL
Total Iron-Binding Capacity (**TIBC**)	500 μg/100 mL	250–410 μg/100 mL

The reference range is the usual range of test values for a healthy population.

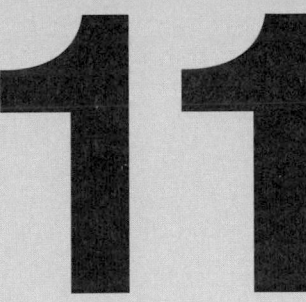

Case Report (CR) 11.1

You are

... a medical assistant working with Susan Lee, MD, a primary care physician at Fulwood Medical Center.

Your patient is

... Mrs. Luisa Sosin, a 47-year-old woman who presented a week ago with fatigue, lethargy, and muscle weakness. Physical examination revealed **pallor** of her skin, a pulse rate of 100, and a respiratory rate of 20. Dr. Lee referred her for extensive blood work. Dr. Lee also determined that the patient had been taking aspirin and **other nonsteroidal anti-inflammatory drugs (NSAIDs)** for the past 6 months for low-back pain.

You are responsible for documenting her investigation and care. She is your next patient, and you are reviewing this laboratory report:

Chapter Learning Outcomes

To understand this report, to be able to communicate intelligently with Dr. Lee about the patient, and to document Mrs. Sosin's medical care, you need to have knowledge of the anatomy, physiology, and medical terminology of **hematology**.

This chapter will provide you with information that enables you to:

LO 11.1 Use the medical terms of hematology to communicate and document in writing accurately and precisely in any health care setting.

LO 11.2 Use the medical terms of hematology to communicate verbally with accuracy and precision in any health care setting.

LO 11.3 Describe the components and functions of blood and the basic laboratory studies that show these.

LO 11.4 Describe the structure and functions of red blood cells (RBCs).

LO 11.5 Discuss disorders of RBCs.

LO 11.6 Describe the types of white blood cells (WBCs) and their functions.

LO 11.7 Discuss disorders of WBCs.

LO 11.8 Explain hemostasis.

LO 11.9 Discuss disorders of coagulation and their pharmacology.

LO 11.10 Identify the different blood groups and their role in transfusions.

Lesson 11.1 Components of Blood

The information in this lesson relates to the composition, functions, and uses of blood and will enable you to use correct medical terminology to:

11.1.1 Identify the components of blood.

11.1.2 Describe plasma and its functions.

11.1.3 Explain the functions of blood.

Abbreviations

dL	deciliter; one-tenth of a liter
fL	femtoliter; one-quadrillionth of a liter
L	liter
Hct	hematocrit
MCH	mean corpuscular hemoglobin; the average amount of hemoglobin in the average red blood cell
MCHC	mean corpuscular hemoglobin concentration; the average concentration of hemoglobin in a given volume of red blood cells
MCV	mean corpuscular volume, the average volume of a red blood cell
mg	microgram; one-millionth of a gram; sometimes written as mcg
NSAID	nonsteroidal anti-inflammatory drug
pg	picogram; one-trillionth of a gram
RBC	red blood cell
TIBC	total iron-binding capacity; the amount of iron needed to saturate transferrin, the protein that transports iron in the blood
WBC	white blood cell

LO 11.3 Components of Blood

Blood is a type of connective tissue and consists of cells contained in a liquid matrix.

Blood volume varies with body size and the amount of adipose tissue. An average-size adult has about 5 L (liters) (10 pints) of blood that represents some 8% of body weight.

If a specimen of blood is collected in a tube and centrifuged, the cells of the blood are packed into the bottom of the tube *(Figure 11.1)*. These cells are called the formed elements of blood and consist of 99% red blood cells (**RBCs**), together with white blood cells (**WBCs**) and platelets. The blood sample is normally about 45% formed elements.

The **hematocrit (Hct)** is the percentage of total blood volume composed of red blood cells. The red blood cells can account for 40% to 54% of the total blood volume in normal males and 38% to 47% in females.

Plasma is the remaining 55% of the blood sample. It is a clear, yellowish liquid that is 91% water. Plasma is the fluid noncellular part of blood. Plasma is a **colloid**, a liquid that contains suspended particles, most of which are the plasma proteins named:

- **Albumin**—makes up 58% of the proteins.
- **Globulin**—makes up 38% of the plasma proteins. Antibodies are globulins *(see Chapter 12)*.
- **Fibrinogen**—makes up 4% of the plasma proteins and is part of the mechanism for blood clotting *(see Lesson 11.4)*.

Nutrients, **waste products**, **hormones**, and **enzymes** are dissolved in plasma for transportation.

When blood is allowed to clot and the solid clot is removed, **serum** is left. Serum is identical to plasma except for the absence of clotting proteins.

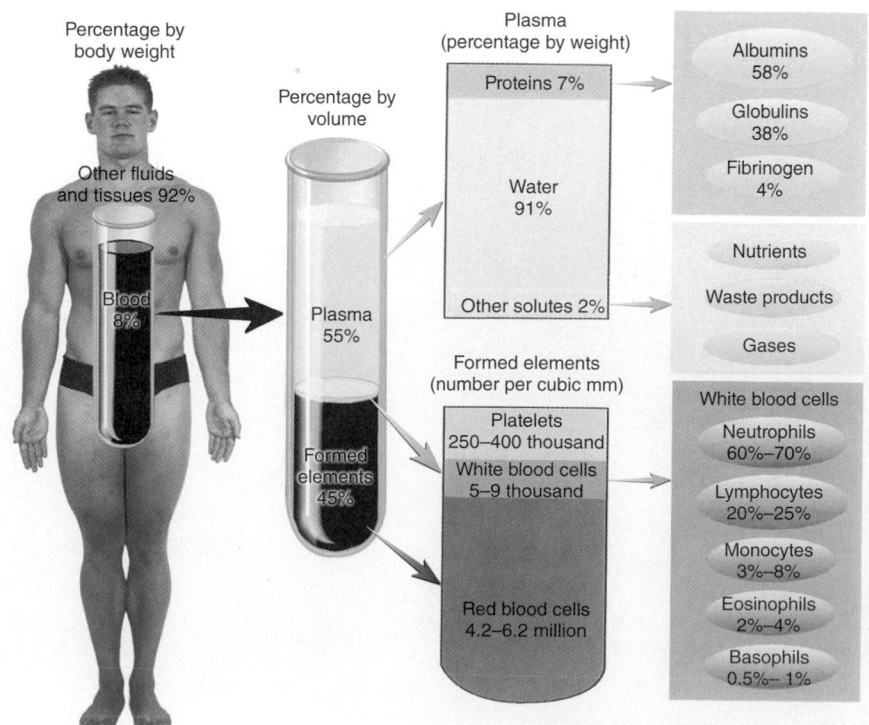

Figure 11.1 Components of Blood. ▶

WORD	PRONUNCIATION		ELEMENTS	DEFINITION
albumin	al-**BYU**-min		Latin *white of an egg*	Simple, soluble protein
colloid	**COLL**-oyd	S/ R/	**-oid** *appearance of* **coll-** *glue*	Liquid containing suspended particles
corpuscle corpuscular (adj)	**KOR**-pus-ul kor-**PUS**-kyu-lar	S/ R/ S/	**-cle** *small (can also be cule)* **corpus-** *body* **-ar** *pertaining to*	A blood cell Pertaining to corpuscle
ferritin	**FER**-ih-tin	S/ R/	**-in** *chemical* **ferrit-** *iron*	Iron-protein complex that regulates iron storage and transport
fibrin fibrinogen	**FIE**-brin fie-**BRIN**-oh-jen	S/ R/CF	Latin *fiber* **-gen** *create, produce* **fibrin/o-** *fibrin*	Stringy protein fiber that is a component of a blood clot Precursor of fibrin in blood-clotting process
globulin	**GLOB**-you-lin		Latin *globule*	Family of blood proteins
hematocrit	**HE**-mat-oh-krit	S/ R/CF	**-crit** *to separate* **hemat/o-** *blood*	Percentage of red blood cells in the blood
hematology hematologist	he-mah-**TOL**-oh-jee he-mah-**TOL**-oh-jist	S/ S/	**-logy** *study of* **-logist** *specialist*	Medical specialty of disorders of the blood Specialist in hematology
hemoglobin	**HE**-moh-**GLOW**-bin	R/CF R/	**hem/o-** *blood* **globin** *protein*	Red-pigmented protein that is the main component of red blood cells
hypochromic	high-poh-**CROW**-mik	S/ P/ R/	**-ic** *pertaining to* **hypo-** *deficient, below* **-chrom-** *color*	Pale in color, as in red blood cells when hemoglobin is deficient
index indices (pl)	**IN**-deks **IN**-dih-seez		Latin *one that points out*	A standard indicator of measurement
microcytic	my-kroh-**SIT**-ik	S/ P/ R/	**-ic** *pertaining to* **micro-** *small* **-cyt-** *cell*	Pertaining to a small cell
pallor	**PAL**-or		Latin *paleness*	Paleness of the skin
plasma	**PLAZ**-mah		Greek *something formed*	Fluid, noncellular component of blood
poikilocytic	**POY**-key-low-**SIT**-ik	S/ P/ R/	**-ic** *pertaining to* **poikilo-** *irregular* **-cyt-** *cell*	Pertaining to an irregular-shaped red blook cell
serum	**SEER**-um		Latin *whey*	Fluid remaining after removal of cells and fibrin clot

Exercises

A. Know your elements—they will increase your medical vocabulary! *This exercise consists of elements taken from the above WAD. Match the element to its correct meaning.* **LO 11.1, 11.3**

_____	1. oid	**a.**	small
_____	2. micro	**b.**	color
_____	3. cyt	**c.**	deficient, below
_____	4. crit	**d.**	iron
_____	5. chrom	**e.**	create, produce
_____	6. hypo	**f.**	appearance of
_____	7. gen	**g.**	to separate
_____	8. ferrit	**h.**	cell

LO 11.3 Functions of Blood

The functions of the blood are to

Keynote

Failure to maintain the normal pH range of the blood between 7.35 and 7.45 can cause paralysis and death.

1. **Maintain the body's homeostasis** *(see Chapter 4)*.

2. **Maintain body temperature**. Warm blood is transported from the interior of the body to its surface, where heat is released from the blood.

3. **Transport nutrients, vitamins, and minerals** from digestive system and storage areas to organs and cells where they are needed. Examples of nutrients are glucose and amino acids *(see Chapter 5)*.

4. **Transport waste products** from cells and organs to the liver and kidneys for detoxification and excretion. Examples are **creatinine**, **urea**, bilirubin, and lactic acid *(see Chapter 5)*.

5. **Transport hormones** from endocrine glands to the target cells. Examples are insulin and thyroxin *(see Chapter 17)*.

6. **Transport gases** to and from the lungs and cells. Examples are oxygen and carbon dioxide *(see Chapter 13)*.

7. **Protect against foreign substances**. Cells and chemicals in the blood are an important part of the immune system for dealing with microorganisms and toxins *(see Chapter 12)*.

8. **Form clots**. Clots provide protection against blood loss and are the first step in tissue repair and restoration of normal function.

9. **Regulate pH and osmosis**.

Abbreviations

CBC	complete blood count
ESR	erythrocyte sedimentation rate
pH	hydrogen ion concentration

Hydrogen ion concentration is measured by using a **pH** scale to show the balance between **acid** and **alkaline** in any solution. Pure water is the neutral solution and has a pH of 7.0. Solutions with a pH less than 7.0 are acidic. Solutions with a pH greater than 7.0 are alkaline (or basic). Blood has a pH between 7.35 and 7.45 and must be maintained within that range for life to continue. **Buffer** systems in the blood are used to maintain the correct pH range. Examples of buffer systems are bicarbonate and phosphate.

Osmosis is the passage of water through a selectively permeable membrane, such as a cell membrane, from the "more watery" side to the "less watery" side. All cells exchange water by osmosis, and red blood cells exchange 100 times their own volume across the cell membrane every second.

Viscosity, the resistance of a fluid to flow, is an important element that affects the blood's ability to flow through blood vessels. Whole blood is five times as viscous as water. If the viscosity decreases because red blood cells are deficient (as in **anemia**), blood flows more easily and puts a strain on the heart because of the increased amount of blood being returned to it in a unit of time.

LO 11.3 Laboratory Studies for Blood

- A **complete blood count** (CBC) is a combination of
  1. Red blood cell (RBC) count and indices.
  2. White blood cell (WBC) count and differential WBC count.
  3. Platelet count. In some laboratories a CBC does not include the differential white blood cell count. This may need to be requested separately. White blood cells are addressed in *Lesson 11.3*.

- **Erythrocyte sedimentation rate** (ESR) is a nonspecific measure of inflammation. This test is falling out of use as other more specific tests are developed.

WORD	PRONUNCIATION		ELEMENTS	DEFINITION
acid	**ASS**-id		Latin *sour*	Substance with a pH below 7.0
alkaline (basic (syn))	**AL**-kah-line	S/ R/	**-ine** *pertaining to, substance* **alkal-** *base*	Substance with a pH above 7.0
anemia	ah-**NEE**-me-ah	P/ R/	**an-** *without, lacking* **-emic** *relating to blood*	Decreased number of red blood cells Suffering from anemia
anemic (adj)	ah-**NEE**-mik	S/	**-ic** *pertaining to*	Pertaining to or suffering from anemia
buffer	**BUFF**-er		Latin *cushion*	Substance that resists a change in pH
creatinine	kree-**AT**-ih-neen	S/ R/	**-ine** *pertaining to, substance* **creatin-** *creatine*	Breakdown product of the skeletal muscle protein creatine
erythrocyte	eh-**RITH**-roh-site	S/ R/CF	**-cyte** *cell* **erythr/o-** *red*	Another name for a red blood cell
homeostasis	ho-mee-oh-**STAY**-sis	R/ R/CF	**-stasis** *stay in one place* **home/o-** *the same*	Stability or equilibrium of a system or the body's internal environment
osmosis	oz-**MO**-sis	S/ R/	**-sis** *process* **osmo-** *push*	The passage of water across a cell membrane
sediment	**SED**-ih-ment		Latin *to settle*	Insoluble material that settles to the bottom of a liquid
sedimentation	**SED**-ih-men-**TAY**-shun	S/ R/	**-ation** *process* **sediment-** *a settling*	Formation of a sediment
urea	you-**REE**-ah		Greek *urine*	End product of nitrogen metabolism
viscous viscosity	**VISS**-kus vis-**KOS**-ih-tee	R/ S/	Latin *sticky* **visco-** *resistance to flow* **-ity** *condition, state*	Sticky; resistant to flowing The resistance of a fluid to flow

Exercises

A. You will help yourself in this exercise if you first slash (/) the bold medical terms into their elements. *Review the above WAD before you start to fill in the blanks.*   **LO 11.1, 11.3**

1. In the term **sedimentation**, the suffix means _____.

2. If something is a buffer, it acts as a _____.

3. **Viscous** is a term meaning _____.

4. In the term **erythrocyte**, the suffix means _____.

5. *A state of equilibrium* means something remains _____.

6. The root in **homeostasis** means _____.

B. Review the above WAD before answering these questions.   LO 11.1, 11.3

1. Urea comes from the Greek meaning _____.

2. The opposite of acid is _____.

3. The prefix in **anemia** means _____.

4. In the term **osmosis**, the root means _____.

5. _____ and _____ are two terms in the WAD that relate to blood.

6. _____ settles to the bottom of a liquid.

Lesson 11.2 Red Blood Cells (Erythrocytes)

LESSON OBJECTIVES

In your bloodstream at this moment are approximately 25 trillion RBCs. Approximately 2.5 million of them are being destroyed every second. This means that 1% of your RBCs are destroyed and replaced every day of your life.

It is crucial to understand the reasons for this dynamic process and to be familiar with the critical role that the RBCs play in maintaining life. This lesson will provide you with the information to use correct medical terminology to:

11.2.1 Match the structure of RBCs to their functions.

11.2.2 Identify the roles of hemoglobin in maintaining homeostasis.

11.2.3 Describe the life history of RBCs.

11.2.4 Discuss some common disorders of RBCs.

Figure 11.2 RBCs. ▶

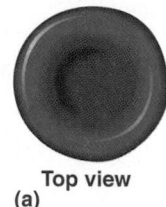

Top view
(a)

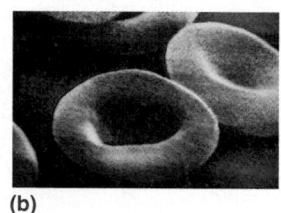

(b)

Abbreviations

CO₂	carbon dioxide
Hb	hemoglobin; may also be written as Hgb
NO	nitric oxide
O₂	oxygen

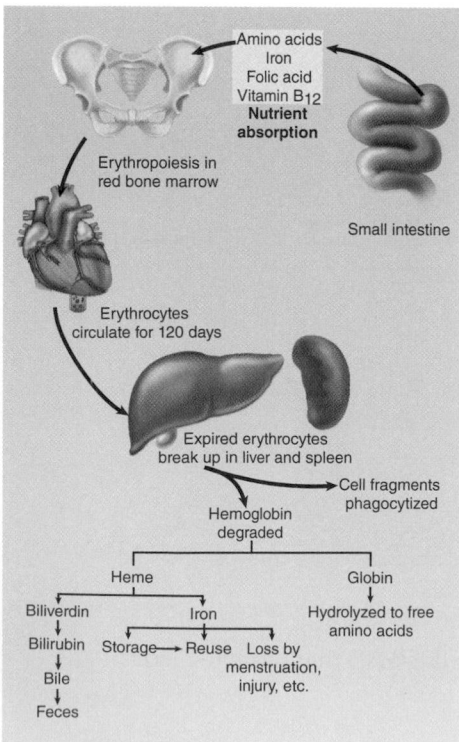

Amino acids
Iron
Folic acid
Vitamin B₁₂
Nutrient absorption

Erythropoiesis in red bone marrow

Small intestine

Erythrocytes circulate for 120 days

Expired erythrocytes break up in liver and spleen

Cell fragments phagocytized

Hemoglobin degraded

Heme   Globin

Biliverdin   Iron   Hydrolyzed to free amino acids

Bilirubin   Storage→ Reuse   Loss by menstruation, injury, etc.

Bile

Feces

▲ **Figure 11.3** Life and Death of RBCs.

LO 11.4 Structure and Function of Red Blood Cells

Structure of Red Blood Cells

The main component of RBCs is **hemoglobin (Hb)**, which gives the cell its red color. Hemoglobin occupies about one-third of the total cell volume and is composed of the iron-containing pigment **heme** bound to a protein called globin. The rest of the red blood cell consists of the cell membrane, water, electrolytes, and enzymes. Mature RBCs do not have a nucleus.

Each RBC is a **biconcave** disc with edges that are thicker than the center (*Figure 11.2*). This biconcave shape gives the disc a larger surface area than if it were a sphere. The biconcave surface area enables a more rapid flow of gases into and out of the RBC.

RBCs are unable to move themselves and are dependent on the heart and blood vessels to move them around the body.

Function of Red Blood Cells

The functions of the RBCs are to

1. **Transport oxygen (O₂)** from the lungs to cells all over the body. Oxygen is transported in combination with hemoglobin (**oxyhemoglobin**).

2. **Transport carbon dioxide (CO₂)** from the tissue cells to the lungs for excretion.

3. **Transport nitric oxide (NO)**, a gas produced by cells lining the blood vessels that signals smooth muscle to relax and is also a transmitter of signals between nerve cells.

Life History of Red Blood Cells

Red blood cell formation (**erythropoiesis**) occurs in the spaces in bones filled with red bone marrow. **Hematopoietic stem cells** become nucleated **erythroblasts** and then nonnucleated erythrocytes, which are released into the bloodstream.

A hormone, **erythropoietin**, produced by the kidneys and liver, controls the rate of RBC production. A lack of oxygen in the body's tissues triggers the release of erythropoietin, which travels in the blood to the red bone marrow to stimulate RBC production.

RBC production is also influenced by the availability of iron, the B vitamins B₁₂ and folic acid, and amino acids through absorption from the digestive tract (*Figure 11.3*).

The average life span of an RBC is 120 days, during which time the cell has circulated through the body about 75,000 times. With age, the cells become more fragile, and squeezing through tiny capillaries ruptures them. **Macrophages** in the liver and spleen take up the hemoglobin that is released and break it down into its components heme and globin. The heme is broken down into iron and into a rust-colored pigment called bilirubin.

WORD	PRONUNCIATION	ELEMENTS		DEFINITION
biconcave	bi-**KON**-cave	P/ R/	**bi-** *two, double* **-concave** *arched, hollow*	Having a hollowed surface on both sides of a structure
erythroblast	eh-**RITH**-ro-blast	S/ R/CF	**-blast** *germ cell* **erythr/o-** *red*	Precursor to a red blood cell
erythropoiesis	eh-**RITH**-ro-poy-**EE**-sis	S/ R/CF	**-poiesis** *to make* **erythr/o-** *red*	The formation of red blood cells
erythropoietin	eh-**RITH**-ro-**POY**-ee-tin	S/ R/CF	**-poietin** *the maker* **erythr/o-** *red*	Protein secreted by the kidney that stimulates red blood cell production
hematopoietic	**HE**-mah-toh-poy-**ET**-ick	S/ S/ R/CF	**-ic** *pertaining to* **-poiet-** *the making* **hemat/o-** *blood*	Pertaining to the making of red blood cells
heme	HEEM		Greek *blood*	The iron-based component of hemoglobin that carries oxygen
macrophage	**MAK**-roh-fayj	P/ R/CF	**macro-** *large* **-phag/e** *to eat*	Large white blood cell that removes bacteria, foreign particles, and dead cells
oxyhemoglobin	**OCK**-see-he-moh-**GLOW**-bin	R/CF R/CF R/	**ox/y-** *oxygen* **hem/o-** *blood* **-globin** *protein*	Hemoglobin in combination with oxygen

Exercises

A. Some of the medical terms from the above WAD are defined for you. *One word in the definition is in bold; find the element in the term that has the same meaning. The first one is done for you.* Fill in the blanks.   **LO 11.4**

1. **macrophage:**   Element _____*macro*_____ = _____*large*_____

   Definition: **large** white blood cell that removes bacteria and dead cells

2. **erythroblast:**   Element _____ = _____

   Definition: **precursor** to red blood cell

3. **biconcave:**   Element _____ = _____

   Definition: having a hollowed surface on **both** sides of a structure

4. **erythropoiesis:**   Element _____ = _____

   Definition: the **formation** of red blood cells

5. **hemoglobin:**   Element _____ = _____

   Definition: red color and oxygen transporter of red **blood** cells

6. **erythropoietin:**   Element _____ = _____

   Definition: protein that is secreted by kidney and stimulates **red blood cell** production

7. **hematopoietic:**   Element _____ = _____

   Definition: **pertaining** to the making of red blood cells

8. The only term in the WAD that does not deconstruct into elements is _____, which means _____.

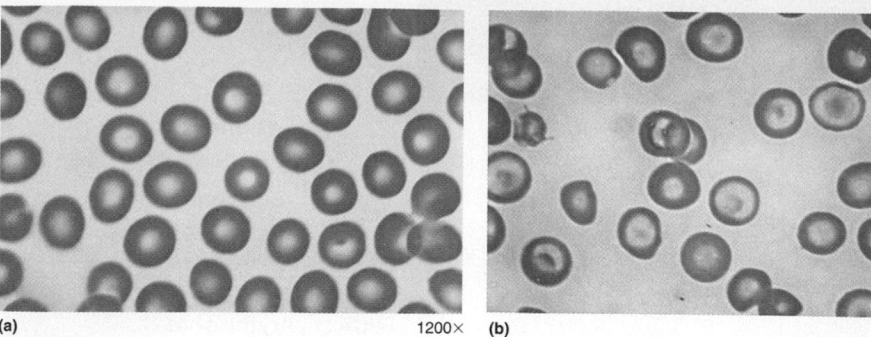

Figure 11.4 Red Blood Cells. ▶
(a) Normal RBCs. (b) Hypochromic RBCs.

(a) 1200×   (b) 1000×

Keynotes

- Anemia reduces the oxygen-carrying capacity of blood.
- Hemolysis liberates hemoglobin from red blood cells.

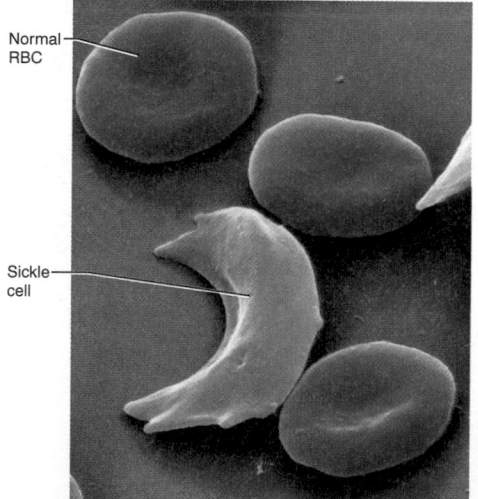

Normal RBC

Sickle cell

▲ **Figure 11.5** Sickle Cell Anemia.

LO 11.5 Disorders of Red Blood Cells

Anemia is a reduction in the number of RBCs or in the amount of hemoglobin each RBC contains *(Figure 11.4)*. Both of these conditions reduce the oxygen-carrying capacity of the blood and produce the symptoms of shortness of breath (**SOB**) and fatigue. They also produce pallor (paleness of the skin) because of the deficiency of the red-colored oxyhemoglobin, the combination of oxygen and hemoglobin, and the red blood cells are **hypochromic** *(Figure 11.4b)*.

There are several types of anemia:

- **Iron-deficiency anemia** is the diagnosis for Mrs. Luisa Sosin. In her case, the cause was chronic bleeding from her gastrointestinal tract due to the aspirin and other painkillers she was taking. Her stools were positive for occult blood. Other causes can be heavy menstrual bleeding or a diet deficient in iron.

- **Pernicious anemia (PA)** is due to vitamin B_{12} deficiency. This is caused by a shortage of *intrinsic factor (see Chapter 5)*, which is normally secreted by cells in the lining of the stomach and binds with vitamin B_{12}; this complex is absorbed into the bloodstream. Without vitamin B_{12}, hemoglobin cannot be formed. The RBCs decrease in number and in hemoglobin concentration and increase in size (**macrocytic**).

- **Sickle cell anemia** (also called *sickle cell disease*) is a genetic disorder found most commonly in African Americans, Africans, and some Mediterranean populations. It results from the production of an abnormal hemoglobin that causes the RBCs to form a rigid sickle cell shape *(Figure 11.5)*. The abnormal cells are sticky, clump together (**agglutinate**), and block small capillaries. This causes intense pain in the **hypoxic** tissues (a sickle cell crisis) and can cause stroke and kidney and heart failure.

  There is a minor form of the disease, sickle cell trait, in which symptoms rarely occur and do not progress to the full-blown disease.

- **Hemolytic anemia** is due to excessive destruction of normal and abnormal RBCs. **Hemolysis** can be caused by such toxic substances as snake and spider venoms, mushroom toxins, and drug reactions. Trauma to RBCs by hemodialysis or heart-lung machines can produce a hemolytic anemia.

- **Aplastic anemia** is a condition in which the bone marrow is unable to produce sufficient new cells of all types—red cells, white cells, and platelets. It can be associated with exposure to radiation, benzene, and certain drugs.

- **Hemoglobinopathies**, such as sickle cell disease and **thalassemia**, with their inherited abnormal hemoglobins, also cause hemolysis.

  Hemolysis can also occur through **incompatible** blood transfusions or maternal-fetal incompatibilities *(see Lesson 11.5)*. Jaundice is a complication.

- **Polycythemia vera** is an overproduction of RBCs and WBCs due to an unknown cause.

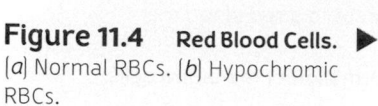

Case Report 11.1 (continued)

    Because Mrs. Luisa Sosin was deficient in iron and hemoglobin, her RBCs were small (microcytic) and lacked the red color of oxyhemoglobin (hypochromic; *Figure 11.5*), and some were irregular-shaped (poikilocytic) rather than the normal, round shape. The volume of each cell, mean corpuscular volume (MCV), and the amount of hemoglobin in each cell, mean corpuscular hemoglobin (MCH), were decreased. The amount of iron in her blood (serum iron) and the amount of ferritin in her serum were decreased. Her total iron-binding capacity was raised because the shortage of iron resulted in an increased availability of the protein to which iron is bound in the bloodstream.

WORD	PRONUNCIATION	ELEMENTS		DEFINITION
agglutinate	ah-**GLUE**-tin-ate	S/ P/ R/	-ate *composed of, pertaining to* ag- *to* -glutin- *stick together, glue*	Stick together to form clumps
aplastic anemia	a-**PLAS**-tik ah-**NEE**-me-ah	S/ P/ R/ P/ R/	-tic *pertaining to* a- *without* -plas- *formation* an- *without, lack of* -emia *blood*	Condition in which the bone marrow is unable to produce sufficient red cells, white cells, and platelets
hemoglobinopathy	**HE**-mo-**GLOW**-bih-**NOP**-ah-thee	S/ R/CF R/CF	-pathy *disease* hem/o- *blood* -globin/o- *protein*	Disease caused by the presence of an abnormal hemoglobin in the red blood cells
hemolysis	he-**MOL**-ih-sis	S/ R/CF	-lysis *destruction* hem/o- *blood*	Destruction of red blood cells so that hemoglobin is liberated
hemolytic (adj)	he-moh-**LIT**-ik	S/ R/	-ic *pertaining to* -lyt- *destroy*	Pertaining to the process of destruction of red blood cells
hypochromic	high-poh-**CROW**-mik	S/ P/ R/	-ic *pertaining to* hypo- *deficient, below* -chrom- *color*	Pale in color, as in RBCs when hemoglobin is deficient
hypoxia	high-**POCK**-see-ah	S/	-ia *condition*	Decrease below normal levels of oxygen in tissues, gases, or blood
hypoxic (**Note:** The surplus "o" is not used.)	high-**POCK**-sik	S/ P/ R/	-ic *pertaining to* hypo- *deficient* -ox- *oxygen*	Deficient in oxygen
incompatible	in-kom-**PAT**-ih-bul	S/ P/ R/	-ible *can do* in- *not* -compat- *tolerate*	Substances that interfere with each other physiologically
macrocyte	**MAK**-roh-site	P/ R/CF	macro- *large* -cyt/e *cell*	Large red blood cell
macrocytic (adj)	mak-roh-**SIT**-ik	S/	-ic *pertaining to*	Pertaining to macrocytes
pernicious anemia (PA)	per-**NISH**-us ah-**NEE**-me-ah	 P/ R/	pernicious *Latin* destructive an- *without, lack of* -emia *blood*	Chronic anemia due to lack of vitamin B$_{12}$
polycythemia vera	**POL**-ee-sigh-**THEE**-me-ah **VEH**-rah	P/ R/ R/	poly- *many, much* -cyth- *cell* -emia *blood* vera *Latin* truth	Chronic disease with bone marrow hyperplasia and increase in number of red blood cells and in blood volume
thalassemia	thal-ah-**SEE**-me-ah	S/ R/	-emia *blood condition* thalass- *sea*	Group of inherited blood disorders that produce a hemolytic anemia, and occur in people living around the Mediterranean Sea.

Exercises

A. After rereading Case Report 11.1, answer the following questions. *Be prepared to discuss your answers in class.*   **LO 11.1, 11.5**

1. If a term means *deficient in*, what element would it start with? (Be specific.) _____

2. What is the opposite of *microcytic*? _____

3. The condition in which the bone marrow is unable to produce sufficient red cells, white cells, and platelets is _____.

4. *Hypochromic* means _____.

5. Why is oxyhemoglobin a red color? (**Hint:** Study the elements.)

    _____

6. Mrs. Sosin's RBCs showed a decrease in _____ and _____.

7. _____ and _____ were raised in Mrs. Sosin's blood, and that resulted in _____

    _____

Lesson 11.3 White Blood Cells (Leukocytes)

The information in this lesson will enable you to use correct medical terminology to:

11.3.1 **Distinguish the different types of WBCs.**
11.3.2 **Describe the functions of the different types of WBCs.**
11.3.3 **Explain white blood cell counts and differential WBC counts.**
11.3.4 **Discuss the effect of common disorders of WBCs on health.**

You are

. . . a laboratory technician reviewing a peripheral blood smear.

Your patient is

. . . Mrs. Latisha Masters, a 27-year-old student.

Case Report 11.2

Mrs. Masters presented with a 5-day history of fatigue, low-grade fever, and sore throat. Physical examination showed tonsillitis with bilateral, enlarged, tender cervical lymph nodes and an enlarged spleen.

The WBC count you performed showed 9200 cells per cubic millimeter. The peripheral smear you are looking at is reported as showing the presence of atypical mononuclear cells with abundant cytoplasm.

LO 11.6 Types of White Blood Cells

Granulocytes

Abbreviation	
PMNL	polymorphonuclear leukocyte

1. **Neutrophils** *(Figure 11.6)* are normally 50% to 70% of the total WBC count. They are also called **polymorphonuclear leukocytes (PMNLs)**. These cells phagocytize bacteria, fungi, and some viruses and secrete a group of enzymes called lysozymes, which destroy some bacteria. In bacterial infections, the number and percentage of neutrophils increase dramatically. In **neutropenia**, the number of neutrophils is diminished below normal.

2. **Eosinophils** *(Figure 11.7)* are normally 2% to 4% of the total WBC count. They are mobile cells that leave the bloodstream to enter tissue undergoing an allergic response. In allergic reactions, the number and percentage of eosinophils increase.

3. **Basophils** *(Figure 11.8)* are normally less than 1% of the total WBC count. Basophils migrate to damaged tissues, where they release histamine (which increases blood flow) and **heparin** (which prevents blood clotting).

Because of their granular cytoplasm surrounding a nucleus, the above three types of WBCs are called **granulocytes**. Their granules are the sites for production of enzymes and chemicals.

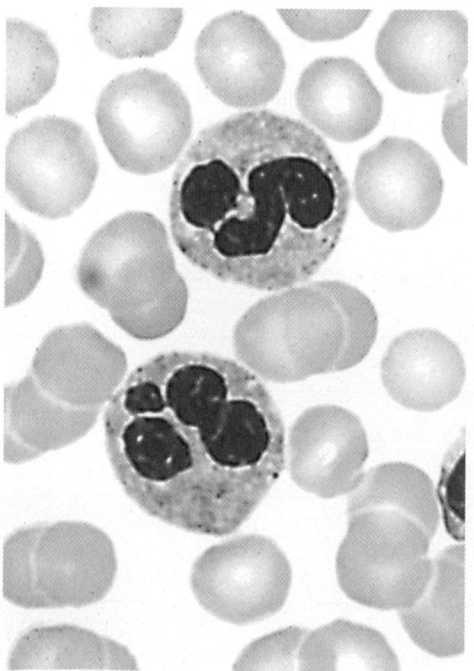

▲ **Figure 11.6** Neutrophils Are Granulocytes.

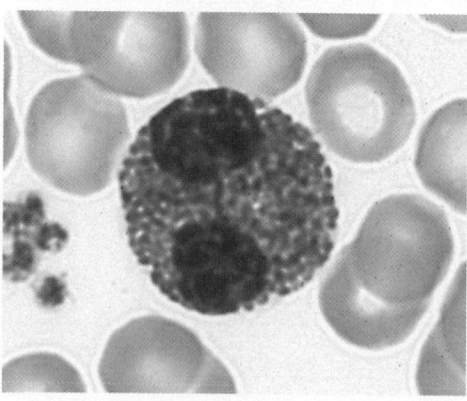

▲ **Figure 11.7** Eosinophils Are Granulocytes.

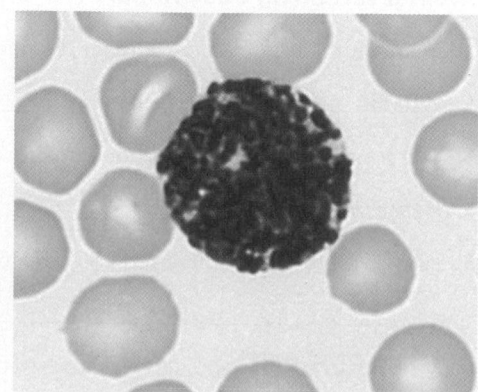

▲ **Figure 11.8** Basophils Are Granulocytes.

WORD	PRONUNCIATION	ELEMENTS		DEFINITION
basophil	BAY-so-fill	S/	-phil *attraction*	A basophil's granules attract a basic blue stain in the laboratory
		R/CF	bas/o- *base*	
differential	dif-er-EN-shal	S/	-ial *pertaining to*	A differential white blood cell count lists percentages of the different leukocytes in a blood sample
		R/	different- *not identical*	
eosinophil	ee-oh-SIN-oh-fill	S/	-phil *attraction*	An eosinophil's granules attract a rosy-red color on staining
		R/CF	eosin/o- *dawn*	
granulocyte	GRAN-you-loh-site	R/	-cyte *cell*	A white blood cell that contains multiple small granules in its cytoplasm
		R/CF	granul/o- *small grain*	
heparin	HEP-ah-rin	S/	-in *chemical*	An anticoagulant secreted particularly by liver cells
		R/	hepar- *liver*	
leukocyte (alternative spelling **leucocyte**)	LOO-koh-site	R	-cyte *cell*	Another term for a white blood cell
		R/CF	leuk/o- *white*	
leukocytosis	LOO-koh-sigh-TOE-sis	S/	-osis *condition*	An excessive number of white blood cells
leukopenia	loo-koh-PEE-nee-ah	S/	-penia *deficiency*	A deficient number of white blood cells
neutrophil	NEW-troh-fill	S/	-phil *attraction*	A neutrophil's granules take up purple stain equally whether the stain is acid or alkaline
		R/CF	neutr/o- *neutral*	
neutropenia	NEW-troh-PEE-nee-uh	S/	-penia *deficiency*	A deficiency of neutrophils
polymorphonuclear	POL-ee-more-foh-NEW-klee-ar	S/	-ar *pertaining to*	White blood cell with a multilobed nucleus
		P/	poly- *many*	
		R/CF	morph/o- *shape*	
		R/	-nucle- *nucleus*	

Exercises

A. Pick the correct suffix to complete the medical term. *One element will remain the same in each group of terms. Review the above WAD before you start the exercise. Fill in the blanks.*   **LO 11.1, 11.6**

-penia   -cyte   -cytosis

1. An excessive number of white blood cells is _____.

2. Another term for a white blood cell is _____.

3. A deficient number of white blood cells is _____.

4. The one element that does not change in each of the preceding terms is _____, which means _____.

B. Using the above WAD as your word bank, match the correct term in column one to its meaning in the second column. LO 11.1, 11.6

1. neutrophil   a. anticoagulant secreted by liver cells

2. leucocyte   b. white blood cell with a multilobed nucleus

3. basophil   c. white blood cell

4. heparin   d. releases histamine in damaged tissues

5. polymorphonuclear   e. secrete a group of enzymes called lysozymes

LO 11.7 Types of White Blood Cells (continued)

Agranulocytes

Because monocytes and lymphocytes have no granules in their cytoplasm, they are called **agranulocytes**.

1. **Monocytes** *(Figure 11.9)* are the largest blood cell and are normally 3% to 8% of the total WBC count. Monocytes leave the bloodstream and become macrophages that phagocytize bacteria, dead neutrophils, and dead cells in the tissues.

2. **Lymphocytes** *(Figure 11.10)* are normally 25% to 35% of the total WBC count. They are the smallest type of WBC. Lymphocytes are produced in red bone marrow and migrate through the bloodstream to lymphatic tissues—lymph nodes, tonsils, spleen, and thymus—where they proliferate.

There are two main types of lymphocyte:

a. **B cells** that differentiate into plasma cells. These are stimulated by bacteria or toxins to produce **antibodies**, or **immunoglobulins (Igs)**.

b. **T cells** that attach directly to foreign antigen-bearing cells such as bacteria, which they kill with toxins they secrete.

In a laboratory report, a **differential white blood cell count (DIFF)** lists the percentages of the different leukocytes in a blood sample.

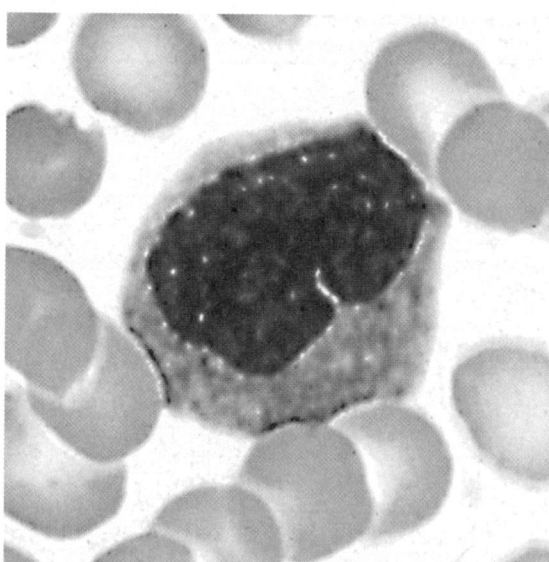

▲ **Figure 11.9**   Monocytes Are Agranulocytes.

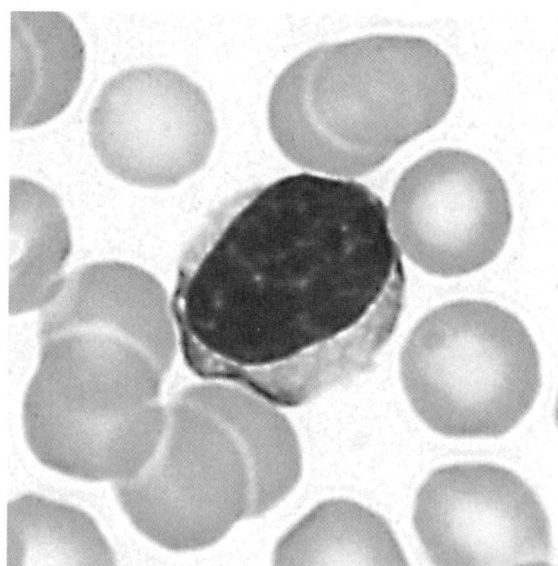

▲ **Figure 11.10**   Lymphocytes Are Agranulocytes.

WORD	PRONUNCIATION	ELEMENTS		DEFINITION
agranulocyte	a-**GRAN**-you-lo-site	P/ S/ R/CF	a- *without, not* -cyte *cell* -granul/o- *granule*	A white blood cell without any granules in its cytoplasm
antibody antibodies (pl)	**AN**-tih-body	P/ R/	anti- *against* body- *substance*	Protein produced in response to an antigen
immunoglobulin	**IM**-you-noh-**GLOB**-you-lin	S/ R/CF R/	-in *chemical* immun/o- *immune response* -globul- *protein*	Specific protein evoked by an antigen; all antibodies are immunoglobulins
lymphocyte	**LIM**-foh-site	S/ R/CF	-cyte *cell* lymph/o *lymph*	Small white blood cell with a large nucleus

Exercises

A. Use the medical terminology learned in this lesson to answer the questions.   LO 11.1, 11.6

1. In the term *agranulocyte,* there is an element meaning

   a. within

   b. alongside

   c. under

   d. without, not

   e. beside

2. In the term *agranulocyte,* there is a term meaning

   a. blue

   b. behind

   c. cell

   d. against

   e. deficient

3. In the term *immunoglobulin,* there is an element meaning

   a. protein

   b. many

   c. against

   d. liquid

   e. black

4. The correct plural of *antibody* is

   a. antibodys

   b. antibodies

   c. antibodyies

   d. antebodyies

   e. antybodies

B. Analyze the following question and circle the only FALSE answer. *Correct the false answer to be true.*   **LO 11.1, 11.6**

1. Because monocytes and lymphocytes have no granules in their cytoplasm, they are called *agranulocytes.*   T   F

2. Monocytes are the largest blood cell.   T   F

3. A lymphocyte is a white blood cell.   T   F

4. B cells and T cells are a type of monocyte.   T   F

5. Lymphocytes are the smallest type of white blood cell.   T   F

6. The false statement is # _____. Write the corrected statement on the lines below.

_____

_____

_____

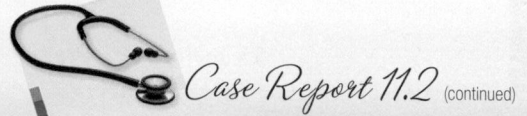

Case Report 11.2 (continued)

Latisha Masters' blood smear indicated a diagnosis of **infectious mononucleosis** caused by the **Epstein-Barr virus (EBV)**. This virus infects white blood cells. A positive **heterophile reaction (Monospot test)** was present. Infectious mononucleosis occurs in the 15- to 25-year-old population. Its cause, the Epstein-Barr virus (EBV), is a very common virus, a member of the herpes virus family. The EBV is transmitted by exchange of saliva, as in kissing. In patients with symptoms compatible with infectious mononucleosis, a positive Monospot test is diagnostic.

Keynotes

- Leukocytosis is the presence of too many white blood cells.
- Leukopenia is the presence of too few white blood cells.
- Pancytopenia is the presence of too few red blood cells, white blood cells, and platelets.
- Acute lymphoblastic leukemia is the most common leukemia in children.

LO 11.7 Disorders of White Blood Cells

Normally a cubic millimeter (**mm³**) of blood contains 5000 to 10,000 white blood cells.

Leukocytosis is defined as a total WBC count of normal cells exceeding 10,000/mm³. When the majority of the increased cells are neutrophils (polymorphonuclear leukocytes), an acute infection is usually present, for example, appendicitis or bacterial pneumonia.

Allergic reactions increase the number of eosinophils. Typhoid fever, malaria, and tuberculosis increase the number of monocytes. Whooping cough and infectious mononucleosis increase the number of lymphocytes.

Leukemia is cancer of the hematopoietic tissues and produces a high number of leukocytes and their **precursors** in the WBC count. As the **leukemic** cells proliferate, they take over the bone marrow and cause a deficiency of normal RBCs, WBCs, and **platelets**. This makes the patient anemic and vulnerable to infection and bleeding.

Myeloid leukemia is characterized by uncontrolled production of granulocytes and their precursors *(Figure 11.11)*. It can be in an acute or chronic form.

Lymphoid leukemia is characterized by uncontrolled production of lymphocytes. It can be in an acute or chronic form. **Acute lymphoblastic leukemia (ALL)** is the most common form of childhood cancer and is curable with modern treatments, such as chemotherapy and bone marrow and umbilical cord **stem cell** transplants.

Leukopenia results when the WBC count drops below 5000 cells/mm³ of blood. Leukopenia is seen in viral infections such as measles, mumps, chickenpox, poliomyelitis, and AIDS.

Pancytopenia occurs when the erythrocytes (RBCs), leukocytes (WBCs), and thrombocytes (**platelets**) in the circulating blood are all markedly reduced. This can occur with cancer chemotherapy.

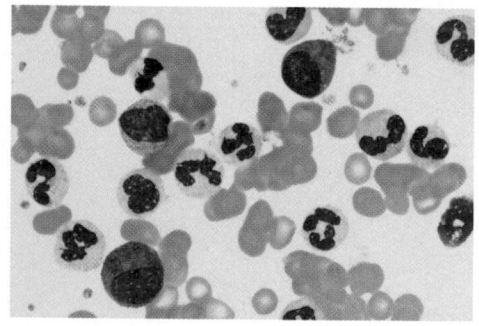

▲ **Figure 11.11**   Myeloid Leukemia.

Procedures

- **Bone marrow biopsy** or **aspiration** is often performed as part of the diagnostic work-up in patients with aplastic anemia, leukemias, lymphomas, and/or multiple myeloma. The specimen is usually taken from the posterior iliac crest of the pelvis *[see Chapter 14]*.

- **Bone marrow transplant** is the transfer of bone marrow from a healthy, compatible donor to a patient with aplastic anemia, leukemia, lymphoma, multiple myeloma, or other diseases. Compatibility requires having the same type of **human leukocyte antigen (HLA)** in a blood sample.

WORD	PRONUNCIATION	ELEMENTS		DEFINITION
aspiration	AS-pih-RAY-shun	S/ R/	-ion *process* aspirat- *to breathe*	Removal by suction of fluid or gas from a body cavity
heterophile (adj)	HET-er-oh-file	S/ R/CF	-phile *attraction* heter/o- *different*	Pertaining to antibodies present during a disease but not directed against the causative agent
leukemia	loo-KEE-mee-ah	S/ R/	-emia *blood* leuk- *white*	Disease in which the blood is taken over by white blood cells and their precursors
leukemic (adj)	loo-KEE-mick	S/	-emic *in the bood*	Pertaining to having the characteristics of leukemia
lymphoid	LIM-foyd	S/ R/	-oid *resembling* lymph- *lymph*	Resembling lymphatic tissue
mononucleosis	MON-oh-nyu-klee-OH-sis	S/ P/ R/	-osis *condition* mono- *single* -nucle- *nucleus*	Presence of large numbers of mononuclear leukocytes
Monospot test	MON-oh-spot TEST		Trade name	Detects heterophile antibodies in infectious mononucleosis
myeloid	MY-eh-loyd	S/ R/	-oid *resembling* myel- *bone marrow*	Resembling cells derived from bone marrow
pancytopenia	PAN-site-oh-PEE-nee-ah	S/ P/ R/CF	-penia *deficiency* pan- *all* -cyt/o- *cell*	Deficiency of all types of blood cells
platelet thrombocyte (syn)	PLAYT-let	S/ R/	-let *small* plate- *flat*	Cell fragment involved in clotting process
precursor	pree-KUR-sir	P/ R/	pre- *before, in front of* -cursor *run*	Cell or substance formed earlier in the development of the cell or substance
stem cell	STEM SELL		stem *Old English* *stalk of a plant*	Undifferentiated cell found in a differentiated tissue that can divide to yield the specialized cells in that tissue

Exercises

A. Test yourself on the *language of hematology* as it appears in the text and Case Report 11.2.   LO 11.1, 11.7

1. Use the glossary or an online medical dictionary to define *infectious*.

_____

2. Rewrite this sentence in your own words: "In patients with symptoms compatible with infectious mononucleosis, a positive Monospot test is diagnostic."

_____

_____

3. "Infectious mononucleosis is caused by the EBV, and this infects WBCs." Explain this sentence to your patient in words she can understand.

_____

_____

B. Continue using the *language of hematology* to answer the following questions.   LO 11.7

1. What is cancer of the hematopoietic tissues called? _____

2. What blood disease appears in viral infections such as measles, mumps, chickenpox, and AIDS? _____

3. "As the leukemic cells proliferate, they take over the bone marrow and cause *deficiency of normal red blood cells, white blood cells, and platelets.*" What one medical word can be substituted for the phrase in italic and mean the same thing? _____

LO 11.9 Disorders of Coagulation (Coagulopathies)

Hemophilia in its classical form (hemophilia A) is a disease males inherit from their mothers and is due to a deficiency of a coagulation factor, called factor VIII. The disorder causes painful bleeding into skin, joints, and muscles. Concentrated factor VIII is given intravenously to reduce the symptoms.

Von Willebrand disease (vWD) is a deficiency of a specific protein of the factor VIII complex that is different from the part involved in hemophilia.

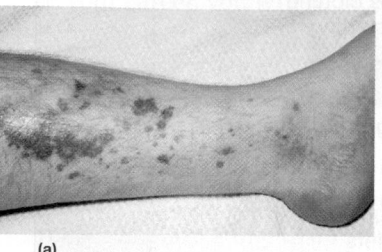 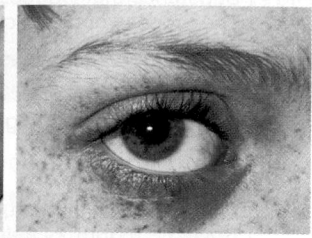

Disseminated intravascular coagulation (DIC) occurs when the clotting mechanism is activated simultaneously throughout the cardiovascular system. The trigger is usually a severe bacterial infection. Small clots form and obstruct blood flow into tissues and organs, particularly the kidney, leading to renal failure. As the clotting mechanisms are overwhelmed, severe bleeding occurs.

Thrombus formation (**thrombosis**) is a clot that attaches to diseased or damaged areas on the walls of blood vessels or the heart. If part of the thrombus breaks loose and moves through the circulation, it is called an **embolus**.

Thrombocytopenia is a low platelet count (below a $100,000/mm^3$ of blood). It occurs when bone marrow is destroyed by radiation, chemotherapy, or leukemia. Small capillary hemorrhages called **petechiae** and bruises can be seen in the skin. **Idiopathic (immunologic) thrombocytopenic purpura (ITP)** is an acute self-limiting form of the disease usually seen in children.

Thrombotic thrombocytopenic purpura (TTP) and **hemolytic-uremic syndrome (HUS)** are acute, potentially fatal disorders in which loose strands of fibrin are deposited in numerous small blood vessels. This causes damage to platelets and RBCs, causing thrombocytopenia and hemolytic anemia.

Henoch-Schönlein purpura (anaphylactoid purpura) is a disorder involving purpura, joint pain, and **glomerulonephritis** (*see Chapter 6*). The etiology is unknown. Most cases resolve spontaneously.

Purpura is bleeding into the skin from small arterioles that produces a larger individual lesion than petechiae from capillary bleeding (*Figure 11.13*). **Bruises** (or **hematomas**) are **extravasations** of blood from all types of blood vessels.

▲ **Figure 11.13**   **Subsurface Bleeding.**
(*a*) Purpura. (*b*) Pinpoint petechiae.
(*c*) Bruises.

Abbreviations

aPTT	activated partial thromboplastin time
DIC	disseminated intravascular coagulation
HUS	hemolytic-uremic syndrome
INR	International Normalized Ratio
ITP	idiopathic (or immunologic) thrombocytopenic purpura
PT	prothrombin time
tPA	tissue plasminogen activator
TTP	thrombotic thrombocytopenic purpura

LO 11.9 Pharmacology of Blood Clotting

- **Aspirin** reduces platelet adherence and aggregation. It is used in 81-mg doses to reduce the incidence of heart attacks.

- **Heparin** is a polysaccharide that prevents prothrombin and fibrin formation. It has to be given **parenterally** (not through the digestive tract), and recently a form of heparin that can be given subcutaneously has been approved. Its dose is monitored by **activated partial thromboplastin time (aPTT)**.

- **Hirudin** is a potent anticoagulant produced by **recombinant DNA technology**. It blocks thrombin formation.

- **Warfarin (Coumadin)** inhibits the synthesis of prothrombin and other coagulation factors, so it acts as an anticoagulant. It is given by mouth, and its dose is monitored by **prothrombin times (PTs)**, which are reported as an **International Normalized Ratio (INR)**.

- **Dabigatran etexilate (Pradaxa)** and **rivaroxaban (Xarelto)** inhibits the synthesis of thrombin and is given by mouth to reduce the risk of stroke and systemic embolism in patients with non-valvular atrial fibrillation *[see Chapter 10]*

- **Streptokinase**, derived from hemolytic streptococci, dissolves the fibrin in blood clots. Given intravenously within 3 to 4 hours of a heart attack, it is often effective in dissolving the clot that has caused the heart attack.

- **Tissue plasminogen activator (tPA)** binds strongly to fibrin and dissolves clots that have caused heart attacks. It is similar in effect and use to streptokinase. Reteplase and urokinase are forms of tPA.

Word Analysis and Definition

S = Suffix   P = Prefix   **R = Root**   **R/CF = Combining Form**

WORD	PRONUNCIATION	ELEMENTS		DEFINITION
coagulopathy coagulopathies (pl)	koh-ag-you-**LOP**-ah-thee	S/ R/CF	-pathy *disease* coagul/o- *clotting*	Disorder of blood clotting
disseminate	dih-**SEM**-in-ate	S/ P/ R/	-ate *composed of, pertaining to* dis- *apart* -semin- *scatter seed*	Widely scatter throughout the body or an organ
embolus	**EM**-boh-lus		Greek *plug, stopper*	Detached piece of thrombus, a mass of bacteria, quantity of air, or foreign body that blocks a blood vessel
extravasate	eks-**TRAV**-ah-sate	S/ P/ R/	-ate *composed of, pertaining to* extra- *out of, outside* -vas- *blood vessel*	To ooze out from a vessel into the tissues
hematoma bruise (syn)	he-mah-**TOH**-mah	S/ R/	-oma *mass, tumor* hemat- *blood*	Collection of blood that has escaped from the blood vessels into tissue
hemophilia	he-moh-**FILL**-ee-ah	S/ R/CF	-philia *attraction* hem/o- *blood*	An inherited disease from a deficiency of clotting factor VIII
petechia petechiae (pl)	peh-**TEE**-kee-ah peh-**TEE**-kee-ee		Latin *spot on the skin*	Pinpoint capillary hemorrhagic spot in the skin
purpura	**PUR**-pyu-rah		Greek *purple*	Skin hemorrhages that are red initially and then turn purple
recombinant DNA	ree-**KOM**-bin-ant dee-en-a	S/ P/ R/	-ant *forming* re- *again* -combin- *combine*	Deoxyribonucleic acid (DNA) altered by inserting a new sequence of DNA into the chain
streptokinase	strep-toe-**KI**-nase	P/ R/	strepto- *curved* -kinase *enzyme*	An enzyme that dissolves clots
thrombocytopenia	**THROM**-boh-site-oh-**PEE**-nee-ah	S/ R/CF R/CF	-penia *deficiency* thromb/o- *clot* -cyt/o- *cell*	Deficiency of platelets in circulating blood
warfarin	**WAR**-fuh-rin		Named after *Wisconsin Alumni Research Foundation*, which funded its discovery	Anticoagulant; also used as rat poison

Exercises

A. Answers to the following questions can be found on this two-page spread. *Fill in the blanks. Be prepared to discuss your answers in class.* **LO 11.1, 11.9**

1. Small, *capillary hemorrhages* are called _____.

2. Bleeding from larger blood vessels called _____ produces *purpura*.

3. What is the difference between an *embolus* and a *thrombus?*

   embolus: _____

   thrombus: _____

4. What is another term for a hematoma? _____

5. Translate the following sentence into language your patient can understand.

   "Aspirin reduces platelet adherence and aggregation. It is used in 81-mg doses to reduce the incidence of myocardial infarction."

   _____

   _____

   _____

6. Deficiency of platelets in circulating blood is called _____.

Lesson 11.5 Blood Groups and Transfusions

To make an appropriate decision, it is critical that you are able to use correct medical terminology to:

11.5.1 **List the different blood groups.**

11.5.2 **Explain what determines a person's ABO blood type and how this relates to transfusion compatibility.**

11.5.3 **Describe the effect of an incompatibility between mother and fetus in the rhesus (Rh) blood type.**

You are

. . . an emergency medical technician–paramedic (EMT-P) working in the Level One Trauma Unit at Fulwood Medical Center.

Your patient is

. . . Ms. Joanne Rodi, an 18-year-old student.

Case Report 11.4

Ms. Rodi has been admitted to the unit from the operating room after surgery for multiple fractures in a car accident. She is receiving a blood transfusion. You document that her temperature has risen to 102°F and her respirations to 24 per minute and she has chills. You take her BP; it has fallen to 90/60. What should you do?

LO 11.10 Red Cell Antigens

On the surfaces of red blood cells are molecules called *antigens.* In the plasma, antibodies are present. Each antibody can combine with only a specific antigen. If the plasma antibodies combine with a red cell antigen, bridges are formed that connect the red cells together. This is called **agglutination**, or clumping, of the cells. Hemolysis (rupture) of the cells also occurs.

The antigens on the surfaces of the cells have been categorized into groups, of which two are the most important. These are the ABO and Rhesus (Rh) blood groups.

ABO Blood Group

The two major antigens on the cell surface are antigen A and antigen B *(Figure 11.14).*

A person with only antigen A has *type A* blood.

A person with only antigen B has *type B* blood.

A person with both antigen A and antigen B has *type AB* blood and is a universal recipient who can receive blood from any other type in the ABO system.

A person with neither antigen has *type O* blood and is a universal donor able to give blood to any other person no matter what that person's blood type is.

Figure 11.14 shows the different combinations of antigens and antibodies in the different blood types.

A **transfusion** of blood or packed red blood cells replaces lost red blood cells to restore the blood's oxygen-carrying capacity. In **autologous** donation and transfusion, people donate their own blood ahead of time to be given to them if necessary during a surgical procedure.

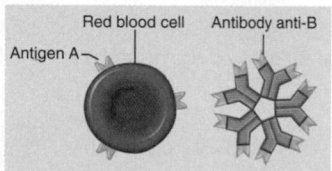

(a) Type A blood

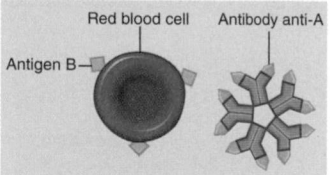

(b) Type B blood

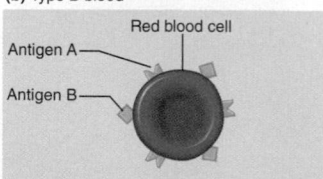

(c) Type AB blood

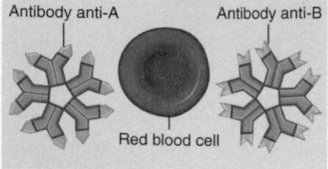

(d) Type O blood

▲ **Figure 11.14** **ABO Blood Types.**

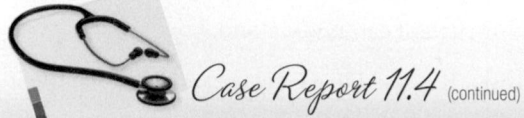

Case Report 11.4 (continued)

In Miss Rodi's case, she has type A blood and, by mistake, received type AB blood, which agglutinated in the presence of her anti-B antibodies. Your immediate response is to stop the transfusion, replace it with a saline **infusion**, call your supervisor, and notify the doctor.

Keynotes

• All blood groups are inherited.

• Rh factor is an antigen on the surface of a red blood cell.

S = Suffix   P = Prefix   R = Root   R/CF = Combining Form

WORD	PRONUNCIATION	ELEMENTS		DEFINITION
agglutination	ah-glue-tih-**NAY**-shun	S/ P/ R/	-ation *process* ag- *to* -glutin- *glue*	Process by which cells or other particles adhere to each other to form clumps
autologous	awe-**TOL**-oh-gus	P/ R/	auto- *self, same* -logous *relation*	Blood transfusion with the same person as donor and recipient
infusion	in-**FYU**-zhun	P/ R/	in- *in* -fusion *to pour*	Introduction intravenously of a substance other than blood
transfusion	trans-**FYU**-zhun	P/ R/	trans- *across* -fusion *to pour*	Transfer of blood or a blood component from donor to recipient

Exercises

A. Review the elements in the above WAD before starting this exercise. *Match the elements in column 1 with the correct meanings in column 2.* **LO 11.1, 11.10**

_____ 1. logous   a. condition

_____ 2. fusion   b. self

_____ 3. trans   c. to pour

_____ 4. blast   d. across

_____ 5. osis   e. relation

_____ 6. auto   f. germ cell

B. Circle the correct medical term from the above WAD in the following statements. LO 11.1, 11.10

1. Chemotherapy drugs would be administered by (infusion/transfusion).

2. (Autologous/Agglutination) would occur if the patient were given the wrong blood type.

3. An (autologous/agglutination) unit of blood is one you donate for later use in your own surgery.

4. Rupture of cells causes (hemolysis/hematemesis).

LO 11.10 Red Cell Antigens (continued)

Rhesus (Rh) Blood Group

If an **Rh** antigen is present on an RBC surface, the blood is said to be Rh-positive (Rh⁺). If there is no Rh antigen on the surface, the blood is Rh-negative (Rh⁻). The presence or absence of Rh antigen is inherited.

If an Rh-negative person receives a transfusion of Rh-positive blood, anti-Rh antibodies will be produced. This can cause RBC agglutination and hemolysis.

If an Rh-negative woman and an Rh-positive man conceive an Rh-positive child *(Figure 11.15a)*, the placenta normally prevents maternal and fetal blood from mixing. However, at birth or during a miscarriage, fetal cells can enter the mother's bloodstream. These Rh-positive cells stimulate the mother's tissues to produce Rh-antibodies *(Figure 11.15b)*.

If the mother becomes pregnant with a second Rh-positive fetus, her Rh-antibodies can cross the placenta and agglutinate and hemolyze the fetal RBCs *(Figure 11.15c)*. This causes hemolytic disease of the newborn (**HDN**, or **erythroblastosis fetalis**).

Hemolytic disease of the newborn due to Rh-incompatibility can be prevented. The Rh-negative mother should be given Rh immune globulin (RhoGAM) during pregnancy, or soon after giving birth to an Rh-positive child.

Other causes of hemolytic disease of the newborn include ABO incompatibility, incompatibility in other blood group systems, hereditary **spherocytosis**, and some infections acquired before birth.

Abbreviations	
EMT-P	emergency medical technician-paramedic
HDN	hemolytic disease of the newborn (erythroblastosis fetalis)
Rh	rhesus
RhoGAM	rhesus immune globulin

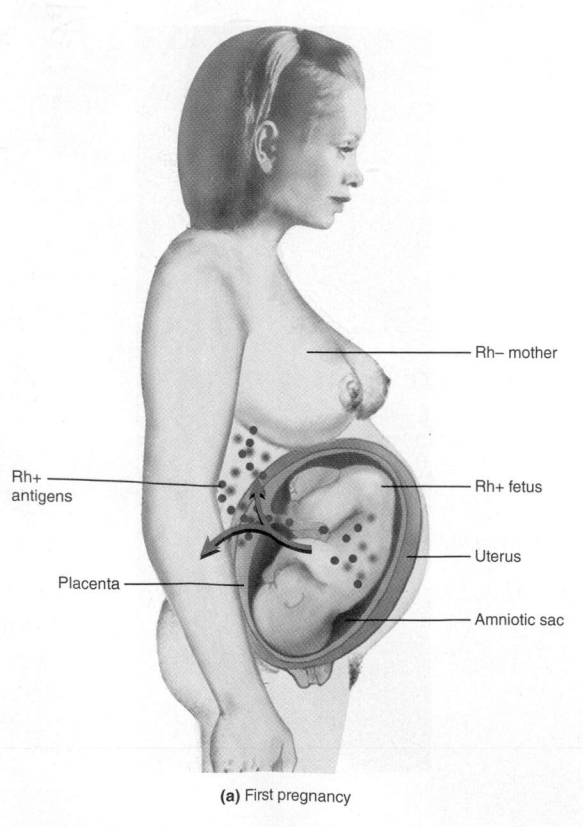

(a) First pregnancy

Rh– mother
Rh+ antigens
Rh+ fetus
Uterus
Placenta
Amniotic sac

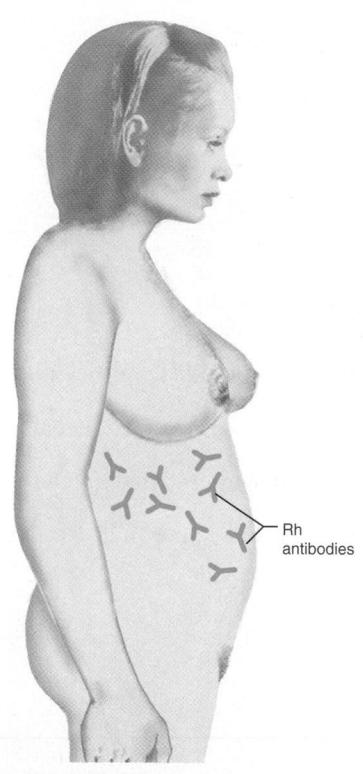

(b) Between pregnancies

Rh antibodies

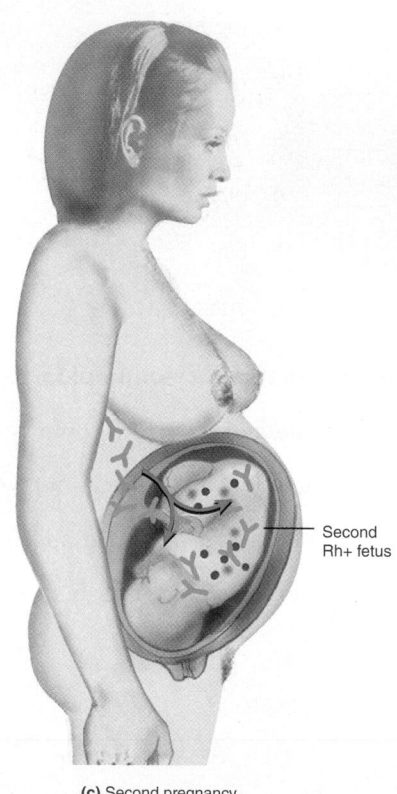

(c) Second pregnancy

Second Rh+ fetus

▲ **Figure 11.15**   Hemolytic Disease of the Newborn.

S = Suffix   P = Prefix   **R = Root   R/CF = Combining Form**

WORD	PRONUNCIATION	ELEMENTS		DEFINITION
erythroblastosis	eh-**RITH**-ro-blast-oh-sis	S/	-osis *condition*	Hemolytic disease of the newborn due to Rh incompatibility
		R/CF	**erythr/o-** *red*	
		R/	**-blast-** *germ cell, immature cell*	
fetalis	fee-**TAH**-lis	S/	-is *belonging to*	
		R/	**fet-** *fetus*	
		S/	-al *pertaining to*	
infusion	in-**FYU**-zhun	P/	in- *in*	Introduction intravenously of a substance other than blood
		R/	**-fusion** *to pour*	
Rhesus factor	**REE**-sus **FAK**-tor		**Greek** *mythical king of Thrace*	Antigen on red blood cells of Rh-positive (Rh+) individuals. It was first identified in the blood of a rhesus monkey
spherocyte	**SFEAR**-oh-site	S/	-cyte *cell*	A spherical cell
		R/CF	**spher/o-** *sphere*	
spherocytosis	**SFEAR**-oh-site-oh-sis	S/	-osis *condition*	Presence of spherocytes in blood

Exercises

A. Use the *language of hematology* to answer the following questions about blood. *Find the only incorrect statement and circle it. Rewrite the sentence to be correct.*   **LO 11.1, 11.10**

1. There are 5 blood types.   T   F

2. Blood is a type of connective tissue.   T   F

3. There are 3 formed elements in blood.   T   F

4. An average adult has about 10 pints of blood.   T   F

5. Blood type O is the universal donor.   T   F

6. Corrected statement # _____ :

   _____

   _____

B. Continue your use of the correct medical terminology to answer the following questions.   **LO 11.1, 11.2, 11.10**

1. Explain the difference between a transfusion and an infusion.

   a. transfusion: _____

   _____

   b. infusion: _____

   _____

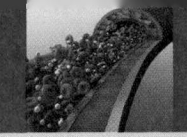
BLOOD

Challenge Your Knowledge

A. Word association. Fill in the blanks. (**LO 11.1**, *Remember, Understand*)

1. The medical term **viscous** means _____.

2. Equate this to something seen in everyday life that has the same consistency. _____

_____

B. Meet the lesson and chapter objectives by testing your knowledge of the blood and its components. *Use this exercise as a study review before a test.* Fill in the blanks. (**LO 11.1, 11.3, 11.4, 11.6**, *Remember, Apply*)

1. Name the functions of blood:

   a. _____

   b. _____

   c. _____

   d. _____

   e. _____

   f. _____

   g. _____

   h. _____

   i. _____

2. List the formed elements of blood and give one function for each:

   a. Component: _____ Function: _____

   b. Component: _____ Function: _____

   c. Component: _____ Function: _____

3. Plasma transports

   a. _____

   b. _____

   c. _____

   d. _____

4. The different types of WBCs are

   a. _____

   b. _____

   c. _____

   d. _____

   e. _____

C. True or false. The following statements about blood are either true or false. Circle the correct answer. Rewrite the false statement(s) correctly on the lines below. (**LO 11.1, 11.3, 11.4, _Understand_**)

1. The formed elements of blood are RBCs, WBCs, platelets, and serum.   T   F

2. Buffer systems in the blood maintain the correct pH range.   T   F

3. Serum is identical to plasma except for the absence of clotting proteins.   T   F

4. Sickle cell anemia is a genetic disorder.   T   F

5. All cells exchange water by thrombosis.   T   F

6. Plasma is the fluid, noncellular part of blood.   T   F

7. The bloodstream is a liquid transport system.   T   F

8. Whole blood is less viscous than water.   T   F

9. Monocytes are the largest blood cells.   T   F

10. Erythropoiesis occurs in bone spaces filled with red bone marrow.   T   F

Corrections:

_____

_____

_____

_____

_____

_____

_____

D. Documentation. Take the patient's own words and translate them into medical language for documentation. (**LO 11.1, 11.2, _Understand_**)

1. "I am always tired, have no energy or 'get up and go,' and my arms and legs ache a lot of the time."

This patient complains of _____

_____.

Take the doctor's words and translate them into language the patient can understand.

2. "In sickle cell disease, the abnormal cells agglutinate and occlude small capillaries, and this causes the intense pain in the hypoxic tissues. This is the sickle cell crisis."

_____

_____

_____

_____

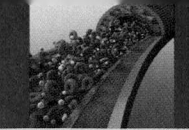

CHAPTER 11 REVIEW

BLOOD

E. Team exercise. Pair with a fellow student or group of students. Choose three medical terms in this chapter that you find the most difficult to remember or understand. Write them, pronounce them, and then use each term in a brief sentence that is a definition. Place a checkmark (✓) on the appropriate line once you have practiced the pronunciations. Take turns quizzing the other students on your terms, and see if you can answer their term questions. Track if there is a pattern of certain terms that you all find difficult. *Use this exercise as a study review.* (**LO 11.1, 11.2,** *Understand*)

1. Term: _____   Pronunciation practiced: _____

   Definition:

   _____

   _____

2. Term: _____   Pronunciation practiced: _____

   Definition:

   _____

   _____

3. Term: _____   Pronunciation practiced: _____

   Definition:

   _____

   _____

F. Patient education. Mrs. Sosin has asked you to interpret the results of her blood work for her. Use your knowledge of blood to explain in your own words her test results. (**LO 11.1, 11.4, 11.5,** *Understand*)

Examination of her peripheral smear reveals her RBCs to be microcytic, hypochromic, and poikilocytic. Laboratory examination reveals a hemoglobin concentration of 10.4 g/dL (normal range 12–16 g/dL).

1. Define the following abbreviation and medical terms for the patient:

   RBC: _____

   microcytic: _____

   hypochromic: _____

   poikilocytic: _____

   hemoglobin: _____

2. In your own words, describe to the patient the role of hemoglobin in the blood.

   _____

   _____

3. Is Mrs. Sosin's hemoglobin concentration within normal limits (WNL)? _____

G. Choose the appropriate meaning of abbreviations to fill in the patient documentation. (**LO 11.1,** *Understand, Apply*)

1. The patient's _____ (Hct) last week was normal, as were her _____ (RBCs), but the (CBC) _____ showed an abnormal number of _____ (WBCs).

2. The patient's _____ (MCV) and _____ (MCH) both showed decreased values on his recent blood test.

3. Laboratory work proved Latisha's mononucleosis to be caused by the _____ (EBV).

4. Orders for this patient's preop testing before her surgery will include a _____ (PT) and an _____ (aPTT).

5. Possible admitting diagnoses for this patient include _____ (vWD) and _____ (ALL).

6. This patient was given a drug containing _____ (tPA) in the Emergency Department following his heart attack.

H. **Medical terminology is a language of small nuances that make a difference.** Determine the difference between the pairs of terms listed below. Underline the element that makes the difference in the term; then provide a brief definition for each term. (**LO 11.1,** *Understand, Apply*)

1. *transfusion* and *infusion*

   _____

   _____

   _____

2. *hemostasis* and *homeostasis*

   _____

   _____

   _____

3. *pancytopenia* and *thrombocytopenia*

   _____

   _____

   _____

4. In the group of terms in questions 1 through 3, in each pair the _____ (type of element) stays the same.

I. **Medical terms may be similar in appearance.** You need to use your knowledge of prefixes, roots, and suffixes to help determine the difference between similar terms. Using the following terms, correctly insert them into the following paragraph. (**LO 11.1, 11.4, 11.5,** *Understand, Apply*)

   erythrocyte   erythroblast   erythroblastosis   erythropoiesis   erythropoietin

   The immature RBC (_____) undergoes the process of formation (_____) in the red bone marrow.

   Too many immature cells result in a condition known as _____. A mature RBC is called an _____.

   The hormone _____ controls the rate of RBC production.

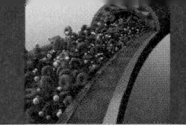

BLOOD

J. **Pharmacology of blood clotting.** Anyone working with patients must know about prescribed drugs and their function. Match the correct drug to its purpose. (**LO 11.9**, *Understand, Apply*)

_____ 1. Dissolves fibrin in blood clots   **a.** heparin

_____ 2. Reduces platelet adherence   **b.** tPA

_____ 3. Prevents prothrombin and fibrin formation   **c.** Coumadin

_____ 4. Inhibits formation of prothrombin   **d.** streptokinase

_____ 5. Inhibits synthesis of coagulation factors   **e.** aspirin

K. **How well do you understand what you read?** First, read the paragraph aloud to check your pronunciation. Then, read the paragraph again and underline the medical terms. Enter the term in the left column of the chart next to its correct meaning. (**LO 11.1, 11.2**, *Understand, Analyze*)

When a lab tech takes a blood sample, he spins it in a centrifuge. Formed elements are separated from the colloidal suspension and are packed into the bottom of the tube. The patient's hematocrit can be determined from this test. Whole blood contains all the formed elements. Transfusions can be done with either whole blood or only certain portions of the formed elements—only transfusing RBCs or platelets, for instance. The remaining part (55%) of a blood sample is the plasma, which is mostly water. Plasma provides the fluid transport for the formed elements as well as nutrients, hormones and enzymes for body cells. Waste cell products dissolve in plasma and are excreted through the kidneys and liver.

Term	Meaning
1.	to dispose of
2.	liquid containing particles that do not settle
3.	introduction of blood or a blood component into a vein
4.	something life sustaining
5.	blood clotting cell
6.	instrument for separating a blood sample
7.	stimulates function of an organ or tissue
8.	erythrocyte
9.	liquid transport system
10.	induces chemical changes in other substances
11.	percentage of RBCs in the blood

L. **Meet a lesson objective and list the different blood types in the ABO blood group.** Be sure to note which type is the "universal donor" and which type is the "universal recipient." *Do you know your own blood type and that of your spouse or children?* (**LO 11.10, Understand, Apply**)

The two major antigens on the cell surface are antigen A and antigen B.

1. A person with only antigen A has type _____ blood.

2. A person with only antigen B has type _____ blood.

3. A person with *both* antigen A and antigen B has type _____ blood.

4. A person with *neither* antigen A nor antigen B has type _____ blood.

5. Because the blood type in question 4 has *neither* antigen, it is compatible with any blood type; therefore, it is the universal

   (donor/recipient) _____.

6. Because the blood type in question 3 has *both* antigens, it is the universal (donor/recipient) _____.

M. **Build medical terms from the following group of elements.** The definition is given to you; fill in the medical term. You will not use every element, and some you may use twice. Fill in the blanks. (**LO 11.1, 11.4, Apply**)

Use a combination of these elements to complete the terms:

ic	micro	auto	osis	hypo	crit	ox
ary	cyte	thrombo	macro	ar	erythro	cyt

1. Another name for an RBC   erythro _____

2. Pertaining to a small cell   _____cyt_____

3. Blood transfusion with the same person as both donor and recipient   _____logous

4. Large RBC   _____cyte

5. Percentage of RBCs in blood   hemato _____

6. Deficient in oxygen   _____/_____/ic

7. Same as a platelet   _____/cyte

8. Formation of a clot   thromb/_____

BLOOD

N. Test your knowledge of blood, blood groups, and Rh factor by choosing the correct answer to the following questions. Circle the best answer. (**LO 11.10,** *Apply, Analyze*)

1. A person with both antigen A and antigen B will have

   a. blood type O

   b. blood type A

   c. blood type B

   d. blood type AB

   e. blood type B−

2. Where are antibodies synthesized after birth?

   a. in the heart

   b. in the blood

   c. in the arteries

   d. in the plasma

   e. in the veins

3. What normally prevents maternal and fetal blood from mixing during pregnancy?

   a. cell membranes

   b. the peritoneum

   c. the placenta

   d. the amniotic sac

   e. the matrix

4. Blood is said to be Rh-positive if

   a. the Rh antigen is present on the RBC surface

   b. the Rh antibody is present in the blood type

   c. the Rh antibody is present in the plasma

   d. the Rh antigen is present on the WBCs

   e. the blood type is AB

5. *Agglutination* occurs when

   a. you have not been vaccinated

   b. you are given the wrong blood type

   c. your antibodies are low

   d. your hematocrit is high

   e. you are Rh-positive

6. The term *transfusion* is used only for

   a. plasma

   b. whole blood

   c. blood or a blood component

   d. saline solution

   e. intravenous (IV) antibiotics

O. Multiple choice. Use the *language of hematology* to answer the following questions. Remember that in the case of multiple choice, there is only one *best* answer. (**LO 11.1, 11.4, 11.6,** *Analyze*)

1. Blood volume varies with

    a. your body size

    b. your weight

    c. the amount of your connective tissue

    d. the amount of your RBCs

    e. your height

2. The percentage of RBCs in a blood sample is called the

    a. hemoglobin

    b. hematocrit

    c. hematemesis

    d. hemolysis

    e. hemostasis

3. In the term **hypochromic**, the root means

    a. blood

    b. center

    c. color

    d. glue

    e. air

4. How many types of WBCs also qualify as granulocytes?

    a. one

    b. two

    c. three

    d. four

    e. five

5. **Myeloid leukemia** is a disorder of

    a. RBCs

    b. WBCs

    c. platelets

    d. plasma

    e. hemoglobin

6. In the term **erythrocyte**, the combining form means

    a. yellow

    b. red

    c. white

    d. black

    e. blue

7. **Heparin** is an

    a. antidepressant

    b. antihistamine

    c. antibody

    d. anticoagulant

    e. antibiotic

8. Which of these terms cannot be connected with blood?

    a. liquid matrix

    b. CBC

    c. formed elements

    d. infusion

    e. transfusion

9. The largest WBC is

    a. monocyte

    b. macrophage

    c. eosinophil

    d. basophil

    e. neutrophil

10. What is plasma minus its protein fibrinogen?

    a. hemoglobin

    b. antithrombin

    c. plasmin

    d. serum

    e. a formed element

BLOCKD

BLOOD

P. Discussion questions. Prepare a brief discussion on either topic—question #1, or question #2. Outline your thoughts briefly on the following lines. (**LO 11.1, 11.2,** *Analyze*)

1. What is the major concern in transfusions? What types of safeguards can be used to prevent a patient getting the wrong blood in a transfusion? Why is it a good thing to know your own blood type?

_____

_____

2. What is the function of buffer systems in the blood? Give some examples. What is the pH range of blood?

_____

_____

Q. There are many diseases associated with the various components of blood. Circle the correct choice in the following descriptions; then, on the blanks, write in which blood component is associated with the disease you circled. Use RBC, WBC, and P (for platelet) for blood component notations. (**LO 11.3, 11.5, 11.7,** *Analyze*)

Blood Component

1. Chronic bleeding from the gastrointestinal tract can cause

   iron-deficiency anemia   pernicious anemia   sickle cell anemia   _____

2. A deficiency of a specific protein of the factor VIII complex is

   thrombus   von Willenbrand disease   iron-deficiency anemia   _____

3. Cancer of the hematopoietic tissues is called

   leukemia   lukemia   lukemmia   _____

4. A disease resulting from vitamin B_{12} deficiency is

   pernicious anemia   hemolytic anemia   polycythemia vera   _____

5. A disease males inherit from their mothers is

   hemmaphilia   hemophilia   hemmophilia   _____

6. A hereditary disease found mostly in people of African descent is

   sickle cell anemia   iron-deficiency anemia   polycythemia vera   _____

7. In this disease numerous small clots form and obstruct blood flow into organs:

   DIC   vWD   tPA   _____

8. This is seen in viral infections such as measles and mumps:

   leukopenia   leukocytosis   leukemia   _____

9. Low blood cell count that produces a tendency to bleed is

   thrombocitopenia   thrombocytopenia   thrombocytopennia   _____

10. Destruction of blood cells by toxic substances is

   polycythemia vera   hemolytic anemia   pernicious anemia   _____

R. Demonstrate your knowledge of word elements by deconstructing the following medical terms. Then write the term next to the appropriate statement that follows. (**LO 11.1, 11.7,** *Analyze*)

Term	Prefix	Root/Combining Form	Suffix
leukocytosis	1.	2.	3.
hypochromic	4.	5.	6.
vasoconstrictor	7.	8.	9.
poikilocytic	10.	11.	12.
precursor	13.	14.	15.
anemia	16.	17.	18.
microcytic	19.	20.	21.
osmosis	22.	23.	24.
hemoglobin	25.	26.	27.
pancytopenia	28.	29.	30.

31. That which comes before something _____

32. Pertaining to a small cell _____

33. Decreased number of RBCs _____

34. Passage of water across a cell membrane _____

35. Pigmented protein in RBCs _____

36. Excessively high WBC count _____

37. Deficiency of all formed elements in the blood _____

38. Agent that causes narrowing of blood vessels _____

39. Pertaining to a RBC of irregular shape _____

40. Pale in color _____

BLOOD

S. **With the possible exception of the appendix, everything in the body has a function.** The functions are listed as follows. Assign each a letter for the blood component that performs the function. (**LO 11.3,** *Analyze*)

Functions

    a. A function of a RBC

    b. A function of a WBC

    c. A function of a platelet

    d. A function of plasma

Assign one of the previous functions to each of the following statements:

  1. Transport oxygen   _____

  2. Help maintain hemostasis   _____

  3. Migrate to damaged tissues and release histamine   _____

  4. Carry nutrients, hormones, and enzymes to cells   _____

  5. Dissolve cellular waste products   _____

  6. Secrete lysozymes   _____

  7. Transport carbon dioxide   _____

  8. Seal off injury and hemorrhage   _____

  9. Provide fluid environment to formed elements   _____

 10. Transport nitric oxide   _____

CHAPTER SUMMARY EXERCISE

A. Spelling comprehension. Circle the correct spelling of the term. (**LO 11.1,** *Remember*)

1. autollogus	autologis	autoligus	autologous	autolagus
2. creatinnine	creatinine	creatynine	creatonin	creatyine
3. erythropoesis	errythropoesis	erythropoisus	erythropuesis	erythropoiesis
4. leukocytusis	leukocytosis	lukocytosis	leukocitosis	lukocitossis
5. feretin	ferrittin	ferriten	ferritin	feriton
6. pitichia	petickia	petechia	petikia	peteckia
7. centrifuje	centerfuge	senterfuge	centrifuge	sentrifuge
8. ossmosis	ossmossis	osmosis	osmoses	osmossus
9. apherises	apheresis	aperisis	aperhisis	apherisus
10. agluetinate	agglutenate	aguentinate	agglutonate	agglutinate

B. Match the number of the correct spelling of the term in Exercise A with the brief description of the term below. (**LO 11.1, 11.4, 11.7,** *Apply*)

_____ **1.** Passage of fluid across a cell membrane

_____ **2.** Removing only platelets and returning the rest to the donor

_____ **3.** Regulates iron storage and transport

_____ **4.** Separates particles in a suspension

_____ **5.** Formation of red blood cells

_____ **6.** Donating your own blood for your surgery

_____ **7.** Minute hemorrhage in the skin

_____ **8.** Clump together

_____ **9.** Excessive number of white blood cells

_____ **10.** Protein found in skeletal muscle

C. Using your knowledge of terms 1–10 in Exercises A and B and their correct spelling, write a brief sentence for each of the terms as it might appear in patient documentation. (**LO 11.1,** *Apply*)

1. _____

2. _____

3. _____

4. _____

5. _____

6. _____

7. _____

8. _____

9. _____

10. _____

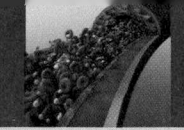

CHAPTER 11 REVIEW

BLOOD

D. **After rereading Case Report 11.4, answer the following questions.** Be prepared to discuss your answers in class. **(LO 11.1, 11.5, 11.7, *Analyze*)**

Case Report 11.4

You are

...an emergency medical technician–paramedic (EMT-P) working in the Level One Trauma Unit at Fulwood Medical Center.

Your patient is

...Miss Joanne Rodi, an 18-year-old student, who has been admitted to the unit from the operating room after surgery for multiple fractures in a car accident.

Miss Rodi is receiving a blood transfusion. You document that her temperature has risen to 102°F and her respirations to 24 per minute and she has chills. You take her blood pressure; it has fallen to 90/60. What should you do?

In Miss Rodi's case, she has type A blood and, by mistake, received type AB blood, which agglutinated in the presence of her anti-B antibodies. Your immediate response is to stop the transfusion, replace it with a saline infusion, call your supervisor, and notify the doctor.

1. If a *transfusion* consists of blood or blood components, what does an *infusion* carry?

_____

2. What is meant by the phrase "blood cells agglutinate"?

_____

3. Can you think of a study hint that will help you remember what *agglutinate* means?

_____

_____

4. What were Miss Rodi's symptoms once the blood started to agglutinate?

_____

_____

5. What specific antigen did Miss Rodi's type A blood react to? _____

6. Define the medical term *incompatible*. _____

7. Write a sentence of documentation in Miss Rodi's case, using the term *incompatible*. _____

_____

_____

E. **Meet the goals of each of the chapter outcomes by using the correct language of hematology for the answers. (LO 11.1–11.10, *Analyze*)**

1. Use the medical terms of hematology to communicate and document in writing accurately and precisely in any health care setting. Explain this sentence: "Plasma is the fluid, noncellular part of blood." (**LO 11.1**)

_____

_____

2. Use the medical terms of hematology to communicate verbally with accuracy and precision in any health care setting. If the doctor tells you the patient is hypoxic, what will he need? (**LO 11.2**)

   a. insulin   **d.** an infusion

   b. a transfusion   **e.** pain medication

   c. oxygen

3. Describe the components and functions of blood and the basic laboratory studies that show them. Circle the correct answer to each question. (**LO 11.3**)

   a. What are the formed elements of blood?

   i. Plasma and WBCs

   ii. Plasma and RBCs

   iii. Platelets, RBCs, and WBCs

   iv. Plasma and platelets

   v. Platelets and serum

   b. Circle the only statement that is NOT a function of blood:

   i. maintains body temperature

   ii. transports hormones

   iii. maintains homeostasis

   iv. regulates Ph and osmosis

   v. aids in digestion

   c. What is "counted" in a complete blood count (CBC)? Circle the correct answer.

   i. RBCs

   ii. RBCs and WBCs

   iii. RBCs, WBCs, and platelets

   iv. RBCs, WBCs, and plasma volume

   v. Plasma volume and platelets

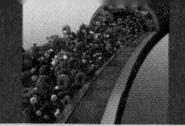

BLOOD

4. Describe the structure and functions of RBCs. (**LO 11.4**)

 a. List three gases that are transported by RBCs: _____, _____, and _____.

 b. What medical term can be used to describe the shape of a RBC? _____

 c. Erythropoiesis is the correct medical term for _____.

5. Discuss disorders of RBCs. Match the definition in the first column to the disorder in the second column. (**LO 11.5**)

 _____ **a.** excessive destruction of normal and abnormal RBCs   **i.** sickle cell anemia

 _____ **b.** overproduction of RBCs and WBCs due to unknown cause   **ii.** pernicious anemia

 _____ **c.** genetic disorder   **iii.** aplastic anemia

 _____ **d.** bone marrow unable to produce new cells   **iv.** hemolytic anemia

 _____ **e.** a disorder due to vitamin B_{12} deficiency   **v.** polycythemia vera

6. Describe the types of WBCs and their functions. Use the language of hematology and fill in the blanks. (**LO 11.6**)

 a. Basophils migrate to damaged tissues and release _____ and _____.

 b. The two basic types of WBCs are _____ and _____.

 c. What type of WBC leaves the bloodstream to enter tissues undergoing an allergic response? _____

 d. What are the two main types of agranulocytes? _____ and _____

 e. B cells and T cells are the two main types of _____.

7. Discuss disorders of WBCs. Circle the correct choice. (**LO 11.7**)

 a. Total WBC count exceeding 10,000/mm3 is

  leukemia   leukocytosis   myeloid leukemia

 b. Cancer of the hematopoietic tissues is

  leukemia   leucopenia   pancytopenia

 c. Which of the following choices is characterized by uncontrolled production of lymphocytes?

  lymphoid leukemia   leukemia   pancytopenia

 d. Which of the following choices is characterized by markedly reduced red blood cells, white blood cells, and platelets in the blood?

  lymphoma   pancytopenia   anemia

8. Explain hemostasis. Use the language of hematology to explain hemostasis. (**LO 11.8**)

   a. Hemostasis is the control of _____.

   b. Hemostasis helps maintain _____.

   c. How does uncontrolled bleeding take the body out of balance?

   _____

   _____

   d. What formed element of blood plays a key role in hemostasis? _____

9. Discuss disorders of coagulation and their pharmacology. Fill in the blanks with the language of hematology. (**LO 11.9**)

   a. Collectively, disorders of coagulation are termed _____.

   b. What is the most common hereditary bleeding disorder? _____

   c. What common over-the-counter drug is used to reduce the incidence of heart attacks? _____

   d. What IV drug should be given within 4 hours of a heart attack to dissolve the clot that caused the heart attack?

   _____

10. Identify the different blood groups and their role in transfusions. Answer the questions with terminology learned in this chapter. (**LO 11.10**)

    a. Name the blood groups:

      1. _____

      2. _____

      3. _____

      4. _____

    b. If you are given the wrong blood type, what occurs?

    _____

    c. Rupture of blood cells is called _____.

    d. What is the difference between a transfusion and an infusion? (Be precise!)

      1. transfusion:

      _____

      _____

      2. infusion:

      _____

      _____

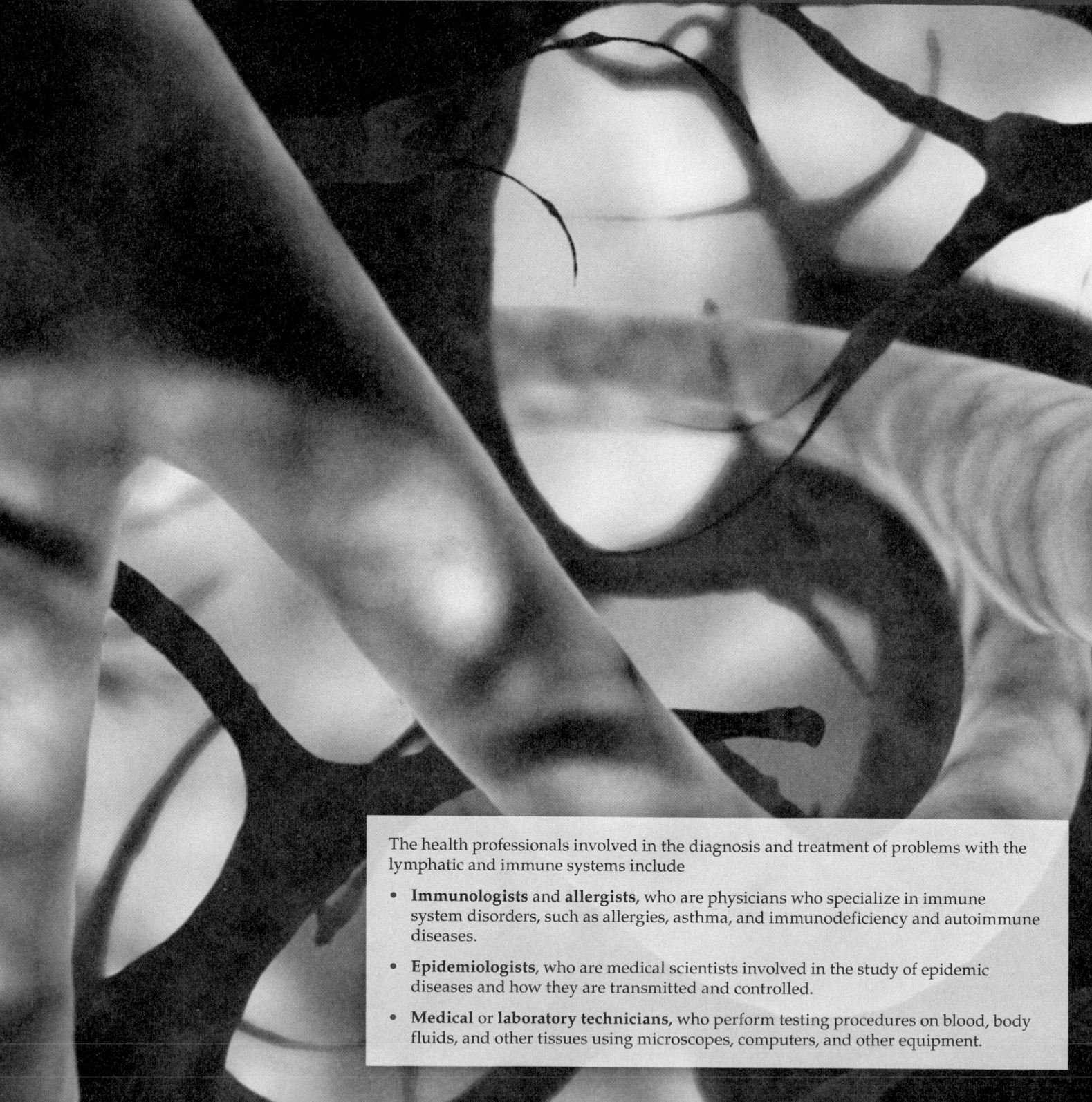

Lymphatic and Immune Systems
The Language of Immunology

The health professionals involved in the diagnosis and treatment of problems with the lymphatic and immune systems include

- **Immunologists** and **allergists**, who are physicians who specialize in immune system disorders, such as allergies, asthma, and immunodeficiency and autoimmune diseases.

- **Epidemiologists**, who are medical scientists involved in the study of epidemic diseases and how they are transmitted and controlled.

- **Medical** or **laboratory technicians**, who perform testing procedures on blood, body fluids, and other tissues using microscopes, computers, and other equipment.

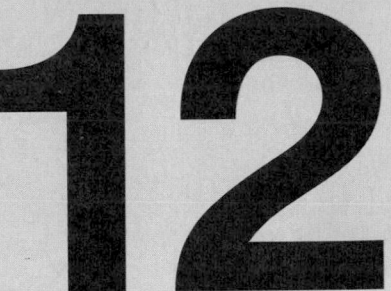

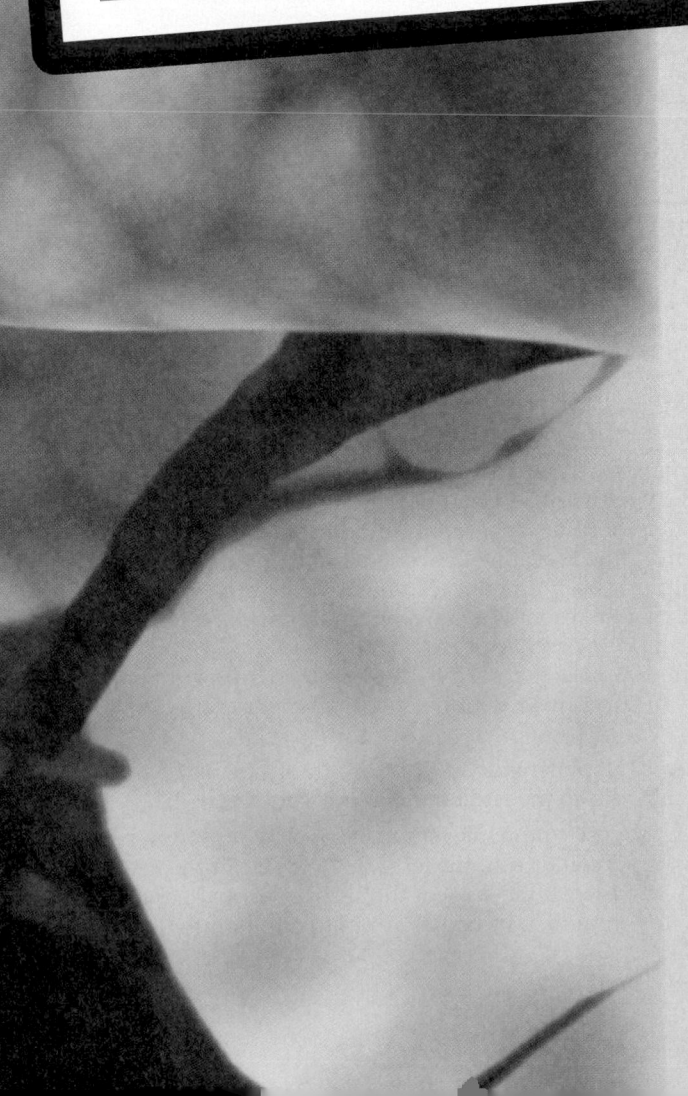

Case Report (CR) 12.1

You are

... a medical assistant working with Susan Lee, MD, in her primary care clinic at Fulwood Medical Center.

Your patient is

... Ms. Anna Clemons, a 20-year-old waitress, who is a new patient. She has noticed a lump in her right neck. On questioning, you find that she has lost about 8 pounds in weight in the past couple of months, has felt tired, and has had some night sweats.

Her vital signs (VS) are normal. There are two firm, enlarged lymph nodes in her right neck. Physical examination is otherwise unremarkable, and there is no evidence of infection in her head, throat, or upper respiratory tract.

Chapter Learning Outcomes

The physical mechanisms of defense are discussed in the individual body system chapters. The lymphatic and immune systems, which are major defenders for the body against disease, form the core of this chapter, the content of which is designed to enable you to:

LO 12.1 Describe the three lines of defense that the body has against foreign organisms, cells and molecules.

LO 12.2 Explain the anatomy and physiology of the lymphatic system.

LO 12.3 Use the medical terms of immunology to communicate and document in writing accurately and precisely in any health care setting.

LO 12.4 Use the medical terms of immunology to communicate verbally with accuracy and precision in any health care setting.

LO 12.5 Define abbreviations that pertain to the lymphatic and immune systems.

LO 12.6 Explain the effects of common disorders of the lymphatic system on health.

LO 12.7 Discuss the specific characteristics that distinguish immunity from the other defense mechanisms of the body.

LO 12.8 Define the two types of immunity and the specialized cells involved.

LO 12.9 Explain the effects of common disorders of the immune system on health.

LESSON OBJECTIVES

As part of your defense mechanisms, the lymphatic system and its fluid provide surveillance and protection against foreign materials.

In this lesson the information provided will enable you to use correct medical terminology to:

12.1.1 **Describe the anatomy and flow of the lymphatic system.**

12.1.2 **List the functions of the lymphatic system.**

12.1.3 **Identify the major cells of the lymphatic system and their functions.**

12.1.4 **Detail the anatomy and functions of the lymph nodes, tonsils, thymus gland, and spleen.**

12.1.5 **Explain the effects of common disorders of the lymphatic system on health.**

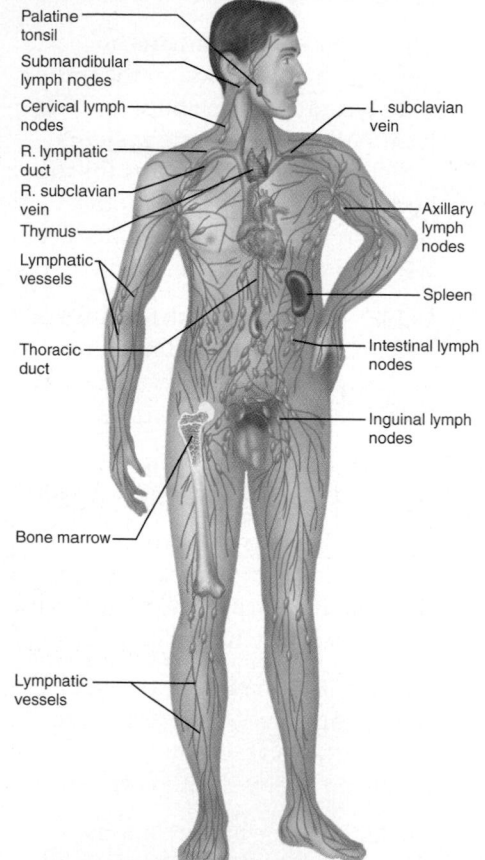

▲ **Figure 12.1** **The Lymphatic System.** (R. = right; L. = left)

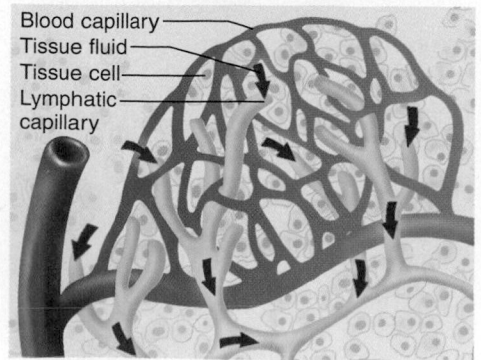

▲ **Figure 12.2** **Lymphatic Flow.**

LO 12.1, 12.2 Lymphatic System

The body has three lines of defense mechanisms against foreign organisms (**pathogens**), cells (**cancer**), and molecules (**pollutants** and **allergens**):

1. **Physical mechanisms**—the skin and mucous membranes, chemicals in perspiration, saliva and tears, hairs in the nostrils, cilia and mucus to protect the lungs. These are described in the individual body system chapters.

2. **Cellular mechanisms**—based on defensive cells (**lymphocytes**) that directly attack suspicious cells such as cancer cells, transplanted tissue cells, or cells infected with viruses or parasites. This is the basis for the lymphatic system.

3. **Humoral defense mechanisms**—based on **antibodies** that are found in body fluids and bind to bacteria, toxins, and extracellular viruses, tagging them for destruction. This is the basis for the **immune** system.

The lymphatic system (Figure 12.1) has three components:

1. A network of thin **lymphatic capillaries and vessels**, similar to blood vessels, that penetrates into the interstitial spaces of nearly every tissue in the body except cartilage, bone, red bone marrow, and the central nervous system (CNS).

2. A group of tissues and organs that produce **immune cells**.

3. **Lymph**, a clear colorless fluid similar to blood plasma but whose composition varies from place to place in the body. It flows through the network of lymphatic capillaries and vessels.

The lymphatic system has three functions:

1. To **absorb** excess interstitial fluid and return it to the bloodstream.

2. To **remove** foreign chemicals, cells, and debris from the tissues.

3. To **absorb** dietary lipids from the small intestine (*see Chapter 5*).

The lymphatic network begins with **lymphatic capillaries** that are closed-ended tubes nestled among blood capillary networks (*Figure 12.2*). The lymphatic capillaries are designed to let interstitial fluid enter, and the interstitial fluid becomes lymph. In addition, bacteria, viruses, cellular debris, and traveling cancer cells can enter the lymphatic capillaries with the interstitial fluid. The lymphatic capillaries converge to form the larger lymphatic collecting vessels. These resemble small veins and have one-way valves in their lumen. They travel alongside veins and arteries.

The larger lymphatic collecting vessels merge into **lymphatic trunks** that drain lymph from a major body region. In turn, these lymphatic trunks merge into two large **lymphatic ducts**:

1. The **right lymphatic duct** receives lymph from the right arm, right side of the thorax, and right side of the head and drains into the **right subclavian vein** (*Figure 12.1*).

2. The **thoracic duct** on the left, the largest lymphatic vessel, receives lymph from both sides of the body below the diaphragm and from the left arm, left side of the head, and left thorax. It begins in the abdomen at the level of the second lumbar vertebra (L2) and passes up through the diaphragm and mediastinum to empty into the **left subclavian vein** (*Figure 12.1*).

WORD	PRONUNCIATION	ELEMENTS		DEFINITION
allergen (*Note:* The duplicate letter "g" is deleted to better form the word.)	AL-er-jen	S/ R/ R/	-gen *to produce* all- *different, strange* -erg- *work*	Substance producing a hypersensitivity (allergic) reaction
allergic	ah-LER-jic	S/	-ic *pertaining to*	Pertaining to or suffering from an allergy
allergy	AL-er-jee	S/	-ergy *process of working*	Hypersensitivity to a particular allergen
antibody	AN-tih-body	P/	anti- *against*	Protein produced in response to an antigen
antibodies (pl)	AN-tih-bod-ees	R/	-body *substance, body*	
humoral	HYU-mor-al	S/ R/	-al *pertaining to* humor- *fluid*	Defense mechanism arising from antibodies in the blood
immune	im-YUNE		Latin *protected from*	Protected from an infectious disease
immunity	im-YUNE-nih-tee	S/ R/	-ity *condition* immun- *immune response*	State of being protected
immunology	im-you-NOL-oh-jee	S/ R/CF	-logy *study of* immun/o- *immune response*	The science and practice of immunity and allergy
immunologist	im-you-NOL-oh-jist	S/	-logist *one who studies, specialist*	Medical specialist in immunology
immunize	IM-you-nize	S/ R/	-ize *affect in a specific way* immun- *immune response*	Make resistant to an infectious disease
immunization	im-you-nih-ZAY-shun	S/	-ization *process of affecting in a specific way*	Administration of an agent to provide immunity
immunoglobulin	IM-you-noh-GLOB-you-lin	R/CF R/ S/	immun/o- *immune response* -globul- *protein* -in *chemical compound*	Specific protein evoked by an antigen; all antibodies are immunoglobulins
lymph	LIMF		Latin *clear spring water*	A clear fluid collected from tissues and transported by lymph vessels to the venous circulation
lymphatic	lim-FAT-ik	S/ R/	-atic *pertaining to* lymph- *lymph*	Pertaining to lymph or the lymphatic system
lymphocyte	LIM-foh-site	R/CF S/	lymph/o- *lymph* -cyte *cell*	Small white blood cell with a nucleus
node	NOHD		Latin *a knot*	A circumscribed mass of tissue
parasite	PAR-ah-site		Greek *a guest*	An organism that attaches itself to, lives on or in, and derives its nutrition from another species
pathogen	PATH-oh-jen	S/ R/CF	-gen *to produce* path/o- *disease*	A disease-causing microorganism
pollutant	poh-LOO-tant	S/ R/	-ant *pertaining to* pollut- *unclean*	Substance that makes an environment unclean or impure
toxin	TOK-sin		Greek *poison*	Poisonous substance formed by a cell or organism
toxic (adj)	TOK-sick	S/ R/	-ic *pertaining to* tox- *poison*	Pertaining to a toxin, poisonous
toxicity (contains two suffixes)	toks-ISS-ih-tee	S/	-ity *state, condition*	The state of being poisonous

Exercises

A. Precision in usage is important if you want to communicate correct information. *These seven terms all contain a common root/combining form. Insert the correct term in each sentence.* **LO 12.1, 12.2, 12.3**

immune	**immunity**	**immunization**	**immunology**
immunologist	**immunoglobulin**		

1. A person who specializes in _____ (the study of the science of immunity and allergy) is called an _____ (type of specialist).

2. An _____ is a class of protein that functions as an antibody.

3. The _____ system is a group of specialized cells in different parts of the body that recognize foreign substances and neutralize them.

4. A prior _____ (vaccination) obtained before she went overseas boosted her _____ (status of being immune) to the disease.

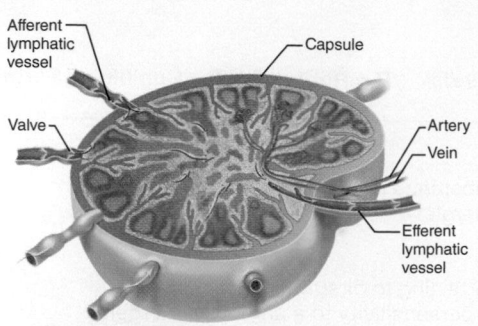

Afferent lymphatic vessel

Capsule

Valve

Artery

Vein

Efferent lymphatic vessel

▲ **Figure 12.3** Lymph Node.

Keynotes

- **Tissues** that are the first line of defense against pathogens—for example, the airway passages—have lymphatic tissue in the submucous layers to help protect against invasion.

- T cells (or T lymphocytes) mature in the thymus, and make up 75% to 85% of the body's lymphocytes.

- B cells (or B lymphocytes) mature in the bone marrow and make up 15% to 25% of the body's lymphocytes.

- Macrophages are produced and stored in the spleen.

Abbreviations	
B cells	B lymphocytes
CD	cluster of differentiation
CNS	central nervous system
Ig	immunoglobulin
T cells	T lymphocytes

LO 12.2 Lymphatic Nodes, Tissues, and Cells

Lymph Nodes

At irregular intervals, the lymphatic collecting vessels enter into the part of the lymphatic network called **lymph nodes** (*Figure 12.3*). There are hundreds of lymph nodes stationed all over the body. They are especially concentrated in the neck, axilla, and groin. Their functions are to filter impurities from the lymph and alert the immune system to the presence of pathogens.

The lymph moves slowly through the node (*Figure 12.3*), which filters the lymph and removes any foreign matter. On its journey back to the bloodstream, lymph passes through several nodes and becomes cleansed of most foreign matter. **Macrophages** in the lymph nodes ingest and break down the foreign matter and display fragments of it to **T cells** (*see the following section*). This alerts the immune system to the presence of an invader. Lymph leaves the nodes again when it enters into the efferent collecting vessels. All these lymph vessels move lymph toward the thoracic cavity.

Lymphatic Tissues and Cells

Many organs have a sprinkling of lymphocytes in their connective tissues and mucous membranes, particularly in passages that open to the exterior—the respiratory, digestive, urinary, and reproductive tracts—where invaders have access to the body.

In some organs, lymphocytes and other cells form dense clusters called **lymphatic follicles**. These are constant features in the tonsils, the adenoids, and the ileum.

Lymphatic tissues are composed of a variety of cells that include

1. **T lymphocytes (T cells).** The "T" stands for *thymus,* where they mature.
   T lymphocytes make up 75% to 85% of body lymphocytes. There are several types of T cells:
   a. **Cytotoxic or "killer" T cells** destroy target cells. Their cell membrane holds a **coreceptor** that can recognize a specific antigen. Coreceptors are named with the letters "**CD**" **(cluster of differentiation)** followed by a number, for these cells, CD8.
   b. **Helper T cells** contain the CD4 coreceptor and are called CD4 cells. They begin the defensive response against a specific antigen.
   c. **Memory T cells** arise from cytotoxic T lymphocytes that have previously destroyed a foreign cell. If they encounter the same antigen, they can now quickly kill it without initiation by a helper T cell.
   d. **Suppressor T cells** suppress activation of the immune system. Failure of these cells to function properly may result in autoimmune diseases.

2. **B lymphocytes (B cells).** These cells mature in the bone marrow. B lymphocytes make up 15% to 25% of lymphocytes. They are activated by helper T cells, respond to a specific antigen, and cause the production of antibodies called **immunoglobulins (Ig)**. The mature B cells are called **plasma cells** and secrete large quantities of antibodies that immobilize, neutralize, and prepare the specific antigen for destruction.

3. **Null cells.** These are large granular lymphocytes that are natural killer cells but lack the specific surface markers of the T and B lymphocytes

4. **Macrophages.** These cells develop from monocytes (*see Chapter 11*) that have migrated from blood. They ingest and destroy tissue debris, bacteria, and other foreign matter **(phagocytosis)**.

WORD	PRONUNCIATION	ELEMENTS		DEFINITION
coreceptor	koh-ree-**SEP**-tor	S/ P/ R/	-or *a doer* co- *with, together* -recept- *receive*	Cell surface protein to enhance the sensitivity of an antigen receptor
cytotoxic (adj)	sigh-toh-**TOX**-ik	S/ R/CF	-toxic- *able to kill* cyt/o- *cell*	Agent able to destroy cells
follicle	**FOLL**-ih-kull		Latin *a small sac*	Spherical mass of cells containing a cavity, or a small cul-de-sac such as a hair follicle
macrophage	**MAK**-roh-fayj	P/ R/CF	macro- *large* -phag/e *to eat*	Large white blood cell (WBC) that removes bacteria, foreign particles, and dead cells
null cells	NULL SELLS		**null** Latin *none*	Lymphocytes with no surface markers, unlike T cells or B cells
phagocyte	**FAG**-oh-site	S/ R/CF	-cyte *cell* phag/o- *to eat*	Blood cell that ingests and destroys foreign particles and cells
phagocytize (verb) phagocytosis	**FAG**-oh-site-ize **FAG**-oh-sigh-**TOE**-sis	S/ S/	-ize *action* -osis *condition*	Ingest foreign particles and cells Process of ingestion and destruction of foreign particles and cells
phagocytic (adj)	fag-oh-**SIT**-ik	S/	-ic *pertaining to*	Pertaining to phagocytes or phagocytosis
plasma cell	**PLAZ**-mah SELL		**plasma** Greek *something formed*	Cell derived from B lymphocytes and active in formation of antibodies

Exercises

A. Elements. *Knowledge of elements is your best key to understanding medical terminology. Reinforce that knowledge with this exercise. Circle the best choice.* **LO 12.2, 12.3**

1. In the term *cytotoxic,* one element means

     to eat   able to kill   large

2. The prefix in *macrophage* identifies

     color   location   size

3. The suffix in *phagocyte* means

     cyst   cell   mass

4. The prefix *co-* means

     next to   with   under

5. The root *-phage* means

     flow   eat   produce

6. This suffix means condition:

     osis   ize   ic

B. Recall from this lesson's text the variety of cells that compose lymphatic tissue and list them below. **LO 12.2, 12.3**

1. _____

2. _____

3. _____

4. _____

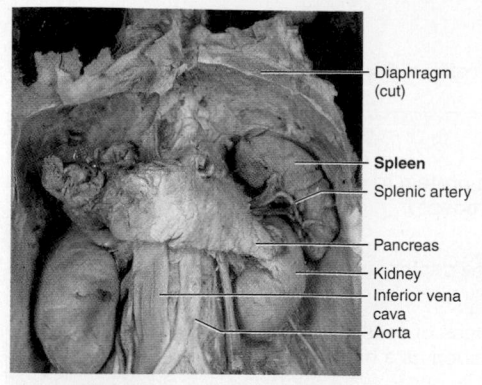

Diaphragm (cut)

Spleen

Splenic artery

Pancreas
Kidney
Inferior vena cava
Aorta

▲ **Figure 12.4**   Position of Spleen.

LO 12.2 Lymphatic Organs

Spleen

The **spleen**, a highly vascular and spongy organ, is the largest lymphatic organ. It is located in the left upper quadrant of the abdomen below the diaphragm and lateral to the kidney *(Figure 12.4)*. It is the only organ the body can live without.

The spleen contains two basic types of tissue:

1. **White pulp**—which is a part of the immune system that produces T cells, B cells, and macrophages. The blood passing through the spleen is monitored for antigens. Antibodies are produced, and the foreign matter is removed.

2. **Red pulp**—which acts as a **reservoir** for erythrocytes, platelets, and macrophages that remove old and defective erythrocytes.

Thus, the functions of the spleen are to

- **Produce** T cells, B cells, and macrophages.
- **Phagocytize** bacteria and other foreign materials.
- **Initiate an immune response** to produce antibodies when antigens are found in the blood.
- **Phagocytize** old, defective erythrocytes and platelets (hemolysis).
- **Serve as a reservoir** for erythrocytes and platelets.

Tonsils

The **tonsils** *(see Chapter 13)* are two masses of lymphatic tissue located at the entrance to the oropharynx, where they entrap inhaled and ingested pathogens. **Adenoids** are similar tissue on the posterior wall of the nasopharynx *(see Chapter 13)*. The tonsils and adenoids form lymphocytes and antibodies, trap bacteria and viruses, and drain them into the tonsillar lymph nodes for elimination. They can become infected themselves.

Thymus Gland

The thymus gland has both endocrine *(see Chapter 17)* and lymphatic functions. T cells develop and mature in it and are released into the bloodstream. The thymus is largest in infancy and childhood *(Figure 12.5a and b)* and reaches its maximum size at puberty. It then regresses and is eventually replaced by fibrous and adipose tissue.

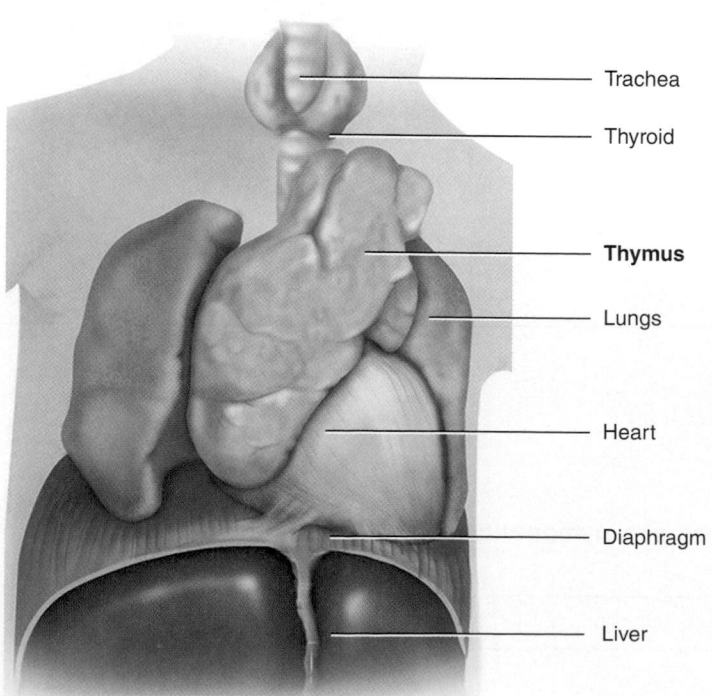

Trachea

Thyroid

Thymus

Lungs

Heart

Diaphragm

Liver

▲ **Figure 12.5a**   Large Thymus in an Infant.

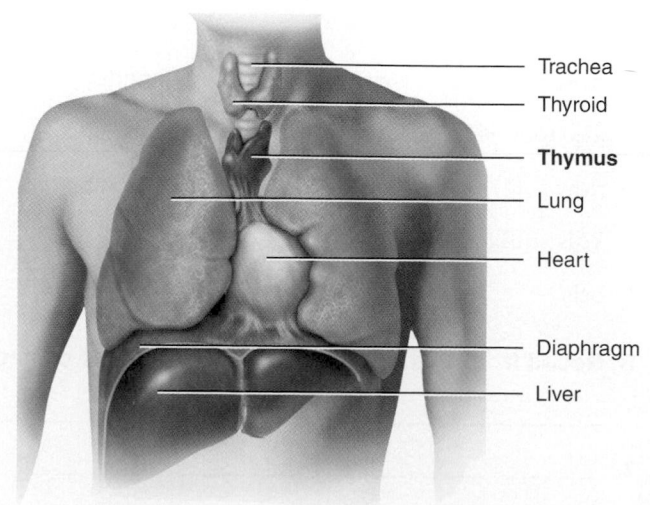

Trachea
Thyroid

Thymus

Lung

Heart

Diaphragm
Liver

▲ **Figure 12.5b**   Adult Thymus.

WORD	PRONUNCIATION	ELEMENTS		DEFINITION
adenoid	ADD-eh-noyd	S/ R/	-oid *resemble* aden- *gland*	Single mass of lymphoid tissue in the midline at the back of the throat
spleen	SPLEEN		Greek *spleen*	Vascular, lymphatic organ in the left upper quadrant of the abdomen
splenectomy splenomegaly (*Note:* The "ee" in **spleen** becomes "e" for easier pronunciation.)	sple-**NECK**-toe-me sple-noh-**MEG**-ah-lee	S/ R/CF S/	-ectomy *surgical excision* splen/o- *spleen* -megaly *enlargement*	Surgical removal of the spleen Enlarged spleen
tonsil	**TON**-sill		Latin *tonsil*	Mass of lymphoid tissue on either side of the throat at the back of the tongue
tonsillectomy	ton-sih-**LEC**-toh-me	S/ R/	-ectomy *surgical excision* tonsill- *tonsil*	Surgical removal of the tonsils
tonsillitis	ton-sih-**LIE**-tis	S/	-itis *inflammation*	Inflammation of the tonsils

Exercises

A. Identify the correct answer which contains all the lymphatic organs. *Circle the best choice.*   **LO 12.2, 12.3**

1. liver, spleen, thyroid gland

2. spleen, lungs, kidney

3. tonsils, spleen, parathyroid gland

4. thymus gland, spleen, lymph vessels and nodes

5. gallbladder, spleen, thyroid gland

B. The spleen is a very important organ in the body. *Select the only false statement about the spleen and rewrite it correctly on the line below.*   **LO 12.2, 12.3**

1. The spleen is a highly vascular and spongy organ.

2. The spleen is the largest of the lymphatic organs.

3. The spleen is located in the right upper quadrant of the body.

4 The spleen contains white pulp and red pulp.

5. The spleen serves as a reservoir for RBCs and platelets.

1. Corrected sentence: _____

C. This exercise describes the "where" of lymphatic tissue—you need to supply the term that is the "what." "What am I?"
Identify the correct medical term for each of the following questions.   **LO 12.2, 12.3**

1. I am located below the diaphragm and lateral to the kidney. _____

2. I am located at the entrance to the oropharynx where I trap pathogens. _____

3. I am located on the posterior wall of the nasopharynx. _____

4. I am located in the chest cavity. _____

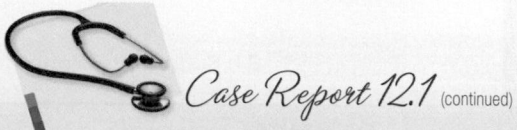

Case Report 12.1 (continued)

Ms. Clemons has cancerous nodes in her neck. They were not caused by metastatic cancer but by a cancer of the lymph nodes called Hodgkin lymphoma *[see the following section]*.

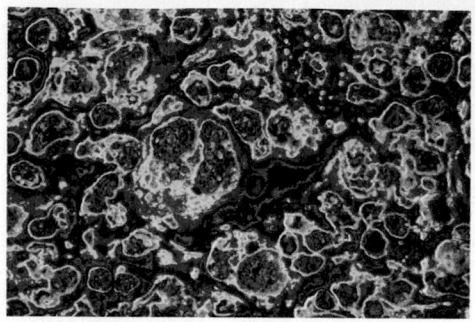

▲ **Figure 12.6** The lymphatic tissues in Hodgkin's disease contain specific cells called Reed-Sternberg cells that are not found in any other cancerous lymphomas or cancers.

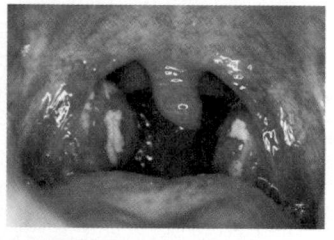

▲ **Figure 12.7** **Tonsillitis.** Open mouth and throat of a 15-year-old girl with inflamed tonsils. They are flecked with infected white patches, due to tonsillitis, an infection usually caused by streptococci bacteria.

LO 12.6 Disorders of the Lymphatic System

Physicians routinely palpate accessible lymph nodes in the neck **(cervical nodes)**, axillae **(axillary nodes)**, and groin **(inguinal nodes)** for enlargement and tenderness. Their presence indicates disease in the tissues drained by the lymph nodes. Cancerous lymph nodes are enlarged, firm, and usually painless.

Infections in the lymph nodes cause them to be swollen and tender to the touch, a condition called **lymphadenitis**. All lymph node enlargements are collectively called **lymphadenopathy**. When lymph nodes are removed, it is called **lymphadenectomy**.

Lymphoma is a malignant neoplasm of the lymphatic organs, usually the lymph nodes. The disorder usually presents as an enlarged, nontender lymph node, often in the neck or axilla.

Lymphomas are grouped into two categories:

1. **Hodgkin lymphoma**—characterized by the presence of abnormal, cancerous B cells called **Reed-Sternberg cells**. These are large cells with two nuclei resembling the eyes of an owl *(Figure 12.6)*. The cancer spreads in an orderly manner to adjoining lymph nodes. This enables the disease to be staged, depending on how far it has spread. Diagnostic procedures include biopsy of an enlarged node to look for Reed-Sternberg cells, x-rays, computed tomography (CT) and magnetic resonance imaging (MRI) scans, **lymphangiogram**, and bone marrow biopsy. Treatment options include radiation, chemotherapy, and an autologous bone marrow transplant.

2. **Non-Hodgkin lymphomas**—occur much more frequently than Hodgkin lymphoma. They include some 30 different disease entities in 10 different subtypes. Treatment depends on the rate of growth of the disease and varies from careful observation to chemotherapy and radiation to bone marrow transplantation.

Tonsillitis, inflammation of the tonsils and adenoids, occurs mostly in the first years of life. The infection can be viral or bacterial (usually streptococcal). It produces enlarged, tender lymph nodes under the jaw *(Figure 12.7)*. A rapid strep test can determine if *Streptococcus* is the cause, in which case a full course of antibiotics is indicated. The infection can be recurrent, and tonsillectomy is sometimes performed.

Splenomegaly, an enlarged spleen, is not a disease in itself but the result of an underlying disorder. However, when the spleen enlarges, it traps and removes an excessive number of blood cells and platelets **(hypersplenism)** and reduces the number of blood cells and platelets in the bloodstream.

The potential causes of splenomegaly are numerous and include infections such as infectious mononucleosis, lymphomas, anemias such as sickle cell anemia, and storage diseases such as Gaucher disease.

Diagnosis and treatment focus on the underlying cause. Occasionally splenectomy is necessary.

Ruptured spleen is a common complication from car accidents or other trauma when the abdomen and rib cage are damaged. Intra-abdominal bleeding from the ruptured spleen can be extensive, with a dramatic fall in blood pressure (BP), and is a surgical emergency requiring splenectomy. After splenectomy, patients are very susceptible to infection but function very well.

Lymphedema is localized, nonpitting fluid retention caused by a compromised lymphatic system, often after surgery or radiation therapy. It can also be primary, where the cause is unknown.

Word Analysis and Definition

WORD	PRONUNCIATION	ELEMENTS		DEFINITION
Hodgkin lymphoma	**HOJ**-kin lim-**FO**-muh		Thomas Hodgkin, 1798–1866, British physician	Disease marked by chronic enlargement of lymph nodes spreading to other nodes in an orderly way
hypersplenism (Note the one "e.")	high-per-**SPLEN**-izm	S/ P/ R/	-ism *condition, process* hyper- *excessive* -splen- *spleen*	Condition in which the spleen removes blood components at an excessive rate
inguinal	**IN**-gwin-al	S/ R/	-al *pertaining to* inguin- *groin*	Pertaining to the groin
lymphadenectomy	lim-**FAD**-eh-**NECK**-toe-me	S/ R/	-ectomy *surgical excision* **lymphaden-** *lymph node*	Surgical excision of a lymph node
lymphadenitis **lymphadenopathy**	lim-**FAD**-eh-neye-tis lim-**FAD**-eh-**NOP**-ah-thee	S/ S/ R/CF	-itis *inflammation* -pathy *disease* **lymphaden/o** *lymph node*	Inflammation of a lymph node Any disease process affecting a lymph node
lymphangiogram	lim-**FAN**-jee-oh-gram	S/ R/CF	-gram *recording* **lymphangi/o-** *lymphatic vessels*	Radiographic images of lymph vessels and nodes following injection of contrast material
lymphedema	**LIMF**-e-dee-mah	R/ R/	**lymph-** *lymph* -edema *edema*	Tissue swelling due to lymphatic obstruction
lymphoma	lim-**FO**-muh	S/ R/	-oma *tumor* **lymph-** *lymph*	Any neoplasm of lymphatic tissue

Exercises

A. Language of immunology. *Work with these six terms from the* language of immunology. *Their roots/combining forms are similar, and their suffixes help define them. First deconstruct each of the terms in the table. Then use those terms to answer the following questions.*   **LO 12.3, 12.6**

Medical Term	Meaning of Prefix	Meaning of Root/ Combining Form	Meaning of Suffix	Meaning of Medical Term
lymphoma	1.	2.	3.	4.
lymphadenectomy	5.	6.	7.	8.
lymphadenopathy	9.	10.	11.	12.
lymphangiogram	13.	14.	15.	16.
lymphedema	17.	18.	19.	20.
lymphadenitis	21.	22.	23.	24.

B. Use the terms from the previous table and answer the following questions.   **LO 12.3, 12.6**

1. List the terms that can be billed as a diagnosis: _____

2. Write the term that is a *surgical* procedure: _____

3. Write the term that is a *radiological* procedure: _____

4. List the terms that concern lymph nodes: _____

5. Find the term that concerns lymphatic vessels. (**Hint:** Check the elements.) _____

LESSON OBJECTIVES

The study of the immune system is called **immunology**. The medical specialist involved in the study and research of the immune system and in treating disorders of the immune system is called an **immunologist**. The information in this lesson will enable you to use correct medical terminology to:

12.2.1 Define the immune system and its specific reactions to stimulation.

12.2.2 Contrast cellular and humoral immunity.

12.2.3 Describe the life histories of B cells and T cells.

12.2.4 Explain the structure and actions of antibodies.

12.2.5 Discuss some common disorders of the immune system, including human immunodeficiency virus (HIV) and acquired immune deficiency syndrome (AIDS).

You are

. . . a laboratory technician working the night shift at Fulwood Medical Center.

Your patient is

. . . Mr. Michael Cowan, a 40-year-old homeless man and drug addict, who has presented to the Emergency Department with a high fever for which no cause is obvious on clinical examination.

Case Report 12.2

You are called to the Emergency Room to take blood from Mr. Cowan. You have inserted the needle into an antecubital vein, and he starts jerking his arm around and trying to get off the gurney. In the struggle, the needle comes out of the vein and pricks your hand through your glove.

As you immediately *flush* and *clean* the wound, *report* the incident, seek *immediate medical attention*, and go through your *initial medical evaluation*, it is essential that you have knowledge about your immune system and its response to the potential infection. Then you can make *informed decisions* about your treatment and future employment.

You will be asked to fill out your incident report at the end of this chapter.

Keynotes

- The immune system is not an organ system but a group of specialized cells.

- Receptors on the surface of T cells and B cells recognize specific nonself (foreign) antigens.

- Antigens are molecules that trigger an immune response. Each antigen has a unique structure that is recognized by the immune system.

- Haptens are small, foreign molecules that attach themselves to host molecules to form large, unique complexes that the immune system can recognize as foreign. Haptens are found in cosmetics, detergents, industrial chemicals, poison ivy, and animal dander.

LO 12.7 The Immune System

The immune system is a group of specialized cells in different parts of the body that recognize foreign substances and neutralize them. It is the third line of defense listed at the beginning of this chapter. When the immune system is functioning correctly, it protects the body against bacteria, viruses, cancer cells, and foreign substances. When the immune system is weak, it allows pathogens (including the viruses that cause common colds and "flu") and cancer cells to successfully invade the body.

Three characteristics distinguish immunity from the first two lines of defense:

1. **Specificity.** The immune response is directed against a particular pathogen. Immunity to one pathogen does not confer immunity to others. Specificity has one disadvantage. If a virus or a bacterium changes a component of its genetic code, it will lead to a change in the structure and/or physiology of the microorganism, which then is no longer recognized by the immune system. This **mutation** occurs, for example, in bacteria in response to antibiotics and in HIV's response to anti-HIV drugs (development of **resistance**).

2. **Memory.** When exposure to the same identical pathogen occurs again, the immune system recognizes the pathogen and has its responses ready to act quickly.

3. **Discrimination.** The immune system learns to recognize agents (**antigens**) that represent "self" and agents that are "**nonself**" (foreign). Most of this recognition is developed prior to birth. A variety of disorders occur when this discrimination breaks down. They are known as **autoimmune** disorders.

WORD	PRONUNCIATION	ELEMENTS		DEFINITION
antigen	AN-tee-gen	P/ R/	anti- *against* -gen *produce, create*	Substance capable of triggering an immune response
autoimmune	aw-toe-im-**YUNE**	P/ R/	auto- *self, same* -immune *immune response*	Immune reaction directed against a person's own tissue
discrimination	DIS-krim-ih-**NAY**-shun	S/ P/ R/	-ation *process* dis- *away from, apart* -crimin- *distinguish*	Ability to distinguish between different things
hapten	HAP-ten		Greek *to fasten or bind*	Small molecule that has to bind to a larger molecule to form an antigen
mutation	myu-**TAY**-shun		Latin *to change*	Change in the chemistry of a gene
resistance	ree-**ZIS**-tants	S/ R/	-ance *state of, condition* resist- *to withstand*	Ability of an organism to withstand the effects of an antagonistic agent
resistant	ree-**ZIS**-tant	S/	-ant *pertaining to*	Able to resist
specific	speh-**SIF**-ik	S/ R/	-ic *pertaining to* specif- *species*	Relating to a particular entity
specificity (**Note:** two suffixes)	spes-ih-**FIS**-ih-tee	S/	-ity *condition, state*	State of having a fixed relation to a particular entity

Exercises

A. Build your knowledge of elements and their meaning by matching the element in the left column with the definition in the right column. LO 12.3, 12.7

_____ 1. crimin

_____ 2. ity

_____ 3. specif

_____ 4. anti

_____ 5. dis

_____ 6. ation

_____ 7. ic

_____ 8. gen

a. species

b. away from

c. distinguish

d. process

e. pertaining to

f. condition, state

g. produce, create

h. against

B. Analyze Case Report 12.2; then answer the following questions. *Be prepared to discuss your answers in class.* **LO 12.3, 12.7**

1. Where is the location of the *antecubital vein*? _____

2. What is the immediate danger after the needle has pricked you through your glove? _____

3. How do you "flush" a wound? _____

4. Why must this incident be reported? _____

• The immune system is thought to be able to produce some 2 million different antibodies.

• Antibodies do not actively destroy an antigen. They render it harmless and mark it for destruction by phagocytes.

• Antibodies can be produced naturally in response to an antigen or artificially in response to immunizations and vaccines.

Abbreviations

IgA	immunoglobulin A
IgD	immunoglobulin D
IgE	immunoglobulin E
IgG	immunoglobulin G
IgM	immunoglobulin M

LO 12.7, 12.8 Immunity

Immunity is classified biologically into two types, though both mechanisms often respond to the same antigen:

1. **Cellular (cell-mediated) immunity** is a direct form of defense based on the actions of lymphocytes to attack foreign and diseased cells and destroy them.

   The many different types of T cells, B cells, and macrophages described in the previous lesson of this chapter are involved in this style of attack.

2. **Humoral (antibody-mediated) immunity** is an indirect form of attack that employs antibodies produced by plasma cells, which have been developed from B cells. The antibodies bind to an antigen and thus tag them for destruction.

These antibodies are called immunoglobulins (Igs), defensive gamma globulins in the blood plasma and body secretions. There are five classes of antibodies (immunoglobulins):

- **IgG** makes up about 80% of the antibodies. It is found in plasma and tissue fluids. It crosses the placenta to give the fetus some immunity.

- **IgA** makes up about 13% of the antibodies. It is found in exocrine secretions such as breast milk, tears, saliva, nasal secretions, intestinal juices, bile, and urine.

- **IgM** makes up about 6% of antibodies. It develops in response to antigens in food or bacteria.

- **IgD** is found on the surface of B cells and acts as a receptor for antigens.

- **IgE** is found in exocrine secretions along with IgA and also in the serum.

Once released by plasma cells, the antibodies function in several ways to make antigens harmless, including

- **Neutralization.** An antibody binds to the antigen and masks it.

- **Agglutination.** An antibody binds to two or more bacteria to prevent them from spreading through the tissues.

- **Precipitation.** Antibodies create an antigen-antibody complex that is too heavy to stay in solution. The complex precipitates (drops out of solution) and can be ingested and destroyed by phagocytes.

- **Complement fixation.** The complement system is a group of 20 or more proteins continually present in blood plasma; IgG and IgM bind to foreign cells, initiating the **binding of complement** to the cell and leading to its destruction. Complement fixation is the major defense mechanism against bacteria and mismatched blood cells.

Based on the production or acquisition of antibodies, four classes of immunity can be described:

1. **Natural active immunity**—the production of your own antibodies as a result of normal maturation, pregnancy, or an infection.

2. **Artificial active immunity**—the production of your own antibodies as a result of **vaccination** or **immunization**. A vaccine consists of either killed or **attenuated** (weakened) pathogens (antigens).

3. **Natural passive immunity**—a temporary immunity that results from acquiring antibodies from another individual. This occurs for the fetus through the placenta (IgG) or for the infant through breast milk (IgA).

4. **Artificial passive immunity**—a temporary immunity that results from the injection of an **immune serum** from another individual or an animal. Immune serum is used to treat snakebite, tetanus, and rabies.

WORD	PRONUNCIATION	ELEMENTS		DEFINITION
agglutination	ah-glue-tih-**NAY**-shun	S/ R/	-ation *process* **agglutin-** *sticking together, clumping*	Process by which cells or other particles adhere to each other to form clumps
agglutinate (verb)	ah-**GLUE**-tin-ate	S/	-ate *composed of, pertaining to*	Stick together to form clumps
attenuate	ah-**TEN**-you-ate	S/ R/	-ate *composed of, pertaining to* **attenu-** *to weaken*	Weaken the ability of an organism to produce disease
attenuated (adj)	ah-**TEN**-you-a-ted	S/	-ated *process*	Weakened
complement	**KOM**-pleh-ment		Latin *that which completes*	Group of proteins in serum that finish off the work of antibodies to destroy bacteria and other cells
humoral immunity	**HYU**-mor-al im-**YOU**-nih-tee	S/ R/ S/ R/	-al *pertaining to* **humor-** *fluid* -ity *condition* **immun-** *immune response*	Defense mechanism arising from antibodies in the blood State of being protected
immune serum (also called **antiserum**)	im-**YUNE SEER**-um		**immune** Latin *protected from* **serum** Latin *whey*	Serum taken from another human or animal that has antibodies to a disease
vaccine vaccinate (verb)	**VAK**-seen **VAK**-sin-ate	S/ R/	-ate *composed of, pertaining to* **vaccin-** *giving a vaccine*	Preparation to generate active immunity To administer a vaccine
vaccination	vak-sih-**NAY**-shun	S/	-ation *process*	Administration of a vaccine

Exercises

A. Organize the important information about immunity. *The* language of immunology *will help you understand the questions and provide the answers. Refer to this exercise for test review. Fill in the blanks.*   **LO 12.3, 12.7, 12.8**

1. Name the two types of immunity, and explain how they function.

    a. _____

    b. _____

2. Which of the types of immunity in question 1 is a direct defense, and which is an indirect form of attack?

    Direct: _____

    Indirect: _____

3. What type of cells produce antibodies? _____

4. Are antibodies produced in direct or indirect defense? _____

5. What is the correct term for these particular antibodies? _____

6. What are the main functions of antibodies?

    a. _____

    b. _____

    c. _____

    d. _____

LO 12.9 Disorders of the Immune System

Hypersensitivity is an excessive immune response to an antigen that would normally be tolerated. Hypersensitivity includes

- **Allergies**, which are reactions to environmental antigens such as pollens, molds, and dusts; to foods such as peanuts, shellfish, and eggs; to plants such as poison ivy; to sunlight *(Figure 12.8)*; and to drugs such as penicillin; as well as asthmatic reactions to inhaled antigens (see following text).
- Abnormal reactions to your *own* tissues (autoimmune disorders).
- Reactions to tissues **transplanted** from *another* person (**alloimmune disorders**).

In most allergic (hypersensitivity) reactions, allergens (antigens) bind to IgE on the membranes of basophils and mast cells *(see Chapter 11)* and, within seconds of exposure, stimulate the cells to produce **histamine**. This triggers vasodilation, increased capillary permeability, and smooth muscle spasms. The symptoms produced by these changes include edema; mucus hypersecretion and congestion; watery eyes; hives (**urticaria**); and sometimes cramps, diarrhea, and vomiting.

Anaphylaxis is an acute, immediate, and severe allergic reaction. It can be relieved by antihistamines.

Anaphylactic shock is more severe and is characterized by dyspnea due to bronchiole constriction, circulatory shock, and sometimes death. It is a life-threatening medical emergency and requires immediate epinephrine and circulatory support.

Asthma is triggered by allergens (as listed earlier) and by air pollutants, drugs, and emotions. These all stimulate plasma cells to secrete IgE, which binds to cells in the respiratory mucosa and releases a mixture of histamine and interleukins. Within minutes, the bronchioles constrict spasmodically (bronchospasm), leading to the wheezing and coughing of asthma.

Autoimmune disorders are an overvigorous response of the immune system in which the immune system fails to distinguish self-antigens from foreign antigens. These self-antigens produce autoantibodies that attack the body's own tissues. This type of response occurs, for example, in lupus erythematosus, type 1 diabetes, multiple sclerosis, rheumatoid arthritis, and psoriasis.

Immunodeficiency disorders are a deficient response of the immune system in which it fails to respond vigorously enough. They are in three categories:

1. **Congenital** (inborn)—caused by a genetic abnormality that is often sex-linked, with boys affected more often than girls. An example from among the 20 or more congenital immunodeficiency diseases is **inherited combined immunodeficiency disease**, in which there is an absence of both T cells and B cells. Affected children are very susceptible to opportunistic infections and must live in protective sterile enclosures.

2. **Immunosuppression**—a common side effect of corticosteroids in treatment to prevent transplant rejection and in chemotherapy treatment for cancer. These drugs reduce the numbers of all lymphocytes, making it possible for opportunistic infections to invade the body.

3. **Acquired immunodeficiency**—a result of diseases such as acquired immunodeficiency syndrome (AIDS) that involve a severely depressed immune system from infection with the human immunodeficiency virus (HIV).

Immunology of Transplantation

The success of any organ transplantation is based on control of the recipient's immune system to prevent rejection of the **allograft**, tissue from another individual of the same species.

Transplant immunity is designed to cause rejection, and both cellular and humoral defense mechanisms are involved. To try to prevent this, the recipient and donor must match at both the human lymphocyte antigen (HLA) and blood group system (ABO) *(see Chapter 11)* types. A combination of immunosuppressive drugs is used to control graft rejection, but the drugs have adverse side effects on the recipient. One combination is corticosteroids with cyclosporine or FK506. Other drugs are in clinical trials.

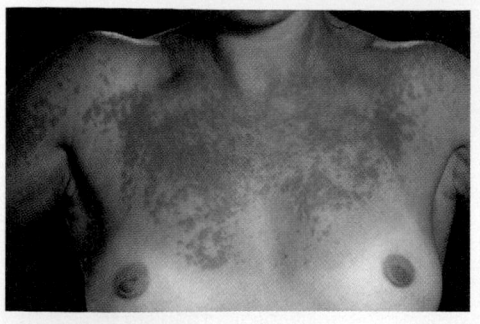

▲ Figure 12.8 Sun allergy.

Keynote

Because of the use of immunosuppressive drugs, 75% of all solid-organ transplants will be newly affected with cytomegalovirus (**CMV**) following organ transplantation.

Abbreviation

CMV cytomegalovirus

WORD	PRONUNCIATION	ELEMENTS		DEFINITION
allogen	AL-oh-jen	P/	allo- *strange, different*	Antigen from someone else in the same species
		R/	-gen *producing*	
allogenic (adj)	al-oh-**JEN**-ik	S/	-ic *pertaining to*	Pertaining to allergen
allograft	AL-oh-graft	R/	-graft *tissue for transplant*	Skin graft from another person or cadaver
alloimmune	AL-oh-im-**YUNE**	P/	allo- *strange, different*	Reaction directed against foreign tissue
		R/	-immune *immune response*	
anaphylaxis	AN-ah-fih-**LAK**-sis	P/	ana- *away from*	Immediate severe allergic response
		R/	-phylaxis *protection*	
anaphylactic (adj)	AN-ah-fih-**LAK**-tik	S/	-tic *pertaining to*	Pertaining to anaphylaxis
		R/	-phylac- *protect*	
histamine	HISS-tah-mean	R/	hist- *derived from histidine*	Compound liberated in tissues as a result of injury or an allergic response
		R/CF	-amin/e *nitrogen compound*	
antihistamine	an-tee-**HISS**-tah-mean	P/	anti- *against*	Drug used to treat allergic symptoms because of its action antagonistic to histamine
hypersensitivity	HIGH-per-sen-sih-**TIV**-ih-tee	S/	-ity *condition*	Exaggerated abnormal reaction to an allergen
		P/	hyper- *excessive*	
		R/	-sensitiv- *feeling*	
immunodeficiency	IM-you-noh-dee-**FISH**-en-see	S/	-ency *quality*	Failure of the immune system
		R/CF	immun/o- *immune response*	
		R/	-defici- *failure*	
immunosuppression	IM-you-noh-suh-**PRESH**-un	S/	-ion *process*	Suppression of the immune response by an outside agent, such as a drug
		R/CF	immun/o- *immune response*	
		R/	-suppress- *pressed under*	
transplant	TRANZ-plant	P/	trans- *across*	The tissue or organ used, or the act of transferring tissue from one person to another
		R/	-plant *plant*	
transplantation	TRANZ-plan-**TAY**-shun	S/	-ation *process, action*	The moving of tissue or an organ from one person or place to another
urticaria	ur-tee-**KARE**-ee-ah		Latin *nettle*	Rash of itchy wheals (hives)

Exercises

A. Build more medical vocabulary for immunology. *Complete the construction of the medical term by using the following elements to fill in the blanks.* **LO 12.3, 12.9**

hyper	defici	phylaxis	auto	suppress	graft
ion	anti	sensitiv	trans	allo	gen

1. Exaggerated, abnormal reaction to an antigen   _____/_____/ity

2. Immune reaction directed against self   _____/immuno

3. Immediate, severe, allergic response   ana/_____

4. Skin from another person or cadaver   allo/_____

5. Failure of the immune system   immuno/_____/ency

6. Transferring tissue or an organ from one person to another   _____/plant

7. Antigen from someone else in the same species   allo/_____

8. Reaction against foreign tissue   _____/immune

9. Drug used to treat allergic symptoms   _____/histamine

10. Suppression of the immune response caused by an outside agent   immuno/_____/_____

Case Report 12.3

In the past couple of months, Mr. Holman has not been taking his medication regularly. In the previous week, he has noticed a progressive shortness of breath and a nonproductive cough. Vital signs are T 102°, P 120, R 32, BP 110/60. He is anxious and dyspneic but not cyanotic. His breath sounds are clear, with no rales or rhonchi heard. You have called Dr. Vandenberg to see him.

Mr. Holman's chest x-ray shows bilateral, diffuse, fluffy infiltrates spreading out from the hila. Bronchial **lavage** with laboratory examination shows *Pneumocystis jiroveci*. His CD4 count is 140. Mr. Holman has developed an opportunistic infection, which is now thought to be due to a fungus.

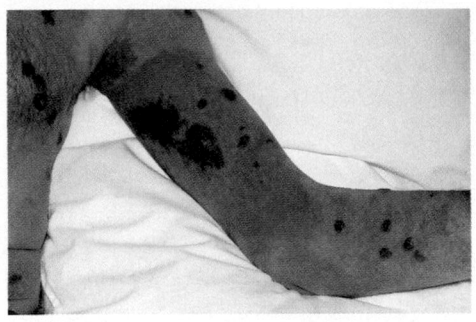

▲ **Figure 12.9** Lesions of Kaposi sarcoma.

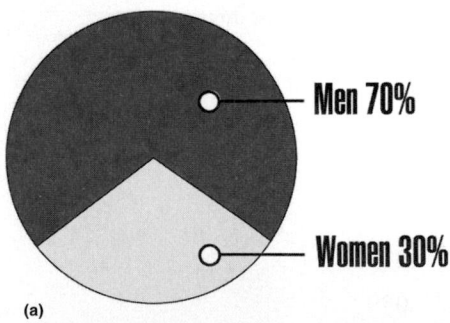

Men 70%

Women 30%

(a)

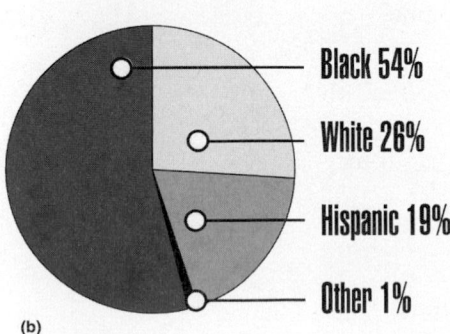

Black 54%

White 26%

Hispanic 19%

Other 1%

(b)

▲ **Figure 12.10** New HIV Infections Each Year in the United States. (*a*) By gender. (*b*) By race.

LO 12.9 HIV and AIDS

Human immunodeficiency virus (HIV) is one of a group of viruses known as **retroviruses**. Like other viruses, it can replicate only inside a living host cell; HIV invades helper T (CD4) cells and cells in the upper respiratory tract and CNS. Inside the cell, the virus generates new deoxyribonucleic acid (DNA) and can stay **dormant** in the cell for months or years. When it is activated, the new viruses emerge from the dying host cell and attack more CD4 cells. This dormant phase (**incubation**) can range from a few months to 12 years.

The CD4 cells are the central coordinators for the immune response. As the virus destroys more and more cells, the CD4 count falls, and antibodies cannot be produced. Symptoms appear, including chills, fever, night sweats, fatigue, weight loss, and lymphadenitis.

When CD4 cells are very low, **opportunistic infections** by bacteria, viruses, and fungi can occur. These infections include toxoplasmosis, pneumocystis, tuberculosis, herpes simplex, cytomegalovirus, and candidiasis. If human immunodeficiency virus (HIV) invades the brain, it causes dementia. Cancers can also invade, and a form of malignancy called **Kaposi sarcoma** (*Figure 12.9*) is often seen in association with autoimmune deficiency syndrome (AIDS).

Human immunodeficiency virus (HIV) is found in blood, semen, vaginal secretions, saliva, tears, and the breast milk of infected mothers.

The most common means of transmission of human immunodeficiency virus (HIV) are

- **Sexual intercourse** (vaginal, oral, anal).
- **Sharing needles** for drug use.
- **Contaminated blood products.** (All donated blood is now tested for HIV.)
- **Transplacental** (from an infected mother to her fetus).

The virus survives poorly outside the human body. It is destroyed by laundering, dishwashing, chlorination, disinfectants, alcohol, and germicidal skin cleansers.

About 1% of HIV's genes mutate every year. This makes the development of natural immunity and the production of a vaccine difficult, so new infections continue to occur (*Figure 12.10*).

Human Immunodeficiency Virus Testing

The **HIV antibody blood test** takes between 3 weeks and 3 months after infection to become positive.

The normal **CD4-cell count** is from 600 to 1200 cells/μL of blood; AIDS patients have counts below 200/μL. Below this figure, opportunistic infections occur, as they did with Mr. Holman.

Viral load count measures the quantity of human immunodeficiency virus (HIV) in the blood. If there are 50 to 200 copies of the virus present, the test will be reported as "undetectable." A 5000 count is very low. The count can rise to several hundred thousand.

There are more than 20 approved anti-HIV (antiretroviral) drugs available and many more in research and development.

WORD	PRONUNCIATION	ELEMENTS		DEFINITION
dormant	**DOR**-mant	S/ R/	**-ant** *forming* **dorm-** *sleep*	Inactive
incubation	in-kyu-**BAY**-shun	S/ R/	**-ation** *process* **incub-** *sit on, hatch*	Process to develop an infection
Kaposi sarcoma	ka-**POH**-see sar-**KOH**-mah		Moritz Kaposi, 1837–1902, Hungarian dermatologist	A malignancy often seen in AIDS patients
lavage	Lah-**VAHZH**		Latin *to wash*	Washing out of a hollow cavity, tube, or organ
opportunistic	**OP**-or-tyu-**NIS**-tik	S/ S/ R/	**-ic** *pertaining to* **-ist-** *agent* **opportun-** *take advantage of*	An organism or a disease in a host with lowered resistance
retrovirus	**REH**-troh-vie-rus	P/ R/	**retro-** *backward* **-virus** *poison*	Virus that replicates in a host cell by converting its ribonucleic acid (RNA) core into deoxyribonucleic acid (DNA)
virus	**VIE**-rus		Latin *poison*	Group of infectious agents that require living cells for growth and reproduction
viral (adj)	**VIE**-ral	S/ R/	**-al** *pertaining to* **vir-** *virus*	Pertaining to or caused by a virus

Exercises

A. Analyze Case Report 12.3 and then answer the following questions. *Be prepared to discuss your answers in class.* **LO 12.3, 12.9**

1. Explain this sentence to Mr. Holman: "Mr. Holman's chest x-ray shows bilateral, diffuse, fluffy infiltrates spreading out from the hila."

   "Mr. Holman, your _____

   _____."

2. What was the purpose of the *bronchial lavage*? _____

   _____

3. What was found on laboratory examination of the *bronchial washings*? _____

   _____

4. What type of *opportunistic infection* do the doctors think Mr. Holman has? _____

5. The diagnosis of *Pneumocystis jiroveci* places this infection in Mr. Holman's (specific organ) _____.

6. Which *vital sign* could indicate that Mr. Holman has an infection going on in his system? _____

7. What does an *opportunistic infection* take advantage of? _____

8. What is the *underlying cause* of this infection occurrence? _____

   _____

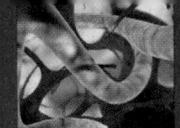

Lymphatic and Immune Systems

Challenge Your Knowledge

A. **Latin and Greek elements cannot be deconstructed into prefix, root, or suffix.** You must know them for what they are. Test your knowledge of these elements with this exercise. Match the meaning in the left column with the correct medical term in the right column. (**LO 12.3,** *Remember*)

_____	**1.** Protected from	**a.** medial
_____	**2.** That which completes	**b.** hapten
_____	**3.** None	**c.** lymph
_____	**4.** To fasten or bind	**d.** lavage
_____	**5.** Divide in the middle	**e.** mutate
_____	**6.** A knot	**f.** complement
_____	**7.** To change	**g.** edema
_____	**8.** To wash	**h.** immune
_____	**9.** Swelling	**i.** null
_____	**10.** Clear fluid	**j.** node

Complete this exercise by using any three medical terms from the above terms A–J in sentences of patient documentation.

11. _____

_____

12. _____

_____

13. _____

_____

B. Language of immunology. Challenge your knowledge of the immune system and employ the *language of immunology* to answer the following questions. Circle the correct choice. (**LO 12.3,** *Remember*)

1. Choose the correct pair of spellings:

   a. tonsel   tonselectomy

   b. tonsil   tonsillectomy

   c. tonssil   tonsilectomy

   d. tonsill   tonsilectomy

   e. tonnsil   tonsillectomy

2. This triggers vasodilation in an allergic response:

   a. interferon

   b. complement fixation

   c. histamine

   d. hormones

   e. antihistamine

3. The largest lymphatic vessel is the

   a. thoracic duct

   b. lymph node

   c. spleen

   d. lymphatic duct

   e. aorta

4. Kaposi sarcoma is a form of

   a. lymphadenitis

   b. malignancy

   c. lymphadenopathy

   d. lung cancer

   e. lymphoma

5. Ingestion and destruction of tissue debris and bacteria is called

   a. lymphadenitis

   b. phagocytosis

   c. lymphadenopathy

   d. agglutination

   e. osmosis

6. A life-threatening medical emergency that cannot be relieved by antihistamines is

   a. asthma

   b. Kaposi sarcoma

   c. anaphylactic shock

   d. urticaria

   e. lymphadenitis

7. An allergic reaction is one of

   a. hypoglycemia

   b. hypersensitivity

   c. hypotension

   d. hyperglycemia

   e. hypertension

8. White pulp and red pulp can be found in the

   a. lymph nodes

   b. spleen

   c. lymph vessels

   d. none of these

   e. all of these

9. *Elevated body temperature* is another name for

   a. pathogen

   b. pyrexia

   c. precipitation

   d. protease

   e. phagocytosis

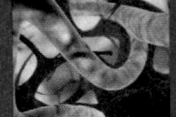

Lymphatic and Immune Systems

C. Language of immunology. Challenge your knowledge of the immune system and employ the *language of immunology* to answer the following questions. Circle the correct choice. (**LO 12.3,** *Remember*)

1. Which disease is likely to cause enlarged lymph nodes under the jaw?

   a. tonsillitis

   b. lymphoma

   c. hypersplenism

   d. asthma

   e. urticaria

2. Abnormal, cancerous B cells are known as

   a. macrophages   d. killer cells

   b. osteoblasts   e. phagocytes

   c. Reed-Sternberg cells

3. Lymph nodes accessible for palpation are in the

   a. neck   d. all of these

   b. axilla   e. only a and c

   c. groin

4. Immunosuppressive drugs are given after

   a. organ transplant

   b. anaphylactic shock

   c. retrovirus

   d. opportunistic infection

   e. viral load count

5. Serum used to treat a snake bite is an example of

   a. natural active immunity

   b. artificial active immunity

   c. natural passive immunity

   d. artificial passive immunity

   e. none of the above

D. Correct spelling of medical terms is *always important*. Listed below are two examples of medical terms for which a variation of the term is not always spelled the same as the original term. Fill in the blanks with the correctly spelled medical terms. (**LO 12. 4,** *Remember*)

Example 1:

Lymphatic organ in LUQ of abdomen   1. _____

Excision/removal of this organ   2. _____

Enlargement of this organ due to an underlying disorder   3. _____

What is the difference you notice in the spelling of these three terms?

4. _____

_____

Example 2:

Lymphoid tissue on either side of the throat   5. _____

Inflammation of this tissue   6. _____

Removal of this tissue   7. _____

What is the difference you notice in the spelling of the previous three terms?

8. _____

_____

E. Translation. First, use your knowledge of medical terminology to understand the statement. Then, organize your thoughts and formulate your answer in layman's terms that a patient could understand. Write an explanation of each sentence on the lines that follow. (**LO 12.3, 12.6,** *Remember, Understand, Apply*)

1. Pyrexia is a defense mechanism because it inhibits reproduction of bacteria and viruses and accelerates tissue repair.

_____

2. Intra-abdominal hemorrhage from a ruptured spleen can be extensive, with dramatic hypotension, and is a surgical emergency requiring splenectomy.

_____

F. Discussion. You may choose from either topic for your discussion/presentation. (**LO 12.3, 12.4, 12.7,** *Understand*)

1. There are four classes of immunity described in this chapter: natural active, artificial active, natural passive, and artificial passive. Pick any two of these classes, and compare and contrast them. How do you acquire these immunities? Give examples. Prepare a 5-minute class presentation on your topic. *You should be able to define any medical terms you use in your presentation.* Hand in your notes and outline of your presentation to the instructor.

_____

_____

_____

_____

2. Your body has three lines of defense mechanisms against foreign organisms that may harm you. Answer these questions: Which types of organisms seek to harm you, and what are the three lines of defense your body puts up? Give examples of each type of defense mechanism, and explain how they act against foreign organisms. Prepare a 5-minute class presentation on your topic. *You should be able to define any medical terms you use in your presentation.* Hand in your notes and outline of your presentation to the instructor.

_____

_____

_____

_____

G. Patient education. Translate for your patients, in words they can understand, the difference among the following terms. (**LO 12.4,** *Understand*)

1. Edema: _____

2. Peripheral edema: _____

3. Pitting edema: _____

4. Lymphedema: _____

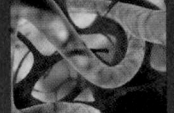

Lymphatic and Immune Systems

H. Incident report. Use the appropriate information for this report to fill in the blanks in the incident report below. You are granted creative license (use your imagination) to fill in the rest of the report in your own words. (**LO 12.3, Apply**)

Case Report 12.2

Your patient is

. . . Mr. Michael Cowan, a 40-year-old homeless man and drug addict, who has presented to the Emergency Department with a high fever for which no cause is obvious on clinical examination.

You are called to the Emergency Room to take blood from Mr. Cowan. You have inserted the needle into an antecubital vein, and he starts jerking his arm around and trying to get off the gurney. In the struggle, the needle comes out of the vein and pricks your hand through your glove.

As you immediately *flush* and *clean* the wound, *report* the incident, seek *immediate medical attention*, and go through your *initial medical evaluation*, it is essential that you have knowledge about your immune system and its response to the potential infection. Then you can make *informed decisions* about your treatment and future employment.

Fulwood Medical Center
3333 Medical Parkway, Fulwood, MI 01234
555-247-6100

Department of Employee Health: Incident Report

Staff member's name: *Jane/John Doe*   Department: _____

Date of occurrence: _____ Date Report filed: _____

Location of incident: _____

Describe the incident in your own words: _____

_____

_____

_____

What is the specific nature of the injury? _____

Was any immediate action taken in the department at the time of the incident?

Yes_____ No_____

If "yes," please describe what action was taken: _____

_____

_____

_____

Were you engaged in patient care at the time of the incident? Yes_____ No_____

If so, give name of patient: _____

Were gloves worn by the employee? Yes_____ No_____

Was the glove penetrated? Yes_____ No_____

Were there any witnesses to the incident? Yes_____ No_____

If yes, please provide their names and departments:

_____

_____

Did you seek immediate medical attention? Yes_____ No_____

If so, where? _____

Name of physician who treated you: _____

Was this incident reported to your immediate supervisor? Yes_____ No_____

Date reported to supervisor: _____

Name of supervisor: _____

Signature of employee: _____ Date: _____

Received by Employee Health Department:

Signature _____ Date _____

I. Use a dictionary or glossary to define the word *reservoir.* Then give a brief explanation as to how the spleen functions as a reservoir. (**LO. 12.2,** *Apply*)

1. Definition of *reservoir:* _____

2. Spleen as a reservoir:

_____

_____

J. Create patient documentation for each of the following abbreviations. Write out the abbreviation's meaning in the sentence. (**LO 12.5,** *Apply*)

1. Ig _____

_____

2. AIDS _____

_____

3. HIV _____

_____

4. T cells _____

_____

K. Construct the entire term by entering the prefix *on* the line, write the meaning of the prefix *under* the line. Fill in the blanks. (**LO 12.3,** *Apply*)

1. Reaction directed against foreign tissue   _____/immune

2. Substance produced in response to an antigen   _____/body

3. Surface protein that enhances sensitivity of antigen receptor _____/recept/or

4. Spleen removes blood components at an excessive rate   _____splen/ism

5. Virus that converts its RNA core to DNA in a host cell   _____/virus

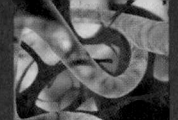

Lymphatic and Immune Systems

C. Using your knowledge of terms 1–10 in Exercises A and B and their correct spelling, write a brief sentence for each of the terms as it might appear in patient documentation. **(LO 12.3, *Apply*)**

1. _____

2. _____

3. _____

4. _____

5. _____

6. _____

7. _____

8. _____

9. _____

10. _____

D. **After rereading Case Report 12.1, answer the following questions.** Be prepared to discuss your answers in class. **(LO 12.6, *Analyze*)**

Case Report 12.1

You are

...a medical assistant working with Susan Lee, MD, in her primary care clinic at Fulwood Medical Center.

Your patient is

...Ms. Anna Clemons, a 20-year-old waitress, who is a new patient. She has noticed a lump in her right neck. On questioning, you elicit that she has lost about 8 pounds in weight in the past couple of months, has felt tired, and has had some night sweats.

Her vital signs (VS) are normal. There are two firm, enlarged lymph nodes in her right neck. Physical examination is otherwise unremarkable, and there is no evidence of infection in her head, throat, or upper respiratory tract.

Ms. Clemons has cancerous nodes in her neck. They were not caused by metastatic cancer but by a cancer of the lymph nodes called Hodgkin lymphoma.

1. What outward sign does the patient have? _____

2. What is the patient's chief complaint? _____

_____

3. Did the patient present with a temperature? _____

4. What is the medical term for *enlarged lymph nodes*? _____

5. What findings were present on physical examination? _____

6. The cancerous nodes were not caused by *metastatic cancer*. What does this mean? _____

_____

7. What are some of the diagnostic tests used to confirm this disease? _____

8. What is the surgical procedure to remove malignant lymph nodes? _____

E. Describe the difference between an allograft and an autograft, then answer the remaining questions. (LO 12.9, *Analyze*)

1. Allograft: _____

2. Autograft: _____

3. Which type of graft is better for the recipient? _____

4. Why is it better? _____

F. Meet the goals of each of the chapter outcomes by using the correct language of immunology for the answers. (LO 12.1–12.9, *Analyze*)

1. What lines of defense does the body have against foreign organisms, cells, and molecules? (**LO 12.1**)

_____

2. What are the three components of the lymphatic system? (**LO 12.2**)

a. _____

b. _____

c. _____

3. Create a sentence using any medical term in this chapter. The sentence cannot be a definition, or directly out of the text. (**LO 12.3**)

_____

4. The doctor has told you the patient is in anaphylactic shock and needs immediate medication. What medication should you

bring? (**LO 12.4**) _____

5. Which of the following abbreviations are the only ones that apply to the immune system? Circle the correct answers. (**LO 12.5**)

a. UTI   f. VS

b. MRI   g. MI

c. PO   h. RUQ

d. CT   i. PTSD

e. AIDS   j. HIV

6. For recurrent tonsillitis, what is sometimes performed? (**LO 12.6**)

a. splenectomy

b. tonsillectomy

c. lymph node biopsy

d. lymphoma

e. splenomegaly

7. What are the characteristics that distinguish immunity from the other defense mechanisms of the body? (**LO 12.7**)

_____

8. Which of the following is NOT a specialized cell involved in cellular immunity? (**LO 12.8**)

a. lymphocytes   d. B cells

b. T cells   e. macrophages

c. autoimmune

9. Which of the following is a life-threatening emergency? (**LO 12.9**)

a. anaphylaxis   d. anaphylactic shock

b. allograft   e. edema

c. urticaria

Respiratory System
The Language of Pulmonology

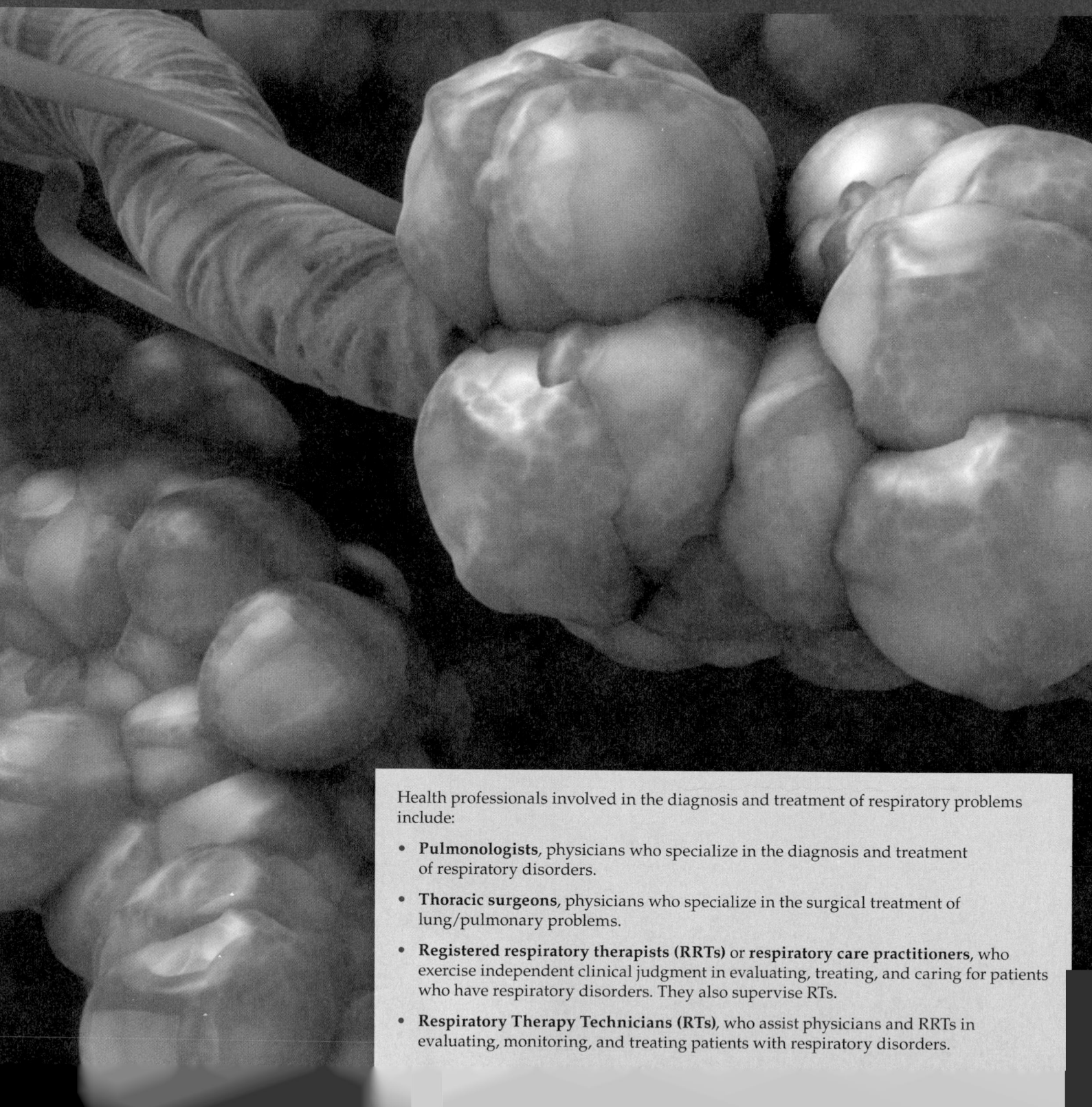

Health professionals involved in the diagnosis and treatment of respiratory problems include:

- **Pulmonologists**, physicians who specialize in the diagnosis and treatment of respiratory disorders.

- **Thoracic surgeons**, physicians who specialize in the surgical treatment of lung/pulmonary problems.

- **Registered respiratory therapists (RRTs)** or **respiratory care practitioners**, who exercise independent clinical judgment in evaluating, treating, and caring for patients who have respiratory disorders. They also supervise RTs.

- **Respiratory Therapy Technicians (RTs)**, who assist physicians and RRTs in evaluating, monitoring, and treating patients with respiratory disorders.

13

Case Report (CR) 13.1

You are

... an advanced-level **registered respiratory therapist (RRT)** working in the Acute Respiratory Care Unit of Fulwood Medical Center with **pulmonologist** Tavis Senko, MD.

Your patient is

... Mr. Jude Jacobs, a 68-year-old retired mail carrier, who is known to have **chronic obstructive pulmonary disease (COPD)** and is on continual oxygen by nasal prongs (cannulae). He has smoked two packs per day for all his adult life.

Last night, he was unable to sleep because of increased **shortness of breath (SOB)** and cough. His cough is productive of yellow **sputum**. He had to sit upright in bed to be able to breathe.

Vital signs **(VS)** are temperature **(T)** 101.6°F, pulse **(P)** 98, respirations **(R)** 36, blood pressure **(BP)** 150/90.

On examination, he is cyanotic and frightened and has nasal prongs. Air entry is diminished in both lungs, and there are **rales** (crackles) at both bases.

You have been ordered to draw blood for arterial blood gases **(ABGs)** and to measure the amount of air entering and leaving his lungs by using **spirometry**.

Chapter Learning Outcomes

To provide optimal care to Mr. Jacobs, to determine what is causing his symptoms and signs, and to communicate with the other health professionals involved in his care, you need to be able to:

LO 13.1 Apply the language of pulmonology to identify the anatomy and physiology of the upper and lower respiratory tracts.

LO 13.2 Apply the language of pulmonology to relate the structures of the upper and lower respiratory tracts to their functions.

LO 13.3 Use the medical terms of pulmonology to communicate and document in writing accurately and precisely in any health care setting.

LO 13.4 Use the medical terms of pulmonology to communicate verbally with accuracy and precision in any health care setting.

LO 13.5 Define abbreviations that relate to the respiratory system.

LO 13.6 Summarize the mechanics of respiration.

LO 13.7 Discuss the significance of the symptoms and signs of respiratory disorders.

LO 13.8 Explain the effects of common upper respiratory tract disorders on health.

LO 13.9 Explain the effects of common lower respiratory tract disorders on health.

LO 13.10 Identify the value of common diagnostic and therapeutic procedures used in disorders of the respiratory system.

LO 13.11 List the classes of drugs used to treat pulmonary disorders.

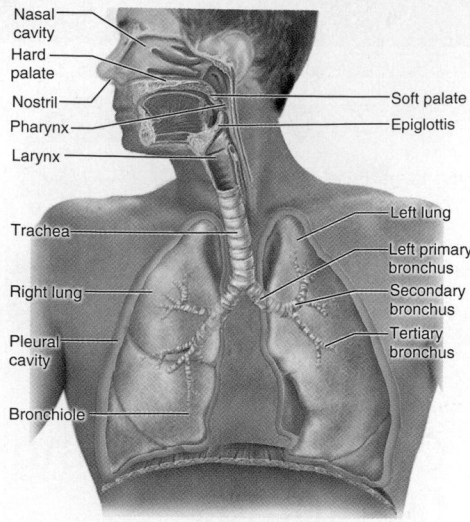

▲ Figure 13.1 The Respiratory System.

Labels (Figure 13.1): Nasal cavity, Hard palate, Nostril, Pharynx, Larynx, Trachea, Right lung, Pleural cavity, Bronchiole, Soft palate, Epiglottis, Left lung, Left primary bronchus, Secondary bronchus, Tertiary bronchus

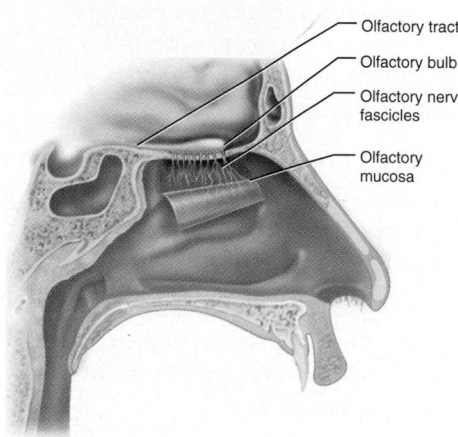

▲ Figure 13.2 Olfactory Region of Nose.

Labels (Figure 13.2): Olfactory tract, Olfactory bulb, Olfactory nerve fascicles, Olfactory mucosa

Abbreviations

ABG	arterial blood gas
BP	blood pressure
CO₂	carbon dioxide
COPD	chronic obstructive pulmonary disease
O₂	oxygen
P	pulse
R	respiration
RRT	registered respiratory therapists
RT	respiratory therapy technicians
SOB	short(ness) of breath
T	temperature
VS	vital signs

LO 13.1, 13.2 Introduction to the Respiratory System

It sounds like a good scheme. Humans and animals can breathe in oxygen (O_2) and breathe out carbon dioxide (CO_2); plants and trees can breathe in CO_2 and breathe out O_2—and nature stays in balance. Unfortunately, we humans have generated increasing amounts of CO_2 in the air by burning coal, oil, and natural gas and cutting down forests. We have disturbed the balance. In addition, we have created organic and inorganic chemicals and small particles of solid matter in the air that can damage the respiratory tract and be taken into our bodies to cause cancer, brain damage, and birth defects. These materials are called **pollutants**.

The **respiratory tract** *(Figure 13.1)* has six connected elements:

1. **Nose**
2. **Pharynx**
3. **Larynx**
4. **Trachea**
5. **Bronchi and bronchioles**
6. **Alveoli**

Respiration is the transport of O_2 from the outside air to tissue cells and the transport of CO_2 in the opposite direction.

Respiration has four components:

1. **Ventilation**, which is the movement of air and its gases into and out of the lungs (inspiration and expiration).
2. **Pulmonary exchange of gases** between air in the alveoli and pulmonary capillaries (external respiration).
3. **Gas transport** from the pulmonary capillaries through the arterial system to the peripheral capillaries in tissues and the transport of gases back to the lung capillaries through the venous system.
4. **Peripheral gas exchange** between tissue capillaries and tissue cells for use in cellular metabolism (internal respiration) *(see Chapter 4).*

The five **functions** of the respiratory system are:

1. **Exchange of gases**. All the body cells need O_2 and produce CO_2. The respiratory system allows O_2 from the air to enter the blood and CO_2 to leave the blood and enter the air.
2. **Regulation of blood pH**. This is accomplished by changing blood CO_2 levels *(see Chapter 4).*
3. **Protection**. The respiratory system uses nasal hair, cilia lining the airways, and mucus formed throughout the system to protect against foreign bodies and against some microorganisms.
4. **Voice production**. Movement of air across the vocal cords makes speech and other sounds possible.
5. **Olfaction**. The 12 million receptor cells for smell are in a patch of epithelium the size of a quarter that is in the extreme superior region of the nasal cavity, the **olfactory region** *(Figure 13.2)*. Each cell has 10 to 20 hairlike structures called **cilia** that project into the nasal cavity covered in a thin mucous film. Because the **olfactory region** is right at the top of the nose, you often have to sniff the air right up there to stimulate the sense of smell. A dog has 4 billion receptor cells, which is why dogs can be trained to sniff for drugs, explosives, and dead bodies.

Many of your sensations of taste are influenced by your sense of smell. For example, without its aroma, coffee tastes only bitter. The same is true for peppermint. This is why, when you have a cold, much of your sense of taste is lost.

WORD	PRONUNCIATION		ELEMENTS	DEFINITION
alveolus alveoli (pl) alveolar (adj)	al-**VEE**-oh-lus al-**VEE**-oh-lee al-**VEE**-oh-lar		Latin *hollow sac*	Tiny air sac terminal element of the respiratory tract
bronchus bronchi (pl) bronchiole	**BRONG**-kuss **BRONG**-key **BRONG**-key-ole	 S/ R/CF	Greek *windpipe* -ole *small* **bronch/i-** *bronchus*	One of two subdivisions of the trachea Increasingly smaller subdivisions of bronchi
cannula cannulae (pl)	**KAN**-you-lah **KAN**-you-lee		Latin *reed*	Tube inserted into a cavity or blood vessel as a channel for fluid or gases
cilium cilia (pl)	**SILL**-ee-um **SILL**-ee-ah		Latin *eyelash*	Hairlike motile projection from the surface of a cell
larynx laryngeal (adj)	**LAIR**-inks lah-**RIN**-jee-al		Greek *larynx*	Organ of voice production
olfaction olfactory (adj)	ol-**FAK**-shun ol-**FAK**-toh-ree		Latin *to smell*	Sense of smell
pharynx pharyngeal (adj)	**FAIR**-inks fair-**IN**-jee-al		Greek *throat*	Air tube from the back of the nose to the larynx
pulmonary (adj)	**PULL**-moh-**NAR**-ee	S/ R/	-ary *pertaining to* **pulmon-** *lung*	Pertaining to the lungs and their blood supply
pulmonology	**PULL**-moh-**NOL**-oh-jee	S/ R/CF	-logy *study of* **pulmon/o-** *lung*	Study of the lungs, or the medical specialty of disorders of the respiratory tract
pulmonologist	**PULL**-moh-**NOL**-oh-jist	S/	-logist *one who studies, specialist*	Medical specialist in pulmonary disorders
rale rales (pl)	RAHL RAHLS		French *rattle*	Crackle heard through a stethoscope when air bubbles through liquid in the lungs
respiration	**RES**-pih-**RAY**-shun	S/ P/ R/	-ation *process* re- *again* **-spir-** *to breathe*	Fundamental process of life used to exchange oxygen and carbon dioxide
respirator respiratory (adj)	**RES**-pir-**AY**-tor **RES**-pir-ah-**TOR**-ee	S/	-ator *person or thing that does something*	Another name for ventilator
spirometer	spy-**ROM**-eh-ter	S/ R/CF	-meter *measure* **spir/o-** *to breathe*	An instrument used to measure respiratory volumes
spirometry	spy-**ROM**-eh-tree	S/	-metry *process of measuring*	Use of a spirometer
sputum	**SPYU**-tum		Latin *to spit*	Matter coughed up and spat out by individuals with respiratory disorders
thorax thoracic (adj)	**THOR**-acks **THOR**-ass-ik	 S/ R/	Greek *breastplate* -ic *pertaining to* **thorac-** *chest*	The trunk between the abdomen and neck Pertaining to the thorax
trachea	**TRAY**-kee-ah		Greek *windpipe*	Air tube from the larynx to the bronchi
ventilation	ven-tih-**LAY**-shun	S/ R/	-ation *process* **ventil-** *wind*	Movement of gases into and out of the lungs
ventilator	**VEN**-tih-**LAY**-tor	S/	-ator *person or thing that does something*	Device that breathes for the patient

Exercises

A. Latin/Greek/Other terms. *Medical terms taken directly from Latin, Greek, or other languages do not deconstruct into prefix, root, or suffix elements the way other medical terms do. You simply have to know them for what they are. Match the medical term in the left column to the correct meaning in the right column. Fill in the blanks.* **LO 13.1, 13.2**

_____ 1. rale

_____ 2. pharynx

_____ 3. sputum

_____ 4. trachea

a. throat

b. spit

c. windpipe

d. crackle

Lesson 13.1 Upper Respiratory Tract

The upper respiratory tract consists of the nose, pharynx, and larynx. It is the first site that brings air and its pollutants inside your body. As a health professional, you must understand the roles of the upper respiratory tract in trying to protect you, as well as enabling you to live by transporting O_2 into and CO_2 out of your body.

The information in this lesson will enable you to use correct medical terminology to:

13.1.1 Trace the flow of air from the nose through the pharynx and larynx.

13.1.2 Relate the function of each segment of the upper airway to its structure.

13.1.3 Define the protective mechanisms of the upper respiratory tract.

13.1.4 Describe how sound is produced.

13.1.5 Explain how smells are recognized.

13.1.6 Describe common disorders of the upper respiratory tract.

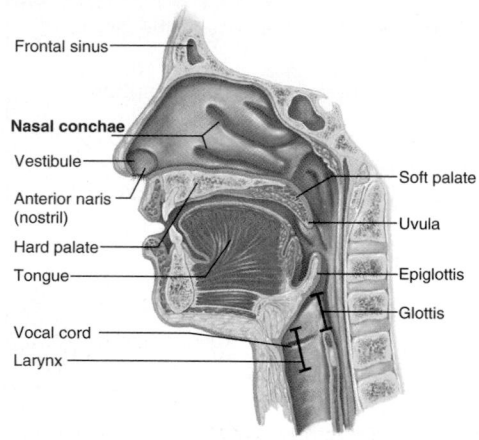

Frontal sinus
Nasal conchae
Vestibule
Anterior naris (nostril)
Hard palate
Tongue
Vocal cord
Larynx
Soft palate
Uvula
Epiglottis
Glottis

▲ **Figure 13.3** **Upper Respiratory Tract.**

Keynotes

- Your nose is the first line of defense against pollutants.

- In a deviated nasal septum, the partition between the two nostrils is pushed to one side, leading to a partially obstructed airway in one nostril.

- **Rhinoplasty** is a surgical procedure to alter the size and/or shape of the nose.

Abbreviation

URI	upper respiratory infection

LO 13.1, 13.2 Nose

When you breathe in air through your nose, the air goes through the nostrils (**nares**) into the **vestibule** of the **nasal cavity**. The nares are guarded by internal (guard) hairs to prevent the entry of large particles.

The nasal cavity is divided by the nasal **septum** into right and left compartments. On the lateral wall of each nasal cavity, three bony ridges called **conchae (turbinate bones)** stick out into each cavity. Beneath each **concha** is a passageway called a **meatus** (*Figure 13.3*). The palate (*see Chapter 14*) forms the floor of the nose.

The nasal cavity is lined with a mucous membrane (mucosa) containing goblet cells that secrete mucus. Mucus forms a protective layer that can trap particles of dust and solid pollutants.

The **paranasal**, frontal, and maxillary **sinuses** open into the nose. Because they are hollow, the functions of these sinuses are to reduce the weight of the skull and to act as resonating chambers for the sounds of the voice. If your sinuses are congested, your voice loses its normal quality.

The following are functions of the nose:

- **Passageway for air.** The palate is the floor of the nasal cavity that separates it from the mouth and enables you to breathe even with food in your mouth.

- **Air cleanser.** The hairs in the vestibule trap some of the large particles in the air.

- **Air moisturizer.** Moisture from nasal mucus and from tears that drain into the cavity through the nasolacrimal duct (*see Chapter 16*) is added to the air.

- **Air warmer.** The blood flowing through the nasal cavity beneath the mucous membrane also warms the air. This prevents damage from the cold to the more fragile lower respiratory passages.

- **Sense of smell (olfaction).** The olfactory region recognizes some 4,000 separate smells.

LO 13.8 Disorders of the Nose

The **common cold** is a viral **upper respiratory infection (URI)**. It is contagious, being transmitted from person to person in airborne droplets from coughing and sneezing. There is no proven effective treatment.

Rhinitis is an inflammation of the nasal mucosa, usually viral in origin. It is also called **coryza**.

Allergic rhinitis affects 15% to 20% of the population. There is swelling of the mucous membranes of the nose, pharynx, and sinuses, with a clear watery discharge.

Sinusitis is an infection of the paranasal sinuses, often following a cold. The infection can be bacterial, producing a **mucopurulent** discharge from the nose. Treatment with **antibiotics** and **decongestants** may be indicated.

Epistaxis is bleeding from the septum of the nose, usually from trauma. If pinching the nose or packing the nostril with gauze does not stop the bleeding, **cautery** (burning and scarring) with silver nitrate or electrical cautery is indicated.

Word Analysis and Definition

S = Suffix   P = Prefix   **R = Root**   **R/CF = Combining Form**

WORD	PRONUNCIATION	ELEMENTS		DEFINITION
cautery	**KAW**-ter-ee		Greek *a branding iron*	Agent or device used to burn or scar a tissue
concha **conchae** (pl)	**KON**-kah **KON**-kee		Latin *shell*	Shell-shaped bone on the lateral wall of the nasal cavity
coryza rhinitis (syn)	ko-**RYE**-zah		Greek *catarrh*	Viral inflammation of the mucous membrane of the nose
decongestant	dee-con-**JESS**-tant	S/ P/ R/	**-ant** *pertaining to* **de-** *take away* **-congest-** *accumulation of fluid*	Agent that reduces the swelling and fluid in the nose and sinuses
epistaxis	ep-ih-**STAK**-sis	S/ P/ R/	**-is** *condition* **epi-** *above, over* **-stax-** *fall in drops*	Nosebleed
meatus	me-**AY**-tus		Latin *a passage*	Passage or channel; also used to denote the external opening of a passage
mucopurulent	myu-koh-**PYUR**-you-lent	S/ R/CF R/	**-ent** *forming* **muc/o-** *mucus* **-purul-** *pus*	Mixture of pus and mucus
naris **nares** (pl) **nasal**	**NAH**-ris **NAH**-rez **NAY**-zal	 S/ R/	 **-al** *pertaining to* **nas-** *nose*	Nostril Pertaining to the nose
paranasal	**PAR**-ah **NAY**-zal	P/	**para-** *adjacent to*	Adjacent to the nose
rhinitis coryza (syn)	rye-**NI**-tis	S/ R/CF	**-itis** *inflammation* **rhin/o-** *nose*	Inflammation of the nasal mucosa
rhinoplasty	**RYE**-no-plas-tee	S/	**-plasty** *surgical repair*	Surgical procedure to change the size or shape of the nose
sinus **sinusitis**	**SIGH**-nus sigh-nyu-**SIGH**-tis	 S/ R/	Latin *cavity* **-itis** *inflammation* **sinus-** *sinus*	Cavity or hollow space in a bone or other tissue Inflammation of the lining of a sinus
turbinate	**TUR**-bin-ate		Latin *shaped like a top*	Another name for the nasal conchae on the lateral walls of the nasal cavity

Exercises

A. Elements. *Work with elements to build your knowledge of the* language of pulmonology. *One element in each of the following medical terms is bold italic. Identify the type of element (P, R, CF, S) in the first column; then write its meaning in the middle column. Fill in the meaning of the term in the last column on the chart.* **LO 13.1, 13.8**

Medical Term	Type of Element (P, R, CF, S)	Meaning of Element	Meaning of Term
epis*tax*is	1.	2.	3.
*rhin*itis	4.	5.	6.
muco*purul*ent	7.	8.	9.
*para*nasal	10.	11.	12.
*nas*al	13.	14.	15.

16. There are two elements in this list with the same meaning. What are they? _____ and _____

17. Both mean _____.

Case Report 13.2

Mr. Gawlinski's wife states that he snores loudly and has 40 or 50 periods in the night when he stops breathing. The snoring is so loud that she cannot sleep even in the adjoining bedroom. Mr. Gawlinski complains of being tired all day and not having the energy he needs for his job. The sleep study is being performed to confirm a diagnosis of obstructive sleep **apnea**.

LO 13.1, 13.2 Pharynx

The **pharynx** is a muscular funnel that receives air from the nasal cavity and food and drink from the oral cavity. It is divided into three regions *(Figure 13.4)*:

1. **Nasopharynx**—located at the back of the nose, above the soft palate and uvula. It is lined with a mucous membrane that includes goblet cells, which produce mucus. Mucus, including any trapped debris, is moved from the nasal cavity through the nasopharynx and swallowed. The posterior surface contains the **pharyngeal tonsil (adenoid)**. Only air moves through this region.
2. **Oropharynx**—located below the soft palate and above the epiglottis. It contains two sets of tonsils called the *palatine* and *lingual* tonsils. Air, food, and drink all pass through this region.
3. **Laryngopharynx**—located below the tip of the epiglottis. This is the pathway to the esophagus. During swallowing, the epiglottis shuts off the trachea so that food cannot enter it. Only food and drink pass through the laryngopharynx.

LO 13.8 Disorders of the Pharynx

Snoring Twenty-five percent of normal adults are habitual snorers. The condition is most frequent in overweight males, and it becomes worse with age. The noises of **snoring** are made at the back of the mouth and nose where the tongue and upper pharynx meet the soft palate and uvula *(Figure 13.5)*. When there is obstruction to the free flow of air, these structures hit each other, and the vibration produces the sounds of snoring.

Obstructive Sleep Apnea This is the condition Mr. Gawlinski has. He has bulky neck tissue from his football training regimen. Obstructive sleep apnea occurs when obstruction by the soft tissues at the back of the nose and mouth causes frequent episodes of gasping for breath followed by complete cessation of breathing (apnea). These episodes of apnea can last for 10 to 30 seconds and occur many times every hour of sleep. The episodes reduce the level of O_2 in the blood **(hypoxemia)**, causing the heart to pump harder. After several years with this problem, hypertension and cardiac enlargement can occur.

Pharyngitis is an acute or chronic infection involving the pharynx, tonsils, and uvula. It is usually of viral origin in children.

Tonsillitis is an infection of the tonsils in the oropharynx by a virus or, in less than 20% of cases, a streptococcus.

Nasopharyngeal carcinoma is a rare form of cancer that occurs mostly in males between the ages of 50 and 60. Radiation and chemotherapy are used in treatment.

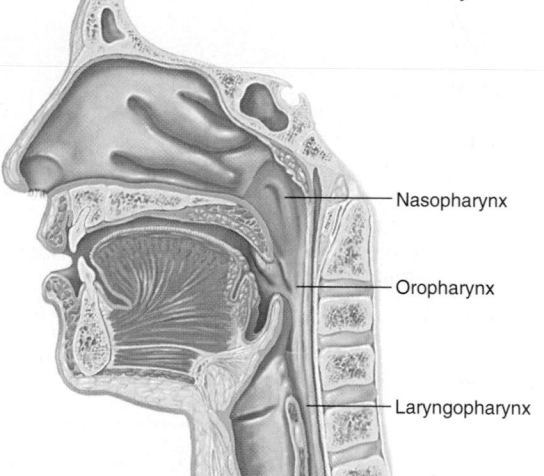

▲ **Figure 13.4** Regions of Pharynx.

Nasopharynx
Oropharynx
Laryngopharynx

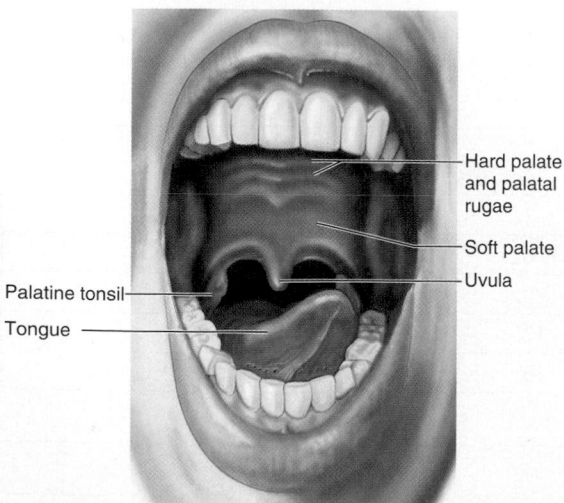

▲ **Figure 13.5** Soft Tissues at Back of Mouth.

Hard palate and palatal rugae
Soft palate
Uvula
Palatine tonsil
Tongue

WORD	PRONUNCIATION	ELEMENTS		DEFINITION
adenoid	ADD-eh-noyd	S/	-oid *resembling*	Single mass of lymphoid tissue in midline at the back of the throat
		R/	aden- *gland*	
apnea	AP-nee-ah	P/	a- *without*	Absence of spontaneous respiration
		R/	-pnea *breathe*	
hypoxia (*Note:* One of the two "o"s in the elements is deleted.)	high-POCK-see-ah	S/	-ia *condition*	Below normal levels of oxygen in the body as a whole or a region of the body
		P/	hypo- *below, deficient*	
		R/	-ox- *oxygen*	
hypoxemia	high-POCK-see-me-ah	S/	-emia *condition in the blood*	Decreased levels of oxygen in the blood
anoxia	an-OX-ee-ah	P/	an- *without*	Complete deprivation of oxygen supply
		R/	-ox- *oxygen*	
		S/	-ia *condition*	
laryngopharynx	lah-RING-oh-FAIR-inks	R/	laryng/o- *larynx*	Region of the pharynx below the epiglottis that includes the larynx
		R/CF	-pharynx *pharynx*	
nasopharynx	NAY-zoh-FAIR-inks	R/	nas/o- *nose*	Region of the pharynx at the back of the nose above the soft palate
		R/CF	-pharynx *pharynx*	
nasopharyngeal (adj)	NAY-zoh-fair-IN-jee-al	S/	-eal *pertaining to*	Pertaining to the nasopharynx
		R/	-pharyng- *pharynx*	
oropharynx	OR-oh-fair-inks	R/	or/o- *mouth*	Region at the back of the mouth between the soft palate and the tip of the epiglottis
oropharyngeal (adj)	OR-oh-fair-IN-jee-al	R/CF	-pharynx *pharynx*	
pharynx	FAIR-inks		Greek *throat*	Air tube from the back of the nose to the larynx
pharyngitis	fair-in-JI-tis	S/	-itis *inflammation*	Inflammation of the pharynx
		R/	pharyng- *pharynx*	
pharyngeal (adj)	fair-IN-jee-al	S/	-eal *pertaining to*	Pertaining to the pharynx
polysomnography	pol-ee-som-NOG-rah-fee	S/	-graphy *process of recording*	Test to monitor brain waves, muscle tension, eye movement, and oxygen levels in the blood as the patient sleeps
		P/	poly- *many*	
		R/CF	-somn/o- *sleep*	
snore	SNOR		Old English *snore*	Noise produced by vibrations in the structures of the nasopharynx
tonsil	TON-sill		Latin *tonsil*	Mass of lymphoid tissue on either side of the throat at the back of the tongue
tonsillitis (note the double "ll")	ton-sih-LIE-tis	S/	-itis *inflammation*	Inflammation of the tonsils
		R/	tonsill- *tonsil*	
tonsillectomy	ton-sih-LEC-toh-me	S/	-ectomy *surgical excision*	Surgical removal of the tonsils

Exercises

A. After reading Case Report 13.2, answer the following questions. *Be prepared to discuss your answers in class.*   **LO 13.3, 13.8**

1. What are Mr. Gawlinski's symptoms? _____

2. Mr. Gawlinski underwent the diagnostic procedure of _____.

3. If left untreated, his chronic obstructive sleep apnea could cause _____.

4. What causes Mr. Gawlinski's obstructive sleep apnea to occur?

_____

_____

5. Why is *polysomnography* done overnight?

_____

_____

LO 13.1, 13.2 Larynx

The flow of inhaled air moves on from the pharynx to the larynx (*Figure 13.6a*), an enlargement of the airway located between the oropharynx and the trachea. The upper opening into it from the oropharynx is called the **glottis**.

The larynx has an outer casing of nine cartilages connected to one another by muscles and ligaments. The uppermost cartilage, the leaf-shaped **epiglottis**, guards the glottis. During the swallowing of food, the epiglottis is pushed down by the tongue to close the glottis and direct food into the esophagus that lies behind it.

The **thyroid cartilage**, or "Adam's apple," is the largest cartilage in the body and forms the anterior and lateral walls of the larynx. Below the thyroid cartilage the ring-shaped **cricoid** cartilage connects the larynx to the trachea (*Figure 13.6b*).

Inside the larynx are the **true vocal cords** (*Figure 13.6b*). **Intrinsic** muscles control the cords.

Functions of the Larynx

- The thyroid and cricoid cartilages maintain an open passage for the movement of air to and from the trachea.
- The epiglottis and vestibular folds prevent food and drink from entering the larynx (*Figure 13.6b*).
- The vocal cords (*Figure 13.6a*) are the source of sound production.

Sound Production

Air moving past the vocal cords makes them vibrate to produce sound. The force of the air moving past the vocal cords determines the loudness of the sound. The intrinsic muscles of the cords pull them closer together with varying degrees of tautness. A high-pitched sound is produced by taut cords (*Figure 13.7b*) and a lower pitch by more relaxed cords (*Figure 13.7a*).

The male vocal cords are longer and thicker than the female, vibrate more slowly, and produce lower-pitched sounds.

The crude sounds produced by the larynx are transformed into words by the actions of the pharynx, tongue, teeth, and lips.

LO 13.8 Disorders of the Larynx

Laryngitis is inflammation of the mucosal lining of the larynx, producing hoarseness and sometimes progressing to loss of voice **(aphonia)**.

Epiglottitis is inflammation of the epiglottis. **Acute epiglottitis** is seen most commonly in children between ages 2 and 7 years and is caused by *Haemophilus influenzae type b* bacteria. Swelling in the epiglottis can cause acute airway obstruction and the need for **intubation**. It is preventable with an available vaccine.

Croup (laryngotracheobronchitis) is a group of viral diseases in children aged 3 months to 5 years. It causes inflammation and obstruction of the upper airway. It produces a characteristic cough that sounds like a seal barking. In severe cases, the child makes a high-pitched, squeaky inspiratory noise called **stridor**. Humidity is the initial treatment.

Papillomas or **polyps** are benign tumors of the larynx that result from overuse or irritation and are treated by surgical excision using a **laryngoscope**.

Carcinoma of the larynx produces a persistent hoarseness. Its incidence peaks in smokers in their fifties and sixties. Treatment can be surgery, radiation, and/or chemotherapy.

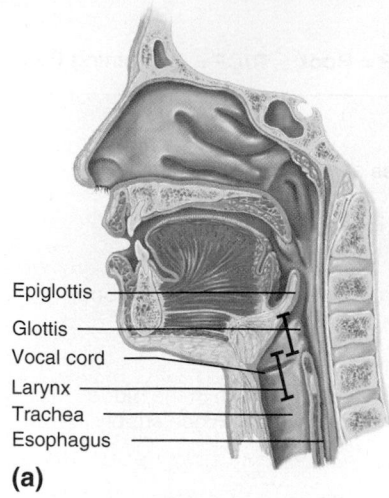

Epiglottis
Glottis
Vocal cord
Larynx
Trachea
Esophagus

(a)

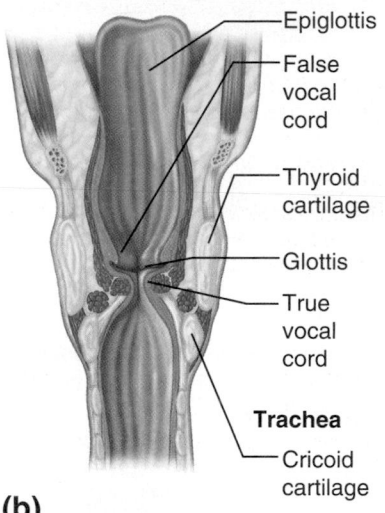

Epiglottis
False vocal cord
Thyroid cartilage
Glottis
True vocal cord
Trachea
Cricoid cartilage

(b)

▲ **Figure 13.6**   **Larynx**
(*a*) Location. (*b*) Structure.

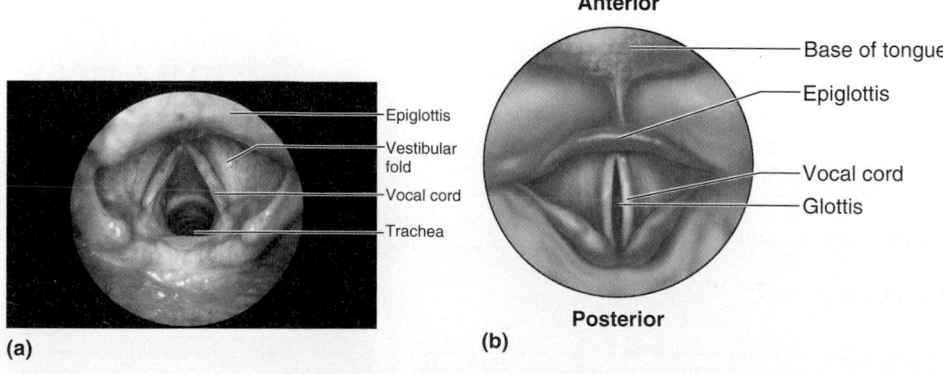

Anterior

Epiglottis
Vestibular fold
Vocal cord
Trachea

Base of tongue
Epiglottis
Vocal cord
Glottis

Posterior

(a)

(b)

▲ **Figure 13.7**   **View of Larynx** (*a*) Using Laryngoscope. (*b*) Vocal Cords Pulled Close and Taut.

S = Suffix   P = Prefix   **R = Root**   R/CF = Combining Form

WORD	PRONUNCIATION	ELEMENTS		DEFINITION
aphonia	a-**FO**-nee-ah	S/ P/ R/	-ia *condition* a- *without* -phon- *voice*	Loss of voice
cricoid	**CRY**-koyd		Latin *a ring*	Ring-shaped cartilage in the larynx
croup laryngotracheobron- chitis (syn)	KROOP		Old English *to cry out loud*	Infection of the upper airways in children; characterized by a barking cough
epiglottis	ep-ih-**GLOT**-is	S/ P/	-is *pertaining to* epi- *above*	Leaf-shaped plate of cartilage that shuts off the larynx during swallowing
epiglottitis glottis	ep-ih-**GLOT**-eye-tis **GLOT**-is	R/	-glott- *mouth of windpipe* Greek *opening of larynx*	Inflammation of the epiglottis The opening from the oropharynx into the larynx
intrinsic	in-**TRIN**-sik		Latin *on the inside*	Any muscle whose origin and insertion are entirely within the structure under consideration, for example, inside the vocal cords or the eye
intubation	**IN**-tyu-**BAY**-shun	S/ P/ R/CF	-tion *process* in- *in* -tub/a- *tube*	Insertion of a tube into the trachea
larynx laryngitis laryngoscope laryngotracheobronchitis croup (syn)	**LAIR**-inks lar-in-**JEYE**-tis lah-**RING**-oh-skope lah-**RING**-oh-**TRAY**-kee-oh-brong-**KI**-tis	R/ S/ R/CF S/ R/CF R/	Greek *larynx* laryng- *larynx* -scope *instrument for viewing* laryng/o- *larynx* -itis *inflammation* -trache/o- *trachea* -bronch- *bronchus*	Organ of voice production Inflammation of the larynx Hollow tube with a light and camera used to visualize or operate on the larynx Inflammation of the larynx, trachea, and bronchi
stridor	**STRY**-door		Latin *a harsh, creaking sound*	High-pitched noise made when there is respiratory obstruction in the larynx or trachea
thyroid	**THIGH**-royd		Greek *an oblong shield*	Gland in the neck, or a cartilage of the larynx
vocal	**VOH**-kal	S/ R/	-al *pertaining to* voc- *voice*	Pertaining to the voice

Exercises

A. Deconstruct. *For long or short medical terms, deconstruction into word elements is your key to solving the meaning of the term. Follow the directions, and fill in the blanks.* **LO 13.3, 13.7**

1. **laryngotracheobronchitis**

   Rewrite this term, and slash all its elements: _____/_____/_____

                                               P   R/CF   S

2. Combine the meanings of the elements, and define the term.

   Laryngotracheobronchitis means

   _____

   _____

3. **vocal**

   Slash this term into all its elements: _____/_____/_____

                                          P   R/CF   S

4. Combine the meanings of the elements, and define the term.

   Vocal means

   _____

Study Hint

Whether the term is 24 letters long or 5 letters long, the principle is the same. Know the meaning of the elements, and you will know the meaning of the term!

Lesson 13.2 Lower Respiratory Tract

Once the air you inhale has passed through the upper airway and many of the pollutants and impurities have been filtered out and swallowed into the digestive system, there still remain the major needs of getting O_2 into the blood and removing CO_2 from the blood. To do these, the inhaled air passes down the trachea, through the bronchi and bronchioles, and into the alveoli of the lungs, where these exchanges can occur. These structures form the lower respiratory tract.

In this lesson, you will learn to use correct medical terminology to:

13.2.1 **Trace the passage of air from the larynx into the alveoli and back.**

13.2.2 **Explain the exchange of O_2 from the air into the blood.**

13.2.3 **Explain the exchange of CO_2 from the blood into the air.**

13.2.4 **Describe the mechanics of ventilation.**

13.2.5 **Match the functions of the different elements of the lower airway with their structure.**

13.2.6 **Discuss the effects of common disorders of the lungs on overall health.**

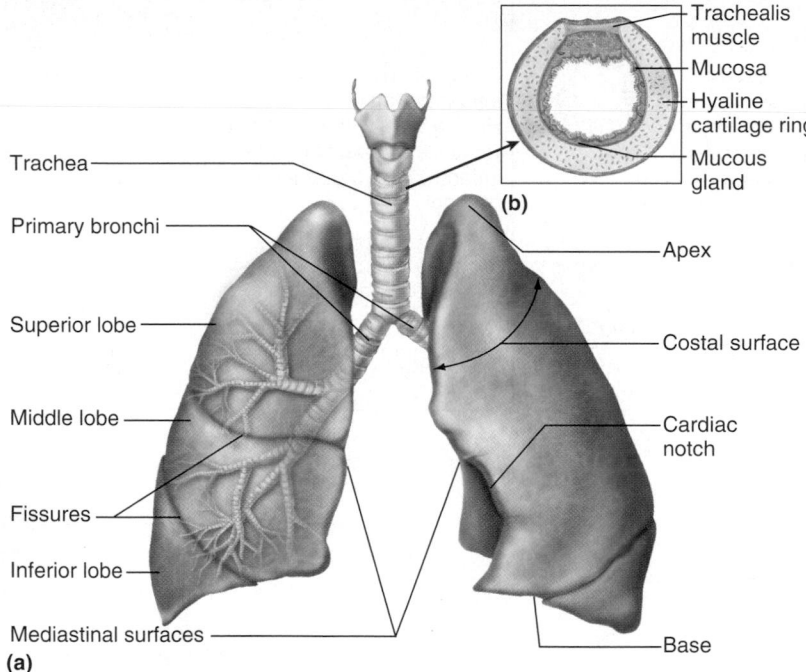

▲ **Figure 13.8** Lower Respiratory Tract.
(a) Gross anatomy.
(b) C-shaped tracheal cartilage.

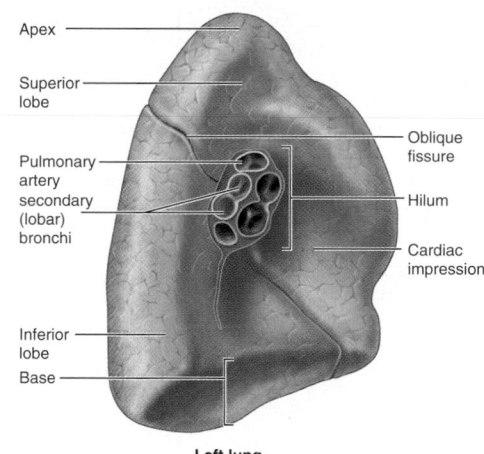

▲ **Figure 13.9** Left Lung Hilum: Medial Surface.

LO 13.1, 13.2 Trachea

The flow of inhaled air now moves into the trachea (windpipe). This is a rigid tube that descends from the larynx to divide into the two main bronchi *(Figure 13.8a)*. The rigidity of the trachea is produced by 16 to 20 C-shaped rings of cartilage that form its anterior and lateral walls *(Figure 13.8b)*. The open part of the "C" faces posteriorly and is closed by the **trachealis** muscle. The trachea divides into the two primary (main) bronchi for the right and left lungs *(Figure 13.8a)*.

LO 13.1, 13.2 Lungs

The two lungs are the main organs of respiration and are located in the thoracic cavity. Each lung is a soft, spongy, conical organ with its base resting on the **diaphragm**. Its apex lies above and behind the clavicle. Its outer, convex costal surface presses against the rib cage. Its inner, concave surface lies alongside the **mediastinum**.

The right lung has three **lobes**—superior, middle, and inferior. The left lung has two lobes, a superior and inferior *(see Figure 13.8a)*. The lobes are separated from each other by **fissures**. The heart makes a concave impression in the left lung, known as the *cardiac notch*.

Each lung receives its bronchus, blood vessels, lymphatic vessels, and nerves through its **hilum** *(Figure 13.9)*. The lung's specific functional cells are called the lung **parenchyma** and are supported by a thin connective tissue framework called the **stroma**. This consists mostly of collagen and elastic fibers, and its elasticity is a factor in the lung's recoil after inhalation.

WORD	PRONUNCIATION	ELEMENTS		DEFINITION
diaphragm	DIE-ah-fram		Greek *diaphragm*	Musculoligamentous partition separating the abdominal and thoracic cavities
diaphragmatic (adj)	DIE-ah-frag-**MAT**-ic	S/ R/CF	**-tic** *pertaining to* **diaphragm/a-** *diaphragm*	Pertaining to the diaphragm
fissure fissures (pl)	FISH-ur	S/ R/	**-ure** *result of* **fiss-** *split*	Deep furrow or cleft
hilum hila (pl)	HIGH-lum HIGH-lah		Latin *small area*	The site where the nerves and blood vessels enter and leave an organ
lobe lobar (adj)	LOBE LOW-bar	S/ R/	Greek *lobe* **-ar** *pertaining to* **lob-** *lobe*	Subdivision of an organ or other part Pertaining to or part of a lobe
mediastinum	ME-dee-ass-**TIE**-num	S/ P/ R/	**-um** *tissue, structure* **media-** *middle* **-stin-** *partition*	Area between the lungs containing the heart, aorta, venae cavae, esophagus, and trachea
mediastinal (adj)	ME-dee-ah-**STIE**-nal	S/	**-al** *pertaining to*	Pertaining to or part of the mediastinum
parenchyma	pah-**RENG**-kih-mah		Greek *to pour in beside*	Characteristic functional cells of a gland or organ that are supported by the connective tissue framework
stroma	STROH-mah		Greek *bed*	Connective tissue framework that supports the parenchyma of an organ or gland
trachealis	tray-kee-**AY**-lis	S/ R/CF	**-alis** *pertaining to* **trach/e-** *trachea*	Pertaining to the trachea

Exercises

A. Precision in communication means using the correct form of the medical term, as well as the correct spelling. *Test your knowledge of plurals, adjectives, and spelling with this exercise. Circle the correct choice.*   **LO 13.1, 13.3**

1. The area between the lungs containing the heart, aorta, venae cavae, esophagus, and trachea is the

   mediastenum   medisternum   mediastinum   midiasternum

2. The patient was diagnosed with _____ pneumonia.

   lobe   lobular   lobar   lumbar

3. _____ is the term for the functional cells of an organ.

   perenchyma   parenchyma   perinchkima   perenkima

4. Since there is a hilum in each lung, collectively they are referred to as the

   hilla   hila   hilia   hilea

5. The muscle separating the abdominal and thoracic cavities is the

   diaphram   diaphragm   diahragm   diapragm

6. Removal of a lobe of a lung would be a

   lobotomy   lobectomy   lobarectomy   lobarotomy

B. Select the correct pronunciation of the following two terms. *Your instructor may call on you to pronounce them in class.*   **LO 13.4**

1. stroma

   a. STROM a

   b. STRO mah

   c. STROH mah

   d. STROH ma

   e. STROM ah

2. diaphragm

   a. DIE a fram

   b. DI a frame

   c. DI ah fram

   d. DIE ah fram

   e. DE a fram

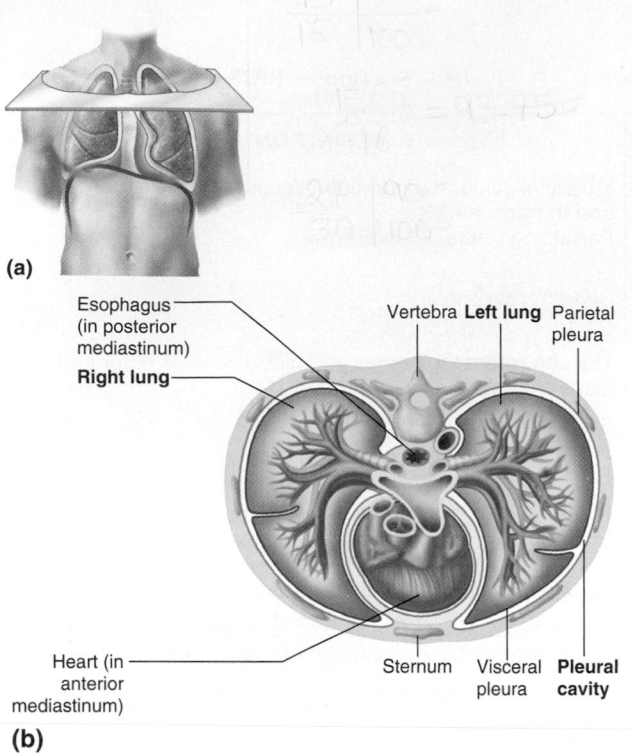

(a)

Esophagus (in posterior mediastinum)

Vertebra **Left lung** Parietal pleura

Right lung

Heart (in anterior mediastinum)

Sternum Visceral **Pleural**
         pleura   **cavity**

(b)

▲ **Figure 13.10** **Pleural Cavity and Membranes**
(a) Site of Cross-section of Superior View.
(b) Pleural Cavity and Membranes in the Superior View.

LO 13.1, 13.2, 13.6 Lower Respiratory Tract (continued)

Pleurae

The surface of each lung is covered with a serous membrane called the **visceral pleura** (*Figure 13.10*). At the hilum, the visceral pleura turns back on itself to form the **parietal pleura**, which lines the rib cage. The space between the visceral and parietal pleurae is called the **pleural cavity**, which contains a thin film of lubricant called the **pleural fluid**.

The functions of the **pleurae** and pleural fluid are to

1. **Reduce friction**. The lubricant quality of the pleural fluid enables the lungs to expand (**inspiration**) and contract (**expiration**) with minimal friction.

2. **Assist in inspiration**. The pressure in the pleural cavity is lower than the pressure of the atmospheric air in the lungs. This assists the **inflation** of the lungs on inspiration.

3. **Separation**. The **pleurae**, **mediastinum**, and **pericardium** protect the organs inside them to prevent infections from spreading easily from one organ to another.

Tracheobronchial Tree

As the inhaled air continues down the respiratory tract, the trachea divides and air flows into the right and left main (primary) bronchi, which enter each lung at the hilum.

In turn, the main bronchi divide into a secondary (lobar) bronchus for each lobe. There are three secondary bronchi in the right lung and two in the left lung. Each secondary bronchus divides into tertiary bronchi that supply segments of each lobe (*Figure 13.11*).

Bronchioles and Alveoli

The tertiary bronchi divide into **bronchioles**, which in turn divide into **terminal bronchioles** and then smaller respiratory bronchioles (*Figure 13.12*). None of these bronchioles has cartilage in the walls, but smooth muscle enables them to dilate or constrict. These bronchioles in turn divide into thin-walled alveoli.

Each alveolus is a thin-walled sac with its cells supported by a thin **respiratory membrane** that allows the exchange of gases with the surrounding pulmonary capillary network (*Figure 13.12*). About 5% of the alveolar cells secrete a detergent-like substance called **surfactant** that keeps the alveolar sacs from collapsing. There are approximately 300 million alveoli in the two lungs.

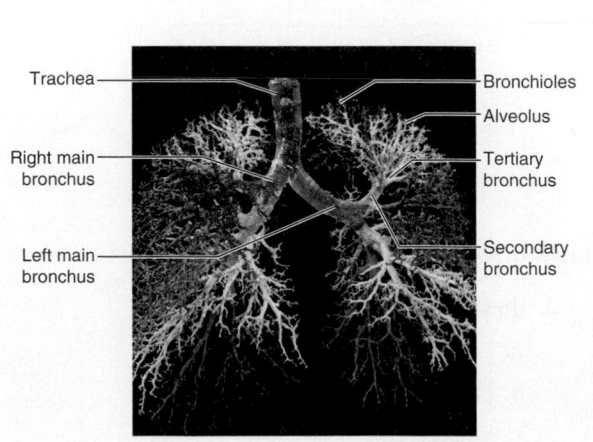

Trachea

Right main bronchus

Left main bronchus

Bronchioles

Alveolus

Tertiary bronchus

Secondary bronchus

▲ **Figure 13.11** Latex Cast of Tracheobronchial Tree.

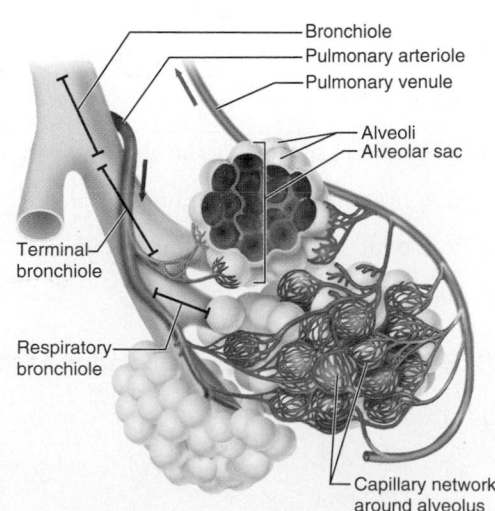

Bronchiole
Pulmonary arteriole
Pulmonary venule

Alveoli
Alveolar sac

Terminal bronchiole

Respiratory bronchiole

Capillary network around alveolus

▲ **Figure 13.12** Bronchioles and Alveoli.

WORD	PRONUNCIATION	ELEMENTS		DEFINITION
expiration (opposite of inspiration) (***Note:*** The "s" is deleted from the root spir- because the prefix ex- already has the "s" sound.)	**EKS**-pih-**RAY**-shun	S/ P/ R/	-ation *process* ex- *out* **-spir-** *to breathe*	Breathe out
inflate (verb) **inflation (noun)** (same as inspiration)	in-**FLAYT** in-**FLAY**-shun	S/ P/ R/	Latin *blow up* -ation *process* in- *into* **-flat-** *blow up*	Expand with air Process of expanding with air
inspiration (opposite of expiration)	in-spih-**RAY**-shun	S/ P/ R/	-ation *process* in- *into* **-spir-** *to breathe*	Breathe in
parietal	pah-**RYE**-eh-tal	S/ R/	-al *pertaining to* **pariet-** *wall*	Pertaining to the outer layer of the pericardium and other body cavities
pericardium	per-ih-**KAR**-dee-um	S/ P/ R/	-um *tissue, structure* peri- *around* **-cardi-** *heart*	The tissue covering the heart
pleura **pleurae (pl)** **pleural (adj)** **pleurisy** **pleuritic (adj)**	**PLUR**-ah **PLUR**-ee **PLUR**-al **PLUR**-ih-see **PLUR**-it-ik	S/ R/ S/ S/	Greek *rib, side* -al *pertaining to* **pleur-** *pleura* -isy *inflammation* -itic *pertaining to*	Membrane covering the lungs and lining the ribs in the thoracic cavity Pertaining to the pleura Inflammation of the pleura Pertaining to pleurisy
surfactant	ser-**FAK**-tant	S/ R/ R/	-ant *pertaining to* **surf-** *surface* **-act-** *to do, perform*	A protein and fat compound that creates surface tension to hold lung alveolar walls apart

Exercises

A. Make the above WAD box work for you. *The following questions can all be answered with information you will find in this WAD. Insert the correct terms in the appropriate space.* **LO 13.1, 13.6**

1. A membrane covering the lung and lining the ribs is the _____. The plural of this term is _____. You need the adjective form of this term to describe the _____ membrane.

2. The two opposite terms that relate to the breathing process are _____, which means _____, and _____, which means _____.

3. The root **spir** means to _____.

4. The purpose of **surfactant** is to _____.

5. **Parietal** pertains to the outer layer of the _____.

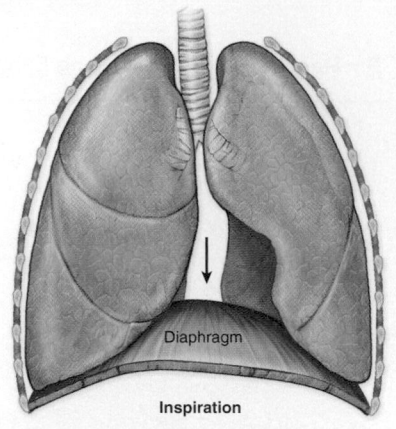

Inspiration

Diaphragm contracts; vertical
dimensions of thoracic cavity increase.

(a)

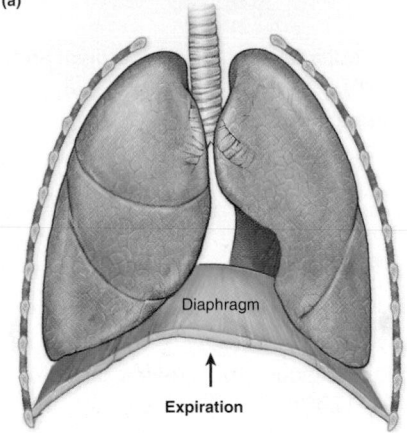

Expiration

Diaphragm relaxes; vertical
dimensions of thoracic cavity decrease.

(b)

▲ **Figure 13.13** Inspiration and
Expiration.

Keynotes

• **Hiccups** are reflex spasms of
the diaphragm, causing an
involuntary inhalation followed
by a sudden closure of the glottis that produces an audible
sound—the "hic." The etiology
is unknown, and there is no
specific medical cure.

• **Yawning** is a reflex that
originates in the brainstem in
response to hypoxia, boredom,
or sleepiness. The exact mechanisms are not known.

LO 13.6 Mechanics of Respiration

A resting adult breathes 10 to 15 times per minute, **inhales** about 500 mL of air during
inspiration, and **exhales** it during expiration. The mission is to get air into and out of the
alveoli so that O_2 can get into the blood and CO_2 can get out of the blood.

The diaphragm does most of the work. In inspiration it drops down and flattens to expand
the volume of the thoracic cavity and reduce the pressure in the airways (*Figure 13.13a*). In
addition, the external intercostal muscles lift the chest wall up and out to further expand
the thoracic cavity.

Expiration is a passive process of letting go. The diaphragm and the intercostal muscles
relax, and the thoracic cavity springs back to its original volume (*Figure 13.13b*).

Not all the inhaled air can get all the way down into the alveoli. The air that does not
get into the alveoli and remains in the mouth, pharynx, trachea, and bronchi down to the
respiratory bronchioles is said to be in the **anatomical dead space.**

LO 13.7 Common Symptoms and Signs of Respiratory Disorders

1. **Coughing** is triggered by irritants in the respiratory tract. You close the glottis and
contract the muscles of expiration to develop high pressure in the lower tract. Then
you suddenly open the glottis to release an explosive blast of air.

   The irritants can be cigarette smoke (as with Mr. Jacobs) or infection or tumors
(as in lung cancer). A productive cough produces sputum that can be swallowed or
expectorated. Bloody sputum is called **hemoptysis**. Thick, yellow (purulent) sputum
indicates infection. A nonproductive cough is dry and hacking. Abnormal amounts of
expectorated clear mucus are called **phlegm.**

2. **Dyspnea**, or shortness of breath (SOB), can be on exertion or, in severe disorders, at
rest when all the respiratory muscles can exchange only a small volume of air.

   Dyspnea can result from airway obstruction. Wheezing associated with dyspnea is
the sound of air being forced through constricted airways, as in asthma. Dyspnea can
also be produced by fibrosis of lung tissues, when the lungs' **compliance** is reduced.
Compliance is the ability of the lungs to expand on inspiration.

3. **Cyanosis** is seen when the blood has increased levels of **unoxygenated hemoglobin**,
which has a characteristic dark gray–blue color. The color is best seen in the lips,
mucous membranes, and nail beds where there is no skin pigmentation to mask it.

   • **Peripheral cyanosis** occurs when there is peripheral vasoconstriction. The
   reduced flow allows hemoglobin to yield more of its O_2, leading to increased
   unoxygenated hemoglobin.

   • **Central cyanosis** occurs with inadequate blood oxygenation in the lungs as a result
   of impaired airflow or impaired blood flow through the lungs.

4. **Changes in rate of breathing. Eupnea** is the normal, easy, automatic respiration—
around 15 breaths per minute in a resting adult. Both **tachypnea** (rapid rate of breathing)
and **hyperpnea** (breathing deeper and more rapidly than normal) are signs of
respiratory difficulty, as is **bradypnea** (slow breathing).

5. **Sneezing** is caused by irritants in the nasal cavity. The glottis stays open while the soft
palate and tongue block the flow of air from getting out. Then they suddenly release to
let air burst out through the nose.

WORD	PRONUNCIATION	ELEMENTS		DEFINITION
bradypnea (opposite of tachypnea)	brad-ip-**NEE**-ah	P/ R/	**brady-** *slow* **-pnea** *breathe*	Slow breathing
compliance	kom-**PLY**-ance	S/ R/	**-ance** *state of, condition* **compli-** *fulfill*	Measure of the capacity of a chamber or hollow viscus to expand, in this case, the lungs
cyanosis	sigh-ah-**NO**-sis	S/ R/	**-osis** *condition* **cyan-** *dark blue*	Blue discoloration of the skin, lips, and nail beds due to low levels of oxygen in the blood
cyanotic (adj)	sigh-ah-**NOT**-ik	S/ R/CF	**-tic** *pertaining to* **cyan/o-** *dark blue*	Marked by cyanosis
dyspnea	disp-**NEE**-ah	P/ R/	**dys-** *bad, difficult* **-pnea** *breathe*	Difficulty breathing
eupnea	yoop-**NEE**-ah	P/ R/	**eu-** *normal* **-pnea** *breathe*	Normal breathing
exhale	**EKS**-hail	P/ R/	**ex-** *out* **-hale** *breathe*	Breathe out
expectorate	ek-**SPEC**-toh-rate	S/ P/ R/	**-ate** *composed of* **ex-** *out* **-pector-** *chest*	Cough up and spit out mucus from the respiratory tract
hemoptysis	he-**MOP**-tih-sis	R/CF R/	**hem/o-** *blood* **-ptysis** *spit*	Bloody sputum
hyperpnea	high-perp-**NEE**-ah	P/ R/	**hyper-** *excessive* **-pnea** *breathe*	Deeper and more rapid breathing than normal
inhale	**IN**-hail	P/ R/	**in-** *in* **-hale** *breathe*	Breathe in
phlegm	FLEM		Greek *flame*	Abnormal amounts of mucus expectorated from the respiratory tract
tachypnea (opposite of bradypnea)	tak-ip-**NEE**-ah	P/ R/	**tachy-** *rapid* **-pnea** *breathe*	Rapid breathing

Exercises

A. Build terms. *Knowing just one element will enable you to build more terms with the addition of other elements. Practice building your pulmonology terms with the following root and various prefixes. Fill in the blanks.* **LO 13.3, 13.6, 13.7**

1. The root -*pnea* means _____.

Add the following prefixes to the root -pnea to form new terms for questions 2 through 6.

tachy   brady   dys   eu   hyper

2. Difficult breathing   _____pnea

3. Deeper breathing than normal   _____pnea

4. Slow breathing   _____pnea

5. Normal breathing   _____pnea

6. Rapid breathing   _____pnea

B. Employ your new medical vocabulary to answer the following questions.   LO 13.3, 13.6, 13.7

Medical Terminology Challenge question:

1. Describe what and where the anatomical dead space is.

   a. What is it? _____

   b. Where is it? _____

> **Study Hint**
> Remember the prefixes in the preceding WAD—they can be applied to many other roots for new terms.

LO 13.9 Disorders of the Lower Respiratory Tract

Acute bronchitis can be viral or bacterial, leading to the production of excess mucus with some obstruction of airflow. A single episode resolves without significant residual damage to the airway.

Chronic bronchitis is the most common obstructive disease, due to cigarette smoking or repeated episodes of acute bronchitis. In addition to excess mucus production, cilia are destroyed. A pattern develops, involving chronic cough, sputum production, dyspnea, and recurrent acute infections.

In advanced chronic bronchitis, hypoxia and **hypercapnia** (excess CO_2) develop and heart failure follows.

Bronchiolitis, inflammation of the small airway bronchioles, occurs in the adult as the early and often unrecognized beginning of airway changes in cigarette smokers or those exposed to "secondhand smoke," inhaling the smoke produced by other peoples' cigarettes.

Bronchiolitis affects children under the age of 2 because their small airways become blocked very easily. The disease is viral and in severe cases can cause marked respiratory distress, with drawing in of the neck and intercostal spaces of the chest with each breath (known as **retractions**).

Pulmonary emphysema is a disease of the respiratory bronchioles and alveoli. These airways become enlarged, and the septa between the alveoli are destroyed, forming large sacs **(bullae)**. There is a loss of surface area for gas exchange. Because the septa contain elastic tissue that assists the lungs' recoil in exhalation, recoil becomes more difficult, and air is trapped in the bullae. This leads to **hyperinflation** of the lungs and the enlarged "barrel chest" shown by many patients with emphysema.

Chronic airway obstruction (CAO) is also called **chronic obstructive pulmonary disease (COPD)**. This is a progressive disease, as Mr. Jacobs' history shows. It involves both chronic bronchitis and emphysema. A history of heavy cigarette smoking, with chronic cough and sputum production, is followed by exertional dyspnea. By the time Mr. Jacobs' dyspnea was severe, irreversible lung damage *(Figure 13.14)* had led to emphysema, recurrent infections, and episodes of respiratory insufficiency. The insufficiency became permanent, and supplementary O_2 is now necessary round the clock. Right-sided heart failure **(cor pulmonale)** is the end-result of pulmonary hypertension and blood backing up into the right ventricle *(see Chapter 10)*.

Bronchiectasis is the abnormal dilatation of the small bronchioles due to repeated infections. The damaged, dilated bronchi are unable to clear secretions, so additional infections and more damage can occur.

Bronchial asthma is a disorder with recurrent acute episodes of bronchial obstruction as a result of constriction of bronchioles **(bronchoconstriction)**, **hypersecretion** of mucus, and inflammatory swelling of the bronchiolar lining. The airflow obstruction these produce is mainly during expiration, and the wheezing exhalation heard in asthma is the result of forcing air out of the lungs through constricted, swollen bronchioles. Between attacks, breathing can be normal. The **etiology** of asthma is an allergic response to substances such as pollen, animal dander, or the feces of house dust mites.

Cystic fibrosis (CF) is caused by an increased viscosity of secretions from the pancreas, salivary glands, liver, intestine, and lungs. In the lungs, a particularly thick mucus obstructs the airways and causes repeated infections. Respiratory failure is the cause of death, often before the age of 30. The disorder is genetic.

Pulmonary edema is the collection of fluid in the lung tissues and alveoli. It is most frequently the result of left ventricular failure or mitral valve disease with **congestive heart failure (CHF)**. Noncardiogenic pulmonary edema can result from sepsis, renal failure, disseminated intravascular coagulation (DIC) *(see Chapter 11)*, and opiate or barbiturate poisoning *(see Chapter 10)*.

In many disorders of the lower respiratory tract, during **auscultation** of the chest the air bubbling through abnormal fluid in the alveoli and small bronchioles (as in pulmonary edema) produces a noise called **rales**. When the bronchi are partly obstructed and air is being forced past an obstruction, a high-pitched noise called a **rhonchus** is heard.

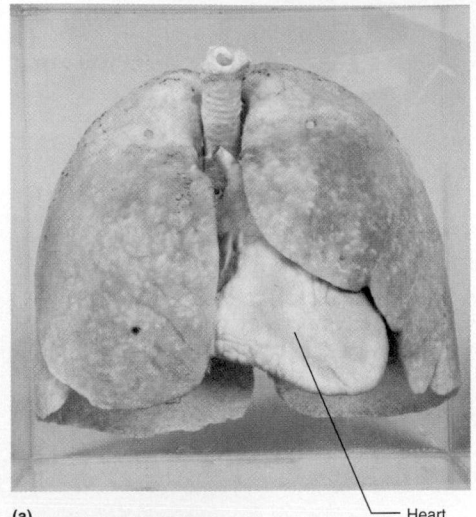

(a)

— Heart

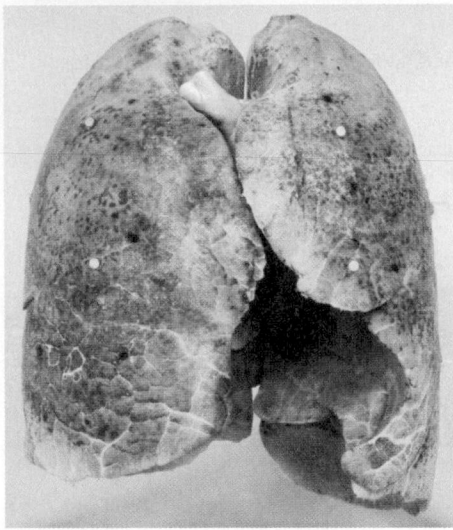

(b)

▲ **Figure 13.14** **Whole Lungs.**
(*a*) Nonsmoker's lungs. (*b*) Smoker's lungs.

Abbreviations

CAO	chronic airway obstruction
CF	cystic fibrosis
CHF	congestive heart failure
COPD	chronic obstructive pulmonary disease
DIC	disseminated intravascular coagulation

S = Suffix   P = Prefix   R = Root   R/CF = Combining Form

WORD	PRONUNCIATION	ELEMENTS		DEFINITION
asthma **asthmatic** (adj)	**AZ**-mah az-**MAT**-ic		Greek *asthma*	Episodes of breathing difficulty due to narrowed or obstructed airways
auscultation	aws-kul-**TAY**-shun	S/ R/	-ation *process* **auscult-** *listen to*	Diagnostic method of listening to body sounds with a stethoscope
bronchiectasis	brong-kee-**ECK**-tah-sis	S/ R/CF	-ectasis *dilation* **bronch/i-** *bronchus*	Chronic dilation of the bronchi following inflammatory disease and obstruction
bronchiolitis (*Note:* This term has two suffixes— the "e" is dropped before the "i" in -itis.)	brong-kee-oh-**LYE**-tis	S/ S/ R/CF	-itis *inflammation* -ole *small* **bronch/i-** *bronchus*	Inflammation of the small bronchioles
bronchoconstriction	**BRONG**-koh-kon-**STRIK**-shun	S/ R/CF R/	-ion *process* **bronch/o-** *bronchus* -constrict- *to narrow*	Reduction in diameter of a bronchus
bulla **bullae** (pl)	**BULL**-ah **BULL**-ee		Latin *bubble*	Bubble-like dilated structure
cor pulmonale	KOR pul-moh-**NAH**-lee	R/ S/ R/	**cor** *heart* -ale *pertaining to* **pulmon-** *lung*	Right-sided heart failure arising from chronic lung disease
cystic fibrosis (CF)	**SIS**-tik fie-**BRO**-sis	S/ R/ S/ R/	-ic *pertaining to* **cyst-** *cyst* -osis *condition* **fibr-** *fiber*	Genetic disease in which excessive viscid mucus obstructs passages, including bronchi
emphysema	em-fih-**SEE**-mah	P/ R/	em- *in, into* -physema *blowing*	Dilation of respiratory bronchioles and alveoli
hypercapnia	**HIGH**-per-**KAP**-nee-ah	S/ P/ R/	-ia *condition* hyper- *excessive* -capn- *carbon dioxide*	Abnormal increase of carbon dioxide in the arterial bloodstream
hyperinflation	**HIGH**-per-in-**FLAY**-shun	S/ P/ P/ R/	-ion *process* hyper- *excessive* in- *in* -flat- *blow up*	Overdistension of pulmonary alveoli with air resulting from airway obstruction
hypersecretion	**HIGH**-per-seh-**KREE**-shun	S/ P/ R/	-ion *process* hyper- *excessive* -secret- *secrete*	Excessive secretion of mucus (or enzymes or waste products)
retraction	ree-**TRAK**-shun	S/ P/ R/	-ion *process* re- *back* -tract- *pull*	A pulling back, as a pulling back of the inter-costal spaces and the neck above the clavicle
rhonchus **rhonchi** (pl)	**RONG**-kuss **RONG**-key		Greek *snoring*	Wheezing sound heard on auscultation of the lungs, made by air passing through a con-stricted lumen

Exercises

A. These elements all appear in the *language of pulmonology*. *Challenge your knowledge of these elements, and make the correct match.*
  Fill in the blanks. **LO 13.3, 13.9**

_____ 1. re

_____ 2. auscult

_____ 3. capn

_____ 4. ole

_____ 5. osis

_____ 6. constrict

_____ 7. ion

_____ 8. tract

_____ 9. ectasis

_____ 10. bronchi

a. to narrow

b. process

c. pull

d. dilation

e. back

f. CO$_2$

g. listen to

h. bronchus

i. small

j. condition

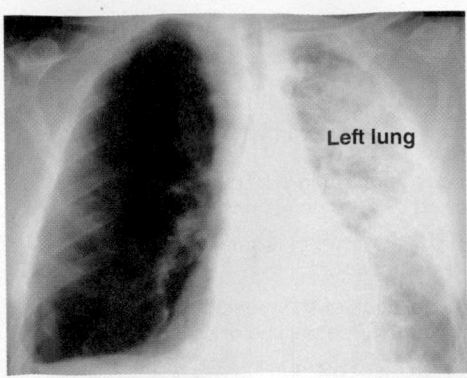

▲ Figure 13.15 **Chest X-Ray of Patient with Pneumonia in the Left Lung.** A normal lung appears as mostly black space but with some lung markings on an x-ray because its spongy structure is filled with air. In contrast, a pneumonic lung appears white or opaque on an x-ray as a result of accumulation of fluid and cells in the alveoli.

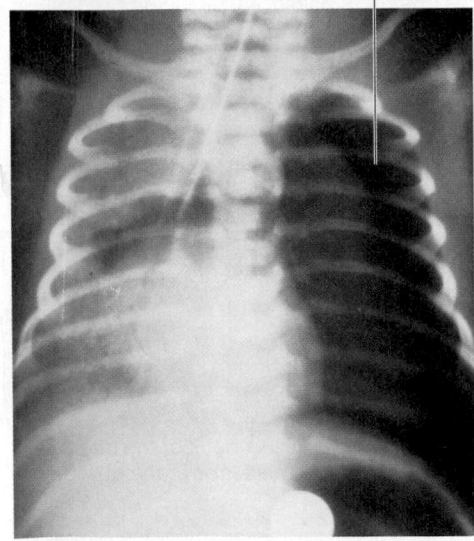

▲ Figure 13.16 **Left Pneumothorax.** There are no lung markings seen in the area of the pneumothorax.

Abbreviations

ARDS acute respiratory distress syndrome
ARF acute respiratory failure
NRDS neonatal respiratory distress syndrome

LO 13.9 Disorders of the Lower Respiratory Tract (continued)

Pneumonia is an acute infection affecting the alveoli and lung parenchyma (*Figure 13.15*). Bacterial infections focus on the alveoli, viral infections on the parenchyma. **Lobar pneumonia** is an infection limited to one lung lobe. **Bronchopneumonia** is used to describe an infection in the bronchioles that spreads to the alveoli.

When an area of the lung (**segment**) or a lobe becomes airless as a result of the infection, the lung is **consolidated**. When an area of the lung collapses as a result of bronchial obstruction, the condition is called **atelectasis**.

Pleurisy, an inflammation of the pleurae, can be a complication of pneumonia. This condition is very painful on breathing. The inflammation often leads to an exudate accumulating in the pleural cavity—a **pleural effusion**. If the pleural effusion contains pus, it is called **empyema**. If it contains blood, it is called **hemothorax**. When pleural fluid is drawn off for therapeutic purposes or for laboratory analysis, the procedure is **aspiration**, or **thoracentesis**.

Lung abscess can be a complication of bacterial pneumonia or cancer. Long-term antibiotics are used, and surgical resection of the abscess may be required.

Pneumothorax is the entry of air into the pleural cavity (*Figure 13.16*). The cause can be unknown (**spontaneous pneumothorax**), but it often results from trauma when a fractured rib, knife blade, or bullet lacerates the parietal pleura.

Thromboembolism is caused by an embolus, usually arising in the deep vein of the calf and lodging in a branch of the pulmonary artery. The symptoms are chest pain, dyspnea, tachypnea (increased respiratory rate), and a reduction in blood O_2 levels.

Acute respiratory distress syndrome (ARDS) is sudden life-threatening lung failure caused by a variety of underlying conditions, from major trauma to sepsis. The alveoli fill with fluid and collapse, and gas exchange is shut down. Hypoxia results. Mechanical ventilation has to be provided. The mortality is from 35% to 50%.

Neonatal respiratory distress syndrome (NRDS) is seen in premature babies whose lungs have not matured enough to produce surfactant. The alveoli collapse, and mechanical ventilation is needed to keep them open.

Chronic infections of the lung parenchyma are the result of prolonged exposure to infection or to occupational irritant dusts or droplets. These disorders are called **pneumoconioses**. Levels of dust inhalation overwhelm the airways' particle-clearing abilities; the dust particles accumulate in the alveoli and parenchyma, leading to fibrosis. **Asbestosis** from inhaling asbestos particles can lead to a cancer (**mesothelioma**) in the pleura. **Silicosis** from silica particles is called *stone mason's lung*. **Anthracosis** from coal dust particles is called *coal miners' lung*. **Sarcoidosis** is an **idiopathic** fibrotic disorder of the lung parenchyma.

Pulmonary tuberculosis is a chronic, infectious disease of the lungs.

Lung cancer, related to tobacco use, used to be a male disease, but now fatalities in women from lung cancer exceed those from breast cancer. Ninety percent of lung cancers arise in the mucous membranes of the larger bronchi and are called **bronchogenic carcinomas**. The tumor obstructs the bronchus, spreads into the surrounding lung tissues, and metastasizes to lymph nodes, liver, brain, and bone.

Acute respiratory failure (ARF) is abnormal respiratory function resulting in inadequate tissue oxygenation or CO_2 elimination that is severe enough to impair vital organ functions. Causes of ARF include congestive heart failure (CHF), chronic obstructive pulmonary disease (COPD,) chest trauma with resultant **flail chest**, spinal cord injury, and neuromuscular disorders in which the muscles of respiration are weak or paralyzed. Endotracheal intubation and mechanical ventilation are used until the underlying cause is treated, if possible.

Word Analysis and Definition

S = Suffix   P = Prefix   R = Root   R/CF = Combining Form

WORD	PRONUNCIATION	ELEMENTS		DEFINITION
anthracosis	an-thra-**KOH**-sis	S/ R/	**-osis** *condition* **anthrac-** *coal*	Lung disease caused by the inhalation of coal dust
asbestosis	as-bes-**TOE**-sis	S/ R/	**-osis** *condition* **asbest-** *asbestos*	Lung disease caused by the inhalation of asbestos particles
atelectasis	at-el-**ECK**-tah-sis	S/ R/	**-ectasis** *dilation* **atel-** *incomplete*	Collapse of part of a lung
bronchogenic	brong-koh-**JEN**-ik	S/ R/CF	**-genic** *creation* **bronch/o-** *bronchus*	Arising from a bronchus
bronchopneumonia	**BRONG**-koh-new-**MOH**-nee-ah	S/ R/ R/CF	**-ia** *condition* **-pneumon-** *air, lung* **bronch/o-** *bronchus*	Acute inflammation of the walls of smaller bronchioles with spread to lung parenchyma
empyema	**EM**-pie-**EE**-mah	S/ P/ R/	**-ema** *result* **em-** *in* **-py-** *pus*	Pus in a body cavity, particularly in the pleural cavity
flail chest	FLAIL CHEST		flail Old English *flapping*	Condition in which three or more consecutive ribs have been fractured, resulting in uncontrolled movement of that segment of the chest
hemothorax	he-moh-**THOR**-ax	R/CF R/	**hem/o-** *blood* **-thorax** *chest*	Blood in the pleural cavity
idiopathic	**ID**-ih-oh-**PATH**-ik	S/ R/CF R/	**-ic** *pertaining to* **idi/o-** *personal, distinct* **-path-** *disease*	Pertaining to a disease of unknown etiology
mesothelioma	**MEZ**-oh-thee-lee-**OH**-mah	S/ P/ R/CF	**-oma** *tumor, mass* **meso-** *middle* **-thel/i-** *lining*	Cancer arising from the cells lining the pleura or peritoneum
pneumonia pneumonitis (syn)	new-**MOH**-nee-ah new-moh-**NI**-tis	S/ R/ S/	**-ia** *condition* **-pneumon-** *air, lung* **-itis** *inflammation*	Inflammation of the lung parenchyma
pneumoconiosis	new-moh-koh-nee-**OH**-sis	S/ R/ R/CF	**-osis** *condition* **-coni-** *dust* **pneum/o-** *air, lung*	Fibrotic lung disease caused by the inhalation of different dusts
pneumothorax	new-moh-**THOR**-ax	R/CF R/	**pneum/o-** *air, lung* **-thorax** *chest*	Air in the pleural cavity
sarcoidosis (***Note:*** Two suffixes.)	sar-koy-**DOH**-sis	S/ S/ R/	**-osis** *condition* **-oid-** *resembling* **sarc-** *sarcoma*	Granulomatous lesions of lungs and other organs; cause is unknown
silicosis	sil-ih-**KOH**-sis	S/ R/	**-osis** *condition* **silic-** *silicon*	Fibrotic lung disease from inhaling silica particles
thoracentesis pleural tap (syn)	**THOR**-ah-sen-**TEE**-sis	S/ R/	**-centesis** *to puncture* **thora-** *chest*	Insertion of a needle into the pleural cavity to withdraw fluid or air
thromboembolism	**THROM**-boh-**EM**-boh-lizm	S/ R/CF R/	**-ism** *condition* **thromb/o-** *blood clot* **-embol-** *plug*	A piece of detached blood clot (embolus) blocking a distant blood vessel
tuberculosis	too-**BER**-kyu-**LOW**-sis	S/ R/	**-osis** *condition* **tubercul-** *nodule, tuberculosis*	Infectious disease that can infect any organ or tissue

Exercises

A. Suffixes. *The above WAD contains a lot of suffixes you will see again in later chapters for other medical terms. Confirm your knowledge of suffixes by filling in the chart with the correct meaning of the element.*   **LO 13.3, 13.9**

Suffix	Meaning of Suffix	Medical Term with This Suffix	Meaning of Term
-centesis	1.	2.	3.
-ectasis	4.	5.	6.
-ema	7.	8.	9.
-genic	10.	11.	12.
-ia	13.	14.	15.

LO 13.10 Pulmonary Function Tests

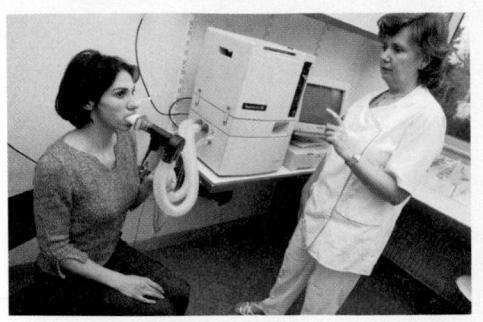

▲ Figure 13.17 Spirometer.

A **spirometer** is a device used to measure the **volume** of air that moves in and out of the respiratory system *(Figure 13.17)*. You ask the patient to breathe in as deeply as possible and then breathe out as rapidly and completely as possible through the spirometer. The volume of air expired at the end of this **pulmonary function test (PFT)** is the patient's **forced vital capacity (FVC)**.

The spirometer also measures **flow rates**. The **forced expiratory volume in 1 second** (FEV_1) is the amount of air expired in the first second of the test.

In obstructive lung disorders such as asthma or COPD, the lumina of the airways are constricted and resistant to airflow. This will cause a reduction in the FEV_1.

In restrictive lung disorders in which the lung tissue is fibrotic or scarred and resists expansion, there will be a reduction in the FVC.

Keynote

Measure pulmonary function with spirometers, peak flow meters, and ABGs.

Abbreviations

FEV_1	forced expiratory volume in 1 second
FVC	forced vital capacity
msec	millisecond
PEFR	peak expiratory flow rate
PFT	pulmonary function test

Keynote

- A **nebulizer** is an electronic device that transforms a liquid medication into a fine mist that can be inhaled deeply into the lungs.
- A nebulizer treatment takes between 10 and 20 minutes.
- A **metered-dose inhaler** (MDI) is a plastic and metal device that delivers a consistent dose of **aerosol** medication that can be inhaled directly into the lungs in 30 seconds.
- An MDI is cheaper, quicker, has fewer side effects and equal effectiveness to a nebulizer.

Case Report 13.1 (continued)

Mr. Jacobs' FEV_1 was only 40% of the predicted value for a man of his age, height, and weight. Mr. Jacobs' FVC was also reduced because of the fibrotic effects of repeated infections on his lung tissues reducing the volume in his airways. When he was off O_2, Mr. Jacobs' O_2 levels were below 50% of normal. Even with nasal prongs and the administration of O_2, his blood O_2 levels were only 75% of normal.

A **peak flow meter** records the greatest flow of air that can be sustained for 10 milliseconds (msec) on forced expiration, the **peak expiratory flow rate (PEFR)**. It is of value in following the course of asthma and, in postoperative care, in monitoring the return of lung function after anesthesia.

Arterial blood gases, the measurement of the levels of O_2 and CO_2 in the blood, are good indicators of respiratory function.

LO 13.11 Pulmonary Pharmacology

- **Bronchodilators** relax the smooth muscles of the bronchioles. Examples are theophylline, beta$_2$-agonists (such as albuterol), and anticholinergics (such as ipratropium bromide).

- **Anti-inflammatory** drugs, such as corticosteroids, are best given by inhalation but can be used orally or intravenously in acute episodes of asthma or COPD.

- **Mucolytics** are agents that break up mucus to allow it to be cleared more effectively from the airways. Examples are guaifenesin (common in over-the-counter cough medications), potassium iodide, and *N*-acetylcysteine taken through a **nebulizer.**

- **Antibiotics** are used when a bacterial infection is present. Penicillin, erythromycin, cefotaxime, and flucloxacillin are frequently used.

- O_2 is used in hypoxia and can be given by nasal **cannulae (prongs)** or by mask and intubation. Patients with severe, chronic COPD can be attached to a portable cylinder of O_2.

WORD	PRONUNCIATION	ELEMENTS		DEFINITION
aerosol	**AIR**-oh sol	R/CF R/	**aer/o** *air* **sol** *solution*	Liquid or particulate material in a stable suspension that can be inhaled
anti-inflammatory	**AN**-tee-in-**FLAM**-ah-tor-ee	S/ P/ R/	**-ory** *having the function of* **anti-** *against* **inflammat-** *set on fire*	Agent that reduces inflammation by acting on the body's response mechanisms without affecting the causative agent
bronchodilator	**BRONG**-koh-die-**LAY**-tor	S/ R/CF R/	**-or** *one who does* **bronch/o-** *bronchus* **-dilat-** *expand*	Agent that increases the diameter of a bronchus
cannula cannulae (pl)	**KAN**-you-lah **KAN**-you-lee		Latin *reed*	Tube inserted into a blood vessel or cavity as a channel for fluid or gas
inhaler	in-**HAIL**-er	S/ P/ R/	**-er** *agent* **in-** *in, into* **-hale-** *breathe*	An instrument to administer medications by inhalation
mucolytic	**MYU**-koh-**LIT**-ik	S/ R/CF R/	**-ic** *pertaining to* **muc/o-** *mucus* **-lyt-** *dissolve*	Agent capable of dissolving or liquefying mucus
nebulizer	**NEB**-you-liz-er	S/ R/	**-izer** *line of action* **nebul-** *cloud*	Device used to deliver liquid medicine in a fine mist
oxygen	**OCK**-see-jen	S/ R/	**-gen** *form, create* **oxy-** *oxygen*	The gas essential for life
spirometer	spy-**ROM**-eh-ter	S/ R/CF	**-meter** *measure* **spir/o-** *to breathe*	An instrument used to measure respiratory volumes

Exercises

A. Deconstruct each of these medical terms into basic elements. *Define the elements; then use each in a sentence that is not a definition to demonstrate that you understand the term's meaning. Fill in the blanks.*   **LO 13.9, 13.10, 13.11**

Medical Term	Meaning of Prefix	Meaning of Root/ Combining Form	Meaning of Suffix	Meaning of Term
nebulizer	1.	2.	3.	4.
spirometer	5.	6.	7.	8.
mucolytic	9.	10.	11.	12.
bronchodilator	13.	14.	15.	16.

1. _____

2. _____

3. _____

4. _____

B. After rereading Case Report 13.1, answer the following questions. *Be prepared to discuss your answers in class.*   **LO 13.9, 13.10, 13.11**

1. Substitute a medical term for the underlined word in the phrase "<u>repeated</u> (_____) infections."

2. Mr. Jacobs' O₂ levels (off supplemental O₂) were below 50% of normal. What medical term would describe this condition?

_____

3. Mr. Jacobs' lung tissue is *fibrotic* because of repeated infections. What limits does fibrosis present to his lung function from now on?

_____

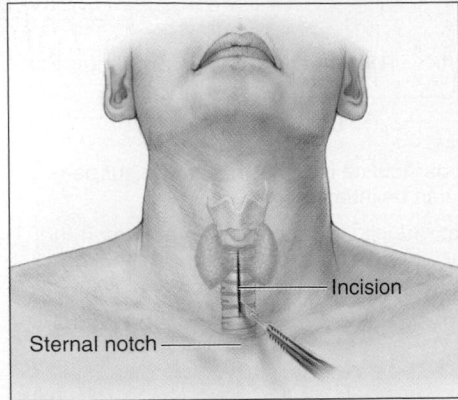

① Tracheotomy incision is made superior to sternal notch.

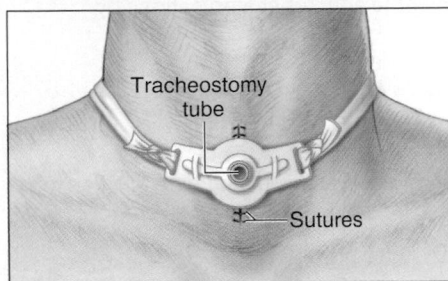

② A tracheostomy tube is inserted, and the remaining incision is sutured closed.

▲ **Figure 13.18** Tracheostomy Procedure.

Abbreviations

AP	anteroposterior
ARDS	adult respiratory distress syndrome
CPAP	continuous positive airway pressure
CT	computed tomography
CXR	chest x-ray
MRA	magnetic resonance angiography
NRDS	neonatal respiratory distress syndrome
PA	posteroanterior
PDT	postural drainage therapy
PEEP	positive end-expiratory pressure
PET	positron emission tomography

Keynotes

- **Pulmonary resection** is the surgical removal of lung tissue.
- **Wedge resection** is the removal of a small localized area of diseased lung.
- **Segmentectomy** is the removal of lung tissue attached to a bronchus.
- **Lobectomy** is the removal of a lobe.
- **Pneumonectomy** is the removal of an entire lung.

LO 13.10 Diagnostic and Therapeutic Procedures

Diagnostic Procedures

Chest x-ray (CXR) is a radiograph image of the chest taken in **anteroposterior (AP)**, **posteroanterior (PA)**, lateral, and sometimes oblique and lateral decubitus positions.

Computed tomography (CT), **angiography** of the pulmonary circulation using contrast materials, **magnetic resonance angiography (MRA)** to define emboli in the pulmonary arteries, and **ultrasonography** of the pleural space are chest imaging techniques in current use. **Positron emission tomography (PET)** can sometimes distinguish benign from malignant lesions.

Bronchoscopy is the insertion of a fiber-optic endoscope into the bronchial tree to visually examine it, take a tissue biopsy, or take a wash for secretions.

Mediastinoscopy is used to stage lung cancer and diagnose mediastinal masses. The mediastinoscope is inserted through an incision in the sternal notch.

Tracheal aspiration uses a soft catheter that allows brushings and washings to be performed to remove cells and secretions from the trachea and main bronchi. It can be passed through a tracheostomy, **endotracheal** tube, or the mouth or nose.

Thoracentesis is the insertion of a needle through an intercostal space to remove fluid from a pleural effusion for laboratory study or to relieve pressure. It is also called a **pleural tap**.

Thoracotomy is used to obtain an open biopsy of tissue from the lung, hilum, pleura, or mediastinum. It is performed through an intercostal incision under general anesthesia.

Therapeutic Procedures

Pulmonary rehabilitation includes education, breathing retraining, exercises for the upper and lower extremities, and psychosocial support.

Nutritional support is critical for patients who have difficulty breathing or who lose a lot of weight.

Immunizations are available against influenza and the pneumococcus bacterium, the most common cause of bacterial pneumonia.

Postural drainage therapy (PDT) uses gravity to promote drainage of secretions from lung segments by positioning and tilting the patient. Chest percussion (tapping) can help loosen, mobilize, and drain the retained secretions.

Continuous positive airway pressure (CPAP) is an attempt to keep the airway open by maintaining a positive pressure. A mask is fitted over the nose and mouth and attached to a ventilator. This can be used at night when a person is sleeping for sleep apnea or in acute situations for COPD.

Positive end-expiratory pressure (PEEP) is a technique in ventilation to keep the alveoli from collapsing in conditions such as **adult respiratory distress syndrome (ARDS)** and **neonatal respiratory distress syndrome (NRDS)**.

Intubation uses an oropharyngeal airway in the unconscious patient during bag-and-mask ventilation to maintain an open airway. A tube is inserted to prevent the tongue from falling back to obstruct the airway and facilitates suctioning the airway.

Endotracheal intubation involves the placement of a tube into the trachea. This allows patients to be placed on a ventilator and their breathing controlled.

Tracheotomy is an incision made into the trachea (windpipe) so that a temporary or permanent opening into the windpipe, called a **tracheostomy**, can be created (*Figure 13.18*). A tracheostomy tube is placed into the opening to provide an airway. A tracheostomy is used to maintain an airway when there is obstruction or paralysis in the respiratory structures above it and for long-term ventilation.

Mechanical ventilation is a process by which gases are moved into and out of the lungs via a device that is set to meet the respiratory requirements of the patient. It requires that a tracheostomy tube or endotracheal tube be attached to the mechanical device (ventilator). It can augment or replace the patient's own ventilatory efforts.

WORD	PRONUNCIATION	ELEMENTS		DEFINITION
bronchoscope	**BRONG**-koh-skope	S/ R/CF	-scope *instrument for viewing* bronch/o- *bronchus*	Endoscope used for bronchoscopy
bronchoscopy	brong-**KOS**-koh-pee	S/	-scopy *to examine*	Examination of the interior of the tracheobronchial tree with an endoscope
endotracheal	en-doh-**TRAY**-kee-al	S/ P/ R/	-al *pertaining to* endo- *inside* -trache- *trachea*	Pertaining to being inside the trachea
lobectomy	low-**BECK**-toe-me	S/ R/	-ectomy *surgical excision* lob- *lobe*	Surgical removal of a lobe of the lungs
mediastinoscopy	**ME**-dee-ass-tih-**NOS**-koh-pee	S/ R/CF	-scopy *to examine* mediastin/o- *mediastinum*	Examination of the mediastinum using an endoscope
pneumonectomy	**NEW**-moh-**NEK**-toe-me	S/ R/	-ectomy *surgical excision* pneumon- *lung, air*	Surgical removal of a lung
resection resect (verb)	ree-**SEK**-shun ree-**SEKT**	S/ P/ R/	-ion *action* re- *back* -sect- *cut off*	Removal of a specific part of an organ or structure
segmentectomy	seg-men-**TEK**-toe-me	S/ R/	-ectomy *surgical excision* segment- *a section*	Surgical excision of a segment of a tissue or organ
thoracotomy	thor-ah-**KOT**-oh-me	S/ R/CF	-tomy *surgical incision* thorac/o- *chest*	Incision through the chest wall
tomography	toe-**MOG**-rah-fee	S/ R/CF	-graphy *process of recording* tom/o- *section*	Radiographic image of a selected slice or section of tissue
tracheostomy tracheotomy	tray-kee-**OST**-oh-me tray-kee-**OT**-oh-me	S/ R/CF S/	-stomy *new opening* trache/o- *trachea* -tomy *surgical incision*	Surgical opening into the windpipe, through which a tube can be inserted to assist breathing Incision made into the trachea to create a tracheostomy
ultrasonography	**UL**-trah-soh-**NOG**-rah-fee	S/ P/ R/CF	-graphy *process of recording* ultra- *beyond* -son/o- *sound*	Delineation of deep structures using sound waves

Exercises

A. Put the following elements into the right combinations to form medical terms for the definitions provided. *Some elements you will use more than once; some elements you will not use at all. Fill in the blanks.* **LO 13.3, 13.10**

endo-	-ectomy	trans-	bronch/o-	-trache/o-	mediastin/o-
lob-	-al	-ator	pharyng/e-	pneumon-	immuniz-
-ation	-son/o-	-tomy	-trache-	in-	-scopy
-sect-	tom/o-	re-	thorac/o-	-stomy	ventil-
-graphy	-ic	-stomy	hyper-	ultra-	-ion

1. Surgical removal of a lung _____

2. Examination of a bronchus _____

3. Radiographic image of a selected slice of tissue _____

4. Image of deep structures using sound waves _____

5. Pertaining to being inside the trachea _____

6. Removal of a specific part of an organ _____

7. Incision through the chest wall _____

8. New opening in the neck to the trachea _____

Respiratory System

Challenge Your Knowledge

A. Plurals. Refresh your memory for the rules of plurals with this exercise. Check (√) whether the given medical term is the singular or plural form. If it is singular, fill in the plural; if it is plural, fill in the singular form. Then write the meaning of the term. Fill in the chart. (**LO 13.3,** *Remember*)

Medical Term	Singular	Plural	Meaning of Medical Term
1. alveolus			2.
3. cilia			4.
5. rale			6.
7. conchae			8.
9. naris			10.

B. Spelling. The following terms come directly from Latin and Greek. Choose the correct spelling based on the definition following the numbers. Circle the best answer. (**LO 13.3,** *Remember*)

1. reed	cannula	canula	canulla
2. passage	miatus	meatis	meatus
3. shell	conca	conka	concha
4. branding iron	cautiry	cautery	cautary
5. lack of breath	apenea	apnea	apnia
6. throat	pharynix	parynix	pharynx
7. ring	cricoid	crickoid	crecoid
8. creaking sound	strideor	stridore	stridor
9. oblong shield	thyrhoid	thiroyd	thyroid
10. nerves enter and leave this area	hylum	hilum	hylim

C. Terminology challenge. Remembering terminology from a body system studied previously, explain the difference between the two terms that follow. (**LO 13.1, 13.3,** *Remember*)

1. hemoptysis:

_____

2. hematemesis:

_____

3. What do both of the preceding terms have in common?

_____

4. What two different body systems do they represent? _____ and _____

D. Pharmacology. For any body system, it is important to know the various types of medications and when they might be prescribed. Demonstrate your knowledge of pharmacology for the respiratory system by assigning the correct drug category in the right column to the statements in the left column. <u>The first one has been done for you.</u> (**LO 13.3, 13.7,** *Understand*)

   D   1. Example: penicillin

_____ 2. Relax smooth muscles of the bronchioles

_____ 3. Corticosteroids

_____ 4. Example: potassium iodide

_____ 5. Used in hypoxia

_____ 6. Used when a bacterial infection is present

_____ 7. Example: theophylline

_____ 8. Best given by inhalation

_____ 9. Administered by nasal cannula

_____ 10. Breaks up mucus

_____ 11. Can be administered with a nebulizer

a. bronchodilators

b. anti-inflammatories

c. mucolytics

d. antibiotics

e. O_2

Respiratory System

E. Interpretation. Use your knowledge of the **language of pulmonology** to understand the Case Report and answer the following questions. Fill in the blanks. (**LO 13.7, 13.8, Understand**)

Case Report 13.1

You are

...an advanced-level RRT working in the Acute Respiratory Care Unit of Fulwood Medical Center with pulmonologist Tavis Senko, MD.

Your patient is

...Mr. Jude Jacobs, a 68-year-old white retired mail carrier, who is known to have COPD and is on continual oxygen by nasal prongs. He has smoked two packs a day for his adult life. Last night, he was unable to sleep because of increased shortness of breath and cough. His cough produced yellow sputum. He had to sit upright in bed to be able to breathe.

VS are T 101.6°F, P 98, R 36, BP 150/90. On examination, he is cyanotic and frightened and has nasal prongs in his nose. Air entry is diminished in both lungs, and there are rales at both bases. You have been ordered to draw blood for ABGs and to measure the amount of air entering and leaving his lungs by using spirometry.

1. What disease appears in Mr. Jacobs' history?

   _____

2. Which particular symptom indicates Mr. Jacobs has an infection?

   _____

3. **Cyanotic** indicates an outward sign the physician can detect. What is it?

   _____

4. Rales heard through a stethoscope indicate the presence of what in the lungs?

   _____

5. What measure has been taken to restore the level of O_2 in Mr. Jacobs' blood?

   _____

6. What will be used to measure Mr. Jacobs' inspiration and expiration volumes?

   _____

7. Where in the Case Report can you substitute an abbreviation for a phrase?

   Abbreviation: _____ Means _____

8. What are Mr. Jacobs' current symptoms and signs? _____

   _____

   _____

9. What is a lay term for *rales*? _____

10. What changes in his lifestyle does Mr. Jacobs need to make to help his breathing?

    _____

F. Roots. Sometimes in medical terminology there can be two roots or combining forms with the same meaning. *Pneum/o-* and *pulmon/o-* are examples. These forms are not interchangeable—the medical term takes either one combining form or the other. Demonstrate your knowledge of the difference between the two elements by choosing the correct form for the terms listed below. (**LO 13.3, 13.5, 13.9,** *Understand*)

> **Study Hint**
> When there are two elements with the same meaning, you must know them both and how to apply them.

1. PFT is the abbreviation for what diagnostic test? _____

2. Acute infection affecting the alveoli and lung parenchyma is called _____.

3. Presence of air in the pleural cavity is called _____.

4. A specialist in the study of the lung is called a _____.

5. Surgical removal of a lung is _____.

6. COPD is the abbreviation for what lung disease? _____

7. Sarcoidosis is a form of which disease? _____

8. Study of the lungs and lung diseases is _____.

G. Understanding. Translate the following sentences into language your patient can understand. (**LO 13.3, 13.5, 13.9,** *Understand*)

1. "The symptoms of a thromboembolism are chest pain, dyspnea, tachypnea, and hypoxia."

_____

_____

2. "Pleurisy, an inflammation of the pleurae, can be a complication of pneumonia."

_____

_____

3. "NRDS is seen in premature babies whose lungs have not matured enough to produce surfactant."

_____

_____

H. Translate from medical language to layman's language. Take the following statement and translate it into layman's language. First, write a simple version of the medical terms in italics. Then reconstruct the following sentence in language a non-medical person could understand. Use your glossary or search online for any terms you can't recall. Fill in the blanks. (**LO 13.3, 13.9,** *Understand*)

1. *Sarcoidosis* is an *idiopathic fibrotic* disorder of the lung *parenchyma*.

sarcoidosis _____

idiopathic _____

fibrotic _____

parenchyma _____

Sentence:

_____

_____

Respiratory System

I. Abbreviations are meant to save time, but you must interpret them correctly. Write out the meaning for the abbreviations in the following sentences. **(LO 13.5, *Understand*)**

1. You have been ordered to draw blood for Mr. Jacobs' ABGs.

   _____

2. Increased viscosity of secretions from the lungs leads to the conclusion that this patient has CF.

   _____

3. PEEP is a technique in ventilation to keep the alveoli from collapsing.

   _____

4. Patient suffers from dyspnea and SOB.

   _____

5. Mrs. White was prescribed medication for her URI.

   _____

6. This patient has been on a ventilator for a week; provisional diagnosis is ARDS or ARF.

   _____

7. PA view of the chest is all that is needed right now.

   _____

8. Mrs. Black is experiencing CAO due to her COPD.

   _____

J. Interpretation. How well do you understand what the physician has written? Translate this physician's order into plain English without any abbreviations. **(LO 13.3, 13.5, *Understand*)**

1. This patient is to have AP and lateral CXRs, followed by a CT, MRI, and PET scan.

   _____

   _____

   _____

K. Translate the following sentence from layman's language into medical language. The words in parentheses need the medical term on the line next to it. Be precise. **(LO 13.3, 13.10, *Understand*)**

1. "A piece of (detached blood clot) _____ that blocks a distant blood vessel is caused by a (clot) _____

   usually arising in the deep vein of the calf and lodging in a branch of the (lung) _____ artery."

   _____

   _____

2. "Magnetic resonance (recording of a blood vessel) _____ is used to define (detached clots) _____

   in the (lung) _____ (blood vessels that carry oxygenated blood) _____."

L. Language of pulmonology. You are a new student in the Respiratory Therapy program. The following questions contain terminology you will use every day on the job. Answer the questions by circling the correct choice. (**LO 13.3, *Understand, Apply***)

1. **Cyanosis** signals deficient oxygenation of blood and will turn nail beds

    a. yellow

    b. red

    c. black

    d. white

    e. blue

2. The shell-shaped bone in the nose is the

    a. meatus

    b. concha

    c. nares

    d. vestibule

    e. choana

3. Which of the following medical terms can be associated with mucopurulent discharge?

    a. pleurisy

    b. sinusitis

    c. epistaxis

    d. pneumonia

    e. nasal polyps

4. A segment of the chest wall separates from the rest of the thoracic cage in

    a. pneumoconiosis

    b. epiglottitis

    c. flail chest

    d. thoracentesis

    e. ARF

5. **Cautery** can be performed electrically or chemically. What is its purpose?

    a. to burn a tissue

    b. to excise a tissue sample for biopsy

    c. to dilate the blood vessels

    d. to sample the blood type

    e. to constrict the blood vessels

Respiratory System

M. Objectives. Meet lesson objectives by briefly explaining the following. (**LO 13.2, 13.3, 13.9,** *Understand, Apply*)

1. Relate the functions of the nose to its structure—in other words—why is the nose constructed the way it is to do the job it's supposed to do?

_____

_____

_____

2. The lungs and the bloodstream work together to get O_2 into and CO_2 out of your body. Explain how this happens, using the terms *inspiration* and *expiration*.

_____

_____

_____

3. Discuss the effects of common disorders of the lungs on overall health. Think of everyday life and how you would manage if your breathing was compromised.

_____

_____

_____

4. Describe how sound is *produced.* What organs are working to help you make sounds and form speech?

_____

_____

_____

5. Explain how smells are recognized. What aids in their recognition? How does the brain get this information? Why are dogs so sensitive to smell and used to sniff out drugs, cadavers, and explosives?

_____

_____

_____

6. Trace the flow of air from the nose to the alveoli. Be sure to include all the major respiratory organs the air travels through.

_____

_____

_____

N. In your own words. Do you understand the following terms well enough to explain the difference to patients if they should ask? (**LO 13.2, 13.3, 13.6,** *Understand, Apply*)

What is the difference between

1. inspiration:

_____

expiration:

_____

aspiration:

_____

2. pneumothorax:

_____

hemothorax:

_____

3. wedge resection:

_____

segmentectomy:

_____

O. Construct terms. The suffix *-itis* is one that you will meet over and over again in this book. Build the correct medical term to match its definition. Fill in the blanks. (**LO 13.8, 13.9,** *Apply*)

1. inflammation of the bronchus   _____itis

2. inflammation of the organ of voice production   _____itis

3. inflammation of the tonsils   _____itis

4. inflammation of the throat   _____itis

5. inflammation of the nose   _____itis

6. inflammation of the epiglottis   _____itis

7. croup   _____itis

8. inflammation of the small bronchioles   _____itis

9. inflammation of the lung parenchyma   _____itis

Respiratory System

P. Analyze. Knowledge of medical terms includes choosing the correct term for the meaning you want to convey either verbally or in documentation. Analyze the suffixes to help you choose the term. Use the following medical terms to fill in the statements, all relating to the bronchus. **(LO 13.1, 13.3, 13.9, 13.10, 13.11,** *Apply, Analyze*)

bronchogenic	bronchi	bronchopneumonia	bronchioles	bronchiolitis
bronchus	bronchial asthma	bronchial	bronchitis	bronchiectasis

1. Greek word for *windpipe*: _____

2. Plural of the word in question 1: _____

3. Pertaining to the windpipe: _____

4. Tertiary bronchi divide into these: _____

5. Inflammation of the bronchus: _____

6. Abnormal dilation of bronchioles due to repeated infections: _____

7. Infection in the bronchioles that usually spreads to the alveoli: _____

8. Inflammation of the bronchioles: _____

9. Recurrent acute episodes of bronchial obstruction due to constriction: _____

10. Arising from a bronchus: _____

> **Study Hint**
>
> In the term **broncho-pneumonia**, the combining form is used, and it is one word. In the term **bronchial asthma**, the suffix *-al* makes it an adjective, and the two words are separated.

Now, using the word elements as follow, build new terms relating to the bronchus. Your root or combining form will still be bronch/o-.

malacia	stenosis	plasty
scope	pathy	pulmonary
staxis	scopy	dilator
dilation	gram	ostomy

11. An instrument used to see into the bronchus: _____

12. Drug meant to open bronchial passages: _____

13. A softening or deficiency in the wall of a bronchus: _____

14. Surgical procedure for plastic repair on a bronchus: _____

15. Any disease of a bronchus: _____

16. Pertaining to the bronchus and the lung: _____

17. Widening the area of the bronchus: _____

18. Bleeding in the bronchus: _____

19. The procedure of looking into the bronchus: _____

20. Constriction or narrowing of the bronchus: _____

21. The record obtained by bronchography: _____

22. Surgical creation of an opening into the bronchus: _____

Q. Discussion question. Describe the process of inspiration and how the lung inflates. Outline your discussion on the following blank lines. Be prepared to name all the organs in the thoracic cavity. (**LO 13.2,** *Analyze*)

1. _____

_____

_____

_____

_____

R. Deconstruct the following terms, and then answer the following questions. (**LO 13.3, 13.8,** *Analyze*)

Medical Term	Prefix	Root/Combining Form	Suffix	Meaning of Term
empyema	1.	2.	3.	4.
pneumoconiosis	5.	6.	7.	8.
tachypnea	9.	10.	11.	12.

Choose the correct preceding terms to complete the following sentences.

13. Rapid breathing is also called _____.

14. Pleural effusion containing pus is also termed _____.

15. Anthracosis is a form of _____.

S. Trace the pathway. The tracheobronchial tree begins with the trachea, which starts air on its pathway all the way down to the alveoli, where gas exchange can occur. Trace this path by sequentially lettering the following choices A through H. (**LO 13.2, 13.6,** *Analyze*)

1. Each secondary bronchus divides into tertiary bronchi. _____

2. Terminal bronchioles divide into several alveoli. _____

3. Bronchi enter the lung at the hilum. _____

4. Bronchioles divide into terminal bronchioles. _____

5. Main bronchi divide into a secondary bronchus for each lobe. _____

6. Tertiary bronchi divide into bronchioles. _____

7. At the carina, the trachea divides into right and left main bronchi. _____

8. The trachea starts air on the pathway to the alveoli _____

Respiratory System

T. Test-taking skills. Employ your test-taking skills when you answer multiple-choice questions. Start by reading the question and ALL the answers. Immediately cross off answers you know to be incorrect. With the choices you have left, one answer will clearly be the *best* choice. Circle the best choice. **(LO 13.1, 13.3, 13.10, *Apply*)**

1. The hairlike structures in the nasal cavity are called

   a. polyps

   b. cilia

   c. adenoids

   d. bullae

   e. trachealis

2. What is the total number of lobes in *both* lungs?

   a. 4

   b. 5

   c. 6

   d. 2

   e. 3

3. What exactly is a lobe?

   a. an opening into an organ

   b. an exit from an organ

   c. a subdivision of an organ

   d. a blood reservoir in an organ

   e. a pathway through an organ

4. An instrument used to measure breathing volume is called

   a. bronchoscope

   b. spirometer

   c. endoscope

   d. tenometer

   e. sphygmomanometer

5. What is a surfactant?

   a. creates surface tension

   b. a mucous membrane

   c. keeps a muscle from collapsing

   d. a subcutaneous lesion

   e. a place where two bones meet to make a joint

U. Use your knowledge of the language of respiration to answer the following questions: Circle the best choice. (**LO 13.3,** *Apply*)

1. The measure of the capacity of a chamber or hollow viscus to expand is called

   a. expectorate

   b. idiopathic

   c. compliance

   d. postural drainage

   e. consolidation

2. Which of the following is another name for the nasal **conchae** on the lateral wall of each nasal cavity?

   a. meatus

   b. choana

   c. nares

   d. turbinates

   e. septum

3. A bubblelike structure is called a

   a. bronchiole

   b. barbiturate

   c. bulla

   d. bronchus

   e. bradypnea

4. The sense of smell is

   a. external respiration

   b. aspiration

   c. internal respiration

   d. exhalation

   e. olfaction

5. Which of the following is another term for heart failure?

   a. cyanosis

   b. conchae

   c. choana

   d. cor pulmonale

   e. chordae tendinae

6. Laryngeal polyps are

   a. benign tumors of the larynx

   b. localized infection of the larynx

   c. papillomas

   d. malignant tumors of the trachea

   e. verucca in the larynx

7. The medical term for the nostrils is

   a. nares

   b. adenoids

   c. polyps

   d. tonsils

   e. papillomas

Respiratory System

CHAPTER SUMMARY EXERCISES

A. Spelling comprehension. Circle the correct spelling of the term. (**LO 13.3,** *Remember*)

1. oldfaction	olefaction	olfaction	olfarction	ofaction
2. hyperpipnea	hyperphnea	hypophnea	hyperpnea	hypopipnia
3. apnea	apenea	apnia	appnea	apneea
4. nubulizer	nebulizer	mebulizer	nebbulizer	nibulizer
5. mucuspurulent	mucousperulent	mucusprulent	mucopurulent	mucoperulent
6. barbiterate	barbiturate	berbiturate	barrbiturate	berbiturite
7. parencyma	parenchyma	parinchyma	parenckyma	peranchyma
8. expectorate	expicterate	expickerate	expextorate	expecturate
9. hyperoxia	hypoxia	hyperoxxia	hypoxxia	hypoxea
10. coriza	coryiza	corryiza	curiza	coryza

B. Match the number of the correct spelling of the terms in Exercise A with the following definitions. (LO 13.3, *Apply*)

1. Reduced O_2 in the blood _____

2. Cough up and spit out _____

3. Connective tissue framework in lungs _____

4. Delivers liquid medicine in a fine mist _____

5. Sense of smell _____

6. Deeper breathing than normal _____

7. Viral URI _____

8. CNS depressant _____

9. Cessation of breathing _____

10. Infected mucus coughed up _____

C. Using your knowledge of terms 1–10 in Exercises A and B and their correct spelling, write a brief sentence for each of the terms as it might appear in patient documentation. (LO 13.3, *Apply*)

1. _____

2. _____

3. _____

4. _____

5. _____

6. _____

7. _____

8. _____

9. _____

10. _____

D. Diagnostic and therapeutic procedures are performed for different reasons. Use the language of pulmonology to identify their medical terminology. Check (√) the appropriate box. Challenge: One term on the chart can be both a diagnostic and therapeutic procedure. Which is it? (**LO 13.10,** *Analyze*)

Medical Term	Diagnostic	Therapeutic
1. intubation		
2. PDT		
3. tracheotomy		
4. CXR		
5. mediastinoscopy		
6. CT		
7. thoracentesis		
8. bronchoscopy		

Respiratory System

E. Meet the goals of each of the chapter outcomes by using the correct language of pulmonology for the answers. (LO 13.1–13.11, *Analyze*)

1. Apply the language of pulmonology to identify the anatomy and physiology of the upper respiratory tracts. Name the three components of the upper respiratory tract: (**LO 13.1**)

   a. _____

   b. _____

   c. _____

2. Apply the language of pulmonology to relate the structures of the upper and lower respiratory tracts to their functions. What are the functions of the larynx? (**LO 13.2**)

   a. _____

   b. _____

   c. _____

3. Use the medical terms of pulmonology to communicate and document in writing accurately and precisely in any health care setting. (**LO 13.3**)

   Proofread the following sentence for errors in fact and spelling. Write the corrected sentence on the following lines.

   "Below the thyroid cartiledge the ring-shaped kricoid cartiledge connects the pharynx to the esophagus."

   _____

   _____

4. Use the medical terms of pulmonology to communicate verbally with accuracy and precision in any health care setting. (**LO 13.4**)

   A patient has called for an appointment because he has a nosebleed he cannot stop. What medical term do you use for his chief complaint? _____

5. Define abbreviations that relate to the respiratory system.

   Match the definition to the correct abbreviation. (**LO 13.5**)

1. common cold	**a.** COPD
2. dyspnea	**b.** CF
3. CAO is also called	**c.** SOB
4. thick mucus in the lungs	**d.** ARDF
5. sudden, life-threatening lung failure	**e.** URI

6. Summarize the mechanics of respiration.

   Trace the flow of air from the nose through the pharynx and larynx. (**LO 13.6**)

   _____

   _____

7. Discuss the significance of the symptoms and signs of respiratory disorders.

Name some of the symptoms and signs that appear with respiratory disorders. (**LO 13.7**)

a. symptoms

_____

_____

b. signs

_____

_____

8. Explain the effects of common upper respiratory tract disorders on health.

Pick one common upper respiratory tract disorder and explain its effects on health. (**LO 13.8**)

_____

_____

_____

9. Explain the effects of a common lower respiratory disorder on health. (**LO 13.9**)

_____

_____

_____

10. Identify the value of common diagnostic and therapeutic procedures used in disorders of the respiratory system.

What tests and procedures might be involved in treatment of lung cancer? (**LO 13.10**)

_____

_____

_____

11. List the classes of drugs used to treat pulmonary disorders.

Choose one category in the table of Pulmonary Pharmacology and discuss its function, giving examples of the drugs and what diagnosis a patient might have who could benefit from using them. (**LO 13.11**)

_____

_____

_____

Musculoskeletal System
The Languages of Orthopedics and Rehabilitation

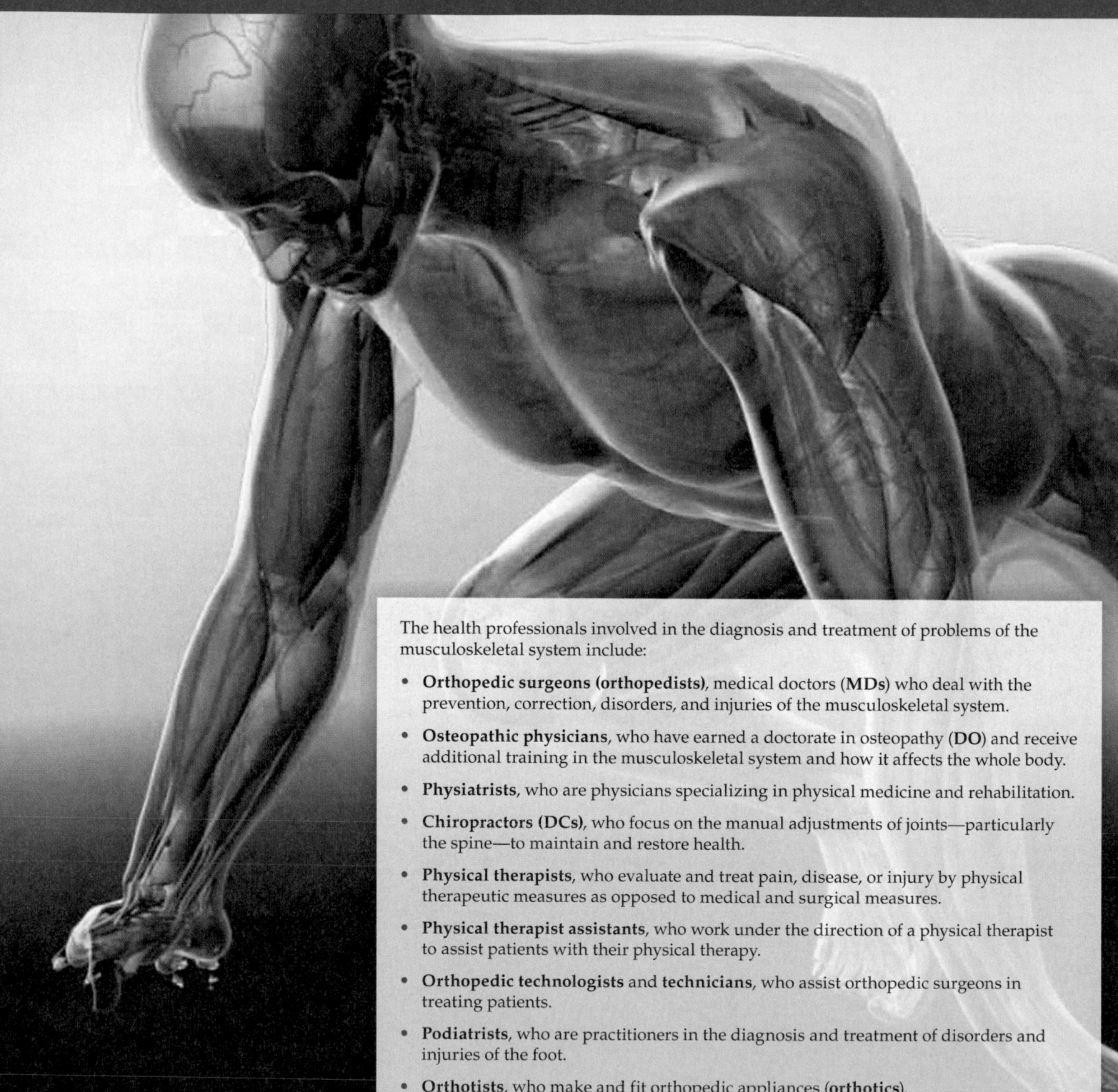

The health professionals involved in the diagnosis and treatment of problems of the musculoskeletal system include:

- **Orthopedic surgeons (orthopedists)**, medical doctors (**MDs**) who deal with the prevention, correction, disorders, and injuries of the musculoskeletal system.

- **Osteopathic physicians**, who have earned a doctorate in osteopathy (**DO**) and receive additional training in the musculoskeletal system and how it affects the whole body.

- **Physiatrists**, who are physicians specializing in physical medicine and rehabilitation.

- **Chiropractors (DCs)**, who focus on the manual adjustments of joints—particularly the spine—to maintain and restore health.

- **Physical therapists**, who evaluate and treat pain, disease, or injury by physical therapeutic measures as opposed to medical and surgical measures.

- **Physical therapist assistants**, who work under the direction of a physical therapist to assist patients with their physical therapy.

- **Orthopedic technologists** and **technicians**, who assist orthopedic surgeons in treating patients.

- **Podiatrists**, who are practitioners in the diagnosis and treatment of disorders and injuries of the foot.

- **Orthotists**, who make and fit orthopedic appliances (**orthotics**).

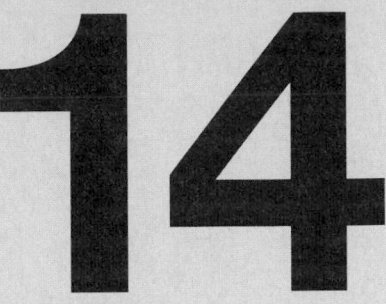

14

Case Report (CR) 14.1

You are

. . . an **orthopedic technologist** working with Kevin Stannard, MD, an **orthopedist** in the Fulwood Medical Group.

Your patient is

. . . Mrs. Amy Vargas, a 70-year-old housewife, who tripped going down the front steps from her house. She has severe pain in her right hip and is unable to stand. An x-ray shows a hip fracture and marked **osteoporosis**. Dr. Stannard examined her in the Emergency Department and has admitted her for a hip replacement.

For you to work with Dr. Stannard to give optimal care to Mrs. Vargas and help her and her family understand the significance of her bone disorder and injury, you will need to be familiar with the terminology of bone structure and function and bone disorders.

Chapter Learning Outcomes

This chapter will review the whole musculoskeletal system and will enable you to:

LO 14.1 Apply the language of orthopedics to the anatomy, growth, and structure of the skeletal system.

LO 14.2 Apply the language of orthopedics to the physiology and functions of the skeletal system.

LO 14.3 Use the medical terms of orthopedics to communicate and document in writing accurately and precisely in any health care setting.

LO 14.4 Use the medical terms of orthopedics to communicate verbally with accuracy and precision in any health care setting.

LO 14.5 Define abbreviations that pertain to the musculoskeletal system.

LO 14.6 Discuss common diseases of bone.

LO 14.7 Explain the causes and types of fractures of bone, their healing, and the procedures for repairing fractures.

LO 14.8 Describe the classes of joints and the movements that they can achieve.

LO 14.9 Identify the common diseases of joints and the surgical procedures used to treat them.

LO 14.10 Match the structure of skeletal muscle to its functions.

LO 14.11 Discuss common disorders of skeletal muscles.

LO 14.12 Describe the structure and functions of the axial skeleton and its associated joints and muscles.

LO 14.13 Identify the structures and functions of the bones, joints, and muscles of the shoulder, arm, and hand.

LO 14.14 Explain common disorders of the shoulder, arm, and hand, and procedures used in their treatment.

LO 14.15 Discuss the structure and functions of the pelvic girdle, hip, thigh, knee, lower leg, ankle, and foot.

LO 14.16 Describe common disorders of the pelvic girdle, hip, thigh, knee, lower leg, ankle, and foot and procedures used in their treatment.

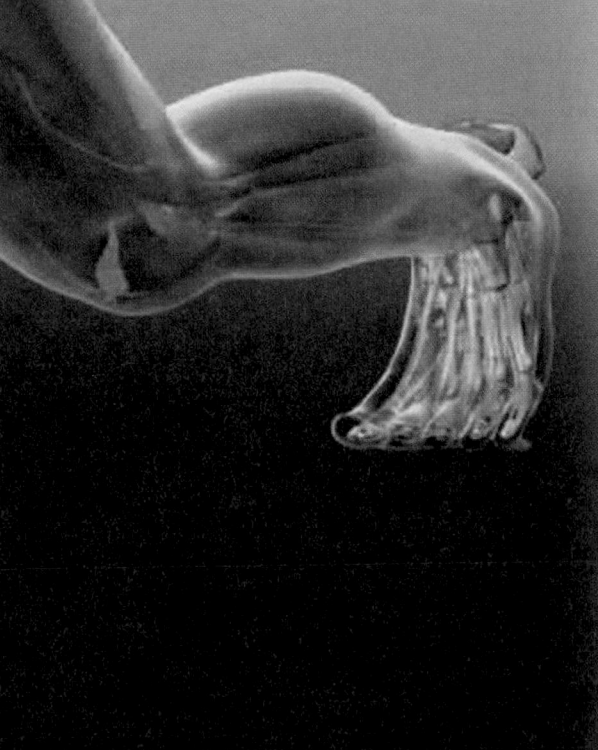

If you didn't have a skeleton, you'd be like a rag doll, shapeless and unable to move. Your skeleton provides support, protects many organ systems, and is the landmark for much of medical terminology. For example, the radial artery you use for taking a pulse is so named because it travels beside the radial bone of the forearm.

In addition, the surface anatomy of bones and their markings enables you to describe and document the sites of symptoms, signs, and clinical, diagnostic, and therapeutic procedures.

The information in this lesson will enable you to use correct medical terminology to:

14.1.1 Recognize the different health professionals involved in the diagnosis and treatment of musculoskeletal problems.

14.1.2 Identify the tissues that form the skeletal system.

14.1.3 Discuss the structures and functions of the skeletal system.

14.1.4 Explain the structure and functions of bones.

14.1.5 Describe the major problems and diseases that occur in the skeletal system.

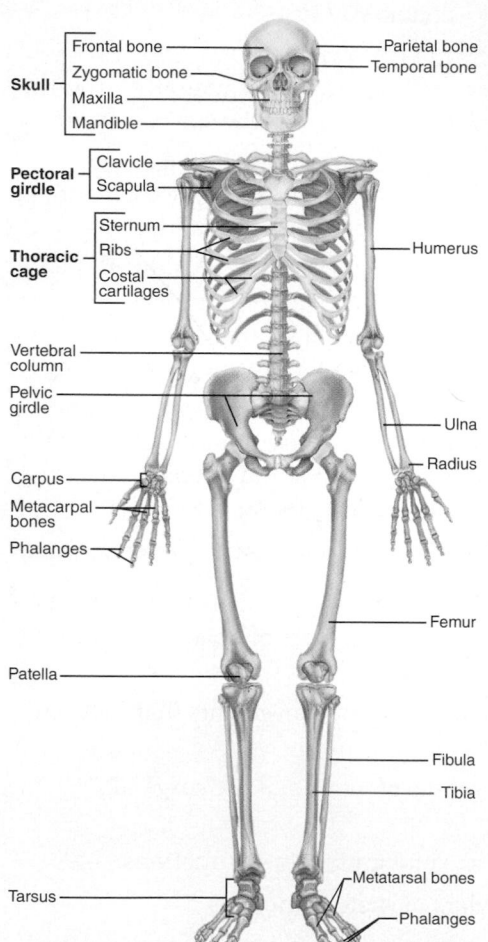

Skull
Frontal bone
Zygomatic bone
Maxilla
Mandible
Parietal bone
Temporal bone

Pectoral girdle
Clavicle
Scapula

Thoracic cage
Sternum
Ribs
Costal cartilages

Humerus

Vertebral column

Pelvic girdle

Ulna

Radius

Carpus
Metacarpal bones
Phalanges

Femur

Patella

Fibula

Tibia

Tarsus

Metatarsal bones

Phalanges

▲ **Figure 14.1** Adult Skeleton: Anterior View.

LO 14.1, 14.2 Functions of the Skeletal System

The four components of the skeletal system (*Figure 14.1*) are

1. *Bones*
2. *Cartilage*
3. *Tendons*
4. *Ligaments*

The bones provide the following functions:

- **Support**. The bones of your vertebral column, pelvis, and legs hold up your body. The jawbone supports your teeth. **Cartilage** supports your nose, ears, and ribs. **Tendons** support and attach your muscles to bone. **Ligaments** support and hold your bones together.

- **Protection**. The skull protects your brain. The vertebral column protects your spinal cord. The rib cage protects your heart and lungs.

- **Movement**. **Muscles** could not function without their attachments to skeletal bones, and muscles are responsible for your movements.

- **Blood formation**. Bone marrow in many bones is the major producer of blood cells, including most of those in your immune system (*see Chapter 12*).

- **Mineral storage and balance**. The skeletal system stores calcium and phosphorus. These are released when your body needs them for other purposes. For example, calcium is needed for muscle contraction, communication between neurons (*see Chapter 9*), and blood clotting (*see Chapter 11*).

- **Detoxification**. Bones remove metals such as lead and radium from your blood, store them, and slowly release them for excretion.

Keynote

Bones are divided into four classes based on their shape: long, short, flat, and irregular.

Abbreviations	
DC	doctor of chiropractic
DO	doctor of osteopathy
MD	doctor of medicine

WORD	PRONUNCIATION	ELEMENTS		DEFINITION
cartilage	**KAR**-tih-lage		Latin *gristle*	Nonvascular, firm connective tissue found mostly in joints
chiropractic	kye-roh-**PRAK**-tik	S/ R/CF R/	-ic *pertaining to* chir/o- *hand* -pract- *efficient*	Diagnosis, treatment, and prevention of mechanical disorders of the musculoskeletal system
chiropractor	kye-roh-**PRAK**-tor	S/	-or *a doer*	Practitioner of chiropractic
detoxification	dee-**TOKS**-ih-fi-**KAY**-shun	S/ P/ R/CF	-fication *remove* de- *from, out of* tox/i- *poison*	Removal of poison from a tissue or substance
ligament	**LIG**-ah-ment		Latin *band, sheet*	Band of fibrous tissue connecting two structures
muscle	**MUSS**-el		Latin *muscle*	Tissue consisting of contractile cells
musculoskeletal	**MUSS**-kyu-loh-**SKEL**-eh-tal	S/ R/CF R/	-al *pertaining to* muscul/o- *muscle* -skelet- *skeleton*	Pertaining to the muscles and the bony skeleton
orthopedic (also spelled orthopaedic)	or-tho-**PEE**-dik	S/ R/CF R/	-ic *pertaining to* orth/o- *straight* -ped- *child*	Pertaining to the correction and cure of deformities and diseases of the musculoskeletal system; originally, most of the deformities treated were in children
orthopedist	or-tho-**PEE**-dist	S/	-ist *specialist*	Specialist in orthopedics
osteopath	**OS**-tee-oh-path	R/ R/CF	-path *disease* oste/o- *bone*	Practitioner of osteopathy
osteopathy	**OS**-tee-**OP**-ah-thee	S/	-pathy *disease*	Medical practice based on maintaining the structural integrity of the musculoskeletal system
radiology	ray-dee-**OL**-oh-jee	S/ R/CF	-logy *study of* radi/o- *radiation, x-rays*	The study of medical imaging
radiologist	ray-dee-**OL**-oh-jist	S/	-logist *one who studies, specialist*	Medical specialist in the use of x-rays and other imaging techniques
tendon	**TEN**-dun		Latin *sinew*	Fibrous band that connects muscle to bone

Exercises

A. This exercise can be answered entirely by using medical terms that appear in the above WAD. *Mastering these terms will start you on your way to learning the language of orthopedics. From the description, identify the correct medical terminology. Fill in the blanks.*
LO 14.1, 14.2

Description   Medical Term(s)

In addition to bones, these three terms are components of the skeletal system: 1. _____

2. _____

3. _____

B. Use the language of orthopedics to fill in the correct answers.   LO 14.1, 14.2

1. Which of the following terms are functions of the skeletal system?

detoxification   movement   temperature control   support   sensory

protection   blood formation   mineral storage   waste excretion   nutrition

Functions of the skeletal system are:

_____

_____

_____

_____

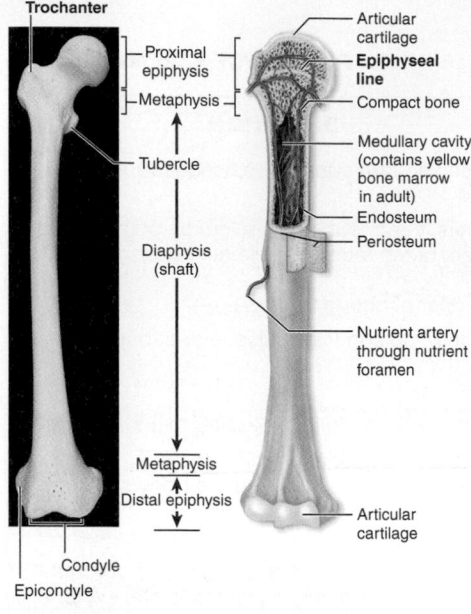

Trochanter

Proximal epiphysis — Articular cartilage
Metaphysis — **Epiphyseal line**
Tubercle — Compact bone
Medullary cavity (contains yellow bone marrow in adult)
Endosteum
Periosteum
Diaphysis (shaft)
Nutrient artery through nutrient foramen
Metaphysis
Distal epiphysis — Articular cartilage
Condyle
Epicondyle

(a) Anterior view   (b) Interior view

▲ **Figure 14.2** Femur: Long Bone of the Thigh.

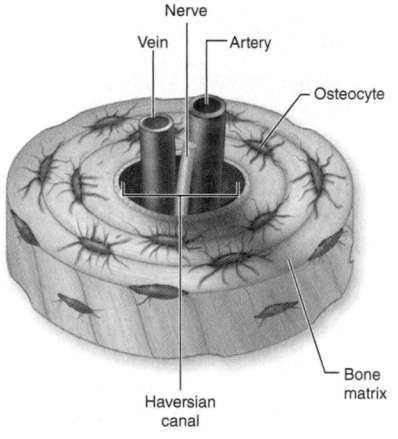

Nerve
Vein — Artery
Osteocyte
Haversian canal
Bone matrix

▲ **Figure 14.3** Blood Supply to Bone.

Keynote

Minerals are deposited in bone when the supply is ample and released when they are needed elsewhere.

LO 14.1 Bone Growth and Structure

Factors that affect bone growth include:

1. **Genes**. Genes determine the size and shape of bones and the ultimate adult height.
2. **Nutrition**. Calcium and phosphorus are needed to develop good bone density.
3. **Exercise**. Exercise increases bone density and total bone mass.
4. **Mineral deposition**. Calcium and phosphate are taken from plasma and deposited in bone.
5. **Mineral resorption**. Calcium and phosphate are released from bone back into the plasma when they are needed elsewhere. For example, calcium is needed for muscle contraction, communication between neurons, and blood clotting. Phosphate is a component of deoxyribonucleic acid (DNA) and ribonucleic acid (RNA).
6. **Vitamins**. Vitamin A activates osteoblasts; vitamin C is essential for collagen synthesis; vitamin D stimulates absorption of calcium and phosphate, its transport, and its deposition into bones.
7. **Hormones**. For example, growth hormone stimulates the epiphyseal plate to calcify, and estrogen and testosterone accelerate bone growth after puberty and maintain bone density (*see Chapter 17*).

LO 14.1, 14.2 Structure and Functions of Bones

Long bones are the most common type of bone in the body (*Figure 14.2*).

The shaft of a long bone is called the **diaphysis**. Each end of the bone is called the **epiphysis** and is expanded to provide extra surface area for the attachment of ligaments and tendons.

Sandwiched between the diaphysis and epiphysis is a thin area called the **metaphysis**. Thin layers of cartilage cells in the **epiphyseal plate** enable the diaphysis (bone shaft) to grow in length. When growth stops, compact bone grows into the epiphyseal plate and forms the **epiphyseal line** (*Figure 14.2b*).

A tough connective tissue sheath called **periosteum** covers the outer surface of all bones and is attached to the compact or **cortical** bone by tough collagen fibers. The periosteum protects the bone and anchors blood vessels and nerves to the surface of the bone.

The hollow cylinder inside the diaphysis is called the **medullary cavity**. It contains bone **marrow** and is lined by a thin membrane called the **endosteum**. The marrow is a fatty tissue that contains blood cells in different stages of development (*see Chapter 11*).

The endosteum and periosteum contain **osteoblasts**, cells that produce the matrix of new bone tissue. This process is called **osteogenesis**. Bone **matrix** consists of cells, collagen fibers, a gel that supports and suspends the fibers, and calcium phosphate crystals that give bone its hardness.

When osteoblasts are incorporated into the new bone, they become **osteocytes**. These cells, which maintain the matrix, reside in small spaces in the matrix called **lacunae**.

Osteoclasts are produced by the bone marrow. They dissolve calcium, phosphorus, and the organic components of the bone matrix. There is a continual balancing act going on as osteoclasts remove matrix and osteoblasts produce matrix. If osteoclasts outperform the osteoblasts, then **osteoporosis** occurs, as with Mrs. Vargas.

All bones are well supplied with blood (*Figure 14.3*). The blood vessels travel through the bone in a system of small **haversian (central) canals**. Because of its good blood supply, bone heals well.

WORD	PRONUNCIATION	ELEMENTS		DEFINITION
cortex **cortical (adj)**	**KOR**-teks **KOR**-tih-cal		Latin *bark*	Outer portion of an organ, such as bone
diaphysis	die-**AF**-ih-sis		Greek *growing between*	The shaft of a long bone
endosteum	en-**DOSS**-tee-um	S/ P/ R/	-um *tissue, structure* end- *within* oste- *bone*	A membrane of tissue lining the inner (medullary) cavity of a long bone
epiphysis	eh-**PIF**-ih-sis	P/ R/	epi- *upon, above* -physis *growth*	Expanded area at the proximal and distal ends of a long bone that provides increased surface area for attachment of ligaments and tendons
epiphyseal plate	eh-**PIF**-ih-see-al PLATE	S/ R/CF	-al *pertaining to* epiphys/e- *growth*	Layer of cartilage between epiphysis and metaphysis where bone growth occurs
haversian canals (also called **central canals**)	hah-**VER**-shan ka-**NALS**		Clopton Havers, English physician, 1655–1702	Vascular canals in bone
lacuna **lacunae (pl)**	la-**KOO**-nah la-**KOO**-nee		Latin *a pit, lake*	Small space or cavity within the matrix of bone
marrow	**MAH**-roe		Old English *marrow*	Fatty, blood-forming tissue in the cavities of long bones
matrix	**MAY**-triks		Latin *mother, womb*	Substance that surrounds cells, is manufactured by cells, and holds them together
medulla **medullary (adj)**	meh-**DULL**-ah **MED**-ul-ah-ree		Latin *marrow*	Central portion of a structure surrounded by cortex
metaphysis	meh-**TAF**-ih-sis	P/ R/	meta- *beyond, after, subsequent to* -physis *growth*	Region between the diaphysis and the epiphysis where bone growth occurs
osteoblast	**OS**-tee-oh-blast	S/ R/CF	-blast *embryo* oste/o- *bone*	Bone-forming cell
osteoclast	**OS**-tee-oh-klast	S/ R/CF	-clast *break down* oste/o- *bone*	Bone-removing cell
osteocyte	**OS**-tee-oh-site	S/ R/CF	-cyte *cell* oste/o- *bone*	Bone-maintaining cell
osteogenesis	**OS**-tee-oh-**JEN**-eh-sis	S/ R/CF	-genesis *creation* oste/o- *bone*	Creation of new bone
osteogenic (adj)	**OS**-tee-oh-**JEN**-ik	S/	-genic *producing*	Relating to the creation of new bone
osteoporosis	**OS**-tee-oh-poh-**ROE**-sis	S/ R/CF R/	-osis *condition* oste/o- *bone* -por- *opening*	Condition in which the bones become more porous, brittle, and fragile and are more likely to fracture
periosteum	**PER**-ee-**OSS**-tee-um	S/ P/ R/	-um *tissue, structure* peri- *around* oste- *bone*	Strong membrane surrounding a bone
periosteal (adj)	**PER**-ee-**OSS**-tee-al	S/	-al *pertaining to*	Pertaining to the periosteum
trochanter	troh-**KAN**-ter		Greek *runner*	One of two bony prominences near the head of the femur

Exercises

A. The combining form oste/o- means bone and is the main element in each of the following terms. *You choose the correct suffix to complete the term. Fill in the blanks.* **LO 14.1, 14.2, 14.3**

blast   cyte   genesis   clast   genic   porosis

The osteo_____ process begins with osteo_____, which produce the matrix of new bone tissue. Osteo_____ has begun. Once these cells incorporate into new bone, they are termed osteo_____. These cells maintain matrix. Osteo_____ are produced by bone marrow. A delicate balance must be maintained between cells that remove matrix and cells that produce matrix. If more matrix is removed than produced, osteo_____ will result.

On questioning, Mrs. Vargas demonstrated many of the risk factors for osteoporosis, including a family history, lack of exercise, cigarette smoking, inadequate diet, postmenopause, and increasing age.

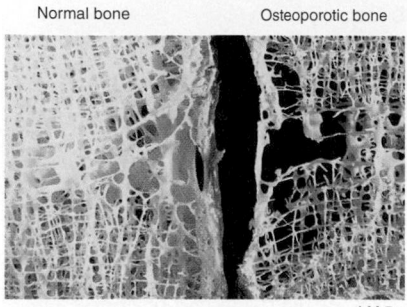

Normal bone   Osteoporotic bone

LM 5×

▲ **Figure 14.4** **Normal Bone and Osteoporotic Bone.**

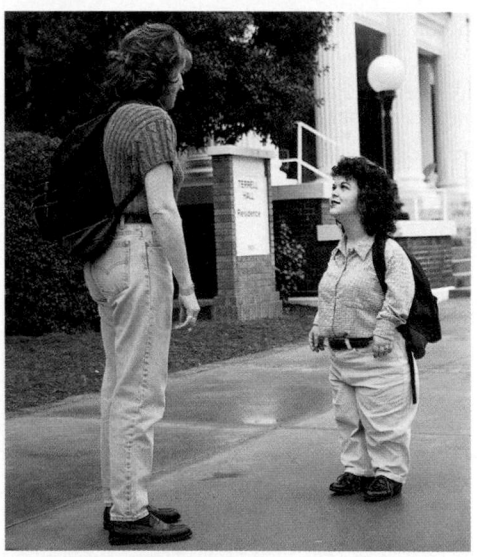

▲ **Figure 14.5** **Achondroplastic Dwarf with College Roommate.**

Abbreviations	
BMD	bone mineral density
DEXA	dual energy x-ray absorptiometry
FDA	U.S. Food and Drug Administration
IU	international unit(s)

LO 14.6 Diseases of Bone

Osteoporosis results from a loss of bone density *(Figure 14.4)* when the rate of bone **resorption** exceeds the rate of bone **formation**. It is more common in women than in men, and its incidence increases with age. Ten million people in the United States already have osteoporosis, and 18 million more have low bone density (**osteopenia**) and are at risk for developing osteoporosis.

In women, production of the hormone estrogen decreases after menopause, and its protection against osteoclast activity is lost. This leads to fragile, brittle bones. In men, reduction in testosterone has a similar but less marked effect.

Women at risk for osteoporosis should have **bone mineral density** (**BMD**) screening using a dual-energy **x-ray absorptiometry** (**DEXA**) scan. Men and women over age 50 should take 1200 mg of calcium daily and 600 to 1,000 **international units** (**IU**) of vitamin D or expose the body to the sun for 15 minutes daily.

Several medications approved by the **U.S. Food and Drug Administration** (**FDA**) are available for the treatment of osteoporosis. Most inhibit osteoclast activity.

Osteomyelitis is an inflammation of an area of bone due to bacterial infection, usually with a staphylococcus. Untreated tuberculosis can spread from its original infection in the lungs to bones via the bloodstream to produce tuberculous osteomyelitis.

Osteomalacia, known as **rickets** in children, is a disease caused by vitamin D deficiency. When bones lack calcium, they become soft and flexible. They are not strong enough to bear weight and become bowed. Osteomalacia occurs in some developing nations and occasionally in this country when children drink soft drinks instead of milk fortified with vitamin D.

Achondroplasia occurs when the long bones stop growing in childhood but the bones of the axial skeleton are not affected *(Figure 14.5)*. This leads to short-stature individuals who are about 4 feet tall. Intelligence and life span are normal. It is caused by a spontaneous gene mutation that then becomes a dominant gene for succeeding generations.

Osteogenic sarcoma is the most common malignant bone tumor. Peak incidence is between 10 and 15 years of age; the tumor often occurs around the knee joint.

Osteogenesis imperfecta is a rare genetic disorder, producing very brittle bones that are easily fractured, often **in utero** (while inside the uterus).

WORD	PRONUNCIATION	ELEMENTS		DEFINITION
achondroplasia	a-kon-droh-**PLAY**-ze-ah	S/ P/ R/CF	-plasia *formation* a- *without* -chondr/o- *cartilage*	Condition with abnormal conversion of cartilage into bone, leading to dwarfism
in utero	IN **YOU**-ter-oh		Latin *uterus*	Within the womb; not yet born
osteogenesis imperfecta	**OS**-tee-oh-**JEN**-eh-sis im-per-**FEK**-tah	S/ R/CF R/	-genesis *creation* oste/o- *bone* imperfecta *unfinished*	Inherited condition in which bone formation is incomplete, leading to fragile, easily broken bones
osteomalacia	**OS**-tee-oh-mah-**LAY**-she-ah	S/ R/CF	-malacia *abnormal softness* oste/o- *bone*	Soft, flexible bones lacking in calcium
osteomyelitis	**OS**-tee-oh-my-eh-**LIE**-tis	S/ R/CF R/	-itis *inflammation* oste/o- *bone* -myel- *bone marrow*	Inflammation of bone tissue
osteopenia	**OS**-tee-oh-**PEE**-nee-ah	S/ R/CF	-penia *deficient* oste/o- *bone*	Decreased calcification of bone
resorption	ree-**SORP**-shun		Latin *to suck back*	Loss of substance, such as bone
rickets	**RICK**-ets		Old English *to twist*	Disease in children due to vitamin D deficiency, producing soft, flexible bones
sarcoma	sar-**KOH**-mah	S/ R/	-oma *tumor, mass* sarc- *flesh*	A malignant tumor originating in connective tissue
osteogenic sarcoma	**OS**-tee-oh-**JEN**-ik sar-**KOH**-mah	S/ R/CF	-genic *creation* oste/o- *bone*	Malignant tumor originating in bone-producing cells

Exercises

A. Bone diseases can strike at any age. *Refer to the above WAD for the correct terminology to identify each disease. Fill in the blanks.*   **LO 14.3, 14.6**

1. Inflammation of an area of bone, usually due to staph infection _____

2. Bone disease in children caused by vitamin D deficiency _____

3. Leads to short stature (height) _____

4. Rare, genetic disorder causing brittle bones _____

5. Decreased calcification of bone _____

6. Most common malignant bone tumor _____

7. Also known as *rickets* in children _____

B. These questions relate to the answers in Exercise A. *Use the language of orthopedics to compose your answers.*   **LO 14.3, 14.6**

1. "Within the womb, not yet born" is documented as _____.

2. What is the medical term for soft, flexible bones lacking in calcium? _____

3. When bone resorption exceeds bone formation, _____ results.

C. Critical thinking: Fill in the blanks.   LO 14.3, 14.6

1. What organic element and vitamin are critical in bone health? _____ and vitamin _____ encourage bone health.

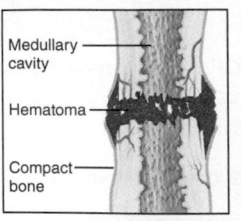

Medullary cavity
Hematoma
Compact bone

(a)

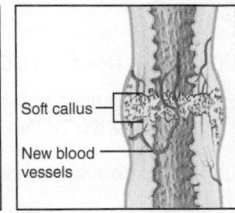

Soft callus
New blood vessels

(b)

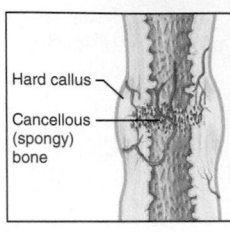

Hard callus
Cancellous (spongy) bone

(c)

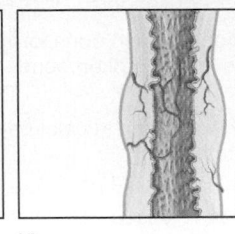

(d)

▲ **Figure 14.6** Healing of Bone Fracture.

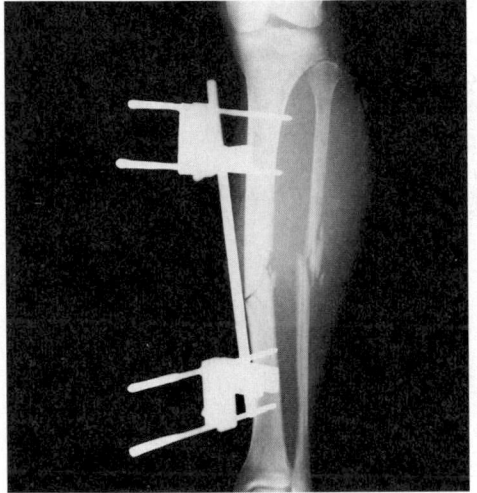

▲ **Figure 14.7** Radiograph of Fractured Limb. X-ray of lower-leg fracture set with steel pins and external plate.

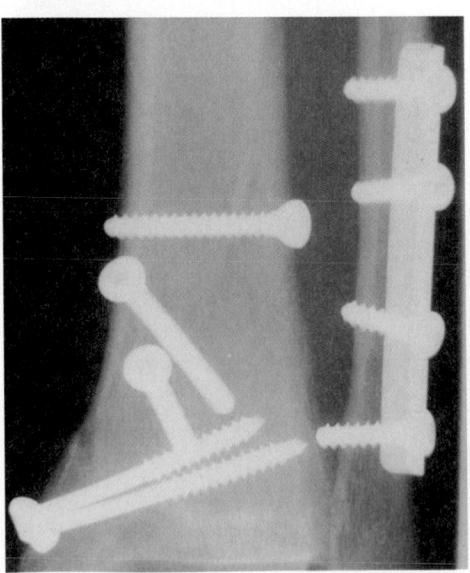

▲ **Figure 14.8** Internal Fixation of Fractures with Screws and Plate.

LO 14.7 Bone Fractures

Healing of Fractures

Step 1: When a bone is fractured, blood vessels bleed into the fracture site, forming a **hematoma** *(Figure 14.6a)*.

Step 2: A few days after the **fracture (Fx),** osteoblasts move into the hematoma and start to produce new bone. This is called a **callus** *(Figure 14.6b)*.

Step 3: Osteoblasts produce immature, lacy, **cancellous** (spongy) bone that replaces the callus *(Figure 14.6c)*.

Step 4: Osteoblasts continue to produce bone cells. They produce compact bone and fuse the bone segments together *(Figure 14.6d)*.

Uncomplicated fractures take 8 to 12 weeks to heal.

Surgical Procedures for Repairing Fractures

The initial goal of fracture treatment is to bring the ends of the bone at the break back opposite each other so that they fit together as they did in the original bone. This is called **alignment**.

External manipulation is used frequently. The bone is pulled from the distal end back into alignment. This process is called **reduction**. Anesthesia may be used.

In external fixation, the alignment is maintained by immobilizing the bone through the use of

- **Plaster and fiberglass casts**.

- **Splints**.

- **Traction**—the gentle but continuous application of a pulling force that can align a fracture, reduce muscle spasm, and relieve pain.

- **External fixators**—by which the bone fragments are secured to a strong external steel rod or plate by means of steel pins that attach the plate or rod to the bone *(Figure 14.7)*.

Internal fixation with materials such as stainless steel and titanium, which are compatible with tissues, enables the patient to return to function quicker and reduces the incidence of **nonunion** and **malunion** (improper healing). The types of internal fixation are

- **Wires**—used as sutures to "sew" the bone fragments together; this method is often used in the hand.

- **Plates**—extended along both or all fragments of bone and held in place by screws.

- **Rods**—can be inserted through the medullary cavity of both fragments to align the bones.

- **Screws**—can be used on their own as well as with plates; they are probably the most common form of internal fixation *(Figure 14.8)*.

- **Pins**—a long, thick metal pin can be driven down the shaft of a bone from one end.

The types of bone fractures are shown in *Figure 14.9* and described in *Table 14.1*, both of which are found on the next two-page spread.

Abbreviation	
Fx	fracture

WORD	PRONUNCIATION	ELEMENTS		DEFINITION
alignment	a-**LINE**-ment	S/ P/ R/	-ment *resulting state* a- (variant of **ad-**) *into* -lign- *line*	A state of being in the correct position in relation to other structures
callus (**Note:** *Callous* is a nonmedical word meaning *insensitive*.)	**KAL**-us		Latin *hard skin*	The mass of fibrous connective tissue that forms at a fracture site and becomes the foundation for the formation of new bone
cancellous	**KAN**-sell-us		Latin *lattice*	Bone that has a spongy or lattice-like structure
hematoma	he-mah-**TOH**-mah	S/ R/	-oma *tumor, mass* hemat- *blood*	Collection of blood that has escaped from the blood vessels into tissue
malunion	mal-**YOU**-nee-un	S/ P/ R/	-ion *action, condition, process* mal- *bad* -un- *one*	Condition in which the two bony ends of a fracture fail to heal together correctly
nonunion	non-**YOU**-nee-un	P/	non- *not*	Total failure of healing of a fracture
reduction	ree-**DUCK**-shun	S/ P/ R/	-ion *action, condition, process* re- *backward* -duct- *lead*	The restoration of a structure to its normal position
traction	**TRAK**-shun		Latin *to pull*	A pulling or dragging force

Exercises

A. After you deconstruct the following medical terms into their basic elements, provide a brief definition for each term. *Fill in the chart; then fill in the blanks at the end of the exercise. The first one is done for you.*   **LO 14.2, 14.3, 14.7**

Medical Term	Prefix	Root/Combining Form	Suffix	Definition of Medical Term
reduction	*re*	*duct*	*ion*	*The restoration of a structure to its normal position*
alignment	1.	2.	3.	4.
malunion	5.	6.	7.	8.
hematoma	9.	10.	11.	12.

B. Demonstrate your understanding of the terms by finishing this exercise. *Refer to the chart in Exercise A for the answers to this exercise.*   **LO 14.2, 14.3, 14.7**

1. Use *both* the terms **reduction** and **alignment** in *one sentence.*

_____

_____

2. The suffix **-oma** means *tumor* as well as *mass*. Briefly explain why a hematoma is not a tumor.

_____

_____

3. Explain the difference between a **malunion** and a **nonunion** of a fracture.

malunion:

_____

nonunion:

_____

LO 14.7 Bone Fractures—continued

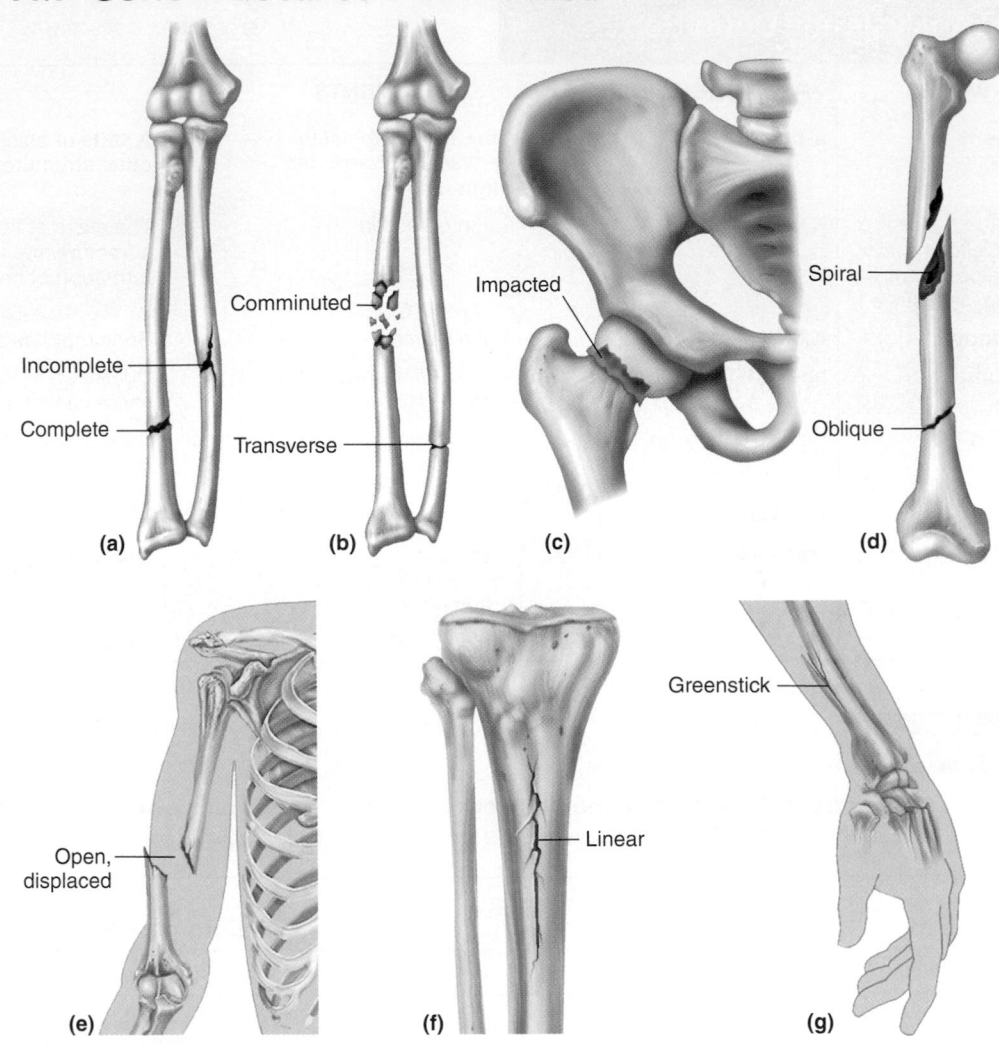

▲ **Figure 14.9** Bone Fractures.

LO 14.7 **Table 14.1** Classification of Bone Fractures

Name	Description	Reference
Closed	A bone is broken, but the skin is not broken.	Figure 14.9a, b, c, d, f, and g
Open	A fragment of the fractured bone breaks the skin, or a wound extends to the site of the fracture.	Figure 14.9e
Displaced	The fractured bone parts are out of alignment.	Figure 14.9e
Complete	A bone is broken into at least two fragments.	Figure 14.9a
Incomplete	The fracture does not extend completely across the bone; it can be **hairline** (as in a stress fracture in the foot when there is no separation of the two fragments).	Figure 14.9a
Comminuted	The bone breaks into several pieces, usually two major pieces and several smaller fragments.	Figure 14.9b
Transverse	The fracture is at a right angle to the long axis of the bone.	Figure 14.9b
Impacted	One bone fragment is driven into the other, with resulting shortening of a limb.	Figure 14.9c
Spiral	The fracture spirals around the long axis of the bone.	Figure 14.9d
Oblique	A diagonal fracture runs across the long axis of the bone.	Figure 14.9d
Linear	The fracture runs parallel to the long axis of the bone.	Figure 14.9f
Greenstick (closed)	This is a partial fracture: one side breaks, the other bends.	Figure 14.9g
Pathologic	The fracture occurs in an area of bone weakened by disease (such as cancer). Also called stress fracture	—
Compression	The fracture occurs in a vertebra from trauma or pathology leading to the vertebra being crushed.	—

WORD	PRONUNCIATION		ELEMENTS	DEFINITION
closed fracture (opposite of open)	KLOSD FRAK-chur	S/ R/	closed Latin *hard skin* -ure *result of* fract- *break*	A bone is broken but the skin over it is intact
comminuted fracture	KOM-ih-nyu-ted	S/ R/	-ed *pertaining to* comminut- *break into small pieces*	A fracture in which the bone is broken into pieces
complete fracture	kom-PLEET		Latin *fill up*	A bone is fractured into two separate pieces
compression fracture	kom-PRESH-un	S/ R/	-ion *condition, action* compress- *press together*	Fracture of a vertebra causing loss of height of the vertebra
displaced fracture	dis-PLAYSD	P/ R/	dis- *apart, away from* -placed *in an area*	A fracture in which the fragments are separated and are not in alignment
greenstick fracture	GREEN-stik	R/ R/	green- *green* -stick *branch twig*	A fracture in which one side of the bone is partially broken and the other side is bent. Occurs mostly in children
hairline fracture	HAIR-line		Old English *hair line* Latin *a mark*	A fracture without separation of the fragments
impacted fracture	im-PAK-ted	S/ P/ R/	-ed *pertaining to* im- *in* -pact- *driven in*	A fracture in which one bone fragment is driven into the other
incomplete fracture	in-kom-PLEET	P/ R/	in- *not* -complete *fill in*	A fracture that does not extend across the bone, as in a hairline fracture
linear fracture	LIN-ee-ar	S/ R/	-ar *pertaining to* line- *a mark*	A fracture running parallel to the length of the bone
oblique fracture	ob-LEEK		Latin *slanting*	A diagonal fracture across the long axis of the bone
open fracture	OH-pen		Old English *not enclosed*	The skin over the fracture is broken
pathologic fracture	path-oh-LOJ-ik	S/ R/CF R/ S/ R/	-ic *pertaining to* path/o- *disease* -log- *to study* -ure *result of* fract- *to break*	Fracture occurring at a site already weakened by a disease process, such as cancer. Also called stress fracture
spiral fracture	SPY-ral	S/ R/	-al *pertaining to* spir- *a coil*	A fracture in the shape of a coil
transverse fracture	trans-VERS	P/ R/	trans- *across* -verse *travel*	A fracture perpendicular to the long axis of the bone

Exercises

A. Fractures. You are working as the new radiology technician in the Radiology Department at the hospital. *You are attempting to identify the types of fractures with the pictures you see on the film. Use the descriptions that follow to identify the types of fracturess. Refer to Table 14.1.* **LO 14.3, 14.7**

Fracture Seen on the Film	Type of Fracture
Fracture at a right angle to the long axis of the radius	
Femur broken into two clean pieces	
Cancer patient with vertebral fracture	
Broken ankle but no broken skin	
Diagonal fracture across the long axis of the femur	
Fractured hand with bone fragments sticking out	

LESSON OBJECTIVES

Without joints you would be a statue. Joints allow you to move, but movable parts that rub together can wear out. Damage or disease in a joint can make movement very difficult and painful. The structure of any joint, or articulation, is directly related to its mobility and function. To understand, describe, and document your patient's joint problems, you need to be able to use correct medical terminology to:

14.2.1 Classify the different types of joints.

14.2.2 Identify the tissues that form the different joints.

14.2.3 Match structures to functions in the different joints.

14.2.4 Describe the major problems and diseases that occur in joints.

You are

. . . an orthopedic technologist working for orthopedic surgeon Kenneth Stannard, MD, at Fulwood Medical Center.

Your patient is

. . . Mr. Hank Johnson, a 63-year-old white male. Mr. Johnson has been active all his life.

Case Report 14.2

In his youth, Mr. Johnson played football and baseball. As an adult, he has played racquetball weekly and jogged 3 to 4 miles most mornings on the streets of his neighborhood. For the past year, he has had lower-back stiffness and pain, particularly in the mornings. Six months ago, while out hiking, he slid down a mountain on his left side for about 100 feet. He is now having pain in his left groin and thigh, with difficulty walking and climbing stairs.

You are responsible for documenting the doctor's diagnostic procedures and treatment and for making sure that Mr. Johnson understands the significance of the diagnostic findings and the recommendations for his treatment.

LO 14.8 Classes of Joints

Joints are classified structurally into three types:

1. **Fibrous** joints are two bones tightly bound together by bands of fibrous tissue with no joint space. They come in three varieties:

   a. **Sutures** occur between the bones of the skull *(Figure 14.10)*; the two opposing bones have interlocking processes to add stability to the joint. The **periosteum** on each of the the outer and inner surfaces of the two bones is continuous and holds the joint together.

   b. **Syndesmosis** is a joining of two bones with fibrous ligaments. Their movement is minimal. An example is the joint above the ankle where the tibia and fibula are attached.

   c. **Gomphoses** are pegs that fit into sockets and are held in place by fine collagen fibers. Examples are the joints between teeth and their sockets.

2. **Cartilaginous** joints join two bones with cartilage:

   a. **Synchondroses** join two bones with **hyaline** cartilage, which allows little or no movement between them, as between your ribs and costal cartilages.

   b. **Symphyses** join two bones with **fibrocartilage**. An example is the symphysis pubis, where your two pubic bones meet at the front of your pelvis.

   3. **Synovial** joints contain synovial fluid as a lubricant and allow considerable movement *(Figure 14.11)*. Most joints in the legs and arms are synovial joints. The ends of the bones are covered with hyaline **articular** cartilage. In some joints, an additional plate of fibrocartilage is located between the two bones. In the knee, this plate is incomplete and is called a **meniscus.**

A **bursa** is an extension of the synovial joint that forms a cushion between structures that otherwise would rub against each other, for example, in the knee joint between the patellar tendon and the patellar and tibial bones *(Figure 14.11)*.

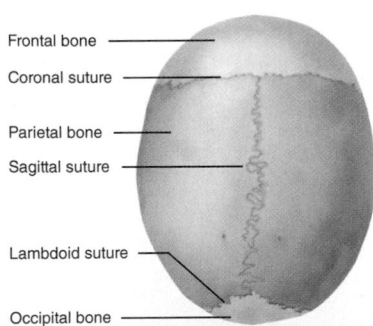

Anterior

Frontal bone
Coronal suture
Parietal bone
Sagittal suture
Lambdoid suture
Occipital bone

Posterior

▲ **Figure 14.10** Sutures of Skull: Superior View.

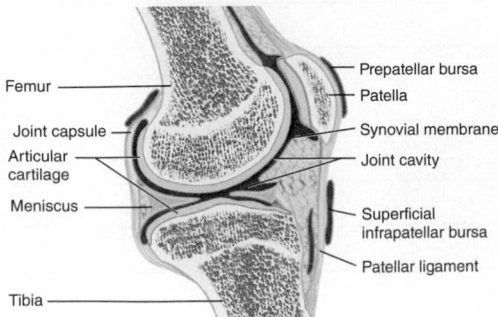

Femur
Joint capsule
Articular cartilage
Meniscus
Tibia

Prepatellar bursa
Patella
Synovial membrane
Joint cavity
Superficial infrapatellar bursa
Patellar ligament

▲ **Figure 14.11** Synovial Joint.

WORD	PRONUNCIATION	ELEMENTS		DEFINITION
articulation articulate (verb) articular (adj)	ar-tik-you-**LAY**-shun ar-**TIK**-you-late ar-**TIK**-you-lar	S/ R/ S/	-ation *process* **articul-** *joint* -ar *pertaining to*	A joint Pertaining to a joint
bursa	**BURR**-sah		Latin *purse*	A closed sac containing synovial fluid
fibrocartilage	fie-bro-**KAR**-til-age	R/CF R/CF	**fibr/o-** *fiber* **-cartilag/e** *cartilage*	Cartilage containing collagen fibers
gomphosis gomphoses (pl)	gom-**FOE**-sis gom-**FOE**-sees	S/ R/	-osis *condition* **gomph-** *bolt, nail*	Joint formed by a peg and socket
hyaline	**HIGH**-ah-line		Greek *glass*	Cartilage that looks like frosted glass and contains fine collagen fibers
meniscus menisci (pl)	meh-**NISS**-kuss meh-**NISS**-key		Greek *crescent*	Disc of connective tissue cartilage between the bones of a joint, for example, in the knee joint
suture sutures (pl)	**SOO**-chur		Latin *a seam*	Place where two bones are joined together by a fibrous band continuous with their periosteum, as in the skull Also means to unite two surfaces by sewing. Also means the material used in the sewing together Also means the seam formed by the sewing together
symphysis symphyses (pl)	**SIM**-feh-sis **SIM**-feh-sees		Greek *growing together*	Two bones joined by fibrocartilage
synchondrosis synchondroses (pl)	sin-kon-**DROH**-sis sin-kon-**DROH**-sees	S/ P/ R/	-osis *condition* syn- *together* -chondr- *cartilage*	A rigid articulation (joint) formed by cartilage
syndesmosis syndesmoses (pl)	sin-dez-**MOH**-sis sin-dez-**MOH**-sees	S/ R/	-osis *condition* **syndesm-** *bind together*	An articulation (joint) formed by ligaments
synovial	si-**NOH**-vee-al	S/ P/ R/CF	-al *pertaining to* syn- *together* -ov/i- *egg*	Pertaining to synovial fluid and synovial membrane

Exercises

A. You must be able to recognize a medical term in its singular and plural forms. *In the following chart, check (√) in the appropriate column whether the given term is singular or plural. If you have checked singular, write the plural form of the term in the appropriate column; if you have checked plural, write the singular form of the term in the appropriate column. Fill in the chart; then write the definitions.*   **LO 14.1, 14.3, 14.8**

Medical Term	Singular	Plural
syndesmoses	1.	2.
suture	3.	4.
gomphosis	5.	6.
menisci	7.	8.

Define any two of these terms in a sentence.

9. _____

10. _____

B. Use the new medical terms in this spread to answer the following questions about joints.   **LO 14.1, 14.3, 14.8**

1. List the types of joints and give an example of each.

a. _____

b. _____

c. _____

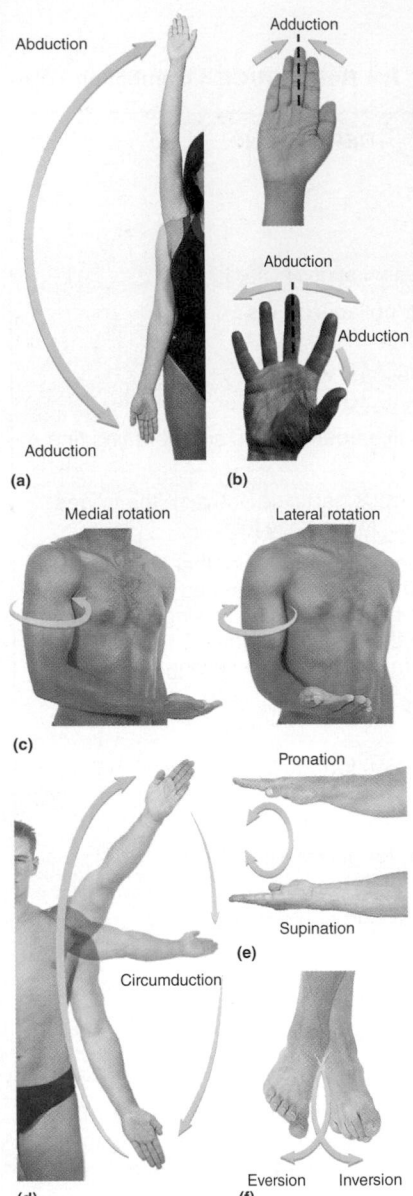

▲ **Figure 14.13** **Movement of the Limbs.** (*a*) Abduction and adduction of the upper limb. (*b*) Abduction and adduction of the fingers. (*c*) Medial and lateral rotation of the arm. (*d*) Circumduction. (*e*) Pronation and supination of the hand. (*f*) Eversion and inversion of the foot.

Keynotes

- **Circumduction of Joints** Circumduction of the shoulder is moving it in a circular movement so that it forms a cone, with the shoulder joint as the apex of the cone (*Figure 14.13d*).

- **Inversion and Eversion** When you turn your ankle so that the sole of your foot faces toward the opposite foot, that is supination or **inversion**. When you turn your ankle so that the sole of the foot faces laterally away from the other foot, that is pronation or **eversion** (*Figure 14.13f*).

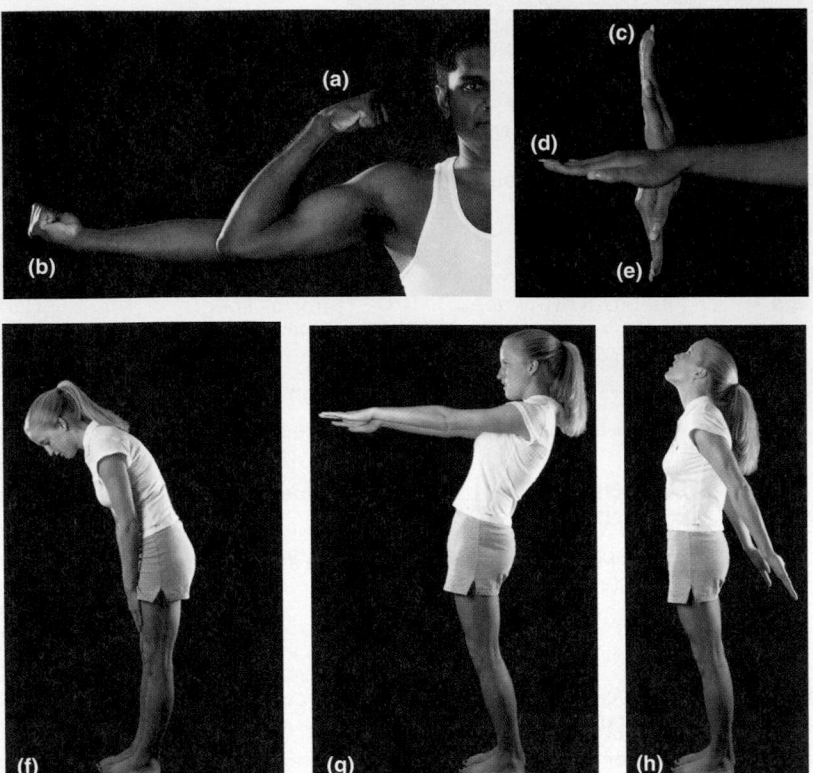

▲ **Figure 14.12** **Joint Flexion and Extension.** (*a*) Flexion of the elbow. (*b*) Extension of the elbow. (*c*) Extension of the wrist. (*d*) Neutral position of the wrist. (*e*) Flexion of the wrist. (*f*) Flexion of the spine. (*g*) Flexion of the shoulder. (*h*) Extension of the shoulder.

LO 14.8 Joint Movement

Flexion and Extension of Joints

The following figures show flexion (bending) and **extension** (straightening) in the elbow joint (*Figure 14.12a and b*), in the wrist joint (*Figure 14.13c, d, and e*), and in the shoulder joint (*Figure 14.12g and h*).

For most of the rest of the body, flexion is movement of a body part *anterior* to the **coronal plane** (*see Chapter 4*). Extension is movement *posterior* to the coronal plane. For example, when you bend your trunk forward, that is flexion (*Figure 14.12f*). When you bend your trunk backward, that is extension (*see Figure 14.12g*). When you bend your trunk sideways to the right or left, that is called *lateral flexion*.

Abduction and Adduction of Joints

Abduction is movement away from the midline. **Adduction** is movement toward the midline. Abduction of your arm is moving it sideways away from your trunk. Adduction is bringing it back to the side of your trunk (*Figure 14.13a*). Abduction of your fingers is spreading them apart, away from the middle finger. Adduction is bringing them back together (*Figure 14.13b*).

Rotation of Joints

Rotation is turning around an axis. Medial rotation of the upper arm bone, the humerus, with the elbow flexed brings the palm of the hand toward the body. Lateral rotation moves the palm away from the body (*Figure 14.13c*).

Pronation and Supination

When you lie flat on the ground facedown on your belly with your palms touching the ground, you are **prone**. When you lie flat on your back with your spine on the floor and your palms facing up, you are **supine**.

When you rotate your forearm so that your palm faces the floor, that is **pronation**. When you rotate the forearm so that your palm is facing upward, that is **supination** (*Figure 14.13e*).

WORD	PRONUNCIATION	ELEMENTS		DEFINITION
abduction abduct (verb)	ab-**DUCK**-shun ab-**DUKT**	S/ P/ R/	-ion *process, action* ab- *away from* -duct- *lead*	Action of moving away from the midline
adduction adduct (verb)	ah-**DUCK**-shun ah-**DUCKT**	S/ P/ R/	-ion *process, action* ad- *toward* -duct- *lead*	Action of moving toward the midline
circumduction circumduct (verb)	ser-kum-**DUCK**-shun ser-kum-**DUCKT**	S/ P/ R/	-ion *process, action* circum- *around* -duct- *lead*	Movement of an extremity in a circular motion
coronal plane	**KOR**-oh-nal PLAIN	S/ R/	-al *pertaining to* coron- *crown* plane Latin *flat*	Vertical plane dividing the body into anterior and posterior portions
eversion evert (verb)	ee-**VER**-shun ee-**VERT**		Latin *overturn*	A turning outward
extension	eks-**TEN**-shun		Latin *stretch out*	When a joint is straightened to increase its angle
flexion	**FLEK**-shun		Latin *to bend*	When a joint is bent to decrease its angle
inversion invert (verb)	in-**VER**-shun in-**VERT**		Latin *to turn about*	A turning inward
prone pronation pronate (verb)	PRONE pro-**NAY**-shun **PRO**-nate	 S/ R/	Latin *prone, lying down* -ion *process, action* pronat- *bend down*	Lying facedown, flat on your belly Process of lying facedown or of turning a hand or foot with the volar (palm or sole) surface down
supine supination	soo-**PINE** soo-pih-**NAY**-shun	 S/ R/	Latin *supine, lying face up* -ion *process, action* supinat- *bend backward*	Lying face up, flat on your spine Process of lying face upward or turning an arm or foot so that the palm or sole is facing up

Exercises

A. Some medical terms can act as both a verb (action) and a noun (person, place or thing). *The following pairs of terms are both verbs and nouns. Write the correct form of each term in the blank.* **LO 14.3, 14.8**

1. circumduct   circumduction

   The baseball pitcher was unable to _____ his arm to wind up his pitch.

2. invert   inversion

   A clubfoot would be an _____ of the foot.

3. abduct   abduction

   Moving away from the midline of the body is called

   _____ .

4. evert   eversion

   The patient was unable to _____ her ankle due to great pain.

5. adduct   adduction

   The patient was asked to _____ his arms from a horizontal plane toward the center of his chest.

B. All of the answers for this exercise can be found in the above WAD. LO 14.3, 14.8

1. What is the difference between *abduct* and *adduct*?

   a. abduct _____

   b. adduct _____

2. Which terms in the WAD are opposites?

   _____

3. A patient is being prepared for back surgery. What would be his position on the operating room **(OR)** table?

   _____

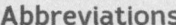

Case Report 14.2 (continued)

By age 65, more than 80% of people have some degree of joint degeneration. Mr. Johnson had always been very physically active, putting a lot of pressure on his weight-bearing joints. At different times in his life he had been overweight, adding to the pressure.

X-rays of his lower back showed **osteoarthritis** of his lower lumbar intervertebral joints and marked osteoarthritis of his left hip joint *(Figure 14.14a and b)*. He received a left total-hip replacement (THR) and physiotherapy (PT) for his lower back.

LO 14.9 Diseases of Joints

Osteoarthritis (OA) is caused by the breakdown and eventual destruction of cartilage in a joint. It develops as a result of wear and tear and is most common in the weight-bearing joints, the knee, hip, and lower back *(Figure 14.14a)*. Because it is a wear-and-tear disease, it is sometimes called **degenerative joint disease (DJD)**. The degenerative process begins in the articular cartilage, which cracks and frays, eventually exposing the underlying bone.

Rheumatoid arthritis (RA) is a chronic, inflammatory disease that can affect many joints, causing deformity and disability. In *Figure 14.14b*, the hand deformities of RA, swelling of the **metacarpophalangeal (MCP)** and **proximal interphalangeal (PIP)** joints with **ulnar deviation** of the fingers, are shown. The disease process initially causes inflammation of the synovial membrane and then spreads to all other parts of the joint. Rheumatoid arthritis is three times as common in women and often begins in the thirties and forties.

Bursitis is inflammation of a **bursa** that can result from overuse of a joint, repeated trauma, or diseases such as RA.

Surgical procedures used to diagnose and treat joint problems are listed in *Table 14.2*.

Abbreviations

DJD	degenerative joint disease
MCP	metacarpophalangeal
OA	osteoarthritis
OR	operating room
PIP	proximal interphalangeal
PT	physiotherapy
RA	rheumatoid arthritis
THR	total-hip replacement

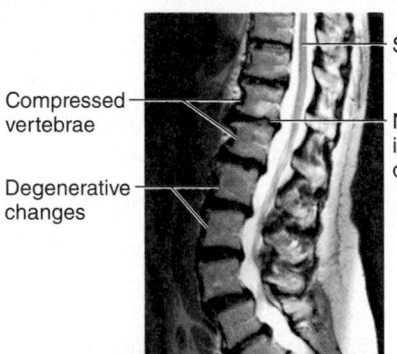

(a) Lumbar vertebrae

Spinal cord
Compressed vertebrae
Narrowed intervertebral disc space
Degenerative changes

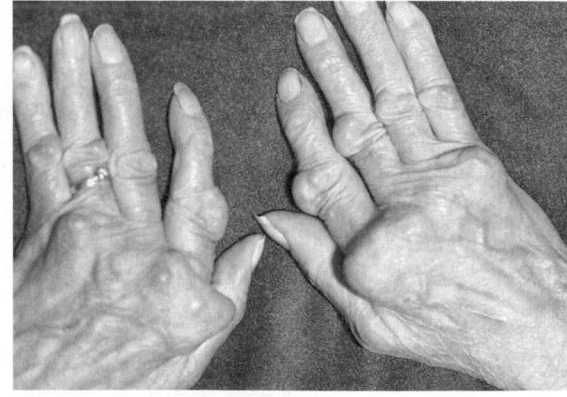

(b)

▲ **Figure 14.14**   **Arthritis.** (*a*) Magnetic resonance imaging (MRI) scan of lumbar vertebrae showing degenerative changes due to osteoarthritis. (*b*) Rheumatoid arthritis of the hands.

Table 14.2 Surgical Procedures for Joints

- **Arthrocentesis**—withdrawal of fluid from a joint through a needle. (The suffix **-centesis** means *to puncture.*)

- **Arthrodesis**—fixation or stiffening of a joint by surgery. (The suffix **-desis** means *to fuse together.*)

- **Arthrography**—an x-ray of a joint taken after the injection of a contrast medium into the joint. A contrast medium makes the inside details of the joint visible. (The suffix **-graphy** means *process of recording.*)

- **Arthroplasty**—surgery to restore as far as possible the function of a joint. It often involves a total replacement of the joint. (The suffix **-plasty** means *surgical repair.*)

- **Arthroscopy**—the visual examination of the interior of a joint using an **arthroscope**. (The suffix **-scopy** means *to view.*)

WORD	PRONUNCIATION	ELEMENTS		DEFINITION
arthrocentesis	AR-throw-sen-TEE-sis	S/ R/CF	-centesis *to puncture* arthr/o	Withdrawal of fluid from a joint through a needle
arthrodesis	ar-THROW-dee-sis	S/ R/CF	-desis *bind together* arthr/o- *joint*	Fixation or stiffening of a joint by surgery
arthrography	ar-THROG-ra-fee	S/ R/CF	-graphy *process of recording* arthr/o- *joint*	X-ray of a joint taken after the injection of a contrast medium into the joint
arthroplasty	AR-throw-plas-tee	S/ R/CF	-plasty *surgical repair* arthr/o- *joint*	Surgery to restore as far as possible the function of a joint
arthroscopy	ar-THROS-koh-pee	S/ R/CF	-scopy *to examine, to view* arthr/o- *joint*	Visual examination of the interior of a joint
arthroscope	AR-thro-skope	S/	-scope *instrument for viewing*	Endoscope used to examine the interior of a joint
bursa bursitis	BURR-sah burr-SIGH-tis	S/ R/	Latin *purse* -itis *inflammation* burs- *bursa*	A closed sac containing synovial fluid Inflammation of a bursa
degenerative	dee-JEN-er-a-tiv	S/ R/	-ive *quality of* degenerat- *deteriorate*	Relating to the deterioration of a structure
deviation	de-ve-A-shun		Latin *turn from straight path*	A turning aside from a normal course
interphalangeal	IN-ter-fay-LAN-jee-al	S/ P/ R/CF	-al *pertaining to* inter- *between* -phalang/e- *phalanx*	Pertaining to the joints between two phalanges
metacarpophalangeal	MET-ah-KAR-poh-fay-LAN-jee-al	S/ R/CF P/ R/CF	-al *pertaining to* -phalang/e- *phalanx* meta- *after, beyond* -carp/o- *bones of the wrist*	Pertaining to the joints between the metacarpal bones and phalanges
osteoarthritis	OS-tee-oh-ar-THRI-tis	S/ R/CF R/	-itis *inflammation* oste/o- *bone* -arthr- *joint*	Chronic inflammatory disease of the joints with pain and loss of function
rheumatoid arthritis	RHU-mah-toyd ar-THRI-tis	S/ R/	-oid *resemble* rheumat- *rheumatism*	Disease of connective tissue, with arthritis as a major manifestation
ulna ulnar (adj)	UL-na UL-nar	R/ S/	Latin *elbow* uln- *forearm bone* -ar *pertaining to*	The medial and larger bone of the forearm Pertaining to the ulna or any of the structures (artery, vein, nerve) named after it

Exercises

A. There are eight terms in the above WAD all using the root or combining form arthr/arthro-. *For questions 1 through 5, match the description of the procedure for which each patient is scheduled in the left column with the name of the procedure the doctor has ordered in the right column. Then fill in the blanks in Exercise B.* **LO 14.3, 14.9**

_____ 1. X-ray of a joint after contrast-medium injection

_____ 2. Withdrawal of fluid from the joint with a needle

_____ 3. Surgery to restore or repair joint function

_____ 4. Surgical fixation of the joint

_____ 5. Visual examination of the interior of the joint

a. arthrodesis

b. arthroplasty

c. arthroscopy

d. arthrography

e. arthrocentesis

B. Fill in the blanks using terms from this spread.   14.3, 14.9

1. The procedure in question 5 will use an arthro _____.

2. The diagnosis for all these patients could be arthr _____.

3. Analyze the terms *interphalangeal* and *metacarpophalangeal*. What is the difference in their location?

    A. interphalangeal _____

    B. metacarpophalangeal _____

In the previous two lessons in this chapter, you have learned how bones of the skeleton support the body and how joints provide mobility. Neither of these functions can occur without muscles and their tendons to provide both posture and movement. Information in this lesson will enable you to use correct medical terminology to:

14.3.1 Describe the structure of skeletal muscle and tendons.

14.3.2 Identify the functions of skeletal muscle and tendons.

14.3.3 Describe the major problems and diseases that occur in muscles and tendons.

You are

... a medical assistant working with Susan Lee, MD, a primary care physician at Fulwood Medical Center.

Your patient is

... Mrs. Mary Carr, a 65-year-old white, retired librarian, who had been in good health until a month ago when she had sudden onset of pain in the muscles of her shoulders and hips.

Case Report 14.3

The pain has become more severe and spread into Mrs. Carr's upper arms, thighs, and lower back. She cannot turn over in bed and cannot get into her car. She has lost 10 pounds in weight and feels constantly tired.

Dr. Lee has diagnosed **polymyalgia rheumatica** and prescribed **prednisone**, 5 mg three times daily (**t.i.d.**). There has been a marked improvement in her symptoms. Your role as Dr. Lee's assistant is to ensure that Mrs. Carr understands the use of her medication and to document changes in her symptoms.

LO 14.10 Functions and Structure of Skeletal Muscle

Functions of Skeletal Muscle

Skeletal muscle is attached to one or more bones. It is also called **voluntary muscle** because it is under conscious control. Because of their length, muscle cells are usually called muscle **fibers**. Each skeletal muscle consists of bundles of muscle fibers, blood vessels, and nerves, with connective tissue sheets that hold the fibers together and connect the muscle to bone.

Skeletal muscle has the following functions:

1. **Movement**. All skeletal muscles are attached to bones, and when a muscle **contracts** it causes movement of the bones to which it is attached *(Figure 14.15)*. This enables you to walk, run, and work with your hands.

2. **Posture**. The **tone** of skeletal muscles holds you straight when sitting, standing, or moving.

3. **Body heat**. When skeletal muscles contract, heat is produced as a by-product of the energy reaction. This heat is essential to maintain your body temperature.

4. **Respiration**. Skeletal muscles move the chest wall as you breathe.

5. **Communication**. Skeletal muscles enable you to speak, write, type, gesture, and grimace.

Structure of Skeletal Muscle

Skeletal **fibers** are narrow and long, up to 1½ inches (approximately 3.7 cm) in length. Each muscle fiber has a thin layer of connective tissue around it. Bundles of muscle fibers are grouped together into **fascicles** that are also surrounded by a layer of connective tissue. Skeletal muscle fibers contain alternating dark and light bands **(striations)** created by the pattern of protein filaments responsible for muscle contraction. Skeletal muscle can be referred to as **striated muscle**.

Bundles of fascicles form a muscle that is separated from adjacent muscles and kept in position by a dense layer of connective tissue called **fascia**. Fascia extends beyond the muscle to form a tendon. The tendon attaches to the periosteum of a bone at the origin and insertion of the muscle.

As an adult, you have the same number of muscle fibers as you had in late childhood. When you exercise and/or lift weights and your muscles enlarge or **hypertrophy**, you have increased the thickness of each muscle fiber. If you do not use your muscles, the reverse happens, and the muscles **atrophy**.

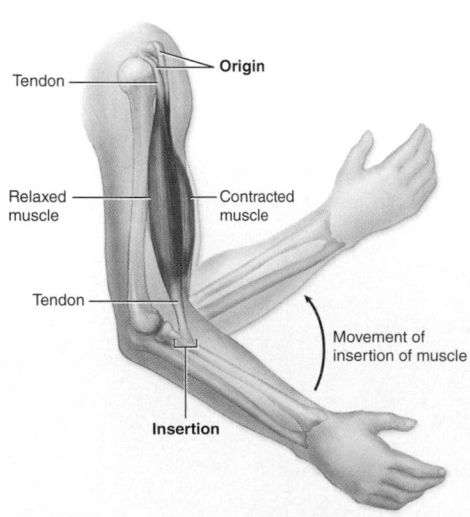

▲ **Figure 14.15**　**Muscle Contraction.**

Abbreviation	
t.i.d.	(Latin *ter in die*) three times a day

Word Analysis and Definition

S = Suffix   P = Prefix   R = Root   R/CF = Combining Form

WORD	PRONUNCIATION	ELEMENTS		DEFINITION
atrophy	AT-roh-fee	P/ R/	a- *without* -trophy *nourishment*	The wasting away or diminished volume of tissue, an organ, or a body part
contract	kon-TRAKT	P/ R/	con- *with, together* -tract *draw*	Draw together or shorten
fascia	FASH-ee-ah		Latin *a band*	Sheet of fibrous connective tissue
fascicle	FAS-ih-kull		Latin *small bundle*	Bundle of muscle fibers
fiber	FIE-ber		Latin *fiber*	A strand or filament
hypertrophy	high-PER-troh-fee	P/ R/	hyper- *excessive* -trophy *nourishment*	Increase in size, but not in number, of an individual tissue element
polymyalgia rheumatica	poll-ee-my-AL-jee-ah rue-MAT-ick-ah	S/ P/ R/ S/ R/	-algia *pain* poly- *many* -my- *muscle* -ica *pertaining to* rheumat- *rheumatism*	Pain in several muscle groups with systemic symptoms
prednisone	PRED-nih-zohn	S/ R/	-isone *cortisone* predn- *a derivative of cholesterol*	A synthetic corticosteroid
striation striated muscle	stri-AY-shun STRI-ay-ted MUSS-el		Latin *stripe*	Stripes Another term for skeletal muscle
tone	TONE		Greek *tone*	Tension present in resting muscles
voluntary muscle	VOL-un-tare-ee MUSS-el	S/ R/	-ary *pertaining to* volunt- *free will*	Another term for skeletal muscle. It is under the control of the will

Exercises

A. Deconstruct the following medical terms from the above WAD into their basic elements; then define each element.
Fill in the chart.   **LO 14.3, 14.10, 14.11**

Medical Term	Prefix	Meaning of Prefix	Root(s)/ Combining Form	Meaning of Root(s)/ Combining Form	Suffix	Meaning of Suffix
hypertrophy	1.	2.	3.	4.	5.	6.
contract	7.	8.	9.	10.	11.	12.
polymyalgia	13.	14.	15.	16.	17.	18.
atrophy	19.	20.	21.	22.	23.	24.
rheumatica	25.	26.	27.	28.	29.	30.

B. Use the *language of orthopedics* to answer the following questions about skeletal muscle.   LO 14.3, 14.10, 14.11

1. Skeletal muscle can also be referred to as _____ muscle.

2. Skeletal muscle attaches to _____.

3. Skeletal muscle is under conscious control; therefore, it is considered a _____ muscle.

4. Skeletal muscle must be used, or _____ (condition) occurs.

LO 14.11 Disorders of Skeletal Muscles

Muscle soreness may be a result of vigorous exercise, particularly if your muscles are not used to it. Exercise causes buildup of lactic acid in muscle fibers, and the resulting inflammation of them and their surrounding connective tissue produces soreness.

Muscle cramps are sudden, painful contractions of a muscle or group of muscles. They are usually of short duration. The etiology of cramp is unknown, but low blood potassium, calcium and magnesium levels, use of caffeine and tobacco, and diminished blood supply are possible causes. There are no effective medications available. The cramp is usually self-limiting.

Muscle strains range from a simple stretch in the muscle or **tendon** to a partial or complete tear in the muscle or muscle-tendon combination. Most strains heal with **RICE** (**r**est, **i**ce, **c**ompression [elastic bandage], and **e**levation) *(Figure 14.16),* followed by simple exercises to relieve pain and restore mobility. A complete tear may require surgical repair.

A **sprain** is a stretch or tear of a ligament, often of the ankle, knee, or wrist. It is also treated by RICE.

Anabolic steroids are related to testosterone but have been altered so that their main effect is to cause skeletal muscle to hypertrophy. They are used illegally in many sports to increase muscle strength. They have marked, often irreversible, side effects, including stunting the height of growing adolescents, shrinking testes and sperm counts, masculinizing women, delusions, and paranoid jealousy. In the long term, there are increased risks of heart attacks and strokes, kidney failure, and liver tumors.

Fibromyalgia affects muscles and tendons all over the body, causing chronic pain associated with fatigue and depression. Its etiology is unknown. There are no laboratory tests for it and no specific treatment except pain management, physiotherapy and stress reduction.

Myasthenia gravis is a chronic autoimmune disease *(see Chapter 12)* characterized by varying degrees of weakness of the skeletal muscles. The weakness increases with activity and decreases with rest. Facial muscles are often involved, causing problems with eye and eyelid movements, chewing, and talking. Antibodies produced by the body's own immune system block the passage of **neurotransmitters** from motor nerves to muscles. **Thymectomy** is usually recommended. **Cholinesterase inhibitors** such as Prostigmin are also used.

Muscular dystrophy is a general term for a group of hereditary, progressive disorders affecting skeletal muscles. **Duchenne muscular dystrophy (DMD)** is the most common, occurring in boys who begin to have difficulty walking around the age of 3. Generalized muscle weakness and atrophy progress, and few live beyond 20 years. There is no effective treatment.

Rhabdomyolysis is the breakdown of muscle fibers. This releases a protein pigment called **myoglobin** into the bloodstream. Myoglobin breaks down into toxic compounds that cause kidney failure. Rhabdomyolysis can be caused by muscle trauma; severe exertion (marathon running); alcoholism; and use of cocaine, heroin, amphetamines, or phencyclidine (**PCP**).

Tenosynovitis is inflammation of the sheath that surrounds a **tendon**. It is usually related to repetitive use and occurs commonly in the wrist and hands. It produces pain, tenderness in the tendon, and difficulty in movement of a joint. Treatment is rest, immobilization, nonsteroidal anti-inflammatory drugs (**NSAIDs**), local corticosteroid injections, and, occasionally, surgery.

Abbreviations

DMD	Duchenne muscular dystrophy
NSAID	nonsteroidal anti-inflammatory drug
PCP	phencyclidine (angel dust)
RICE	rest, ice, compression and elevation

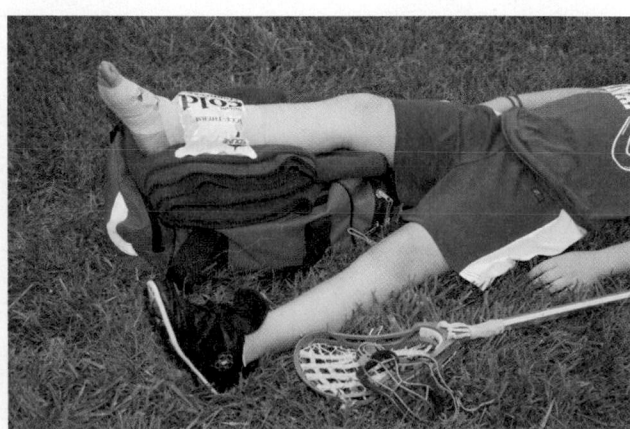

▲ **Figure 14.16** RICE Treatment.

WORD	PRONUNCIATION	ELEMENTS		DEFINITION
Duchenne muscular dystrophy	**DOO**-shen **MUSS**-kyu-lar **DISS**-troh-fee	P/ R/	Guillaume Benjamin Duchenne, French neurologist, 1806–1875 dys- *bad, difficult* -**trophy** *nourishment*	A condition with symmetrical weakness and wasting of pelvic, shoulder, and proximal limb muscles
fibromyalgia	fie-bro-my-**AL**-jee-ah	S/ R/CF R/	-algia *pain* **fibr/o-** *fiber* -**my-** *muscle*	Pain in the muscle fibers
myoglobin	**MY**-oh-**GLOW**-bin	S/ R/CF R/	-in *substance* **my/o-** *muscle* -**glob-** *globe*	Protein of muscle that stores and transports oxygen
neurotransmitter (*Note: Transmitter* is a word in itself and begins with a prefix.)	**NYUR**-oh-trans-**MIT**-er	S/ R/CF P/ R/	-er *agent* **neur/o-** *nerve* -**trans-** *across* -**mitt-** *to send*	Chemical agent that relays messages from one nerve cell to the next
rhabdomyolysis	**RAB**-doh-my-oh-**LIE**-sis	S/ R/CF R/CF	-lysis *destruction* **rhabd/o-** *rod shaped* -**my/o-** *muscle*	Destruction of muscle to produce myoglobin
sprain	SPRAIN		root unknown	A wrench or tear in a ligament
strain	STRAIN		Latin *to bind*	Overstretch or tear in a muscle or tendon
tendon **tendinitis** (also spelled **tendonitis**)	**TEN**-dun ten-dih-**NYE**-tis	S/ R/	Latin *sinew* -**itis** *inflammation* **tendin-** *tendon*	Fibrous band that connects muscle to bone Inflammation of a tendon
tenosynovitis	**TEN**-oh-sine-oh-**VIE**-tis	S/ R/CF R/	-itis *inflammation* **ten/o-** *tendon* -**synov-** *synovial membrane*	Inflammation of a tendon and its surrounding synovial sheath
thymectomy	thigh-**MEK**-toe-me	S/ R/	-ectomy *surgical excision* **thym-** *thymus gland*	Surgical removal of the thymus gland

Exercises

A. The following elements are all contained in the above WAD. *Circle the best answer.*   **LO 14.3, 14.11**

1. **Dys** is a   suffix   prefix   root
2. **Fibro** is a   combining form   root   suffix
3. The suffix **-algia** means   inflammation   pain   swelling
4. **Ectomy** means   fixation   repair   excision

B. Using the medical terms in the above WAD answer the following questions.   LO 14.3, 14.11

1. List all the terms that are diagnoses.

_____

_____

2. List any terms that are procedures.

_____

_____

3. List any other terms that do not fall in the categories in questions 1 and 2 and give a definition for each.

_____

_____

_____

_____

Lesson 14.4 Axial Skeleton

LESSON OBJECTIVES

The vertebral column is part of the axial skeleton. In this lesson, information about the axial skeleton, with its joints and the muscles that function in an integrated manner, will enable you to use correct medical terminology to:

14.4.1 Define the regions and bones of the vertebral column.

14.4.2 Describe the structure and functions of an intervertebral joint.

14.4.3 Identify the major muscles that hold the vertebral column erect.

14.4.4 Describe the major problems and diseases that affect the vertebral column.

14.4.5 Identify the bones of the skull.

14.4.6 Identify the major muscles of mastication and respiration.

You are

. . . a physical therapist assistant working in the Physical Therapy Department of Fulwood Medical Center.

Your patient is

. . . Ms. Nancy Cardenas, a 27-year-old jeweler. Ms. Cardenas was waiting in her car at a traffic light 3 days ago when her car was rear-ended.

Case Report 14.4

Ms. Cardenas now has severe neck pain radiating down her left arm, with dizziness and headaches. She is unable to go to work. Dr. Stannard has examined her and diagnosed her condition as a **whiplash** injury. A magnetic resonance image (MRI) shows **herniation** of intervertebral discs between C5–C6 and C6–C7. Your role is to implement a regime of physiotherapy, including range-of-motion (ROM) exercises for her neck joints.

LO 14.12 Structure of Axial Skeleton

The axial skeleton comprises the

1. Vertebral column
2. Skull
3. Rib cage

The axial skeleton is the upright axis of the body and protects the brain, spinal cord, heart, and lungs—most of the major centers of our physiology.

The **vertebral column** has 26 bones divided into five regions *(Figure 14.17):*

1. **Cervical** region, with seven vertebrae, labeled C1 to C7 and curved anteriorly.
2. **Thoracic** region, with 12 vertebrae, labeled T1 to T12 and curved posteriorly.
3. **Lumbar** region, with five vertebrae, labeled L1 to L5 and curved anteriorly.
4. **Sacral** region, with one bone curved posteriorly.
5. **Coccyx** (tailbone), with one bone curved posteriorly.

The **spinal cord** lies protected in the vertebral canal. Spinal nerves leave the spinal cord through the **intervertebral foramina** to travel to other parts of the body.

Intervertebral discs consist of fibrocartilage and inhabit the intervertebral space between the bodies of adjacent vertebrae. They provide additional support and cushioning for the vertebral column. The center of the disc is a gelatinous nucleus pulposus.

Abnormal spinal curvatures can result from disease, poor posture, or congenital defects in the vertebrae. The defect that is most common is called **scoliosis**, an abnormal lateral curve in the thoracic region *(Figure 14.18a).* In older people, particularly with osteoporosis, an exaggerated thoracic curvature is called **kyphosis** *(Figure 14.18b).* An exaggerated lumbar curve is called **lordosis** *(Figure 14.18c).*

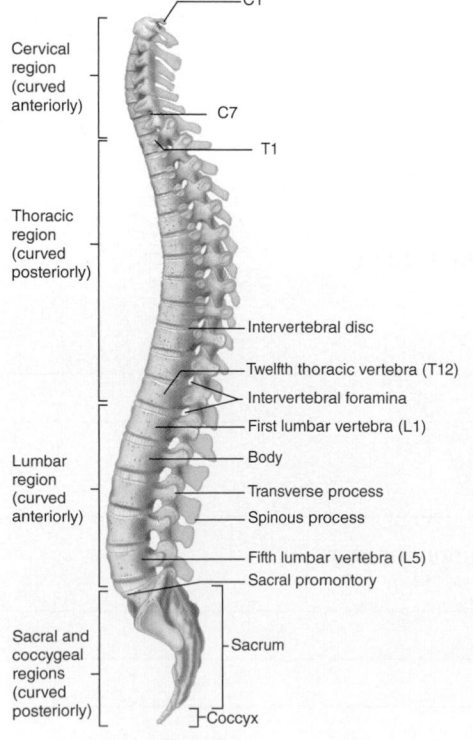

Cervical region (curved anteriorly)

C1

C7

T1

Thoracic region (curved posteriorly)

Intervertebral disc

Twelfth thoracic vertebra (T12)

Intervertebral foramina

First lumbar vertebra (L1)

Body

Lumbar region (curved anteriorly)

Transverse process

Spinous process

Fifth lumbar vertebra (L5)

Sacral promontory

Sacral and coccygeal regions (curved posteriorly)

Sacrum

Coccyx

Lateral view

▲ **Figure 14.17** Vertebral Column.

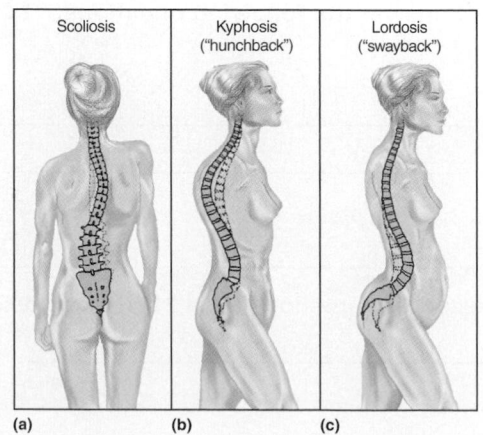

Scoliosis | Kyphosis ("hunchback") | Lordosis ("swayback")

(a) | (b) | (c)

▲ **Figure 14.18** Abnormal Spinal Curvatures. (*a*) Scoliosis. (*b*) Kyphosis. (*c*) Lordosis.

S = Suffix   P = Prefix   R = Root   R/CF = Combining Form

WORD	PRONUNCIATION	ELEMENTS		DEFINITION
cervical	**SER**-vih-kal	S/ R/	-al *pertaining to* **cervic-** *neck*	Pertaining to the neck region
coccyx	**KOK**-sicks		Greek *coccyx*	Small tailbone at the lowest end of the vertebral column
foramen foramina (pl)	fo-**RAY**-men fo-**RAM**-in-ah		Latin *an aperture*	An opening through a structure
herniation herniate (verb)	**HER**-nee-ay-shun **HER**-nee-ate	S/ R/CF	-tion *process, being* **herni/a-** *rupture*	Protrusion of an anatomical structure from its normal position
intervertebral	**IN**-ter-**VER**-teh-bral	S/ P/ R/	-al *pertaining to* **inter-** *between* **-vertebr-** *vertebra*	Located between two vertebrae
kyphosis kyphotic (adj)	ki-**FOH**-sis ki-**FOT**-ik		French *humpbacked*	A normal posterior curve of the thoracic spine that can be exaggerated in disease
lordosis lordotic (adj)	lore-**DOH**-sis lore-**DOT**-ik		Greek *bend backward*	An exaggerated forward curvature of the lumbar spine
lumbar (adj)	**LUM**-bar		Latin *loin*	Relating to the region in the back and sides between the ribs and pelvis
sacrum sacral (adj)	**SAY**-crum **SAY**-kral		Latin *sacred*	Segment of the vertebral column that forms part of the pelvis
scoliosis scoliotic (adj)	skoh-lee-**OH**-sis **SKOH**-lee-**OT**-ik		Greek *crooked*	An abnormal lateral curvature of the vertebral column
spine spinal (adj)	SPINE **SPY**-nal		Latin *spine*	Vertebral column, *or* a short projection from a bone
thorax thoracic (adj)	**THO**-racks **THOR**-ass-ik		Greek *breastplate*	The part of the trunk between the abdomen and neck
vertebra vertebrae (pl) vertebral (adj)	**VER**-teh-brah **VER**-teh-bray **VER**-teh-bral		Latin *spinal joint*	One of the bones of the spinal column
whiplash	**WHIP**-lash	R/ R/	**whip-** *to swing* **-lash** *end of whip*	Symptoms caused by sudden, uncontrolled extension and flexion of the neck, often in an automobile accident

Exercises

A. After reading Case Report 14.4, answer the following questions. *Be prepared to discuss your answers in class.*   **LO 14.3, 14.12**

1. What are Ms. Cardenas' presenting symptoms? _____

2. What medical term means *the space between two vertebrae*? _____

3. What caused the patient's whiplash injury? _____

4. Herniation of a disc means _____.

B. Using the *language of orthopedics*, continue answering questions related to Case Report 14.4.   LO 14.3, 14.12

1. What is the meaning of the phrase *radiating pain*?

_____

2. What diagnostic test did Ms. Cardenas undergo?

_____

3. What is the exact location of her pain?

_____

4. What is her treatment plan as prescribed by Dr. Stannard?

_____

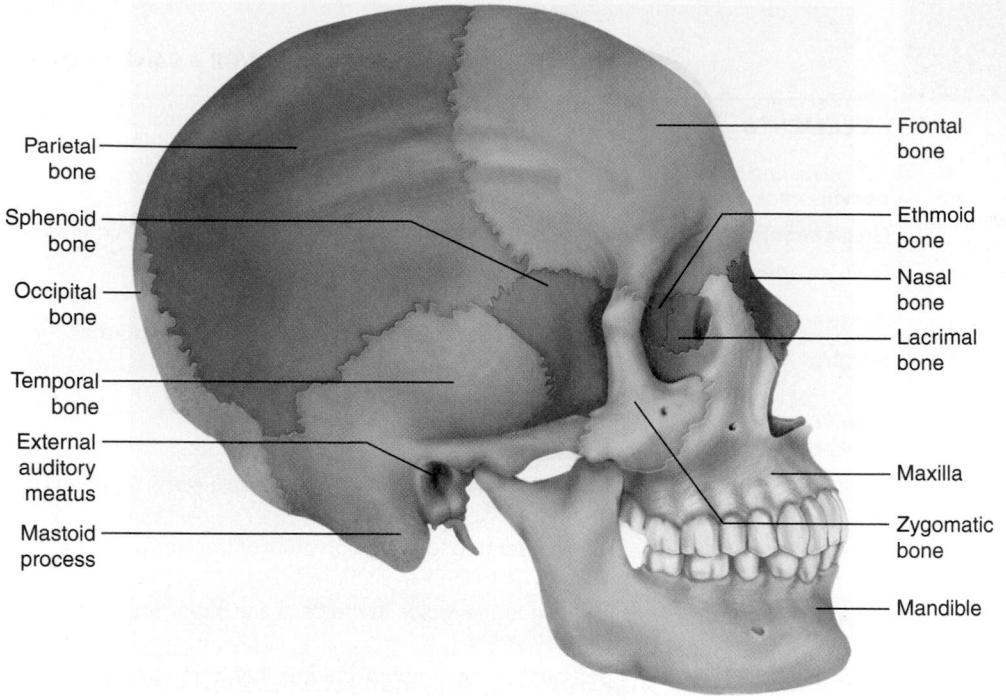

▲ Figure 14.19 Skull: Right Lateral View.

Labels: Parietal bone, Sphenoid bone, Occipital bone, Temporal bone, External auditory meatus, Mastoid process, Frontal bone, Ethmoid bone, Nasal bone, Lacrimal bone, Maxilla, Zygomatic bone, Mandible

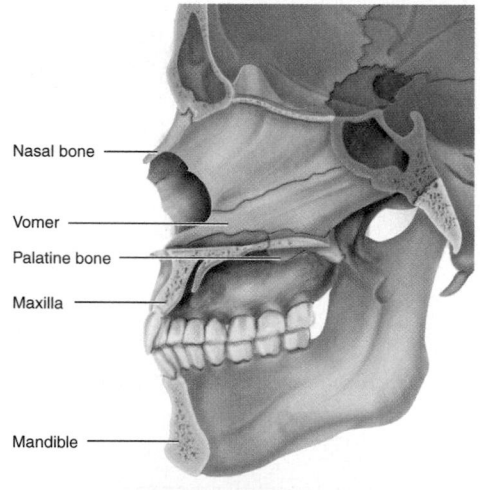

▲ Figure 14.20 Facial Bones.

Labels: Nasal bone, Vomer, Palatine bone, Maxilla, Mandible

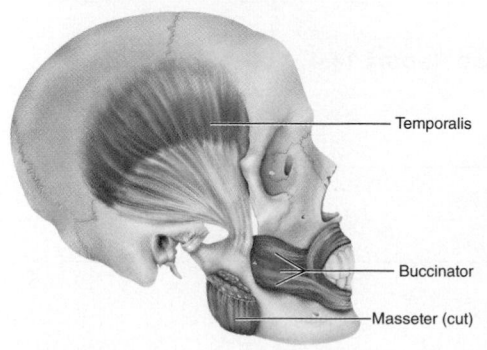

▲ Figure 14.21 Muscles of Chewing.

Labels: Temporalis, Buccinator, Masseter (cut)

LO 14.12 The Skull

The human skull has 22 bones, 8 of which make up the **cranium**, the upper part of the skull that encloses the **cranial cavity** and protects the brain (*Figure 14.19*). The bones of the cranium are

1. **Frontal** bone—forms the forehead and the roofs of the orbits and contains a pair of right and left frontal sinuses above the orbits.
2. **Parietal** bones (2)—form the bulging sides and roof of the cranium.
3. **Occipital** bone—forms the back of and part of the base of the cranium.
4. **Temporal** bones (2)—form the sides and part of the base of the cranium.
5. **Sphenoid** bone—forms part of the base of the cranium and the orbits.
6. **Ethmoid** bone—forms parts of the nose and the orbits and is hollow, forming the ethmoid sinuses.

The bones of the cranium are joined together by sutures, joints that appear as seams, covered on the inside and outside by a thin layer of connective tissue.

The lower anterior part of the skull comprises the 14 bones of the facial skeleton (*Figure 14.20; see also Figure 14.19*):

1. **Maxillary** bones (2)—form the upper jaw, hold the upper teeth, and are hollow, forming the maxillary sinuses.
2. **Palatine** bones (2)—are located behind the maxilla.
3. **Zygomatic** bones (2)—form the prominences of the cheeks below the eyes.
4. **Lacrimal** bones (2)—form the medial wall of each eye orbit.
5. **Nasal** bones (2)—form the sides and bridge of the nose.
6. **Vomer** bone—separates the two nasal cavities (*Figure 14.20*).
7. Inferior nasal **conchae** (2)—are fragile bones in the lower nasal cavity.
8. **Mandible**—is the lower jawbone, which holds the lower teeth.

The third component of the axial skeleton, the rib cage, is discussed in *Chapter 13*.

Bones, Joints, and Muscles of Mastication

The **temporomandibular joint (TMJ)** connects the condyle of the mandible to a fossa in the temporal bone at the base of the skull. The joint acts like a hinge when you open and close your mouth.

The muscles you use to chew food include

1. The **masseter**, which raises the jawbone and controls the rate at which you lower it (*Figure 14.21*).
2. The **temporalis**, a fan-shaped muscle that raises the jawbone (*Figure 14.21*).
3. The **medial pterygoid**, which closes the jaw and moves it from side to side.
4. The **lateral pterygoid**, which opens the mouth and moves the jawbone from side to side. The pterygoid muscles are hidden behind the mandible in *Figure 14.21*.
5. The **buccinator**, which compresses the cheek against the teeth during chewing (*Figure 14.21*)

Abbreviations	
TMJ	temporomandibular joint

WORD	PRONUNCIATION	ELEMENTS		DEFINITION
concha conchae (pl)	**KON**-kah **KON**-key		Latin *a shell*	Shell-shaped bone on medial wall of nasal cavity
cranium cranial (adj)	**KRAY**-nee-um **KRAY**-nee-al		Greek *skull*	The upper part of the skull that encloses and protects the brain Pertaining to the skull
ethmoid	**ETH**-moyd	S/ R/	-oid *resemble* ethm- *sieve*	Bone that forms the back of the nose and encloses numerous air cells
mandible mandibular (adj)	**MAN**-di-bel man-**DIB**-you-lar	 S/ R/	Latin *jaw* -ar *pertaining to* mandibul- *the jaw*	Lower jawbone Pertaining to the mandible
masseter	**MASS**-eh-ter		Greek *to chew*	Muscle that closes the mouth
maxilla maxillary (adj)	mak-**SILL**-ah mak-**SILL**-ary		Latin *jawbone*	Upper jawbone, containing right and left maxillary sinuses
occipital	ock-**SIP**-it-al		Latin *occiput*	The back of the skull
palatine	**PAL**-ah-tine		Latin *palate*	Bone that forms the hard palate and parts of the nose and orbits
parietal	pah-**RYE**-eh-tal	S/ R/	-al *pertaining to* pariet- *wall*	The two bones forming the sidewalls and roof of the cranium
pterygoid	**TER**-ih-goyd	S/ R/	-oid *resemble* pteryg- *wing*	Pterygoid muscles are two wing-shaped muscles that open and close the mouth
sphenoid	**SFEE**-noyd	S/ R/	-oid *resemble* sphen- *wedge*	Wedge-shaped bone at the base of the skull
temporal	**TEM**-por-al	S/ R/	-al *pertaining to* tempor- *temple, side of head*	Bone that forms part of the base and sides of the skull
temporalis muscle	tem-poh-**RAHL**-is **MUSS**-el	S/ R/	-alis *pertaining to* tempor- *temple, side of head*	Muscle attached to temporal bone that opens and closes the jaw
temporomandibular joint (TMJ)	**TEM**-por-oh-man-**DIB**-you-lar JOYNT	S/ R/CF R/	-ar *pertaining to* tempor/o- *temple, side of head* -mandibul- *the jaw*	The joint between the temporal bone and the mandible
vomer	**VOH**-mer		Latin *ploughshare*	Lower nasal septum
zygoma zygomatic (adj)	zye-**GOH**-mah zye-goh-**MAT**-ic		French *yoke*	Bone that forms the prominence of the cheek

Exercises

A. The human skull has 22 bones. *Meet a lesson objective by listing the eight bones of the cranium (upper skull), with a brief description of their location. Fill in the blanks.* **LO 14.3, 14.12**

The eight bones of the cranium are:

1. _____

2. _____

3. _____

4. _____

5. _____

6. _____

7. _____

8. _____

Lesson 14.5 Appendicular Skeleton, Joints, and Muscles

Attached to the axial skeleton through joints and muscles is the appendicular skeleton, the bones of the upper limbs and the shoulder girdle and those of the lower limbs and the pelvic girdle. These limbs carry out many of the commands issued by your brain in response to changes in your body and in your external environment, particularly in terms of mobility and the manipulation of objects.

Information in this lesson will enable you to use correct medical terminology to:

14.5.1 Describe the structure and functions of the bones, joints, and muscles of the shoulder girdle and upper limbs.

14.5.2 Describe the structure and functions of the bones, joints, and muscles of the pelvic girdle and lower limbs.

14.5.3 Discuss the major problems and diseases that affect mobility and other functions of the limbs.

You are

... an emergency technician working in the Emergency Department at Fulwood Medical Center.

Your patient is

... Mr. Bruce Adams, a 55-year-old construction worker.

Case Report 14.5

Mr. Adams presents with severe pain in his right shoulder that has made him leave work and seek relief. The pain began 3 or 4 months ago; it is worse at the end of the workday and when he has to work with his arm above the shoulder. In the past week, the pain has awakened him from sleep.

The company physician has diagnosed a shoulder bursitis and treated Mr. Adams with anti-inflammatory medication and a heating pad. Mr. Adams has no previous history of work injuries. Physical examination shows marked limitation by pain of all passive and active movements of the right shoulder and weakness in all lifting movements.

LO 14.13 Shoulder Girdle and Upper Arm

The **pectoral** (shoulder) **girdle** connects the axial skeleton to the upper limbs and helps with movements of the upper limb.

The bones of the pectoral girdle are the **scapulae** (shoulder blades) and **clavicles** *(Figure 14.22)*. The scapula extends over the top of the joint to form a roof called the **acromion**. The acromion is attached to the clavicle at the **acromioclavicular (AC)** joint. This also provides a connection between the axial skeleton, pectoral girdle, and upper arm.

The joint that connects the pectoral girdle to the upper limb is the shoulder joint, located between the scapula and the **humerus** bone of the upper arm *(see Figure 14.22)*. This joint is a ball-and-socket joint in which the head of the humerus allows the greatest range of motion of any joint in the body. Because of this, the shoulder joint also is the most unstable joint and is liable to **dislocation**.

Several ligaments hold together the articulating surfaces of the humerus and scapula.

Muscles around the shoulder joint are essential for its stability. Four muscles that originate on the scapula wrap around the joint and fuse to form one large tendon, the **rotator cuff**, which is inserted into the humerus. This tendon keeps the ball of the humerus tightly in the socket of the scapula and provides the strength that baseball pitchers need. The rotator cuff muscles are

1. Subscapularis   2. Supraspinatus   3. Infraspinatus   4. Teres minor

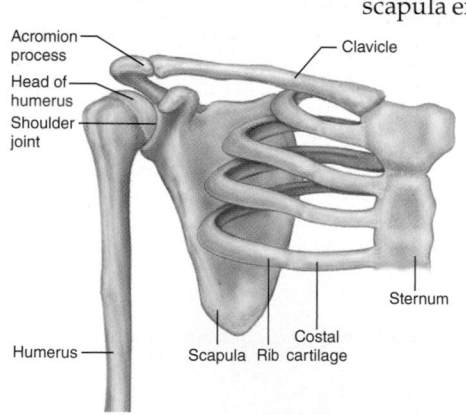

Acromion process
Head of humerus
Shoulder joint
Humerus
Clavicle
Sternum
Costal cartilage
Scapula   Rib

▲ **Figure 14.22**   Pectoral Girdle.

Case Report 14.5 (continued)

When Mr. Adams was evaluated by Dr. Stannard, an x-ray (which looks for bony abnormalities) revealed no shoulder abnormality. An MRI, which shows slices of all tissues, revealed a full-thickness tear of the rotator cuff.

LO 14.4 Common Disorders of the Shoulder

Rotator cuff tears are the result of the wear and tear of overuse in work situations or in sports actions such as the throwing done by baseball pitchers. The tears can be partial or complete and usually require surgical repair.

Shoulder separation is a dislocation of the acromioclavicular joint, usually due to a fall on the point of the shoulder.

Keynotes

- **Shoulder dislocation** occurs when the ball of the humerus slips out of the socket of the scapula, usually anteriorly.

- **Shoulder subluxation** occurs when the ball of the humerus slips partially out of position and then moves back in.

WORD	PRONUNCIATION	ELEMENTS		DEFINITION
acromion	ah-**CROW**-mee-on	S/ R/	-ion *action* **acrom-** *acromion*	Lateral end of the scapula, extending over the shoulder joint
acromioclavicular	ah-**CROW**-mee-oh-klah-**VICK**-you-lar	S/ R/CF R/	-ar *pertaining to* **acromi/o-** *acromion* **-clavicul-** *clavicle*	Pertaining to the joint between the acromion and the clavicle
clavicle **clavicular (adj)**	**KLAV**-ih-kul klah-**VICK**-you-lar		Latin *collarbone*	Curved bone that forms the anterior part of the pectoral girdle
dislocation	dis-low-**KAY**-shun	S/ P/ R/	-ion *action* **dis-** *apart* **-locat-** *a place*	The state of being completely out of joint
humerus	**HYU**-mer-us		Latin *shoulder*	Single bone of the upper arm
pectoral **pectoral girdle**	**PEK**-tor-al **PEK**-tor-al **GIR**-del	S/ R/	-al *pertaining to* **pector-** *chest* **girdle** Old English *encircle*	Pertaining to the chest Incomplete bony ring that attaches the upper limb to the axial skeleton
rotator cuff	roh-**TAY**-tor CUFF	S/ R/	-or *a doer* **rotat-** *rotate* **cuff** Old English *band*	Part of the capsule of the shoulder joint
scapula **scapulae (pl)** **scapular (adj)**	**SKAP**-you-lah **SKAP**-you-lee **SKAP**-you-lar	S/ R/	Latin *shoulder blade* -ar *pertaining to* **scapul-** *scapula*	Shoulder blade Pertaining to the shoulder blade
separation	sep-ah-**RAY**-shun	S/ R/	-ion *action* **separat** *move apart*	A shoulder separation is a dislocation of the acromioclavicular joint
subluxation	sub-luck-**SAY**-shun	S/ P/ R/	-ion *action* **sub-** *under, slightly* **-luxat-** *dislocate*	An incomplete dislocation in which some contact between the joint surfaces remains

Exercises

A. Use your knowledge of the *language of orthopedics* to complete the following medical terms.   LO 14.3, 14.14

1. Incomplete dislocation   _____/_____/_____

2. Joint between acromion and clavicle   _____/_____/_____

3. Completely out of joint   _____/_____/_____

4. Pertaining to the chest   _____/_____/_____

B. Implement the *language of orthopedics* to answer the following questions.   LO 14.1, 14.14

1. X-rays and MRIs are diagnostic tools that look at parts of the body differently. What is the difference?

   a. X-rays look at

   _____

   b. MRIs look at

   _____

2. Write medical terms for the following:

   a the shoulder girdle _____

   b. shoulder blades _____

   c. collarbones _____

3. What is the difference between a shoulder separation and shoulder dislocation?

   a. separation _____

   b. dislocation _____

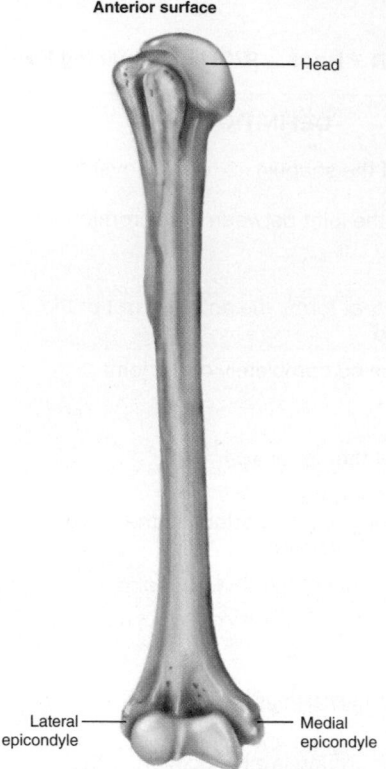

Anterior surface

Head

Lateral epicondyle

Medial epicondyle

▲ **Figure 14.23** Humerus.

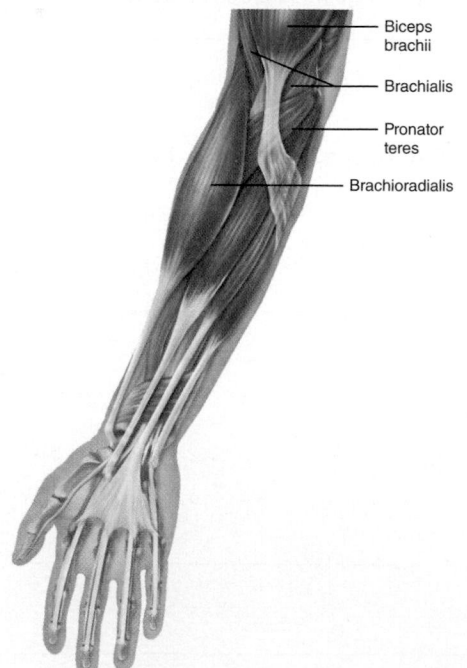

Biceps brachii

Brachialis

Pronator teres

Brachioradialis

▲ **Figure 14.25** Muscles of Elbow Joint.

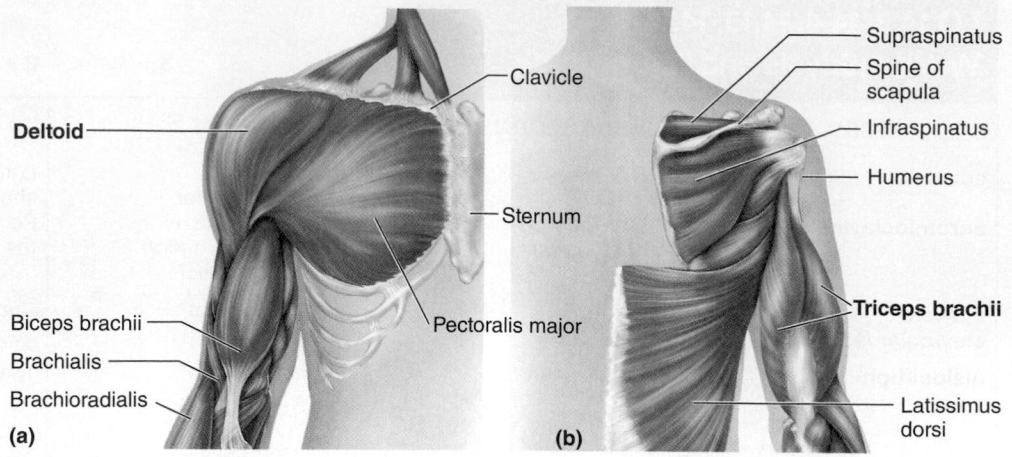

Clavicle

Deltoid

Sternum

Biceps brachii

Brachialis

Brachioradialis

Pectoralis major

(a)

Supraspinatus

Spine of scapula

Infraspinatus

Humerus

Triceps brachii

Latissimus dorsi

(b)

▲ **Figure 14.24** **Muscles Joining Arm to Body.** [*a*] Anterior view. [*b*] Posterior view.

LO 14.13 Upper Arm and Elbow Joint

The **humerus** is the long bone of the upper arm *(Figure 14.23)*. It extends from the scapula to the elbow joint. Muscles connect it to the pectoral girdle, vertebral column, and ribs. These muscles enable the arm to be freely movable at the shoulder joint. The major anterior muscles are the **deltoid** and **pectoralis major** *(Figure 14.24a)*, and among the major posterior muscles is the **latissimus dorsi** *(Figure 14.24b)*.

The elbow joint has two **articulations**:

1. A hinge joint between the humerus and **ulna** bone of the forearm, which allows flexion and extension of the elbow.
2. A gliding joint between the humerus and **radius** bone of the forearm, which allows pronation and supination of the forearm and hand.

A joint capsule and ligaments hold the two articulations together.

Muscles that move the elbow joint and forearm have their **origins** on the humerus or pectoral girdle and are **inserted** into the bones of the forearm. On the front of the arm, a group of three muscles (the **biceps brachii**, **brachialis**, and **brachioradialis**) flexes the forearm at the elbow joint and rotates the forearm and hand laterally (supination) *(Figure 14.25)*. On the back of the arm, a single muscle, the **triceps brachii**, extends the elbow joint and forearm *(Figure 14.24b)*.

LO 14.14 Common Disorders of the Elbow

Tennis elbow is caused by overuse of the elbow joint or poor techniques in playing tennis or golf. Tendons of upper-arm and forearm muscles are inserted into the medial and lateral **epicondyles** of the humerus just above the elbow joint *(Figure 14.24)*. Small tears in the tendons at their attachments occur with overuse, and eventually enough tears accumulate to cause pain and restrict elbow movement. The pain occurs when straightening the elbow or opening and closing the fingers. Treatment is rest, ice, pain medication, massage, and stretching exercises.

Ligament strains and **bone fractures** due to a heavy fall or a blow to the elbow are also common injuries.

WORD	PRONUNCIATION	ELEMENTS		DEFINITION
biceps brachii	**BYE**-sepz **BRAY**-key-eye	P/ R/ R/	bi- *two* -ceps *head* brachii *of the arm*	A muscle of the upper arm that has two heads or points of origin on the scapula
brachialis	**BRAY**-kee-al-is	S/ R/	-alis *pertaining to* brachi- *arm*	Muscle that lies underneath the biceps and is the strongest flexor of the forearm
brachioradialis	**BRAY**-kee-oh-**RAY**-dee-al-is	S/ R/CF R/	-is *belonging to* brachi/o- *arm* -radial- *radius*	Muscle that helps flex the forearm
deltoid	**DEL**-toyd	S/ R/	-oid *resembling* delt- *Greek letter delta*	Large, fan-shaped muscle connecting the scapula and clavicle to the humerus
epicondyle	ep-ih-**KON**-dile	P/ R/	epi- *above* -condyle *knuckle*	Projection above the condyle for attachment of a ligament or tendon
insertion	in-**SIR**-shun	S/ R/	-ion *process* insert- *put together*	The insertion of a muscle is the attachment of a muscle to a more movable part of the skeleton, as distinct from the origin
latissimus dorsi	la-**TISS**-ih-muss **DOOR**-sigh	S/ R/ R/	-imus *most* latiss- *wide* dorsi *back*	The widest (broadest) muscle in the back
origin	**OR**-ih-gin		Latin *source of*	Fixed source of a muscle at its attachment to bone
radius	**RAY**-dee-us		Latin *spoke of a wheel*	The forearm bone on the thumb side
triceps brachii	**TRY**-sepz **BRAY**-key-eye	P/ R/ R/	tri- *three* -ceps *head* brachii *of the arm*	Muscle of the arm that has three heads or points of origin

Exercises

A. There would be no movement without bones and muscles. *Reduce the terminology of the following muscles to the basic elements.*
Fill in the chart; then fill in the blanks with the terms from the chart. **LO 14.3, 14.13**

Muscle	Prefix	Root/Combining Form	Suffix
biceps brachii	1.	2.	3.
brachialis	4.	5.	6.
brachioradialis	7.	8.	9.
deltoid	10.	11.	12.
latissimus dorsi	13.	14.	15.
triceps brachii	16.	17.	18.

B. Using the terms from the preceding chart, write the name of the correct muscle on the line next to its description.
LO 14.3, 14.13

1. Three heads or points of origin   _____

2. Strongest flexor of the forearm   _____

3. Fan-shaped muscle   _____

4. Helps flex the forearm   _____

5. Two points of origin on the scapula   _____

6. Broadest muscle of the back   _____

The office accounting system is computerized, and Ms. Baker works at a keyboard all day, inputting charges and payments. For the past 3 months, she has had constant pain in her right hand, arm, and shoulder. She has numbness and tingling in her fingers and drops things out of her right hand. She is now unable to work.

Dr. Stannard has diagnosed tenosynovitis of the wrist. He has prescribed an anti-inflammatory medication, physiotherapy, and a brace for the wrist. Ms. Baker is to ask for an **ergonomic** keyboard for her computer.

She requires help in filling out her worker's compensation form. (This task is an exercise at the end of the chapter.)

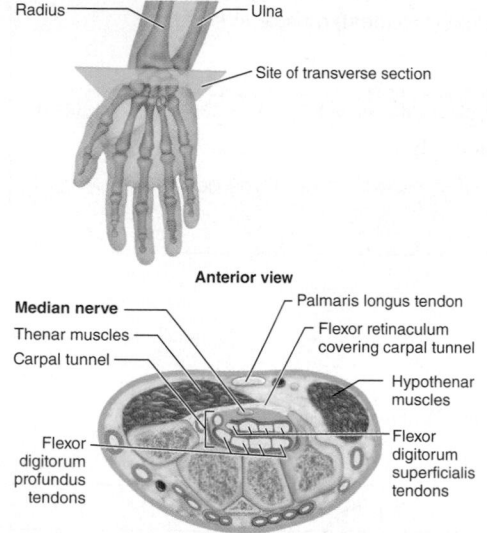

▲ Figure 14.26 Carpal Tunnel: Transverse Section.

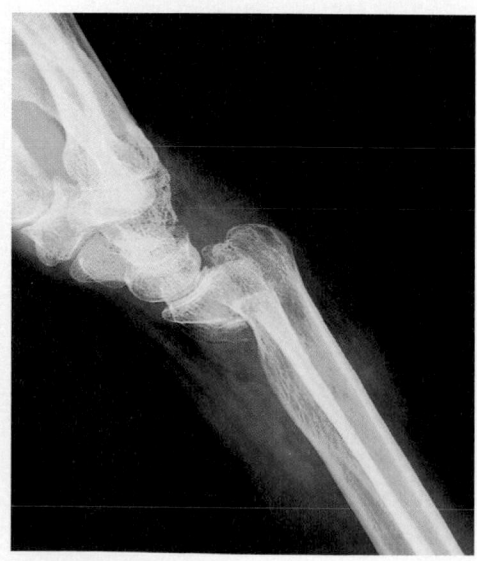

LO 14.13 Forearm and Wrist

The forearm has two bones, the **radius** on the thumb side and the **ulna** on the little-finger side. They articulate at the wrist joint with the small **carpal** bones. The muscles of the forearm **supinate** and **pronate** the forearm, flex and extend the wrist joint and hand, and move the hand medially and laterally.

Your forearm is bigger near the elbow because the fleshy bellies of the forearm muscles are bulky. Your wrist is much thinner because the muscles have become tendons that pass over the wrist on the way to being inserted into the bones of the fingers. As the tendons pass over the wrist, they are surrounded by sheaths of synovial membrane and held in place on the wrist by a transverse, thick fibrous band called a **retinaculum** (*Figure 14.26*).

LO 14.14 Common Disorders of the Wrist

Ganglion cysts are fluid-filled cysts arising when the synovial tendon sheaths that run over the back of the wrist are irritated or inflamed. They often disappear spontaneously.

Stenosing tenosynovitis is inflammation of the synovial sheaths on the back of the wrist that causes pressure to develop under the retinaculum, producing pain in the wrist. This is what happened to Ms. Baker.

Carpal tunnel syndrome (*Figure 14.26*) develops similarly on the front of the wrist as a result of inflammation and swelling of tendon sheaths arising from overuse of repetitive movements, such as those in computer keyboard operation. The swelling compresses the **median nerve** between the carpal bones and the retinaculum. This causes "pins and needles" or pain and loss of muscle power in the thumb side of the hand. The retinaculum may need to be incised and released (**fasciotomy**).

Colles fracture is a common fracture of the radius just above the wrist joint. It occurs when a person tries to break a fall with an outstretched hand. The distal radius just proximal to the wrist is broken. In some cases, the distal ulnar is also fractured and the wrist joint dislocated. The fracture is diagnosed with an x-ray (*Figure 14.27*).

◀ Figure 14.27 X-Ray of Colles Fracture with Radius and Ulna Involved.

WORD	PRONUNCIATION	ELEMENTS		DEFINITION
carpus carpal (adj)	KAR-pus KAR-pal	S/ R/	Greek *wrist* -al *pertaining to* carp- *bones of the wrist*	Collective term for the eight carpal bones of the wrist Pertaining to the wrist
Colles fracture	KOL-ez FRAK-chur		Abraham Colles, Irish surgeon, 1773–1843	Fracture of the distal radius at the wrist
cyst	SIST		Greek *bladder*	An abnormal, fluid-containing sac
ergonomic	err-go-NOM-ick	S/ R/CF R/	-ic *pertaining to* erg/o- *work* -nom- *law*	Pertaining to a workplace tool or equipment designed to prevent worker injury and discomfort
fascia fasciotomy fasciectomy	FASH-ee-ah fash-ee-OT-oh-me fash-ee-EK-toe-me	S/ R/CF S/	Latin *band* -otomy *incision* fasc/i- *fascia* -ectomy *excision*	Sheet of fibrous connective tissue An incision through a band of fascia, usually to relieve pressure on underlying structures Surgical removal of fascia
ganglion ganglionic (adj)	GANG-lee-on gang-LEE-on-ik		Greek *swelling*	Fluid-containing swelling attached to the synovial sheath of a tendon
pronate	PRO-nate		Latin *bend forward*	Rotate the forearm so that the surface of the palm faces posteriorly in the anatomical position
retinaculum	ret-ih-NACK-you-lum	S/ R/	-um *structure* retinacul- *hold back*	Fibrous ligament that keeps the tendons in place on the wrist so that they do not "bowstring" when the forearm muscles contract
stenosis	steh-NOH-sis		Greek *narrowing*	Narrowing of a passage
supinate	SOO-pih-nate		Latin *face up*	Rotate the forearm so that the surface of the palm faces anteriorly in the anatomical position

Exercises

A. Insert the correct orthopedic terminology from the above WAD in the following sentences. *You may use a term only one time.*
Fill in the blanks. **LO 14.3, 14.13, 14.14**

1. Because the patient has _____ tunnel syndrome, she will require a(n) _____ keyboard for her computer at work.

2. The two terms in this WAD that are opposites are _____ and _____.

3. Inflammation of a tendon is tendinitis, but inflammation of a cyst is _____.

4. Constriction produces the narrowing of a passage; _____ will do the same.

5. A fasciectomy is removal of the _____; a cystectomy would be removal of a _____.

B. Insert the correct orthopedic terminology from the above WAD in the following sentences. *You can use a term only one time.*
Fill in the blanks. **LO 14.3, 14.13, 14.14**

1. A _____ is attached to the synovial sheath of a tendon.

2. The _____ is the fibrous ligament that keeps the tendons in place on the wrist.

These questions can be answered using the information in Case Report 14.6 and the text on the opposite page.

3. What type of repetition injury does Ms. Baker have? _____

_____

4. What is the treatment plan for Ms. Baker? _____

_____

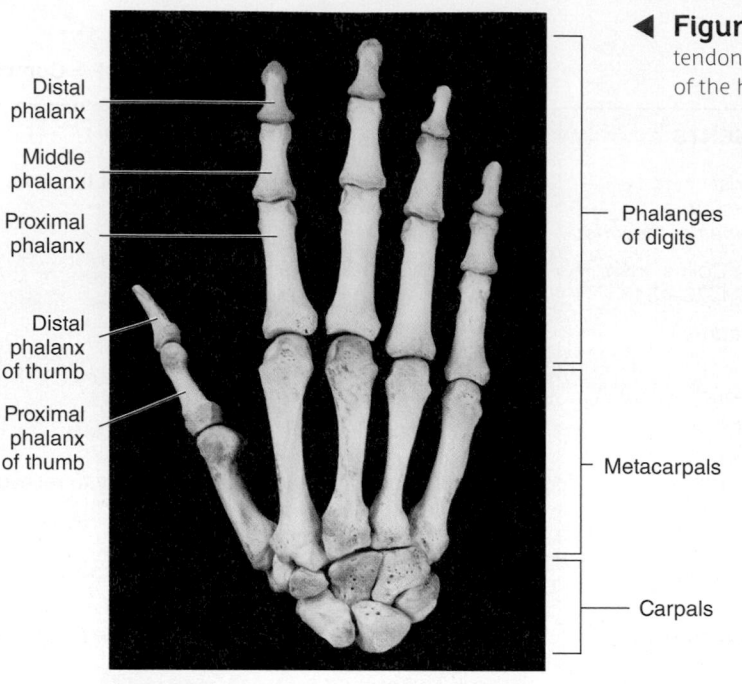

Distal phalanx

Middle phalanx

Proximal phalanx

Distal phalanx of thumb

Proximal phalanx of thumb

Phalanges of digits

Metacarpals

Carpals

(a)

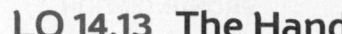

◀ **Figure 14.28** **The Hand.** (*a*) Bones of the hand. (*b*) Muscles and tendons of the palm of the hand. (*c*) Muscles and tendons of the dorsum of the hand.

LO 14.13 The Hand

Disorders of and injuries to the hand are among the most common reasons for office and Emergency Department visits and for ambulatory surgical procedures.

The complex structure of the hand (*Figure 14.28*) has evolved in response to the complicated and often very fine movements that modern-day activities require the hand to perform. Examples are making jewelry, repairing a watch, and sewing an artery or nerve back together.

When you look at the **palmar** surface of your hand, at the base of the thumb is a prominent pad of muscles called the **thenar eminence**. A smaller pad of muscles at the base of the little finger is called the **hypothenar eminence** (*Figure 14.29*). The back of the hand is called the **dorsum**.

The five fingers of one hand together have 14 bones called **phalanges**. The thumb has two phalanges. The remaining four fingers have three each (*Figure 14.28a*).

In the palm of the hand, the five bones proximal to the fingers are **metacarpals**, which connect at the wrist to eight small **carpal** bones. These in turn connect the hand to the bones of the forearm (*Figure 14.28*).

All these bones require numerous joints with ligaments to connect and stabilize them. The movements of the hand are accomplished by three sets of muscles and tendons:

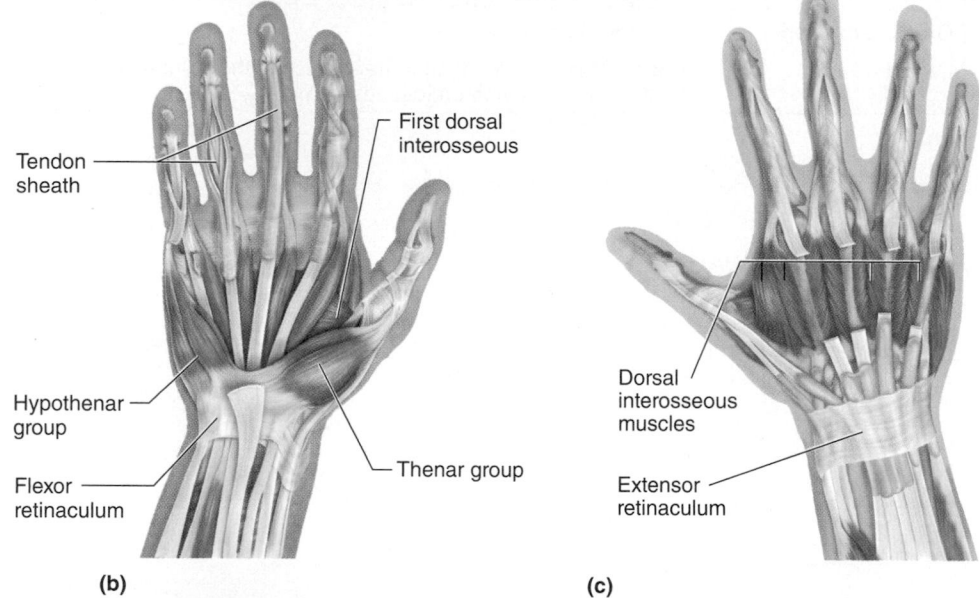

Tendon sheath

First dorsal interosseous

Hypothenar group

Flexor retinaculum

Thenar group

Dorsal interosseous muscles

Extensor retinaculum

(b)

(c)

1. The flexor muscles that bend the fingers are located on the front of the forearm and are attached by tendons to the phalanges on the palmar surfaces (*Figure 14.28b*).

2. The extensor muscles are located on the back of the forearm and are attached by tendons to the dorsal surfaces of the phalanges (*Figure 14.28c*).

3. Small muscles that originate and insert on the hand are located entirely within the palm and include the **interosseous muscles** between the metacarpals (*see Figure 14.28b and c*). These muscles assist in flexion and extension of the fingers but also adduct and abduct them and enable the thumb to touch the tips of the other fingers, a movement called **opposition**.

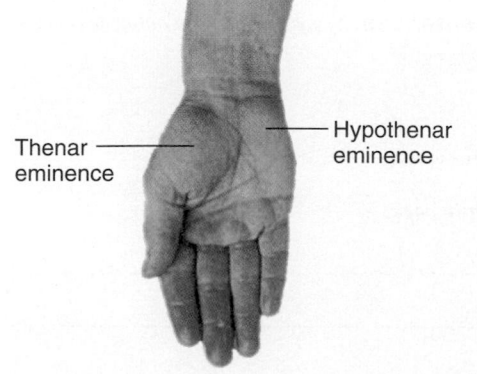

Thenar eminence

Hypothenar eminence

▲ **Figure 14.29** Palmar Surface of Hand.

WORD	PRONUNCIATION	ELEMENTS		DEFINITION
dorsum dorsal (adj)	**DOR**-sum **DOR**-sal		Latin *back*	Upper, posterior, or back surface
eminence	**EM**-ih-nens		Latin *stand out*	A higher place or part
hypothenar	high-poh-**THAY**-nar	P/ R/	hypo- *below, smaller* -thenar *palm*	Fleshy eminence at the base of the little finger
interosseous	in-ter-**OSS**-ee-us	S/ P/ R/CF	-ous *pertaining to* inter- *between* -oss/e- *bone*	A structure between bones, such as the muscles between the metacarpals
metacarpal	**MET**-ah-**KAR**-pal	S/ P/ R/	-al *pertaining to* meta- *after* -carp- *bones of the wrist*	The five bones between the carpus and the fingers
opposition	op-oh-**SIH**-shun		Old English *to set against*	The movement of the thumb across the palm of the hand to touch the tips of the other fingers
palm palmar (adj)	PAHLM **PAHL**-mah		Latin *palm*	The flat anterior surface of the hand
phalanx phalanges (pl)	**FAY**-lanks **FAY**-lan-jeez		Greek *line of soldiers*	A bone of a finger or toe
thenar	**THAY**-nar		Greek *palm*	The thenar eminence is the fleshy mass at the base of the thumb

Exercises

A. Because the body has 206 bones, there is an extensive amount of orthopedic vocabulary. *Build your knowledge of hand terminology with this exercise. Circle your best choice.* **LO 14.3, 14.13**

1. The term **dorsum** means   front   back   middle   end

2. The prefix **inter-** means   between   before   behind   beneath

3. The suffix **-ous** means   process   action   full of   pertaining to

4. The prefix **hypo-** means   smaller   larger   twisted   excess

5. The suffix **-al** means   pertaining to   one who does   study of   condition

6. The prefix **meta-** means   before   during   after   middle

7. The root **thenar-** means   finger   hand   palm   wrist

8. The term **metacarpal** refers to   arm   elbow   forearm   hand

9. The element **osse** refers to   blood   wrist   knuckle   bone

10. The bone of a finger *or* toe is   carpus   fascia   eminence   phalanx

11. Flesh at the base of the thumb is   thenar   metacarpal   hypothenar   phalanges

12. A higher place or part is   emmenince   emminence   eminence   emenince

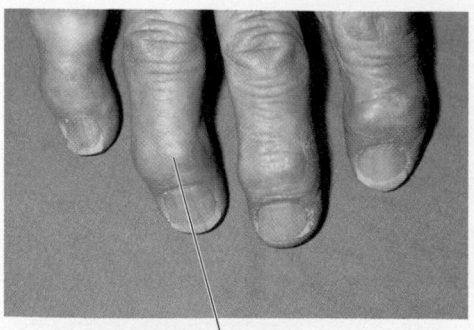

Heberden node

▲ **Figure 14.30 Hand with Osteoarthritis.** Osteoarthritis of hands showing Heberden nodes.

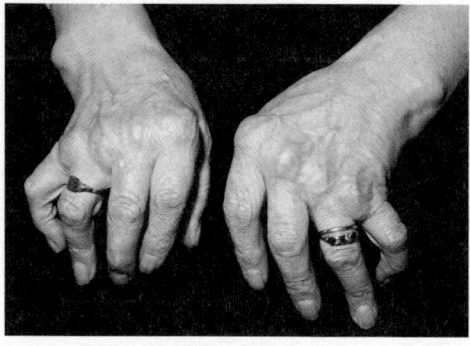

▲ **Figure 14.31 Hands with Rheumatoid Arthritis.**

Abbreviations	
JRA	juvenile rheumatoid arthritis
RA	rheumatoid arthritis

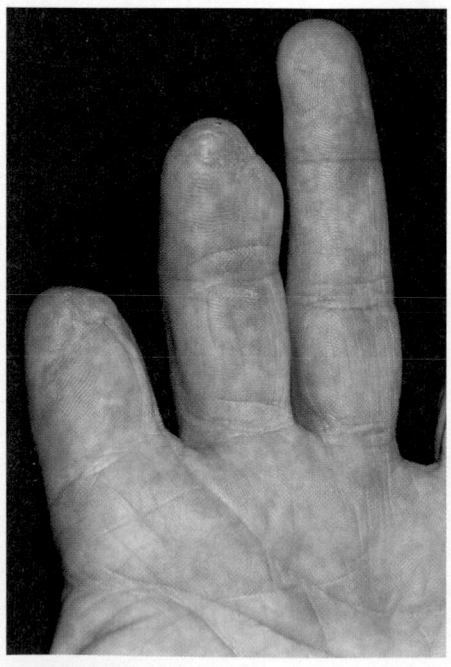

▲ **Figure 14.32 Healed Partial Amputation of Two Fingers.**

LO 14.14 Disorders of the Hand

Osteoarthritis in the hand joints occurs from wear and tear, particularly in the joint at the base of the thumb. It occurs mostly in the elderly. As a finger joint deteriorates, small bony spurs called **Heberden nodes** form over it *(Figure 14.30)*. William Heberden (1710–1801), a surgeon in Cambridge, England, first described these nodes.

Rheumatoid Arthritis (RA), with destruction of joint surfaces, joint capsule, and ligaments, leads to marked **deformity** and joint **instability** *(Figure 14.31)*. It occurs mostly in women, with onset between ages 20 and 50.

The great majority of patients have involvement of the hands, where the disease affects the synovial membrane that lines joints and tendons. The abnormal synovial membrane can invade the smooth, gliding joint surfaces and destroy them, or it can invade the surrounding joint capsule and ligaments and cause deformity and joint instability. Lumps known as **rheumatic nodules** form over the small joints of the hand and wrist. The metacarpophalangeal joints can be affected, and this leads to drift of the fingers away from the thumb, called **ulnar deviation**.

Juvenile rheumatoid arthritis (JRA) affects children under the age of 17 with inflammation and stiffness of joints. Many children grow out of it.

Dupuytren contracture is a progressive thickening and contracture of the skin and connective tissues of the palm of the hand.

Injuries of the Hand

Flexor tendon injuries occur as a result of lacerations. Because the flexor tendons lie just beneath the skin on the palmar surfaces of the fingers, they are very **susceptible** to injury even with a shallow laceration. Even after repair, there can be **residual** stiffness and limited motion of the fingers.

Open fractures of hand bones, when the skin is broken and the broken bone penetrates through the break in the skin, can lead to infection of hand tissues.

Partial amputation of a fingertip is a common type of injury, particularly in people who work with sharp tools *(Figure 14.32)*. This type of wound also produces an open phalangeal fracture.

Surgical Procedures of the Hand

Fasciectomy is the surgical removal of the hypertrophied connective tissue to release a contracture.

Tendon reconstruction stitches the two ends of a lacerated tendon back together or inserts a tendon graft.

Arthrodesis is the surgical fixation of a joint to prevent motion. Bone graft, wires, screws, or a plate can be used to stabilize the joint.

Arthroplasty in this setting is the complete replacement of a damaged finger joint with an artificial joint made of silicone rubber.

Reattachment of amputated fingers is performed frequently. The bones are rejoined with plates, wires, or screws. The tendons are reconstructed. Nerves and blood vessels are joined back together by using microsurgical instruments.

WORD	PRONUNCIATION	ELEMENTS		DEFINITION
amputation **amputate (verb)** **amputee (noun)**	am-pyu-**TAY**-shun **AM**-pyu-tate **AM**-pyu-tee		Latin *cut, prune*	Process of removing a limb, a part of a limb, a breast, or some other projecting part A person with an amputation
contracture	kon-**TRAK**-chur	S/ R/	-ure *process* **contract-** *draw together*	Muscle shortening due to spasm or fibrosis
deformity	de-**FOR**-mih-tee	S/ P/ R/	-ity *condition* de- *change of* -form- *form, appearance*	A permanent structural deviation from the normal
Dupuytren contracture	du-pwe-**TRAHN** kon-**TRAK**-chur		Guillaume Dupuytren, French surgeon, 1777–1835	A thickening and shortening of fibrous bands in the palm of the hand
flexor **flex (verb)**	**FLEK**-sor FLEKS		Latin *to bend*	Muscle or tendon that flexes a joint To bend a joint so that the two parts come together
Heberden node	**HEH**-ber-den NOHD		William Heberden, English physician, 1710–1801	Bony lump on the terminal phalanx of the fingers in osteoarthritis
instability	in-stah-**BIL**-ih-tee	S/ P/ R/	-ity *condition* in- *not* -stabil- *stand firm*	Abnormal tendency of a joint to partially or fully dislocate
juvenile	**JU**-ven-ile		Latin *youthful*	Between the ages of 2 and 17 years
nodule	**NOD**-yule		Latin *small knot*	Small node or knotlike swelling
residual **residue (noun)**	re-**ZID**-you-al **REZ**-ih-dyu	S/ R/CF	-al *pertaining to* **resid/u-** *what is left over*	Pertaining to anything left over
rheumatism **rheumatic (adj)** **rheumatoid arthritis**	**RU**-mat-izm ru-**MAT**-ik **RHU**-mah-toyd ar-**THRI**-tis	S/ R/ S/ S/	-ism *condition* **rheumat-** *a flow* -ic *pertaining to* -oid *resembling*	Pain in various parts of the musculoskeletal system Relating to or characterized by rheumatism Disease of connective tissue, with arthritis as a major manifestation
susceptible	suh-**SEP**-tih-bill		Latin *to take up*	Capable of being affected by

Exercises

A. Demonstrate your knowledge of the difference between these similar terms. *Use the correct form of the term in the appropriate place. Fill in the blanks.* **LO 14.3, 14.4, 14.9, 14.14**

1. **amputation**   **amputate**   **amputee**

   The surgeon has decided to _____ the patient's left leg below the knee. The _____ will be performed as soon as possible. Following the surgery, the _____ will be fitted for a new leg prosthesis.

2. **flex**   **flexor**

   The _____ tendons _____ a joint so that the two parts of the joint can come together.

3. **residual**   **residue**

   The _____ in the bottom of the test beaker can be referred to as the _____.

4. **rheumatic**   **rheumatoid arthritis**   **rheumatism**

   _____ is a generic term for _____ pain in various parts of the musculoskeletal system.

   However, _____ is a specific systemic disease affecting many joints.

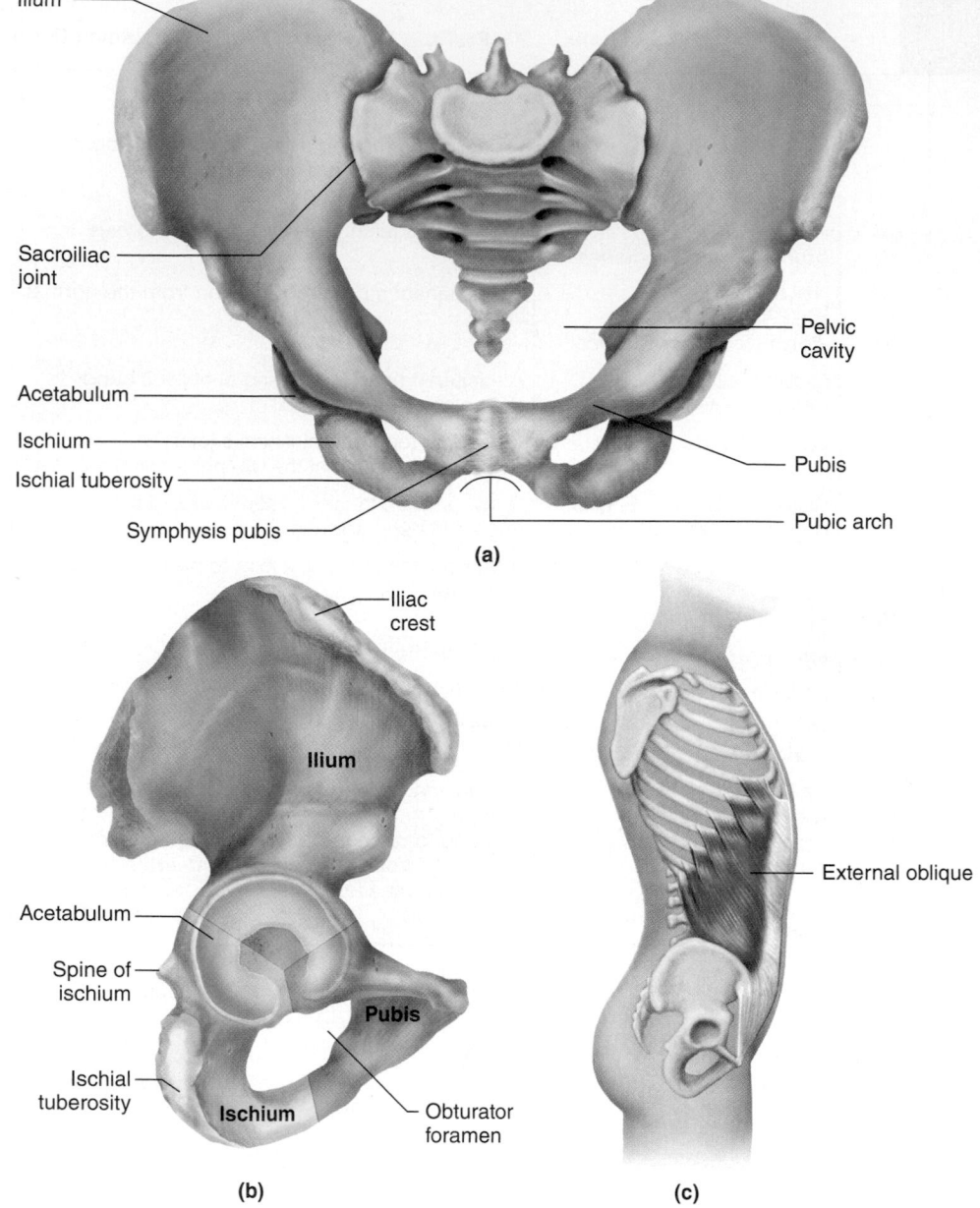

Ilium

Sacroiliac
joint

Acetabulum

Ischium

Ischial tuberosity

Symphysis pubis

Pelvic
cavity

Pubis

Pubic arch

(a)

Iliac
crest

Ilium

Acetabulum

Spine of
ischium

Pubis

Ischial
tuberosity

Ischium

Obturator
foramen

(b)

External oblique

(c)

▲ **Figure 14.33** **Pelvic Girdle.** (*a*) Front view. (*b*) Side view. (*c*) Abdominal muscles supporting the pelvic girdle.

LO 14.15 Pelvic Girdle

The pelvic girdle (*Figure 14.33*) is the two hip bones that articulate anteriorly with each other at the **symphysis pubis** and posteriorly with the **sacrum** to form the bowl-shaped **pelvis**. The two joints between the hip bones and the sacrum are the **sacroiliac (SI) joints**.

The pelvic girdle has the following functions:

1. Supports the axial skeleton.
2. Transmits the body's weight through to the lower limbs.
3. Provides attachments for the lower limbs.
4. Protects the internal reproductive organs, urinary bladder, and distal end of the large intestine.

Each hip bone is a fusion of three bones, the **ilium**, **ischium**, and **pubis** (*Figure 14.33a*). The fusion takes place in the region of the **acetabulum**, a cup-shaped cavity on the lateral surface of each hip bone that receives the **head** of the **femur** (thigh bone, *Figure 14.33b*).

The lower part of the pelvis is formed by the lower ilium, ischium, and pubic bones that surround a short canal-like cavity. This opening is larger in females than males to allow the infant to pass through during childbirth. The outlet from the cavity is spanned by strong muscular layers through which the rectum, vagina, and urethra pass.

Muscles anchor the pelvic girdle to the vertebrae and ribs of the axial skeleton. Anteriorly, these are the external oblique abdominal muscles that are inserted into the ilium and pubis (*Figure 14.33c*).

LO 14.16 Disorders of the Pelvic Girdle

SI joint strain is a common cause of lower-back pain. Unlike most joints, the sacroiliac joint is only designed to move ¼ inch (approximately 6 mm) during weight bearing and forward flexion. Its main function is to provide shock absorption for the spine.

During pregnancy, hormones enable connective tissue to relax so that the pelvis can expand enough to allow birth. The stretching in the sacroiliac joint ligaments makes it excessively mobile and susceptible to wear-and-tear painful arthritis.

Another cause of pain in the sacroiliac joint is trauma, with tearing of the joint ligaments generating too much motion and pain. The pain is felt in the low back, in the buttock, and sometimes in the back and front of the thigh.

A diagnosis of sacroiliac pain can be made by clinical examination, joint x-ray, and CT scan. **Fluoroscopic** injection of local anesthetic into the joint can relieve the pain temporarily. Treatment is usually **stabilization** of the joint with a **brace** and physical therapy to strengthen the low-back muscles. Occasionally, **arthrodesis** of the joint is necessary.

Diastasis symphysis pubis is another result of the stretching of pelvic ligaments during pregnancy. The softening and stretching of the ligaments of the symphysis pubis stretches the joint between the two pubic bones and leads to pain over the joint and difficulty in walking, climbing stairs, and turning over in bed.

WORD	PRONUNCIATION	ELEMENTS		DEFINITION
acetabulum	ass-eh-**TAB**-you-lum		Latin *vinegar cup*	The cup-shaped cavity of the hip bone that receives the head of the femur to form the hip joint
brace	BRACE		Old English *to fasten*	Appliance to support a part of the body in its correct position
diastasis	die-**ASS**-tah-sis		Greek *separation*	Separation of normally joined parts
femur femoral (adj)	**FEE**-mur **FEM**-oh-ral		Latin *thigh*	The thigh bone
fluoroscopy	flor-**OS**-koh-pee	S/ R/CF	**-scopy** *to examine, to view* **fluor/o-** *x-ray beam*	Examination of structures of the body by x-rays
fluoroscopic (adj)	flor-oh-**SKOP**-ik	S/	**-ic** *pertaining to*	Relating to or effected by fluoroscopy
head	HED		Old English *head*	The rounded extremity of a bone
ilium (**Note:** The ileum is a section of the small intestine [Chapter 6].) ilia (pl)	**ILL**-ee-um **ILL**-ee-ah		Latin *groin*	Large wing-shaped bone at the upper and posterior part of the pelvis
ischium ischial (adj) ischia (pl)	**ISS**-kee-um **ISS**-kee-al **ISS**-kee-ah		Greek *hip*	Lower and posterior part of the hip bone
pelvis pelvic (adj)	**PEL**-vis **PEL**-vic		Latin *basin*	A cup-shaped ring of bone; also a cup-shaped cavity, as in the pelvis of the kidney
pubis	**PYU**-bis		Latin *pubis*	Bony front arch of the pelvis of the hip; also called *pubic bone*
pubic (adj)	**PYU**-bik	S/ R/	**-ic** *pertaining to* **pub-** *pubis*	Pertaining to the pubis
sacrum	**SAY**-crum		Latin *sacred*	Segment of the vertebral column that forms part of the pelvis
sacral (adj)	**SAY**-kral	S/ R/	**-al** **sacr**	In the neighborhood of the sacrum
sacroiliac	say-kroh-**ILL**-ih-ak	S/ R/CF R/	**-ac** **sacr/o-** **-ili-**	The joint between the sacrum and ilium

Exercises

A. Match the language of the pelvic girdle to the correct definitions. *Fill in the blanks.*   **LO 14.15, 14.16**

_____ 1. receives head of femur

_____ 2. cup-shaped ring of bones

_____ 3. posterior part of hip bone

_____ 4. separation of normally joined parts

_____ 5. wing-shaped bone, upper part of pelvis

_____ 6. segment of vertebral column

_____ 7. thigh bone

a. sacrum

b. ilium

c. diastasis

d. femur

e. pelvis

f. ischium

g. acetabulum

B. Use the *language of orthopedics* associated with the pelvic girdle to answer the following questions.   **LO 14.15**

1. What is the meaning of the term *articulate*? (If you don't know this term, look it up in the glossary or an online dictionary.)

_____

2. What are the joints between the hip bones and sacrum called? _____

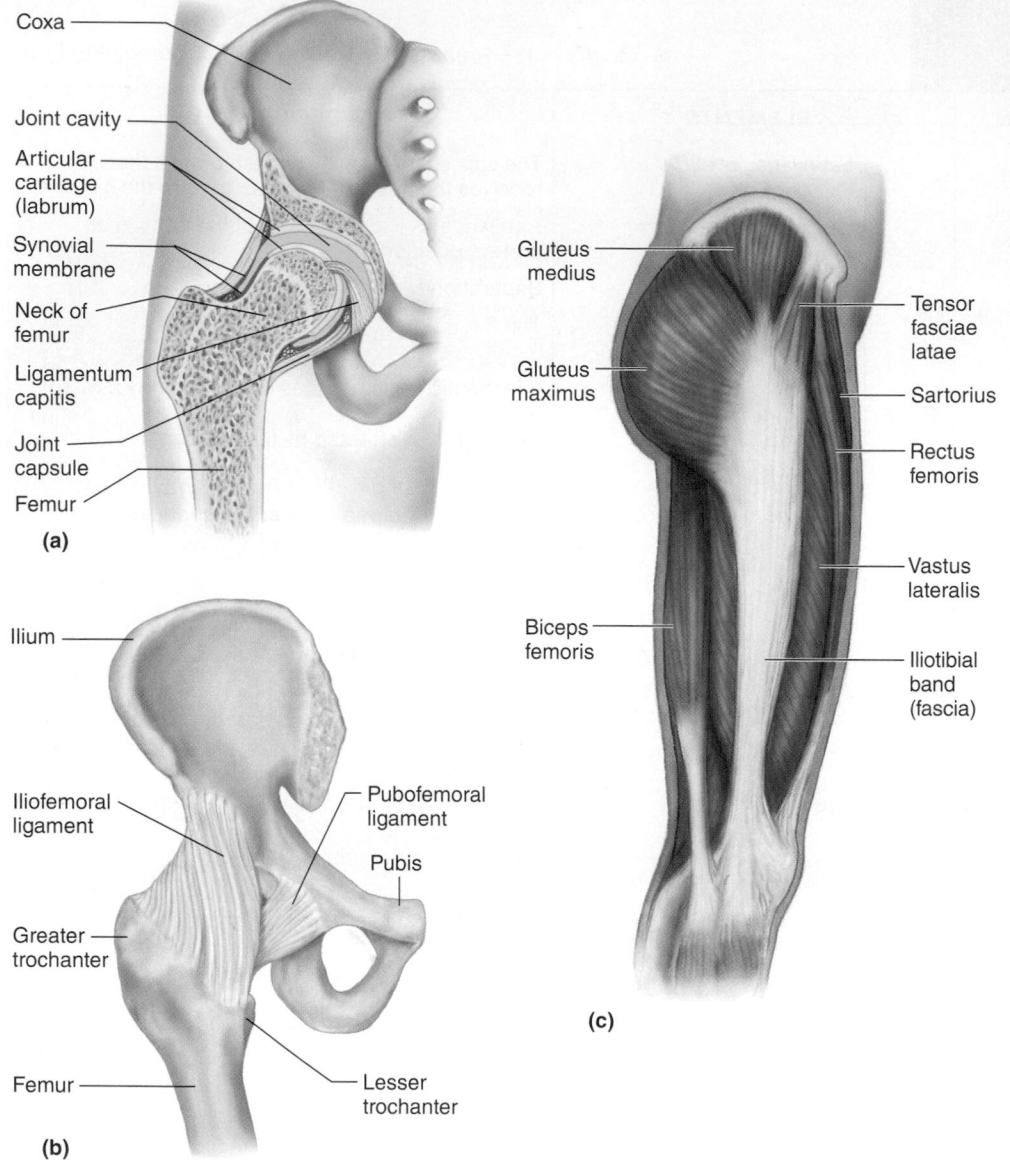

Figure 14.34 (a) Labels:
- Coxa
- Joint cavity
- Articular cartilage (labrum)
- Synovial membrane
- Neck of femur
- Ligamentum capitis
- Joint capsule
- Femur

(a)

(b) Labels:
- Ilium
- Iliofemoral ligament
- Pubofemoral ligament
- Pubis
- Greater trochanter
- Femur
- Lesser trochanter

(b)

(c) Labels:
- Gluteus medius
- Gluteus maximus
- Biceps femoris
- Tensor fasciae latae
- Sartorius
- Rectus femoris
- Vastus lateralis
- Iliotibial band (fascia)

(c)

▲ **Figure 14.34** **Hip Joint.** (*a*) Right frontal view of a section of hip joint. (*b*) Ligaments of hip joint. (*c*) Muscles of hip and thigh (lateral view).

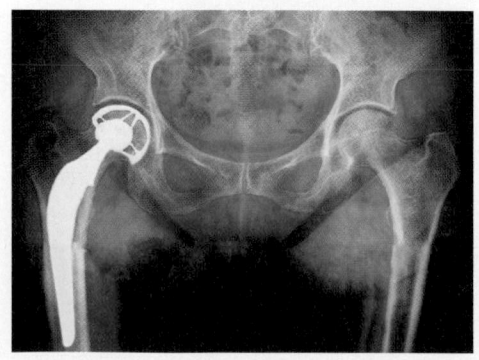

▲ **Figure 14.35** **Total-Hip Replacement.** Colored x-ray of prosthetic hip.

LO 14.15 Bones, Joints, and Muscles of the Hip and Thigh

The **hip joint** is a **ball-and-socket** synovial joint between the head of the femur and the cup-shaped **acetabulum** of the hip bone (*Figure 14.34a*). A ligament (ligamentum capitis) attached to the head of the femur from the lining of the acetabulum carries blood vessels to the head of the femur to nourish it.

The joint is held in place by a thick joint **capsule** reinforced by strong ligaments that connect the neck of the femur to the rim of the acetabulum (*Figure 14.34b*).

The **labrum** is the cartilage that forms a rim around the socket of the joint; it cushions the joint and helps keep the head of the femur in place in the socket. Recent improvements in diagnostic techniques have shown that with injury the labrum can tear and cause pain. The tear is diagnosed on MRI and may need surgery to be repaired.

Powerful muscles that support the hip joint and move the thigh have their **origins** on the pelvic girdle and their **insertions** into the femur. Prominent among them are the three **gluteus** muscles, **maximus, medius,** and **minimus** (*Figure 14.34c*), and the **adductor** muscles that run down the inner thigh.

LO 14.16 Disorders and Injuries of the Hip Joint

Hip pointer, usually a football-related injury, is a blow to the rim of the pelvis that leads to bruising of the bone and surrounding tissues.

Osteoarthritis is common in the hip as a result of aging, weight bearing, and repetitive use of the joint. The cartilage on both the acetabulum and the head of the femur degenerates, and eventually there is total loss of the cartilage cushion. The resulting friction between the bones of the head of the femur and the acetabulum leads to pain and loss of mobility.

Rheumatoid arthritis (RA) can also affect the hip, beginning in the synovial membrane and progressing to destroy cartilage and bone.

Avascular necrosis of the femoral head is the necrosis (death) of bone tissue when the blood supply becomes avascular (is cut off), usually as a result of trauma.

Fractures of the neck of the femur occur as a result of falls, most commonly in elderly women with osteoporosis.

LO 14.16 Surgical Procedures

Arthroplasty, a total replacement of the hip joint with a metal **prosthesis**, is the most common hip surgery today; 150,000 total-hip replacements are performed each year in the United States, mostly for osteoarthritis of the hip joint. The diseased parts of the joint are removed and replaced with artificial parts made of titanium, other metals, and ceramics (*Figure 14.35*).

Arthrocentesis, the aspiration of fluid from the hip joint and replacement of the fluid with a steroid solution, is also performed frequently for osteoarthritis.

LO 14.3, 14.4, 14.15, 14.16
Word Analysis and Definition

S = Suffix   P = Prefix   R = Root   R/CF = Combining Form

WORD	PRONUNCIATION		ELEMENTS	DEFINITION
arthritis	ar-**THRY**-tis	S/ R/	-itis *inflammation* **arthr-** *joint*	Inflammation of a joint or joints
avascular	a-**VAS**-cue-lar	S/ P/ R/	-ar *pertaining to* **a-** *without* **vascul-** *blood vessel*	Without a blood supply
gluteus maximus	**GLU**-tee-us **MAKS**-ih-mus		Greek *buttocks* Latin *the biggest or the greatest*	Refers to a muscle in the buttocks The gluteus maximus muscle is the largest muscle in the body, covering a large part of each buttock
medius	**ME**-dee-us		Latin *middle*	The gluteus medius muscle is partly covered by the gluteus maximus; it originates on the ilium and is inserted into the femur
minimus	**MIN**-ih-mus		Latin *smallest*	The gluteus minimus is the smallest of the gluteal muscles and lies under the gluteus medius
gluteal (adj)	**GLU**-tee-al	S/ R/	-eal *pertaining to* **glut-** *buttocks*	Pertaining to the buttocks
labrum	**LAY**-brum		Latin *lip-shaped*	Cartilage that forms a rim around the socket of the hip joint
necrosis necrotic (adj)	neh-**KROH**-sis neh-**KROT**-ik		Greek *death*	Pathologic death of cells or tissue Affected by necrosis
prosthesis	**PROS**-thee-sis		Greek *addition*	Manufactured substitute for a missing part of the body

Exercises

A. Continue working with the *language of orthopedics*. *Demonstrate your knowledge of the terms by circling the best answer to each of the following questions.*   **LO 14.3, 14.15, 14.16**

1. Maximus, medius, and minimus are all

   bones   muscles   tendons   ligaments   phalanges

2. Gluteus refers to the

   wrist   hand   buttocks   hip   spine

3. If tissue is dead, it is

   necrotic   sacral   rheumatic   degenerative   fibrotic

4. Avascular means no

   living tissue   tendon support   movement   blood supply   inflammation

5. A prosthesis is a(n)

   procedure   cast   diagnostic test   brace   artificial body part

B. Determine the correct medical term to complete the sentence. *Fill in the blanks.*   **LO 14.15, 14.16**

1. _____ is the cartilage that forms a rim around the hip joint.

2. Who is most likely to fall as a result of osteoporosis? _____

3. Name three likely causes of osteoarthritis in the hip joint.

   a. _____

   b. _____

   c. _____

4. Artificial hips and knees are medically termed a _____.

5. If a part of the body is *avascular*, it has no _____.

Case Report 14.7

Preoperative Diagnosis: Traumatic ACL tear and tear of medial meniscus right knee.

Postoperative Diagnosis: Same.

Procedure Performed: Repair of medial collateral ligament, ACL reconstruction, repair of torn medial meniscus, right knee.

Operative Findings: An avulsed anterior cruciate ligament off the femoral condyle, with a tear of the posterior horn of the medial meniscus and a tear of the medial collateral ligament.

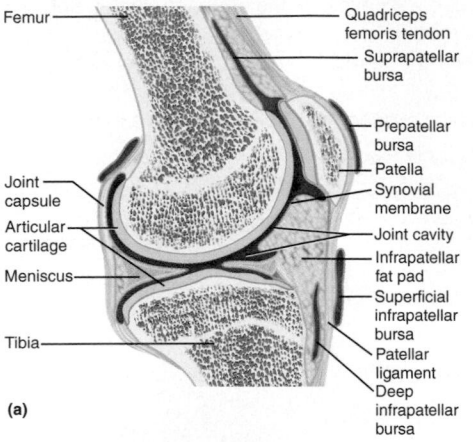

(a)

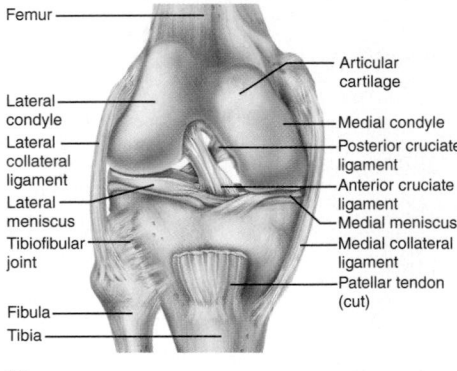

(b)

▲ **Figure 14.36** **Knee Joint** (*a*) Section of knee joint. (*b*) Right knee joint: anterior view.

Abbreviations	
ACL	anterior cruciate ligament
PCL	posterior cruciate ligament

LO 14.15 Bones, Joints, and Muscles of the Knee and Thigh

Knee Joint

The knee is a hinged joint formed with four bones:

1. The lower end of the **femur**, shaped like a horseshoe. The two ends of the horseshoe are the medial and lateral femoral **condyle**s (*Figure 14.36b*).

2. The flat upper end of the **tibia**.

3. The **patella** (kneecap), a flat triangular bone embedded in the **patellar tendon**. The patella articulates with the femur between its two **condyles** (*Figure 14.36a*).

4. The **fibula**, which forms a separate joint by articulating with the tibia. This is called the **tibiofibular joint** (*see Figure 14.36b*).

Mechanically, the role of the patella is to provide an increase of about 30% in the strength of extension of the knee joint.

Within the knee joint, two crescent-shaped pads of cartilage lie on top of the tibia to articulate with the femoral condyles. They are the **medial** and **lateral menisci**. Their function is to distribute weight more evenly across the joint surface to minimize wear and tear. They play a crucial role in joint stability, lubrication, and transmission of force.

The knee joint has a **fibrous capsule** lined with **synovial membrane** to secrete **synovial fluid**, which provides lubrication for the joint. The joint is held together by **ligaments**. The two ligaments outside the joint are the **medial** and **lateral collateral ligaments**. Two other ligaments are located inside the joint cavity and are called the **anterior cruciate ligament** **(ACL)** and the **posterior cruciate ligament (PCL)**. They cross over each other to form an "X" (*Figure 14.36b*). There are numerous bursae associated with the knee joint (*Figure 14.36a*). Their function is to aid the movement of the patella and the patellar tendon over the bones of the joint.

Thigh Muscles

The thigh muscles move the knee joint and lower leg. The anterior thigh is composed of the large **quadriceps femoris** muscle, which has four heads and is the most powerful muscle in the body. The four muscles converge into the **quadriceps tendon**, which contains the patella, and continue as the patellar tendon to insert into the tibia (*Figure 14.36a*). The quadriceps muscle extends (straightens) the knee joint and, because of the weight of the lower leg, has to be a powerful muscle.

The posterior thigh is composed mostly of the three **hamstring muscles**: the **biceps femoris**, **semimembranosus**, and **semitendinosus**. They flex (bend) the knee joint and rotate the leg. The hollow at the back of the knee between the hamstring tendons is called the **popliteal fossa**.

WORD	PRONUNCIATION	ELEMENTS		DEFINITION
collateral	koh-**LAT**-er-al	S/ P/ R/	-al *pertaining to* co- *together* -later- *side*	Situated at the side, often to bypass an obstruction
condyle	**KON**-dile		Latin *knuckle*	Large, smooth rounded expansion of the end of a bone that forms a joint with another bone
cruciate	**KRU**-she-ate		Latin *cross*	Shaped like a cross
fibula fibular (adj)	**FIB**-you-lah **FIB**-you-lar		Latin *clasp or buckle*	The smaller of the two bones of the lower leg
lateral (opposite of medial)	**LAT**-er-al	S/ R/	-al *pertaining to* later- *side*	Situated at the side of a structure
meniscus menisci (pl)	meh-**NISS**-kuss meh-**NISS**-key		Greek *crescent*	Disc of connective tissue cartilage between the bones of a joint, for example, in the knee joint
patella (kneecap) patellae (pl) patellar (adj)	pah-**TELL**-ah pah-**TELL**-ee pah-**TELL**-ar		Latin *small plate*	Thin, circular bone in front of the knee joint and embedded in the patellar tendon
popliteal fossa	pop-**LIT**-ee-al **FOSS**-ah	S/ R/CF	-al *pertaining to* poplit/e- *ham* fossa Latin *ditch*	The hollow at the back of the knee
quadriceps femoris	**KWAD**-rih-seps **FEM**-or-is	P/ R/ S/ R/	quadri- *four* -ceps *head* -is *belonging to* femor- *femur*	An anterior thigh muscle with four heads
tibia tibial (adj)	**TIB**-ee-ah **TIB**-ee-al		Latin *large shinbone*	The larger bone of the lower leg

Exercises

A. A medical term must be spelled correctly. *Work with a fellow student on this exercise. Cover the above WAD while the other student dictates four of the terms in this WAD to you. Do your best to spell them correctly in the left column. When you are finished, uncover the WAD and check your spelling. If you have made any errors, rewrite the correct spelling in the right column.*   **LO 14.3, 14.15, 14.16**

Spelling   Corrections

1. _____   _____

2. _____   _____

3. _____   _____

4. _____   _____

B. After reading Case Report 14.7 on the opposite page and on the next page, answer the following questions. *Be prepared to discuss your answers in class.*   **LO 14.15, 14.16**

1. The adjective *fibular* means *pertaining to the* _____.

2. What does the term *unstable* mean in relation to the knee? _____

3. If a ligament is described as *collateral*, where is it located? _____

4. Is *anterior* in the front or the back of the knee? _____

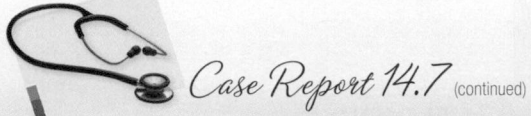
Gail Griffith, a 17-year-old, landed awkwardly after jumping for a ball during a basketball game. "My knee kinda popped as I landed." She had to be assisted off the court. In the Emergency Room, the knee was swollen and unstable. An MRI showed a complete tear of the medial collateral ligament, a complete tear of the **anterior cruciate ligament (ACL)**, and a partial tear (**avulsion**) of the medial meniscus (*Figure 14.37*). Gail decided to have surgery, even though full recovery would take 6 months to 1 year of rehabilitation.

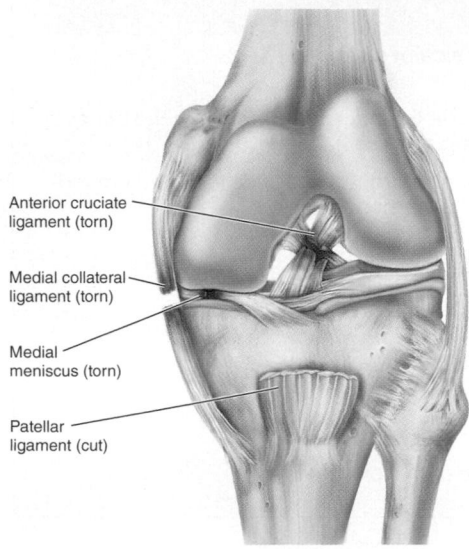

Anterior cruciate ligament (torn)

Medial collateral ligament (torn)

Medial meniscus (torn)

Patellar ligament (cut)

▲ **Figure 14.37** **Gail Griffith's Knee Injuries.**

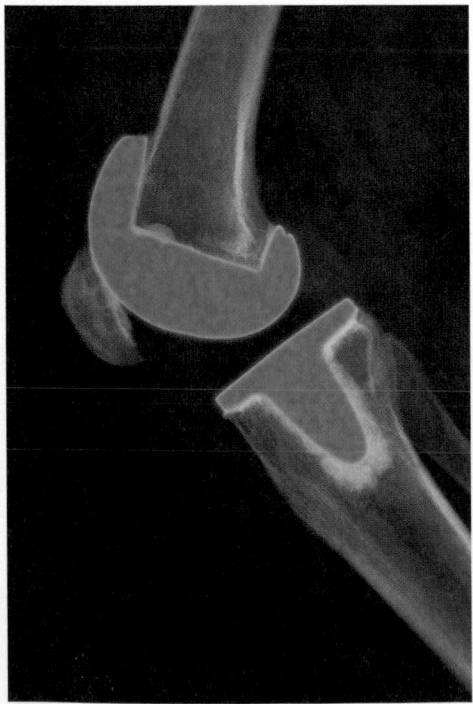

▲ **Figure 14.38** **Total Knee Replacement.** Colored x-ray of total knee replacement of left knee.

LO 14.16 Injuries to the Knee Joint

The **anterior cruciate ligament** (ACL) is the most commonly injured ligament in the knee (*Figure 14.37*), particularly in female athletes. The injury is often caused by a sudden **hyperflexion** of the knee joint when landing awkwardly on flat ground as in Gail's injury. Because of its poor vascular supply, once torn the ligament does not heal. The knee becomes unstable, risking further joint damage and arthritis. If the ACL has been torn away from its bony insertions, the surgeon will harvest a thin portion of a hamstring or patellar tendon and screw the ends into the tibia and femur. This is a **tendon autograft**. If donated tissue from a tissue bank is used for the graft, it is called an **allograft**. If tissue from another species is used for a graft, it is called a **xenograft** or a **heterograft**.

Other major ligaments that are commonly injured are the medial and lateral collateral ligaments and the posterior cruciate ligament.

Meniscus injuries result from a twist to the knee. Pain and locking are the result of the torn meniscus flipping in and out of the joint as it moves. Because loss of a meniscus leads to arthritic changes, repair of the meniscus, as in Gail's case, rather than removal is preferred. Removal of a meniscus is a **meniscectomy**.

Patellar problems produce pain that is noticed particularly when descending stairs. The force on the patella when descending stairs is about seven times body weight compared to about two times body weight when ascending stairs.

Chondromalacia patellae (runner's knee) is caused by irritation of the undersurface of the patella.

Patellar subluxation or **dislocation** produces an unstable painful kneecap.

Prepatellar bursitis (housemaid's knee) produces painful swelling over the bursa at the front of the knee and is seen in people who kneel for extended periods of time, such as carpet layers.

Tendinitis of the patellar tendon is produced by overuse during such activities as cycling, running, or dancing. Pain is felt where the tendon is inserted into the tibia. It is treated by RICE.

Rupture of the patellar tendon can occur in the elderly when trying to break a fall or in athletes such as basketball players with their repeated jumping. An MRI can confirm the tear, which may need to be repaired surgically.

LO 14.16 Surgical Procedures of the Knee Joint

Arthrocentesis, aspiration of fluid from the knee joint, is used to establish a diagnosis by laboratory examination of the fluid and to drain off infected fluid.

Diagnostic arthroscopy is an exploratory procedure performed using an arthroscope to examine the internal compartments of the knee joint.

Surgical arthroscopy, performed through an arthroscope, can be a **debridement** or removal of torn tissue such as a meniscus or a ligament. It can also be repair of a torn ligament by suturing, tendon autograft, or repair of a torn meniscus.

Arthroplasty involves a total replacement of the knee joint (*Figure 14.38*), usually because of osteoarthritis of the joint. The lower end of the femur is replaced with a metal shell. The upper end of the tibia is replaced with a metal trough lined with plastic, and the back of the patella can be replaced with a plastic button.

WORD	PRONUNCIATION	ELEMENTS		DEFINITION
allograft	**AL**-oh-graft	P/ R/	allo- *different* -**graft** *splice*	Tissue graft from another person or cadaver
autograft	**AWE**-toe-graft	P/ R/	auto- *self, same* -**graft** *splice*	A graft using tissue taken from the individual who is receiving the graft
avulsion	a-**VUL**-shun		Latin *to tear away*	Forcible separation or tearing away, often of a tendon from bone
chondromalacia	**KON**-dro-mah-**LAY**-she-ah	S/ R/CF	-**malacia** *abnormal softness* **chondr/o-** *cartilage*	Softening and degeneration of cartilage
debridement	day-**BREED**-mon	S/ P/ R/	-**ment** *action* de- *take away* -**bride-** *rubble*	The removal of injured or necrotic tissue
heterograft xenograft (syn)	**HET**-er-oh-graft	P/ R/	hetero- *different* -**graft** *splice*	A graft using tissue taken from another species
hyperflexion	high-per-**FLEK**-shun	S/ P/ R/	-**ion** *action, condition, process* hyper- *excess* -**flex-** *bend*	Flexion of a limb or part beyond the normal limits
meniscectomy	men-ih-**SEK**-toh-me	S/ R/	-**ectomy** *excision* **menisc-** *crescent, meniscus*	Excision (cutting out) of all or part of a meniscus
prepatellar	pree-pah-**TELL**-ar	S/ P/ R/	-**ar** *pertaining to* pre- *before, in front of* -**patell-** *patella*	In front of the patella
rupture	**RUP**-tyur		Latin *break*	Break or tear of any organ or body part
tendinitis (also spelled **tendonitis**)	ten-dih-**NYE**-tis	S/ R/	-**itis** *inflammation* **tendin-** *tendon*	Inflammation of a tendon
xenograft heterograft (syn)	**ZEN**-oh-graft	R/CF R/	**xen/o-** *foreign material* -**graft** *splice*	A graft from another species

Exercises

A. Recognition of word elements will help you understand the medical term. *In each of the following terms, a specific element is in bold. Identify the type of element, and then define that element on the lines provided. Fill in the chart.*   **LO 14.3, 14.16**

Medical Term	Type of Element (P, R, CF, S)	Definition of Element
pre*patellar*	1.	2.
*tend*initis	3.	4.
*hyper*flexion	5.	6.
*debride*ment	7.	8.
auto*graft*	9.	10.
chondro*malacia*	11.	12.
menisc*ectomy*	13.	14.
hetero*graft*	15.	16.
*allo*graft	17.	18.

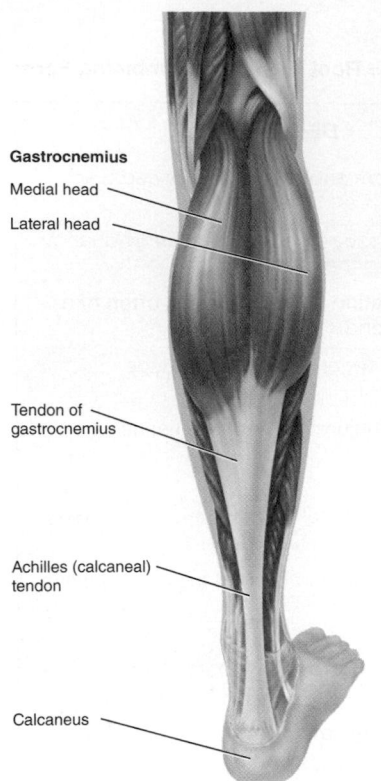

Gastrocnemius
Medial head
Lateral head

Tendon of gastrocnemius

Achilles (calcaneal) tendon

Calcaneus

▲ **Figure 14.39** Muscles of Back of Right Lower Leg.

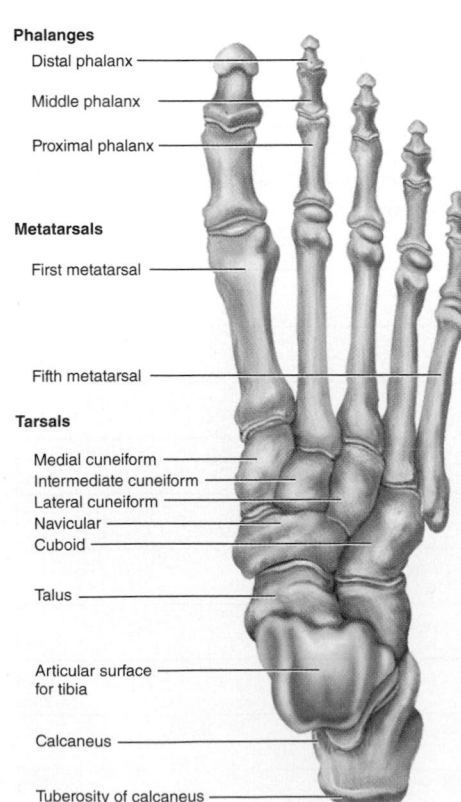

Phalanges
Distal phalanx
Middle phalanx
Proximal phalanx

Metatarsals
First metatarsal

Fifth metatarsal

Tarsals
Medial cuneiform
Intermediate cuneiform
Lateral cuneiform
Navicular
Cuboid

Talus

Articular surface for tibia

Calcaneus

Tuberosity of calcaneus

▲ **Figure 14.40** Twenty-Six Bones and 33 Joints of Right Foot.

LO 14.15 Bones, Joints, and Muscles of the Lower Leg, Ankle, and Foot

The two bones of the lower leg are the larger and medial **tibia** and the thinner and lateral **fibula**. The lower end of the tibia on its medial border forms a prominent process called the medial **malleolus**. The lower end of the fibula forms the lateral malleolus. You can **palpate** both these prominences at your own ankle.

The muscles of the lower leg move the ankle, foot, and toes. Those on the front of the leg are in a compartment between the tibia and fibula. They **dorsiflex** the foot at the ankle and extend the toes. Those on the lateral side of the leg **evert** the foot.

Those on the back of the leg **plantar flex** the foot at the ankle, flex the toes, and **invert** the foot (*Figure 14.39*). The **gastrocnemius** muscle forms a large part of the calf. The distal end of it joins with the tendon of the **soleus** muscle to form the **Achilles (calcaneal) tendon**, which is attached to the heel bone (**calcaneus**). The gastrocnemius muscle and the Achilles tendon enable you to "push off" and start running or jumping.

The ankle has two joints:

1. One between the lateral malleolus of the fibula and the talus.

2. One between the medial malleolus of the tibia and the talus.

The **talus** is the most superior of the seven **tarsal** bones of the ankle and proximal foot (*Figure 14.40*), and its trochlear surface articulates with the tibia. The tarsal bones help the ankle bear the body's weight. Strong ligaments on both sides of the ankle joint hold it together.

Attached to the tarsal bones are the five parallel **metatarsal** bones that form the instep and then fan out to form the ball of the foot, where they bear weight. The toes each have three **phalanges**, except for the big toe, which has only two. This is identical to the thumb and its relation to the hand. The tendons of the leg muscles are inserted into the phalanges.

LO 14.16 Disorders and Injuries of the Ankle and Foot

Podiatry is a health care specialty concerned with the diagnosis and treatment of disorders and injuries of the foot.

Bunions occur usually at the base of the big toe and are swellings of the bones that cause the metatarsophalangeal joint to be misaligned and stick out medially. This deformity is called **hallux valgus**.

Strains and sprains are more common in the ankle than in any other joint in the body. A strain is an acute injury resulting from overstretching or overcontraction of a muscle or tendon. A sprain is the result of an abnormal stretch or tear of a ligament. Some severe sprains with tearing of the ligament may require surgical repair.

Pott fracture is a term applied to a variety of fractures in which there is a fracture of the fibula near the ankle, often accompanied by a fracture of the medial malleolus of the tibia.

Achilles tendinitis results from a small stretch injury that causes the tendon to become swollen and painful. A larger partial or complete **tear** leads to loss of function with difficulty in walking and no ability to "push off."

Plantar fasciitis is the overstretching or tearing of the dense sheet of fascia that supports the arch of the foot. If the plantar fascia is weak, **pes planus** (flatfoot) can be present.

Ingrown toenails are nails that grow into the skin folds on either side of the toe. They are often infected and painful and may need surgical repair.

Gout is an extremely painful arthritis of the big toe and other joints caused by a buildup of uric acid in the blood, which forms needlelike crystals that accumulate in the joints. Treatment is with allopurinol; some newer drugs are currently being tested.

WORD	PRONUNCIATION	ELEMENTS		DEFINITION
Achilles tendon calcaneal tendon (syn)	ah-**KILL**-eeze		a Greek warrior	A tendon formed from gastrocnemius and soleus muscles and inserted into the calcaneus
bunion	**BUN**-yun		French *bump*	A swelling at the base of the big toe
calcaneus calcaneal (adj)	kal-**KAY**-knee-us kal-**KAY**-knee-al		Latin *the heel*	Bone of the tarsus that forms the heel
fasciitis (note spelling)	fash-ee-**I**-tis	S/ R/CF	**-itis** *inflammation* **fasc/i-** *fascia*	Inflammation of the fascia
gastrocnemius	gas-trok-**NEE**-me-us	S/ R/	**-ius** *pertaining to* **gastrocnem-** *calf of leg*	Major muscle in back of the lower leg (the calf)
gout	GOWT		Latin *drop*	Painful arthritis of the big toe and other joints
hallux valgus	**HAL**-uks **VAL**-gus		**hallux** *big toe* **valgus** *turn out*	Deviation of the big toe toward the lateral side of the foot
metatarsus	**MET**-ah-**TAR**-sus	P/ R/CF	**meta-** *behind* **-tars/us** *flat surface*	A collective term referring to the five parallel bones of the foot between the tarsus and the phalanges
metatarsal (adj)	**MET**-ah-**TAR**-sal	R/ S/	**-tars-** *flat surface* **-al** *pertaining to*	Pertaining to the metatarsus
pes planus	PES **PLAY**-nuss		**pes** *foot* **planus** *flat surface*	A flat foot with no plantar arch
podiatry	po-**DIE**-ah-tree	S/ R/	**-iatry** *treatment* **pod-** *foot*	Specialty concerned with the diagnosis and treatment of disorders and injuries of the foot
podiatrist	po-**DIE**-ah-trist	S/	**-iatrist** *practitioner*	Practitioner of podiatry
Pott fracture	POT **FRAK**-chur		Percival Pott, London surgeon, 1714–1788	Fracture of lower end of fibula, often with fracture of tibial malleolus
soleus	**SO**-lee-us		From Latin for "sole of foot"	Large muscle of the calf
talipes	**TAL**-ip-eze	R/ R/	**-pes** *foot* **tali-** *ankle bone*	Deformity of the foot involving the talus
talus	**TAY**-luss		Latin *heel bone*	The tarsal bone that articulates with the tibia to form the ankle joint
tarsus tarsal (adj)	**TAR**-sus **TAR**-sal		Latin *flat surface*	The collection of seven bones in the foot that form the ankle and instep

Exercises

A. Complete your knowledge of the skeleton by matching the statement in the left column to the appropriate term in the right column.   LO 14.15, 14.16

_____ 1. forms ankle joint

_____ 2. flatfoot

_____ 3. forms ankle and instep

_____ 4. heel bone

_____ 5. large muscle of calf

_____ 6. deviation of big toe

_____ 7. swelling at base of big toe

_____ 8. five parallel bones in the foot

_____ 9. foot deformity involving talus

a. hallux valgus

b. gastrocnemius

c. tarsus

d. talipes

e. pes planus

f. metatarsus

g. talus

h. calcaneus

i. bunion

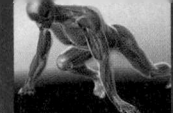

Musculoskeletal System

Challenge Your Knowledge

A. **The following medical terms contain only roots, combining forms, and suffixes.** Identify each element, and then give a brief definition of the medical term. Fill in the chart. (**LO 14.1,** *Remember*)

Medical Term	Root(s)/Combining Form(s)	Suffix	Definition of Term
chiropractic	1.	2.	3.
insertion	4.	5.	6.
osteoporosis	7.	8.	9.
hematoma	10.	11.	12.
pronation	13.	14.	15.
carpal	16.	17.	18.

B. **Terminology challenge.** One term in this chapter has an alternative spelling—either one is acceptable professionally. Find the term. Fill in the blanks with the alternative spelling and definition. (**LO 14.3,** *Remember*)

1. One term is an inflammation: _____

2. Meaning of the term: _____

C. **Knowing the exact number of certain body parts, and their relative positions, will ensure precision in your medical documentation.** Match the correct number to the correct term. Use one answer twice. (**LO 14.3,** *Remember*)

1. Number of lumbar vertebrae: _____   **a.** 7

2. Number of bones in the vertebral column: _____   **b.** 5

3. Number of cervical vertebrae: _____   **c.** 4

4. Number of components in the skeletal system: _____   **d.** 12

5. Number of regions in the vertebral column: _____   **e.** 26

6. Number of thoracic vertebrae: _____

D. **Match the health professional in the second column with his or her job description in the first column.** (**LO 14.3,** *Remember, Understand, Apply*)

_____ 1. Practitioner in the diagnosis and treatment of disorders and injuries of the foot   **a.** orthotist

_____ 2. Practitioner who evaluates and treats pain, disease, or injury by measures other than medical or surgical   **b.** physiatrist

_____ 3. Practitioner who makes and fits orthopedic appliances   **c.** podiatrist

_____ 4. Physician who specializes in physical medicine and rehabilitation   **d.** chiropractor

_____ 5. Practitioner who focuses on manual adjustment of joints to maintain and restore health   **e.** physical therapist

E. Correct spelling and formation of plurals are important in medical documentation. Improve your skill with this exercise. Circle the correct spelling of the singular term, and then form the plural. Use either the singular or the plural form in a sentence. **(LO 14.3, *Remember, Apply*)**

1. **epiphysis**   **epipisis**   **ephysis**   **epyisis**

   Plural: _____

   Sentence: _____

2. **laccuna**   **lacuna**   **lecuna**   **lacunna**

   Plural: _____

   Sentence: _____

3. **thoraax**   **torax**   **thorax**   **thoraxx**

   Plural: _____

   Sentence: _____

4. **palanx**   **phalanx**   **phalynx**   **palanyx**

   Plural: _____

   Sentence: _____

F. Identify the element by placing a check (√) in the appropriate column, define the element, and then give an example of a medical term using that element. Fill in the chart. **(LO 14.1, 14.2, *Remember, Apply*)**

	Prefix	Root/Combining Form	Suffix	Meaning of Element	Medical Term Using This Element
algia	_____	_____	_____	_____	_____
circum	_____	_____	_____	_____	_____
malacia	_____	_____	_____	_____	_____
dys	_____	_____	_____	_____	_____
inter	_____	_____	_____	_____	_____

G. The following prefixes have all appeared in this chapter. The meaning of the prefix is given to you—identify the prefix, and give an example of a medical term that starts with that prefix. Fill in the chart. **(LO 14.3, 14.4, *Remember, Apply*)**

Prefix	Meaning of Prefix	Medical Term
1.	*from, out of*	2.
3.	*beyond, making change*	4.
5.	*many*	6.
7.	*without*	8.
9.	*bad*	10.
11.	*backward*	12.
13.	*together*	14.
15.	*away from*	16.
17.	*toward*	18.
19.	*around*	20.

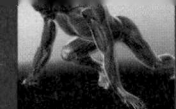

Musculoskeletal System

H. Demonstrate your knowledge of the upper-body bones and joints by circling the correct answer to these questions. (LO 14.13, *Remember, Apply*)

1. What is the long bone of the upper arm called?

   radius   ulna   humerus   carpal   scapula

2. What is a likely shoulder injury?

   separation   ACL tear   Colles Fx   ganglion   tenosynovitis

3. What structures hold an articulation together?

   ligaments   tendons   muscles   joint capsule   all of these

4. Incision through a band of fascia is called

   arthrotomy   fasciectomy   arthrodesis   arthroplasty   fasciotomy

5. What connects the humerus to the pectoral girdle?

   ligaments   tendons   muscles   joints   bones

6. The broadest muscle in the back is the

   biceps   triceps   brachii   latissimus dorsi   ulna

7. Ganglion cysts are fluid-filled cysts arising from the

   muscles   joints   synovial tendon sheaths   articulations   bursa

8. Where does a Colles fracture occur?

   arm   leg   shoulder   elbow   wrist

9. Carpal tunnel syndrome develops as a result of inflammation and swelling of

   bones   ligaments   tendon sheaths   cysts   muscles

10. Four muscles that originate on the scapula, wrap around the joint, and fuse to form one large tendon are called the

    articulation   rotator cuff   brachialis   scapulae   pectoral

I. Many medical terms come directly from Greek or Latin. Test your knowledge of these terms with this exercise. Be sure to add a brief definition for the term in the last column. The first one is done for you. Fill in the chart. (**LO 14.1, 14.3, *Remember, Apply***)

Medical Term	Meaning of Greek or Latin	Definition
bursa	*purse*	*closed sac containing synovial fluid*
callus	1.	2.
cartilage	3.	4.
condyle	5.	6.
cortex	7.	8.
lacuna	9.	10.
ligament	11.	12.
matrix	13.	14.

Use any two terms from the preceding chart to create a sentence of patient documentation.

15. _____

_____

_____

16. _____

_____

_____

J. Explain the difference among these abnormal spinal curvatures to a patient. (**LO 14.1, 14.4, *Understand***)

1. lordosis _____

2. scoliosis _____

3. kyphosis _____

4. Which one is the most common defect? _____

5. Which defect is seen in patients with osteoporosis? _____

K. Functions of skeletal muscles. Bones and joints would get us nowhere without the muscles to move them. Illustrate how each of these functions is accomplished with skeletal muscles. (**LO 14.10, *Understand***)

Function	How Function Is Affected
Movement	_____
Posture	_____
Body heat	_____
Respiration	_____
Communication	_____

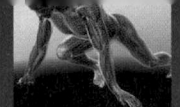

Musculoskeletal System

L.   Employ the language of orthopedics to answer the following questions about muscles. (LO 14.10, 14.11, *Understand*)

   1. What is muscle tone?

   _____

   _____

   2. What is muscle contraction?

   _____

   _____

   3. What is the difference between muscle atrophy and hypertrophy?

   _____

   _____

M.   Some medical terms have common layman's terms associated with them. Write the layman's term for the following terms. (**LO 14.3,** *Understand*)

   1. femur _____

   2. patella _____

N.   Physical therapists instruct patients in range-of-motion (ROM) exercises to improve mobility. The exercises are described for you—determine the correct medical term. (**LO 14.3, 14.8,** *Understand, Apply*)

abduction	lateral rotation	rotation	pronation	supination
inversion	circumduction	medial rotation	adduction	eversion

   1. Rotating the humerus with the elbow flexed while bringing the palm of the hand toward the

      body: _____

   2. Elbow flexed at 90 degrees, rotating forearm so that palm is facing the floor: _____

   3. Sole of the foot facing toward the opposite foot: _____. This is also called _____.

   4. Action of moving toward the midline: _____

   5. Turning a joint on its axis: _____

   6. Sole of the foot facing laterally away from the other foot: _____ or _____

   7. Moving the shoulder so that it forms a cone with the shoulder joint as the apex of the cone: _____

   8. Spreading fingers apart, away from the middle finger: _____

   9. Moving the palm away from the body: _____

   10. Lying flat on your back, palms facing up: _____

O. **How well do you understand what you read?** Could you explain it to a patient? First read the paragraph; then translate the medical terms that are written in bold into layman's language for a patient explanation. Use a dictionary or the glossary for terms you don't recognize. (**LO 14.15,** *Understand, Apply*)

The two bones of the lower leg are the larger and **medial tibia** and the thinner and **lateral fibula**. The **distal** end of the tibia on its medial border forms a prominent process called the *medial* **malleolus**. The lower end of the fibula forms the lateral malleolus. You can **palpate** both these **prominences** on your ankle.

1. medial _____

_____

_____

2. tibia _____

_____

_____

3. lateral _____

_____

_____

4. fibula _____

_____

_____

5. distal _____

_____

_____

6. malleolus _____

_____

_____

7. palpate _____

_____

_____

8. prominence _____

_____

_____

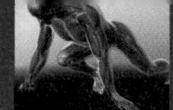

Musculoskeletal System

P. **Choose the correct medical term(s) from the list to complete the sentence.** You will not use all the terms. (**LO 14.3,** *Understand, Apply*)

striation	symphysis	detoxification	intervertebral discs
DMD	orthotic	opposition	pelvis
retinaculum	shoulder girdle	fascicle	acetabulum
popliteal fossa	traction	steroids	fibromyalgia

1. line or streak across a muscle is called a _____.

2. A transverse, fibrous band on the wrist is called a _____.

3. _____ support and cushion the vertebral column.

4. _____ has no known etiology, no laboratory tests for it, and no known treatment except pain management.

5. Movement that enables the thumb to touch the tips of the other fingers is called _____.

6. Cartilaginous joint between two bones is called _____.

7. A bundle of muscle fibers is called _____.

8. Dr. Stannard ordered continuous application of weight to the patient's broken leg. The patient has been placed in _____.

9. _____ cause skeletal muscle to hypertrophy.

10. The hollow at the back of the knee is called the _____.

Q. Show your understanding of orthopedic terminology by providing the meaning of the elements for the terms that follow and then using the term in a sentence. Slash (/) the terms into elements before you start the exercise. **(LO 14.1, 14.3,** *Understand, Apply***)**

1. **orthopedic**   The combining form is _____ and means _____.

   Sentence:

   _____

   _____

2. **endosteum**   The prefix is _____ and means _____.

   Sentence:

   _____

   _____

3. **epiphysis**   The root is _____ and means _____.

   Sentence:

   _____

   _____

4. **articulation**   The suffix is _____ and means _____.

   Sentence:

   _____

   _____

5. **degenerative**   The root is _____ and means _____.

   Sentence:

   _____

   _____

6. **arthrodesis**   The suffix is _____ and means _____.

   Sentence:

   _____

   _____

7. **fibromyalgia**   The combining form is _____ and means _____.

   Sentence:

   _____

   _____

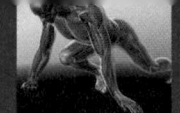

Musculoskeletal System

R. **Many professional certification exams are given in multiple-choice format.** Decide on the answer by quickly eliminating the answers you know to be incorrect. Then decide which of the remaining answers is the *best* choice. (**LO 14.1, 14.2, 14.3,** *Understand, Apply*)

1. Which of the following terms is NOT surgical hardware used to repair a fracture?
   - **a.** wires
   - **b.** rods
   - **c.** plates
   - **d.** screws
   - **e.** batteries

2. Bone growth occurs at the
   - **a.** origin
   - **b.** epiphyseal plate
   - **c.** diaphysis
   - **d.** epicondyle
   - **e.** lacuna

3. An inherited condition in which bone formation is incomplete is
   - **a.** osteoarthritis
   - **b.** osteomalacia
   - **c.** osteomyelitis
   - **d.** osteogenesis imperfecta
   - **e.** osteopenia

4. Lubricant for joint movement is
   - **a.** mucin
   - **b.** mucus
   - **c.** mucous
   - **d.** synovial
   - **e.** meniscus

5. The following is where two bones come together at a joint:
   - **a.** articulation
   - **b.** reduction
   - **c.** mastication
   - **d.** striation
   - **e.** herniation

6. An extension of synovial membrane that forms a cushion to prevent structures from rubbing together is
   - **a.** tendon
   - **b.** periosteum
   - **c.** ligament
   - **d.** bursa
   - **e.** muscle

7. Pulling a bone from the distal end back into alignment is
   - **a.** subluxation
   - **b.** dislocation
   - **c.** reduction
   - **d.** resorption
   - **e.** external fixation

8. The process of lying face-upward, flat on your spine is
   - **a.** pronation
   - **b.** abduction
   - **c.** adduction
   - **d.** supination
   - **e.** inversion

9. Overstretching or tearing of the dense sheet of tissue that supports the arch of the foot is
   - **a.** pes planus
   - **b.** plantar fasciitis
   - **c.** hallux valgus
   - **d.** Achilles tendinitis
   - **e.** exostosis

10. Joints between the teeth and their sockets are called
    - **a.** symphyses
    - **b.** gomphoses
    - **c.** sutures
    - **d.** syndesmoses
    - **e.** synchondroses

S. **Fill out the disability form for Ms. Lara Baker.** Use the information provided in Case Report 14.6, with the additional facts provided in the sentences following the form. (**LO 14.3**, *Apply*)

1. Ms. Baker must complete her physiotherapy first, and then return to see Dr. Stannard.

2. Ms. Baker is to remain off work until she has completed PT and returned to see Dr. Stannard in 3 weeks.

3. Dr. Stannard is an MD.

4. Ms. Baker has no other current medical problems.

5. The disability insurance carrier is Empire Insurance Company.

6. On examination, Dr. Stannard has found pain, swelling, numbness, tingling, and reduced grip in Ms. Baker's right hand.

7. The office phone number is on the letterhead, and Dr. Stannard takes calls from 8 to 9 a.m. and again from 3 to 4 p.m., Monday through Friday.

Fulwood Medical Center
3333 Medical Parkway, Fulwood, MI 01234
555-247-6100

Department of Orthopedics
Dr. Stannard 555-247-6100

Doctor's report of occupational injury or illness

Patient name: _____
Patient address: _____
Occupation: _____
Employer: _____
Employer's insurance company: _____
(Please provide insurance claim form to billing manager) _____
Date of onset of illness: (*back date from date seen*) _____
Date seen: (*use current date*) _____
Date last worked: (*use current date*) _____

_____
Patient's description of how injury occurred: _____
Patient's chief complaints: _____
Doctor's findings: _____
Diagnosis: _____
Treatment Plan _____
_____

Any special equipment ordered? No_____Yes_____
If yes, describe equipment: _____
Is there any other current condition that will delay recovery from this injury/illness?
No _____ Yes _____ If yes, describe_____
Is further treatment required? No _____ Yes _____
Follow-up appointment?   No _____ Yes _____
When _____
Can patient return to work at this time?

YES	NO
No modifications _____	Still in treatment _____
With modification _____	Unable to return to this job _____
Describe restrictions: No lifting _____ No standing _____ No sitting for extended periods of time _____ Other_____	
Full time_____	
Part time only _____	

May we call you concerning this patient? No _____Yes_____ Best time:_____
Doctor's name and degree:_____
License number:_____ Tax ID#_____
Doctor's signature: (stamped signature not acceptable)
_____

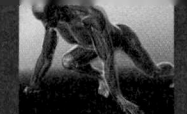

Musculoskeletal System

T. **Build your orthopedic terminology by completing the medical terms defined here.** After you fill in the element on the line, write the type of element (prefix, root, combining form, suffix) you have used below the lines. Fill in the blanks. (**LO 14.1, 14.2,** *Apply*)

1. Removing poison from tissue   de/ _____ / _____

2. Bone disease   osteo/_____/_____

3. Projection above the condyle   _____ /condyle/_____

4. Membrane surrounding a bone   peri/ _____ / _____

5. Region between diaphysis and epiphysis _____ /physis/_____

6. Bones lacking in calcium   osteo/ _____ / _____

7. Inflammation of bone tissue   osteo/ _____ /itis

8. Collection of blood in tissues   _____ /oma/ _____

9. Moving toward the midline   _____ / _____ /ion_____

10. Fixation of a joint with surgery   arthro/ _____ / _____

U. **Post the OR schedule for the Orthopedic Department.** Convert the description into a medical term for billing the procedure. Fill in the chart. (**LO 14.3, 14.9,** *Analyze*)

Description	Medical Term
insertion right-hip prosthesis	1.
removing dead tissue from an open wound of the leg	2.
scope examination of left shoulder	3.
surgical removal of torn meniscus of left knee	4.
withdrawal of fluid from the right knee	5.
removal of gangrenous right leg	6.
surgical removal of hypertrophied connective tissue to release a contracture	7.

V. **The skeleton effects movement and provides support and protection for the entire body.** Help build your knowledge of the skeleton and orthopedic terminology with this mini-outline. (**LO 14.3, 14.10,** *Analyze*)

The four components of the skeletal system are

1. _____

2. _____

3. _____

4. _____

These components have the following functions:

5. _____

6. _____

7. _____

8. _____

9. _____

10. _____

Factors that affect bone growth are

11. _____

12. _____

13. _____

14. _____

15. _____

16. _____

17. _____

The most common type of bone in the body is the long bone. Define these terms related to long bones:

18. epiphysis _____

19. diaphysis _____

20. metaphysis _____

21. Covers outer surface of all bones: _____

22. Cartilage cells in the _____ enable the bone shaft to grow in length.

23. The _____ contains the bone marrow and is lined with the membrane called

the _____.

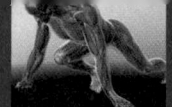

Musculoskeletal System

W. Short answers. Patients will ask for a layman's explanation of medical terms. If a patient asks, could you explain the difference between the following? (**LO 14.7, 14.11, 14.14,** *Analyze*)

1. Malunion and nonunion of a fracture: _____

2. A muscle strain and a muscle sprain: _____

3. Shoulder separation, dislocation, and subluxation: _____

_____

X. Challenge your knowledge of bones, joints, muscles, tendons, and ligaments by attributing the medical term to the correct category. Place a check (√) in the appropriate column. (**LO 14.4,** *Analyze*)

Medical Term	Bone	Joint	Muscle	Tendon	Ligament
1. ball and socket					
2. TMJ					
3. DMD					
4. gastrocnemius					
5. rotator cuff					
6. ACL					
7. rickets					
8. dislocation					
9. compact or cortical					
10. tenosynovitis					
11. hinge					
12. marrow					
13. acetabulum					
14. DJD					
15. Achilles					

Y. The practice needs to hire an additional doctor due to patient volume. The business manager has asked you to run a computer report that will give you the 10 most frequently billed diagnoses in the orthopedic clinic. You must analyze the report to give the manager the information she needs. The 10 most frequently billed diagnoses are shown as follows (not in any special order). Determine the meaning of the key terms and which body part is affected. <u>The first one is done for you.</u> (**LO 14.6, 14.9,** *Analyze*)

Diagnosis	Meaning	Body Part
osteoarthritis of the patella	*arthritis of the knee*	*knee*
repair of AC joint	1.	2.
herniated discectomy	3.	4.
rotator cuff repair	5.	6.
ACL repair	7.	8.
meniscectomy	9.	10.
THR	11.	12.
patellar arthroplasty	13.	14.
L3–L5 discectomy	15.	16.

17. According to this chart, the practice should hire a specialist in _____ surgery.

Z. Discussion question. Amy Vargas has six different risk factors for osteoporosis. What exactly is a "risk factor"? List each risk factor; then discuss what can or cannot be done to counteract that risk. What steps could Amy have taken to improve her lifestyle and lessen her risk for osteoporosis? (**LO 14.9,** *Analyze, Evaluate*)

A. _____

_____

_____

B. _____

_____

_____

C. _____

_____

_____

D. _____

_____

_____

E. _____

_____

_____

F. _____

_____

_____

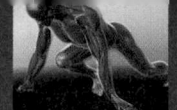
Musculoskeletal System

CHAPTER SUMMARY EXERCISES

A. **Spelling comprehension.** Circle the correct spelling of the term. (**LO 14.1, 14.2, 14.3,** *Remember*)

1. ephiseal   epiphyseal   epificeal   epyhiseal   epyiseal

2. fastiotomy   fasciotomy   fassiotomy   faseotomy   faciotomy

3. fibromyalgia   febromialgia   fibromialga   febromealga   fibrromialgia

4. peterygoid   pterygoid   terygoid   peterigoid   terigoid

5. interoseus   interossius   interosseous   interosseus   intraosseus

6. syndismosis   syndesmosis   sindesmosis   syndemosis   sindismosis

7. ischium   eschium   eschiom   ischeum   iseum

8. kiposis   kyposis   khyposis   kyphosis   kiphosis

9. coccix   cocyx   coccyx   cockyx   cockix

10. scapulay   scapuae   scalpulay   scappulae   scapulae

B. **Match the number of the correct spelling of the terms in Exercise A with the following brief descriptions of the terms.** (**LO 14.3,** *Apply*)

1. Incision and release of retinaculum   _____

2. Tail bone   _____

3. Opens and closes mouth   _____

4. Joint formed by ligaments   _____

5. Lower/posterior part of the hip bone   _____

6. Pain in muscle fibers   _____

7. Compact bone grows in and forms this line   _____

8. Structure between bones   _____

9. Shoulder blades   _____

10. Posterior spinal curve   _____

C. Using your knowledge of terms 1–10 in Exercises A and B and their correct spelling, write a brief sentence for each of the terms as it might appear in patient documentation. (LO 14.4, *Apply*)

1. _____

2. _____

3. _____

4. _____

5. _____

6. _____

7. _____

8. _____

9. _____

10. _____

D. After rereading all of Case Report 14.2, answer the following questions. Be prepared to discuss your answers in class. (LO 14.3, 14.9, *Analyze*)

Case Report 14.2

In his youth, Mr. Johnson played football and baseball. As an adult, he has played racquetball weekly and jogged 3 to 4 miles most mornings on the streets of his neighborhood. For the past year he has had lower-back stiffness and pain, particularly in the mornings. Six months ago, while out hiking, he slid down a mountain on his left side for about 100 feet. He is now having pain in his left groin and thigh, with difficulty walking and climbing stairs.

By age 65, more than 80% of people have some degree of joint degeneration. Mr. Johnson had always been very physically active, putting a lot of pressure on his weight-bearing joints. At different times in his life he had been overweight, adding to the pressure.

X-rays of his lower back showed osteoarthritis of his lower lumbar intervertebral joints and marked osteoarthritis of his left hip joint. He received a left total-hip replacement (THR) and physiotherapy (PT) for his lower back.

1. Explain to your patient in layman's terms what is meant by "joint degeneration."

   _____

   _____

2. Describe what is meant by a "weight-bearing" joint and where it is located on the body. _____

   _____

3. What physical condition complicated Mr. Johnson's joint problems? _____

   _____

4. What is the chronic inflammatory disease of the joints that causes pain and loss of function? _____

5. Where are the "lower lumbar" intervertebral joints located? _____

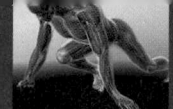

Musculoskeletal System

E. **Meet the goals of each of the chapter outcomes by using the correct language of the musculoskeletal system for the answers. (LO 14.1-14.15, *Analyze*)**

1. Apply the language of orthopedics to the anatomy, growth, and structure of the skeletal system. (**LO 14.1**)

    Bones are divided into _____ classes on the basis of their _____. Name them:

    _____

2. Apply the language of orthopedics to the physiology and functions of the skeletal system. (**LO 14.2**)

    Explain the bone function of detoxification. What is removed from the body?

    _____

3. Use the medical terms of orthopedics to communicate and document in writing accurately and precisely in any health care setting. (**LO 14.3**)

    Construct the sentence with the appropriate medical language.

    "Mrs. Baker has (softening of her bones) _____ and is probably going to (break) _____ her hip."

4. Use the medical terms of orthopedics to communicate verbally with accuracy and precision in any health care setting. Fill in the blank. (**LO 14.4**)

    If a surgeon tells you the procedure will require a *heterograft*, he could have also said it would require a _____.

5. Define abbreviations that pertain to the musculoskeletal system. Which of the following abbreviations is the only one that applies to the musculoskeletal system? (**LO 14.5**)

    a. RUQ   **c.** STAT   **e.** VCUG

    b. BMD   **d.** URI

6. Discuss common diseases of bone. (**LO 14.6**)

    a. The medical term for rickets is _____.

    b. Inflammation of an area of bone due to bacterial infection is _____.

    c. _____ results from loss of bone density.

7. Explain the causes and types of fractures of bone, their healing, and the procedures for repairing fractures. (**LO 14.7**)

    a. If a fracture is reduced by external manipulation, is an incision necessary? _____

    b. What is the initial goal of fracture treatment? _____

8. Describe the classes of joints and the movements that they can achieve. (**LO 14.8**)

    a. Which type of joint contains a lubricant that allows for considerable movement? _____

    b. _____ is a joining of two bones with fibrous ligaments; their movement is minimal.

    c. _____ occur between the bones of the skull; there is virtually no movement.

9. Identify the common diseases of joints and surgical procedures used to treat them. Describe the difference between an arthrocentesis and an arthroplasty. (**LO 14.9**)

    a. arthrocentesis _____

    b. arthroplasty _____

10. Match the structure of skeletal muscle to its functions. How is movement achieved by the body? (**LO 14.10**)

_____

_____

11. Discuss common disorders of skeletal muscles. What is the difference between a strain and a sprain? (**LO 14.11**)

a. strain _____

b. sprain _____

12. Describe the structure and functions of the axial skeleton and its associated joints and muscles. What is the axial skeleton, and what does it protect? (**LO 14.12**)

_____

_____

13. Identify the structures and functions of the bones, joints, and muscles of the shoulder, arm, and hand. Identify the correct statements with a circle, and rewrite the false one on the following lines. (**LO 14.13**)

a. The scapulae are bones in the shoulder.   T   F

b. The shoulder joint allows the greatest motion of any joint in the body.   T   F

c. The knee joint is the most unstable joint because of its ROM.   T   F

d. The rotator cuff is a fusion of 3 muscles.   T   F

e. The rotator cuff is a large tendon.   T   F

Corrections:

_____

_____

14. Explain common disorders of the shoulder, arm, and hand, and procedures used in their treatment. What is the treatment for each of the following disorders of the shoulder, arm, and hand? (**LO 14.14**)

a. rotator cuff tear _____

b. carpal tunnel syndrome _____

c. tennis elbow _____

15. Discuss the structure and functions of the pelvic girdle, hip, thigh, knee, lower leg, ankle, and foot. What three bones fuse to form the hip bone? (**LO 14.15**)

a. _____

b. _____

c. _____

16. Describe common disorders of the pelvic girdle, hip, thigh, knee, lower leg, ankle, and foot. (**LO 14.16**)

a. What is the medical term for the Achilles tendon? _____

b. The medical term for the deformity commonly called a _bunion_ is _____.

c. Arthritis of the big toe caused by uric acid is called _____.

d. _Flatfoot_ in medical language is _____.

Integumentary System
The Language of Dermatology

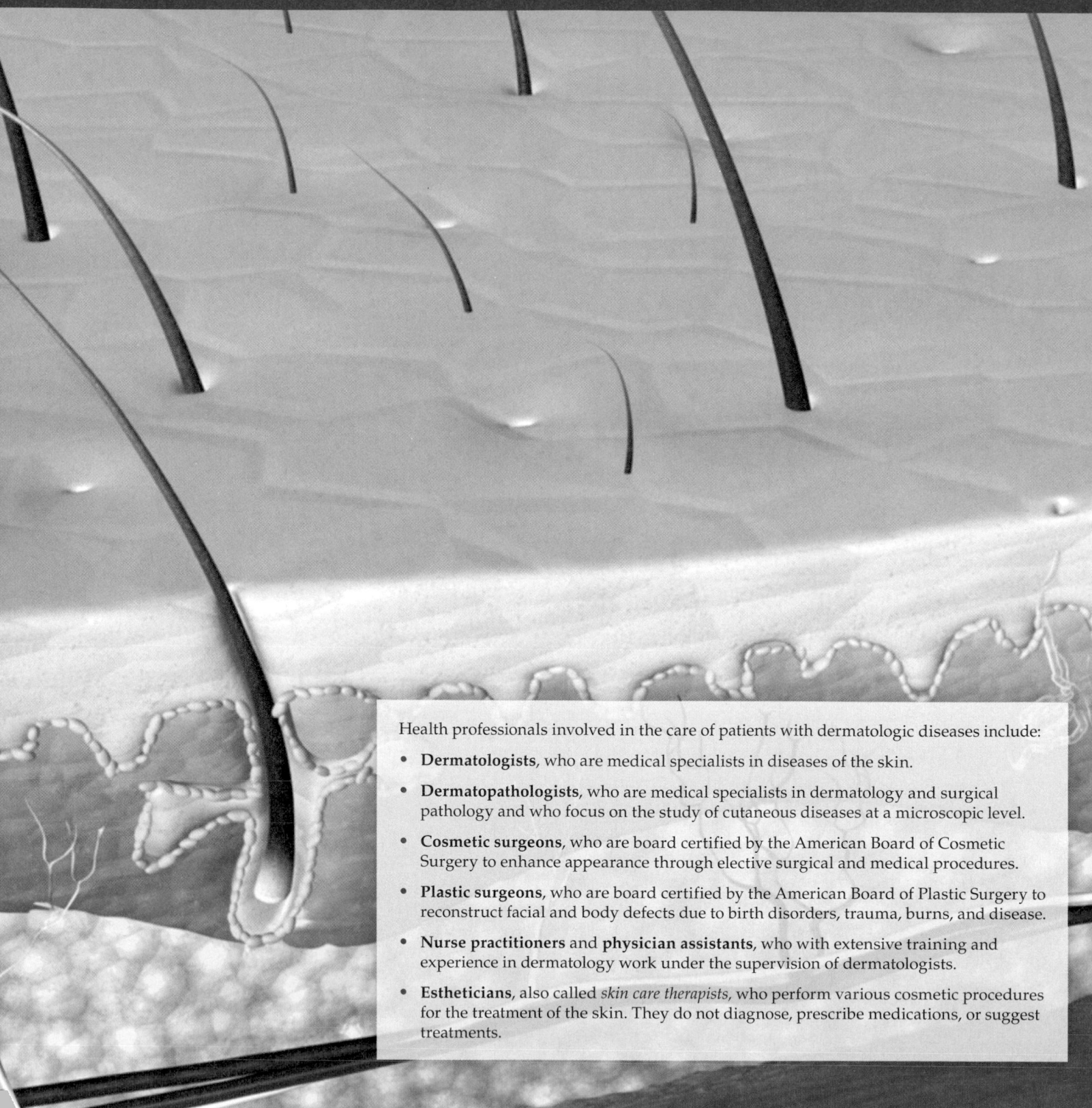

Health professionals involved in the care of patients with dermatologic diseases include:

- **Dermatologists**, who are medical specialists in diseases of the skin.

- **Dermatopathologists**, who are medical specialists in dermatology and surgical pathology and who focus on the study of cutaneous diseases at a microscopic level.

- **Cosmetic surgeons**, who are board certified by the American Board of Cosmetic Surgery to enhance appearance through elective surgical and medical procedures.

- **Plastic surgeons**, who are board certified by the American Board of Plastic Surgery to reconstruct facial and body defects due to birth disorders, trauma, burns, and disease.

- **Nurse practitioners** and **physician assistants**, who with extensive training and experience in dermatology work under the supervision of dermatologists.

- **Estheticians**, also called *skin care therapists*, who perform various cosmetic procedures for the treatment of the skin. They do not diagnose, prescribe medications, or suggest treatments.

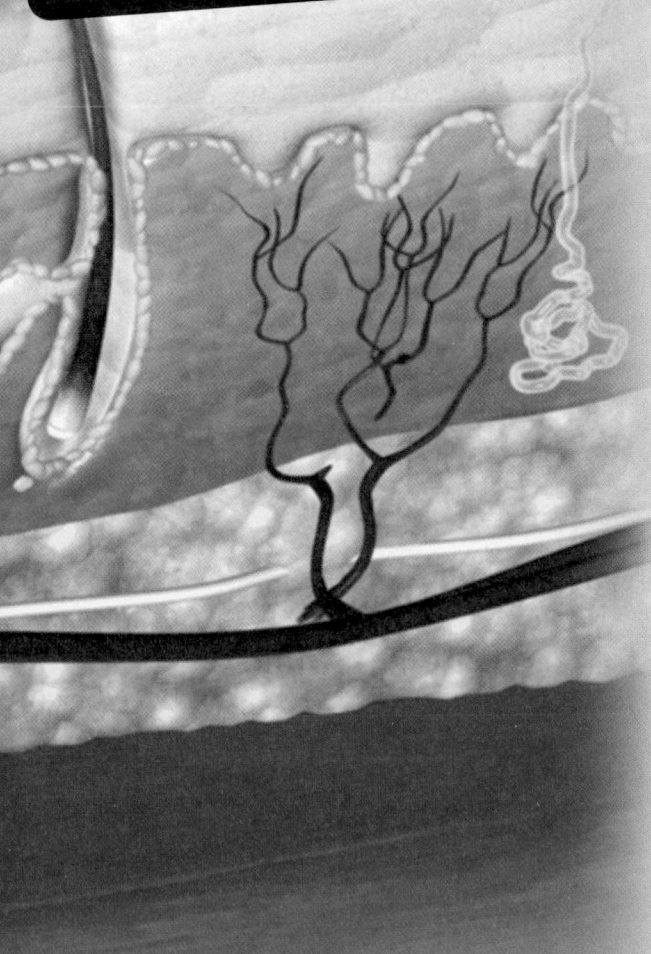

Case Report (CR) 15.1

You are

. . . a clinical medical assistant working in the office of dermatologist Dr. Lenore Echols, a member of the Fulwood Medical Group.

Your patient is

. . . Mr. Rod Andrews, a 60-year-old man, who shows you three skin lesions—two on his left forearm and one on the back of his left hand. On questioning him, you learn that he has been living for the past 10 years in Arizona and has returned to the area to be near his daughter and young grandchildren. You find no other skin lesions on his body.

Chapter Learning Outcomes

In addition to anticipating Dr. Echols' needs for equipment to **biopsy**, diagnose, and treat the **lesions**, you also have to be able to communicate clearly with her in medical terms and to understand her language as she communicates with you and the patient about the **etiology** (cause) and structure of the lesions. You will then need to document the medical history and treatment and communicate clearly with Mr. Andrews about the treatment of his lesions and their **prognosis**.

To perform these tasks, you must be able to:

LO 15.1 Describe the overall structure, functions, and regions of the skin.

LO 15.2 Discuss the different layers of the skin and their functions.

LO 15.3 Differentiate the different sites for injections in the skin and their effect.

LO 15.4 Describe the common disorders, diseases, and infections of the skin.

LO 15.5 Use the medical terms of dermatology to communicate and document in writing accurately and precisely in any health care setting.

LO 15.6 Use the medical terms of dermatology to communicate verbally with accuracy and precision in any health care setting.

LO 15.7 Define the types of topical agents used in the treatment of skin disorders.

LO 15.8 Match the accessory skin organs to their functions.

LO 15.9 Describe disorders of the accessory skin organs.

LO 15.10 Discuss burns and injuries to the skin.

LO 15.11 Describe the healing of wounds to the skin.

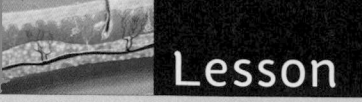

Lesson 15.1 Functions and Structure of the Skin

INTEGUMENTARY SYSTEM

The three lesions on Mr. Andrews' arm and hand developed in the superficial layer of the skin called the epidermis. This lesson looks at the structure and functions of the skin and at diseases of the epidermis so that you will be able to:

15.1.1 Discuss the functions and structure of the skin.

15.1.2 Describe the Rule of Nines for estimating the surface area of the six different regions of the skin.

15.1.3 List the layers of the skin.

15.1.4 Name the tissues in the different layers of the skin.

15.1.5 Identify the functions of the different layers of the skin.

15.1.6 Describe disorders affecting the superficial layers of the skin, including cancers.

15.1.7 Apply correct medical terminology to the anatomy, physiology, and disorders of the superficial layers of the skin.

Keynotes

- The skin is the largest and most vulnerable organ in the body.

- There are four combining forms for skin:
  - cutane/o
  - derm/a
  - dermat/o
  - derm/o

Case Report 15.1 (continued)

When Dr. Echols examined Mr. Andrews, she determined clinically that two of his lesions were basal cell **carcinomas** and she treated them with **cryosurgery**. She believed that the third lesion was a **squamous cell** carcinoma, and she performed a **biopsy removal** of that **lesion**. You sent it to the laboratory with a request for **pathological** diagnosis and determination of whether the lesion had been completely removed. This is done by ensuring that a normal skin margin completely surrounds the lesion when it is examined under the **microscope**.

LO 15.1 Functions of the Skin

The **integumentary system** consists of the skin and its associated organs *(Figure 15.1)*. The study and treatment of the integumentary system is called **dermatology**. This organ system receives more medical and personal attention than any other organ system. Your understanding of its structures and functions will be used every day in your professional and personal life.

The skin is the largest organ in your body and accounts for 7% to 8% of your body weight. The skin is the most vulnerable of all your organs because it is continually exposed to chemicals, trauma, infection, radiation, temperature change, humidity variation, and all the pollution of modern life. Your skin is an important part of your own self-image and an important part of total patient care.

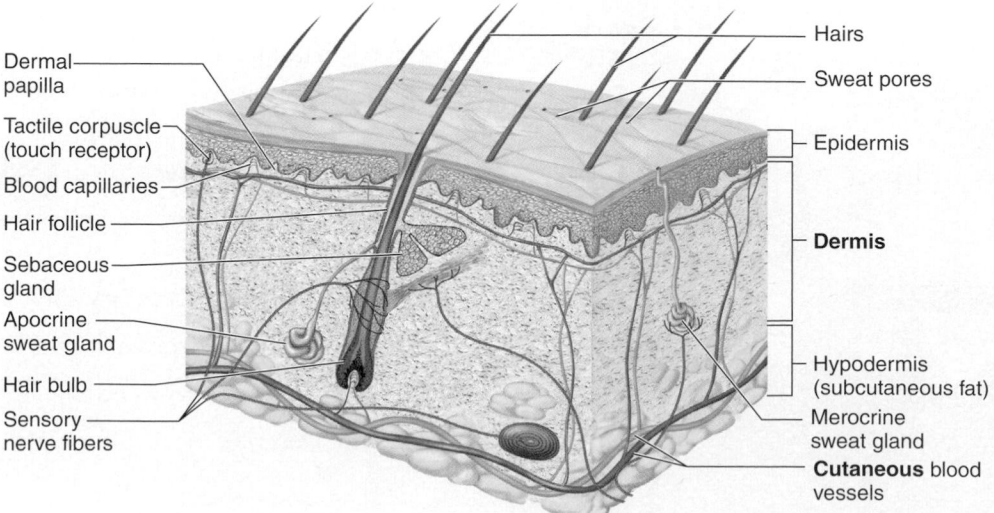

▲ **Figure 15.1** Structure of the Skin and Subcutaneous Tissue.

WORD	PRONUNCIATION	ELEMENTS		DEFINITION
biopsy	**BI**-op-see	S/	**-opsy** *to view*	Removing tissue from a living person for laboratory examination
		R/CF	**bi/o-** *life*	
biopsy removal (also called excisional biopsy)	**BI**-op-see re-**MUV**-al			Used for small tumors when complete removal provides tissue for a biopsy and cures the lesion
excision	ek-**SIZH**-un	S/	**-ion** *action*	Surgical removal of part or all of a structure
		R/	**excis-** *cut out*	
carcinoma	kar-sih-**NOH**-mah	S/	**-oma** *tumor, mass*	A malignant and invasive **epithelial** tumor
		R/	**carcin-** *cancer*	
cosmetic	koz-**MET**-ik		Greek *an adornment*	A concern for appearance
cryosurgery	cry-oh-**SUR**-jer-ee	S/	**-ery** *process of*	Use of liquid nitrogen or argon gas in a probe to freeze and kill abnormal tissue
		R/CF	**cry/o-** *icy cold*	
		R/	**-surg-** *operate*	
cutaneous	kyu-**TAY**-nee-us	S/	**-us** *pertaining to*	Pertaining to the skin
		R/CF	**cutane/o-** *skin*	
dermis	**DER**-miss		Greek *skin*	Connective tissue layer of the skin beneath the epidermis
dermal (adj)	**DER**-mal			
dermatology	der-mah-**TOL**-oh-jee	S/	**-logy** *study of*	Medical specialty concerned with disorders of the skin
		R/CF	**dermat/o-** *skin*	
dermatologist	der-mah-**TOL**-oh-jist	S/	**-logist** *one who studies*	Medical specialist in diseases of the skin
epidermis	ep-ih-**DER**-miss	P/	**epi-** *upon*	Top layer of the skin
		R/	**-dermis** *skin*	
epithelium	ep-ih-**THEE**-lee-um	S/	**-um** *tissue*	Tissue that covers surfaces or lines cavities
		P/	**epi-** *upon*	
		R/CF	**thel/i-** *nipple*	
epithelial (adj)	ep-ih-**THEE**-lee-al	S/	**-al** *pertaining to*	Relating to or consisting of epithelium
esthetics	es-**THET**-iks		Greek *sensation*	Concerned with beauty
esthetician	es-**THET**-ish-un	S/	**-ician** *specialist*	A therapist who enhances the beauty of the skin
		R/	**esthet-** *beauty*	
integument	in-**TEG**-you-ment		Latin *a covering*	Organ system that covers the body, the skin being the main organ within the system
integumentary (adj)	in-**TEG**-you-**MEN**-tah-ree	S/	**-ary** *pertaining to*	Pertaining to the covering of the body
		R/	**integument-** *covering of the body*	
lesion	**LEE**-zhun		Latin *injury*	Pathological change or injury in a tissue
microscope	**MY**-kroh-skope	P/	**micro-** *small*	Instrument for viewing something small that cannot be seen in detail by the naked eye
		R/	**-scope** *instrument for viewing*	
microscopic (adj)	**MY**-kroh-**SKOP**-ik	S/	**-ic** *pertaining to*	Visible only with the aid of a microscope
pathology	pa-**THOL**-oh-jee	S/	**-logy** *study of*	Medical specialty dealing with the structural and functional changes of a disease process or the cause, development, and structural changes in disease
		R/CF	**path/o-** *disease*	
pathologic (adj)	path-oh-**LOJ**-ik	S/	**-ic** *pertaining to*	Pertaing to the changes in the body induced by disease
prognosis	prog-**NO**-sis	P/	**pro-** *projecting forward*	Forecasting of the probable course of a disease
		R/	**-gnosis** *knowledge*	
squamous cell	**SKWAY**-mus **SELL**		Latin *scaly*	Flat, scalelike epithelial cell

Exercises

A. Review the above WAD before starting this exercise. *Build your knowledge of the elements in the* language of dermatology. *Circle the best answer.* **LO 15.1, 15.5**

1. The suffix **-oma** can mean tumor or

   gland   mass   cancer

2. Circle the term that means *study of*:

   dermatology   dermatologist   dermatitis

3. **Cryo-** is a combining form that signifies

   color   temperature   location

4. The term **cutaneous** means *pertaining to*

   skin   mass   tumor

Keynote
_____

The skin provides protection, contains sensory organs, and helps control body temperature.

LO 15.1 Functions of the Skin

- **Protection**. The skin is physical barrier against injury, chemicals, ultraviolet rays, microbes, and toxins.
- **Water resistance**. You don't swell up every time you take a bath because your skin is water resistant. It also prevents water from leaking out from the body tissues.
- **Temperature regulation**. A network of **capillaries** in the skin opens up or dilates **(vasodilation)** when your body is too hot so that the blood flow increases and the heat from the blood dissipates through your skin. When your body is cold, the capillary network narrows **(vasoconstriction)**, blood flow decreases, and heat is retained in your body.
- **Vitamin D synthesis**. As little as 15 to 30 minutes of sunlight daily allows your skin cells to initiate the metabolism of vitamin D, which is essential for bone growth and maintenance.
- **Sensation**. Nerve endings that detect touch, pressure, heat, cold, pain, vibration, and tissue injury are particularly numerous on your face, fingers, palms, soles, nipples, and genitals.
- **Excretion and secretion**. Water and small amounts of waste products from cell metabolism are lost through the skin by **excretion** (the process of removal of waste products from the body) and by **secretion** (the process of producing and releasing a substance by a tissue or organ of the body) from your sweat glands.
- **Social functions**. The skin reflects your emotions, blushing when you are self-conscious, going pale when you are frightened, wrinkling when you dislike something.

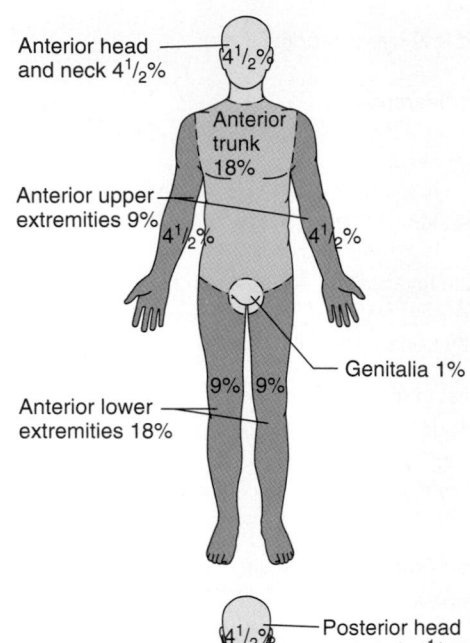

Anterior head and neck 4½%
Anterior trunk 18%
Anterior upper extremities 9%
4½% 4½%
Genitalia 1%
Anterior lower extremities 18%
9% 9%

LO 15.1 Skin as a Barrier

The skin is a barrier that is not easily broken. Few infectious organisms can penetrate the skin on their own. Those that do use accidental breaks in the skin or rely on animals such as mosquitoes, fleas, or ticks to puncture the skin to allow access for the infectious organisms. The skin is also a barrier to solar radiation, including ultraviolet (UV) rays.

Blood receives 1% to 2% of its oxygen from diffusion through the skin, and it releases through the skin some carbon dioxide and organic chemicals that attract mosquitoes and other insects to people.

LO 15.1 Regions of Skin Surface Area

The skin's surface area can be divided into six regions, each one of which is a fraction or multiple of 9% of the total surface area. This is called the Rule of Nines *(Figure 15.2)*.

The treatment and prognosis for a burn patient depend, in part, on the extent of the body surface that is affected. This is estimated by applying the Rule of Nines to determine the percentage of the skin's surface affected by burns:

- Head and neck are assigned 9% (4½% anterior and 4½% posterior).
- Each arm is 9% (4½% anterior and 4½% posterior).
- Each leg is 18% (9% anterior and 9% posterior).
- The anterior trunk is 18%.
- The posterior trunk is 18%.
- The genitalia are 1%.

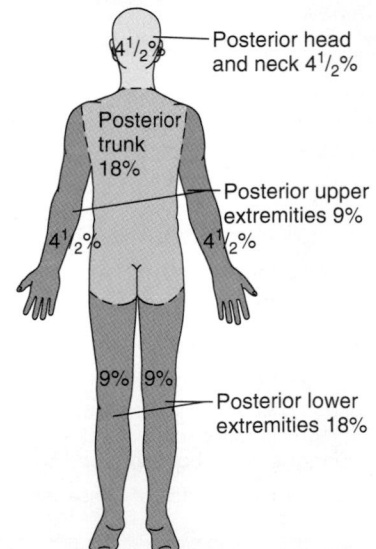

Posterior head and neck 4½%
Posterior trunk 18%
Posterior upper extremities 9%
4½% 4½%
9% 9%
Posterior lower extremities 18%

▲ **Figure 15.2**   Rule of Nines.

WORD	PRONUNCIATION	ELEMENTS		DEFINITION
excrete (verb)	eks-**KREET**		Latin *remove*	To pass out of the body waste products of metabolism
excretion (noun)	eks-**KREE**-shun			Removal of waste products of metabolism out of the body
function	**FUNK**-shun		Latin *to perform*	The ability of an organ or tissue to perform its special work
protection (noun)	pro-**TEK**-shun	S/	**-ion** *action, condition*	Defense against attack or invasion
protect (verb)		P/	**pro-** *before*	To shield from attack or invasion
		R/	**-tect-** *to shelter*	
regulation (noun)	reg-you-**LAY**-shun	S/	**-ation** *process*	Control of the way in which a process progresses
	REG-you-late	R/	**regul-** *to rule*	
regulate (verb)		S/	**-ate** *pertaining to*	To control the way in which a process progresses
resistance (noun)	ree-**ZIS**-tants	S/	**-ance** *state of*	Ability of an organism to withstand the effects of an antagonistic
resist (verb)		R/	**resist-** *to withstand*	agent
secrete (verb)	se-**KREET**		Latin *to separate*	To produce a chemical substance in a cell and release it from
secretion (noun)	se-**KREE**-shun			the cell
sensation (noun)	sen-**SAY**-shun	S/	**-ation** *process*	The conscious feeling of the effects of a stimulation
sense (verb)		R/	**sens-** *to feel*	
synthesis (noun)	**SIN**-the-sis	P/	**syn-** *together*	The process of building a compound from different elements
synthesize (verb)	**SIN**-the-size	R/	**-thesis** *to arrange*	

Exercises

A. The following are functions of the skin—assign one to each statement by filling in the blanks.   LO 15.1, 15.5

protection   water resistance   temperature regulation   vitamin D synthesis

sensation   excretion   secretion   social function

1. water and waste products lost through the skin: _____

2. detection by nerve endings of touch, pressure, heat: _____

3. prevention of leakage from body tissues: _____

4. vasoconstriction or vasodilation: _____

5. production of sweat glands: _____

6. metabolism with sunlight: _____

7. physical barrier against toxins: _____

B. Choose any pair of noun-verb medical terms in the above WAD, and use each term in a sentence of medical documentation.   LO 15.1, 15.5

1. Noun: _____

_____

_____

2. Verb: _____

_____

_____

Dr. Echols learned that Mr. Andrews had driven extensively in Arizona while wearing a short-sleeved shirt. His left forearm and hand were exposed to sunlight through the untinted car window to his left. This was an important factor in causing his skin cancers, all of which responded to the appropriate treatment.

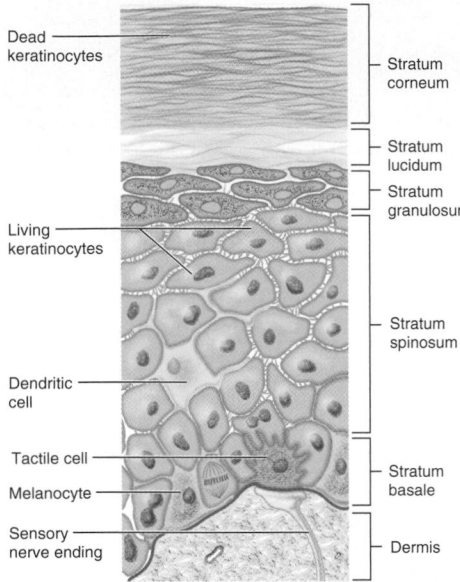

Dead keratinocytes

Stratum corneum

Stratum lucidum

Stratum granulosum

Living keratinocytes

Stratum spinosum

Dendritic cell

Tactile cell

Melanocyte

Stratum basale

Sensory nerve ending

Dermis

▲ **Figure 15.3** Epidermis.

Keynotes
___

- The stratum granulosum waterproofs the skin.
- The stratum spinosum holds the epidermis together.

LO 15.2 Structure of the Skin: Epidermis

The three lesions that Mr. Andrews had were present in the **epidermis**, the most superficial layer of his skin. This layer

- **Protects** underlying structures.
- **Withstands** the toxic pollution of modern life.
- **Sheds** its superficial cells and renews them continually throughout life.
- **Provides** a waterproof barrier.

The outer layer of the epidermis, the **stratum corneum** *(Figure 15.3)*, is a layer of compact, dead cells packed with **keratin**. These dead cells have no nuclei and are continually shed. **Dandruff** is clumps of these cells stuck together with **sebum**, oil from **sebaceous** glands. Keratin is a tough, scaly protein that is also the basis for hair and nails.

Underneath the stratum corneum on the thick skin of the palms, soles, fingers, and toes is a thin translucent layer of cells, the **stratum lucidum**. These cells are filled with a protein that becomes keratin and are called **keratinocytes**.

In the next layer down, the **stratum granulosum**, these keratinocytes produce a fatty mixture that covers the surface of the cells and waterproofs them. This waterproof barrier not only stops water from getting in and out but also cuts off the supply of nutrients to the keratinocytes above it and they die.

In the next layer, the **stratum spinosum**, the keratinocytes contain nuclei and are firmly attached to each other by numerous spines (hence "spinosum"). This enables the epidermis to be firm and strong.

The **squamous cell carcinoma** *(Figure 15.4)* that Mr. Andrews had on his hand arose from keratinocytes in the stratum spinosum in skin on the back of the hand, face, and ears, areas exposed to sunlight. It responds well to surgical removal but can **metastasize** (spread) to lymph glands if neglected.

The bottom layer of the epidermis, the **stratum basale**, is a single layer of cells that form the keratinocytes. This layer also contains **melanocytes**, which produce the dark pigment **melanin**, and **tactile** (touch) cells attached to sensory nerve fibers. The process by which keratinocytes migrate from this layer to the skin's surface, where they are shed as dead cells, takes about a month.

Mr. Andrews' **basal cell carcinoma** *(Figure 15.5)* began in the cells of the stratum basale and invaded the dermis and epidermis. It is the most common skin cancer and is also the least dangerous because it does not metastasize.

Malignant melanoma *(Figure 15.6)* is the least common skin cancer but is the most deadly. It arises from the melanocytes in the stratum basale. It metastasizes quickly and is fatal if neglected.

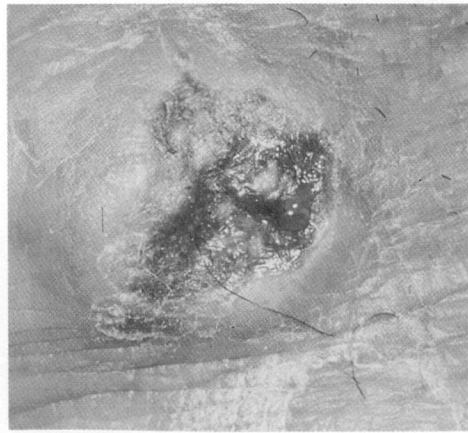

▲ **Figure 15.4** Squamous Cell Carcinoma.

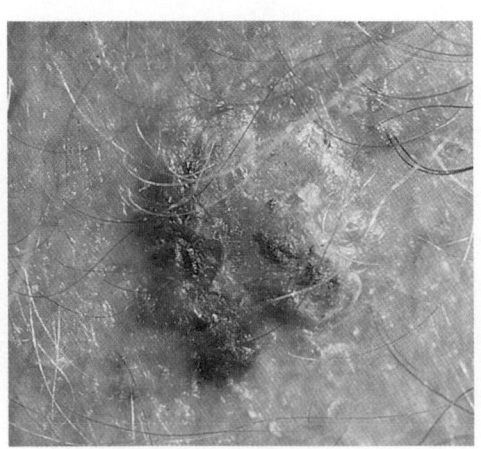

▲ **Figure 15.5** Basal Cell Carcinoma.

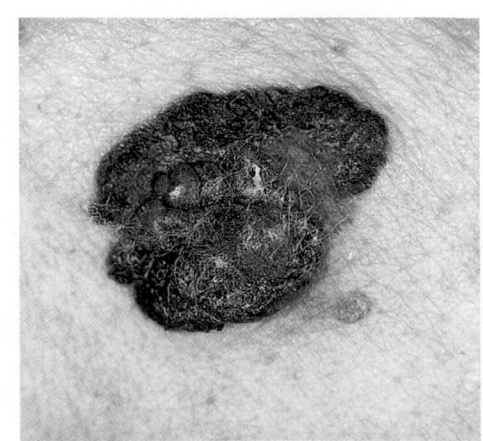

▲ **Figure 15.6** Malignant Melanoma.

WORD	PRONUNCIATION	ELEMENTS		DEFINITION
keratin	**KER**-ah-tin		**Greek** *keratin*	Protein found in the dead outer layer of skin and in nails and hair
keratinocyte	ke-**RAT**-in-oh-site	S/ R/CF	-cyte *cell* keratin/o- *keratin*	Cell producing a tough, horny protein (keratin) in the process of differentiating into the dead cells of the stratum corneum
macule (noun) macular (adj)	**MAK**-yul **MAK**-yu-lar		Latin *spot*	Small, flat spot or patch on the skin
malignancy (noun) malignant (adj)	mah-**LIG**-nan-see mah-**LIG**-nant	S/ R/ S/	-ancy *state of* malign- *harmful* -ant *pertaining to*	Tumor that invades surrounding tissues and metastasizes to distant organs Having the properties of being locally invasive and metastasizing
melanin melanocyte melanoma	**MEL**-ah-nin **MEL**-ann-oh-cyte **MEL**-ah-**NO**-mah	S/ R/CF S/	Greek *black* -cyte *cell* melan/o- *black* -oma *tumor, mass*	Black pigment found in skin, hair, retina Cell that synthesizes (produces) melanin Malignant neoplasm formed from cells that produce melanin
metastasis (noun) metastasize (verb) metastatic (adj)	meh-**TAS**-tah-sis meh-**TAS**-tah-size meh-tah-**STAT**-ik	P/ R/ S/ R/ S/	meta- *beyond, subsequent to* -stasis *stagnate, stay in one place* -ize *affect in a specific way* stat- *stationary* -ic *pertaining to*	Spread of a disease from one part of the body to another To spread to distant parts. Pertaining to the character of cells that can metastasize.
sebaceous glands sebum	se-**BAY**-shus **GLANZ** **SEE**-bum	S/ R/CF	-us *pertaining to* sebace/o- *wax* Latin *tallow*	Glands in the dermis that open into hair follicles and secrete an oily fluid called sebum Waxy secretion of the sebaceous glands
stratum basale strata (pl)	**STRAH**-tum ba-**SAL**-eh	S/ R/ R/	-um *tissue* strat- *layer* basal/e *deepest part*	Deepest layer of the epidermis, from which the other cells originate and migrate
tactile	**TAK**-tile		Latin *to touch*	Relating to touch

Exercises

A. Apply the correct rule for plurals in question 2, and form the plural of the term stratum. *Demonstrate that you know the difference in terms by using each form in a sentence.*   **LO 15.2, 15.5**

1. Singular: *stratum*

   Sentence:

   _____

2. Plural: _____

   Sentence:

   _____

B. Medical terms that are nouns can also have an adjectival form, as seen in macule **and** macular. *Use the correct form of each of these terms in the following sentences.*   **LO 15.2, 15.5**

1. The report from pathology diagnosed the lesion as a _____.

2. The _____ tissue was removed in the biopsy.

C. Medical terms that are nouns can also have an adjectival form, as seen in *metastasis* **and** *metastatic*. *Use the correct form of each of these terms in the following sentences.*   **LO 15.2, 15.5**

1. The chest x-ray revealed a large _____ to the right lung.

2. Her _____ breast cancer had spread to her lung.

Abbreviations	
IM	intramuscular
SC	subcutaneous
TB	tuberculosis

LO 15.2 Structure of the Skin: Dermis

Figure 15.7 shows that the **dermis** is a much thicker connective tissue layer than the epidermis. It consists mostly of **collagen**, with fibers and fibroblasts. It is well supplied with blood vessels and nerves and contains the other **skin organs**: **sweat glands**, **sebaceous glands**, **hair follicles**, and **nail roots**. The boundary between the dermis and the epidermis is distinct and irregular.

LO 15.2 Structure of the Skin: Hypodermis

The hypodermis, the layer beneath the dermis, is the site of **subcutaneous** fat (**adipose** tissue). It is also called the **subcutaneous tissue layer**.

LO 15.3 Clinical Applications

Giving Injections

Another important reason you should be able to identify the layers of the skin is to understand the different sites for giving injections. The three types of injection are

- **Intradermal** *(Figure 15.8)*. A short, thin needle is introduced into the dermis between the stratum corneum and the stratum basale. Injected into this site, the medication raises a small **wheal**. This site is used for allergy testing or a **tuberculosis (TB)** test.
- **Subcutaneous (SC)** *(Figure 15.8)*. A longer needle pierces the epidermis and dermis to reach the hypodermis, or subcutaneous layer. This site is used for insulin injections.
- **Intramuscular (IM)** *(Figure 15.8)*. A long needle pierces the epidermis, dermis, and subcutaneous layer into the muscles underneath. Some antibiotics can be given by this route.

Transdermal Applications

Some medications can be administered through the skin by an adhesive **transdermal** patch that is applied to the skin. In the patch, a small reservoir contains medication that leaves the reservoir at a known rate through a **semipermeable membrane**. The medication diffuses across the epidermis and enters the blood vessels in the dermis. Medications for motion sickness and cardiac problems, testosterone, birth control hormones, and the chemical nicotine are administered by transdermal patches.

▲ **Figure 15.7** **Dermis and Its Organs.**

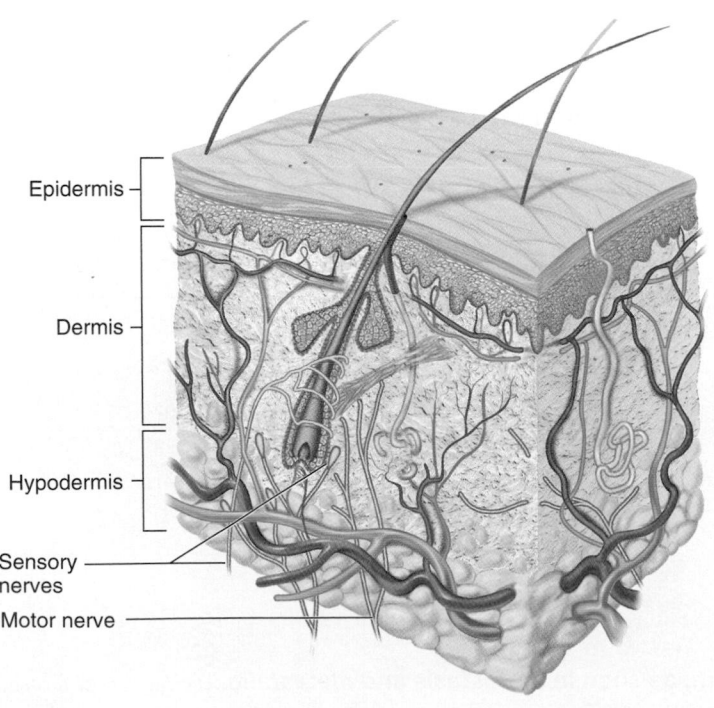

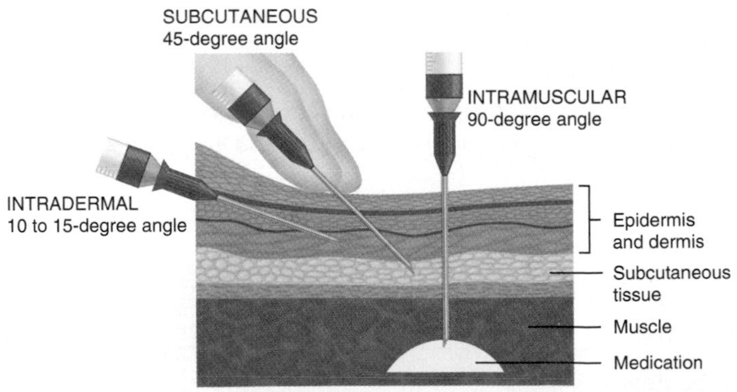

▲ **Figure 15.8** **Intradermal, Subcutaneous, and Intramuscular Injection.**

WORD	PRONUNCIATION	ELEMENTS		DEFINITION
adipose	**ADD**-i-pose	S/ R/	-ose *condition* **adip-** *fat*	Containing fat
collagen	**KOL**-ah-jen	S/ R/	gen *producing* **coll/a-** *glue*	Major protein of connective tissue, cartilage, and bone
follicle	**FOLL**-ih-kull		Latin *small sac*	Spherical mass of cells containing a cavity or a small cul-de-sac, such as a hair follicle
hypodermis	high-poh-**DER**-miss	P/ R/	hypo- *below* -dermis *skin*	Tissue layer below the dermis
hypodermic (adj)	high-poh-**DER**-mik	S/ R/	-ic *pertaining to* -derm *skin*	Beneath the skin
intradermal	in-trah-**DER**-mal	S/ P/ R/	-al *pertaining to* intra- *within* -derm- *skin*	Within the dermis
intramuscular	in-trah-**MUSS**-kew-lar	S/ P/ R/	-ar *pertaining to* intra- *within* -muscul- *muscle*	Within the muscle
papilla papillae (pl) papilloma	pah-**PILL**-ah pah-**PILL**-ee pap-ih-**LOH**-mah	S/ R/CF	Latin *small pimple* -oma *tumor, mass* **papill/o-** *pimple*	Any small projection Benign projection of epithelial cells
semipermeable membrane	sem-ee-**PER**-me-ah-bull **MEM**-brain	S/ P/ R/CF R/	-able *capable of* semi- *half* -perm/e- *pass through* membrane *cover, skin*	A membrane that allows only certain substances to pass through it
subcutaneous hypodermic (syn)	sub-kew-**TAY**-nee-us	S/ P/ R/CF	-ous *pertaining to* sub- *below* -cutan/e- *skin*	Below the skin
transdermal	trans-**DER**-mal	S/ P/ R/	-al *pertaining to* trans- *across, through* -derm- *skin*	Going across or through the skin
wheal hives (syn)	WHEEL		Old English *wheal*	Small, itchy swelling of the skin. Wheals raised by an injection do not itch

Exercises

A. The following definitions represent medical terms found in the above WAD. *Find the missing elements and build the terms. Fill in the blanks.* **LO 15.2, 15.3, 15.5**

1. pertaining to below the skin: _____/derm/_____

2. containing fat: _____/adip/_____

3. pertaining to within muscle: _____/_____/ar

4. pertaining to below the skin: _____/cutane/_____

5. pertaining to going across the skin: trans/_____/_____

Study Hint

Whenever there are two or more terms with the same meaning, you must know all of them.

B. Answer the following questions regarding terms in the above WAD. *Fill in the blanks.* **LO 15.2, 15.3, 15.5**

1. What is another term for hives? _____

2. What is the difference between *transdermal* and *intradermal*?

    Transdermal: _____

    Intradermal: _____

3. What term in the WAD has an element meaning *fat*? _____

4. Is a papilloma benign or malignant? _____

5. The term *folllicle* can be associated with what part of the body? _____

LESSON OBJECTIVES

This lesson will enable you to use correct medical terminology to:

15.2.1 Describe common disorders of the skin.

15.2.2 Identify the different types of infections of the skin.

15.2.3 Define the types of pharmacologic agents used in the treatment of skin disorders.

Case Report 15.2

Fulwood Medical Center

Mrs. Rose McGinnis, a 72-year-old widow, was in a nursing home for the past 6 months. She was unable to get out of bed since surgery to repair a broken hip. She was depressed and difficult to feed and nurse. Two months ago, she developed **decubitus ulcers** over her buttocks and left heel. The ulcer over her buttocks became infected with a methicillin-resistant *Staphylococcus aureus* (MRSA). Staphylococcal septicemia ensued, and she died.

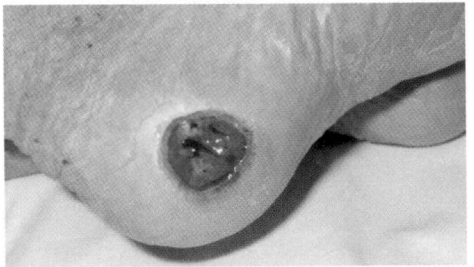

▲ **Figure 15.9** Decubitus Ulcer on Heel.

LO 15.4 Disorders of the Skin

When a patient lies in one position for a long period, the pressure between the bed and bony body projections, like the lower spine or heel, cuts off the blood supply to the skin and **decubitus (pressure) ulcers** can appear *(Figure 15.9)*. The protective function of the skin is broken, and germs can enter the body.

Other major factors in the breakdown of Rose's skin were that it was thin and dry because of aging. Also, her poor nutritional status had depleted the fatty protective layer in the hypodermis under the skin.

Case Report 15.3

Fulwood Medical Center

Ms. Cheryl Fox is a 37-year-old nursing assistant working in a surgical unit in Fulwood Medical Center. Recently her fingers became red and itchy, with occasional **vesicles**. She also noticed irritation and swelling of her earlobes and a generalized **pruritus**. Over the weekends, both the itching and the rash on her hands worsened. A patch test by her dermatologist showed her to be **allergic** to nickel in rings that she wore on both hands and in her earrings. She wore these only on weekends and not during her workdays.

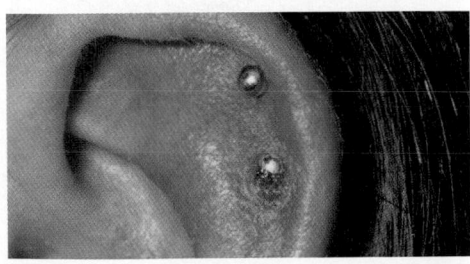

▲ **Figure 15.10** Dermatitis of Ear due to Nickel Sensitivity.

Abbreviation

MRSA	methicillin-resistant *Staphylococcus aureus*

Ms. Fox had a **dermatitis** *(Figure 15.10)*, resulting from direct exposure to an irritating agent. In her case, it was not just a reaction to an irritant. Her form of **atopic (allergic) dermatitis** develops when the body becomes sensitive to an **allergen** such as **latex**, nickel in jewelry, or poison ivy. This whole-body involvement was shown by her systemic symptoms of pruritus distant from the local irritant site. She has stopped wearing the rings and earrings at any time.

Eczema is a general term used for inflamed, itchy skin conditions. When the itchy skin is scratched, it becomes **excoriated** and produces the dry, red, scaly patches characteristic of eczema. The **atopic** dermatitis that Ms. Fox developed to nickel is a common form of eczema.

Sunlight can also be an irritant to the skin, not only by burning it but by leading to cancer when there is excessive exposure, as it did for Mr. Andrews.

Any congenital lesion of the skin, including various types of birthmarks and all **moles**, is referred to as a **nevus**.

WORD	PRONUNCIATION	ELEMENTS		DEFINITION
allergen allergenic (adj) allergy allergic (adj)	**AL**-er-jen al-er-**JEN**-ik **AL**-er-jee ah-**LER**-jik	S/ R/	**-gen** *producing* **allerg-** *allergy* Greek *other work*	Substance producing a hypersensitivity (allergic) reaction Hypersensitivity to an allergen Pertaining to or suffering from an allergy.
atopy atopic (adj)	**AY**-toh-pee ay-**TOP**-ik		Greek *strangeness*	State of hypersensitivity to an allergen; allergic
decubitus ulcer	de-**KYU**-bit-us **UL**-ser	P/ R/ R/	**de-** *from* **-cubitus** *lying down* **ulcer** *sore*	Sore caused by lying down for long periods of time
dermatitis	der-mah-**TYE**-tis	S/ R/	**-itis** *inflammation* **dermat-** *skin*	Inflammation of the skin
eczema eczematous (adj)	**EK**-zeh-mah **EK**-zem-ah-tus	 S/ R/	Greek *to boil or ferment* **-tous** *pertaining to* **eczema-** *eczema*	Inflammatory skin disease often with a serous discharge Pertaining to or resembling eczema
excoriate	eks-**KOR**-ee-ate	S/ P/ R/	**-ate** *composed of,* *pertaining to* **ex-** *away from, out of* **-cori-** *skin*	To scratch
excoriation (noun)	eks-**KOR**-ee-**AY**-shun	S/	**-ation** *process*	Scratch mark
latex	**LAY**-tecks		Latin *liquid*	Manufactured from the milky liquid in rubber plants; used for gloves in patient care
mole	MOLE		Latin *spot*	Benign localized area of melanin-producing cells
nevus nevi (pl)	**NEE**-vus **NEE**-vie		Latin *mole, birthmark*	Congenital or acquired lesion of the skin
pruritus pruritic (adj)	proo-**RYE**-tus proo-**RIT**-ik		Latin *to itch*	Itching Itchy
serous	**SEER**-us		Latin *serum*	Thicker and less transparent than water
vesicle	**VES**-ih-kull		Latin *small sac*	Small sac containing liquid, for example, a blister

Exercises

A. Medical terms can have small differences that make them entirely new words. *Underline the root of these terms, which stays the same; then focus on how they are different. Insert the correct term in the blanks.* **LO 15.4, 15.5, 15.6**

allergen   allergenic   allergy   allergic

1. After many _____ tests, it was determined that she was _____ to mold.

2. There were too many _____ substances in the carpet, and it was removed from the room.

3. Dust mites, peanuts, and pollen are _____.

B. One of the following terms is a noun (person, place, or thing), and the other term is a verb (action). *Identify the noun and verb; then use each term in a sentence.* **LO 15.5**

1. Excoriate   Noun or verb: _____

2. Sentence: _____

3. Excoriation   Noun or verb: _____

4. Sentence: _____

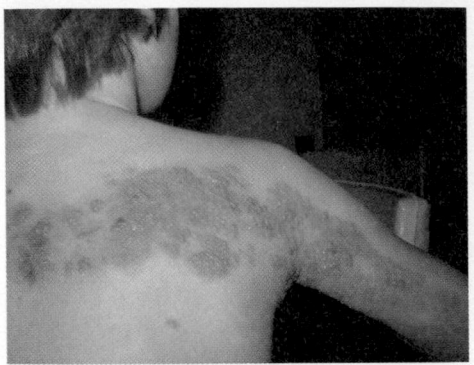

▲ **Figure 15.11**   Shingles.

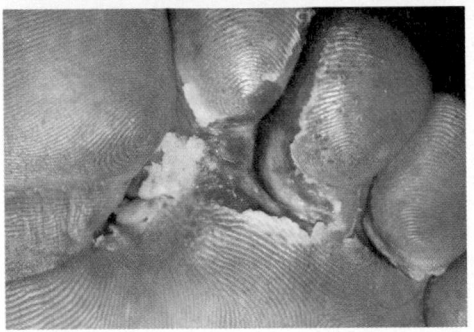

▲ **Figure 15.12**   Tinea Pedis between Toes.

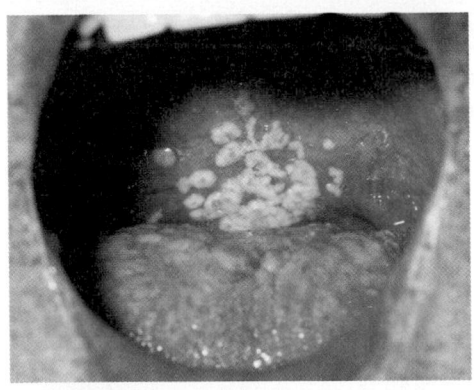

▲ **Figure 15.13**   Oral Thrush.

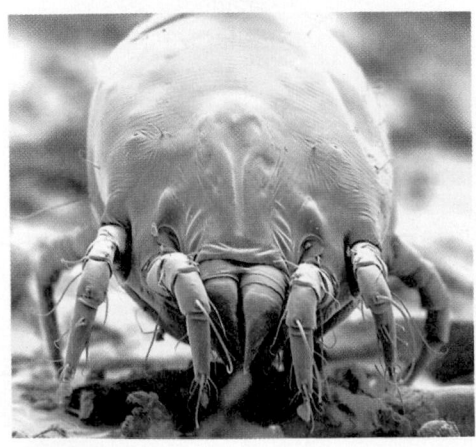

▲ **Figure 15.14**   House Dust Mite.

LO 15.4 Infections of the Skin

The skin is also susceptible to the many different types of infections. The following are examples.

Viral Infections

Warts (verrucas) are caused by the human papillomavirus invading the epidermis and causing the outer epidermal cells to produce a roughened projection from the skin surface. Human papillomavirus is discussed extensively in *Chapter 8.*

Varicella-zoster virus causes **chickenpox** in unvaccinated people, forming macules, papules, and vesicles. The virus can then remain dormant in the peripheral nerves for decades before erupting as the painful vesicles of **herpes zoster (shingles)** *(Figure 15.11).*

Fungal Infections

Tinea is a general term for a group of related skin infections caused by different species of fungi. The fungi live on, and are strictly confined to the nonliving stratum corneum and its derivatives, hair and nails, where keratin provides their food. The different types of tinea take their name from the location of the infection.

Tinea pedis, athlete's foot, causes itching, redness, and peeling of the foot, particularly between the toes *(Figure 15.12).* **Tinea capitis** describes infection of the scalp (ringworm); **tinea corporis** is the name for infections of the body. **Tinea cruris** ("jock itch") is the name for infections of the groin. The fungus spreads from animals, from the soil, and by direct contact with infected individuals. **Tinea versicolor** is characterized by brown and white patches on the trunk.

A yeastlike fungus, *Candida,* can produce recurrent infections of the skin, nails, and mucous membranes. The first sign can be a recurrent diaper rash or thrush in infants. Older children can show recurrent or persistent lesions on the scalp. In adults, chronic **candidiasis** can affect the mouth (**thrush**) *(Figure 15.13)* and vagina, as well as the skin. It can also be associated with diseases of the immune system *(see Chapter 12).*

Parasitic Infestations

A **parasite** is an organism that lives in contact with and feeds off another organism (host). This process is called an **infestation**. It is different from an **infection**.

Lice are small, wingless, blood-sucking parasites that produce the disease **pediculosis** by attaching their eggs (nits) to hair and clothing *(Table 15.1).*

Scabies ("itch mites") produce an intense, itching rash, often in the genital area, waist, breast, and armpits. The mites live and lay eggs under the skin.

The skin normally sheds its cells. These tiny specks form some of the dust on our furniture, floors, and carpets. The house **dust mite** *(Figure 15.14)* thrives on the keratin of these cells and lives well on carpets, upholstery, pillows, and mattresses. Many people are allergic to the inhaled feces of these parasites.

Bacterial Infections

Staphylococcus aureus (commonly called *staph*) is the most common bacterium to invade the skin and is the cause of pimples, boils, **carbuncles**, and **impetigo**. It can infect hair follicles and the surrounding tissues to produce **furuncles** and carbuncles. Staph can cause a **cellulitis** of the epidermis and dermis.

Necrotizing fasciitis is caused when some strains of staph and strep produce enzymes that are very toxic and digest the connective tissues and spread into muscle layers.

Table 15.1 Pediculosis

Louse (lice, pl)	Attachment of Eggs	Disease
Pediculus capitis	Hair of scalp	Pediculosis capitis
Phthirus pubis (crab-shaped)	Pubic hair	Pediculosis cruris (crabs)
Pediculus humanus	Clothing, body hair	Pediculosis corporis

WORD	PRONUNCIATION	ELEMENTS		DEFINITION
Candida	**KAN**-did-ah		Latin *dazzling white*	A yeastlike fungus
candidiasis thrush	can-dih-**DIE**-ah-sis THRUSH	S/ R/	**-iasis** *condition, state of* **candid-** *Candida*	Infection with the yeastlike fungus *Candida* Infection with *Candida albicans*
carbuncle	**KAR**-bunk-ul		Latin *carbuncle*	Infection composed of many furuncles in a small area, often on the back of the neck
cellulitis	sell-you-**LIE**-tis	S/ R/	**-itis** *inflammation* **cellul-** *small cell*	Infection of subcutaneous connective tissue
furuncle	**FU**-rung-kel		Latin *a boil*	An infected hair follicle that spreads into the tissues around the follicle
herpes zoster shingles (syn)	**HER**-pees **ZOS**-ter		**herpes** *to creep or spread* **zoster** *belt, girdle*	Painful eruption of vesicles that follows a dermatome or nerve root on one side of the body
impetigo	im-peh-**TIE**-go		Latin *scabby eruption*	Infection of the skin that produces thick, yellow crusts
infection	in-**FEK**-shun	S/ R/	**-ion** *process* **infect-** *tainted, internal invasion*	Invasion of the body by disease-producing microorganisms
infestation	in-fes-**TAY**-shun	S/ R/	**-ation** *process* **infest-** *invade*	Act of being invaded on the skin by a troublesome other species, such as a parasite
louse lice (pl)	LOWSE LICE		Old English *louse*	Parasitic insect
necrotizing fasciitis	neh-kroh-**TIZE**-ing fash-eh-**EYE**-tis	S/ R/CF S/ S/ R/CF	**-ing** *quality of* **necr/o-** *death* **-tiz-** *pertaining to* **-itis** *inflammation* **fasc/i** – *fascia*	Inflammation of fascia, producing death of the tissue
parasite	**PAR**-ah-site		Greek *guest*	An organism that attaches itself to, lives on or in, and derives its nutrition from another species
pediculosis	peh-dick-you-**LOH**-sis	S/ R/	**-osis** *condition* **pedicul-** *louse*	An infestation with lice
scabies	**SKAY**-bees		Latin *to scratch*	Skin disease produced by mites
tinea	**TIN**-ee-ah		Latin *worm*	General term for a group of related skin infections caused by different species of fungi
verruca	ver-**ROO**-cah		Latin *wart*	Wart caused by a virus

Exercises

A. Make the WADs work for you. *As you read each WAD, notice any elements that may have the same meaning; highlight them, or keep a separate list in the back of your book. The preceding WAD contains two pairs of elements that each have the same meaning. Find the elements, and define them.*
LO 15.4, 15.5

1. _____ and _____ both mean _____.

2. _____ and _____ both mean _____.

B. Match the correct Latin or Greek term to its medical meaning. *Circle the best answer.*   **LO 15.4, 15.5**

1. impetigo: carbuncle   boil   scabby eruption

2. verruca: ulcer   furuncle   wart

3. vesicle: carbuncle   blister   boil

4. scabies: to bleed   to cut   to scratch

LO 15.4 Diseases of the Skin

Collagen Diseases

Collagen, a fibrous protein, accounts for 30% of total body protein. Therefore, collagen diseases can have a dramatic effect all over the body. Collagen diseases, **autoimmune** or otherwise, attack collagen or other components of connective tissue.

Systemic lupus erythematosus (SLE), an autoimmune disease, occurs most commonly in women and produces characteristic skin lesions. A butterfly-shaped red rash on both cheeks joined across the bridge of the nose is commonly seen *(Figure 15.15)*. It is associated with fever, fatigue, joint pains, and multiple internal organ involvement.

Rosacea produces a facial rash similar to that of SLE, and the underlying capillaries become enlarged and show through the skin. It is thought to be worsened by alcohol and spicy food. Its etiology is unknown. It has no **systemic** complications.

Scleroderma is a chronic, persistent autoimmune disease, occurring more often in women and characterized by hardening and shrinking of the skin that makes it feel leathery *(Figure 15.16)*. Joints show swelling, pain, and stiffness. Internal organs such as the heart, lungs, kidneys, and digestive tract can be involved in a similar process. The etiology is unknown, and there is no effective treatment.

Other Skin Diseases

Psoriasis *(Figure 15.17)* is marked by itchy, flaky, red patches of skin of various sizes covered with white or silvery scales. It appears most commonly on the scalp, elbows, and knees. Its cause is unknown.

Vitiligo produces pale, irregular patches of skin. It is thought to have an auto-immune etiology.

> ### Study Hint
> There are many different suffixes that mean *pertaining to.* Some have been introduced in the next WAD. Start keeping a list of them in the back of your book, with an example of each in a medical term.

Skin Manifestations of Internal Disease

Signs of the presence of cancer inside the body are often shown by skin lesions, even before the cancer has produced **symptoms** or been diagnosed.

Dermatomyositis *(Figure 15.18)* is often associated with ovarian cancer, which can appear within 4 to 5 years after the skin disease is diagnosed.

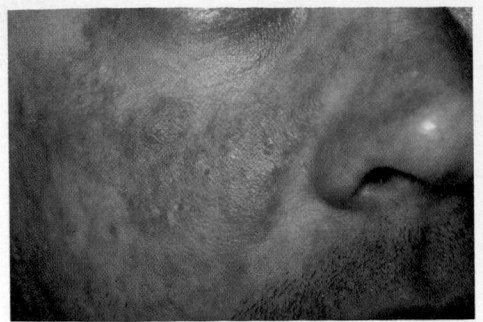

▲ **Figure 15.15**   Systemic Lupus Erythematosus.

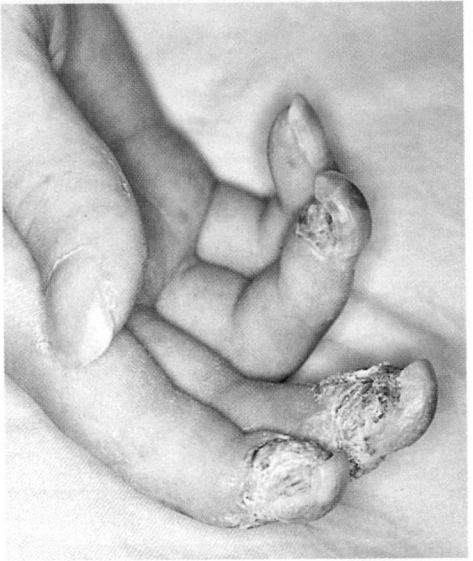

▲ **Figure 15.16**   Scleroderma.

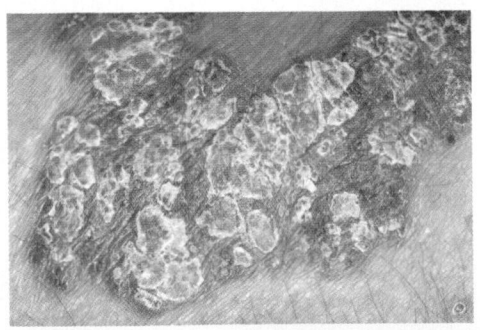

▲ **Figure 15.17**   Psoriasis.

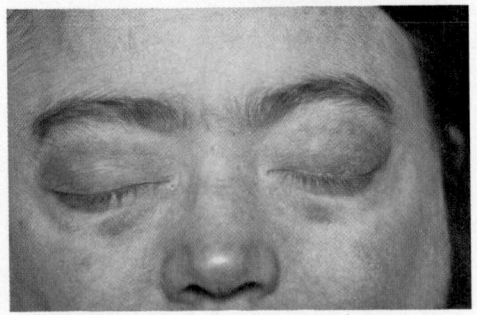

▲ **Figure 15.18**   Periorbital Rash of Dermatomyositis.

LO 15.7 Pharmacology

No matter what the cause of skin lesions, a wide range of **topical pharmacologic agents** of different types can be used in their treatment, either to relieve symptoms or to cure the disease.

- **Antipruritics**—topical lotions, ointments, creams, or sprays that relieve itching. **Corticosteroids** such as hydrocortisone are most frequently used.

- **Antibacterials**—topical agents that eliminate the bacteria that cause epidermal infections. The antibiotic neomycin is frequently used in ointments for this purpose.

- **Antifungals**—topical agents that eliminate or inhibit the growth of fungi. Lamisil is used as a cream, gel, or spray.

- **Parasiticides**—topical agents that kill parasites living on the skin. Lindane 1% is in a lotion or shampoo used to kill lice.

- **Keratolytics**—topical agents that peel the stratum corneum away from the other epidermal layers. Salicylic acid is used for this purpose.

- **Anesthetics**—topical agents that relieve pain or itching on the skin's surface. Benzocaine is used for this purpose.

- **Retinoids**—derivatives of **retinoic acid** that are used in the treatment of acne.

WORD	PRONUNCIATION	ELEMENTS		DEFINITION
anesthetic anesthesia (noun)	an-es-**THET**-ic an-es-**THEE**-zee-ah	S/ P/ R/	-ic *pertaining to* an- *without* -esthet- *sensation*	Substance that takes away feeling and pain Complete loss of sensation

antipruritic
  pruritus (noun)
  pruritic (adj)
	AN-tee-pru-**RIT**-ik
	proo-**RYE**-tus
	proo-**RIT**-ik
		S/
		P/
		R/
			-ic *pertaining to*
			anti- *against*
			-prurit- *itch*
				Medication against itching
				Itching
				Itchy

corticosteroid	**KOR**-tih-koh-**STEHR**-oyd	S/ R/CF R/	-oid *resembling* cortic/o- *cortisone* ster- *steroid*	A hormone produced by the adrenal cortex
dermatomyositis	**DER**-mah-toe-**MY**-oh-site-is	S/ R/CF R/	-itis *inflammation* dermat/o- *skin* -myos- *muscle*	Inflammation of the skin and muscles
pharmacology pharmacologic (adj) pharmacist pharmacy	far-mah-**KOLL**-oh-jee far-mah-ko-**LOJ**-ik **FAR**-mah-sist **FAR**-mah-see	S/ R/CF S/	-logy *study of* pharmac/o- *drug* -ist *specialist*	Science of the preparation, uses, and effects of drugs Person licensed by the state to prepare and dispense drugs Facility licensed to prepare and dispense drugs
psoriasis	so-**RYE**-ah-sis		Greek *the itch*	Rash characterized by reddish, silver-scaled patches
retinoid	**RET**-ih-noyd		Derived from retinoic acid	A class of keratolytic agents
rosacea	roh-**ZAY**-she-ah		Latin *rosy*	Persistent erythematous rash of the central face
scleroderma	sklair-oh-**DERM**-ah	S/ R/CF	-derma *skin* scler/o- *hard*	Thickening and hardening of the skin due to new collagen formation
sign (objective) symptom (subjective) symptomatic (adj)	SINE **SIMP**-tum simp-toe-**MAT**-ik	 S/ R/	Latin *mark* Greek *sign* -ic *pertaining to* symptomat- *symptoms*	Physical evidence of a disease process Departure from normal health experienced by the patient Pertaining to the symptoms of a disease
systemic lupus erythematosus	sis-**TEM**-ik **LOO**-pus er-ih-**THEE**-mah-toe-sus	S/ R/ S/ R/	-ic *pertaining to* system- *body system* lupus *wolf* -osus *condition* erythemat- *redness*	Inflammatory connective tissue disease affecting the whole body
topical	**TOP**-ih-kal	S/ R/	-al *pertaining to* topic- *local*	Medication applied to the skin to obtain a local effect
vitiligo	vit-ill-**EYE**-go		Latin *skin blemish*	Nonpigmented white patches on otherwise normal skin

Exercises

A. Building medical terms and taking them apart force you to focus on the elements they contain. *Understanding elements is the key to increasing your medical vocabulary. Deconstruct the following terms to increase your knowledge of their elements. Fill in the chart.* **LO 15.4, 15.5, 15.7**

Medical Term	Meaning of Prefix	Meaning of Root/Combining Form	Meaning of Suffix
anesthetic	1.	2.	3.
antipruritic	4.	5.	6.
corticosteroid	7.	8.	9.
pharmacology	10.	11.	12.
scleroderma	13.	14.	15.

LESSON OBJECTIVES

Hair follicles and their associated sebaceous glands, sweat glands, and nails are organs located in your skin. They each have specific anatomical and physiologic characteristics. You must understand their roles in the different functions of the skin and in diseases that affect the skin. This lesson will enable you to use correct medical terminology to:

15.3.1 Name the associated skin organs.

15.3.2 Identify the anatomy and physiology of the associated skin organs.

15.3.3 Match the structures of the different organs to their functions.

15.3.4 Describe disorders affecting the associated skin organs.

15.3.5 Explain the etiology of disorders affecting the associated skin organs.

You are

. . . a medical assistant working with Lenore Echols, MD, a dermatologist in Fulwood Medical Center.

Your patient is

. . . Wayne Winter, an 18-year-old man, who has been accepted to college in the fall.

Case Report 15.4

He has had acne since the age of 15 and has tried numerous over-the-counter products. Retinoic acid has also been unsuccessful. He has numerous **comedones**, **papules**, **pustules**, and scars on his face and forehead with severe **cystic** lesions and scars on his back. His social life is nonexistent, and he is teased by his peers. He wishes to change all this before he gets to college.

Your role is to document his care and explain to him how to use the medications Dr. Echols prescribes, what their effects will be, and his prognosis.

LO 15.8 Hair Follicles and Sebaceous Glands

Each hair follicle has a **sebaceous gland** opening into it *(Figure 15.19)*. The gland secretes into the follicle a mixture of oily, acidic **sebum** and broken-down cells from the base of the gland.

Around puberty, **androgens** are thought to trigger excessive production of sebum from the glands, which then brings excessive numbers of broken-down cells toward the skin surface. This blocks the follicle, forming a **comedo** (whitehead or blackhead). Comedones can stay closed, leading to **papules**, or can **rupture**, allowing bacteria to get in and produce **pustules**. These are the classic signs of **acne**, which is said to affect, in different degrees, about 85% of people between 12 and 25 years *(Figure 15.20)*. For many acne patients, treatment is difficult during puberty and the face can be scarred.

A different skin problem involving the sebaceous glands is **seborrheic dermatitis**. The glands are thought to be inflamed and to produce a different sebum. The skin around the face and scalp is reddened and covered with yellow, greasy scales. In infants, this condition is called cradle cap. Seborrheic dermatitis of the scalp produces **dandruff**.

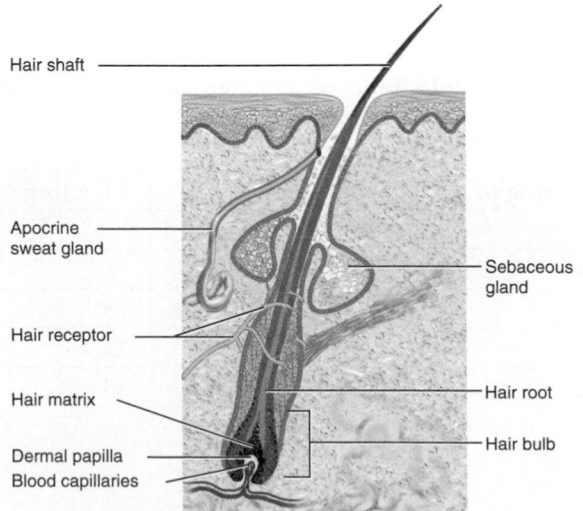

Hair shaft

Apocrine sweat gland

Hair receptor

Hair matrix

Dermal papilla
Blood capillaries

Sebaceous gland

Hair root

Hair bulb

▲ **Figure 15.19** Hair Follicle and Sebaceous Gland.

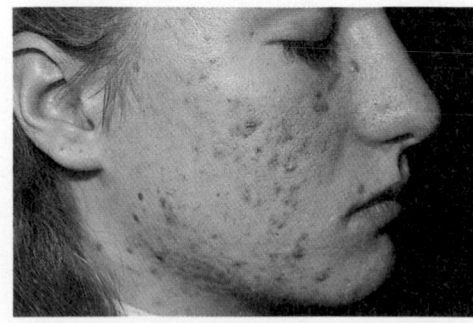

▲ **Figure 15.20** Acne.

WORD	PRONUNCIATION	ELEMENTS		DEFINITION
acne	**AK**-nee		Greek *point*	Inflammatory disease of sebaceous glands and hair follicles
androgen	**AN**-droh-jen	S/ R/CF	-gen *to produce* andr/o- *male*	Hormone that promotes masculine characteristics
comedo comedones (pl)	**KOM**-ee-doh		Latin *eat up*	A whitehead or blackhead caused by too much sebum and too many keratin cells blocking the hair follicle
cyst cystic (adj)	SIST **SIS**-tik	S/ R/	Greek *sac, bladder* -ic *pertaining to* cyst- *cyst, bladder*	An abnormal, fluid-containing sac Relating to a cyst
dandruff	**DAN**-druff		Old English *scurf*	Seborrheic scales from the scalp
papule	**PAP**-yul		Latin *pimple*	Small, circumscribed elevation on the skin
pustule	**PUS**-tyul		Latin *pustule*	Small protuberance on the skin that contains pus
rupture	**RUP**-tyur		Latin *break*	Break or tear of any organ or body part
sebum	**SEE**-bum		Latin *wax*	Waxy secretion of the sebaceous glands
seborrhea	seb-oh-**REE**-ah	S/ R/CF	-rrhea *flow* seb/o- *sebum*	Excessive amount of sebum
seborrheic (adj)	seb-oh-**REE**-ik	S/	-ic *pertaining to*	Pertaining to seborrhea

Exercises

A. Make an extra effort to learn the correct spelling of the terms seborrhea and seborrheic. *The "rrh" combination occurs in other medical terms as well—diarrhea, hemorrhage, menorrhagia, herniorrhaphy, etc. Be alert to this combination of letters in terms. You can be sure these terms will appear on a test. Match the Greek or Latin term to its medical meaning.* **LO 15.5, 15.8**

_____ 1. sebum   **a.** point

_____ 2. cyst   **b.** containing pus

_____ 3. pustule   **c.** whitehead, blackhead

_____ 4. acne   **d.** wax

_____ 5. comedo   **e.** sac, bladder

_____ 6. dandruff   **f.** hormone that promotes masculine characteristics

_____ 7. rupture   **g.** excessive amount of sebum

_____ 8. androgen   **h.** break or tear of any organ or part

_____ 9. papule   **i.** seborrheic scales from the scalp

_____ 10. seborrhea   **j.** small, circumscribed elevation of the skin

Study Hint

An easy way to remember the meaning of the word **pustule** is the word **pus**. A pustule is a small protuberance on the skin that contains pus.

B. Read Case Report 15.4 on the opposite page, and circle the best answer for each statement. **LO 15.7, 15.8, 15.9**

1. A *pustule* is filled with pus.   T   F

2. *Acne* is a degenerative disease of the skin.   T   F

3. A *cystic lesion* is filled with hard, packed cells.   T   F

4. An "over-the-counter" product is available without a prescription.   T   F

5. A *comedo* can be either a whitehead or a blackhead.   T   F

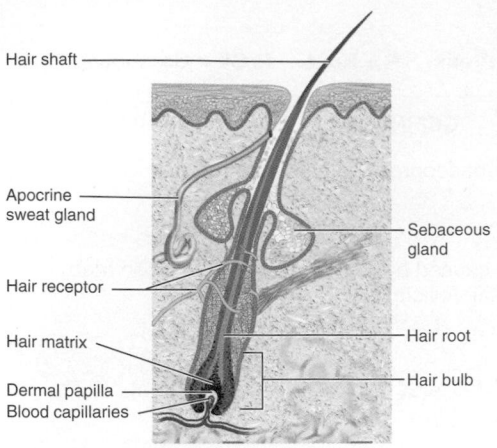

Hair shaft

Apocrine sweat gland

Hair receptor

Hair matrix

Dermal papilla
Blood capillaries

Sebaceous gland

Hair root

Hair bulb

▲ **Figure 15.21** **Hair Follicle.**

Keynotes

- Genes, hormones, and pigment determine hair characteristics.
- Body hair has no specific function.

LO 15.8, 15.9 Accessory Skin Organs

Hair

Each hair, no matter where it is on your body or scalp, originates from epidermal cells at the base (matrix) of a hair follicle. As these cells divide and grow, they push older cells upward away from the source of nutrition in the hair papilla *(Figure 15.21)*. The cells become keratinized and die. They rest for a while; and when a new hair is formed, the old, dead hair is pushed out and drops off.

In cross-section, each hair has three layers *(Figure 15.22a)*. Its core, the **medulla**, is composed of loosely arranged cells containing a flexible keratin. The **cortex** is composed of densely packed cells with a harder keratin that gives hair its stiffness. These cells also contain pigment. The outer **cuticle** is a single layer of scaly, dead keratin cells.

Straight hair is round in cross-section *(Figure 15.22a and b)*. Curly hair is oval *(Figure 15.22c and d)*. Two pigments derived from **melanin** (**eumelanin** and **pheomelanin**) give hair its natural color. Black and dark brown hair has a lot of a dark form of the pigment eumelanin in the cells of the cortex *(Figure 15.22b)*. Blonde hair has little of this dark pigment but a moderate amount of the lighter form of pheomelanin *(Figure 15.22a)*. Red hair has a lot of the lighter pigment *(Figure 15.22c)*. White or gray hair has little pigment *(Figure 15.22d)*.

A problem with the scalp hair follicle occurs in men when a combination of genetic influence and excess testosterone produces "top of the head" baldness. In most people, aging causes **alopecia**, thinning of the hair and baldness as the follicles shrink and produce thin, wispy hairs.

Scalp hair is thick enough to retain heat. Body hair has no specific function in our present evolution because, in most people, it is too thin to retain heat. Beard, pubic, and **axillary** (armpit) hair reflect sexual maturity. Stronger hairs guard the nostrils and ears to prevent foreign particles from entering. Similarly, eyelashes protect the eyes, and eyebrows help keep perspiration from running into the eyes.

Melanin is in the black skin melanocytes of dark-skinned people and is the pigment generated by sunbathing and tanning. The absence of melanin produces **albinism**.

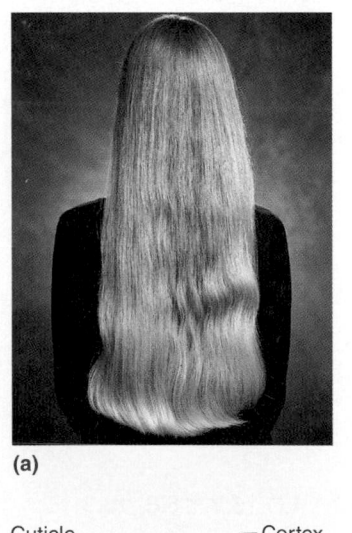
(a)

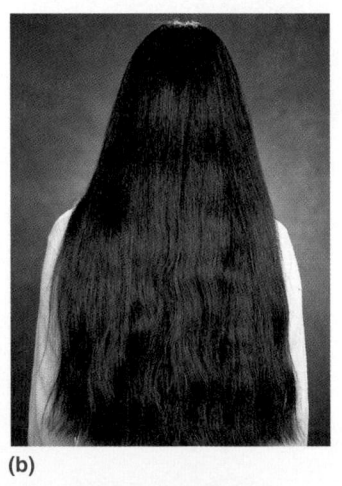
(b)

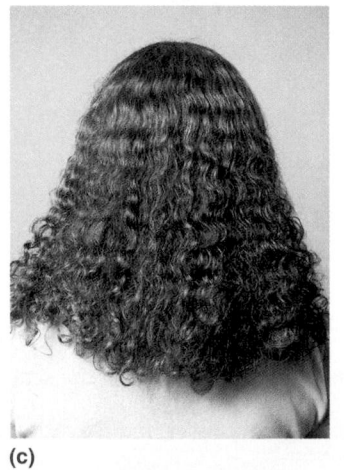
(c)

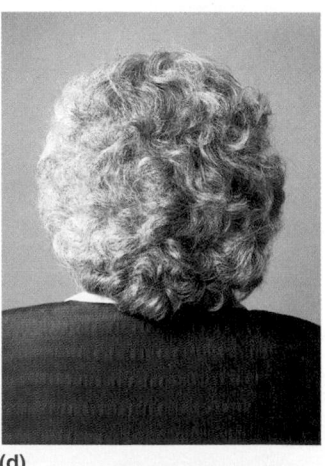
(d)

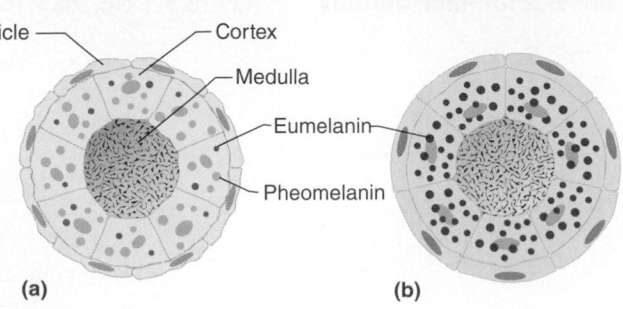

Cuticle

Cortex

Medulla

Eumelanin

Pheomelanin

(a)

(b)

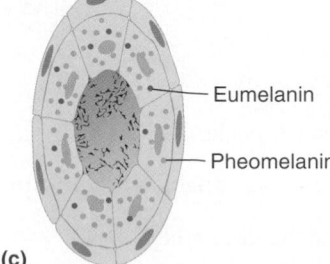

Eumelanin

Pheomelanin

(c)

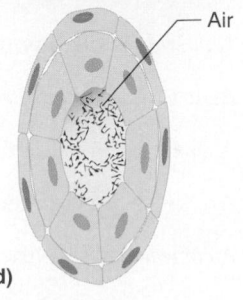

Air

(d)

▲ **Figure 15.22** **Basis of Hair Color and Texture.**

WORD	PRONUNCIATION	ELEMENTS		DEFINITION
albinism albino	AL-bih-nizm al-BY-no	S/ R/CF	-ism *condition* albin/o- *white*	Genetic disorder with lack of melanin Person with albinism
alopecia	al-oh-PEE-shah		Greek *mange*	Partial or complete loss of hair, naturally or from medication
axilla axillae (pl) axillary (adj)	AK-sill-ah AK-sill-ee AK-sill-air-ee		Greek *region under a bird's wing*	Medical name for the armpit Pertaining to the axilla
cortex cortical (adj) cortices (pl)	KOR-teks KOR-tih-kal KOR-tih-sees		Latin *outer covering*	Outer portion of an organ, such as bone Gray covering of cerebral hemispheres
cuticle	KEW-tih-cul		Diminutive of cutis *skin*	Nonliving epidermis at the base of the fingernails and 4 toenails, and the outer layer of hair
medulla medullary (adj)	meh-DULL-ah meh-DULL-eh-ree		French *middle*	Central portion of a structure surrounded by cortex
melanin eumelanin pheomelanin	MEL-ah-nin YOU-mel-ah-nin FEE-oh-mel-ah-nin	 P/ R/ P/	Greek *black* eu- *good, normal* -melanin *black* pheo- *gray*	Black pigment found in skin, hair, retina The dark form of the pigment melanin The lighter form of melanin

Exercises

A. A good review of the above WAD will aid you in answering the following questions about the *language of dermatology*. *Fill in the blanks.*   **LO 15.5, 15.8, 15.9**

1. The root _____ denotes the color _____.

2. The medical term for **armpit** is _____.

3. The plural form of **cortex** is _____.

4. The central portion of a structure is the _____, which means _____.

5. The outer portion of an organ is the _____.

6. The medical term for baldness is _____.

7. **Alopecia** can result from natural causes or from _____.

B. The following nouns all have an adjectival form. *Fill in the blanks.*   **LO 15.5, 15.6**

1. Noun: axilla   Adjective: _____

2. Noun: cortex   Adjective: _____

3. Noun: medulla   Adjective: _____

4. Use any one of these adjectives in a sentence.

_____

_____

_____

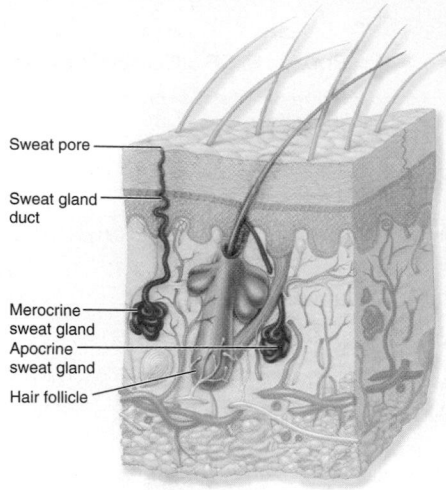

▲ Figure 15.23 **Sweat Glands.**

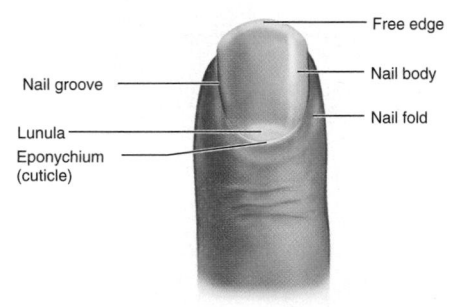

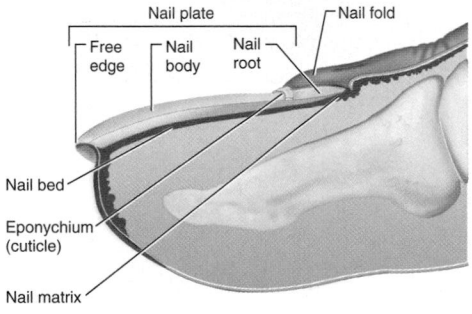

▲ Figure 15.24 **Anatomy of a Fingernail.**

Sweat Glands

You have 3 million to 4 million **eccrine (merocrine)** sweat glands *(Figure 15.23)* scattered all over your skin, with higher concentrations on your palms, soles, and forehead.

Their main function is to produce the watery perspiration (sweat) that cools your body. Your sweat is 99% water; the rest is made up of electrolytes such as sodium chloride, which gives the sweat its salty taste. Some waste products of cell metabolism are also secreted.

In the dermis the sweat gland is a coiled tube lined with epithelial cells that secrete the sweat. Around the tube, muscle cells contract to squeeze the sweat up the tube directly to the surface of the skin.

In your armpits (**axillae**), around your nipples, in your groin, and around your anus, **apocrine** sweat glands produce a thick, cloudy secretion that interacts with normal skin bacteria to produce a distinct, noticeable smell. The ducts of these glands lead directly into hair follicles *(see Figure 15.23)*. They respond to sexual stimulation and stress and secrete chemicals called **pheromones**, which have an effect on the sexual behavior of other people.

Ceruminous glands are found in the external ear canal, where their secretions combine with sebum and dead epidermal cells to form earwax. This wax waterproofs the external ear canal and kills bacteria.

Sweat gland functions are severely affected in a group of diseases termed *ectodermal dysplasia*, manifested in the reduction or absence of sweat. They can be involved in the infections that engulf the nearby hair follicles and sebaceous glands.

Mammary glands, a type of modified sweat gland, serve a distinct purpose in reproduction and are therefore discussed in *Chapter 8* under the female reproductive system.

Nails

Nails are formed from the stratum corneum of the epidermis. They consist of closely packed, thin, dead cells that are filled with parallel fibers of hard keratin.

Fingernails grow about 1 mm per week. New cells are added by cell division in the nail **matrix**, which is protected by the nail fold of skin and the cuticle at the base of the nail *(Figure 15.24)*. The nail rests on the nail bed, which consists of the living layers of the epidermis, the strata basale, spinosum, and granulosum.

Diseases of Nails Fifty percent of all nail disorders are caused by fungal infections and are labeled **onychomycosis** *(Figure 15.25)*. They begin in nails constantly exposed to moisture and warmth; for example, in warm shoes when associated with poor foot hygiene, in the hands of a restaurant dishwasher, under artificial fingernails, and in pedicure bowls if they are not sanitized. The fungus grows under the nail and leads to brittle cracked nails that separate from the underlying nail bed.

Paronychia *(Figure 15.26)* is a bacterial infection, usually staphylococcal, of the base of the nail. The nail fold and cuticle become swollen, red, and painful, and pus forms under the nail and can escape at the side of the nail.

The nail of the big toe can grow into the skin at the side of the nail, particularly if pressured by tight, narrow shoes. Infection can then get underneath this ingrown toenail.

The nails can reflect systemic illness. In anemia, the nail bed is pale, and the nails can become spoon-shaped. In conditions producing chronic **hypoxia**, the fingers, toes, and nails become clubbed. **Malnutrition** or severe illness can produce horizontal white lines in the nails.

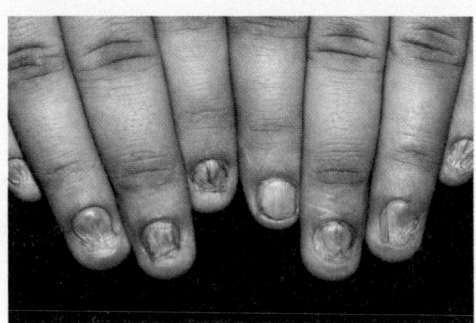

▲ Figure 15.25 **Onychomycosis (Fungal Infection).**

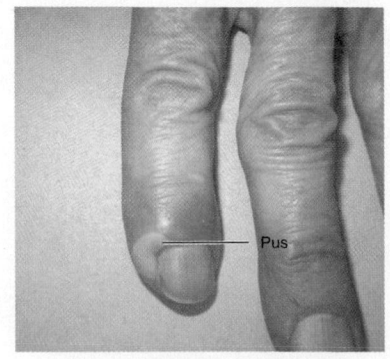

▲ Figure 15.26 **Paronychia, with Pus at the Corner of the Nail Bed.**

WORD	PRONUNCIATION	ELEMENTS		DEFINITION
apocrine	AP-oh-krin	P/ R/	apo- *different from* -crine *secrete*	Apocrine sweat glands open into the hair follicle
cerumen ceruminous (adj)	seh-**ROO**-men seh-**ROO**-mih-nus		Latin *wax*	Waxy secretion of the ceruminous glands of the external ear
eccrine	**EK**-rin		Greek *to secrete*	Coiled sweat gland that occurs in skin all over the body
hypoxia	high-**POCK**-see-ah	S/ P/ R/	-ia *condition* hyp- *below* -ox- *oxygen*	Decrease below normal levels of oxygen in tissues, gases, or blood
hypoxic (adj)	high-**POCK**-sik	S/	-ic *pertaining to*	Deficient in oxygen
malnutrition	mal-nyu-**TRISH**-un	S/ P/ R/	-ion *process* mal- *bad, inadequate* -nutrit- *nourishment*	Inadequate nutrition from poor diet or inadequate absorption of nutrients
matrices (pl)	**MAY**-triks		Latin *womb*	Substance that surrounds cells, is manufactured by the cells, and holds them together
merocrine	**MARE**-oh-krin	P/ R/	mero- *partial* -crine *secrete*	Another name for eccrine
onychomycosis	oh-ni-koh-my-**KOH**-sis	S/ R/CF R/	-osis *condition* onych/o- *nail* -myc- *fungus*	Condition of a fungus infection in a nail
paronychia	par-oh-**NICK**-ee-ah	S/ P/ R/	-ia *condition* para- *alongside* -onych- *nail* (**Note:** The vowel "a" at the end of para- is dropped to make the composite word flow more easily.)	Infection alongside the nail
pheromone	**FER**-oh-moan	P/ R/	pher- *carrying* -omone *excite, stimulate*	Substance that carries and generates a physical attraction for other people

Exercises

A. Work on understanding the meanings of the elements. *Deconstruct the medical terms into their elements, and show that you know their meanings. Fill in the blanks.* **LO 15.5, 15.8, 15.9**

Medical Term	Prefix	Meaning of Prefix	Root/ Cmbining Form	Meaning of Root/ Combining Form	Suffix	Meaning of Suffix
pheromone	1.	2.	3.	4.	5.	6.
apocrine	7.	8.	9.	10.	11.	12.
hypoxia	13.	14.	15.	16.	17.	18.
merocrine	19.	20.	21.	22.	23.	24.
onychomycosis	25.	26.	27.	28.	29.	30.
paronychia	31.	32.	33.	34.	35.	36.

B. Answer the following questions about the medical terms in the above WAD. **LO 15.5, 15.9**

A plural form of a term that relates to cells has been intentionally left out of this WAD box. Find the term, form its plural, and write the rule that applies to that ending.

1. Singular term: _____ Plural term: _____

2. Rule: _____. *Note:* Go back and write the plural form in the WAD box under the singular term.

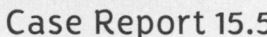

Lesson 15.4 Burns and Injuries to the Skin

INTEGUMENTARY SYSTEM

You have learned that a major role of the skin is protection of your internal organs. In the previous lessons, you have seen the effects of infectious agents on the skin. In this lesson, you will learn the effects of direct injury to the skin, and you will be able to use correct medical terminology to:

15.4.1 Distinguish the four types of burns.

15.4.2 Describe the inflammatory process of the skin when it is injured.

15.4.3 Explain the process of healing and repair of the skin.

15.4.4 Describe wounds, burns, and the process of healing and repair.

You are

. . . a burn technologist employed in the Burn Unit at Fulwood Medical Center.

Your patient is

. . . Mr. Steven Hapgood, a 52-year-old man, admitted to the Fulwood Burn Unit with severe burns over his face, chest, and abdomen.

Study Hint

Pay special attention to the graft prefixes.

Case Report 15.5

After an evening of drinking, Mr. Hapgood was smoking in bed and fell asleep. His next-door neighbors in the apartment building smelled smoke and called 911. In the Burn Unit, his initial treatment included large volumes of intravenous (IV) fluids to prevent **shock**.

Your role will be to participate in Mr. Hapgood's care as a member of the Burn Unit team and to document the care and his response to it. Mr. Hapgood's burns were mostly third-degree. The protective ability of the skin to prevent water loss had been removed, as had the skin barrier against infection. The burned, dead tissue forms an **eschar** that can have toxic effects on the digestive, respiratory, and cardiovascular systems. The eschar was surgically removed by **debridement**.

LO 15.10 Burns

Burns are the leading cause of *accidental* death. The immediate threats to life are from fluid loss, infection, and the systemic effects of burned dead tissue.

Burns are classified according to the depth of tissue involved *(Figure 15.27)*:

- **First-degree (superficial) burns** involve only the epidermis and produce inflammation with redness, pain, and slight **edema**. Healing occurs in 3 to 5 days without scarring.

- **Second-degree (partial-thickness) burns** involve the epidermis and dermis but leave some of the dermis intact. They produce redness, blisters, and more severe pain. Healing occurs in 2 to 3 weeks with minimal scarring.

- **Third-degree (full-thickness) burns** involve the epidermis, dermis, and subcutaneous tissues, which are often completely destroyed. Healing takes a long time and involves using skin grafts.

- **Fourth-degree burns** destroy all layers of the skin and involve tendons, muscles, and sometimes bones.

Burn injury to the lungs through damage from heat or smoke inhalation is responsible for 60% or more of fatalities from burns.

In partial-thickness burns, **regeneration** of the skin can occur from remaining cells in the stratum basale, from residual hair follicles and sweat glands, and from the edges of the burned area. In full-thickness burns there is no dermal tissue left for regeneration, and skin grafts are needed. The ideal graft is an **autograft** taken from another location on the patient. It is not rejected by the immune system. Mr. Hapgood had autografts taken from his unburned legs and back.

If the patient's burns are too extensive, **allografts** from another person are needed. These are provided by skin banks and are taken from deceased people (cadavers). A **homograft** is another name for an allograft. A **xenograft**, or **heterograft**, is a graft from another species, for example, pigs.

Artificial skin is being developed commercially and can stimulate the growth of connective tissues from the patient's underlying tissue.

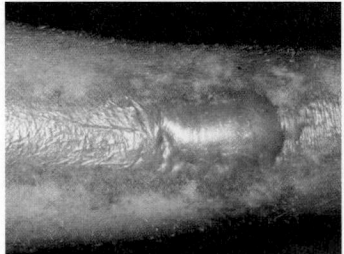

(a) First degree (superficial) **(b)** Second degree (partial thickness)

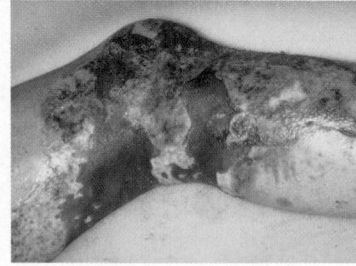

(c) Third degree (full thickness)

▲ **Figure 15.27** Degrees of Burns.

WORD	PRONUNCIATION	ELEMENTS		DEFINITION
allograft	AL-oh-graft	P/ R/	allo- *other* -graft *transplant*	Skin graft from another person or cadaver
homograft (syn)	HOH-moh-graft	P/	homo- *same, alike*	
autograft	AWE-toe-graft	P/ R/	auto- *self* -graft *transplant*	A graft using tissue taken from the individual who is receiving the graft
debridement	day-BREED-mon	S/ P/ R/	-ment *resulting state* de- *take away* -bride- *rubbish*	The removal of injured or necrotic tissue
edema	ee-DEE-mah		Greek *swelling*	Excessive collection of fluid in cells and tissues
edematous (adj)	ee-DEM-ah-tus	R/ S/	edema- *excess spacing watery fluid* -tous *pertaining to*	Marked by edema
eschar	ESS-kar		Greek *scab of a burn*	The burned, dead tissue lying on top of third-degree burns
regenerate	ree-JEN-eh-rate	S/ P/ R/	-ate *composed of,* re- *again* -gener- *produce*	To reconstitute a lost part
regeneration (noun)	ree-JEN-eh-RAY-shun	S/	-ation *process*	Reconstitution of a lost part
shock	SHOCK		German *to clash*	Sudden physical or mental collapse or circulatory collapse
xenograft	ZEN-oh-graft	P/ R/	xeno- *foreign* -graft *transplant*	A graft from another species
heterograft (syn)	HET-er-oh-graft	P/	hetero- *different*	

Exercises

A. Continue your work with elements from the *language of dermatology*. *Match the element in 1–12 to its correct meaning in A–L.* *Fill in the blanks.* **LO 15.5, 15.10**

_____ 1. homo-   a. again

_____ 2. -bride-   b. foreign

_____ 3. -ate   c. produce

_____ 4. allo-   d. same, like

_____ 5. -ment   e. different

_____ 6. xeno-   f. other

_____ 7. -gener-   g. composed of, pertaining to

_____ 8. -graft   h. resulting state

_____ 9. auto-   i. rubbish

_____ 10. de-   j. transplant

_____ 11. re-   k. self

_____ 12. hetero-   l. take away

B. Apply your knowledge of burns to the following questions. *Fill in the blanks.* **LO 15.5, 15.10**

1. Burns are the leading cause of _____ death.

2. The ideal skin graft comes from _____.

3. Burns are classified according to _____.

4. The burned, dead tissue lying on top of third-degree burns is termed _____.

5. If bone is involved, that classifies as a _____-degree burn.

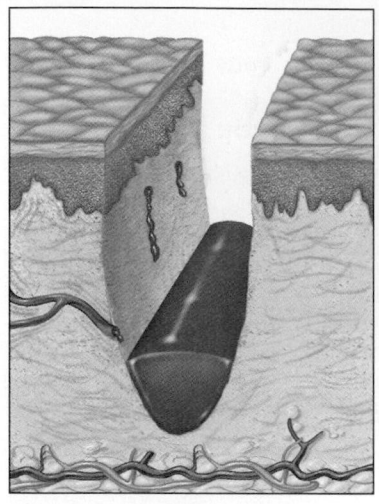

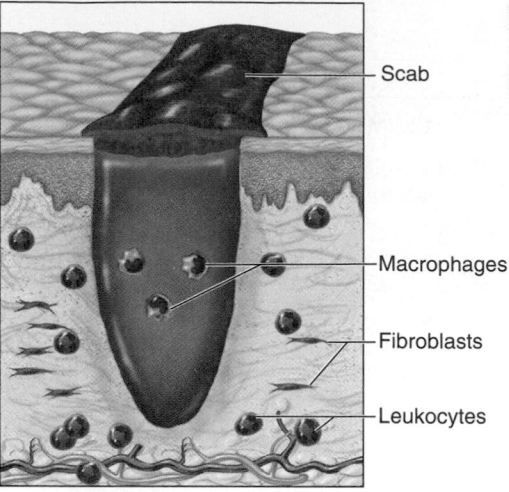

(a) Bleeding into the wound

(b) Scab formation and macrophage activity

▲ **Figure 15.28** Wound Healing.

Scab —

Macrophages

Fibroblasts

Leukocytes

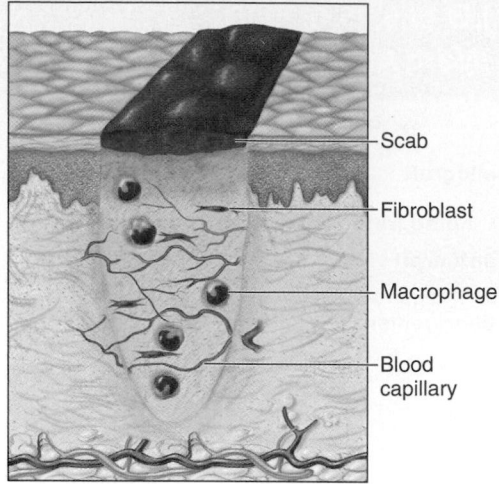

Scab

Fibroblast

Macrophage

Blood
capillary

▲ **Figure 15.29** Formation of Granulation Tissue.

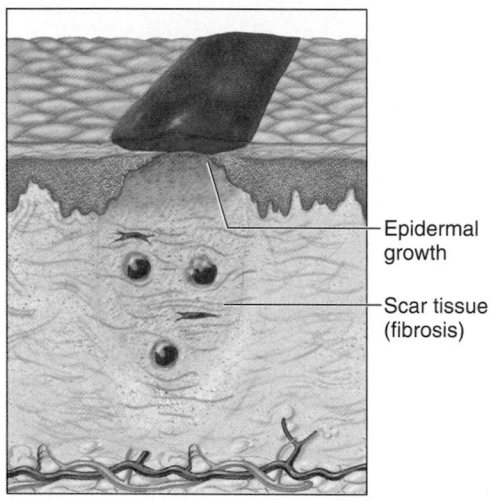

Epidermal growth

Scar tissue (fibrosis)

▲ **Figure 15.30** Scar Formation.

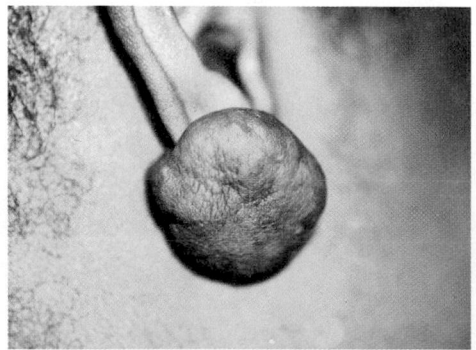

▲ **Figure 15.31** A Keloid of the Earlobe.
This scar resulted from piercing the ear for earrings.

LO 15.11 Wounds and Tissue Repair

If you cut yourself with paper and produce a shallow **laceration** primarily in the epidermis, the epithelial cells along its edges will divide rapidly and fill in the gap. An adhesive bandage helps the process by pulling the edges together.

If you cut yourself more deeply, extending the **wound** into the dermis or hypodermis, or if a surgeon makes an **incision**, then blood vessels in the dermis break and blood escapes into the wound *(Figure 15.28a)*.

This escaped blood forms a **clot** in the wound. The clot consists of the protein (**fibrin**) together with **platelets**, blood cells, and dried tissue fluids trapped in the fibers. **Macrophages** come into the wound with the escaped blood. They digest and clean up the tissue debris. The surface of the clot dries and hardens in the air to form a **scab**. The scab seals and protects the wound from becoming infected *(Figure 15.28b)*.

The clot begins to be invaded by new capillaries from the surrounding dermis. Three or four days after the injury, fibroblasts migrate into the wound and form new collagen fibers that pull the wound together. This soft tissue in the wound is called **granulation tissue** and in unsutured wounds takes a couple of weeks to completely form *(Figure 15.29)*.

As healing continues, surface epithelial cells from the edges of the wound migrate into the area underneath the scab. As this new epithelium thickens, the scab loosens and falls off. Inside the wound, new collagen fibers formed by the fibroblasts form a **scar** to replace the granulation tissue *(Figure 15.30)*. In unsutured wounds, this takes up to a month to complete.

Suturing brings together the edges of the wound to enhance tissue healing. It also reduces the risk of infection and the amount of scarring. A liquid skin adhesive can sometimes be used in place of sutures. Some sutures eventually dissolve, avoiding the need for suture removal. The scar formation and remodeling process may go on for more than a year.

In some people, there is excessive fibrosis and scar tissue formation, producing raised, irregular, lumpy, shiny scars called **keloids** *(Figure 15.31)*. They can extend beyond the edges of the original wound and often return if they are surgically removed. They are most common on the upper body and earlobes.

Surgery on the skin is now being performed using light beams called **lasers**. These beams of light can be focused precisely to vaporize specific lesions on the superficial layers of the skin. The beams remove lesions and create a fresh surface over which new skin can grow. Healing takes 10 to 15 days and goes through the process described above, with clotting and scabbing.

A superficial scraping of the skin, a mucous membrane, or the cornea *(see Chapter 16)* is called an **abrasion**.

Word Analysis and Definition

S = Suffix   P = Prefix   **R = Root   R/CF = Combining Form**

WORD	PRONUNCIATION		ELEMENTS	DEFINITION
abrasion	ah-**BRAY**-shun		Latin *to scrape*	Area of skin or mucous membrane that has been scraped off
clot	KLOT		German *to block*	The mass of fibrin and cells that is produced in a wound
fibrin **fibrous (adj)**	**FIE**-brin **FIE**-brus	S/ R/	Latin *fiber* -ous *pertaining to* **fibr-** *fiber*	Stringy protein fiber that is a component of a blood clot Tissue containing fibroblasts and fibers
granulation	gran-you-**LAY**-shun	S/ R/	-ation *process* **granul-** *small grain*	New fibrous tissue formed during wound healing
incision	in-**SIZH**-un	S/ R/	-ion *action, condition* **incis-** *cut into*	A cut or surgical wound
keloid	**KEY**-loyd		Greek *stain*	Raised, irregular, lumpy, shiny scar due to excess collagen fiber production during healing of a wound
laceration	lass-eh-**RAY**-shun	S/ R/	-ation *process* **lacer-** *to tear*	A tear of the skin
laser	**LAY**-zer		acronym for **L**ight **A**mplification by **S**timulated **E**mission of **R**adiation	Intense, narrow beam of monochromatic light
macrophage	**MAK**-roh-fayj	P/ R/	**macro-** *large* **-phage** *to eat*	Large white blood cell that removes bacteria, foreign particles, and dead cells
platelet (also called **thrombocyte**)	**PLAYT**-let		Greek *small plate*	Cell fragment involved in clotting process
scab	SKAB		Old English *crust*	Crust that forms over a wound or sore during healing
scar	SKAR		Greek *scab*	Fibrotic seam that forms when a wound heals
suture	**SOO**-chur		Latin *seam*	Stitch to hold the edges of a wound together
wound	WOOND		Old English *wound*	Any injury that interrupts the continuity of skin or a mucous membrane

Exercises

A. Review the above WAD before starting this exercise—the elements and definitions will help you work out the answers. *Put on your thinking cap. Fill in the blanks.*   **LO 15.5, 15.11**

1. Reorder these terms into the order of their occurrence.

   scab   scar   clot   wound

   _____

2. How are a *keloid* and a *scar* different?

   _____

3. What is the soft tissue in the wound-healing process called?

   _____

4. What's the relationship between a *clot* and a *scab*?

   _____

5. What is another name for a stitch used to close a wound?

   _____

Congratulations! You have mastered these terms.

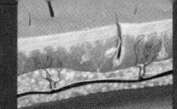

Integumentary System

Challenge Your Knowledge

A. **Name the five different types of skin grafts and where they come from. (LO 15.4, 15.5, 15.10,** *Remember*)

1. _____ comes from _____.

2. _____ comes from _____.

3. _____ comes from _____.

4. _____ comes from _____.

5. _____ comes from _____.

B. **Medical vocabulary is filled with terms taken directly from Greek and Latin.** The medical term is given to you—write the definition beside it. (**LO 15.5,** *Remember*)

1. dermis _____

2. integument _____

3. mole _____

4. squamous _____

5. collagen _____

6. follicle _____

7. vesicle _____

8. edema _____

9. nevus _____

10. boil _____

C. **Label exercise.** Identify the integumentary term in phrases 1–6, and write the terms on the correct lines A–F in the illustration. (**LO 15.2, 15.5,** *Remember, Apply*)

1. Open into hair follicles

2. Also called *subcutaneous tissue layer*

3. Top layer of the skin

4. Concentrated on palms, soles of feet, and forehead

5. Layer of skin below epidermis

6. Secrete chemicals called *pheromones*

B. _____

D. _____

F. _____

A. _____

E. _____

C. _____

D. Plurals. Follow the rules and form the plurals for the following terms. (**LO 15.4, 15.5,** *Remember, Apply*)

1. papilla   Plural: _____

2. matrix   Plural: _____

3. cortex   Plural: _____

4. axilla   Plural: _____

E. Abbreviations appear in written documentation and must be used correctly. Rewrite the following sentences with the correct abbreviation(s) in the appropriate place. (**LO 15.5,** *Remember, Apply*)

1. This patient is suffering from septicemia and tuberculosis.

_____

2. Is this an intramuscular or subcutaneous injection?

_____

3. Rheumatoid arthritis and systemic lupus erythematosus are classified as autoimmune diseases.

_____

_____

F. Skin diseases can affect any and all parts of the body. Some skin diseases are an early manifestation of a more serious internal problem. Match the symptom or association in the left column with the correct medical term in the right column. You have more answer choices than you need. (**LO 15.4,** *Understand*)

_____ 1. cause unknown; silvery scales   **a.** pemphigus vulgaris

_____ 2. butterfly rash   **b.** vitiligo

_____ 3. associated with ovarian cancer   **c.** rosacea

_____ 4. enlarged capillaries show through skin   **d.** psoriasis

_____ 5. pale patches of skin   **e.** seborrheic lesions

_____ 6. shrinking of skin; hardening   **f.** scleroderma

     g. SLE

     h. herpes zoster

     i. dermatomyositis

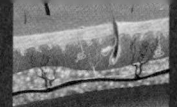

Integumentary System

G. To have a better understanding of the integumentary system, you must know the layers of skin and its tissue components, as well as its functions. Fill in the following blanks. (**LO 15.2, 15.5,** *Understand*)

Name the three layers of skin, the type of tissue found in each layer, and the function of each layer of skin.

1. Skin layer: _____

   Tissue(s): _____

   Function(s): _____

2. Skin layer: _____

   Tissue(s): _____

   Function(s): _____

3. Skin layer: _____

   Tissue(s): _____

   Function(s): _____

H. Translate to layman's terms. Expressing yourself verbally is something you will have to do every day on the job. Your patient is asking about the following procedures. In the space given, briefly define each procedure in terms the patient will understand. (**LO 15.6,** *Understand*)

1. Cryosurgery: _____

   _____

2. Biopsy removal: _____

   _____

3. Debridement: _____

   _____

I. Also known as. Some medical terms may be known by a more common term. You need to know both. Fill in the blanks with the alternate terms. (**LO 15.4, 15.5,** *Understand*)

1. pressure ulcer = _____

2. cradle cap = _____

3. shingles = _____

4. staph = _____

5. armpit = _____

6. baldness = _____

7. wax = _____

8. whitehead or blackhead = _____

9. athlete's foot = _____

10. hives = _____

11. lice eggs = _____

12. ringworm = _____

J. Aid your memory by making a connection from a medical term to an English word.
Fungal infections that cause human disease are named *tinea*. Which three body areas host this fungus? Fill in the following chart. (**LO 15.4, 15.5, 15.6,** *Understand*)

💡 *Study Hint*
Try to match the term to an English word with the same sense or meaning.

Body Area	Medical Term Is	Correlate to an English Word
1.	tinea pedis	
2.	tinea capitis	
3.	tinea corporis	

K. Discussion. Explain this sentence: "The skin is the largest and most vulnerable organ in the body." (**LO 15.1, 15.6,** *Understand*)
In your discussion of this with your classmates, you must answer these questions:

1. What does *vulnerable* mean? (Look it up in an online dictionary.)

_____

_____

2. Why is skin vulnerable?

_____

_____

3. What makes skin an organ?

_____

_____

L. Patient education (in your own words). Philip was involved in a motor vehicle accident and was burned over 60% of his body when his car caught fire. The plastic surgeon has just told Philip he will need extensive grafting to repair his third-degree burns. Pain and nervousness kept Philip from entirely understanding what the surgeon told him. He is asking you for more explanation. (**LO 15.6, 15.10,** *Understand*)
You need to explain to the patient:

1. What an autograft is, and where it will come from.

_____

_____

2. How this procedure will help his skin regenerate.

_____

_____

M. Use your knowledge of the language of dermatology to make the connection with the following medical terms. Match the medical terms in the left column with the descriptions in the right column. (**LO 15.4, 15.5,** *Understand, Apply*)

_____ 1. pruritus   **a.** can infiltrate or metastasize

_____ 2. edema   **b.** body as a whole

_____ 3. malignancy   **c.** swelling

_____ 4. systemic   **d.** infection of the scalp

_____ 5. ringworm   **e.** itching

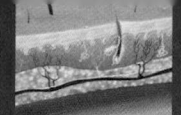
Integumentary System

N. **The previous exercises should help you apply your knowledge of the integumentary system and correctly answer the following questions.** Circle the answer. (**LO 15.4, 15.5,** *Understand, Apply*)

1. Use of liquid nitrogen to freeze or kill abnormal tissue is called

   a. biopsy

   b. patch test

   c. cryosurgery

   d. hypodermic injection

   e. infestation

2. A laceration that is *superficial* is not very

   a. swollen

   b. edematous

   c. deep

   d. purulent

   e. infected

3. Keratinized stratified squamous epithelium is

   a. stratum spinosum

   b. dandruff

   c. hair follicle

   d. sweat

   e. dermatitis

4. An ointment, cream, or spray prescribed to relieve itching is called

   a. antifungal

   b. keratolytic

   c. antipruritic

   d. retinoid

   e. antibacterial

5. Subcutaneous fat is another name for

   a. epidermis

   b. hypodermis

   c. dermis

   d. adipose tissue

   e. follicles

O. **Burn treatment is a highly specialized area of care.** Use the language of burn terminology to fill in the blanks. (**LO 15.5, 15.10,** *Apply*)

1. A superficial burn is _____-degree.

2. What degree burns require skin grafts? _____

3. Burn injury can involve other body systems. Name one. _____

4. The immediate threats to life are from _____, _____, and _____.

5. Name three occupations that risk burn injury on the job. _____, _____, and _____

P. **Continue applying your knowledge of the language of dermatology to the integumentary system.** Circle the best choice. **(LO 15.4, 15.5, Apply)**

1. A congenital lesion of the skin, including birthmarks and moles, is called a

   a. macule

   b. papule

   c. vesicle

   d. nevus

   e. melanoma

2. Another name for a pressure ulcer is

   a. eczema

   b. excoriation

   c. decubitus

   d. edematous

   e. serous

3. Strep enzymes digest connective tissue and spread into muscle layers in

   a. lesions

   b. atopic dermatitis

   c. cellulitis

   d. ulcers

   e. necrotizing fasciitis

4. The medical term for shingles is

   a. erysipelas

   b. herpes zoster

   c. impetigo

   d. candidiasis

   e. pediculosis

5. Kaposi sarcoma is associated with

   a. SC

   b. HIV

   c. SLE

   d. TB

   e. MRSA

Integumentary System

Q. Medical terms that are nouns can also have an adjectival form that must be used in some cases. Test your knowledge of the correct form of the term to use in the following sentences. Circle the best choice. (**LO 15.5, Apply**)

1. This puncture wound has completely penetrated the (dermis/dermal).

2. This burn wound has completely penetrated the (dermis/dermal) layer of skin.

3. Please take this specimen to the (pathological/pathology) department.

4. The (pathology/pathological) diagnosis has not been determined yet.

5. The (anesthesia/anesthetic) properties of the aloe lotion reduced the pain in the sunburn.

R. Some terms can function as a noun and a verb. To *suture* (verb) means *to stitch the edges of a wound together.* A *suture* (noun) is the material used to make the stitch itself. Demonstrate your understanding of both terms by creating a sentence of patient documentation for each term. (**LO 15.5, Apply**)

1. Sentence (verb)

_____

_____

2. Sentence (noun)

_____

_____

S. Build your medical language of dermatology. Complete the medical terms by filling in the blanks. The first one is done for you. (**LO 15.5, Apply**)

1. Study of disorders of the skin   /dermato/*logy*

2. To scratch the skin   ex/_____/ate

3. Sore caused by lying in bed   de/_____/_____

4. Infestation with lice   _____/_____/osis

5. Takes away feeling and pain   an/_____/_____

6. Medication against itching   _____/_____ic

7. Infection alongside a nail   _____/_____/ia

8. Deficient in oxygen   _____/_____ /oxia

9. Forecast of probable course of disease   pro/_____/_____

T. **Apply your knowledge of the language of dermatology to the following Case Report.** Read the report out loud for pronunciation practice. Underline the medical terms, and be sure you understand them. Answer the questions. (**LO 15.4, 15.5, Apply**)

Case Report 15.3

Ms. Cheryl Fox is a 37-year-old nursing assistant working in a surgical unit in Fulwood Medical Center. Recently her fingers have become red and itchy, with occasional vesicles. She has also noticed irritation and swelling of her earlobes and a generalized pruritus. Over the weekends, both the itching and the rash on her hands worsened. A patch test by her dermatologist showed her to be allergic to nickel in rings that she wears on both hands and in her earrings. She wore these on weekends and not during her workdays.

1. What diagnostic test did Ms. Fox have to determine the cause of her condition?

   _____

2. List Ms. Fox's symptoms.

   _____

   _____

3. What part of her body was *edematous*?

   _____

4. **Pruritus** is a medical term for _____.

5. Describe a vesicle. _____

6. What is the *allergen* that Ms. Fox is allergic to? _____

7. A likely diagnosis for Ms. Fox would be (circle one):

   melanoma   dermatitis   vitiligo   candidiasis

U. **The terms in each of the following groups of medical terms have something in common.** Use your knowledge of the *language of dermatology* to determine what links them together. The first one is done for you. Fill in the blanks. (**LO 15.2, 15.4, 15.5, Analyze**)

1. Epidermis, dermis, and hypodermis <u>are all layers of skin</u>_____

2. Melanoma, malignancy, and metastasis _____.

3. Bee stings, peanuts, cats, and pollen _____.

4. Intradermal, subcutaneous, and intramuscular _____.

5. Merocrine, apocrine, and ceruminous _____.

6. Mole, papule, and macule _____.

7. Parasite, pediculosis, and lice _____.

8. Scleroderma, rosacea, and SLE _____.

9. Paronychia, onychomycosis, and matrix _____.

10. Eschar, debridement, and xenograft _____.

Integumentary System

V. Diagnoses. Identifying the root(s) of the following diagnoses will help you understand the meaning of the medical term. First, determine the root/combining form(s), then give the meaning of the root/combining form(s), and then provide a brief description of the meaning of the term. Fill in the chart below. (**LO 15.2, 15.4, 15.5,** *Analyze*)

Diagnosis	Root/CF(s)	Meaning of Root/ Combining Form	Meaning of Term
candidiasis	1.	2.	3.
carcinoma	4.	5.	6.
decubitus ulcer	7.	8.	9.
dermatitis	10.	11.	12.
dermatomyositis	13.	14.	15.
hypoxia	16.	17.	18.
onychomycosis	19.	20.	21.
paronychia	22.	23.	24.
pediculosis	25.	26.	27.
scleroderma	28.	29.	30.

W. Terminology challenge. Many medical terms can appear in several different forms—a noun (person, place, thing), a verb (action), or an adjective (description). Use the following medical terms to complete the sentences. Note at the end of the sentence whether you have used the noun, verb, or adjectival form of the term. Fill in the blanks. (**LO 15.5,** *Analyze*)

metastasis   **metastasize**   **metastatic**

1. The surgeon predicted that the lesion would _____ to the liver.

   Form used: _____

2. The _____ lesion received radiation therapy, while the primary lesion was surgically removed.

   Form used: _____

3. The pathology report confirmed that there was no _____ of the lesion.

   Form used: _____

Apply your rule for plural endings and make the plural form of the medical term used in question 3.

4. Plural: _____

5. The rule for forming this plural is _____

X. Fine-tune your knowledge. Being able to explain something to someone else means *you* understand it. Explain to your class-mates the differences in the following terms. (**LO 15.5, 15.6,** *Analyze*)

1. What is the difference between an *infestation* and an *infection?* Using correct medical terms, give an example of each.

   Infestation: _____

   _____

   Infection: _____

   _____

2. What is the difference between a *viral* and a *bacterial* infection? Using correct medical terms, give an example of each.

   Viral infection _____

   _____

   Bacterial infection _____

   _____

3. What is the difference between *vasoconstriction* and *vasodilation?* What is the purpose of each?

   Vasoconstriction: _____

   Purpose: _____

   Vasodilation: _____

   Purpose: _____

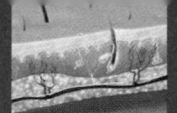

Integumentary System

CHAPTER SUMMARY EXERCISE

A. **Spelling comprehension.** Circle the correct spelling of the term. (**LO 15.5,** *Remember*)

1. ediology	etiology	eteology	iteology	etelogy
2. eczema	eksema	ecczemia	ecczema	ekzema
3. furruncle	furunckle	ferunkle	faruncle	furuncle
4. squamous	squamus	squuamus	sguamus	squamis
5. skleroderma	skeloderma	scleroderma	sccleroderma	sclerroderma
6. wheel	weal	wheil	weel	wheal
7. decubbitus	dicubitus	dekcubitus	decubeitus	decubitus

B. **Match the number of the correct spelling of the term in Exercise A with the following brief description of the term.** (**LO 15.2, 15.5,** *Apply*)

1. Wart _____

2. Means *to itch* _____

3. Hardening and shrinking of the skin _____

4. Secretes a greasy substance called sebum _____

5. From lying down too long _____

6. Inflammatory skin disease with serous discharge _____

7. Layer of scaly cells _____

C. **Using your knowledge of terms 1–7 in Exercises A and B and their correct spelling, write a brief sentence for each of the terms as it might appear in patient documentation.** (**LO 15.5,** *Apply*)

1. _____

2. _____

3. _____

4. _____

5. _____

6. _____

7. _____

After rereading Case Report 15.5, answer the following questions. Be prepared to discuss your answers in class. **(LO 15.5, 15.6, 15.10,** *Analyze*)

Case Report 15.5

You are

...a burn technologist employed in the Burn Unit at Fulwood Medical Center.

Your patient is

...Mr. Steven Hapgood, a 52-year-old man, admitted to the Fulwood Burn Unit with severe burns over his face, chest, and abdomen. After an evening of drinking, Mr. Hapgood was smoking in bed and fell asleep. His next-door neighbors in the apartment building smelled smoke and called 911. In the Burn Unit, his initial treatment included large volumes of intravenous fluids to prevent shock.

Your role will be to participate in Mr. Hapgood's care as a member of the Burn Unit team and to document the care and his response to it. Mr. Hapgood's burns were mostly third-degree. The protective ability of the skin to prevent water loss had been removed, as had the skin barrier against infection. The burned, dead tissue forms an eschar that can have toxic effects on the digestive, respiratory, and cardiovascular systems. The eschar was surgically removed by debridement.

1. Where are Mr. Hapgood's burns located? _____

2. Because of the extent of his burns, Mr. Hapgood has lost a large volume of body fluids. This could lead to what potentially

   life-threatening condition? _____

3. How are the fluids replaced? _____

4. Third-degree burns are also known as _____ and involve which layers of skin? _____

5. What two functions of skin have been eliminated due to Mr. Hapgood's large burn area?

   a. _____

   b. _____

6. _____ is the medical term for the burned, dead tissue lying on top of third-degree burns, and _____

   is the surgical procedure that removes this dead tissue.

7. This burned, dead tissue can have toxic effects on which other body systems? _____

8. Why are burn patients in a special unit and not in rooms with other patients with various diseases and conditions?

   _____

9. What other surgical procedure is necessary to promote the growth of new skin for Mr. Hapgood? _____

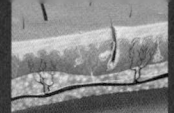

Integumentary System

E. **Meet the goals of each of the chapter outcomes by using the correct language of dermatology for the answers. (LO 15.1–15.11, *Analyze*)**

1. Describe the overall structure, functions, and regions of the skin. (**LO 15.1**)

   Describe the functions of the skin:

   _____

   _____

2. Discuss the different layers of the skin and their functions. (**LO 15.2**)

   Name the function of the epidermal layer of skin:

   _____

   _____

3. Differentiate the various sites for injections in the skin. (**LO 15.3**)

   Name the various sites for injections in the skin:

   a. _____

   b. _____

   c. _____

4. Describe the common disorders, diseases, and infections of the skin. Choose any type of skin infection and describe its symptoms. (**LO 15.4**)

   a. Infection: _____

   b. Symptoms: _____

5. Comprehend, spell, and write the medical terms of dermatology so that you communicate and document accurately and precisely in any health care setting. Insert into the following sentence the correctly spelled medical term from the following pairs. (**LO 15.5**)

   benine/benign   melignant/malignant

   _____ melanoma is the least common form of skin cancer, but the most deadly.

6. Recognize and pronounce the medical terms of dermatology so that you can communicate verbally with accuracy and precision in any health care setting. Choose the correct pronunciation for the term *paronychia*. (**LO 15.6**)

   a. PAR-o-nic-ia

   b. PAR-o-nick-ea

   c. par-oh-**NICK**-ia

   d. par-oh-**NICK**-ee-ah

   e. par-oh-**NIC**-ia

7. Define the types of topical agents used in the treatment of skin disorders. (**LO 15.7**)

What types of topical agents are used in the treatment of skin disorders?

a. _____

b. _____

c. _____

d. _____

8. Match the accessory skin organs to their functions. (**LO 15.8**)

Choose one of the accessory skin organs and describe its functions.

a. Accessory skin organ: _____

b. Functions: _____

9. Describe disorders of the accessory skin organs. (**LO 15.9**)

Pick one disorder of an accessory skin organ and describe its symptoms.

disorder: _____

symptoms: _____

10. Discuss burns and injuries to the skin. (**LO 15.10**)

List the degrees of burns and describe their appearance.

_____

_____

_____

_____

11. Describe the healing of wounds to the skin. (**LO 15.11**)

Wounds heal from the inside out. Describe the process of wound healing, using the correct medical terminology.

_____

_____

_____

_____

_____

Special Senses of the Eye and Ear
The Languages of Ophthalmology and Otology

In your future career, you may work directly and/or indirectly with the following health professionals in the area of ophthalmology:

- Ophthalmologists, who are medical specialists (MDs) in the diagnosis and treatment of diseases of the eye.

- Optometrists (ODs), who are professionals skilled in the measurement of vision. They are not medical doctors and cannot prescribe medication.

- Opticians, who are licensed to make corrective lenses, adjust and repair spectacles, and fit contact lenses.

The health professionals in the following list perform specific assigned procedures and support ophthalmologists according to the depth of their training:

- Certified ophthalmic medical technicians

- Certified ophthalmic assistants

- Certified ophthalmic technicians

- Certified ophthalmic technologists

- Registered ophthalmic ultrasound biometrists

- Diagnostic ophthalmic sonographers

In the area of otology, you may work directly and/or indirectly with the following health professionals:

- Otologists, who are medical specialists in diseases of the ear.

- Otorhinolaryngologists, who are medical specialists in disease of the ear, nose, and throat (ENT).

- Audiologists, who evaluate hearing function.

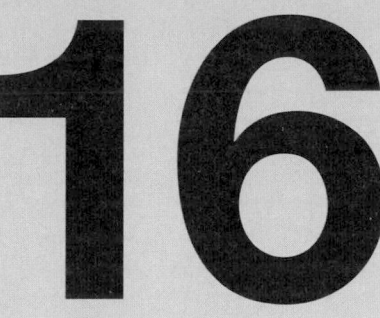

Case Report (CR) 16.1

You are

> . . . an **ophthalmic** technician **(OT)** working in the office of **ophthalmologist** Angela Chun, MD, a member of the Fulwood Medical Group.

Your patient is

> . . . Mrs. Jenny Hughes, a 30-year-old computer software consultant, who walked into the office with painful, red, swollen eyelids and a sticky, **purulent** discharge from both eyes. The administrative medical assistant did not hold her in the reception area but brought her directly in to you.
>
> Mrs. Hughes complains of headache and **photophobia**, and her eyelids were stuck together when she woke up this morning. She tells you that, a couple of days earlier, she had gone into a small business office to install software at 10 work-stations. One of the employees was absent with "**pink eye**." She wants to know if she could have contracted the disease from that employee's keyboard and how to prevent her husband and two children from getting it.
>
> You have in your hand a clipboard, pen attached, with the office Notice of Privacy Practices and sign-in sheet for her to sign. How do you proceed?

Chapter Learning Outcomes

In order to make correct decisions when you see patients with eye or ear problems, to communicate with other health professionals about the patient, to participate in patient education, and to document the patient's care, you need to be able to:

LO 16.1 Use the medical terms of ophthalmology and otology to communicate and document in writing accurately and precisely in any health care setting.

LO 16.2 Use the medical terms of ophthalmology and otology to communicate verbally with accuracy and precision in any health care setting.

LO 16.3 Describe the accessory structures of the eye and their common disorders.

LO 16.4 Identify the common conditions of the eye due to imbalance of the extrinsic muscles of the eye.

LO 16.5 Discuss the structure and functions of the eyeball and its different components.

LO 16.6 Map the visual pathway from the lens to the visual cortex of the brain.

LO 16.7 Describe the disorders of refraction.

LO 16.8 Describe the cause, appearance, diagnosis, and treatment of common disorders of the eye and its accessory structures.

LO 16.9 Define the purpose of certain ophthalmic procedures.

LO 16.10 Describe the anatomy of the external ear and its disorders.

LO 16.11 Discuss the structure and functions of the middle ear and its disorders.

LO 16.12 Discuss the structure and functions of the inner ear for hearing and balance and its disorders.

LO 16.13 Identify the value of hearing test procedures.

Note: The sense of smell is discussed as an integral part of the respiratory system (Chapter 13), the sense of taste as an integral part of the digestive system (Chapter 5), and the sense of touch as an integral part of the nervous system (Chapter 9).

LESSON OBJECTIVES

Mrs. Jenny Hughes's "**pink eye**" involved her **conjunctiva** and **eyelids**, two of the **periorbital** accessory structures of the eye, located around the **orbit** and in front of the **eyeball**. The other accessory structures are the **eyebrows and eyelashes** and the **lacrimal (tear) apparatus** *(Figure 16.1)*. All these structures support and protect the exposed front surface of the eye.

An understanding of the terminology, anatomy, and physiology of these accessory structures is an essential step to acquire an understanding of how they function to maintain the integrity of the eye.

The information in this lesson will enable you to:

16.1.1 Link the structure of the accessory structures of the eye to their appropriate functions.

16.1.2 Explain the roles of the accessory structures in protecting the eye.

16.1.3 Describe some common abnormalities and disorders of the accessory structures.

16.1.4 Apply the correct medical terminology to the anatomy, physiology, and disorders of the accessory structures.

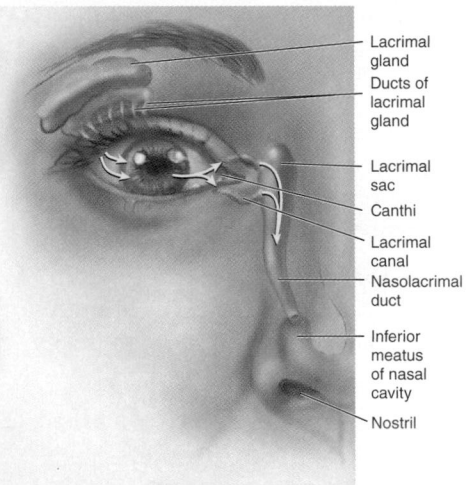

Lacrimal gland
Ducts of lacrimal gland
Lacrimal sac
Canthi
Lacrimal canal
Nasolacrimal duct
Inferior meatus of nasal cavity
Nostril

▲ **Figure 16.1** Lacrimal Apparatus and Accessory Structures.

Abbreviations

OD	doctor of optometry
OT	ophthalmic technician

LO 16.3 Accessory Structures

Eyebrows keep sweat from running into the eye and function in nonverbal communication.

Eyelids protect the eye from foreign objects. They blink to move tears across the surface of the eye and sweep debris away. They close in sleep to keep out visual stimuli. They are covered in the body's thinnest layer of skin. They consist mostly of muscle that fans out from each eyelid onto the forehead and cheek to open and close the eyelids.

In the eyelids, a flat, fibrous connective tissue layer (**tarsus**) holds 20 to 25 **tarsal glands**, whose ducts open along the edge of the eyelid. These glands secrete an oily fluid that keeps the eyelids from sticking together. The two corners where the upper and lower eyelids meet are called **canthi** (singular, **canthus**).

Eyelashes are strong hairs that help keep debris out of the eyes. They arise on the edge of the lids from hair follicles *(see Chapter 15)*.

The **conjunctiva** is a transparent **mucous membrane** that lines the inside of both eyelids and covers all of the front of the eye except the central portion, the **cornea**. In the conjunctiva, numerous goblet cells secrete a thin film of **mucin** that prevents the surface of the eyeball from dehydrating.

The conjunctiva is freely movable over the eyeball. It has numerous small blood vessels and is richly supplied with nerve endings that make it very sensitive to pain.

The **lacrimal apparatus** *(Figure 16.1)* consists of four structures. The **lacrimal (tear) gland**, located in the upper, lateral corner of the orbit, secretes tears. Short **lacrimal ducts** carry the tears to the surface of the conjunctiva. After washing across the conjunctiva, the tears leave the eye at the medial corner of the eye by draining into the **lacrimal sac**. They then flow through the **nasolacrimal duct** into the nose, from where they are swallowed.

The functions of tears are to

- *Clean and lubricate* the surface of the eye.
- *Deliver* nutrients and oxygen to the conjunctiva.
- *Prevent infection* through a bactericidal enzyme called **lysozyme**.

WORD	PRONUNCIATION	ELEMENTS		DEFINITION
canthus canthi (pl)	**KAN**-thus **KAN**-thi		Greek *corner of the eye*	Corner of the eye where upper and lower lids meet
conjunctiva conjunctivitis conjunctival (adj)	kon-junk-**TIE**-vah kon-junk-tih-**VI**-tis kon-junk-**TIE**-val	S/ R/ S/	Latin *inner lining of eyelids* -itis *inflammation* **conjunctiv-** *conjunctiva* -al *pertaining to*	Inner lining of the eyelids Inflammation of the conjunctiva Pertaining to the conjunctiva
cornea corneal (adj)	**KOR**-nee-ah **KOR**-nee-al		Latin *web, tunic*	The central, transparent part of the outer coat of the eye covering the iris and pupil
lacrimal nasolacrimal duct	**LAK**-rim-al **NAY**-zoh-**LAK**-rim-al DUKT	S/ R/ R/CF R/	-al *pertaining to* **lacrim-** *tears* **nas/o-** *nose* **duct** *to lead*	Pertaining to tears Passage from the lacrimal sac to the nose
lysozyme	**LIE**-soh-zime	R/ R/CF	-zyme *enzyme* **lys/o-** *decomposition*	Enzyme that dissolves the cell walls of bacteria
ophthalmology ophthalmologist ophthalmic (adj)	off-thal-**MALL**-oh-jee off-thal-**MALL**-oh-jist off-**THAL**-mik	S/ R/CF S/ S/	-logy *study of* **ophthalm/o-** *eye* -logist *one who studies, specialist* -ic *pertaining to*	Medical specialty that diagnoses and treats diseases of the eye Medical specialist in ophthalmology Pertaining to the eye
orbit orbital (adj)	**OR**-bit **OR**-bit-al		Latin *circle*	The bony socket that holds the eyeball
periorbital	per-ee-**OR**-bit-al	S/ P/ R/	-al *pertaining to* **peri-** *around* -orbit- *orbit*	Pertaining to tissues around the orbit
photophobia photophobic (adj)	foh-toe-**FOH**-bee-ah foh-toe-**FOH**-bik	S/ R/CF S/	-phobia *fear* **phot/o-** *light* -ic *pertaining to*	Fear of the light because it hurts the eyes Relating to or suffering from photophobia
pink eye	PINK EYE		lay term for conjunctivitis	Conjunctivitis
purulent	**PURE**-you-lent	S/ R/	-ulent *abounding in* **pur-** *pus*	Showing or containing a lot of pus
tarsus (**Note:** *Tarsus* also is used to refer to the seven bones in the instep of the foot.) tarsal (adj)	**TAR**-sus **TAR**-sal		Greek *flat*	The flat fibrous plate that gives shape to the outer edges of the eyelids

Exercises

A. Your work with elements is important to build your medical vocabulary. *Many of the prefixes and suffixes you see in this chapter you will meet in later chapters and use to build your knowledge of additional medical terms. Fill in the chart.*   **LO 16.1, 16.3**

Medical Term	Prefix	Meaning of Prefix	Root(s)/ Combining Form	Meaning of Root(s)/ Combining Form	Suffix	Meaning of Suffix
purulent	1.	2.	3.	4.	5.	6.
conjunctivitis	7.	8.	9.	10.	11.	12.
lysozyme	13.	14.	15.	16.	17.	18.
periorbital	19.	20.	21.	22.	23.	24.
ophthalmology	25.	26.	27.	28.	29.	30.
nasolacrimal	31.	32.	33.	34.	35.	36.
ophthalmologist	37.	38.	39.	40.	41.	42.

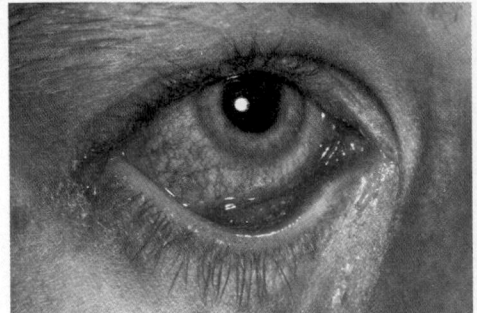

▲ **Figure 16.2**   Conjunctivitis.

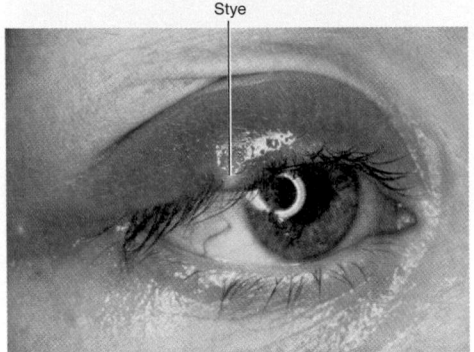

▲ **Figure 16.3**   Stye Showing Pus-Filled Cyst.

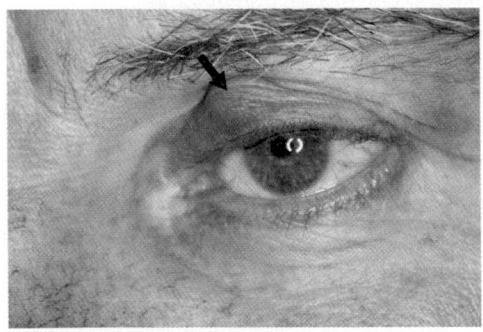

▲ **Figure 16.4**   Chalazion in Upper Eyelid.

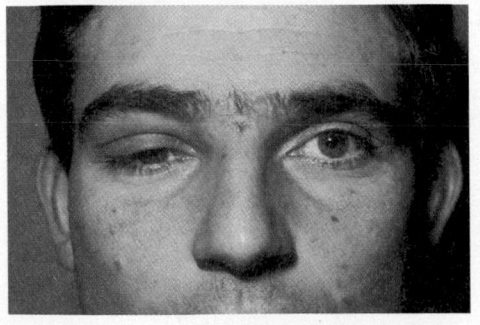

▲ **Figure 16.5**   Ptosis of Right Eyelid.

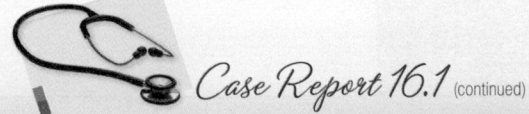

Case Report 16.1 (continued)

Mrs. Jenny Hughes's "pink eye" is called acute **contagious** conjunctivitis [see Figure 16.3]. It responds well to **antibiotic** eyedrops. Her hands were **contaminated** from the keyboard of the employee who had left work and gone home with "pink eye." Mrs. Hughes transmitted the infection from her fingers to her eyes by touching or rubbing.

Your documentation of Mrs. Hughes's office visit could read

Progress Note 04/10/13

Mrs. Jenny Hughes was brought directly into the clinical area at 1030 hrs with what appeared to be conjunctivitis, "pink eye." Both eyelids were red and swollen with a purulent discharge. She complained of headache and photophobia. Dr. Chun prescribed Neosporin eyedrops, three drops every four hours (q.4.h). A swab was sent to the laboratory. I instructed and watched Mrs. Hughes wash her hands and use an alcohol-based hand gel. I then had her sign in and sign our Notice of Privacy Practices. I instructed her in the use of the drops and emphasized home care and hand care measures to prevent the infection from spreading to her family. She was given a return appointment in 1 week and told to call the office if the drops did not help. Daphne Butras, OT. 1055 hrs.

Abbreviation	
q.4.h.	every four hours

LO 16.3 Disorders of the Accessory Glands

Conjunctivitis (*Figure 16.2*), inflammation of the conjunctiva, is more commonly viral than bacterial and can also be caused by irritants such as chlorine, soaps, fumes, and smoke.

Eyelid edema, generalized swelling of the eyelids, is often produced by an allergic reaction due to cosmetics, pollen in the air, or stings and bites from insects.

A **stye**, or **hordeolum**, is an infection of an eyelash follicle producing an abscess (*Figure 16.3*), with localized pain, swelling, redness, and pus formation at the edge of the eyelid.

A **chalazion** is a small, painless, localized, whitish swelling inside the lid when a tarsal gland becomes blocked (*Figure 16.4*). It can disappear spontaneously or require surgical removal.

Blepharitis occurs when multiple eyelash follicles and tarsal glands become infected. The margin of the eyelid shows persistent redness and crusting and may become ulcerated. The infection is usually staphylococcal. It is treated with antibiotic ointments.

Dacryostenosis is blockage of the drainage of tears, usually due to narrowing of the nasolacrimal ducts.

Dacryocystitis is an infection of the lacrimal sac, with swelling and pus at the medial corner of the eye.

Ptosis occurs when the upper eyelid is constantly drooped over the eye due to **paresis** (partial paralysis) of the muscle that raises the upper lid (*Figure 16.5*). It can be associated with diabetes, myasthenia gravis, brain tumor, and muscular dystrophy, all of which are described in subsequent chapters. The term **blepharoptosis** is used for sagging of the eyelids due to excess skin. The plastic surgery procedure of **blepharoplasty** is used for the repair of the eyelid.

WORD	PRONUNCIATION	ELEMENTS		DEFINITION
antibiotic	AN-tih-bye-OT-ik	S/ P/ R/	-tic *pertaining to* anti- *against* -bio- *life*	A substance that has the capacity to destroy bacteria and other microorganisms
blepharitis	blef-ah-RYE-tis	S/ R/	-itis *inflammation, infection* blephar- *eyelid*	Inflammation of the eyelid
blepharoptosis	BLEF-ah-ROP-toe-sis	S/ R/CF	-ptosis *drooping* blephar/o- *eyelid*	Drooping of the upper eyelid
blepharoplasty	BLEF-ah-ro-plas-tee	S/	-plasty *surgical repair*	Surgical repair of the eyelid
chalazion	kah-LAY-zee-on		Greek *lump*	Cyst on the outer edge of an eyelid
contagious	kon-TAY-jus		Latin *touch closely*	Able to be transmitted, as infections transmitted from person to person or from person to air or surface to person
contaminate (verb)	kon-TAM-in-ate	S/ P/ R/	-ate *composed of,* *pertaining to* con- *together* -tamin- *touch*	To cause the presence of an infectious agent to be on any surface
contamination (noun)	KON-tam-ih-NAY-shun	S/	-ation *process*	Presence of an infectious agent on a surface or in substances
dacryocystitis	DAK-re-oh-sis-TIE-tis	S/ R/CF R/	-itis *inflammation, infection* dacry/o- *tears* -cyst- *sac*	Inflammation of the lacrimal sac
dacryostenosis	DAK-re-oh-ste-NO-sis	S/ R/	-osis *condition* -sten- *narrowing*	Narrowing of the nasolacrimal duct
hordeolum stye (syn)	hor-DEE-oh-lum		Latin *stye in the eye*	Abscess in an eyelash follicle
paresis	par-EE-sis		Greek *paralysis*	Partial paralysis
ptosis (**Note:** When a word begins with two consonants, the first is silent.)	TOE-sis		Greek *drooping*	Sinking down of an eyelid or an organ

Exercises

A. Disorders: The accessory structures of the eye have their own disorders. *The patient conditions are described in the left column; match the condition with the correct medical term (right column) from this lesson. Fill in the blanks.* **LO 16.3**

_____ 1. allergic reaction to pollen

_____ 2. drooping of upper eyelid over eye

_____ 3. infection of the lacrimal sac

_____ 4. produced by a blocked tarsal gland

_____ 5. blockage of the drainage of tears

_____ 6. red, crusted, and ulcerated eyelid

_____ 7. pus at the edge of the eyelid

a. chalazion

b. hordeolum

c. dacryostenosis

d. blepharitis

e. eyelid edema

f. dacryocystitis

g. ptosis

You are

...an ophthalmic technician (OT) working with Angela Chun, MD, an ophthalmologist at Fulwood Medical Center.

Your patient is

...Sam Hughes, a 2-year-old boy, who has been referred by his pediatrician to Dr. Chun.

Case Report 16.2

His mother, Mrs. Jenny Hughes, states that she has noticed for the past couple of months that his right eye has turned in. The only visual difficulty she has noticed is that he sometimes misses a Cheerio when he tries to grab it. Otherwise, he is healthy.

You are responsible for documenting Sam's diagnostic and therapeutic procedures and explaining the significance of these to his mother.

LO 16.4 Extrinsic Muscles of the Eye

Humans, with their two eyes working closely together, have developed very good three-dimensional perception (**stereopsis**) and hand-eye coordination. Stereopsis depends on an accurate alignment of the two eyes.

This alignment is held in place by the coordination of six **extrinsic eye muscles** in each eye that are attached to the inner wall of the orbit and to the outer surface of the eyeball (*Figure 16.6*). These muscles move the eye in all directions.

When there is muscle imbalance in one eye, as in Sam's case, the alignment breaks down, and the resulting condition is called **strabismus**, also known in lay terms as "squinting" or "cross-eyed."

Esotropia is the eye turned in toward the nose. In **congenital** or infantile **esotropia**, both eyes look in toward the nose—the right eye looks to the left, and the left eye looks to the right. These children require surgical intervention.

Accommodative esotropia is an inward eye turn, usually noticed around 2 years of age in 1% to 2% of children (*Figure 16.7*). In Sam's case, he had an accommodative esotropia in one eye. He will probably respond to treatment using glasses and perhaps a patch over the stronger eye to encourage use of the weaker eye.

Exotropia, an outward turning of one eye, is noticed around 2 to 4 years of age. It will often respond to vision therapy, which includes eye exercises and glasses, from an **optometrist**. Eye muscle surgery may be necessary to establish good **ocular** alignment.

Strabismus is not the same as **amblyopia**, or "lazy eye," which occurs in children when vision in one eye has not developed as well as in the other. It occurs because the eye and the brain are not cooperating for the one eye. Treatment involves getting the child to develop the vision in the weaker eye. This can be done by putting a patch over the stronger eye full-time or part-time or using **atropine** eyedrops to blur the vision in the stronger eye.

Keynote

Amblyopia is the failure or incomplete development of the pathways of vision to the brain.

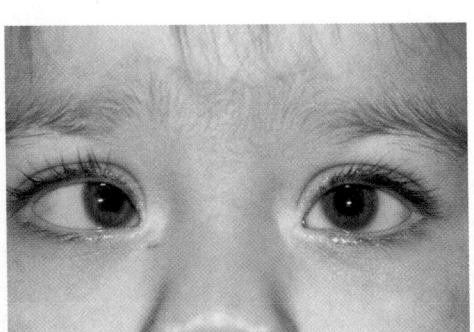

▲ **Figure 16.7** Strabismus with Right Eye Turned Inward.

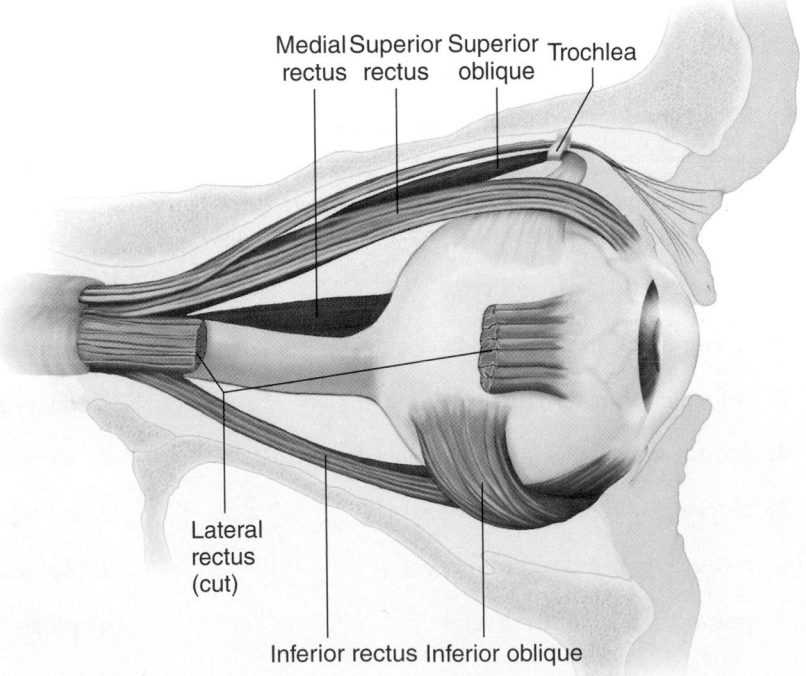

▲ **Figure 16.6** Extrinsic Muscles of the Right Eye. Lateral View.

WORD	PRONUNCIATION	ELEMENTS		DEFINITION
accommodation	ah-kom-oh-**DAY**-shun	S/	-ion *action*	The act of adjusting something to make it fit the needs; in the case of the eye, the lens adjusts itself
accommodate (verb)	ah-**KOM**-oh-date	S/ P/ R/	-ion *action process* ac- *toward* **-commodat-** *adjust*	
amblyopia	am-blee-**OH**-pee-ah	P/ R/	ambly- *dull* -opia *sight*	Failure or incomplete development of the pathways of vision to the brain
atropine	**AT**-ro-peen		Greek *belladonna*	Pharmacologic agent used to dilate pupils
congenital	kon-**JEN**-ih-tal	S/ P/ R/	-al *pertaining to* con- *together, with* **-genit-** *bring forth*	Present at birth, either inherited or due to an event during gestation up to the moment of birth
esotropia	es-oh-**TROH**-pee-ah	S/ P/ R/	-ia *condition* eso- *inward* **-trop-** *turn*	A turning of the eye inward toward the nose
exotropia	ek-soh-**TROH**-pee-ah	S/ P/ R/	-ia *condition* exo- *outward* **-trop-** *turn*	A turning of the eye outward away from the nose
extrinsic **intrinsic**	eks-**TRIN**-sik in-**TRIN**-sik		Latin *on the outer side* Latin *on the inner side*	Extrinsic eye muscles are located on the outside of the eye, as opposed to intrinsic muscles, which are located inside the eye
ocular	**OCK**-you-lar	S/ R/	-ar *pertaining to* **ocul-** *eye*	Pertaining to the eye
optometrist	op-**TOM**-eh-trist	R/CF S/	opt/o- *vision* -metrist *skilled in measurement*	Someone who is skilled in the measurement of vision but cannot treat eye diseases or prescribe medication
stereopsis	ster-ee-**OP**-sis	S/ R/	-opsis *vision* **stere-** *three-dimensional*	Three-dimensional vision
strabismus	strah-**BIZ**-mus	S/ R/	-ismus *take action* **strab-** *squint*	A turning of an eye away from its normal position

Exercises

A. Notice in this exercise that not every medical term needs a prefix and/or a suffix. *However, every medical term does contain one or more roots and/or combining forms.* **Deconstruct** *the following medical terms into their elements. Fill in the chart.* **LO 16.1, 16.4**

Medical Term	Prefix	Root(s)/Combining Form	Suffix
strabismus	1.	2.	3.
exotropia	4.	5.	6.
accommodation	7.	8.	9.
optometrist	10.	11.	12.
esotropia	13.	14.	15.
amblyopia	16.	17.	18.
stereopsis	19.	20.	21.

B. Use the terms in Exercise A to fill in the blanks in the statements in Exercise B.   LO 16.1, 16.4

1. skilled in the measurement of vision _____

2. a turning of the eye outward away from the nose _____

3. failure or incomplete development of the pathways of vision to the brain _____

4. turning of the eye inward toward the nose _____

5. a turning of an eye away from its normal position _____

6. three-dimensional vision _____

7. the adjustment of the lens by itself _____

The eyeball is a fluid-filled globe about 1 inch in diameter. Knowledge of its terminology, structure, and function enables you to understand how we see and what major problems and disorders of the eyeball can arise.

In this lesson, the information will enable you to:

16.2.1 Identify the principal components of the eyeball.

16.2.2 Explain the role of the cornea and the problems that can occur in that structure.

16.2.3 Describe the structure and functions of the lens and its associated structures.

16.2.4 Link the different components of the retina to their functions.

16.2.5 Discuss common disorders of the eyeball and its components.

16.2.6 Apply correct medical terminology to the anatomy, physiology, and disorders of the eyeball.

Keynotes

- The cornea protects the eye and, by changing shape, provides about 60% of the eye's focusing power.

- The pupil controls the amount of light entering the eye.

- The lens changes its shape to focus rays of light onto the retina.

- Both the cornea and the lens refract light rays. Neither has a blood supply, which compromises healing from injury or disease.

LO 16.5 The Eyeball (Globe)

The functions of the eyeball are to

- *Adjust* continuously the amount of light it lets in to reach the retina.

- *Focus* continuously on near and distant objects.

- *Produce images* continuously of those objects and instantly transmit them to the brain.

The front of the eyeball (except for the cornea) is covered by the conjunctiva, a thin layer of tissue that covers the inside of the eyelids and curves over the eyeball to meet the **sclera**, the tough, white outer layer of the eye.

The center of the front of the eye is a transparent, dome-shaped membrane called the **cornea**. The cornea has no blood supply and obtains its nutrients from tears and from fluid in the **anterior chamber** behind it.

When light rays strike the eye, they pass through the cornea. Because of its domed curvature, those rays striking the edge of the cornea are bent toward its center. The light rays then go through the **pupil**, the black opening in the center of the colored area (the **iris**) in the front of the eye.

The pupil controls the amount of light entering the eye. When you are in a dark place, the pupil opens (dilates) to allow more light to enter. When you are in bright light, the pupil closes (constricts) to admit less light. The **sphincter pupillae muscle** (*Figure 16.8*) opens and closes the pupil.

After passing through the pupil, the light rays pass through the transparent **lens**. The ciliary muscle of the **ciliary body** makes the lens thicker and thinner, enabling it to bend the light rays and focus them on the **retina** at the back of the eye. This process of changing focus is called **accommodation**. The process of bending the light rays by the cornea and lens is called **refraction**.

The lens has no supply of blood vessels or nerves. With increasing age, the lens loses its elasticity. When you reach your forties, your eyes may have difficulty focusing on near objects, and the telephone directory can become unreadable without spectacles, a condition called **presbyopia**.

Medical shorthand for a quick normal eye examination can be **PERRLA**, which means *p*upils *e*qual, *r*ound, *r*eactive to *l*ight and *a*ccommodation.

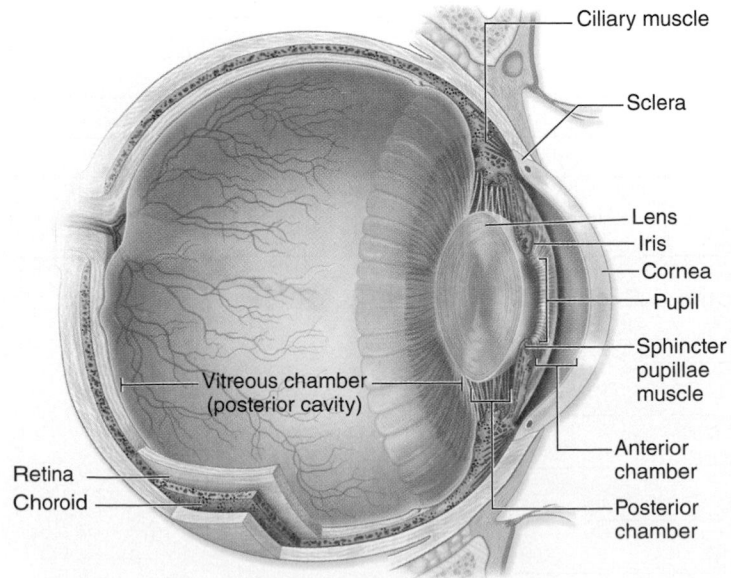

▲ Figure 16.8   Anatomy of the Eyeball.

Labels: Ciliary muscle · Sclera · Lens · Iris · Cornea · Pupil · Sphincter pupillae muscle · Anterior chamber · Posterior chamber · Vitreous chamber (posterior cavity) · Retina · Choroid

Abbreviation	
PERRLA	pupils equal, round, reactive to light and accommodation

WORD	PRONUNCIATION	ELEMENTS		DEFINITION
ciliary body	SILL-ee-ary BOD-ee	S R/ R/	-ary *pertaining to* cili- *eyelid* body *mass*	Muscles that make the eye lens thicker and thinner
iris	EYE-ris		Greek *diaphragm of the eye*	Colored portion of the eye with the pupil in its center
lens	LENZ		Latin *lentil shape*	Transparent refractive structure behind the iris
presbyopia	prez-bee-OH-pee-ah	R/ R/	-opia *sight* presby- *old person*	Difficulty in nearsighted vision occurring in middle and old age
pupil pupillae (pl) pupillary (adj)	PYU-pill pyu-PILL-ee PYU-pill-AH-ree		Latin *pupil*	The opening in the center of the iris that allows light to reach the lens
refract (verb) refraction (noun)	ree-FRACT ree-FRAK-shun		Latin *break up*	Make a change in direction of, or bend, a ray of light
retina retinal (adj)	RET-ih-nah RET-ih-nal		Latin *net*	Light-sensitive innermost layer of eyeball
sclera	SKLAIR-ah		Greek *hard*	Fibrous outer covering of the eyeball and the white of the eye
scleral (adj)	SKLAIR-al	S/ R/	al *pertaining to* scler- *hard, white of eye*	Pertaining to the sclera
scleritis	sklair-RI-tis	S/	-itis *inflammation*	Inflammation of the sclera
sphincter	SFINK-ter		Greek *band*	Band of muscle that encircles an opening; when it contracts, the opening squeezes closed

Exercises

A. Components of the eyeball: Enhance your knowledge of the components of the eyeball and their functions. *This will help you to understand the vision process. Match the phrase in the left column with the appropriate medical term in the right column.*   **LO 16.5**

_____ 1. Colored portion of the eye

_____ 2. Change direction of a ray of light

_____ 3. Opening in the iris

_____ 4. Band of muscle that encircles an opening

_____ 5. Transparent, refractive structure

_____ 6. Difficulty in nearsighted vision

_____ 7. Innermost layer of eyeball

_____ 8. White of the eye

_____ 9. Operate the lens

_____ 10. Normal eye examination

a. lens

b. retina

c. sphincter

d. pupil

e. ciliary body

f. PERRLA

g. refract

h. iris

i. presbyopia

j. sclera

B. Review the text and the above WAD to find the answers to the following questions. *Fill in the blanks.*   **LO 16.1, 16.2**

1. Critical thinking: The eye has a sphincter muscle. What other part of the body has a sphincter muscle?

_____

2. Use the correct grammatical form of the medical terms in the WAD to fill in the blanks.

   a. The patient has an abrasion on her _____. This _____ injury has caused her _____.

   b. The doctor has examined both _____ and confirms a _____ injury.

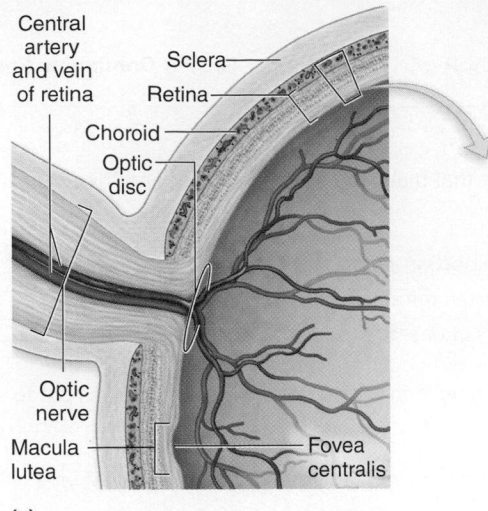

(a)

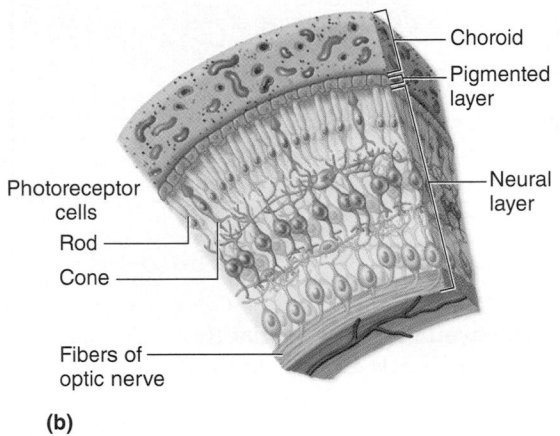

(b)

▲ **Figure 16.9** Structure of the Retina.

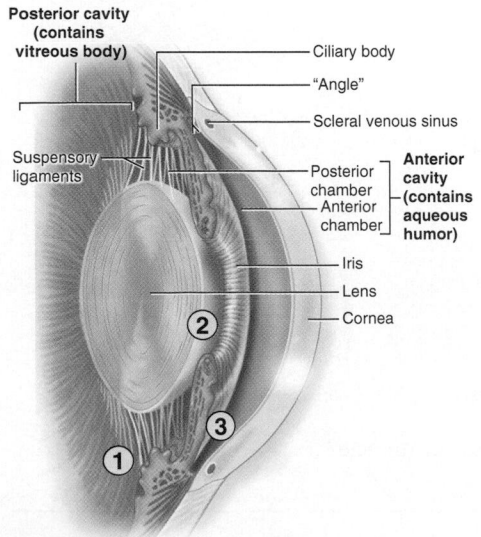

▲ **Figure 16.10** Circulation of Aqueous Humor.

LO 16.5 The Eyeball (Globe) (continued)

The Retina

The final destination of the light rays is the **retina**, the thin lining at the back of your eye *(Figure 16.9a)*. It's an area the size of a small postage stamp that has 10 layers of cells. The retina has 130 million **rods** *(Figure 16.9b)*, which perceive only light, not color, and function mostly when the light is dim. There are 6.5 million **cones** *(see Figure 16.10b)*, which are activated by light and color and have precise **visual acuity**. Different cones respond to red, blue, and green light. Your perception of color is based on the intensity of different mixtures of colors from the three types of cones.

Some people have a hereditary lack of response by one or more of the three types of cones and show **color blindness**. The most common form is red-green color blindness, in which these colors and related shades cannot be distinguished from each other.

Rods and cones are called **photoreceptor** cells. The rods and cones convert the energy of the light rays into electrical impulses, and the **optic nerve**, a bundle of more than a million nerve fibers, transmits these impulses to the **visual cortex** at the back of the brain. The area where the optic nerve leaves the retina is called the **optic disc**. Because it has no rods and cones, the optic disc cannot form images and is called the **blind spot**.

Night blindness is the inability to see in poor light. It is a symptom of an underlying problem that can be

- Uncorrected nearsightedness.
- Cataracts.
- Retinitis pigmentosa.
- Vitamin A deficiency.
- Glaucoma medications (such as pilocarpine) that constrict the pupil.

Just lateral to the optic disc at the back of the retina is a circular, yellowish region called the **macula lutea** *(see Figure 16.9a)*. In the center of the macula is a small pit called the **fovea centralis**, which has 4000 tiny cones and no rods. Each cone has its own nerve fiber, and this makes the fovea the area of sharpest vision. As you read this text, the words are precisely focused on your fovea centralis.

Behind the photoreceptor layer of the retina is a very **vascular** layer called the **choroid**. This layer, together with the iris and **ciliary body**, is called the **uvea**.

Segments of the Eye

The eyeball is divided into two fluid-filled segments separated by the lens and the ciliary muscle. The fluids maintain the shape of the eyeball. In the back, the **posterior cavity** extends from the back of the lens to the retina and contains a transparent jelly called the **vitreous body**, which helps maintain the shape of the eyeball.

In front, the **anterior cavity** extends from the cornea to the lens and is divided into two chambers. The **anterior chamber** extends from the cornea to the iris, and the **posterior chamber** extends from the iris to the lens *(Figure 16.10)*. **Aqueous humor** is produced in the posterior chamber as a filtrate from plasma (Step 1). It passes through the pupil into the anterior chamber (Step 2) where it is continually reabsorbed into a vascular space called the **scleral venous sinus** (Step 3) and taken into the venous bloodstream. The aqueous humor also removes waste products and helps maintain the internal chemical environment of the eye.

Keynotes

- Rods of the retina perceive only dim light and not color.
- Cones of the retina perceive bright light and color.
- Rods and cones are called photoreceptor cells.

WORD	PRONUNCIATION	ELEMENTS		DEFINITION
aqueous humor	ACHE-we-us HEW-mor	S/ R/CF	-ous *pertaining to* aqu/e- *watery* humor *Greek liquid*	Watery liquid in the anterior and posterior chambers of the eye
choroid	KOR-oid		Greek *membrane*	Region of the retina and uvea
fovea centralis	FOH-vee-ah sen-TRAH-lis		fovea Latin *a pit*	Small pit in the center of the macula that has the highest visual acuity
macula lutea	MAK-you-lah LOO-tee-ah		macula *small spot* lutea *yellow*	Yellowish spot on the back of the retina; contains the fovea centralis
optic optical (adj)	OP-tick OP-tih-kal	S/ R/	Greek *eye* -ical *pertaining to* opt- *eye*	Pertaining to the eye
photoreceptor	foh-toe-ree-SEP-tor	S/ R/CF R/	-or *that which does something* phot/o- *light* -recept- *receive*	A photoreceptor cell receives light and converts it into electrical impulses
uvea	YOU-vee-ah		Greek *layer of eyeball*	Middle coat of eyeball; includes iris, ciliary body, and choroid
uveitis	you-vee-I-tis	S/ R/	-itis *inflammation* uve- *uvea*	Inflammation of the uvea
visual acuity	VIH-zhoo-wal ah-KYU-ih-tee	S/ R/	-al *pertaining to* visu- *sight* acuity Latin *sharpen*	Sharpness and clearness of vision
vitreous humor	VIT-ree-us HEW-mor		Latin *glass*	A gelatinous liquid in the posterior cavity of the eyeball with the appearance of glass

Exercises

A. The medical terms contained in these two pages will be the answers in the following exercise on the retina and segments of the eye. *Review the above WAD and text before you begin the exercise. Circle the best answer.* **LO 16.1, 16.5**

1. Sharpness and clearness of vision is called

   a. optical

   b. acuity

   c. vascular

   d. aqueous

   e. choroid

2. The term **photoreceptor** has

   a. two combining forms and a suffix

   b. a prefix, root, and suffix

   c. a root, a combining form, and a suffix

   d. two roots and a suffix

   e. a suffix and a root

3. The choroid, iris, and ciliary body make up the

   a. optic disc

   b. blind spot

   c. uvea

   d. visual cortex

   e. optic nerve

4. The gel contained in the posterior cavity is called

   a. vitreous humor

   b. ciliary body

   c. visual cortex

   d. aqueous humor

   e. macula lutea

5. This helps maintain the shape of the eyeball:

   a. vitreous body

   b. rods

   c. fovea centralis

   d. cones

   e. macula lutea

6. The area of sharpest vision is the

   a. cornea

   b. rods

   c. macula lutea

   d. fovea centralis

   e. choroid

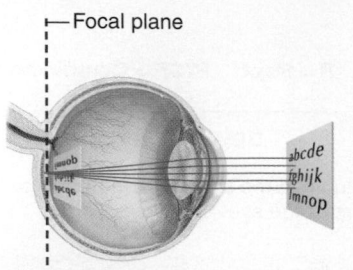

▲ **Figure 16.12**　Emmetropia, Normal Vision.

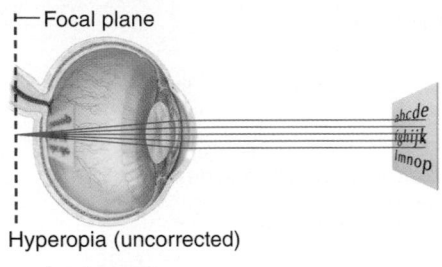

Hyperopia (uncorrected)

Corrected focal plane　Convex corrective lens

▲ **Figure 16.13**　Hyperopia (Farsightedness).

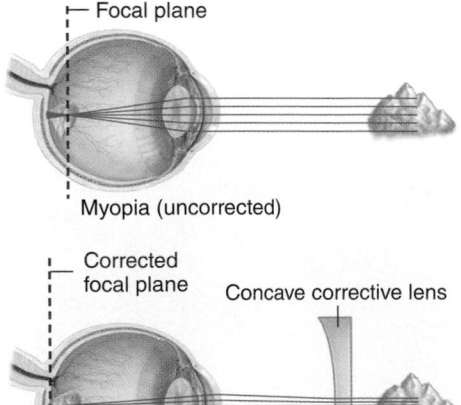

Myopia (uncorrected)

Corrected focal plane　Concave corrective lens

▲ **Figure 16.14**　Myopia (Nearsightedness).

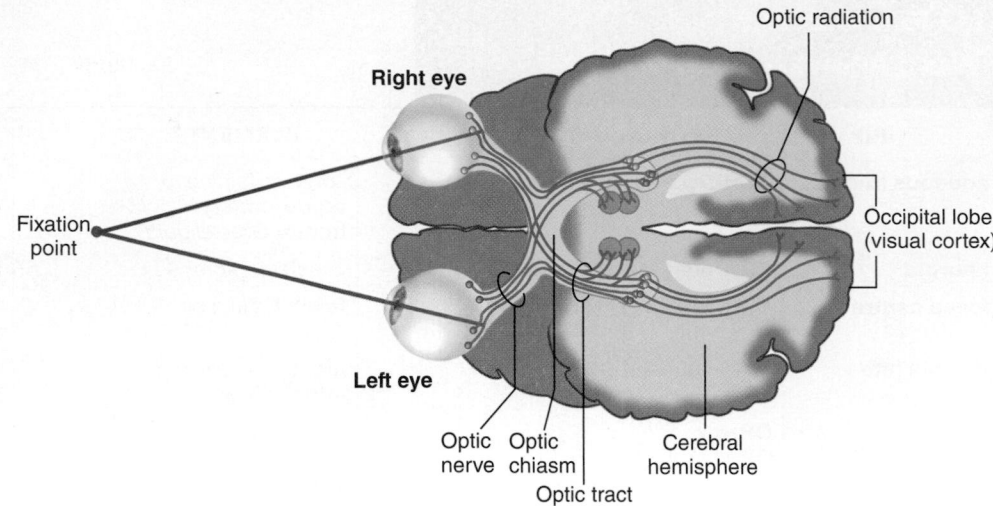

▲ **Figure 16.11**　Visual Pathway.

LO 16.6　Visual Pathway

After the optic nerves leave the back of your retina and eyeball, they leave each orbit through the **optic foramen**. They converge into an "X" called the **optic chiasm** (*Figure 16.11*). Here, the fibers from the medial half of each retina cross to the opposite side of the brain.

After leaving the chiasm, the fibers form the **optic tract** and then the **optic radiation** to take the nerve impulses to the **visual cortex** in the **occipital lobes** at the back of your brain. Here the incoming visual stimuli are interpreted.

Refraction

Light is traveling at a speed of 186,000 miles per second when it hits your eye. Light rays that hit the center of your cornea pass straight through, but because of the curvature of the cornea, rays that hit away from center are bent toward the center. The light rays then hit your lens, are bent again, and, in normal vision, the image is focused sharply on your retina (*Figure 16.12*). This normal vision is called **emmetropia**.

Farsighted people are said to have **hyperopia** (*Figure 16.13*). Because the eyeball is shortened, objects close to the eye are focused behind the retina and vision is blurred. Convex lenses are needed to correct the problem.

Nearsighted people are said to have **myopia** (*Figure 16.14*). Because the eyeball is elongated, faraway objects are focused in front of the retina. Vision is blurred. Concave lenses are needed to correct the problem.

In **presbyopia**, the lens loses its flexibility, so there is difficulty focusing for near vision. This happens when you reach your forties. Convex bifocal or transitional lenses are needed for this problem.

In **astigmatism**, unequal curvatures of the cornea cause unequal focusing and blurred images. Cylindrical lenses, which refract light more in one plane than another, are needed to correct this problem.

A surgical procedure, **radial keratotomy**, is used to treat myopia. Radial cuts, like the spokes of a wheel, flatten the cornea and enable it to refract the light rays to focus on the retina.

Laser surgery can also change the shape of the cornea. It can flatten it to correct myopia or alter the outer edges of the cornea to correct hyperopia.

Laser-assisted in situ keratomileusis (LASIK) is being used to treat myopia, hyperopia, and astigmatism. A hinged flap of cornea is reflected (laid back) surgically to expose the midsection of the cornea. A computer-controlled laser, using a cold beam of ultraviolet light, alters the shape of the cornea by vaporizing the tissue.

S = Suffix   P = Prefix   R = Root   R/CF = Combining Form

WORD	PRONUNCIATION	ELEMENTS		DEFINITION
astigmatism	ah-**STIG**-mah-tism	S/ P/ R/	-ism *action* a- *without* -stigmat- *focus*	Inability to focus light rays that enter the eye in different planes
chiasm chiasma (alternative term)	**KYE**-asm **KYE**-az-mah		Greek *cross*	X-shaped crossing of the two optic nerves at the base of the brain
emmetropia	emm-eh-**TROH**-pee-ah	P/ R/	emmetr- *measure* -opia *sight*	Normal refractive condition of the eye
foramen foramina (pl)	fo-**RAY**-men fo-**RAM**-ih-nah		Latin *hole*	An opening through a structure
hyperopia	high-per-**OH**-pee-ah	P/ R/	hyper- *beyond* -opia *sight*	Able to see distant objects but unable to see close objects
in situ	IN **SIGH**-tyu		Latin *in its original place*	In the correct place
keratomileusis	ker-ah-**TOE**-mill-oo-sis	R/ R/CF	-mileusis *lathe* kerat/o- *cornea*	A surgical procedure that involves cutting and shaping the cornea
keratotomy	ker-ah-**TOT**-oh-mee	S/ R/CF	-tomy *surgical incision* kerat/o- *cornea*	Incision in the cornea
myopia (**Note:** An "o" is removed from the elements.)	my-**OH**-pee-ah	P/ R/	myo- *to blink* -opia *sight*	Able to see close objects but unable to see distant objects
presbyopia	prez-bee-**OH**-pee-ah	R/ R/	presby- *old person* -opia *sight*	Difficulty in nearsighted vision occurring in middle and old age in both sexes
radiation	ray-dee-**AY**-shun	S/ R/	-ation *process* radi- *radius, radiation*	A spreading out, as of anatomical parts
tract	TRAKT		Latin *path*	Bundle of nerve fibers with a common origin and destination

Exercises

A. Create new medical terms by applying different prefixes to the root opia. *The definition of each term is provided; you construct the medical term. Fill in the blanks.* **LO 16.6, 16.7**

1. Meaning of **opia:** _____.

2. Difficulty in nearsighted vision occurring in middle and old age: _____/opia

3. Normal refractive condition of the eye: _____/opia

4. Able to see close objects but unable to see distant ones: _____/opia

5. Able to see distant objects but unable to see close objects: _____/opia

6. *Challenge question:* If **dipl/o** means *double* and *two*, what then is diplopia? _____

B. Circle the correct answer, using the *language of ophthalmology*. **LO 16.1, 16.2, 16.6**

1. Which of the following medical terms does not apply to the visual pathway?

   a. visual cortex

   b. occipital lobes

   c. optic foramen

   d. labyrinth

   e. optic tract

2. What eye condition requires cylindrical lenses for correction?

   a. astigmatism

   b. myopia

   c. hyperopia

   d. emmetropia

   e. presbyopia

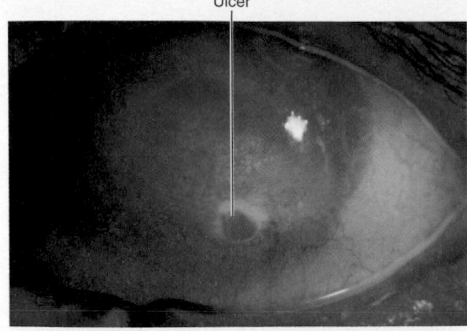

▲ **Figure 16.15**　Fluorescein-Stained Corneal Ulcer.

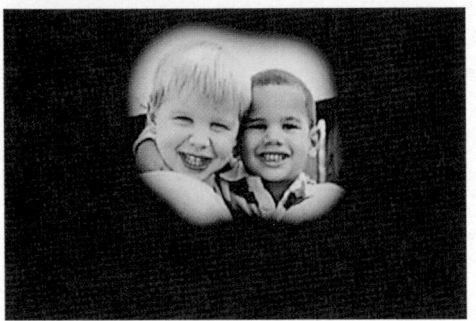

▲ **Figure 16.16**　Vision with Glaucoma.

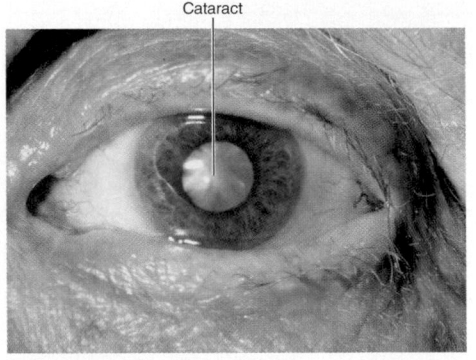

▲ **Figure 16.17**　Cataract.

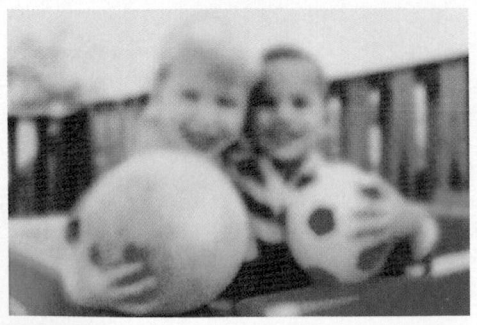

▲ **Figure 16.18**　Vision with Cataract.

LO 16.8　Disorders of the Anterior Eyeball

Conjunctivitis is the **infectious**, contagious condition that Mrs. Jenny Hughes had in the first Case Report in this chapter. It can be caused by viruses, many different bacteria, and organisms that cause sexually transmitted diseases (STDs, see *Chapter 8*). It is a cause of "bloodshot" eyes.

Allergic conjunctivitis can be part of seasonal **hay fever** or be produced by year-round **allergens** such as animal dander and dust mites (*see Chapter 12*). **Irritant conjunctivitis** can be caused by air **pollutants** (smoke and fumes) and by chemicals such as chlorine and those found in soaps and cosmetics.

Neonatal conjunctivitis (ophthalmia neonatorum) can be caused by a blocked tear duct in the baby, by the antibiotic eyedrops given routinely at birth, or by sexually transmitted bacteria in an infected mother's birth canal.

Corneal abrasions can be caused by foreign bodies, by direct trauma (such as being poked by a fingernail), or by badly fitting contact lenses. The abrasion can grow into an ulcer. The lesions can be stained with drops of the green dye **fluorescein** to make them more easily visible on examination (*Figure 16.15*).

Scleritis, inflammation of the sclera (the white outer covering of the eyeball) can affect one or both eyes. It causes dull pain and intense redness and is often associated with rheumatoid arthritis (*see Chapter 14*) and the digestive disorder Crohn disease (*see Chapter 5*).

Uveitis, inflammation of the iris, ciliary body, and choroid, produces pain, intense photophobia, blurred vision, and constriction of the pupil. There is usually an underlying disease, such as rheumatoid arthritis.

Glaucoma

The circulation of aqueous humor was described earlier in this chapter. If the aqueous humor cannot escape from the eye into the bloodstream, the fluid continues to be produced and pressure builds up inside the eye. The pressure interferes with the blood supply to the retina, causing death of retinal cells. Eventually the optic nerve fibers are damaged. This condition is called **glaucoma** and is a major cause of blindness (*Figure 16.16*). Treatment is lifelong use of eyedrops to arrest the advance of glaucoma, but lost vision cannot be restored.

Cataracts

A **cataract** is a cloudy or opaque area in the lens (*Figure 16.17*). It is typically caused by deterioration of the lens due to aging and may be associated with diabetes and with cigarette smoke. It presents with blurring of vision and **photosensitivity** or may be discovered on routine eye examination. It is another major cause of blindness.

The majority of cataracts occur in the center of the lens, but those associated with diabetes can be cortical (around the outside of the lens). Cortical cataracts can cause diminished **peripheral vision** and photosensitivity.

When a cataract interferes with vision (*Figure 16.18*), the lens needs to be removed and replaced with an artificial **intraocular** lens, which becomes a permanent part of the eye. A surgical technique called **phacoemulsification** uses ultrasonic waves to fragment the cataract, making its removal much easier.

WORD	PRONUNCIATION		ELEMENTS	DEFINITION
abrasion	ah-**BRAY**-shun		Latin *to scrape off*	Area of skin or mucous membrane that has been scraped off
allergen	**AL**-er-jen	S/	-gen *create*	Substance producing a hypersensitivity (allergic) reaction
		S/	-er- *agent*	
		R/	**all-** *other, strange*	
allergy	**AL**-er-jee	S/	-ergy *process of working*	Hypersensitivity to an allergen
allergic (adj)	ah-**LER**-jik	S/	-ic *pertaining to*	Pertaining to being hypersensitive
cataract	**KAT**-ah-ract		Greek *waterfall*	Complete or partial opacity of the lens
fluorescein	flor-**ESS**-ee-in	P/	fluo- *fluorine*	Dye that produces a vivid green color under a blue light to diagnose corneal abrasions and foreign bodies in the eye
		R/	-rescein *resin*	
glaucoma	glau-**KOH**-mah	S/	-oma *mass, tumor*	Increased intraocular pressure
		R/	**glauc-** *lens opacity*	
infectious	in-**FEK**-shus	S/	-ous *pertaining to*	Capable of being transmitted, or caused by infection by a microorganism
		R/CF	**infect/i-** *internal invasion*	
intraocular	in-trah-**OCK**-you-lar	S/	-ar *pertaining to*	Pertaining to the inside of the eye
		P/	intra- *inside*	
		R/	-ocul- *eye*	
ophthalmia	off-**THAL**-me-ah	S/	-ia *condition*	Conjunctivitis of the newborn
neonatorum	ne-oh-nay-**TOR**-um	R/	**ophthalm-** *eye*	
		S	-orum *function of*	
		P/	neo- *new*	
		R/	**-nat-** *born*	
neonatal	**NEE**-oh-**NAY**-tal	S/	-al *pertaining to*	Pertaining to the newborn infant
peripheral vision	peh-**RIF**-er-al **VIZH**-un	S/	-al *pertaining to*	Ability to see objects as they come into the outer edges of the visual field
		R/	**peripher-** *external boundary*	
phacoemulsification	fake-oh-ee-**MUL**-sih-fih-**KAY**-shun	S/	-ation *process*	Technique used to fragment the center of the lens into very tiny pieces and suck them out of the eye
		P/	phaco- *lens*	
		R/	**-emulsific-** *to milk out*	
photosensitivity	foh-toe-**SEN**-sih-tiv-ih-tee	S/	-ity *condition*	Condition in which light produces pain in the eye
photosensitive (adj)	foh-toe-**SEN**-sih-tiv	R/CF	**phot/o-** *light*	
		R/	**-sensitiv-** *sensitive*	
pollution	poh-**LOO**-shun	S/	-ion *condition*	Condition that is unclean, impure, and a danger to health
		R/	**pollut-** *to defile*	
pollutant	poh-**LOO**-tant	S/	-ant *pertaining to*	Substance that makes the environment unclean or impure

Exercises

A. Review the medical terms in the above WAD. *Use the* language of ophthalmology *to complete the sentences. You may use a term only one time. Fill in the blanks.*   **LO 16.1, 16.8**

1. Dust mites and pollen are _____.

2. Scratching your eye with a tree branch produces a(n) _____.

3. _____ produces increased intraocular pressure.

4. Phacoemulsification is a treatment for _____.

5. Sensitivity to light that produces eye pain is _____.

6. Another name for conjunctivitis of the newborn is _____.

7. _____ refers to anything pertaining to the inside of the eye.

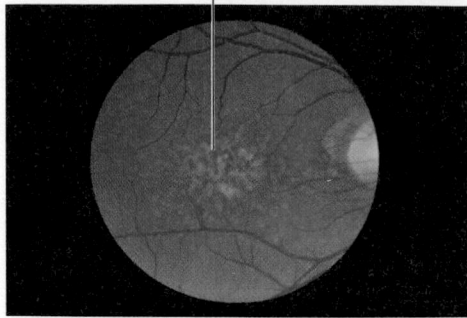

▲ **Figure 16.19** Ophthalmoscopic View of Macular Degeneration.

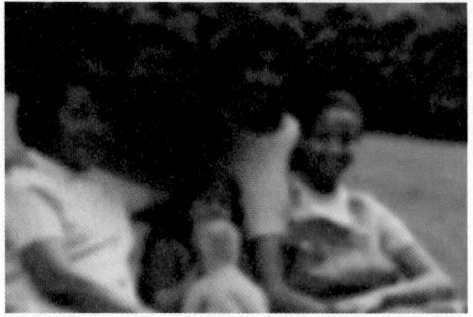

▲ **Figure 16.20** Vision with Macular Degeneration.

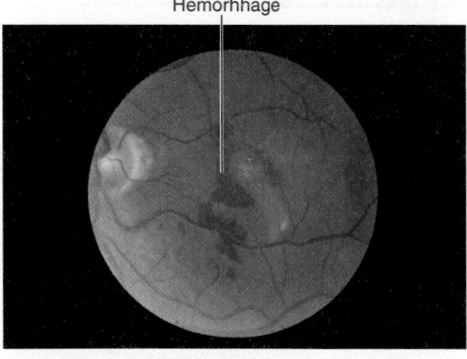

▲ **Figure 16.21** Ophthalmoscopic View of Diabetic Retinopathy.

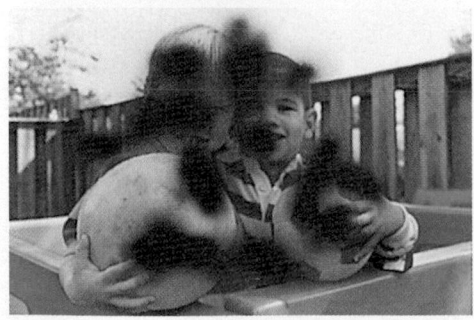

▲ **Figure 16.22** Vision with Diabetic Retinopathy.

LO 16.8 Diseases of the Retina

Macular Degeneration

Degeneration of the central macula results in loss of visual acuity, with a dark blurry area of vision loss in the center of the visual field *(Figures 16.19 and 16.20)*.

There is photoreceptor cell loss and bleeding, with capillary proliferation and scar formation. The condition can progress to blindness. Most cases occur in people over age 55.

At this time, there is no known cure, but laser **photocoagulation** destroys the abnormal capillaries, thereby slowing the pace of the visual loss.

Retinal Detachment

Separation of the retina from its underlying choroid layer may be partial or complete and produces a retinal tear or hole. The detachment can happen suddenly, without pain. The patient sees a dark shadow invading his peripheral vision. The detachment can be seen on **ophthalmoscopic** examination.

When the retina is detached, photoreceptor cells can die; this condition is a surgical emergency. Treatment of small lesions is by **laser surgery**. The laser creates tiny burns around the tear to "weld" the retina back in place. Another form of treatment, **cryopexy**, freezes the area around the hole to help it reattach to the surrounding retina.

Diabetic Retinopathy

This disease occurs most frequently in diabetics whose blood sugar levels are not controlled. Some 50% of diabetics have **retinopathy**.

In the early stages, **microaneurysms** of the small retinal blood vessels form. There are usually no symptoms. Later, hemorrhages can occur, leading to destruction of the photoreceptor cells (rods and cones) and visual difficulties.

Ophthalmoscopic examination shows the disease *(Figure 16.21)*, and **fluorescein angiography** with pictures taken as the dye passes through the retina reveals more details.

Laser photocoagulation is usually effective in controlling the lesions; but once vision is lost from an area of the retina, it usually does not return *(Figure 16.22)*.

Papilledema

Papilledema is swelling of the optic disc due to increased **intracranial** pressure. It is not a diagnosis; it is a sign of some underlying pathology. It is seen on ophthalmoscopic examination.

Cancer of the Eye

Tumors of the skin of the eyelids include the **squamous cell** and **basal cell carcinomas** and **melanoma** described in *Chapter 15*.

Retinoblastoma is the most common cancer in children and is diagnosed most commonly around 18 months of age. Twenty percent have the cancer in both eyes. The condition can be hereditary.

The first symptom is a white appearance of the pupil (**leukocoria**). With early detection and aggressive treatment based on chemotherapy and laser surgery, 90% of cases are cured.

In adults, the most common cancers are **metastases** to the eye from cancer of the lung in men and the breast in women.

WORD	PRONUNCIATION	ELEMENTS		DEFINITION
angiography	an-jee-**OG**-rah-fee	S/	-**graphy** *process of recording*	Radiography of vessels after injection of contrast material
angiogram	**AN**-jee-oh-gram	R/CF S/	**angi/o-** *blood vessel* -**gram** *a record*	Radiograph obtained after injection of radiopaque contrast material into blood vessels
cryopexy	cry-oh-**PEX**-ee	S/ R/CF	-**pexy** *fixation* **cry/o-** *cold*	Repair of a detached retina by freezing it to surrounding tissue
intracranial	in-trah-**KRAY**-nee-al	S/ P/ R/	-**al** *pertaining to* **intra-** *inside* -**crani-** *skull*	Within the cranium (skull)
laser surgery	**LAY**-zer **SUR**-jer-ee	R/ S/ R/	**laser** *acronym for* **L**ight **A**mplification by **S**timulated **E**mission of **R**adiation -**ery** *process of* **surg-** *operation*	Use of a concentrated, intense narrow beam of electromagnetic radiation for surgery
leukocoria	loo-koh-**KOH**-ree-ah	S/ R/CF R/	-**ia** *condition* **leuk/o-** *white* **cor-** *pupil*	Reflection in pupil of white mass in the eye
metastasis metastases (pl)	meh-**TAS**-tah-sis meh-**TAS**-tah-sees	P/ R/	**meta-** *beyond* -**stasis** *stay in one place*	Spread of disease from one part of the body to another
microaneurysm	my-kroh-**AN**-yu-rizm	P/ R/	**micro-** *small* -**aneurysm** *dilation*	Focal dilation of retinal capillaries
ophthalmoscope	off-**THAL**-moh-skope	S/ R/CF	-**scope** *instrument for viewing* **ophthalm/o-** *eye*	Instrument for viewing the retina
ophthalmoscopy ophthalmoscopic	**OFF**-thal-**MOS**-koh-pee **OFF**-thal-**MOS**-koh-pik	S/ S/	-**scopy** *to examine, to view* -**ic** *pertaining to*	The process of viewing the retina Pertaining to the use of an ophthalmoscope
papilledema	pah-pill-eh-**DEE**-mah	R/ R/	-**edema** *swelling* **papill-** *pimple*	Swelling of the optic disc in the retina
photocoagulation	**FOH**-toe-koh-**AG**-you-**LAY**-shun	S/ R/CF R/	-**ation** *process* **phot/o-** *light* -**coagul-** *clot*	The use of light (laser beam) to form a clot
retinoblastoma	**RET**-in-oh-blas-**TOE**-mah	S/ S/ R/CF	-**oma** *tumor, mass* -**blast** *germ cell* **retin/o-** *retina*	Malignant neoplasm of primitive retinal cells
retinopathy	ret-ih-**NOP**-ah-thee	S/	-**pathy** *disease*	Degenerative disease of the retina

Exercises

A. Continue your work with elements to help build your knowledge of the *language of ophthalmology*. *One element in each of the following medical terms is in bold letters in the left column. Identify the type of element (P, R, CF, S) in the middle column, and then write the meaning of the element in the right column. Fill in the chart.* **LO 16.8**

Medical Term	Type of Element	Meaning of Element
retino**blast**oma	1.	2.
metastasis	3.	4.
intracranial	5.	6.
cryo**pexy**	7.	8.
microaneurysm	9.	10.
ophthalmoscope	11.	12.
angiography	13.	14.
photo**coagul**ation	15.	16.
retino**pathy**	17.	18.

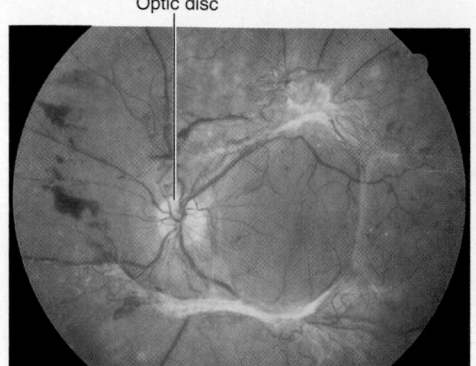

Optic disc

▲ **Figure 16.23** Ophthalmoscopic Examination of the Eye.

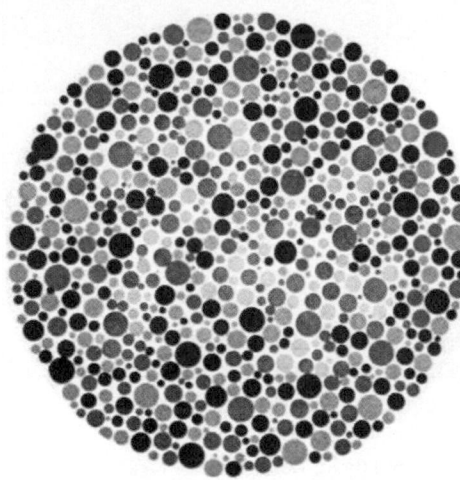

▲ **Figure 16.24** **Test for Color Blindness.** Reproduced with permission from *Ishihara's Tests for Color Deficiency*, published by Kanehara Trading Inc., Tokyo, Japan. Tests for color deficiency cannot be conducted with this figure. For accurate testing, the original plates should be used.

Abbreviations	
O.D.	right eye
O.S.	left eye
O.U.	both eyes

Figure 16.25 **Visual Acuity Tests.** ▶
(*a*) Snellen letter chart for distance vision.
(*b*) Jaeger reading card.

LO 16.9 Ophthalmic Procedures

As an ophthalmic assistant, you may be trained to perform the following procedures.

Examination of the Retina

When you perform a **fundoscopy** and examine the retina with an **ophthalmoscope**, you can first identify the **optic disc** (*Figure 16.23*). This is where the optic nerve leaves the back of the eye. The optic disc has no receptor cells and therefore produces a blind spot in the visual field of each eye. In the middle of the disc, a retinal artery enters to supply the **intraocular** structures, and a retinal vein leaves the eye.

Lateral to the optic disc is a yellowish area called the **macula lutea**. In the center of the macula is the tiny pit called the **fovea centralis**. This pit is the area of sharpest vision. The arteries and veins of the retina can also be seen and provide clues about vascular diseases (*see Chapter 10*).

Color Vision

As an ophthalmic assistant, you may use illustrations such as those from the **Ishihara color system**. In the example shown in *Figure 16.24*, people with red-green color blindness would not be able to see the number 24 among the colored dots.

Distance Vision

As an ophthalmic assistant, you may use the **Snellen letter chart** to test distance vision (*Figure 16.25a*). The results are recorded as a fraction. For example, when the chart is viewed from 20 feet, line 8 is the smallest line a person with standard vision can read. This is recorded as 20/20. If the patient using her left eye misses two letters on line 8, document it as OS 20/20 -2²

Near Vision

As an ophthalmic assistant, you may use handheld charts or **Jaeger reading cards** with printed paragraphs of different sizes of print to test near vision (*Figure 16.25b*).

Visual Fields

As an ophthalmic assistant, you will sit 2 feet in front of your patient, who covers one eye. Cover your own opposite eye and bring a pencil into the horizontal and vertical fields. The field is mapped on a visual field grid.

Glaucoma

As an ophthalmic assistant, you will measure the intraocular pressure with a **tonometer**, which determines the eyeball's resistance to indentation or tension.

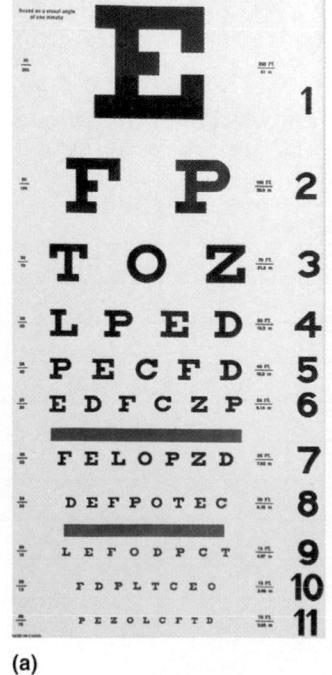

(a)

(b)

WORD	PRONUNCIATION	ELEMENTS		DEFINITION
fundus	**FUN**-dus		Latin *bottom*	Part farthest from the opening of a hollow organ
fundoscopy	fun-**DOS**-koh-pee	S/ R/CF	-scopy *to examine* fund/o- *fundus*	Examination of the fundus (retina) of the eye
fundoscopic (adj)	fun-do-**SKOP**-ik	S/	-ic *pertaining to*	As a result of fundoscopy
Ishihara color system	ish-ee-**HAR**-ah		Shinobu Ishihara, Japanese ophthalmologist, 1879–1963	Test for color vision defects
Jaeger reading cards	**YA**-ger		Edward Jaeger, Austrian ophthalmologist, 1818–1884	Printed in different sizes of print for testing near vision
peripheral vision	peh-**RIF**-er-al **VIZH**-un	S/ R/	-al *pertaining to* peripher- *external boundary*	Ability to see objects as they come into the outer edges of the visual field
Snellen letter chart	**SNEL**-en		Hermann Snellen, Dutch ophthalmologist, 1834–1908	Test for acuity of distant vision
tonometer	toe-**NOM**-eh-ter	S/ R/CF	-meter *measure* ton/o- *pressure, tension*	Instrument for determining intraocular pressure
tonometry	toe-**NOM**-eh-tree	S/	-metry *process of measuring*	The measurement of intraocular

Exercises

A. The ophthalmic technician (OT) in Dr. Chun's office needs to be familiar with all these terms in order to communicate with Dr. Chun and her patients. *Show your understanding of the terms by circling the correct answers.* **LO 16.9**

1. An instrument used in an ophthalmologist's office is the

   a. cystoscope

   b. endoscope

   c. tonometer

   d. bronchoscope

   e. stethoscope

2. The test used to measure color blindness is

   a. Snellen

   b. Jaeger

   c. Ishihara

   d. visual fields

   e. otoscope

3. Peripheral vision measures the outer edge of the

   a. anterior segment

   b. vitreous body

   c. aqueous humor

   d. posterior segment

   e. visual field

4. A test for near vision is the

   a. Snellen chart

   b. ophthalmoscope

   c. Jaeger cards

   d. Ishihara

   e. visual fields

5. Tonometry measures

   a. interocular pressure

   b. arterial pressure

   c. venous pressure

   d. intraocular pressure

   e. capillary pressure

6. The part farthest from the opening of a hollow organ is the

   a. apex

   b. base

   c. fundus

   d. intraocular

   e. peripheral

LESSON OBJECTIVES

In order to understand what is going on with Eddie, to communicate with Dr. Lee about him, to respond to the mother's concerns, and to document the office visit, you need to be able to:

16.3.1 Describe the structures and functions of the three regions of the ear.

16.3.2 Explain how sound waves progress through the ear and are transferred to the brain and recognized as sounds.

16.3.3 Identify how common diseases of the ear interfere with the process of hearing.

16.3.4 Apply the correct medical terminology to the anatomy, physiology, and disorders of the ear.

You are

. . . a medical assistant working with **primary care** physician Susan Lee, MD, of the Fulwood Medical Group on March 16, 2012.

Your patients are

. . . 3-year-old Eddie Cardenas and his mother, Mrs. Carmen Cardenas.

Case Report 16.3

Mrs. Cardenas has brought in her son, Eddie. She tells you that he has had a cold for a couple of days. Early this morning he woke up screaming, felt hot, and was tugging his ears. She gave him **acetaminophen** with some orange juice, and he threw up. This is the third similar episode in the past year. Since the last time, she is concerned that he is not hearing normally. You see a worried mother and a very unhappy, restless toddler with a green nasal discharge. His oral temperature taken with an electronic digital thermometer is 102.4°F, pulse 100. Dr. Lee examines Eddie and finds that he has an **upper respiratory infection (URI)** with a **bilateral otitis media (BOM)**. She prescribes amoxicillin 250 mg four times a day (q.i.d) for 10 days, and acetaminophen 160 mg when necessary (p.r.n.) for pain, after which she will see Eddie again. After the acute infection subsides, if there remains an effusion in the middle ear, she will refer Eddie to an otologist. I explained this to Mrs. Cardenas. —Luisa Guittierez, CMA. 1115 hrs. 3/16/12.

Abbreviations

mg	milligram
p.r.n.	when necessary
q.i.d.	four times each day
URI	upper respiratory infection
BOM	bilateral otitis media

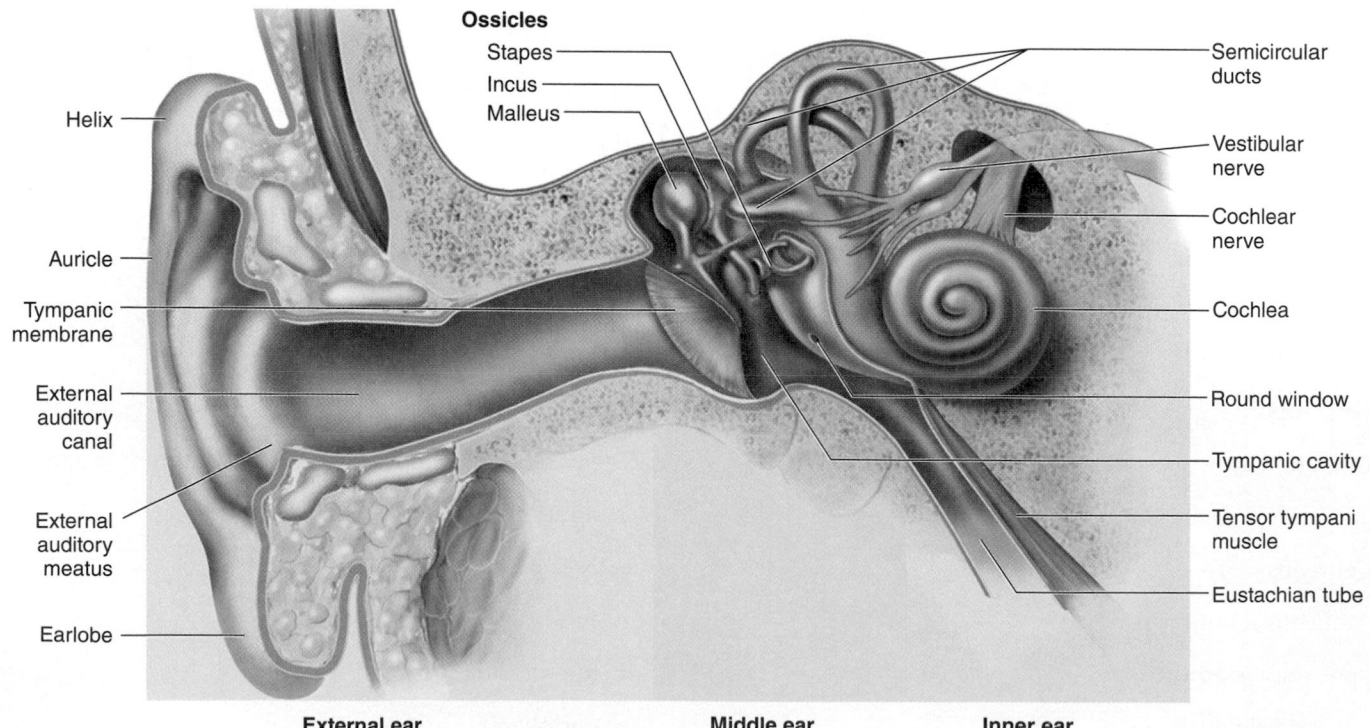

▲ **Figure 16.26**   Anatomical Regions of the Ear.

Labels: Ossicles — Stapes, Incus, Malleus; Helix; Auricle; Tympanic membrane; External auditory canal; External auditory meatus; Earlobe; Semicircular ducts; Vestibular nerve; Cochlear nerve; Cochlea; Round window; Tympanic cavity; Tensor tympani muscle; Eustachian tube; External ear; Middle ear; Inner ear

WORD	PRONUNCIATION		ELEMENTS	DEFINITION
acetaminophen	ah-seat-ah-**MIN**-oh-fen		generic drug name	Medication that is an **analgesic** and an **antipyretic**
acute	ah-**KYUT**		Latin *sharp*	Describes a disease of sudden onset that is usually severe and of short duration
analgesia	an-al-**JEE**-ze-ah	S/ P/ R/	-ia *condition* an- *without* -alges- *sensation of pain*	State in which pain is reduced Substance that reduces the response to pain
analgesic	an-al-**JEE**-zic	S/	-ic *pertaining to*	Capable of producing anesthesia or characterized by a reduced response to painful
antipyretic	**AN**-tee-pie-**RET**-ik	S/ P/ R/	-ic *pertaining to* anti- *against* -pyret- *fever*	Agent that reduces fever or capable of reducing fever
bilateral	by-**LAT**-er-al	S/ P/ R/	-al *pertaining to* bi- *two, twice* -later *side*	On two sides, for example, in both ears
chronic	**KRON**-ik		Greek *time*	Describes a persistent, long-term disease
effusion	eh-**FYU**-shun		Latin *pouring out*	Collection of fluid that has escaped from blood vessels into a cavity or tissues
otitis media	oh-**TIE**-tis **ME**-dee-ah	S/ R/ R/	-itis *inflammation* ot- *ear* media *middle*	Inflammation of the middle ear
otologist	oh-**TOL**-oh-jist	S/ R/CF	-logist *one who studies, specialist* ot/o- *ear*	Medical specialist in diseases of the ear
otology otorhinolaryngologist	oh-**TOL**-oh-jee oh-toe-rhino-lah-rin-**GOL**-oh-jist	S/ R/CF R/CF	-logy *study of* -rhin/o- *nose* -laryng/o- *larynx*	Study of the function and diseases of the ear Ear, nose, and throat medical specialist
primary care	**PRY**-mah-ree KAIR		**primary** Latin *first* **care** Greek *concern*	Comprehensive and preventive health care services that are the first point of care for a patient

Exercises

A. Break down these medical terms into their basic elements. *Analyzing each term will help you answer the following questions. Fill in the blanks.*   **LO 16.1, 16.11**

Medical Term	Prefix	Root(s)/Combining Form	Suffix
analgesia	1.	2.	3.
bilateral	4.	5.	6.
otitis media	7.	8.	9.
otologist	10.	11.	12.
otorhinolaryngologist	13.	14.	15.

16. A medication that is an analgesic reduces _____.

17. Name another body part that is bilateral. _____

18. What is the difference between an otologist and an otorhinolaryngologist?

_____

19. Where in the ear does otitis media occur? _____

20. In the above WAD, which element is a prefix referring to a number? _____ means _____.

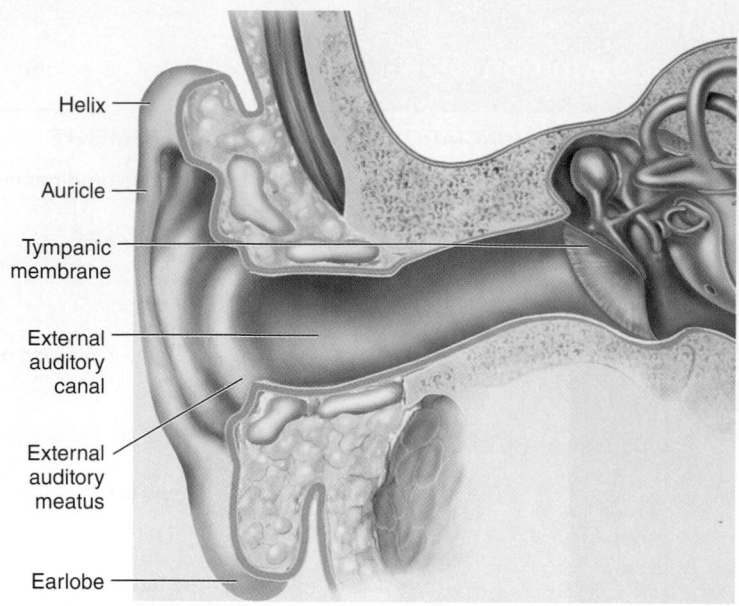

▲ **Figure 16.27** External Ear.

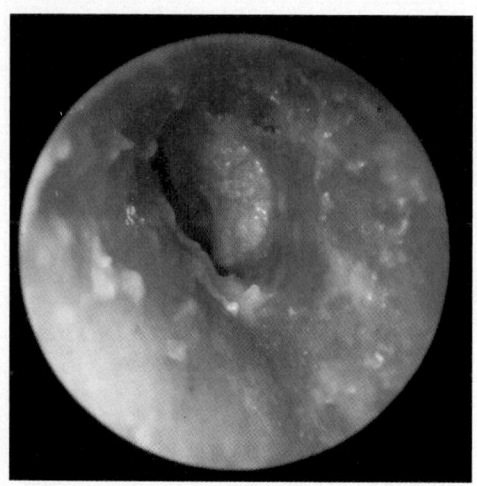

▲ **Figure 16.28** Otoscopic View of Otitis Externa with Purulent Exudate *(shown in yellow)*.

LO 16.10 External Ear

The **auricle**, or **pinna**, is a wing-shaped structure that directs sound waves coming through the air into the **external auditory meatus** and **external auditory canal**. This in turn ends at the **tympanic membrane** *(Figure 16.27)*. The external auditory canal not only protects the middle and inner ears but also acts as a resonator to augment the transmission of sound to the middle and inner ears.

The external auditory canal is the only skin-lined cul-de-sac in the body. Its interior is dark, warm, and prone to become moist. These are ideal conditions for bacterial and fungal growth.

The meatus and canal are lined with skin that contains many modified sweat glands called ceruminous glands, which secrete **cerumen**. The cerumen and hairs growing in the meatus help to keep out foreign objects. Cerumen combines with dead skin cells to form **earwax**. Overproduction of cerumen can completely block the external canal, causing hearing loss and preventing examination of the tympanic membrane with an **otoscope**.

If a foreign body, such as a small bead, does get into the canal, or if cerumen becomes **impacted** in the canal, then hearing loss can result.

LO 16.10 Disorders of External Ear

Otitis externa *(Figure 16.28)* is an infection of the lining of the external auditory canal. It produces a painful, red, swollen ear canal, sometimes with purulent drainage. The infection can be bacterial or fungal. Fungal infections are responsible for 10% of otitis externa cases and are called **otomycoses**.

Conditions helping to cause otitis externa include trauma to the canal during attempts to self-clean it; use of unclean earplugs, earphones, or hearing aids; and the presence of other skin diseases, such as seborrhea and psoriasis *(see Chapter 15)*.

Treatment entails thorough cleansing of the canal, acidification with a topical solution of 2% acetic acid in a hydrocortisone solution, and the use of antibiotic drops. Occasionally a wick is needed to enable the topical medications to penetrate down the canal.

Swimmer's ear is a form of otitis externa that comes after swimming, particularly if the water is polluted.

Excessive earwax can be removed in your physician's office by ear **irrigation** or with a **curette**, a small metal ring at the end of a handle.

WORD	PRONUNCIATION	ELEMENTS		DEFINITION
auditory	**AW**-dih-tor-ee		Latin *hearing*	Pertaining to the sense or organs of hearing
audiology	aw-dee-**OL**-oh-jee	S/	**-logy** *study of*	Study of hearing disorders
		R/CF	**audi/o-** *hearing*	
audiologist	aw-dee-**OL**-oh-jist	S/	**-logist** *one who studies*	Specialist in evaluation of hearing function
auricle	**AW**-ri-kul		Latin *ear*	The shell-like external ear
cerumen	seh-**ROO**-men		Latin *wax*	Waxy secretion of ceruminous glands of external ear canal
curette	kyu-**RET**	S/	**-ette** *little*	Scoop-shaped instrument for scraping the interior of a cavity or removing new growths
		R/	**cur-** *cleanse, cure*	
curettage	kyu-reh-**TAHZH**	S/	**-age** *related to*	Scraping the interior of a cavity
(**Note:** The final "e" of **curette** is dropped because the suffix -age begins with a vowel.)				
impacted	im-**PAK**-ted		Latin *driven in*	Immovably wedged, as with earwax blocking the external ear canal
irrigation	ih-rih-**GAY**-shun	S/	**-ation** *process*	Use of water to clean wax out of the external ear canal
		P/	**-ir** *in*	
		R/	**-rig** *water*	
meatus	me-**AY**-tus		Latin *passage*	Passage or channel; also used to denote the external opening of a passage
meatal (adj)	me-**AY**-tal	S/	**-al** *pertaining to*	
		R/	**meat-** *passage or channel*	
otomycosis	**OH**-toe-my-**KOH**-sis	S/	**-sis** *abnormal condition*	Fungal infection of the external ear canal
		R/CF	**ot/o-** *ear*	
		R/CF	**-myc/o-** *fungus*	
otoscope	**OH**-toe-skope	S/	**-scope** *instrument for viewing*	Instrument for examining the ear
		R/CF	**ot/o-** *ear*	
otoscopic (adj)	oh-toe-**SKOP**-ik	S/	**-ic** *pertaining to*	Pertaining to examination with an otoscope
otoscopy	oh-**TOS**-koh-pee	S/	**-scopy** *to examine*	Examination of the ear
pinna	**PIN**-ah		Latin *wing*	Another name for auricle
pinnae (pl)	**PIN**-ee			
tympanic	tim-**PAN**-ik	S/	**-ic** *pertaining to*	Pertaining to the tympanic membrane or tympanic cavity
		R/	**tympan-** *eardrum, tympanic membrane*	

Exercises

A. Every part of the body has its own specialized vocabulary. *Test your knowledge of the language of otology by matching correct answers. Match the phrase in the left column with the appropriate medical term in the right column.* **LO 16.10**

_____ 1. External ear fungal infection

_____ 2. External opening of a passage

_____ 3. Instrument for viewing the ear

_____ 4. Procedure for scraping or removing growths

_____ 5. Shell-like external ear

_____ 6. "Driven in"

_____ 7. Another name for auricle

_____ 8. Pertaining to the sense or organs of hearing

_____ 9. Earwax

_____ 10. Pertaining to the eardrum

a. pinna

b. auditory

c. auricle

d. tympanic

e. otomycosis

f. curettage

g. meatus

h. otoscope

i. impacted

j. cerumen

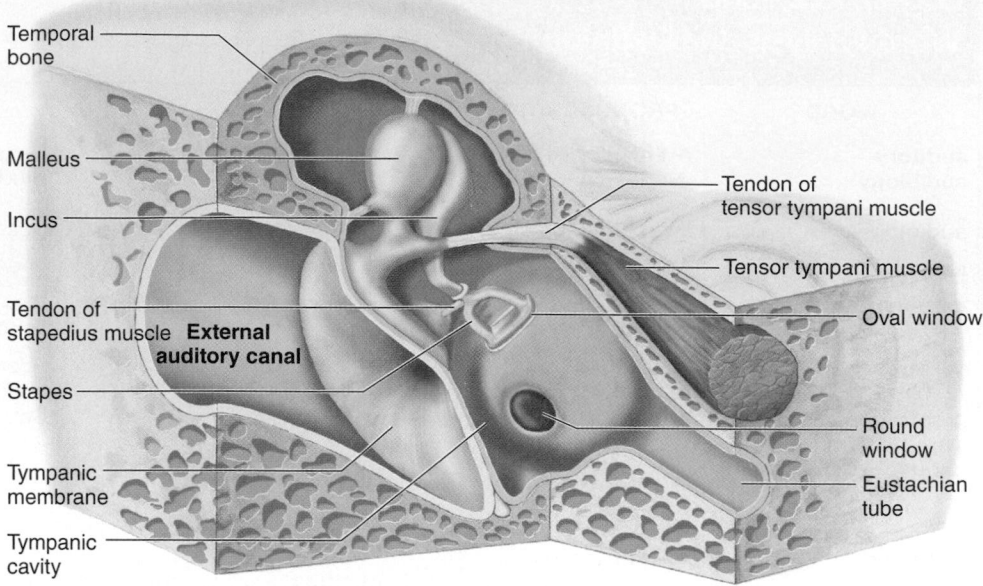

▲ Figure 16.29 Middle Ear.

LO 16.11 Middle Ear

The middle ear has four components: the tympanic membrane, the tympanic cavity, the **eustachian** (auditory) **tube**, and the ossicles *(Figure 16.29)*.

1. The **tympanic membrane (eardrum)** is located at the inner end of the external auditory canal. It is suspended in a bony groove, is concave on its outer surface, and vibrates freely as sound waves hit it. It has a good nerve supply and is very sensitive to pain. When examined through the otoscope, it is transparent and reflects light *(Figure 16.30)*.

2. The **tympanic cavity** is immediately behind the tympanic membrane. It is filled with air that enters through the eustachian (auditory) tube, and the cavity is continuous with the **mastoid** air cells in the bone behind it. The presence of air in the cavity maintains equal air pressure on both sides of the tympanic membrane, which is essential for normal hearing. The cavity contains the ossicles.

3. The eustachian (auditory) tube *(Figure 16.30)* connects the middle ear with the **nasopharynx** (throat), into which it opens close to the pharyngeal **tonsil (adenoid)** *(Figure 16.31)*. In children under 5 years, the tube is not fully developed. It is short and horizontal, and the valvelike flaps in the throat that protect it are not developed. When you are landing in an airplane and moving from a high altitude to a lower one, the air pressure in the external auditory canal increases and pushes the tympanic membrane inward. If your eustachian (auditory) tube is blocked, no air can get into the middle ear to equalize the pressure, and your eardrum is painful. If you can force some air up the eustachian (auditory) tube by chewing or swallowing, then your ear "pops" as the tympanic membrane moves back to its normal position.

4. The three **ossicles**, the **malleus**, **incus**, and **stapes** *(Figure 16.29)*, are attached to the wall of the tympanic cavity by tiny ligaments that are covered by a mucous membrane. The malleus is attached to the tympanic membrane and vibrates with the membrane when sound waves hit it. The malleus is also attached to the incus, which also vibrates and passes the vibrations onto the stapes. The stapes is attached to the oval window, an opening that transmits the vibrations to the inner ear. The stapes is the smallest bone in the body.

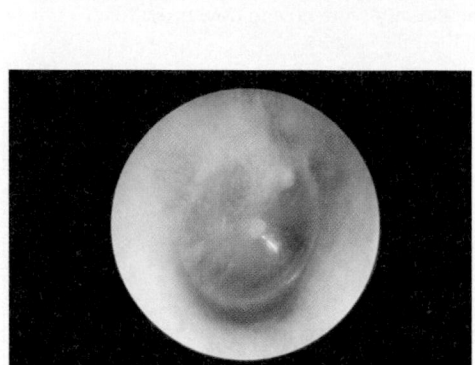

▲ Figure 16.30 Otoscopic View of Normal Tympanic Membrane.

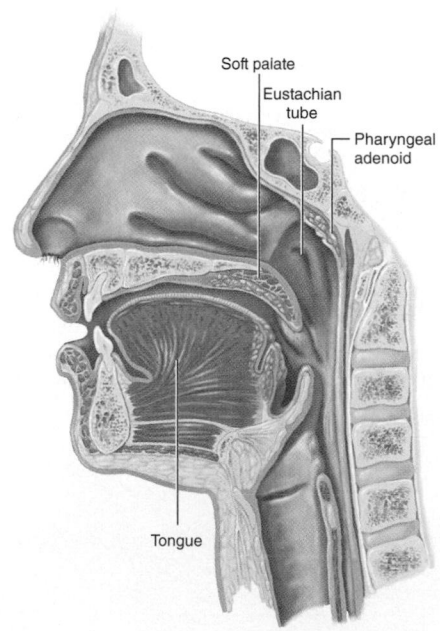

▲ Figure 16.31 Nasopharynx (Throat).

Keynote

The three ossicles amplify sound so that soft sounds can be heard.

Word Analysis and Definition

S = Suffix   P = Prefix   R = Root   R/CF = Combining Form

WORD	PRONUNCIATION	ELEMENTS		DEFINITION
adenoid	**ADD**-eh-noyd	S/ R/	-oid *resembling* aden- *gland*	Single mass of lymphoid tissue in the midline at the back of the throat
eustachian tube auditory tube (syn)	you-**STAY**-shun TYUB		Bartolommeo Eustachio, Italian anatomist, 1524–1574	Tube that connects the middle ear to the nasopharynx
incus	**IN**-cuss		Latin *anvil*	Middle one of the three ossicles in the middle ear; shaped like an anvil
malleus	**MAL**-ee-us		Latin *hammer*	Outer (lateral) one of the three ossicles in the middle ear; shaped like a hammer
mastoid	**MASS**-toyd	S/ R/	-oid *resembling* mast- *breast*	Small bony protrusion immediately behind the ear
nasopharynx	**NAY**-zoh-**FAIR**-inks	R/CF R/	nas/o- *nose* -pharynx *throat*	Region of the pharynx at the back of the nose and above the soft palate
ossicle	**OS**-ih-kel	S/ R/CF	-cle *small* oss/i- *bone*	A small bone, particularly relating to the three bones in the middle ear
stapes	**STAY**-peas		Latin *stirrup*	Inner (medial) one of the three ossicles of the middle ear; shaped like a stirrup
tonsil tonsillar (adj)	**TON**-sill **TON**-sih-lar		Latin *tonsil*	Mass of lymphoid tissue on either side of the throat at the back of the tongue

Exercises

A. Answers to the following questions can all be found in the above WAD. *Review the terms before you start this exercise. Pay special attention to the spelling. Circle the best choice.* **LO 16.1, 16.11**

1. In the term **mastoid**, the suffix means

   condition   resembling   inflammation

2. The element **mast** means

   throat   breast   ear

3. The **stapes** is a(n)

   gland   ossicle   mastoid

4. The element **pharynx** means

   throat   nose   gland

5. The term **nasopharynx** is composed of

   prefix + suffix   root + root   combining form + root

6. This type of tissue is found in an adenoid:

   mucoid   connective   lymphoid

7. The _____ is shaped like a hammer.

   malleus   malleolus   maleus

8. The element **aden** in adenoid is a

   prefix   root   combining form

9. One of the names for the tube that connects the middle ear to the nasopharynx is the _____ tube.

   eusstachian   eustashian   eustachian

10. The _____ is shaped like an anvil.

   incus   stapes   adenoid

B. This exercise pertains to the ossicles. *Use the language of otology for your answers.* **LO 16.1, 16.11**

1. How many bones are in the ossicles? _____ Name them: _____

   _____

2. Which of them is the smallest bone in the body? _____

3. Which bone is attached to the tympanic membrane and the incus? _____

4. Are the ossicles in the external ear, the middle ear, or the inner ear? _____

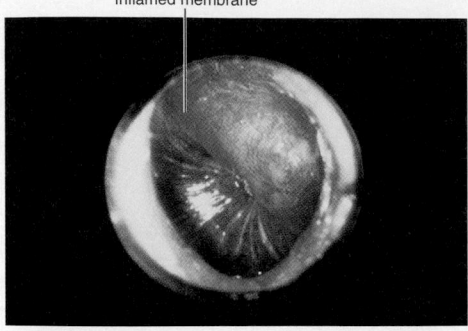

▲ **Figure 16.32** Otoscopic View of Otitis Media (Acute), Showing Inflamed Tympanic Membrane.

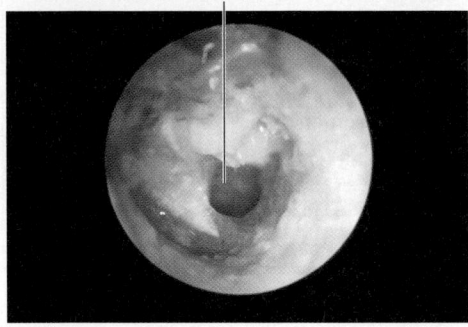

▲ **Figure 16.33** Otoscopic View of Otitis Media (Chronic) with Perforated Tympanic Membrane.

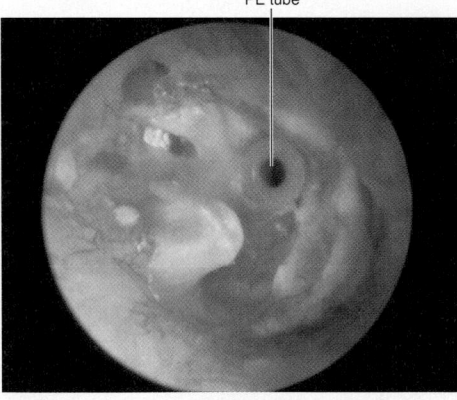

▲ **Figure 16.34** Pressure Equalization (PE) Tube in Tympanic Membrane.

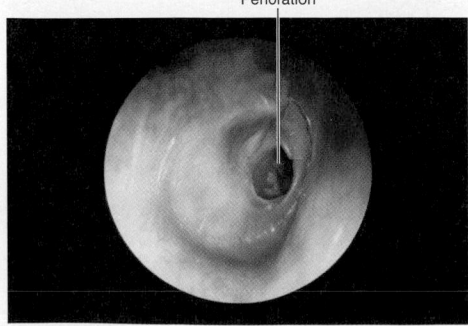

▲ **Figure 16.35** Perforated Tympanic Membrane.

Case Report 16.3 (continued)

Eddie Cardenas' ear problems began with his eustachian (auditory) tube. His cold (**URI**, or **coryza**) inflamed the mucous membranes of his throat and auditory tube. Because a young child's auditory tube is short and horizontal, the inflammation spread easily into the middle ear, causing Eddie's acute otitis media (**AOM**). The inflammatory process produced fluid (**effusion**) in the middle ear. His tympanic membrane became painful and inflamed, which you could see through an otoscope *(Figure 16.32)*.

LO 16.11 Disorders of Middle Ear

Acute otitis media (AOM) is the presence of pus in the middle ear with pain in the ear, fever, and redness of the tympanic membrane. This occurs most often in the first 2 to 4 years of age because:

- Eustachian tubes in children are shorter and more horizontal than in adults, making it easier for bacteria and viruses to find their way into the middle ear from the nasopharynx.

- Adenoids at the back of the nasopharynx near the eustachian tubes can block the opening of the eustachian tubes.

- Children's immune systems are not fully developed until 7 years of age, and they have difficulty fighting infections.

If the infections are viral, they will go away on their own. If bacterial, oral antibiotics may be necessary.

Chronic otitis media (COM) occurs when the acute infection subsides but the eustachian tube is still blocked. The **effusion** (fluid) in the middle ear cannot drain out and gradually becomes stickier. This is called **chronic otitis media with effusion (OME)** and produces hearing loss because the sticky fluid prevents the ossicles from vibrating. You can see the fluid through the otoscope *(Figure 16.33)*. Dr. Lee was concerned that this had happened to Eddie in his previous ear infection.

If the sticky fluid persists, a **myringotomy** can be performed and a small, hollow plastic tube can be inserted through the tympanic membrane to allow the effusion to drain. The ear tubes have several names: **tympanostomy tubes**, **pressure-equalization tubes**, or, most commonly, **PE tubes** *(Figure 16.34)*. The tube is inserted under general anesthesia as an outpatient surgery. It remains in the ear for 6 to 18 months before it drops out on its own.

A **perforated tympanic membrane** can occur in acute otitis media when pus in the middle ear cannot escape down the eustachian tube. It builds up pressure and perforates the eardrum *(Figures 16.33, 35)*. Other causes of perforation include a puncture by a cotton swab, an open-handed slap to the ear, or large pressure changes (as may be induced in scuba diving). Most perforations will heal spontaneously in a month, leaving a small scar.

Cholesteatoma is a complication of chronic otitis media with effusion or of poor eustachian tube function. Chronically inflamed cells in the middle ear multiply and collect into a tumor. They damage the ossicles and can spread to the inner ear. Surgical removal is required.

Otosclerosis is a middle-ear disease that usually affects people between 18 and 35 years of age. It can affect one ear or both and produces a gradual hearing loss for low and soft sounds. Its etiology is unknown. Spongy bone forms around the junction of the oval window and stapes, preventing the stapes from conducting the sound vibrations to the inner ear. The only treatment is to replace the stapes with a metal or plastic **prosthesis**.

Abbreviations

AOM	acute otitis media
COM	chronic otitis media
OME	otitis media with effusion
PE	pressure equalization (tubes)
URI	upper respiratory infection

WORD	PRONUNCIATION	ELEMENTS		DEFINITION
cholesteatoma	koh-less-tee-ah-**TOE**-mah	S/ R/CF R/	-oma *tumor, mass* **chol/e-** *bile* **-steat-** *fat*	Yellow, waxy tumor arising in the middle ear
coryza rhinitis (syn)	ko-**RYE**-zah		Greek *catarrh*	Viral inflammation of the mucous membrane of the nose
effusion	eh-**FYU**-shun		Latin *pouring out*	Collection of fluid that has escaped from blood vessels into a cavity or tissues
myringotomy	mir-in-**GOT**-oh-me	S/ R/CF	-tomy *surgical incision* **myring/o-** *tympanic membrane*	Incision in the tympanic membrane
otosclerosis	oh-toe-sklair-**OH**-sis	S/ R/CF R/CF	-sis *abnormal condition* **-scler/o-** *hardening* **ot/o-** *ear*	Hardening at the junction of the stapes and oval window that causes loss of hearing
perforated	**PER**-foh-ray-ted		Latin *to bore through*	Punctured with one or more holes
prosthesis	**PROS**-thee-sis		Greek *addition*	Manufactured substitute for a missing part of the body
tympanic	tim-**PAN**-ik	S/ R/	-ic *pertaining to* **tympan-** *eardrum, tympanic membrane*	Pertaining to the tympanic membrane or tympanic cavity
tympanostomy	tim-pan-**OS**-toe-me	S/ R/CF	-stomy *new opening* **tympan/o-** *eardrum, tympanic membrane*	Surgically created new opening in the tympanic membrane to allow fluid to drain from the middle ear

Exercises

A. Build medical terms. *This is a two-step exercise. Fill in the blanks with the correct element to complete the terms in questions 1–5. Then match the terms in questions 6–9 to their meanings.* **LO 16.1, 16.11**

1. Pertaining to the eardrum: _____ /ic

2. Hardening at the junction of the stapes and oval window:

   oto/_____ /sis

3. Another name for coryza: _____ /itis

4. Incision into the tympanic membrane: myringo/_____

5. Yellow, waxy tumor in the middle ear:

   _____ / _____oma

Step 2. Match the following terms to their meanings.

_____ 6. Manufactured body part   **a.** coryza

_____ 7. Fluid in a cavity   **b.** perforated

_____ 8. Common cold   **c.** prosthesis

_____ 9. Punctured   **d.** effusion

B. Circle the correct answer to each statement.   **LO 16.11**

1. The term *effusion* implies

   a. tumor   **d.** tear

   b. mass   **e.** blockage

   c. liquid

2. The term *rhinitis* has a root/combining form that refers to the nose. What other root/combining form also means nose?

   a. ren   **d.** uro

   b. nephro   **e.** gyneco

   c. naso

3. What surgical procedure is performed to insert PE tubes?

   a. appendectomy

   b. myringotomy

   c. blepharoplasty

   d. phaecoemulsion

   e. cryopexy

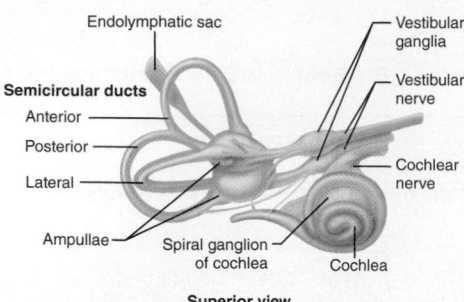

Endolymphatic sac

Semicircular ducts
Anterior
Posterior
Lateral

Ampullae

Spiral ganglion of cochlea

Vestibular ganglia

Vestibular nerve

Cochlear nerve

Cochlea

Superior view

▲ **Figure 16.36**   Inner Ear.

Abbreviations

A.D.	right ear
A.S.	left ear
A.U.	both ears
JC	Joint Commission

Keynotes

- Repeated exposure to loud noise causes hearing loss in young people as well as in older people.

- A **conductive hearing loss** occurs when sound is not conducted efficiently through the external auditory canal to the tympanic membrane and the ossicles. Causes include

  - Middle ear pathology, such as acute otitis media, otitis media with efffusion, or a perforated eardrum.

  - Impacted cerumen.

  - An infected external auditory canal.

  - A foreign body in the external canal.

LO 16.12 Inner Ear for Hearing

The inner ear is a **labyrinth** (*Figure 16.36*) of complex, intricate systems of passages. The passages in the **cochlea**, a part of the labyrinth, contain receptors to translate vibrations into nerve impulses so that the brain can interpret them as different sounds.

The membrane of the oval window separates the middle ear from the **vestibule** of the inner ear. From the tympanic membrane (① *in Figure 16.37*), the stapes ② moves the oval membrane to generate pressure waves in the fluid inside the cochlea ③. The pressure waves cause **vestibular** and **basilar membranes** inside the cochlea to vibrate ④ and sway fine hair cells attached to the basilar membrane ⑤. The hair cells convert this motion into nerve impulses, which travel via the **cochlear nerve** to the brain. The excess pressure waves in the cochlea escape the inner ear via the round window ⑥.

Today, the most common cause of hearing loss is damage to the fine hairs in the cochlea by exposure to repeated loud noise, either related to work (for example, jackhammers, leaf blowers) or to leisure activities (such as amplified music at concerts, personal listening devices, and motorcycles). This is a **sensorineural hearing loss**.

Hearing aids are becoming more sophisticated and smaller, but they do not help people with cochlear damage. **Cochlear implants** are used to bypass the damaged hair cells and directly stimulate cochlear nerve endings.

Hearing Test Procedures

Whispered Speech Testing: Ask the patient to cover one ear. Stand 2 feet away from the uncovered ear, whisper words, and ask the patient to repeat them. If the patient cannot repeat them, say the words more loudly. This is a simple screening method.

Weber Test: Strike the tuning fork against your elbow to make a tone, place the tuning fork in the middle of the patient's forehead, and ask whether the tone is louder in one ear or equal on both sides. This determines on which side a hearing loss is located.

Rinne Test: Place the vibrating tuning fork on the mastoid process behind the opening of the ear canal. Then hold it opposite the ear canal. Ask the patient where the tone was louder and/or lasted longer. Normally, sound is heard longer by air conduction at the ear canal than by bone conduction at the mastoid process. The reverse indicates a conductive hearing loss.

Audiometer: After proper training, use an audiometer to test for hearing loss. The audiometer is an electronic device that generates sounds in different frequencies and intensities and can print out the patient's responses.

When recording the results of hearing testing, **A.D.** is shorthand for the right ear, **A.S.** for the left ear, and **A.U.** for both ears. (*Note:* To avoid confusion with similar abbreviations, the **Joint Commission [JC]** recommends writing out the full terms.)

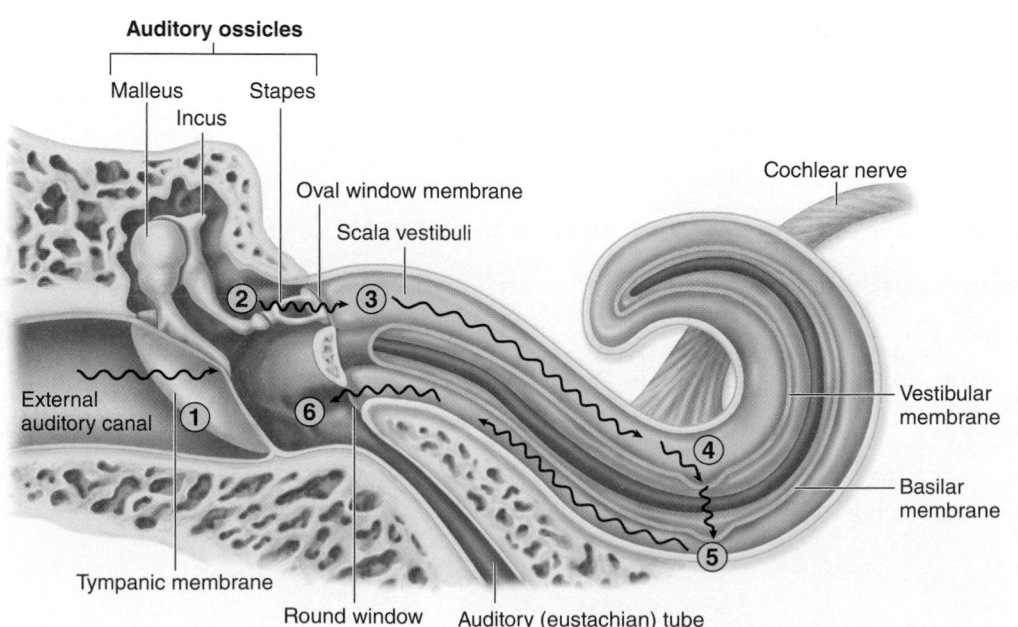

Auditory ossicles

Malleus
Incus
Stapes

Oval window membrane

Scala vestibuli

Cochlear nerve

External auditory canal

Vestibular membrane

Basilar membrane

Tympanic membrane

Round window   Auditory (eustachian) tube

▲ **Figure 16.37**   Hearing Process in the Inner Ear.

WORD	PRONUNCIATION	ELEMENTS		DEFINITION
audiometer	aw-dee-**OM**-ee-ter	S/ R/CF	-meter *measure* audi/o- *hearing*	Instrument to measure hearing
audiometric (adj)	**AW**-dee-oh-**MET**-rik	S/ R/	-ic *pertaining to* metr- *measure*	Pertaining to the measurement of hearing
basilar	**BAS**-ih-lar	S/ R/	-ar *pertaining to* basil- *base, support*	Pertaining to the base of a structure
cochlea cochlear (adj)	**KOK**-lee-ah **KOK**-lee-ar		Latin *snail shell*	An intricate combination of passages; used to describe the part of the inner ear used in hearing
conductive hearing loss	kon-**DUK**-tiv		Latin *to lead*	Hearing loss caused by lesions in the outer ear or middle ear
implant	im-**PLANT**		Latin *to plant*	To insert material into tissues, or the material inserted into tissues
labyrinth labyrinthitis	**LAB**-ih-rinth **LAB**-ih-rin-**THI**-tis	R/ S/	labyrinth- *inner ear* -itis *inflammation*	The inner ear Inflammation of the inner ear
Rinne test	**RIN**-eh TEST		Friedrich Rinne, German otologist, 1819–1868	Test for conductive hearing loss
sensorineural hearing loss	**SEN**-sor-ih-**NYUR**-al	S/ R/CF R/	-al *pertaining to* sensor/i- *sensory* -neur- *nerve*	Hearing loss caused by lesions of the inner ear or the auditory nerve
vestibule vestibular (adj)	**VES**-tih-byul ves-**TIB**-you-lar		Latin *entrance*	Space at the entrance to a canal
Weber test	**VA**-ber TEST		Ernst Weber, German physiologist, 1794–1878	Test for sensorineural hearing loss

Exercises

A. Increase your knowledge of the *language of otology* by correctly answering the following questions. *Review the above WAD; then circle the best answer.* **LO 16.1, 16.12, 16.13**

1. In the term **basilar, basil-** is a

   prefix   root   combining form

2. The **entrance to the inner ear** is the

   vestibule   labyrinth   cochlea

3. **Labyrinthitis** is a(n)

   procedure   condition   inflammation

4. The element **neur** means

   never   nerve   nose

5. An **audiometer** is used to

   measure   scan   examine

6. An **intricate combination of passages** in the ear is the

   cochlea   vestibule   labyrinth

7. The root meaning **hearing** can be found in the word

   vestibule   audiometric   otology

8. **Hearing loss** caused by lesions of the inner ear is called _____ hearing loss.

   auditory   basilar   sensorineural

9. The suffix meaning **pertaining to** is found in the term

   vestibular   labyrinthitis   audiometer

Case Report 16.4

Mr. Santiago complains of **recurrent** attacks of nausea and vomiting, a sense of spinning or whirling, and ringing in his ears. The attacks last about 24 hours and are getting more frequent. He has been having trouble hearing quiet speech on his left side.

Your role is to document his investigation, diagnosis, and care and to act as translator between Mr. Santiago and Dr. Thompson.

LO 16.12 Inner Ear for Equilibrium and Balance

The **vestibule** and the three **semicircular canals** *(Figure 16.38)* are the organs of balance.

Inside the fluid-filled vestibule are two raised, flat areas (**maculae**) covered with hair cells and a gelatinous material. This gelatinous material contains crystals of calcium and protein called **otoliths**. The position of the head alters the pressure applied to the hair cells by the gelatinous mass. The hair cells respond to horizontal and vertical changes and send impulses to the brain indicating the position to which the head has tilted.

Each of the three fluid-filled semicircular canals has a dilated end called an **ampulla** that contains a mound of hair cells embedded in a gelatinous material that together are called a **crista ampullaris** *(Figure 16.39)*. They detect rotational movements of the head that distort the hair cells and lead to stimulation of connected nerve cells. The nerve impulses travel via the vestibular nerve and go to the brain. From the brain, nerve impulses travel to the muscles to maintain **equilibrium** and balance.

The sensation of spinning or whirling that Mr. Santiago experiences is called **vertigo**, often described by patients as dizziness. The ringing in his ears is called **tinnitus**. Both sensations arise in the inner ear.

Acute labyrinthitis is an acute viral infection of the labyrinth, producing extreme vertigo, nausea, and vomiting. It usually lasts 1 to 2 weeks.

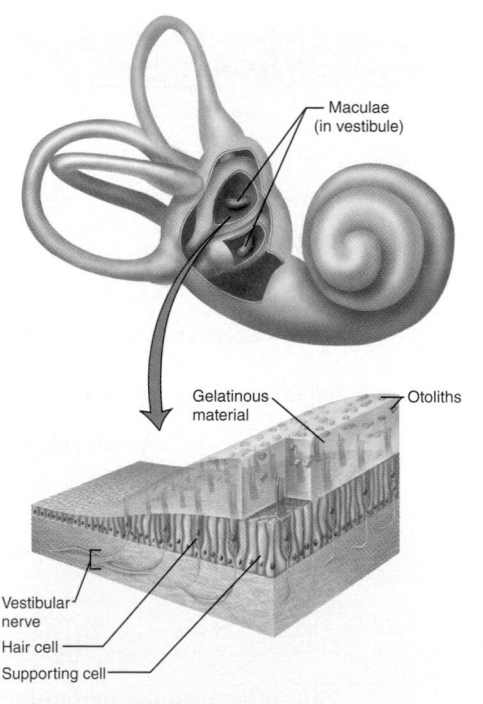

▲ **Figure 16.38** Vestibule and Maculae.

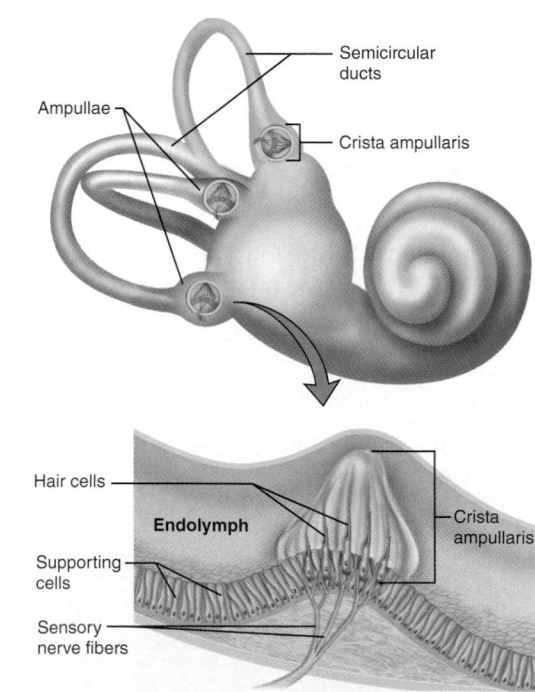

▲ **Figure 16.39** Semicircular Ducts.

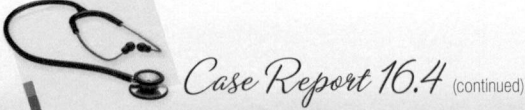

Case Report 16.4 (continued)

The recurrent attacks that Mr. Santiago suffered are called Ménière disease. The disease involves the destruction of inner-ear hair cells, but the etiology is unknown, and there is no cure. Dr. Thompson prescribed medication to control his nausea and vomiting.

WORD	PRONUNCIATION	ELEMENTS		DEFINITION
ampulla crista ampullaris	am-**PULL**-ah **KRIS**-tah am-**PULL**-air-is	R/ S/ R/	Latin *two-handled bottle* **crista** *crest* -aris *pertaining to* **ampull-** *bottle-shaped*	Dilated portion of canal or duct Mound of hair cells and gelatinous material in the ampulla of a semicircular canal
equilibrium	ee-kwi-**LIB**-ree-um	P/ R/	equi- *equal* **-librium** *balance*	Being evenly balanced
macula maculae (pl)	**MAK**-you-lah **MAK**-you-lee		Latin *small spot*	Small area of special function: in the ear, a sensory receptor
Ménière disease	men-**YEAR** diz-**EEZ**		Prosper Ménière, French physican, 1799–1862	Disorder of inner ear with cluster of symptoms of acute attacks of tinnitus, vertigo, and hearing loss
otolith	**OH**-toe-lith	S/ R/CF	-lith *stone* **ot/o-** *ear*	A calcium particle in the vestibule of the inner ear
paroxysmal	par-ock-**SIZ**-mal	S/ R/	-al *pertaining to* **-paroxysm-** *irritation*	Occurring in sharp, spasmodic episodes
recurrent	ree-**KUR**-ent	S/ P/ R/	-ent *pertaining to* re- *back* **curr-** *to run*	Symptoms or lesions returning after an intermission
tinnitus	**TIN**-ih-tus		Latin *jingle*	Persistent ringing, whistling, clicking, or booming noise in the ears
vertigo	**VER**-tih-go		Latin *dizziness*	Sensation of spinning or whirling

Exercises

A. Challenge your knowledge of the ear by filling in the correct terms for the following definitions. *Demonstrate your understanding of the terms by using any one of them correctly in a sentence of your choice. Fill in the blanks.* **LO 16.1, 16.12**

Definition	Medical Term
1. Persistent ringing in the ears	_____
2. Sensation of spinning or whirling	_____
3. Occurring in sharp, spasmodic episodes	_____
4. Evenly balanced	_____
5. Dilated portion of a canal or duct	_____
6. Small area of special function	_____
7. Calcium particle in the vestibule	_____
8. Mound of hair cells found in ampulla	_____

Use any one of these terms in a sentence of your choice that is not a definition.

9. _____

_____

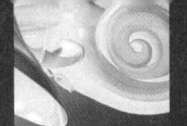

Special Senses of the Eye and Ear

Challenge Your Knowledge

A. Apply your knowledge of medical terminology to change this report from layman's terms into medical communication. Then practice reading the entire paragraph aloud. (**LO 16.1, 16.2, 16.8,** *Remember*)

Preoperative Diagnosis: Diabetic _____ (disorder of the retinal blood vessels) with vitreous _____ (sudden discharge of blood), left eye.

Procedure Performed: Laser _____ (clotting together with light) _____ with (surgical removal of vitreous), left eye.

After suitable anesthesia, the patient was prepped and draped in the usual manner. The _____ (inner lining of the eyelid) was well irrigated to remove any debris from the field. A slit _____ (cutting into) was made at four different sites on the _____ (white outer covering of the eyeball), and the central vitreous cavity was entered. The origin of the bleeding was confined to the _____ (area of sharpest vision). The blood vessels were cauterized with the laser. Fortunately, the _____ (inner lining of the eye) had not become detached, although the vitreous had separated. This was removed in pieces. All operative sites were closed routinely. Ointment, patch, and shield were applied to the affected eye. Patient returned to the postanesthesia care unit for discharge. Patient will be given prescriptions for _____ (medication to destroy bacteria) to be filled when she leaves the hospital. She will follow up with me in the office in 1 week.

B. Recall and review. How well do you remember these word elements from previous chapters? Try to answer without first looking back to check. Fill in the blanks. (**LO 16.2,** *Remember*)

Element	Type of Element (P, R, CF, S)	Meaning of Element
dermat/o	1. _____	2. _____
itis	3. _____	4. _____
nephr/o	5. _____	6. _____
super	7. _____	8. _____
um	9. _____	10. _____

C. Suffixes. The following terms all have a suffix with a common meaning. Circle the suffix; then identify the common meaning, and define each term. (**LO 16.1, 16.2,** *Remember*)

1. periorbital _____

2. lacrimal _____

3. bactericidal _____

4. intraocular _____

5. neural _____

6. optic _____

7. tarsal _____

8. macular _____

9. retinal _____

10. corneal _____

These suffixes all mean _____.

D. Prefixes. Use your knowledge of prefixes to deconstruct the following terms; then write the definition of the term. (**LO 16.1, 16.2, 16.7, 16.8,** *Remember, Understand*)

Term	Prefix	Meaning of Prefix	Definition of Term
periorbital	1.	2.	3.
esotropia	4.	5.	6.
astigmatism	7.	8.	9.
contaminate	10.	11.	12.
accommodation	13.	14.	15.
exotropia	16.	17.	18.
bilateral	19.	20.	21.
analgesic	22.	23.	24.
intraocular	25.	26.	27.

E. Diagnosis. You are preparing to code the claim forms for various patients seen in the clinic today. The doctor has given each diagnosis in general terms on the charge slip. Not every term in the *ICD-9-CM Index* is cross-referenced, so you must know the medical term to find the code. Write the correct medical term for each general term. (**LO 16.1, 16.2,** *Remember, Understand*)

1. Pink eye _____

2. Sensitivity to light _____

3. Nearsighted _____

4. Scratched cornea _____

5. Inflammation of the iris _____

6. "Lazy eye" _____

7. Farsighted _____

8. Inflamed eyelash and tarsal gland _____

9. Droopy eyelid _____

10. Cross-eyed _____

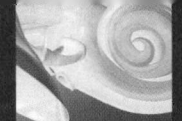

Special Senses of the Eye and Ear

F. Match the Latin and Greek terms in the left column to their meanings in the right column. (LO 16.2, 16.8, *Remember, Understand*)

_____ 1. orbit	**a.** flat
_____ 2. extrinsic	**b.** drooping
_____ 3. chalazion	**c.** on the outer side
_____ 4. cornea	**d.** paralysis
_____ 5. cortex	**e.** lump
_____ 6. ptosis	**f.** corner of the eye
_____ 7. canthus	**g.** web
_____ 8. contagious	**h.** circle
_____ 9. tarsus	**i.** outer shell
_____ 10. paresis	**j.** touch closely

Use any two terms from this exercise as they would appear in patient documentation.

11. _____

_____

_____

12. _____

_____

_____

G. **Patient documentation.** You must be precise in your use of abbreviations for documentation. Demonstrate your knowledge of abbreviations by filling in the blanks. You are given the medical language—translate it into an abbreviation. (**LO 16.1, 16.2, 16.11,** *Remember, Understand*)

1. The prescription read 150 _____ (milligrams) of Cipro, _____ (four times a day).

2. The patient was diagnosed with _____ (otitis media with effusion) secondary to an _____ (upper respiratory infection).

3. Since the _____ (acute otitis media) was resolving, the pain medication was used _____ (when necessary).

H. Master your documentation—it is a legal record. Circle the most appropriate choice, and insert the correct abbreviation where indicated on the line. (**LO 16.2, 16.8,** *Remember, Understand, Apply*)

1. Patient complains of sticky eyelids with (purulent/perulent) discharge, both eyes (_____[abbreviation])

   Diagnosis: (scleritis/conjunctivitis)

2. (Refraction/Accommodation) reveals patient's vision now 20/40 in the right eye, with correction.

3. The (diagnosis/prognosis) for Mr. Baker is continued decreasing vision in his right eye (_____[abbreviation])

   if his diabetes remains uncontrolled and his (retinopathy/retinoblastoma) worsens.

4. (Opthalmoscopic/Ophthalmoscopic) examination of the left eye (_____[abbreviation]) reveals (microaneurisms/

   microaneurysms) forming. (Fluoreseen/Fluorescein) angiography is ordered for more details.

I. Terminology challenge. The following medical terms are associated with either an eye specialist or an ear specialist. Check (√) the appropriate specialist for the term. (**LO 16.1, 16.2,** *Remember, Apply*)

Term	Otologist	Ophthalmologist
1. uveitis		
2. otolith		
3. vertigo		
4. cholesteatoma		
5. conjunctivitis		
6. glaucoma		
7. labyrinthitis		
8. papilledema		
9. canthus		
10. audiologist		
11. hordeolum		
12. dacryostenosis		
13. LASIK		
14. ptosis		

Special Senses of the Eye and Ear

J. **Word elements.** Learning word elements is your most valuable tool for increasing your medical vocabulary. Use your knowledge of word elements to answer the following questions. Circle the correct answer. (**LO 16.1, 16.2, *Remember, Apply***)

1. The root for *tear* is

    a. blephar

    b. tamin

    c. commodat

    d. strab

    e. lacrim

2. The root of this word means *letting go* and is used to indicate partial paralysis:

    a. parietal

    b. periorbital

    c. paresis

    d. ptosis

    e. presbyopia

3. On the basis of its suffix, you can tell that a *keratotomy* is a

    a. body part

    b. procedure

    c. diagnosis

    d. medication

    e. infection

4. The prefix in *microaneurysm* tells you that this aneurysm is

    a. large   **d.** painful

    b. black   **e.** red

    c. small

5. In the term *amblyopia, opia* means

    a. sound   **d.** movement

    b. light   **e.** pain

    c. sight

6. *In situ* is a Latin phrase that means *(Be precise!)*

    a. in this place

    b. in another place

    c. in its original place

    d. in the place

    e. in place of

7. In the terms *retinoblastoma* and *retinopathy,* the combining form tells you that both these terms concern the

    a. cornea

    b. iris

    c. lens

    d. vitreous body

    e. retina

8. *Angiography* is a diagnostic test of a(n)

    a. organ

    b. bone

    c. blood vessel

    d. muscle

    e. gland

9. In the term *antibiotic, anti* is a prefix that means

    a. within

    b. outside

    c. on top of

    d. against

    e. around

K. Build terms from the language of otology. Identify the following elements by checking the appropriate column. Give the meaning of the element; then give an example of a medical term containing that element. Fill in the chart. (**LO 16.1, 16.2, *Remember, Apply***)

Element	Prefix	Root/ Combining Form	Suffix	Meaning of Element	Medical Term
1. algesia				2.	3.
4. anti				5.	6.
7. ette				8.	9.
10. bi				11.	12.
12. ot				13.	14.
15. rhino				16.	17.
18. laryngo				19.	20.
21. tympan				22.	23.
24. aden				25.	26.
27. stomy				28.	29.
30. sclero				31.	32.
33. audio				34.	35.

L. Abbreviations. The following abbreviations are all part of the *language of otology*. Match the abbreviation in the left column with its meaning in the right column. (**LO 16.1, *Remember, Apply***)

_____	1. PE	a. ear infection with fluid collection
_____	2. BPPV	b. both ears
_____	3. A.S.	c. four times each day
_____	4. p.r.n.	d. right ear
_____	5. q.i.d.	e. common cold
_____	6. OME	f. sensation of spinning or whirling
_____	7. A.U.	g. every 4 hours
_____	8. q.4.h.	h. pressure-equalization tubes
_____	9. URI	i. left ear
_____	10. A.D.	j. when necessary

Special Senses of the Eye and Ear

M. **Match the Greek and Latin terms in the left column with their meanings in the right column.** Expand your knowledge of the *language of otology*. Fill in the blanks. (**LO 16.2**, *Remember, Apply*)

_____ 1. chronic		**a.** pouring out
_____ 2. impacted		**b.** wing
_____ 3. auricle		**c.** sharp
_____ 4. vertigo		**d.** stirrup
_____ 5. meatus		**e.** driven in
_____ 6. effusion		**f.** time
_____ 7. cerumen		**g.** dizziness
_____ 8. pinna		**h.** ear
_____ 9. stapes		**i.** wax
_____ 10. acute		**j.** go through

N. **Schedule your patients.** The following doctors and ancillary personnel are seeing patients in the clinic today. Based on the patient's needs, schedule the patient for the correct physician or technician. (In some cases, there may be two possible answers.) (**LO 16.1, 16.2, 16.8, 16.13**, *Remember, Apply, Analyze*)

ophthalmologist   **optometrist**   **ophthalmic technician**

otologist   **otorhinolaryngologist**

Patient Needs/Has	Schedule With
refraction	1.
PE tubes	2.
phacoemulsification	3.
instruction in using eyedrops	4.
cholesteatoma	5.
patient hit in eye with tree branch	6.
removal of tonsils and adenoids	7.
LASIK surgery	8.
child has bubble gum in nose	9.
runny nose, stopped-up ears, sore throat	10.
broken eyeglasses	11.

O. Patient education. Your patient is confused by some medical terms the doctor has used. Translate for her into simple language the difference between the following terms. (**LO 16.1, 16.2, 16.8, *Understand***)

1. *hyperopia* and *myopia* _____

    Hyperopia: _____

    Myopia: _____

2. *dacryocystitis* and *dacryostenosis* _____

    Dacryocystitis: _____

    Dacryostenosis: _____

P. Teamwork. You are helping with the orientation of a new medical assistant in the otorhinolaryngologist's office where you work. Can you describe to her the office use for the following tools? (**LO 16.1, 16.2, 16.13, *Understand, Apply***)

1. otoscope _____

_____

2. audiometer _____

_____

3. tonometer _____

_____

Q. Deconstruct the following medical terms into their word elements and meanings. This group of terms has something in common. What is it? Fill in the blanks. (**LO 16.8, 16.9, *Understand, Apply***)

Medical Term	Prefix	Root/Combining	Suffix	Meaning of Medical Term
phacoemulsification	1.	2.	3.	4.
photocoagulation	5.	6.	7.	8.
cryopexy	9.	10.	11.	12.

13. This group of terms is similar because _____.

R. Terminology challenge. *Acute* and *chronic* are two opposite descriptions. Define each term, give an example of an acute condition and a chronic one, and then explain how they are different. (**LO 16.1, *Understand, Apply***)

1. Definition of *acute:* _____

2. Acute condition: _____

3. Definition of *chronic:* _____

4. Chronic condition: _____

5. How are acute and chronic different?

_____

_____

Chapter 16 Review

Special Senses of the Eye and Ear

S. Apply what you know about the middle ear to choose the answer. Circle the best choice. (**LO 16.2, 16.11,** *Understand, Apply*)

1. Which of these is NOT a component of the middle ear?

   a. tympanic membrane

   b. eustachian (auditory) tube

   c. malleus, incus, stapes

   d. nasopharynx

   e. tympanic cavity

2. The eustachian (auditory) tube connects the

   a. tonsils and nasopharynx

   b. middle ear and nasopharynx

   c. nasopharynx and ossicles

   d. nasopharynx and tympanic membrane

   e. tympanic cavity and tympanic membrane

3. Identify the three ossicles:

   a. pinna, auricle, stapes

   b. eustachian (auditory) tube, mastoid cells, tonsils

   c. nasopharynx, tonsils, middle ear

   d. malleus, incus, stapes

   e. tonsils, stapes, incus

4. What is a complication of chronic otitis media with effusion?

   a. vertigo

   b. acute infection

   c. cholesteatoma

   d. dizziness

   e. nausea

5. Which of these would NOT cause a perforated eardrum?

   a. puncture by a cotton swab

   b. open-handed slap to the ear

   c. scuba diving

   d. pus from acute otitis media

   e. sinusitis

T. Patient education. Patients will ask you for clarification of certain terms they do not understand or for more explanation of body processes. Be prepared to answer the following questions for your patients. (**LO 16.1, 16.2, 16.12,** *Understand, Analyze*)

1. Andrew Baker has severe otosclerosis in his left ear. Dr. Lee has recommended replacement of his stapes with a plastic prosthesis. Explain to Mr. Baker what a prosthesis is, and compare it with other body part replacements he may already have.

   a. Look up **prosthesis** in the glossary. Define **prosthesis**. _____

   b. Name three other types of prostheses that can be inserted into the body. _____, _____,

   and _____

   c. Why can a prosthesis also be considered a "foreign body"? _____

   _____

2. Caroline Mason has had many ear problems since she was a child. Frequent infections necessitated PE tubes at a young age. Even after tube removal, she continued to have frequent upper respiratory infections, tonsillitis, middle-ear infections, impacted cerumen, labyrinthitis, and vertigo later in life.

   a. Can you explain to her the cumulative effect all these previous conditions have had on her hearing loss?

   _____

   _____

   b. Trace for her the pathway of sound waves through the ear to the brain, in order to be recognized as sounds.

   _____

   _____

   c. How have her previous ear problems interfered with this process?

   _____

   _____

   d. Is Ms. Mason's condition an acute or chronic condition?

   _____

U. Regions of the ear. Identify whether the statement references the external, middle, or inner ear by placing a check (√) in the correct column. (**LO 16.10, 16.11, 16.12,** *Analyze*)

Reference	External Ear	Middle Ear	Inner Ear
1. swimmer's ear			
2. otosclerosis			
3. labyrinthitis			
4. tympanic membrane			
5. PE tubes			
6. otitis externa			
7. eustachian (auditory) tube			
8. ossicles			
9. cochlear implants			

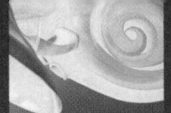

Special Senses of the Eye and Ear

V. **Discussion question.** Prepare a brief discussion that will address the following questions about CR 16.1. (**LO 16.1, 16.3, 16.8,** *Analyze*)

Case Report 16.1

Mrs. Jenny Hughes's "pink eye" is called acute **contagious** conjunctivitis *[See Figure 16.3]*. It responds well to **antibiotic** eyedrops. Her hands were **contaminated** from the keyboard of the employee who had left work and gone home with "pink eye." Mrs. Hughes transmitted the infection to her eyes by touching or rubbing.

Your documentation of Mrs. Hughes's office visit could read:

Progress Note 04/10/13

Mrs. Jenny Hughes was brought directly into the clinical area at 1030 hrs with what appeared to be conjunctivitis, "pink eye." Both eyelids were red and swollen with a purulent discharge. She complained of headache and **photophobia**. Dr. Chun prescribed Neosporin eyedrops, three drops every four hours (q.4.h.). A swab was sent to the laboratory. I instructed and watched Mrs. Hughes wash her hands and use an alcohol-based hand gel. I then had her sign in and sign our Notice of Privacy Practices. I instructed her in the use of the drops and emphasized home care and hand care measures to prevent the infection from spreading to her family. She was given a return appointment in 1 week and told to call the office if the drops did not help. Daphne Butras, OT. 1055 hrs.

1. Why was Mrs. Hughes asked to wash her hands before signing the sign-in sheet?

_____

_____

2. If she hadn't washed her hands, what could possibly happen?

_____

_____

3. What sanitary precautions must you take when you work with patients?

_____

_____

4. What types of precautions could Mrs. Hughes use at home to keep her contagious disease from spreading to the rest of her family?

_____

_____

W. Deconstruct the following medical terms. A portion of the term is in bold. Identify that element and give its meaning. <u>The first one is done for you.</u> Fill in the blanks. (**LO 16.1, 16.2, Analyze**)

Medical Term	Element	Meaning of Element
otitis	*root*	*ear*
oto**scopy**	1.	2.
mast**oid**	3.	4.
cholesteatoma	5.	6.
myringotomy	7.	8.
oto**sclerosis**	9.	10.
neur**al**	11.	12.
equilibrium	13.	14.
oto**lith**	15.	16.
par**oxysm**al	17.	18.

X. Visual pathway. In order to better understand the visual pathway, trace its route by putting the following terms in the correct order. (**LO 16.6, Analyze**)

visual cortex   optic chiasm   optic radiation   optic tract   optic foramen   cerebral hemisphere

1. _____

2. _____

3. _____

4. _____

5. _____

6. _____

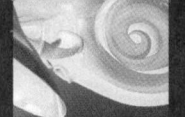

Chapter 16 Review

Special Senses of the Eye and Ear

CHAPTER SUMMARY EXERCISE

A. Spelling comprehension. Circle the correct spelling of the term. (**LO 16.1,** *Remember*)

1. optholmologist   ophtalmologist   optolmologist   ophthalmologist   optalmologist

2. strebissmus   strabbismus   strubismis   strabismus   strabithmus

3. petosis   putosis   ptosis   ptysosis   phytosis

4. yustachian   eustachian   eustacian   eusstacyan   yustachien

B. Match the number of the correct spelling of the term in Exercise A with the brief description of the term below. (**LO 16.1,** *Understand, Apply*)

1. The turning of an eye away from its normal position   _____

2. Connects middle ear to nasopharynx   _____

3. Treats diseases of the eye and prescribes medication   _____

4. Falling or drooping of an eyelid (or organ)   _____

C. Using your knowledge of terms 1–4 in Exercises A and B and their correct spelling, write a brief sentence for each of the terms as it might appear in patient documentation. (**LO 16.1, 16.2,** *Apply*)

1. _____

2. _____

3. _____

4. _____

D. After rereading the progress note from Case Report 16.1, answer the following questions. Be prepared to discuss your answers in class. (**LO 16.1, 16.2, 16.8,** *Analyze*)

Progress Note 04/10/12

Mrs. Jenny Hughes was brought directly into the clinical area at 1030 hrs with what appeared to be conjunctivitis, "pink eye." Both eyelids were red and swollen with a purulent discharge. She complained of headache and **photophobia**. Dr. Chun prescribed Neosporin eyedrops, three drops q.4.h. A swab was sent to the laboratory. I instructed and watched Mrs. Hughes wash her hands and use an alcohol-based hand gel. I then had her sign in and sign our Notice of Privacy Practices. I instructed her in the use of the drops and emphasized home care and hand care measures to prevent the infection from spreading to her family. She was given a return appointment in 1 week and told to call the office if the drops did not help. Daphne Butras, OT. 1055 hrs.

1. Define the term *conjunctivitis*. _____

2. What were the patient's chief complaints? _____

3. Describe Mrs. Hughes's symptoms. _____

4. How often is Mrs. Hughes supposed to use the eyedrops? _____

5. Photophobia is _____ of the light because _____.

6. If an infection can be spread from person to person, it is considered _____.

E. **Meet the goals of each of the chapter outcomes by using the correct language of the study of the eye and ear for the answers. (LO 16.1–16.13, *Analyze*)**

1. Use the medical terms of ophthalmology and otology to communicate and document in writing accurately and precisely in any health care setting. Circle the only term in the following list that does not relate to ophthalmology. (**LO 16.1**)

   a. stereopsis

   b. strabismus

   c. labyrinth

   d. ocular

   e. sclera

2. Use the medical terms of ophthalmology and otology to communicate verbally with accuracy and precision in any health care setting. The doctor has told you to write on the patient's chart the acronym "PERRLA" during today's visit. What does that mean? (**LO 16.2**)

   _____

   _____

3. Describe the accessory structures of the eye and their common disorders. Pick any one accessory structure of the eye and describe one of its disorders. (**LO 16.3**)

   a. structure:

   _____

   b. disorder:

   _____

4. Identify the common conditions of the eye due to imbalance of the extrinsic muscles of the eye. Circle the only incorrect statement about the extrinsic muscles of the eye. (**LO 16.4**)

   a. Stereopsis depends on an accurate alignment of the two eyes.   T   F

   b. There are 8 extrinsic eye muscles.   T   F

   c. Esotropia is a condition of the extrinsic eye muscles.   T   F

   d. Extrinsic eye muscles move the eye in all directions.   T   F

   e. Extrinsic eye muscles are attached to the inner wall of the eye orbit and to the outer surface of the eyeball.   T   F

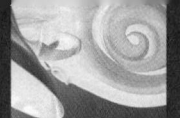

Special Senses of the Eye and Ear

5. Discuss the structure and functions of the eyeball and its different components. (**LO 16.5**)

   a. structure:

   _____

   _____

   b. functions:

   _____

   _____

   c. components:

   _____

   _____

6. Map the visual pathway from the lens to the visual cortex of the brain. (**LO 16.6**)

   Start your map after the first sentence.

   After passing through the pupil, the light rays pass through the transparent lens. Then,

   _____

   _____

   _____

   _____

   _____

   _____ to the visual cortex at the back of the brain.

7. Describe the disorders of refraction. (**LO 16.7**)

   a. What exactly is refraction? _____

   b. A normal refraction can be abbreviated as _____

   c. Pick any one disorder of refraction and describe it.

      i. disorder:

      _____

      ii. description:

      _____

      _____

8. Describe the cause, appearance, diagnosis, and treatment of common disorders of the eye and its accessory structures. Conjunctivitis is a common diagnosis for the eye. Describe its cause, appearance, and treatment. Write your answers on the following lines. (**LO 16.8**)

   a. cause:

   _____

   b. appearance:

   _____

   c. treatment:

   _____

9. Define the purpose of certain ophthalmic procedures. Match the medical terms in the first column to the statements in the second column. (**LO 16.9**)

   _____ a. Snellen letter chart   i. tests normal vision

   _____ b. tonometer   ii. tests distance vision

   _____ c. fundoscopy   iii. tests near vision

   _____ d. Jaeger reading cards   iv. measures intraocular pressure

   _____ e. refraction   v. examines the retina of the eye

Special Senses of the Eye and Ear

10. Describe the anatomy of the external ear and its disorders. Which of the following is not a term pertaining to the external ear? Circle the correct choice below. **(LO 16.10)**

    a. auricle

    b. meatus

    c. pinna

    d. canthus

    e. tympanic membrane

11. Discuss the structure and functions of the middle ear and its disorders. **(LO 16.11)**

    a. List the four components of the middle ear:

        i. _____

        ii. _____

        iii. _____

        iv. _____

    b. Give a brief description of each of these middle ear disorders:

        i. cholesteatoma _____

        ii. AOM _____

        iii. OME _____

        iv. otosclerosis _____

12. Discuss the structure and functions of the inner ear for hearing and balance and its disorders. **(LO 16.12)**

    a. Vertigo and tinnitus are conditions that arise in the inner ear. Describe their differences.

        i. vertigo _____

        ii. tinnitus _____

    b. Which pair of terms are the organs of balance? Circle the correct choice.

        i. otolith   cholesteatoma

        ii. vestibule   semicircular canals

        iii. meatus   labyrinth

        iv. ampullaris   ptosis

        v. chiasm   uvea

13. Identify the value of hearing test procedures.

Choose any two hearing test procedures. Describe them and state what their results confirm. (**LO 16.13**)

1. hearing test

description: _____

results confirm: _____

2. hearing test

description: _____

results confirm: _____

Endocrine System
The Language of Endocrinology

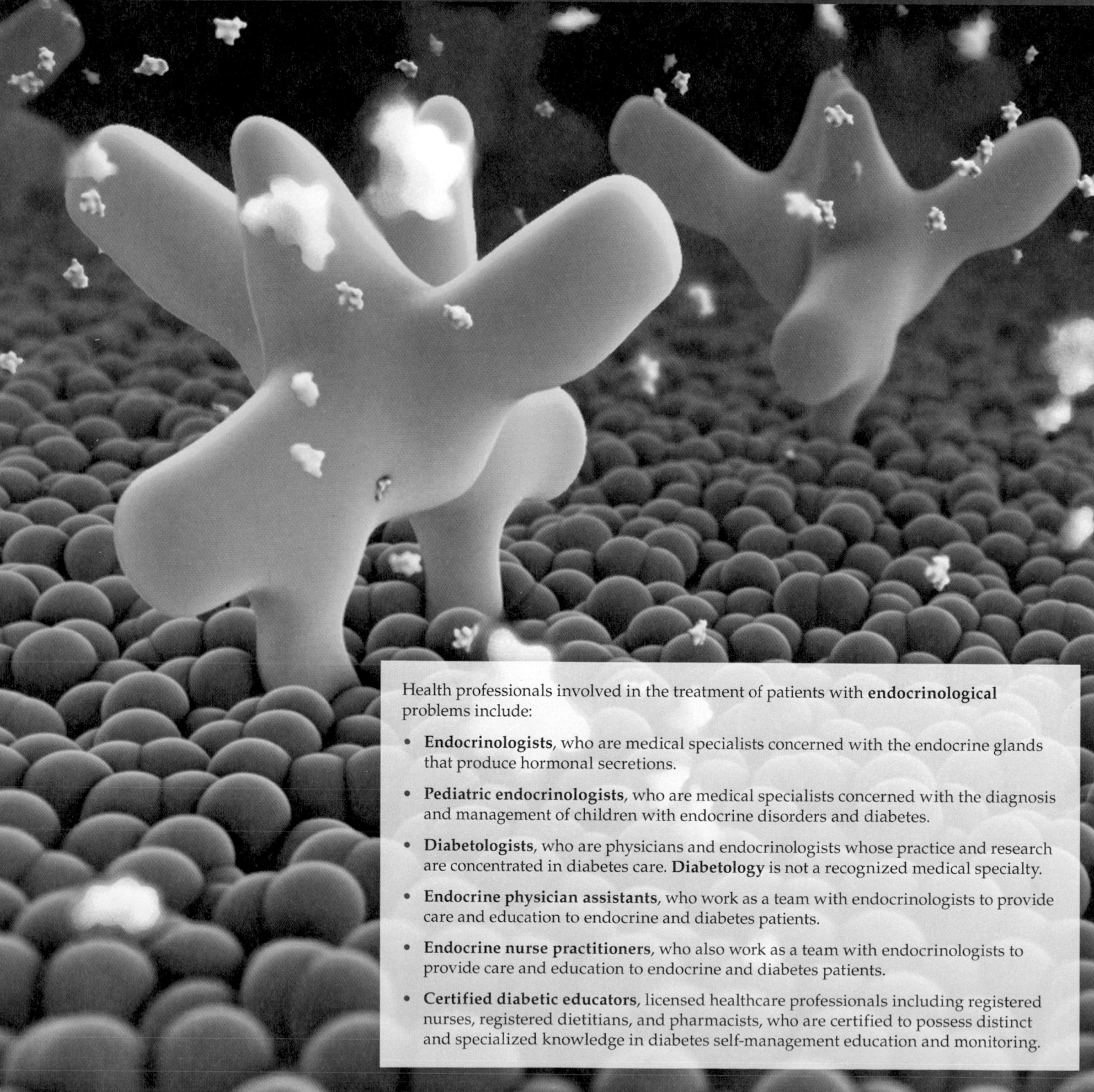

Health professionals involved in the treatment of patients with **endocrinological** problems include:

- **Endocrinologists**, who are medical specialists concerned with the endocrine glands that produce hormonal secretions.

- **Pediatric endocrinologists**, who are medical specialists concerned with the diagnosis and management of children with endocrine disorders and diabetes.

- **Diabetologists**, who are physicians and endocrinologists whose practice and research are concentrated in diabetes care. **Diabetology** is not a recognized medical specialty.

- **Endocrine physician assistants**, who work as a team with endocrinologists to provide care and education to endocrine and diabetes patients.

- **Endocrine nurse practitioners**, who also work as a team with endocrinologists to provide care and education to endocrine and diabetes patients.

- **Certified diabetic educators**, licensed healthcare professionals including registered nurses, registered dietitians, and pharmacists, who are certified to possess distinct and specialized knowledge in diabetes self-management education and monitoring.

17

You are

> ...a registered nurse (**RN**) working with endocrinologist Sabina Khalid, MD, in the Endocrinology Clinic at Fulwood Medical Center.

Your patient is

> ...Mrs. Gina Tacher, a 33-year-old schoolteacher. She complains of coarsening of her facial features and enlargement of the bones of her hands. Over the past 10 years her nose and jaw have increased in size, and her voice has become husky. She brought photos of herself at ages 9 and 16. She has no other health problems.

Chapter Learning Outcomes

The **endocrine system** is a communication system. The **hormones** it produces circulate in the bloodstream, giving them access to all other cells of the body. Hormones are bloodborne messengers secreted by endocrine glands. They are distributed anywhere that blood goes but affect only the target cells that have receptors for them; they alter the metabolism of these cells.

The information in this chapter enables you to:

LO 17.1 Identify the endocrine glands and the hormones each gland secretes.

LO 17.2 Locate the anatomical position of each endocrine gland in the body.

LO 17.3 Describe the functions of the different hormones in the body.

LO 17.4 Identify the disorders resulting from excessive and deficient production of the different hormones.

LO 17.5 Use the medical terms of endocrinology to communicate and document in writing accurately and precisely in any health care setting.

LO 17.6 Use the medical terms of endocrinology to communicate verbally with accuracy and precision in any health care setting.

LO 17.7 Explain the clinical and laboratory tests used to determine the presence or absence of a specific hormone.

LO 17.8 Describe agents used in the treatment of endocrine disorders.

LO 17.9 Discuss the body's reaction to stress.

LO 17.10 Identify the different types, symptoms, and signs of diabetes.

LO 17.11 Describe the criteria used to diagnose diabetes.

LO 17.12 Discuss the different forms of treatment of diabetes.

Keynotes

- A hormone is secreted by an organ and carried by the bloodstream to act at distant target sites.

- The medical specialty concerned with the hormonal secretions of the endocrine glands, their physiology, and pathology is called *endocrinology*.

Endocrine System Overview: Hypothalamus, Pituitary, and Pineal Glands

LESSON OBJECTIVES

The information in this lesson will enable you to use correct medical terminology to:

17.1.1 Identify the glands that make up the endocrine system.
17.1.2 List the hormones produced by the hypothalamus and pituitary gland.
17.1.3 Explain the interactions between the hypothalamus and pituitary gland.
17.1.4 Describe the controls the hypothalamus and pituitary exert over other endocrine glands.
17.1.5 Identify the roles of the pineal gland.
17.1.6 Describe disorders of the hypothalamus, pituitary gland, and pineal gland.

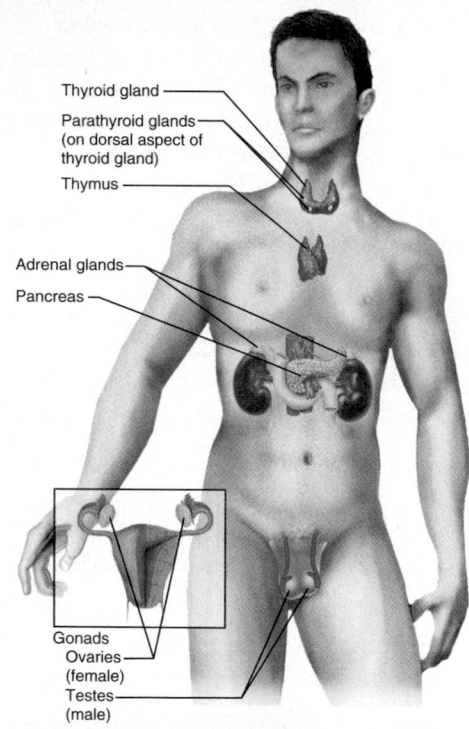

Thyroid gland

Parathyroid glands (on dorsal aspect of thyroid gland)

Thymus

Adrenal glands

Pancreas

Gonads
Ovaries (female)
Testes (male)

▲ **Figure 17.1** Major Endocrine Glands.

LO 17.1, 17.2 Endocrine System

The endocrine system comprises a number (14) of major glands (*Figure 17.1*):

- Pituitary gland and the nearby hypothalamus
- Pineal gland
- Thyroid gland
- Parathyroid glands (4)
- Thymus gland
- Adrenal glands (2)
- Pancreas
- Gonads: testes (2) in the male; ovaries (2) in the female

In addition, endocrine cells found in tissues all over the body secrete hormones. Examples are

- **Cells in the upper GI tract** that secrete the hormone **gastrin**, which stimulates gastric secretions and the hormone **cholecystokinin**, which contracts the gallbladder (*see Chapter 5*).
- **Cells in the kidney** that secrete **erythropoietin**, which stimulates erythrocyte production (*see Chapter 6*).
- **Fat cells** that secrete **leptin**, which helps suppress appetite. Lack of it can lead to overeating and obesity.
- **Cells in tissues throughout the body** that secrete **prostaglandins**, which act locally to dilate blood vessels, relax airways, stimulate uterine contractions in menstrual cramps or labor, and lower acid secretion in the stomach. When tissues are injured, prostaglandins promote an inflammatory response.

Hypothalamus

The hypothalamus (*Figure 17.2*) forms the floor and walls of the brain's third ventricle (*see Chapter 9*) and produces eight hormones. Six of them are local hormones that regulate the production of hormones by the anterior pituitary gland (*see page XXX*). Two of them, oxytocin and **antidiuretic hormone (ADH)**, are transported to the posterior pituitary, where they are stored until they are needed elsewhere in the body.

Pineal Gland

The pineal gland is located on the roof of the third ventricle of the brain, posterior to the hypothalamus (*Figure 17.2*). It secretes **serotonin** by day and converts it to **melatonin** at night. The gland reaches its maximum size in childhood and may regulate the timing of puberty. It may also play a role in **seasonal affective disorder (SAD)**, in which people are depressed in the dark days of winter.

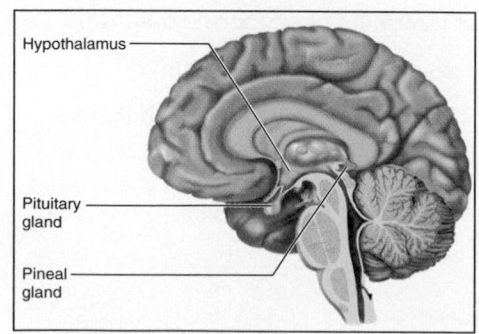

Hypothalamus

Pituitary gland

Pineal gland

▲ **Figure 17.2** Hypothalamus, Pituitary Gland, and Pineal Gland.

Abbreviations

ADH	antidiuretic hormone
RN	registered nurse
SAD	seasonal affective disorder

Word Analysis and Definition

S = Suffix   P = Prefix   R = Root   R/CF = Combining Form

WORD	PRONUNCIATION	ELEMENTS		DEFINITION
antidiuretic (**Note:** This term has two prefixes.)	**AN**-tih-die-you-**RET**-ik	S/ P/ P/ R/	-ic *pertaining to* anti- *against* -di- *complete* -uret- *urination*	An agent that decreases urine production
endocrine	**EN**-doh-krin	P/ R/CF	endo- *within* -crin/e *secrete*	Pertaining to a gland that produces an internal or hormonal secretion
endocrinology (**Note:** The "e" in -crine changes to "o" for easier pronunciation.)	**EN**-doh-krih-**NOL**-oh-jee	R/CF S/	-crin/o *secrete* -logy *study of*	Medical specialty concerned with the production and effects of hormones
endocrinologist	**EN**-doh-krih-**NOL**-oh-jist	S/	-logist *one who studies, specialist*	A medical specialist in endocrinology
gland	**GLAND**		Latin *glans* acorn	A collection of cells functioning as a secretory or excretory organ
hormone	**HOR**-mohn		Greek *to set in motion*	Chemical formed in one tissue or organ and carried by the blood to stimulate or inhibit a function of another tissue or organ
hormonal (adj)	hor-**MOHN**-al	S/ R/	-al *pertaining to* hormon- *chemical messenger*	Pertaining to a hormone(s) or the endocrine system
leptin	**LEP**-tin	S/ R/	-in *chemical compound* lept- *thin, small*	Hormone secreted by adipose tissue
melatonin	mel-ah-**TONE**-in	S/ R/ R/	-in *chemical compound* mela- *black* -ton- *tension, pressure*	Hormone formed by the pineal gland
oxytocin	**OCK**-see-toe-sin	S/ P/ R/	-in *chemical compound* oxy- *quick* -toc- *labor, birth*	Hypothalamic hormone, stored in the posterior pituitary, that stimulates the uterus to contract
parathyroid	par-ah-**THIGH**-royd	S/ P/ R/	-oid *resemble* para- *beside* -thyr- *thyroid*	Endocrine glands embedded in the back of the thyroid gland
pineal	**PIN**-ee-al		Latin *like a pine cone*	Pertaining to the pineal gland
pituitary	pih-**TOO**-ih-tary	S/ R/	-ary *pertaining to* pituit- *pituitary*	Pertaining to the pituitary gland
prostaglandin	**PROS**-tah-**GLAN**-din	S/ R/CF R/	-in *chemical compound* prost/a- *prostate* -gland- *gland*	Hormone present in many tissues, but first isolated from prostate gland
seasonal affective disorder (**Note:** The abbreviation for this is SAD, which is how you feel with this disorder.)	see-**ZON**-al af-**FEK**-tiv dis-**OR**-der			Depression that occurs at the same time every year, often in winter
serotonin	ser-oh-**TOE**-nin	S/ R/CF R/	-in *substance* ser/o- *serum* -ton- *tension, pressure*	A neurotransmitter in the central and peripheral nervous systems

Exercises

A. Elements are listed in the left column. *Place a checkmark (√) in the column identifying the type of element. Finish the exercise by writing the meaning of the element in the right column.* **LO 17.5**

Element	Prefix	Root/Combining Form	Suffix	Meaning of Element
1. di	_____	_____	_____	_____
2. anti	_____	_____	_____	_____
3. endo	_____	_____	_____	_____
4. mela	_____	_____	_____	_____

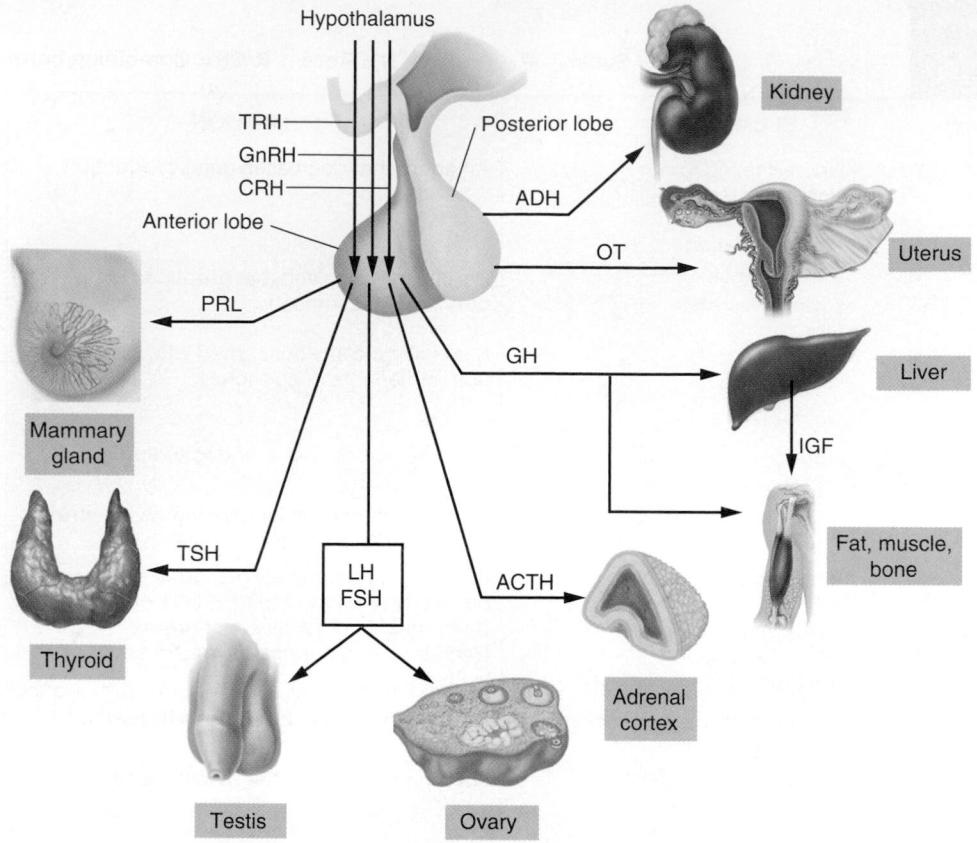

▲ Figure 17.3 Hormones of the Pituitary Gland and Their Target Organs.

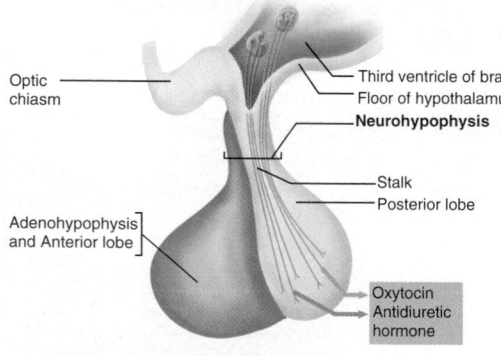

▲ Figure 17.4 Hormones of the Posterior Lobe of the Pituitary Gland.

Abbreviations	
ACTH	adrenocorticotropic hormone
ADH	antidiuretic hormone
FSH	follicle-stimulating hormone
GH	growth hormone
GnRH	gonadotropin-releasing hormone
LH	luteinizing hormone
OT	oxytocin
PRL	prolactin
TSH	thyroid-stimulating hormone

LO 17.1, 17.2, 17.3 Pituitary Gland

While there is no single conductor of the endocrine orchestra in which each hormone plays its part in maintaining homeostasis, the pituitary gland and the hypothalamus work together and often influence the production of hormones in the other endocrine glands.

The pituitary gland (**hypophysis**) is suspended from the hypothalamus. The gland has two components:

1. A large anterior lobe called the **adenohypophysis**.

2. A smaller posterior lobe called the **neurohypophysis**.

Anterior lobe hormones are six in number *(Figure 17.3)*:

- **Follicle-stimulating hormone (FSH)** stimulates target cells in the ovaries to develop eggs and stimulates sperm production in the testes.

- **Luteinizing hormone (LH)** stimulates ovulation and the formation of a corpus luteum in the ovary *(see Chapter 8)* to secrete estrogen and progesterone. In the male, LH stimulates production of testosterone *(see Chapter 17)*.

(FSH and LH are gonadotropins and are released under the control of gonadotropin-releasing hormone [GnRH] of the hypothalamus *[see page XXX]*.)

- **Thyroid-stimulating hormone (TSH)**, or **thyrotropin**, stimulates the growth of the thyroid gland and the production of **thyroxine**.

- **Adrenocorticotropic hormone (ACTH)**, or **corticotropin**, stimulates the adrenal glands to produce hormones called **corticosteroids**.

- **Prolactin (PRL)** stimulates the mammary glands after pregnancy to produce milk.

- **Growth hormone (GH)**, or **somatotropin**, is produced in quantities at least a thousand times as great as any other pituitary hormone. It stimulates cells to enlarge and divide to produce growth, particularly in childhood and adolescence.

Tropic (also spelled **trophic**) **hormones** are hormones that stimulate other endocrine glands to produce their hormones. All of the anterior lobe hormones except PRL and GH are tropic hormones.

Posterior lobe hormones, which are produced by nuclei in the hypothalamus and then stored in and released by the pituitary posterior lobe, are of two types *(Figure 17.4)*:

- **Oxytocin (OT)** in childbirth stimulates uterine contractions and in lactation forces milk to flow down ducts to the nipple. In both sexes, its production increases during sexual intercourse to help give the feelings of satisfaction and emotional bonding.

- **Antidiuretic hormone (ADH)** reduces the volume of urine produced by the kidneys. It is also called **vasopressin**.

WORD	PRONUNCIATION	ELEMENTS		DEFINITION
adenohypophysis (***Note:*** The prefix hypo- is part of **hypophysis**, which is a term in itself.)	**AD**-en-oh-hi-**POF**-ih-sis	R/ R/CF P/	**-physis** *growth* **aden/o-** *gland* **-hypo-** *below*	Anterior lobe of the pituitary gland
adrenal gland	ah-**DREE**-nal GLAND	S/ P/ R/	**-al** *pertaining to* **ad-** *near, toward* **-ren-** *kidney*	The suprarenal, or adrenal, gland on the upper pole of each kidney
adrenocorticotropic hormone	ah-**DREE**-noh-**KOR**-tih-koh-**TROH**-pik **HOR**-mohn	S/ R/CF R/CF	**-tropic** *stimulator* **adren/o-** *adrenal gland* **-cortic/o-** *cortisone, cortex*	Hormone of the anterior pituitary that stimulates the cortex of the adrenal gland to produce its own hormones
antidiuretic hormone (ADH) (also called **vasopressin**)	**AN**-tih-die-you-**RET**-ik **HOR**-mohn	S/ P/ P/ R/CF R/CF	**-tic** *pertaining to* **anti-** *against* **-di-** *complete* **-ur/e-** *urinary system* **hormon/e** *chemical messenger, hormone*	Posterior pituitary hormone that decreases urine output by acting on the kidney
corticosteroid	**KOR**-tih-koh-**STEHR**-oyd	S/ R/CF	**-steroid** *steroid* **cortic/o-** *cortisone, cortex*	A hormone produced by the adrenal cortex
corticotropin	**KOR**-tih-koh-**TROH**-pin	S/ R/CF	**-tropin** *stimulation* **cortic/o-** *cortisone, cortex*	Pituitary hormone that stimulates the cortex of the adrenal gland to secrete cortisone
hypophysis	high-**POF**-ih-sis	P/ R/	**hypo-** *below* **-physis** *growth*	Another name for the pituitary gland
neurohypophysis	**NYUR**-oh-high-**POF**-ih-sis	R/ R/CF P/	**-physis** *growth* **neur/o-** *nervous tissue* **-hypo-** *below*	Posterior lobe of the pituitary gland
prolactin	pro-**LAK**-tin	S/ P/ R/	**-in** *chemical compound* **pro-** *before* **-lact-** *milk*	Pituitary hormone that stimulates the production of milk
somatotropin (also called **growth hormone**)	**SO**-mah-toh-**TROH**-pin	S/ R/CF	**-tropin** *stimulation* **somat/o-** *the body*	Hormone of the anterior pituitary that stimulates growth of body tissues
thyroid	**THIGH**-royd		Greek *an oblong shield*	Endocrine gland in the neck, or a cartilage of the larynx
thyrotropin	thigh-roe-**TROH**-pin	S/ R/CF	**-tropin** *stimulation* **thyr/o-** *thyroid*	Hormone from the anterior pituitary gland that stimulates function of the thyroid gland
thyroxine	thigh-**ROCK**-sin	S/ R/ R/CF	**-ine** *pertaining to* **thyr** **thyr-** *thyroid*	Thyroid hormone T$_4$, tetraiodothyronine
tropic (adj) **tropin (noun)**	**TROH**-pik **TROH**-pin		Greek *a turning*	Tropic hormones stimulate other endocrine glands to produce hormones
vasopressin (also called **antidiuretic hormone ADH**)	vay-soh-**PRESS**-in	S/ R/CF R/	**-in** *chemical compound* **vas/o-** *blood vessel* **-press-** *press, close*	Pituitary hormone that constricts blood vessels and decreases urine output

Exercises

A. Many hormones are known by their abbreviation. *Match the description in the left column to the correct abbreviation in the right column.*
   LO 17.3

_____ 1. Stimulates formation of corpus luteum   **a.** PRL   _____ 5. Reduces volume of urine   **e.** TSH

_____ 2. Stimulates production of corticosteroids   **b.** LH   _____ 6. Stimulates milk production   **f.** OT

_____ 3. Stimulates uterine contractions   **c.** GH   _____ 7. Stimulates production of thyroxin   **g.** FSH

_____ 4. Stimulates ovaries to develop eggs   **d.** ACTH   _____ 8. Stimulates cells to enlarge and divide   **h.** ADH

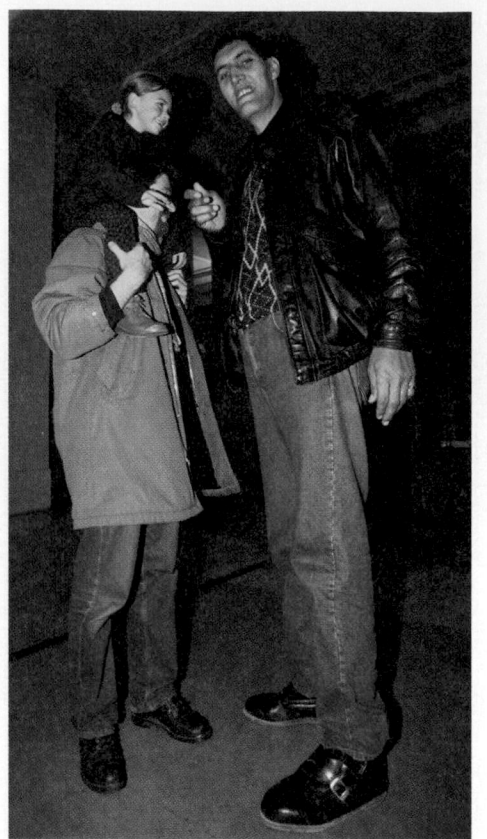

▲ **Figure 17.5** Pituitary Gigantism.

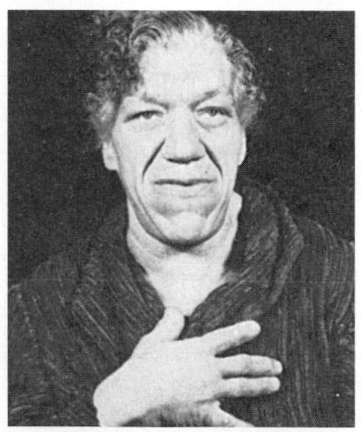

▲ **Figure 17.6** Woman with Acromegaly, Age 52.

Abbreviations	
BP	blood pressure
CT	computed tomography
DI	diabetes insipidus
IGF	insulinlike growth factor
MRI	magnetic resonance imaging

Case Report 17.1 (continued)

Dr. Khalid's examination of Mrs. Gina Tacher showed a protruding mandible (**prognathism**) and an enlarged, deeply grooved tongue. Her feet and hands were enlarged. She had noticed an increase in her shoe size and an inability to remove her wedding band. Her ribs were thickened, her heart was enlarged, and her blood pressure (**BP**) was 140/90. Her body hair was dark and coarse, and she was sweating freely.

X-rays showed a thickened skull with enlarged nasal sinuses and thickened terminal phalanges of her hands. A diagnosis of **acromegaly** was made.

Computed tomography (**CT**) and magnetic resonance imaging (**MRI**) scans showed a tumor in the pituitary that occupies most of the sella turcica *(see Chapter 5)*.

Blood tests showed high levels of growth hormone and **insulin-like growth factor (IGF)**.

LO 17.4 Disorders of Pituitary Hormones

Overproduction of Pituitary Hormones

Overproduction of growth hormone stimulates excessive growth of bones and muscles. It is almost always caused by a benign pituitary adenoma.

In children, the excessive production starts before the growth plates of the long bones have closed. The long bones grow enormously, producing **gigantism** *(Figure 17.5)*. Puberty can be delayed, genitalia may not develop fully, and diabetes can be a problem.

In adults, excessive growth hormone produces **acromegaly** *(Figure 17.6)*. This is the condition Mrs. Gina Tacher has.

Treatment of acromegaly is difficult. In Mrs. Tacher's case, surgery was able to remove much of the pituitary adenoma and was followed by radiation therapy.

A **prolactinoma** is a benign prolactin-secreting tumor of the pituitary gland in both men and women. It can lead to breast milk production in women who are not breast-feeding and produce scanty menstrual periods. In men it leads to breast milk production and impotence. The abnormal production of breast milk is called galactorrhea *(see Chapter 13)*.

Underproduction of Pituitary Hormones

Underproduction of growth hormone can be present at birth and leads to **pituitary dwarfism** *(Figure 17.7)*. The short stature becomes evident at around 1 year of age and is associated with episodes of hypoglycemia.

Hypopituitarism is uncommon. It can be caused by a pituitary tumor and cause a decline in the production of several hormones at the same time, a condition called **panhypopituitarism**.

Diabetes insipidus (DI) results from a decreased production of ADH, which helps regulate the amount of water in the body. (Diabetes mellitus is an entirely different disorder; *see Lesson 17.4.*) Antidiuretic hormone is produced in the hypothalamus and stored in the posterior pituitary lobe. Diabetes insipidus can result from insufficient production of ADH in the hypothalamus or failure of the pituitary gland to release it.

Symptoms begin with excessive urine production (polyuria) by day and by night. This leads to thirst and the need to drink up to 40 quarts of fluid per day.

In contrast to diabetes mellitus, urine in diabetes insipidus is dilute and does not contain sugar.

Treatment of diabetes insipidus is with vasopressin or desmopressin, synthetic modified forms of ADH. They are taken as a nasal spray several times daily, the dose being adjusted to maintain a normal urine output.

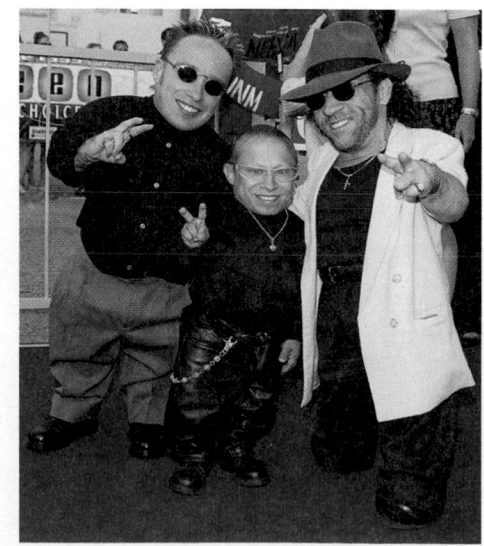

▲ **Figure 17.7** Pituitary Dwarfism.

WORD	PRONUNCIATION	ELEMENTS		DEFINITION
acromegaly	ak-roe-**MEG**-ah-lee	P/	**acro-** *highest point, extremity*	Enlargement of the head, face, hands, and feet due to excess growth hormone in an adult
		R/	**-megaly** *enlargement*	
diabetes insipidus	dye-ah-**BEE**-teez in-**SIP**-ih-dus		**diabetes** Greek *siphon*	Excretion of large amounts of dilute urine as a result of inadequate ADH production
		S/	**-us** *pertaining to*	
		P/	**in-** *not, without*	
		R/	**-sipid-** *flavor*	
dwarfism	**DWORF**-izm	S/	**-ism** *condition*	Short stature due to underproduction of growth hormone
		R/	**dwarf-** *miniature*	
gigantism	**JI**-gan-tizm	S/	**-ism** *condition*	Abnormal height and size of entire body
		R/	**gigant-** *giant*	
hypopituitarism	**HIGH**-poh-pih-**TYU**-ih-tah-rizm	S/	**-ism** *condition*	Condition of one or more deficient pituitary hormones
		P/	**hypo-** *deficient*	
		R/	**-pituitar-** *pituitary*	
panhypopituitarism	pan-**HIGH**-poh-pih-**TYU**-ih-tah-rizm	S/	**-ism** *condition*	Deficiency of all the pituitary hormones
		P/	**-hypo-** *deficient*	
		P/	**pan-** *all*	
		R/	**-pituitar-** *pituitary*	
prognathism	**PROG**-nah-thizm	S/	**-ism** *condition*	Condition of a forward-projecting jaw
		P/	**pro-** *before, in front*	
		R/	**-gnath-** *jaw*	
prolactinoma	pro-lak-tih-**NO**-muh	S/	**-oma** *tumor*	Prolactin-producing tumor
		P/	**pro-** *before, in front*	
		R/	**-lact-** *milk*	
		S/	**-in-** *chemical compound*	

Exercises

A. After reading Case Report 17.1 on the opposite page, answer the following questions. *Be prepared to discuss your answers in class.*   **LO 17.4, 17.5**

1. Describe a *protruding mandible*. _____

2. What is the correct medical term for this condition? _____

3. What are the *signs* and *symptoms* Mrs. Tacher presented with?

   Signs (observable on the outside):

   _____

   Symptoms (felt by the patient on the inside):

   _____

4. Was her blood pressure elevated? _____

5. What diagnostic tests has Mrs. Tacher had? _____

6. In the diagnosis *acromegaly,* which element means *enlargement*? _____

7. What hormone does Mrs. Tacher have in excess? _____

8. Where are the *terminal phalanges*? _____

9. How has this condition affected her other body systems? (Be specific.) _____

Thyroid, Parathyroid, and Thymus Glands

LESSON OBJECTIVES

To understand what is happening in Case Report 17.2 and what treatment is being given, you will need to be able to use correct medical terminology to:

17.2.1 Describe the location and anatomy of the thyroid gland.

17.2.2 Explain how the three thyroid hormones are produced and secreted.

17.2.3 Specify the functions of the thyroid hormones.

17.2.4 Discuss common disorders of the thyroid gland.

17.2.5 Locate the positions of the parathyroid and thymus glands.

17.2.6 List the hormones produced by the parathyroid and thymus glands and state their functions.

You are

. . . an emergency medical technician (**EMT**) working in the Emergency Room at Fulwood Medical Center at 0200 hours.

Your patient is

. . . Ms. Norma Leary, a 22-year-old college student living with her parents for the summer.

Case Report 17.2

Ms. Leary is **emaciated**, extremely agitated, restless, and at times disoriented and confused. Her parents tell you that, in the past 3 or 4 days, she has been coughing and not feeling well. In the past 12 hours she has become feverish and been complaining of a left-sided chest pain. With questioning, the parents reveal that prior to this acute illness she had lost about 20 pounds in weight, although she was eating voraciously. Her vital signs (VS) are T 105.2°F, P 180 and irregular, R 24, BP 160/85.

You call for Dr. Hilinski **STAT** (immediately) On his initial examination, he believes that the patient is in **thyroid storm**. This is a medical emergency. There are no immediate laboratory tests that can confirm this diagnosis.

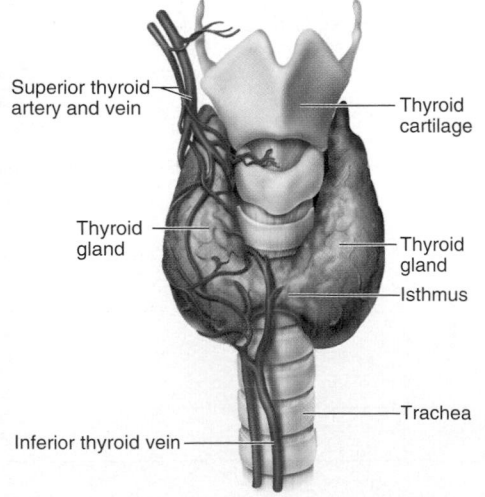

Superior thyroid artery and vein

Thyroid cartilage

Thyroid gland

Thyroid gland

Isthmus

Trachea

Inferior thyroid vein

▲ **Figure 17.8** Anatomy of the Thyroid Gland.

Abbreviations

EMT	emergency medical technician
STAT	immediately
T₃	triiodothyronine
T₄	thyroxine (tetraiodothyronine)
TSH	thyroid-stimulating hormone

LO 17.2, 17.3 Thyroid Gland

The thyroid gland lies just beneath the skin of the neck and below the thyroid cartilage (Adam's apple). It is about 2 inches (5 cm) across and shaped like a bow tie. Two lobes extend up on either side of the trachea and are joined by an isthmus *(Figure 17.8)*.

The thyroid is a soft, very vascular organ composed mostly of small follicles lined with epithelial cells. These cells secrete the two thyroid hormones **triiodothyronine (T_3)** and **thyroxine (T_4)**. The term **thyroid hormone** refers to T_3 and T_4 collectively.

Thyroid hormone acts in three interrelated ways:

- **Stimulates** almost every tissue in the body to produce proteins.
- **Increases** the amount of oxygen that cells use.
- **Controls** the speed at which the body's chemical functions proceed (metabolic rate).

The thyroid gland extracts **iodine** from the blood to produce T_3 and T_4. The hormones are produced in response to **thyroid-stimulating hormone (TSH)** from the anterior pituitary gland. The pituitary gland, in turn, increases or slows the release of TSH in response to the level of thyroid hormone in the blood.

The thyroid also produces the hormone **calcitonin** from the **C cells** found between the follicles. Calcitonin stimulates osteoblastic activity *(see Chapter 14)* to promote calcium deposition and bone formation. It is secreted in response to **hypercalcemia**.

WORD	PRONUNCIATION	ELEMENTS		DEFINITION
calcitonin	kal-sih-**TONE**-in	S/ R/CF R/	-in *chemical compound* **calc/i-** *calcium* **-ton-** *pressure, tension*	Thyroid hormone that moves calcium from blood to bones
emaciation emaciated (adv)	ee-may-see-**AY**-shun	S/ R/CF S/	-ation *process* **emac/i-** *make thin* -ated *composed of*	Abnormal thinness Abnormally thin and wasted
hypercalcemia	**HIGH**-per-cal-**SEE**-me-ah	S/ P/ R/	-emia *condition of the blood* **hyper-** *above, excessive* **-calc-** *calcium*	Excessive level of calcium in the blood
iodine	**EYE**-oh-dine or **EYE**-oh-deen	S/ R/	-ine *pertaining to* **iod-** *violet, iodine*	Chemical element, the lack of which causes thyroid disease
thyroid hormone	**THIGH**-royd **HOR**-mohn		**thyroid** *thyroid gland* **hormone** *chemical messenger*	Collective term for the two thyroid hormones, T_3 and T_4
thyroid storm	**THIGH**-royd STORM		**thyroid** *thyroid gland* **storm** *crisis*	Medical crisis and emergency due to excess thyroid hormones
thyroxine	thigh-**ROCK**-sin	S/ R/ R/CF	-ine *pertaining to* **-ox-** *oxygen* **thyr/o** *thyroid*	Thyroid hormone T_4, tetraiodothyronine
triiodothyronine	tri-**EYE**-oh-doh-**THY**-roh-neen	S/ P/ R/CF R/CF	-ine *pertaining to* **tri-** *three* **-iod/o-** *violet, iodine* **-thyr/o-** *thyroid gland*	Thyroid hormone T_3

Exercises

A. After reading Case Report 17.2 on the opposite page, answer the following questions. *Be prepared to discuss your answers in class.* **LO 17.2, 17.3, 17.4, 17.5**

1. Describe someone who looks *emaciated.* _____

2. What *signs* are observable with this patient? _____
_____

3. What are Ms. Leary's *symptoms*? _____
_____

4. What additional symptoms developed in the last 24 hours before she came to the emergency room? _____
_____

5. What is unusual about her current weight? _____
_____

6. What is happening in Ms. Leary's body that makes it a *medical emergency*? _____
_____

7. Which other body systems are involved in her response in the preceding question 1? _____
_____

8. What does the abbreviation *STAT* mean? _____
_____

9. *Thyroid storm* is due to what? _____
_____

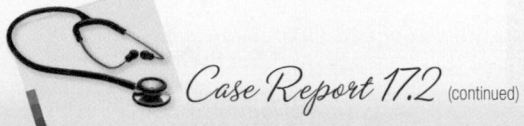

Case Report 17.2 (continued)

Thyroid storm is the condition Ms. Norma Leary presented with in the Emergency Department. It shows severely exaggerated effects of the thyroid hormones. This explains her hyperpyrexia, tachycardia, agitation, and delirium. The weight loss before her illness became acute was part of her undiagnosed Graves disease. Ms. Leary's immediate treatment included supplemental oxygen, intravenous (IV) fluids with dextrose solutions, ice packs and cooling blanket, propranolol, **antithyroid** medications, and oral iodine compounds.

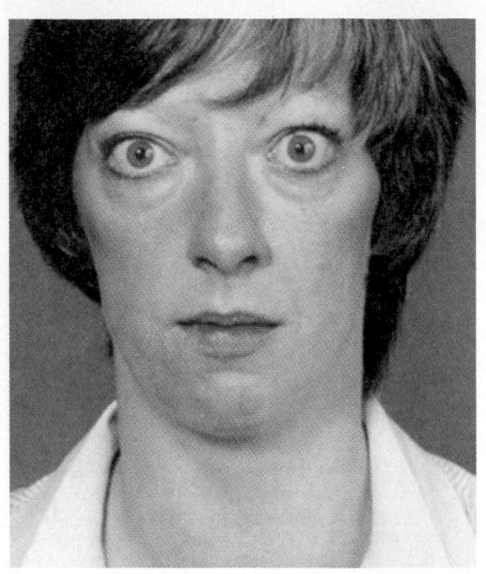

▲ **Figure 17.9** Hyperthyroidism May Cause the Eyes to Protrude (Exophthalmos).

LO 17.4 Disorders of the Thyroid Gland

Hyperthyroidism (Thyrotoxicosis)

Whatever the cause of **hyperthyroidism**, the symptoms are those of increased body metabolism. These include tachycardia, hypertension, sweating, shakiness, anxiety, weight loss despite increased appetite, and diarrhea.

Graves disease is an autoimmune disorder *(see Chapter 12)* in which an antibody stimulates the thyroid to produce and secrete excessive quantities of thyroid hormones into the blood. It is associated with one or more symptoms of **goiter** (enlarged thyroid gland), **exophthalmos**, and pretibial **myxedema**.

Exophthalmos, in which the eyes bulge outward *(Figure 17.9)*, is caused by a substance that builds up behind the eyes. The same substance is occasionally deposited in the skin over the shins and called *pretibial myxedema*.

Thyroiditis is an inflammation of the thyroid gland. It presents in three forms:

- **Silent lymphocytic thyroiditis** is characterized by some thyroid enlargement and a **self-limiting** hyperthyroid phase of a few weeks, followed by recovery to the normal **euthyroid** state.

- **Subacute thyroiditis** has a history of an antecedent viral upper respiratory infection (URI) followed by signs of hyperthyroidism with a diffusely enlarged thyroid gland. It is self-limiting.

- **Hashimoto disease** is an autoimmune disease with lymphocytic infiltration of the thyroid gland. Hypothyroidism results, necessitating lifelong synthetic thyroid hormone replacement therapy.

Toxic thyroid adenoma is a nodule in the gland that produces thyroid hormones without stimulation by the pituitary's TSH. The nodule can be removed surgically.

Goiter *(Figure 17.10)* is an enlargement of the thyroid gland that, as it enlarges, can cause difficulty in swallowing and breathing. It can occur in any of the disorders listed previously and also in pregnancy.

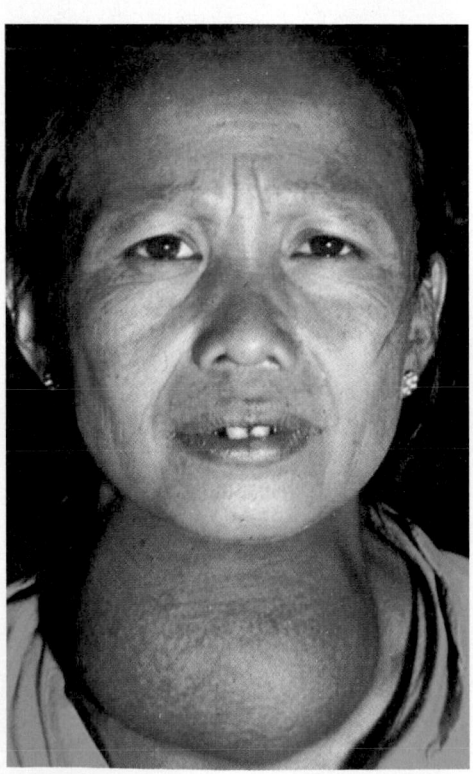

▲ **Figure 17.10** Woman with Goiter.

WORD	PRONUNCIATION	ELEMENTS		DEFINITION
antithyroid	an-tee-**THIGH**-royd	P/ R/	anti- *against* -thyroid *thyroid*	A substance that inhibits production of thyroid hormones
euthyroid	you-**THIGH**-royd	P/ R/	eu- *good, normal* -thyroid *thyroid*	Normal thyroid function
exophthalmos	ek-sof-**THAL**-mos	P/ R/	ex- *out, out of* -ophthalmos *eye*	Protrusion of the eyeball
goiter	**GOY**-ter		Latin *throat*	Enlargement of the thyroid gland
Graves disease	GRAVZ **DIZ**-eez		Robert Graves, 1796–1853, Irish physician	Hyperthyroidism with toxic goiter
Hashimoto disease Hashimoto thyroiditis (syn)	hah-shee-**MOH**-toe diz-**EEZ**		Hakaru Hashimoto, 1881–1934, Japanese surgeon	Autoimmune disease of the thyroid gland
hyperthyroidism	high-per-**THIGH**-royd-ism	S/ P/ R/	-ism *condition, process* hyper- *excessive* -thyroid- *thyroid*	Excessive production of thyroid hormones
myxedema	miks-eh-**DEE**-muh	P/ R/	myx- *mucus* -edema *swelling*	Severe hypothyroidism
thyroidectomy	thigh-roy-**DEK**-toe-me	S/ R/	-ectomy *surgical excision* thyroid- *thyroid*	Surgical removal of the thyroid gland
thyroiditis	thigh-roy-**DIE**-tis	S/ R/	-itis *inflammation* thyroid- *thyroid*	Inflammation of the thyroid gland
thyrotoxicosis	**THIGH**-roe-toks-ee-**KOH**-sis	S/ R/CF R/CF	-sis *abnormal condition* thyr/o- *thyroid* -toxic/o- *poison*	Disorder produced by excessive thyroid hormone production

Exercises

A. Elements: One word or phrase in each of the descriptions in the following questions is in bold. *This is your clue to finding the correct medical term in the word bank. Fill in the blanks with the language of endocrinology.* **LO 17.4, 17.5**

Word Bank:

thyroiditis   euthyroid   antithyroid   exophthalmos   thyroidectomy

thyrotoxicosis   hyperthyroidism

1. **Excessive production** of thyroid hormones: _____

2. **Removal** of the thyroid gland: _____

3. **Inhibition** of production of thyroid hormone: _____

4. **Normal** thyroid function: _____

5. **Inflammation** of the thyroid gland: _____

6. **Protrusion** of the eyeball: _____

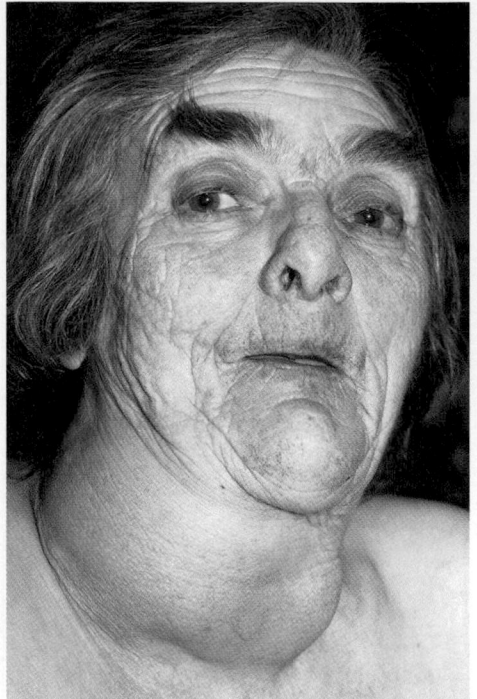

▲ **Figure 17.11** **Elderly Woman with Hypothyroidism.**

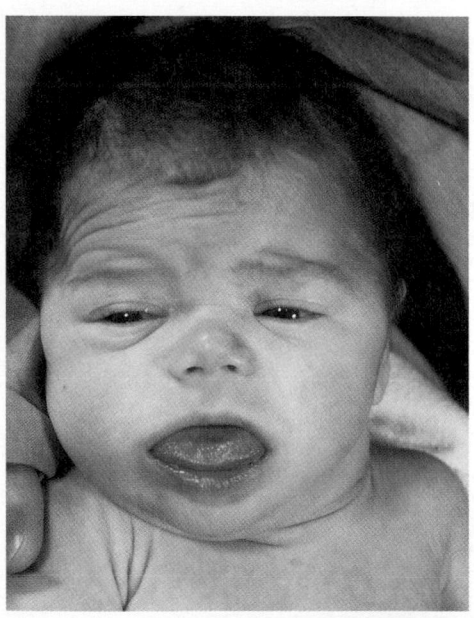

▲ **Figure 17.12** **Infant with Cretinism.**

LO 17.4 Disorders of the Thyroid Gland (continued)

Hypothyroidism

Hypothyroidism results from an inadequate production of thyroid hormone, leading to a slowing of the body's metabolism. Primary hypothyroidism, in which no specific cause is found, affects 10% of older women. Severe hypothyroidism is called *myxedema*. In developing countries, a common cause is lack of iodine in the diet. In the United States, iodine is added to table salt to prevent hypothyroidism, and iodine is also found in dairy products and seafood.

Hypothyroidism causes the body to function slowly. Symptoms develop gradually. They include loss of hair; dry, scaly skin; puffy face and eyes; slow, hoarse speech; weight gain; constipation; and inability to tolerate cold *(Figure 17.11)*. If untreated, hypothyroidism can progress to coma, triggered by severe cold or other physical stresses.

Diagnosis of primary hypothyroidism is confirmed with a TSH blood level that is high. Treatment is to replace the thyroid hormone with synthetic T_4 (L-thyroxine), which is started in small doses.

Cretinism *(Figure 17.12)* is a congenital form of thyroid deficiency that severely retards mental and physical growth. If it is diagnosed and treated early with thyroid hormones, significant improvement can be achieved.

Thyroid cancer usually presents as a symptomless nodule in the thyroid gland.

LO 17.7 Thyroid Diagnostic Tests

TSH level in the blood: If the thyroid gland is overactive, the level of TSH is low.

Thyroid hormone levels in blood detail the activity of the gland: If the thyroid gland is overactive, thyroid hormones are generally high.

Antithyroid antibodies are associated with autoimmune inflammatory diseases of the thyroid.

Isotopic thyroid scans detail the nature of the thyroid enlargement and the function of the gland.

Serum calcitonin level is elevated in medullary carcinoma.

Fine needle aspiration biopsy distinguishes benign from malignant nodules.

Ultrasonography reveals the size of the gland and the presence of nodules.

LO 17.8 Thyroid Pharmacology

Antithyroids prevent formation of thyroid hormones:

- Propylthiouracil inhibits the uptake of iodine and the conversion of T_4 to T_3.

- Methimazole inhibits the uptake of iodine.

Radioactive iodine taken orally reaches the thyroid through the bloodstream and destroys thyroid cells.

Thyroid replacements are

- L-thyroxine—this synthetic T_4 is a preferred replacement.

- Liothyronine sodium—this synthetic T_3 has a rapid turnover and has to be monitored frequently.

Word Analysis and Definition

S = Suffix   P = Prefix   **R = Root**   **R/CF = Combining Form**

WORD	PRONUNCIATION		ELEMENTS	DEFINITION
cretin cretinism	**KREH**-tin **KREH**-tin-izm	S/ R/	French *cretin* -ism *condition, process* cretin- *cretin*	A person with severe congenital hypothyroidism Condition of severe congenital hypothyroidism
hypothyroidism	high-poh-**THIGH**-royd-ism	S/ P/ R/	-ism *condition, process* hypo- *deficient* -thyroid- *thyroid*	Deficient production of thyroid hormones
isotope isotopic (adj)	I-so-tope	P/ R/ S/	iso- *equal* -tope *part* -ic *pertaining to*	Radioactive element; some of these elements are used in diagnostic procedures Of identical chemical composition
nodule	**NOD**-yule		Latin *small knot*	Small node or knotlike swelling
radioactive iodine	**RAY**-dee-oh-**AK**-tiv **EYE**-oh-dine	S/ R/CF R/	-ive *pertaining to* radi/o- *radiation* -act- *performance* iodine *nonmetallic element*	Any of the various tracers that emit alpha, beta, or gamma rays
ultrasonography	**UL**-trah-soh-**NOG**-rah-fee	S/ P/ R/CF	-graphy *recording* ultra- *beyond* son/o- *sound*	Delineation of deep structures using sound waves

Exercises

A. Certain kinds of tests are performed for the purpose of arriving at the correct diagnosis for treatment. *Employ the language of endocrinology to fill in the blanks with the name of the test that is described.* **LO 17.4, 17.5, 17.7, 17.8**

1. Is associated with autoimmune inflammatory disease of the thyroid: _____

2. Blood test to measure activity of the thyroid gland: _____

3. Level becomes elevated in medullary carcinoma: _____

4. Levels in the blood are generally low if the thyroid gland is overactive: _____

5. Reveals the size of the gland and the presence of nodules: _____

6. Distinguishes benign from malignant nodules: _____

7. Details the nature of the thyroid enlargement and the function of the gland: _____

B. Meet a lesson objective by correctly answering the following questions on a common disorder of the thyroid gland. *Fill in the blanks.* **LO 17.4, 17.5**

1. What is the opposite of *hypothyroidism*? _____

2. What is the body's *metabolism*? _____

_____

3. Is *hypothyroidism* the result of an overactive or underactive thyroid gland? _____

_____

4. What confirms the diagnosis of *primary hypothyroidism*? _____

_____

5. What is the *congenital form of thyroid deficiency* that severely retards physical and mental growth? _____

_____

6. What is the *etiology* of *Hashimoto disease*? _____

_____

7. What is the medical term for *severe hypothyroidism*? _____

_____

LO 17.1, 17.2, 17.3, 17.4 Other Endocrine Glands

Parathyroid Glands

The **parathyroid glands** are usually four in number and are partially embedded in the posterior surface of the thyroid gland *(Figure 17.13)*. They secrete **parathyroid hormone (PTH)** in response to hypocalcemia. Calcitonin and PTH are antagonistic: PTH stimulates osteoclasts to reabsorb bone and bring calcium back into the blood while calcitonin takes calcium from the blood and stimulates osteoblasts to lay down bone *(see Chapter 14)*.

Disorders of Parathyroid Glands

Hypoparathyroidism is a deficiency of parathyroid hormone that lowers levels of blood calcium (hypocalcemia). Most symptoms are neuromuscular, ranging from tingling in the fingers to muscle cramps and the painful muscle spasms of **tetany** (*not* **tetanus**). A genetically engineered recombinant form of parathyroid hormone is now available, but classic treatment for hypoparathyroidism still involves high-dose calcium and vitamin D supplements.

    Hyperparathyroidism is an excess of parathyroid hormone. It is seen more often than hypoparathyroidism and is usually caused by one of the four glands enlarging and secreting excess parathyroid hormone in an unregulated manner. It leads to four major abnormalities:

1. Bones are depleted of calcium (osteopenia) and become brittle.

2. High blood calcium levels (hypercalcemia) lead to decreased bowel motility and constipation and to increased gastric acidity and heartburn.

3. Extra excretion of calcium in the urine leads to kidney stones (nephrolithiasis).

4. High blood calcium leads to mental symptoms such as depression and fatigue and can lead to coma.

    Surgical removal of the enlarged gland is **curative**.

Thymus Gland

The **thymus gland** is located in the mediastinum behind the sternum between the lungs and above the heart *(Figure 17.14)*. It is large in children and decreases in size until, in the elderly, it is mostly fibrous tissue. It secretes a group of hormones that stimulate the production of T lymphocytes *(see Chapter 12)*.

Disorders of Thymus Gland

DiGeorge syndrome is a genetic immunodeficiency disorder *(see Chapter 12)* in which the thymus is underdeveloped or absent at birth. Abnormalities of the thymus and parathyroid glands, heart, and facial structure are present, with few or no T lymphocytes. Transplantation of stem cells or thymus tissue can cure the immunodeficiency.

    Thymomas, benign tumors, and **thymic carcinomas** are rare tumors that can be associated with myasthenia gravis *(see Chapter 9)* and other autoimmune syndromes, such as lupus erythematosus and rheumatoid arthritis. Treatment is usually surgical removal of the tumor or the gland **(thymectomy)**, followed by **adjuvant** radiotherapy.

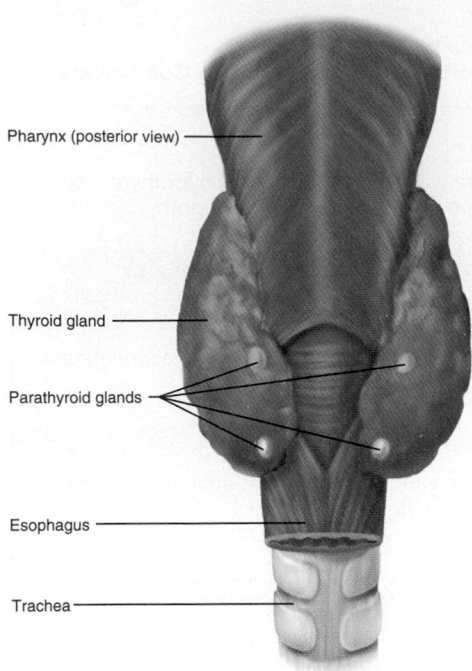

Pharynx (posterior view)

Thyroid gland

Parathyroid glands

Esophagus

Trachea

▲ **Figure 17.13** Site of Parathyroid Glands: Posterior View.

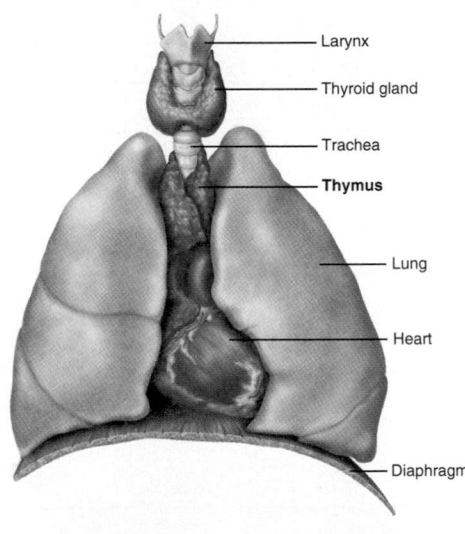

Larynx

Thyroid gland

Trachea

Thymus

Lung

Heart

Diaphragm

▲ **Figure 17.14** Position of Thymus Gland in the Mediastinum.

Abbreviation	
PTH	parathyroid hormone

WORD	PRONUNCIATION	ELEMENTS		DEFINITION
adjuvant	**AD**-joo-vant	S/ R/	-ant *pertaining to* adjuv- *give help*	Additional treatment after a primary treatment has been used
antagonist	an-**TAG**-oh-nist	S/ P/ R/	-ist *agent* ant- *against* -agon- *to fight*	An opposing structure, agent, disease, or process
antagonistic (adj) (*Note:* Two suffixes.)	an-**TAG**-oh-nist-ik	S/	-ic *pertaining to*	Having an opposite function
curative	**KYUR**-ah-tiv	S/ R/	-ive *quality of* curat- *to care for*	That which heals or cures
DiGeorge syndrome	dee-**JORJ SIN**-drome		Angelo M. DiGeorge, U.S. pediatrician, described syndrome in 1921	Congenital absence of the thymus gland
parathyroid	par-ah-**THIGH**-royd	P/ R/	-para- *adjacent* -thyroid- *thyroid*	Endocrine glands embedded in the back of the thyroid gland
hyperparathyroidism	**HIGH**-per-para-**THIGH**-royd-ism	S/ P/	-ism *condition, process* hyper- *excessive*	Excessive levels of parathyroid hormone
hypoparathyroidism	**HIGH**-poh-para-**THIGH**-royd-ism	S/ P/ P/ R/	-ism *condition, process* hypo- *deficient* -para- *adjacent* -thyroid- *thyroid*	Deficient levels of parathyroid hormone
tetany tetanic (adj)	**TET**-ah-nee teh-**TAN**-ik		Greek *convulsive tension*	Severe muscle twitches, cramps, and spasms
thymectomy	thigh-**MEK**-toe-me	S/ R/	-ectomy *surgical excision* thym- *thymus gland*	Surgical removal of the thymus gland
thymoma	thigh-**MOH**-mah	S/ R/	-oma *tumor, mass* thym- *thymus gland*	Benign tumor of the thymus
thymus	**THIGH**-mus		Greek *sweetbread*	Endocrine gland located in the mediastinum

Exercises

A. Meet a lesson objective by employing the *language of endocrinology* to answer the following questions. LO 17.1, 17.2, 17.3, 17.5

1. Locate the positions of the parathyroid and thymus glands.

   Parathyroid location: _____

   Thymus location: _____

2. List the hormone(s) produced by each gland, and state their function(s).

   Parathyroid gland:

   _____

   Function of the hormone(s) from the *parathyroid* gland:

   _____

   _____

   Thymus gland:

   _____

   Function of the hormone(s) from the *thymus gland:*

   _____

   _____

Lesson 17.3 Adrenal Glands and Hormones

The information in this lesson will enable you to use correct medical terminology to:

17.3.1 Locate the adrenal glands.

17.3.2 Differentiate between the adrenal cortex and medulla.

17.3.3 Identify the functions of the hormones produced by the cortex and medulla.

17.3.4 Describe how the body adapts to stress.

17.3.5 Explain common disorders of the adrenal glands.

Case Report 17.3

John Fitzgerald Kennedy (1917–1963) was elected president of the United States of America in 1960 at the age of 43, the youngest person elected to that office *(Figure 17.15)*. Since the age of 13, when he was diagnosed as having colitis, he had had health problems. At age 27, he had low-back pain necessitating lower-back surgery, and he was then diagnosed as having adrenal gland insufficiency **(Addison disease)** with osteoporosis of his lumbar spine. This required lower-back surgery on three more occasions. Kennedy received adrenal hormone replacement therapy for the rest of his life, together with pain medication for his low-back pain, until his assassination in Dallas, Texas, in 1963.

In medical retrospect, instead of colitis, he probably had celiac disease *(see Chapter 5)*, which has strong associations with Addison disease.

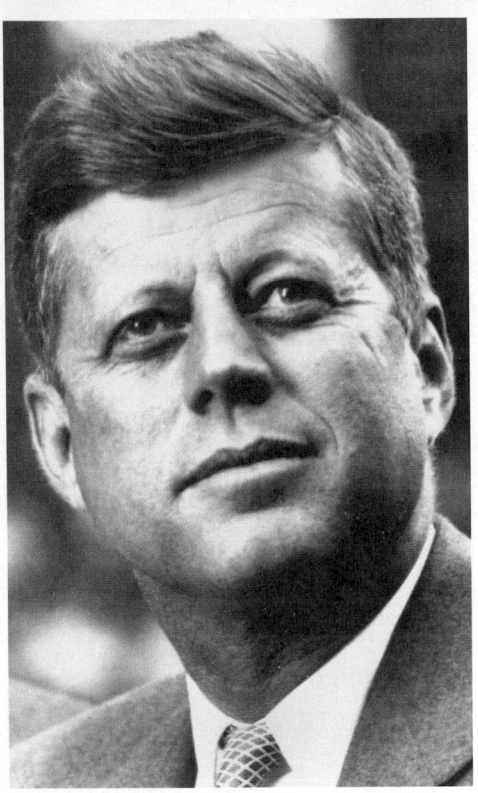

▲ **Figure 17.15**   John F. Kennedy.

LO 17.1, 17.2, 17.3, 17.4   Adrenal Glands

An **adrenal (suprarenal) gland** is anchored like a cap on the upper pole of each kidney *(Figure 17.16)*.

The outer layer of the gland, the **adrenal cortex**, synthesizes more than 25 steroid hormones known collectively as **adrenocortical hormones, corticosteroids**, or **corticoids**. There are three groups of corticosteroids:

1. **Glucocorticoids**—particularly **hydrocortisone (cortisol)**. These hormones stimulate fat and protein catabolism and help regulate blood glucose levels, particularly as the body resists stress *(see next lesson)*. Hydrocortisone also has an anti-inflammatory effect and is used in ointments to relieve inflammation.

2. **Mineralocorticoids**—the principal one of which is called **aldosterone**. This hormone promotes sodium retention and potassium excretion by the kidneys.

3. **Sex steroids**:

    a. **Androgens**—principally **dehydroepiandrosterone (DHEA)**, which is a weak androgen but is converted by other tissues into testosterone *(see Chapter 7)*.

    b. **Estrogens**—principally estradiol, which is produced in much smaller quantities than in the ovaries *(see Chapter 8)*.

The inner layer of the adrenal gland, the **adrenal medulla**, secretes hormones called **catecholamines**, principally **epinephrine (adrenaline)** and **norepinephrine**. These hormones prepare the body for physical activity. They raise blood pressure, increase circulation to muscles, increase pulmonary blood flow, and stimulate gluconeogenesis.

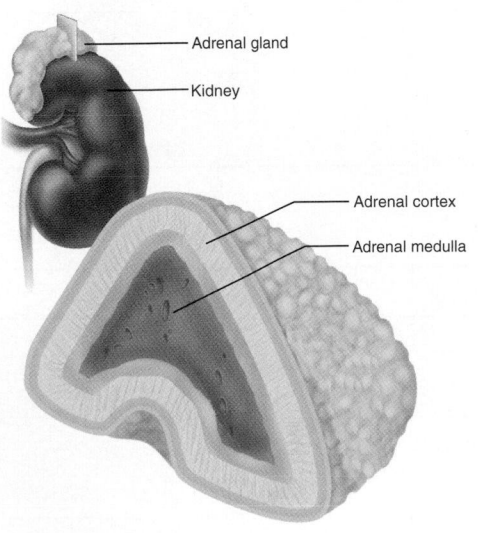

Adrenal gland

Kidney

Adrenal cortex

Adrenal medulla

▲ **Figure 17.16**   Adrenal Gland.

WORD	PRONUNCIATION	ELEMENTS		DEFINITION
Addison disease	**ADD**-ih-son **DIZ**-eez		Thomas Addison, English physician, 1793–1860	An autoimmune disease leading to decreased production of adrenocortical steroids
adrenal gland	ah-**DREE**-nal GLAND	S/ P/ R/	-al *pertaining to* ad- *to* -ren- *kidney*	The suprarenal, or adrenal, gland on the upper pole of each kidney
adrenaline **epinephrine (syn)**	ah-**DREN**-ah-lin	S/	-ine *pertaining to*	One of the catecholamines
adrenocortical	ah-dree-noh-**KOR**-tih-kal	S/ R/CF R/	-al *pertaining to* adren/o- *adrenal gland* -cortic- *cortex, cortisone*	Pertaining to the cortex of the adrenal gland
aldosterone	al-**DOS**-ter-own	S/ R/CF R/	-one *hormone* ald/o- *organic compound* -ster- *steroid*	Mineralocorticoid hormone of the adrenal cortex
catecholamine	kat-eh-**COAL**-ah-meen	S/ R/	-amine *nitrogen-containing* catechol- *benzene derivative*	Any major hormones in stress response; includes epinephrine and norepinephrine
corticoid **corticosteroid (syn)**	**KOR**-tih-koyd	S/ R/	-oid *resemble* cortic- *cortex, cortisone*	One of the steroid hormones produced by the adrenal cortex
cortisol **hydrocortisone (syn)**	**KOR**-tih-sol	S/ R/	-ol *chemical substance* cortis- *cortisone*	One of the glucocorticoids produced by the adrenal cortex; has anti-inflammatory effects
dehydroepian- **drosterone (DHEA)**	de-**HIGH**-droh-epee-an-**DROS**-ter-own	S/ P/ R/CF P/ R/CF R/	-one *hormone* de- *without, change of* -hydr/o- *water* -epi- *above* -andr/o -ster-	Precursor to testosterone; produced in the adrenal cortex
epinephrine **adrenaline (syn)**	ep-ih-**NEF**-rin	S/ P/ R/	-ine *pertaining to* epi- *above* -nephr- *kidney*	Main catecholamine produced by the adrenal medulla
glucocorticoid	glu-co-**KOR**-tih-koyd	S/ R/ R/CF	-oid *resemble* -cortic- *cortex, cortisone* gluc/o- *glucose*	Hormone of the adrenal cortex that helps regulate glucose metabolism
hydrocortisone **cortisol (syn)**	high-droh-**KOR**-tih-sohn	S/ R/CF R/	-one *hormone* hydr/o- *water* -cortis- *cortisone*	Potent glucocorticoid with anti-inflammatory properties
mineralocorticoid	**MIN**-er-al-oh-**KOR**-tih-koyd	S/ R/ R/CF	-oid *resemble* -cortic- *cortex, cortisone* mineral/o- *inorganic materials*	Hormone of the adrenal cortex that influences sodium and potassium metabolism
norepinephrine **noradrenaline (syn)**	**NOR**-ep-ih-**NEFF**-rin	S/ P/ P/ R/	-ine *pertaining to* nor- *normal* -epi- *above* -nephr- *kidney*	Parasympathetic neurotransmitter that is a catecholamine hormone of the adrenal gland

Exercises

A. Elements are the building blocks of medical terms. *Match the elements in 1–10 to their correct meanings in A–J. Review the above WAD table before you begin the exercise.* **LO 17.1, 17.5**

_____ 1. hydro

_____ 2. adren/o

_____ 3. oid

_____ 4. epi

_____ 5. ster

a. normal

b. resemble

c. hormone

d. glucose

e. water

_____ 6. andr/o

_____ 7. gluc/o

_____ 8. nor

_____ 9. one

_____ 10. nephr

f. steroid

g. kidney

h. adrenal

i. above

j. male

LO 17.4 Disorders of Adrenal Glands

Adrenal cortical hypofunction can be primary when the disorder is in the adrenal cortex (Addison disease) or secondary when there is a lack of ACTH from the pituitary gland.

Addison disease is caused mostly by idiopathic atrophy of the adrenal cortex. Production of the three groups of adrenocortical steroids is diminished or absent.

Decreased cortisol production leads to weakness, fatigue, diminished resistance to stress, increased susceptibility to infection, and weight loss.

Decreased aldosterone production leads to dehydration, decreased circulatory volume, hypotension, and circulatory collapse.

Replacement therapy in Addison disease is daily hydrocortisone **by mouth (PO)**. Additionally, fluorocortisone is given PO to replace aldosterone. **Intercurrent** infections require that the hydrocortisone dose be doubled. John F. Kennedy received replacement therapy from his late twenties until he died.

Acute adrenocortical insufficiency in patients with Addison disease is called an **adrenal crisis**. It can be precipitated by an infection or trauma and leads to peripheral vascular collapse and kidney failure. Treatment is with IV fluids and IV hydrocortisone.

Adrenal cortical hyperfunction is due to excessive production of the groups of the corticosteroids.

Hypersecretion of glucocorticoids produces **Cushing syndrome** (*Figure 17.17*). Clinical manifestations include "moon" **facies**, obesity of the trunk, muscle wasting and weakness, osteoporosis, kidney stones, and reduced resistance to infection. Most cases of Cushing syndrome are due to a pituitary tumor secreting too much ACTH, thereby causing the normal adrenal glands to produce too much cortisol.

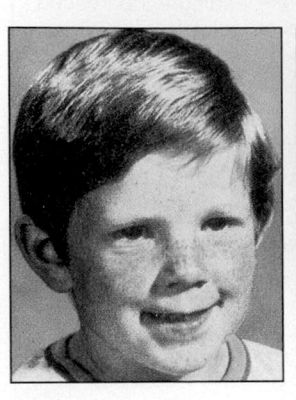 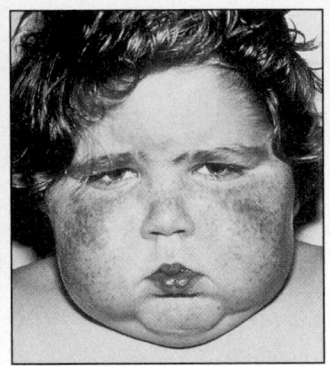

(a)   **(b)**

▲ **Figure 17.17**   Cushing Syndrome.
(*a*) Patient before onset of the syndrome. (*b*) The same boy, only 4 months later, showing the "moon face" characteristic
of Cushing syndrome.

Often, the symptoms of Cushing syndrome can result from therapeutic administration of excess cortisol medications.

Hypersecretion of aldosterone (aldosteronism, or Conn syndrome) leads to sodium retention and potassium loss with increased blood volume, hypertension, excessive thirst, and excessive urination. A benign adenoma **(aldosteronoma)** is the most common cause and can be removed by laparoscopic adrenalectomy.

Hypersecretion of androgens is called **adrenal virilism** or **adrenogenital syndrome**. In adult women, manifestations include **hirsutism**, baldness, acne, deepened voice, decreased breast size, and other signs of masculinization. If a tumor is found by CT or MRI scan, it can be removed surgically.

Pheochromocytoma is a tumor of the adrenal medulla that overproduces the catecholamines epinephrine and norepinephrine. It produces marked hypertension that is difficult to control, with severe headaches, tachycardia, palpitations, and feelings of impending death.

Keynotes

• Prolonged or repeated stress can cause physical illness.

• Stress reduction techniques are an important part of modern life.

LO 17.9 Stress

Is there an exam at the end of the week? Is the babysitter sick? You know what stress is and how it affects your physical and emotional well-being.

Your body reacts to stress in a consistent way called *the stress response* or *general adaptation syndrome.*

The initial stage of the stress response is an **alarm reaction** ("fight or flight") initiated by catecholamines that raise blood pressure and increase glucose production from stored glycogen. This source of glucose is soon exhausted, and the feelings of anxiety, irritability, and insecurity are replaced by headache and back and neck pain. If the stress is allowed to persist, the physical priority is to provide alternative fuels to provide energy. In the second stage of the stress reaction, the adrenal gland increases its output of cortisol to stimulate glucose synthesis. Fatigue, indigestion, and diminished sex drive become dominant.

The third stage of a prolonged stress response is exhaustion when glycogen and fat stores have gone. The immune system cannot find the energy to continue functioning. This is when deep physical illness takes over. Body muscle wastes away, and heart and kidney failure or overwhelming infection are the end result.

WORD	PRONUNCIATION	ELEMENTS		DEFINITION
adrenalectomy	ah-dree-nal-**ECK**-to-me	S/ S/ P/ R/	-ectomy *surgical excision* -al- *pertaining to* ad- *to* -ren- *kidney*	Removal of part or all of an adrenal gland
adrenogenital syndrome	ah-**DREE**-no-**JEN**-it-al **SIN**-drome	S/ R/CF R/	-al *pertaining to* adren/o- *adrenal gland* -genit- *androgen*	Hypersecretion of androgens from the adrenal gland
aldosteronism	al-**DOS**-ter-on-izm	S/ R/CF R/	-ism *condition, process* ald/o- *organic compound* -steron- *steroid*	Condition caused by excessive secretion of aldosterone
aldosteronoma Conn syndrome (syn)	al-**DOS**-ter-on-oma KON **SIN**-drom	S/	-oma *tumor, mass* Jerome W. Conn, U.S. endocrinologist, 1907–1981	Benign adenoma of the adrenal cortex
Cushing syndrome	**KUSH**-ing **SIN**-drom		Harvey Cushing, American neurosurgeon, 1869–1939	Hypersecretion of cortisol (hydrocortisone) by the adrenal cortex
facies	**FASH**-eez		Latin *appearance*	Facial expression and features characteristic of a specific disease
hirsutism	**HER**-sue-tizm		Latin *shaggy*	Excessive body and facial hair
intercurrent	**IN**-ter-**KUR**-ent	S/ P/ R/	-ent *end result, pertaining to* inter- *among, between* -curr- *to run*	A disease attacking a person who already has another disease
pheochromocytoma	fee-oh-**KRO**-moh-sigh-**TOE**-muh	S/ P/ R/CF R/	-oma *tumor* pheo- *gray* -chrom/o- *color* -cyt- *cell*	Adenoma of the adrenal medulla secreting excessive catecholamines
virilism	**VIR**-ih-lizm	S/ R/	-ism *condition, process* viril- *masculine*	Development of masculine characteristics by a woman or girl

Exercises

A. Language of Endocrinology: The meaning of a word element never changes, regardless of the term that contains it. *Demonstrate your knowledge of word elements by making the correct choice in the following multiple-choice questions.* **LO 17.4, 17.5**

1. On the basis of its suffix, an *aldosteronoma* is a

   a. condition

   b. facial hair

   c. tumor

   d. facial expression

   e. gland

2. In the term *pheochromocytoma*, the prefix is one of

   a. size

   b. shape

   c. direction

   d. color

   e. gender

3. Circle the term with a root that means *masculine*:

   a. hirsutism

   b. aldosteronism

   c. facies

   d. virilism

   e. aldosteronoma

4. The suffix in this term means *surgical excision*:

   a. adrenalectomy

   b. virilism

   c. aldosteronoma

   d. facies

   e. pheochromocytoma

B. In your own words, describe the three stages of a body's response to stress.   LO 17.5, 17.9

1. first stage: _____

2. second stage: _____

3. third stage: _____

Lesson 17.4 Pancreas

LESSON OBJECTIVES

The information provided in this lesson will enable you to:

17.4.1 Distinguish between the different cells of the pancreas and their secretions.

17.4.2 Identify the functions of the hormones produced by the pancreas.

17.4.3 Explain common disorders of the pancreatic hormones.

You are

. . . a medical assistant working with Susan Lee, MD, in her primary care clinic at Fulwood Medical Center.

Your patient is

. . . Mrs. Martha Jones, who is here for her monthly checkup.

Case Report 17.4

Mrs. Martha Jones is a 53-year-old type 2 diabetic on insulin, with diabetic retinopathy and diabetic neuropathy of her feet. Bariatric surgery has enabled her to reduce her weight from 275 to 156 pounds. The time is 0930 hrs. She is complaining of having a cold and cough for the past few days. Now she is feeling drowsy and nauseous and has a dry mouth. As you talk with her, you notice that her speech is slurred. She cannot remember if she gave herself her morning insulin. Examination of her lungs reveals rales at her right base. Her vital signs are T 97.8°F, P 120, R 20, BP 100/50. You perform her blood glucose measurement. The reading is 525 mg/dL (a recommended value 2 hours after breakfast is < 145 mg/dL).

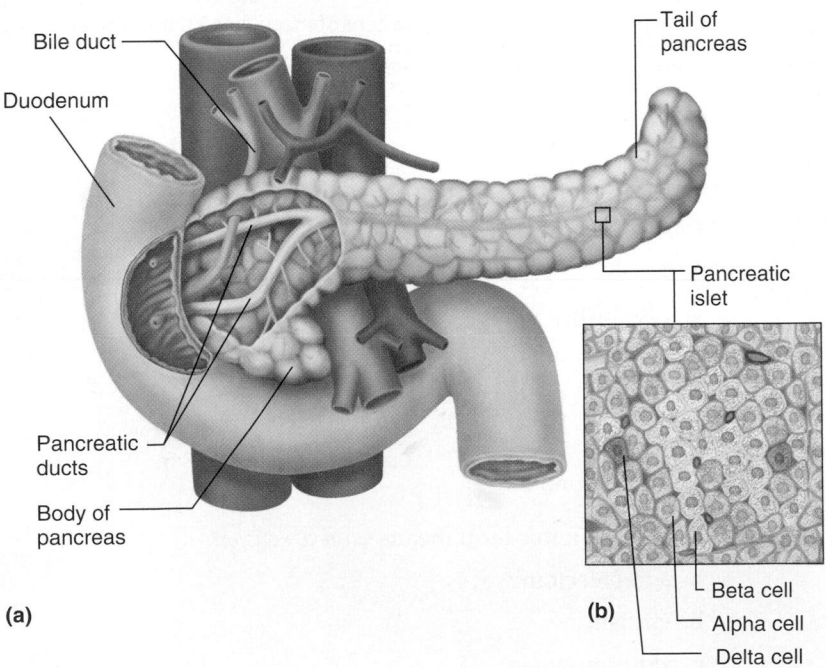

▲ **Figure 17.18** **Pancreas.** (*a*) General anatomy. (*b*) Alpha, beta, and delta cells.

Keynote

Glucagon is not the only hormone that raises blood glucose; epinephrine, cortisol, and growth hormone also have that effect. Insulin is the only hormone that lowers blood glucose.

LO 17.1, 17.2, 17.3 Pancreas

The location and structure of the pancreas are detailed in *Chapter 5*. Most of the pancreas is an exocrine gland that secretes digestive juices into the duodenum through a duct (*Figure 17.18*). Scattered throughout the pancreas are clusters of endocrine cells grouped around blood vessels. These clusters are called **pancreatic islets (islets of Langerhans)**. Within the islets are three distinct cell types:

1. **Alpha cells**—secrete the hormone **glucagon** in response to a low blood glucose. Glucagon's actions are

   a. In the liver, to stimulate **gluconeogenesis, glycogenolysis**, and the release of glucose into the bloodstream.

   b. In adipose tissue, to stimulate fat catabolism and the release of free fatty acids.

2. **Beta cells**—secrete **insulin** in response to a high blood glucose. Insulin has the opposite effects of glucagon:

   a. In muscle and fat cells, to encourage absorption of glucose and to store glycogen and fat.

   b. In the liver, to stimulate the conversion of glucose to glycogen and to inhibit the conversion of noncarbohydrates to glucose.

3. **Delta cells**—secrete **somatostatin**, which acts within the pancreas to inhibit the secretion of glucagon and insulin.

These three types of cell secrete their hormones directly into the bloodstream.

WORD	PRONUNCIATION	ELEMENTS		DEFINITION
glucagon	**GLU**-kah-gon	S/ R/	-agon *contest* gluc- *glucose*	Pancreatic hormone that supports blood glucose levels
gluconeogenesis	**GLU**-ko-nee-oh-**JEN**-eh-sis	S/ P/ R/CF	-genesis *creation* -neo- *new* gluc/o- *glucose*	Formation of glucose from noncarbohydrate sources
glycogenolysis	**GLYE**-koh-jen-oh-**LYE**-sis	S/ R/CF R/CF	-lysis *break down* glyc/o- *glycogen* -gen/o- *to create*	Conversion of glycogen to glucose
insulin	**IN**-syu-lin	S/ R/	-in *chemical compound* insul- *island*	A hormone secreted by the islet cells of the pancreas
islets of Langerhans	**EYE**-lets of **LAHNG**-er-hahnz		Paul Langerhans, German anatomist, 1847–1888	Areas of pancreatic cells that produce insulin and glucagon
pancreas	**PAN**-kree-ass		**Greek** *sweetbread*	Lobulated gland, the head of which is tucked into the curve of the duodenum
pancreatic (adj)	pan-kree-**AT**-ik	S/ R/	-ic *pertaining to* pancreat- *pancreas*	Pertaining to the pancreas
somatostatin	**SO**-mah-toe-**STAT**-in	S/ R/CF	-statin *inhibit* somat/o- *body*	Hormone that inhibits release of growth hormone and insulin

Exercises

A. After reading Case Report 17.4 on the opposite page, answer the following questions. *Be prepared to discuss your answers in class.*   **LO 17.2, 17.3, 17.4, 17.6**

1. What conditions appear in Mrs. Jones's medical history?

_____

_____

2. What was the diagnosis that prompted Mrs. Jones to have *bariatric* surgery?

_____

_____

3. What are the patient's chief complaints?

_____

_____

4. What *signs* are observable to the medical assistant and doctor?

_____

B. Continue using the *language of endocrinology* to answer the following questions. *Be prepared to discuss your answers in class.*
   LO 17.2, 17.3, 17.4, 17.5

1. Where is insulin produced? _____

_____

2. Where is glucagon produced? _____

_____

3. What can be said about Mrs. Jones's current blood glucose level? _____

_____

Abbreviations

DM	diabetes mellitus
IDDM	insulin-dependent diabetes mellitus
MODY	mature-onset diabetes of youth
NIDDM	non-insulin-dependent diabetes mellitus

Keynotes

- Type 2 diabetes used to occur primarily after the age of 30 but is now seen also in children, adolescents, and young adults.

- Stress can raise blood glucose levels in type 2 diabetes by having a direct effect on insulin response and effectiveness but also by disturbing the patient's pattern of disease management.

- The brain is the first organ affected by hypoglycemia.

- Diabetics should always carry candy or glucose tablets and an identification card, bracelet, or neck chain indicating they are diabetic.

LO 17.10, 17.11 Disorders of Pancreatic Hormones: Diabetes Mellitus

Diabetes mellitus (DM) is a syndrome characterized by hyperglycemia resulting from an absolute or relative impairment of insulin secretion and/or insulin action. This leads to a disruption of carbohydrate, fat, and protein metabolism. It is the world's most prevalent metabolic disease and the leading cause of blindness, renal failure, and gangrene. There are four categories of diabetes mellitus:

1. **Type 1 diabetes**, also called **insulin-dependent diabetes mellitus (IDDM)**, accounts for 10% to 15% of all cases of DM but is the predominant type of DM under the age of 30. When symptoms become apparent, 90% of the pancreatic insulin-producing cells have been destroyed by **autoantibodies**. The incidence of type 1 diabetes is increased in patients with Graves disease, Hashimoto disease, and Addison disease.

2. **Type 2 diabetes**, also called **non-insulin-dependent diabetes mellitus (NIDDM)**, accounts for 85% to 90% of all cases of DM. Almost 7% of U.S. residents are diagnosed with type 2 diabetes, and the incidence is increasing rapidly. Not only is there some impairment of insulin response, but there is decreased insulin effectiveness in stimulating glucose uptake by tissues and in restraining hepatic glucose production. This is called **insulin resistance**. In addition to type 2 diabetes, insulin resistance leads to other common disorders such as obesity, hypertension, hyperlipidemia, and coronary artery disease. Type 2 diabetes can be secondary to Cushing syndrome, acromegaly, pheochromocytoma, and aldosteronism.

3. **Gestational diabetes** is seen in the latter half of 5% of pregnancies. While most cases of gestational diabetes resolve after the pregnancy, a woman who has this complication of pregnancy has a 30% chance of developing type 2 diabetes within 10 years.

4. **Mature-onset diabetes of youth (MODY)** is genetically inherited, occurs in thin individuals who are in their teens and twenties, and is comparable to type 2 diabetes in its severity.

Hypoglycemia is present when blood glucose is below 70 mg/dL. Hormonal defense mechanisms (glucagon and adrenaline) are activated as the blood glucose drops below 55mg/dL. Because brain metabolism depends primarily on glucose, the brain is the first organ affected by hypoglycemia. Impaired mental efficiency starts to be seen when the blood glucose falls below 65 mg/dL. It becomes very obvious (shakiness, anxiety, confusion, tremor) around 40 mg/dL, and below that figure seizures can occur. If the blood glucose falls below 10 mg/dL, the neurons become electrically silent, resulting in diabetic **coma**. Symptomatic hypoglycemia is sometimes called **insulin shock**.

Low blood glucose can be raised to normal in minutes by taking 3 to 4 ounces of orange, apple, or grape juice. Symptoms should begin to improve in 5 minutes, with full recovery in 10 to 15 minutes. In an emergency, if the patient is not able to take oral sugar, treatment is begun with a rapid IV **bolus** of 25 mL of 50% glucose solution, followed by an intravenous infusion of glucose.

WORD	PRONUNCIATION	ELEMENTS		DEFINITION
autoantibody	aw-toe-**AN**-tee-bod-ee	P/ P/ R/	**auto-** *self, same* **-anti-** *against* **-body** *body*	Antibody produced in response to an antigen from the host's own tissue
bolus	**BOH**-lus		Greek *a lump*	Single mass of a substance
coma	**KOH**-mah		Greek *deep sleep*	State of deep unconsciousness
diabetes mellitus	dye-ah-**BEE**-teez **MEL**-ih-tus		**diabetes** Greek *a siphon* **mellitus** Latin *sweetened with honey*	Metabolic syndrome caused by absolute or relative insulin deficiency and/or insulin ineffectiveness
diabetic (adj)	dye-ah-**BET**-ik	S/ R/	**-ic** *pertaining to* **diabet-** *diabetes*	Pertaining to or suffering from diabetes
hypoglycemia	**HIGH**-poh-glie-**SEE**-me-ah	S/ P/ R/	**-emia** *blood condition* **hypo-** *below, deficient* **-glyc-** *glucose*	Low level of glucose (sugar) in the blood
hypoglycemic (adj)	**HIGH**-poh-glie-**SEE**-mik	S/	**-emic** *in the blood*	Pertaining to or suffering from hypoglycemia

Exercises

A. Diabetes is the world's most prevalent metabolic disease. *Many patients have diabetes as a concurrent condition with other health problems—which always makes it a consideration in treatment and prescribing medications. Test your knowledge of this disease by answering the following questions. Circle the correct choice.* **LO 17.10, 17.11**

1. Diabetes mellitus is the leading cause of

    blindness   hypotension   hemorrhage   kidney stones   reflux disease

2. The first organ affected by hypoglycemia is the

    kidney   heart   pancreas   brain   liver

3. The predominant type of diabetes mellitus in patients under the age of 30 is

    type 1   type 2   non-insulin-dependent DM   gestational diabetes type 3

4. Impairment of insulin response and decreased insulin effectiveness are termed insulin

    production   resistance   autoantibodies   control   conversion

5. Most cases of gestational diabetes resolve after

    medication   treatment   testing   delivery   surgery

B. Circle the correct choice to answer the questions. **LO 17.10, 17.11**

1. Symptomatic hypoglycemia is sometimes called

    insulin resistance   coma   insulin shock   glucolysis   bolus

2. Type 1 diabetes is also known as

    IDDM   NIDDM   hypoglycemia   hyperglycemia   coma

3. Insulin resistance can lead to

    obesity   aldosteronoma   hirsutism   myxedema   virilism

4. Low blood glucose can be raised to normal with a

    vitamin   hormone   enzyme   carbohydrate   electrolyte

5. What can raise blood glucose levels in type 2 diabetes?

    stress   dehydration   nausea   coughing   vomiting

LO 17.10, 17.11 Disorders of Pancreatic Hormones: Diabetes Mellitus (continued)

- Hyperglycemia causes damage to vascular endothelial cells at the microvascular and macrovascular levels.
- Untreated hyperglycemia can progress to coma.
- Diabetic ketoacidosis is a medical emergency.

Abbreviation

DKA   diabetic ketoacidosis

Hyperglycemia

The classic symptoms of hyperglycemia are *poly*uria (excessive urination), *poly*dipsia (excessive thirst), and *poly*phagia (excessive hunger), with unexplained weight loss.

Symptomatic hyperglycemia is how type 1 diabetes usually presents. Type 2 diabetes can be symptomatic or asymptomatic and is often found during a routine health examination.

Because of high glucose levels, hyperglycemia damages capillary endothelial cells in the retina and renal glomerulus and neurons and Schwann cells in peripheral nerves. Of all diabetics, 85% develop some degree of diabetic retinopathy, while 30% develop diabetic nephropathy, which can progress to end-stage renal disease *(see Chapter 6)*. Diabetic neuropathy causes sensory defects with numbness, tingling, and **paresthesias** in the stocking-glove (feet-hands) distribution.

In larger blood vessels, the hyperglycemia contributes to endothelial cell lining damage and atherosclerosis. Coronary artery disease and peripheral vascular disease with claudication *(see Chapter 10)* are complications. Hyperglycemia is the most common cause of foot ulcers followed by gangrene of the lower extremity, sometimes necessitating amputation. The risk of infection is increased by the cellular hyperglycemia and the circulatory deficits.

The complications of hyperglycemia can be kept at bay by strict control of blood glucose levels.

Diabetic ketoacidosis (DKA) is a state of marked hyperglycemia with dehydration, **metabolic acidosis**, and **ketone formation**. It is seen mostly in type 1 diabetes and is usually the result of a lapse in insulin treatment, acute infection, or trauma that renders the usual insulin treatment inadequate.

It presents with polyuria, vomiting, and lethargy and can progress to coma. **Acetone** (a ketone) can be smelled on the breath. Diabetic ketoacidosis is a medical emergency and requires rapid fluid volume expansion, correction of hyperglycemia, prevention of hypokalemia, and treatment of any infection. There is a 2% to 5% mortality from circulatory collapse.

Diabetic coma, a severe medical emergency, has three causes, which have been described earlier:

- **Diabetic ketoacidosis (DKA).**

- **Hyperglycemia** with dehydration, but not the ketosis and acidosis of DKA. This condition is called **hyperosmolar coma.** This is the condition that Mrs. Jones presented with. She was on the verge of going into a coma.

- **Hypoglycemic coma.** A blood glucose test will differentiate hypoglycemia from the other two causes.

Case Report 17.4 (continued)

Mrs. Martha Jones is in the early stages of a hyperglycemic, nonketotic (hyperosmolar) coma, probably initiated by a right-lower-lobe pneumonia. A urine specimen is obtained. Dr. Lee is notified. Blood is taken for a full chemistry panel, and arterial blood gases were drawn. An IV infusion bolus of 550 mL of isotonic sodium chloride is given, followed by 1.5 L of isotonic **saline** over the next 2 hours. Mrs. Jones is given 10 units of regular insulin IV and admitted to the hospital.

WORD	PRONUNCIATION	ELEMENTS		DEFINITION
acetone	**ASS**-eh-tone		Latin *vinegar*	Ketone that is found in blood, urine, and breath when diabetes mellitus is out of control
hyperglycemia	**HIGH**-per-gly-**SEE**-me-ah	S/ P/ R/	-emia *blood condition* hyper- *above* -glyc- *glucose*	High level of glucose (sugar) in blood
hyperglycemic (adj)	**HIGH**-per-gly-**SEE**-mik	S/	-emic *in the blood*	Pertaining to high blood sugar
hyperosmolar	**HIGH**-per-os-**MOH**-lar	S/ P/ R/	-ar *pertaining to* hyper- *above* -osmol- *concentration*	Marked hyperglycemia without ketoacidosis
ketoacidosis	**KEY**-toe-ass-ih-**DOE**-sis	S/ R/ R/CF	-osis *condition* -acid- *acid* **ket/o-** *ketone*	Excessive production of ketones, making the blood acid
ketone ketosis (**Note:** With the "o" in ket/o- preceding the "o" in -osis, one "o" drops out for simpler pronunciation.)	**KEY**-tone key-**TOE**-sis	S/ R/	Greek *acetone* -osis *condition* **ket-** *ketone*	Chemical formed in uncontrolled diabetes or in starvation Excessive production of ketones
metabolic acidosis	met-ah-**BOL**-ik ass-ih-**DOE**-sis	S/ R/ S/ R/	-ic *pertaining to* **metabol-** *change* -osis *condition* **acid-** *acid*	Decreased pH in blood and body tissues as a result of an upset in metabolism
paresthesia paresthesias (pl)	par-es-**THEE**-ze-ah par-es-**THEE**-ze-as	S/ P/ R/	-ia *condition* par- *abnormal* **-esthes-** *sensation*	An abnormal sensation, for example, tingling, burning, pricking
polydipsia	pol-ee-**DIP**-see-ah	S/ P/ R/	-ia *condition* poly- *many, much* **-dips-** *thirst*	Excessive thirst
polyphagia	pol-ee-**FAY**-jee-ah	S/ P/ R/	-ia *condition* poly- *many, much* **-phag-** *to eat*	Excessive eating
polyuria	pol-ee-**YOU**-ree-ah	S/ P/ R/	-ia *condition* poly- *many, much* **-ur-** *urine*	Excessive production of urine
saline	**SAY**-leen		Latin *salt*	Salt solution, usually sodium chloride

Exercises

A. After reading Case Report 17.4 on the opposite page, answer the following questions. *Be prepared to discuss your answers in class.*   **LO 17.5, 17.10, 17.11, 17.12**

1. *Hyperglycemic* means that the level of _____ is too high in the patient's blood.

2. *Hyperosmolar coma* is the same thing as _____.

3. What are the three classic symptoms of *diabetes mellitus*, and what do they describe?

   a. _____ is _____.

   b. _____ is _____.

   c. _____ is _____.

Abbreviations	
BUN	blood urea nitrogen
ECG	electrocardiogram
Hb A1c	glycosylated hemo-globin (hemoglobin A one-C)
OGTT	oral glucose toler-ance test
U	unit

LO 17.11, 17.12 Diagnosis and Treatment of Diabetes Mellitus

Criteria for the Diagnosis of Diabetes Mellitus

The accepted **criteria** for the diagnosis of diabetes mellitus (DM) include either a fasting (8 hours) plasma glucose of 126 mg/dL or greater or symptoms (polyuria, polydipsia, polyphagia, unexplained weight loss) and a random plasma glucose of 200 mg/dL or higher.

An **oral glucose tolerance test (OGTT)** is used occasionally in diagnosing type 2 diabetes.

Treatment of Diabetes Mellitus

The basic principle of diabetes treatment is to avoid hyperglycemia and hypoglycemia. The following are the areas of treatment:

- **Diet and exercise**. To achieve weight reduction of 2 pounds per week in overweight type 2 patients is essential. For insulin-treated diabetics, detailed diet management restricts variations in timing, size, and content of meals.

- **Patient education**. Patients are taught to understand the disease process, to recognize the indications for seeking immediate medical care, and to follow a regimen of foot care.

- **Plasma glucose monitoring**. This is an essential skill that all diabetics must learn. Patients on insulin must learn to adjust their insulin doses. Home glucose analyzers use a drop of blood obtained by a spring-powered lancet from the fingertip or forearm. The frequency of testing is varied individually. As a rule, insulin-treated patients should test their plasma glucose before meals, 2 hours after meals, and at bedtime.

- **Routine physician visits**. The patient is assessed for symptoms or signs of complications. Skin condition, pulses, and sensation in feet are tested. Urine is tested for **microalbuminuria** by using **immunoassays**. This detects smaller increases in urinary albumin than does conventional urine testing.

- **Periodic laboratory evaluation**. This includes **blood urea nitrogen (BUN)** and serum creatinine (kidney function), lipid profile, electrocardiogram (ECG), and an annual complete ophthalmologic evaluation.

Glycosylated hemoglobin (Hb A1c) is used to monitor plasma glucose control during the preceding 1 to 3 months. It is formed at rates that increase with plasma glucose levels. Normal Hb A1c is less than 6%. In poor control, the value is 9% to 12%. It is also part of a periodic laboratory evaluation.

Fructosamine is formed by glucose combining with plasma protein and reflects plasma glucose control over the preceding 1 to 3 weeks. A standard reference range for this test is not available.

Insulin preparations routinely contain 100 units (U/mL) **(U-100 insulin)**. The insulin is injected subcutaneously by using disposable syringes that hold 0.5 mL. In addition, already prepared mixtures of intermediate and regular insulins in different ratios are available. An **insulin pen** is an injection device that holds several days' dosage.

Continuous subcutaneous insulin infusion is given by a battery-powered, programmable pump that provides continuous insulin through a small needle in the abdominal wall.

Keynotes

- Maintaining normal plasma glucose levels is the basis for good management of DM.

- Many insulin-dependent diabetics need multiple subcutaneous insulin injections each day.

- Oral antidiabetic drugs are used for type 2 but not type 1 diabetes. These drugs include

  ○ Metformin, which acts by decreasing hepatic glucose production. It also promotes weight loss and decreases lipid levels. It is synergistic in combination with sulfonylureas.

  ○ Sulfonylureas, which act by stimulating the beta cells to secrete insulin.

  ○ Thiazolidinediones, such as pioglitazone, which improve insulin sensitivity in skeletal muscle and suppress hepatic glucose production. They are used in type 2 DM patients to help insulin work more effectively.

LO 17.12 Pharmacology: Classes of Insulin

Insulin Type	Onset of Action*	Peak of Action*	Duration of Action*	Examples
Rapid acting	15 min	30–60 min	3–5 hr	Humalog, NovoLog
Regular acting	30–60 min	100–120 min	5–8 hr	Humulin R, Novolin R
Intermediate acting (NPH)	1–3 hr	7–8 hr	18–24 hr	Humulin N, Novolin N
Long acting	4–8 hr	minimal peak effects	16–24 hr	Lantus, Levemir

*min = minutes; hr = hours.

WORD	PRONUNCIATION	ELEMENTS		DEFINITION
criterion criteria (pl)	kri-**TEER**-ee-on kri-**TEER**-ee-ah		**Greek** *a standard*	Standard or rule for judging
fructosamine	**FRUK**-toe-sah-meen	S/ R/	**-amine** *nitrogen-containing* **fructos-** *fruit sugar*	Organic compound with fructose as its base
glycosylated hemoglobin (Hb A1c)	**GLYE**-koh-sih-lay-ted **HE**-moh-**GLOW**-bin	R/CF S/	**glyc/o-** *glucose* **-sylated** *linked*	Hemoglobin A fraction linked to glucose; used as index of glucose control
immunoassay	**IM**-you-noh-**ASS**-ay	R/ R/CF	**-assay** *evaluate* **immun/o-** *immune response*	Biochemical test that uses the reaction of an antibody to its antigen to measure the amount of a substance in a liquid
microalbuminuria	**MY**-kroh-al-byu-min-**YOU**-ree-ah	S/ P/ R/ R/	**-ia** *condition* **micro-** *small* **-albumin-** *albumin* **-ur-** *urine*	Presence of very small quantities of albumin in urine that cannot be detected by conventional urine testing
synergist	**SIN**-er-jist	S/ P/ R/	**-ist** *specialist* **syn-** *together* **-erg-** *work*	Agent or process that aids the action of another
synergistic (adj)		S/	**-ic** *pertaining to*	Working together

Exercises

A. Medications: Diabetics will deal with medications for the rest of their lives. *Match the statement to the correct drug by placing a check mark (√) in the column with the appropriate drug name.* **LO 17.12**

Statement	Metformin	Sulfonylureas	Thiazolidinedione
1. Acts by stimulating the beta cells to secrete insulin			
2. Improves insulin sensitivity in skeletal muscle			
3. Suppresses hepatic glucose production			
4. Can be used in combination with other drugs			
5. Promotes weight loss			
6. Allows insulin to work more effectively in type 2 DM patients			
7. Decreases lipid levels			
8. Pioglitazone is an example			

B. Answering the following questions correctly will reinforce your knowledge of diabetes. *Fill in the blanks.* **LO 17.12**

1. Oral antidiabetic drugs are used for type _____ diabetes but not type _____.

2. Name the four major types of insulin preparations:

    a. _____

    b. _____

    c. _____

    d. _____

Endocrine System

Challenge Your Knowledge

A. **Diseases and disorders.** Identify the diseases and disorders of the endocrine system as described in the following statements. Special attention to the prefixes will aid you in matching your correct choice. (**LO 17.4, 17.5,** *Remember*)

_____	1. Autoimmune disease with lymphocytic infiltration manifesting with hypothyroidism	**a.** Graves disease
_____	2. Congenital form of thyroid deficiency	**b.** thyroid cancer
_____	3. Excess of PTH	**c.** hypoparathyroidism
_____	4. Severe hypothyroidism	**d.** thyroiditis
_____	5. Presents as symptomless thyroid nodule	**e.** Hashimoto disease
_____	6. Inflammation of the thyroid gland	**f.** goiter
_____	7. Hyperthyroidism associated with a goiter	**g.** exophthalmos
_____	8. Deficiency of PTH	**h.** hyperparathyroidism
_____	9. Enlargement of the thyroid gland	**i.** myxedema
_____	10. Eyes bulging outward	**j.** cretinism

B. **Latin and Greek terms.** Latin and Greek terms cannot be further deconstructed into prefix, root, or suffix. You must know them for what they are. Test your knowledge of these terms with the following exercise. Match the meaning in the left column with the correct medical term in the right column. Use any one medical term (A–J) in a sentence of patient documentation. (**LO 17.5,** *Remember, Apply*)

_____	1. Oblong shield	**a.** tetany
_____	2. Island	**b.** coma
_____	3. Deep sleep	**c.** tropic
_____	4. Stimulation, change	**d.** thyroid
_____	5. Insulin deficiency	**e.** insulin
_____	6. A lump	**f.** facies
_____	7. Convulsive tension	**g.** hirsutism
_____	8. Appearance	**h.** bolus
_____	9. Shaggy or hairy	**i.** hormone
_____	10. To set in motion	**j.** diabetes

Sentence:

11. _____

_____

_____

C. Translation. Rewrite the following sentence—without any abbreviations—into language a patient can understand. Review any terms you need to before you start writing. (**LO 17.1, 17.5, *Understand***)

"ADH, also called vasopressin, causes vasoconstriction in small arterioles, usually insufficient to cause hypertension."

Translation: _____

_____

_____

_____

D. Language of endocrinology. Knowing the endocrine system will aid you in understanding the overall body process of *homeostasis*. Apply the *language of endocrinology* to the following questions about the anatomy and physiology of the endocrine system; circle the correct answer. (**LO 17.4, 17.5, *Understand, Apply***)

1. Which of the following is not a part of the endocrine system?

   a. pancreas

   b. pituitary

   c. pineal

   d. parathyroid

   e. palatine

2. The abnormal production of breast milk is called

   a. dysmenorrhea

   b. polydipsia

   c. galactorrhea

   d. dysphagia

   e. menorrhagia

3. The speed at which the body's chemical functions proceed is called

   a. cardiac rate

   b. vasoconstriction

   c. metabolic rate

   d. blood pressure

   e. homeostasis

4. The only hormone that lowers blood glucose is

   a. glucagon

   b. cortisol

   c. aldosterone

   d. corticosterone

   e. insulin

Endocrine System

E. Language of endocrinology. Apply the *language of endocrinology* to the following questions about the anatomy and physiology of the endocrine system; circle the correct answer. **(LO 17.4, 17.5, *Understand, Apply*)**

1. A congenital form of thyroid deficiency that severely retards mental and physical growth is

   a. goiter

   b. thyroid adenoma

   c. cretinism

   d. pretibial myxedema

   e. hyperthyroidism

2. *Tetany* is

   a. lockjaw

   b. painful muscle spasm

   c. protrusion of the eyeball

   d. enlargement of the thyroid gland

   e. excessive production of thyroid hormones

3. A condition produced by a pituitary tumor that causes a decline in the production of several hormones at the same time is called

   a. hypopituitarism

   b. hyperpituitarism

   c. panhypopituitarism

   d. prolactinoma

   e. diabetes mellitus

4. Another name for *epinephrine* is

   a. corticosteroid

   b. corticosterone

   c. adrenalin

   d. hydrocortisone

   e. cortisol

5. The pineal gland secretes *serotonin* by day and converts it to _____ at night.

   a. melatonin

   b. a vasodilator

   c. vasopressin

   d. prolactin

   e. an enzyme

F. Hormones. Hormones are bloodborne messengers secreted by endocrine glands. Each has a specific purpose. Correctly use the following terms or abbreviations to fill in the blanks after each definition. **(LO 17.1, 17.3, *Understand, Apply*)**

ACTH	FSH	somatotropin	PRL	tropic
insulin	glucocorticoid	melatonin	LH	thyrotropin

1. Hormone that stimulates the growth of the thyroid gland: _____

2. Hormones that stimulate other endocrine glands to produce hormones: _____

3. Hormone that stimulates ovulation and testosterone production: _____

4. Hormone of the adrenal cortex that helps regulate glucose metabolism: _____

5. Hormone that stimulates cells to enlarge and divide: _____

6. Hormone that regulates blood sugar: _____

7. Hormone of the anterior pituitary that stimulates cortex of adrenal gland to produce its own hormones: _____

8. Hormone that stimulates target cells in the ovaries and testes: _____

9. Hormone that replaces serotonin at night: _____

10. Hormone that stimulates the mammary glands after pregnancy to produce milk: _____

G. Plurals. Enhance your command of plurals in medical terminology by completing this exercise. Circle the best choice for the correct form of the plural in the sentence. **(LO 17.5, *Understand, Apply*)**

1. Patient complains of multiple (paresthesiae/paresthesias) on her left side.

2. There are several (criterion/criteria) by which to judge this patient's recovery.

3. (Catecholamines/Catecholamina) are major elements in stress response.

4. Insulin sensitivity in skeletal muscle is improved by (thiazolidinediones/thiazolidinedionia).

H. Terminology construction. Construct the *language of endocrinology*. Build the term for the definition provided. Fill in the blanks. **(LO 17.1, 17.5, *Apply*)**

1. Hormone formed by the pineal gland _____/_____/_____

2. Protrusion of the eyeball _____/_____/_____

3. Hormone produced by the adrenal cortex _____/_____/_____

4. Deficiency of all the pituitary hormones _____/_____/_____

5. Another name for the pituitary gland _____/_____/_____

6. Hormone that stimulates the uterus to contract _____/_____/_____

7. Removal of part or all of the adrenal gland _____/_____/_____

8. Prolactin-producing tumor _____/_____/_____

9. Waxy, nonpitting edema of skin _____/_____/_____

10. Excess of growth hormone that produces enlarged hands and feet _____/_____/_____

Endocrine System

I. Elements. Use your knowledge of word elements to answer the following questions about hormones in other body systems. Fill in the blanks. (**LO 17.1, 17.3, Apply**)

1. Based on its root, the hormone gastrin would have a connection with which body organ? _____

2. Based on its root, the hormone cholecystokinin has an effect on which body organ? _____

3. Both of the above organs are part of which body system that you have already studied? _____

4. Based on its root, the hormone erythropoietin stimulates production of _____. This hormone is secreted by the (organ) _____, which is part of the _____ system.

Continue working with elements as clues in the following terms. From among this bank of terms, choose the correct terms to fit the descriptions. Some blanks may need more than one term, and there are extra terms you will not use. Fill in the blanks.

Word Bank:

acromegaly	iodine	microalbuminuria	serotonin	hypoglycemia
thyroidectomy	prolactinoma	galactorrhea	adrenalectomy	antidiuretic
prolactin	panhypopituitarism	melatonin	gigantism	pheochromocytoma

5. Term(s) connected to urine:

_____

6. Blood condition:

_____

7. Procedure(s):

_____

8. Term(s) connected to milk:

_____

9. Excessive growth:

_____

10. Term(s) that contain a color:

_____

J. Abbreviations. This exercise contains all the letters you need to form the correct abbreviations for the terms described. Fill in the blanks. (**LO 17.5,** *Apply, Analyze*)

A   D   G   H   I   K   M   N   O   P   S   T

1. Stored in the posterior pituitary: _____

2. Type 2 diabetes: _____

3. Thyrotropin: _____

4. Somatotropin: _____

5. Secreted in response to hypocalcemia: _____

6. Type 1 diabetes: _____

7. Winter depression: _____

8. Marked hyperglycemia with dehydration: _____

9. Used occasionally to diagnose type 2 diabetes: _____

10. Disorder caused by insulin deficiency: _____

K. Terminology challenge. An element may have more than one meaning. For example, **hypo-** can mean either *below* (location) or *deficient* (less in quantity or number). The following five terms all start with **hypo-**. Place a check mark (√) in the correct column to indicate whether the prefix in this case means *below* or *deficient*, and then write in the definition of each term in the last column. Fill in the chart. (**LO 17.2,** *Analyze*)

Medical Term	Prefix Means *below*	Prefix Means *deficient*	Meaning of Term
1. hypoglycemia			2.
3. hypodermic			4.
5. hypothalamus			6.
7. hypophyseal			8.
9. hypophysis			10.

Endocrine System

L. Brain teaser. The alarm reaction ("fight or flight") triggers other body systems to kick into action along with the endocrine response. Based on the chapters you have already read, what other systems come into action, and how do they perform? Write your thoughts on the following lines. (**LO 17.5,** *Analyze*)

_____

_____

_____

M. Deconstruction. Deconstruct these medical terms into the meanings of their basic elements. Demonstrate that you understand the meanings by using one term in a sentence of patient documentation. Fill in the chart. (**LO 17.5,** *Analyze*)

Medical Term	Meaning of Prefix	Meaning of Root(s)/CF	Meaning of Suffix	Meaning of Medical Term
polyuria	1.	2.	3.	4.
parathyroid	5.	6.	7.	8.
vasopressin	9.	10.	11.	12.
panhypopituitarism	13.	14.	15.	16.
prognathism	17.	18.	19.	20.
polydipsia	21.	22.	23.	24.
euthyroid	25.	26.	27.	28.

Sentence:

29. _____

   _____

N. Precision in communication. Because of errors in communication, these patients were sent to the wrong specialists! Find the errors and correct the sentences. **(LO 17.5, *Analyze*)**

Underline the incorrect medical terminology in the following sentences.

1. Because of this patient's *neuropathy*, I am referring him to a kidney specialist.

   This sentence should have read

   Because of _____.

   _____

2. Because of this patient's *diabetic retinopathy*, I am referring her to an orthopedist.

   This sentence should have read

   Because of _____.

   _____

You are ultimately responsible for everything you communicate regarding patient care!

Endocrine System

CHAPTER SUMMARY EXERCISE

A. Spelling comprehension. Circle the correct spelling of the term. (**LO 17.5,** *Remember*)

1. hypophysis	hypopersis	hypopisis	hypophsis	hypophses
2. hersutism	hirsutism	herrsutism	hirssutism	hirsutesm
3. emaciated	emmaciated	imaciated	immaciated	emacciated
4. prolacktinomma	prolactinoma	prolictinoma	proliktinoma	prolacktinnoma
5. gooter	gutter	goiter	goiiter	guiter
6. isotope	issotope	eisotope	eissotope	isutope
7. thyroidtoxicosis	thyrotoxicosis	thyroidtoxicossis	thyrodtoxicosis	throidtoxicosis
8. myxxedema	mixxedema	mexidema	myxedema	mixedema
9. uthyroid	euthyroid	euuthroid	uthroid	utthryoid
10. insepidus	insippidus	inseppidus	insipidus	insipides

B. Match the number of the correct spelling of each term in Exercise A with the following brief descriptions. (**LO 17.4, 17.5,** *Apply*)

1. Normal thyroid function _____

2. Excessive body and facial hair _____

3. Enlargement of thyroid gland _____

4. Another term for pituitary gland _____

5. Radioactive element used in diagnostic procedures _____

6. Nonpitting edema _____

7. Can appear in both men and women _____

8. Abnormally thin _____

9. Results from decreased production of ADH _____

10. Disorder produced by excessive thyroid hormone production _____

C. Using your knowledge of terms 1–10 in Exercises A and B and their correct spelling, write a brief sentence for each of the terms as it might appear in patient documentation. (LO 17.5, *Apply*)

1. _____

2. _____

3. _____

4. _____

5. _____

6. _____

7. _____

8. _____

9. _____

10. _____

D. After rereading Case Report 17.3, answer the following questions. Be prepared to discuss your answers in class. (LO 17.5, 17.6, *Analyze*)

Case Report 17.3

John Fitzgerald Kennedy (1917–1963) was elected president of the United States of America in 1960 at the age of 43, the youngest person elected to that office. Since the age of 13, when he was diagnosed as having colitis, he had had health problems. At age 27, he had low-back pain necessitating lower-back surgery, and he was then diagnosed as having adrenal gland insufficiency (**Addison disease**) with osteoporosis of his lumbar spine. This required lower-back surgery on three more occasions. Kennedy received adrenal hormone replacement therapy for the rest of his life, together with pain medication for his low-back pain, until his assassination in Dallas, Texas, in 1963. In medical retrospect, instead of colitis, he probably had celiac disease, which has strong associations with Addison disease.

Fill in the blanks, using the language of endocrinology:

1. Define *colitis.* _____

2. What is another term for *adrenal gland insufficiency?* _____

3. The disease in question 2 falls under which generalized group of diseases?

_____

4. Where are the adrenal glands located?

_____

5. What is *osteoporosis?*

_____

Endocrine System

6. Describe the location of the *lumbar spine*. _____

_____

7. What was John F. Kennedy's treatment plan? _____

_____

8. What diagnosis most likely was the correct one, and what body system does it represent?

Diagnosis: _____

Body system: _____

E. **Meet the goals of each of the chapter outcomes by using the correct language of the endocrine system for the answers. (LO 17.1–17.12, *Analyze*)**

1. Identify the endocrine glands and the hormones each gland secretes. Which of the following is NOT an endocrine gland? Circle the correct choice. (**LO 17.1**)

   a. pancreas

   b. gonads

   c. thymus

   d. adrenal

   e. spleen

2. Circle the false statement about the location of an endocrine gland. (**LO 17.2**)

   a. The hypothalamus forms the floor and the walls of the third ventricle of the brain.   T   F

   b. The pituitary gland is suspended from the hypothalamus.   T   F

   c. The parathyroid glands are partially embedded in the posterior surface of the thyroid gland.   T   F

   d. The pineal gland is located posterior to the hypothalamus.   T   F

   e. The thyroid gland lies just below the skin of the abdomen.   T   F

3. Describe the functions of the different hormones in the body. The function of a hormone is given to you; name the hormone it pertains to. (**LO 17.3**)

   a. stimulates erythrocyte production: _____

   b. helps suppress appetite: _____

   c. stimulates stomach secretions: _____

   d. when tissues are injured, this hormone promotes an inflammatory response: _____

   e. contracts the gallbladder: _____

4. Identify the disorders resulting from excessive and deficient production of the different hormones. Use the correct medical terminology to identify the appropriate answer. (**LO 17.4**)

   a. In adults, excessive growth hormone produces _____.

   b. Underproduction of growth hormone can be present at birth and leads to _____.

   c. What results from decreased production of ADH? _____

5. Use the medical terms of endocrinology to communicate and document in writing accurately and precisely in any health care setting. What is the medical term for an excessive level of calcium in the blood? Circle the correct choice. (**LO 17.5**)

   a. hypocalsemia

   b. hypercalcemia

   c. hypocalcemia

   d. hypercalsemia

   e. hypocallsemia

6. Use the medical terms of endocrinology to communicate verbally with accuracy and precision in any health care setting. What is the correct pronunciation of the medical term that means a condition of severe congenital hypothyroidism? (**LO 17.6**)

   a. KREH-ten-ism

   b. CRE-ten-izm

   c. cre-TEN-ism

   d. KREH-tin-izm

   e. CREE-ten-izm

Endocrine System

7. Explain the clinical and laboratory tests used to determine the presence or absence of a specific hormone. Briefly explain each of the following thyroid diagnostic tests. Fill in the blanks. (**LO 17.7**)

   a. TSH level in the blood:

   _____

   b. thyroid hormone levels in the blood:

   _____

   c. serum calcitonin level in the blood:

   _____

8. Which of the following agents would NOT be used in the treatment of endocrine disorders? (**LO 17.8**)

   a. insulin

   b. transplantation of stem cells

   c. arthroplasty

   d. surgery

   e. blood tests

9. Discuss the body's reaction to stress. (**LO 17.9**)

   a. What is another word for the term *stress response*? _____

   b. What stage of response to stress is the alarm reaction? _____

   c. Exhaustion occurs in which stage of stress response? _____

   d. What is responsible for raising blood presure and increasing glucose production in a stress response? _____

10. Identify the different types, symptoms, and signs of diabetes. Which of the following groups of medical terms represent the classic symptoms of diabetes? Circle the correct answer. (**LO 17.10**)

   a. diarrhea   hypertension   heartburn

   b. hematuria   pyrexia   migraine headache

   c. polydipsia   polyuria   polyphagia

   d. dyspnea   pallor   hypotension

   e. hypoglycemia   retinopathy   nausea

11. Describe the criteria used to diagnose diabetes. (**LO 17.11**)

Fill in the blanks with the criteria used to diagnose diabetes

a. _____

b. _____

c. _____

12. Discuss the different forms of treatment of diabetes. Which of the following is an accepted form of treatment for diabetes? Circle the correct choice. (**LO 17.12**)

a. radiation therapy

b. chemotherapy

c. plasma glucose monitoring

d. physical therapy

e. transfusions

Mental Health
The Languages of Psychology and Psychiatry

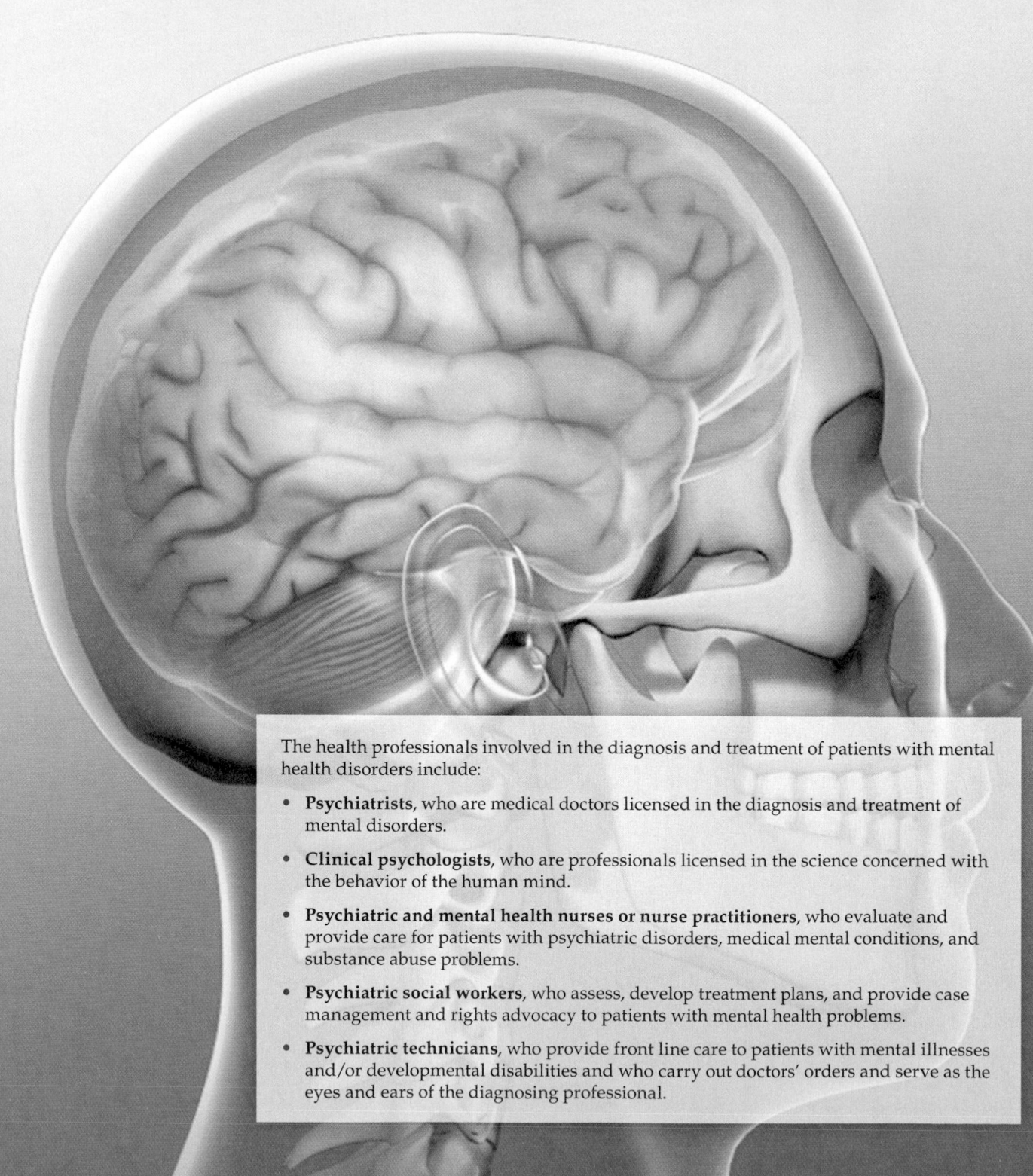

The health professionals involved in the diagnosis and treatment of patients with mental health disorders include:

- **Psychiatrists**, who are medical doctors licensed in the diagnosis and treatment of mental disorders.

- **Clinical psychologists**, who are professionals licensed in the science concerned with the behavior of the human mind.

- **Psychiatric and mental health nurses or nurse practitioners**, who evaluate and provide care for patients with psychiatric disorders, medical mental conditions, and substance abuse problems.

- **Psychiatric social workers**, who assess, develop treatment plans, and provide case management and rights advocacy to patients with mental health problems.

- **Psychiatric technicians**, who provide front line care to patients with mental illnesses and/or developmental disabilities and who carry out doctors' orders and serve as the eyes and ears of the diagnosing professional.

Case Report (CR) 18.1

You are

... a **psychiatric technician** employed in the Psychiatric Department of Fulwood Medical Center. Your patient has been referred from the Emergency Department, where he was seen earlier this morning.

Your patient is

... Mr. Harlan Diment, a 40-year-old construction worker. He was brought to the Emergency Department by his roommate, who says that Mr. Diment has slept only a couple of hours each night for the past 3 weeks. He stays up most of the night, cleaning their apartment and drinking beer. He has bought a new home entertainment set, including a big-screen plasma TV, that he cannot afford. He is very irritable and explosive when challenged about his behavior. His roommate has seen no signs of drugs and is not aware of any medical problems. Mr. Diment is usually very quiet, thoughtful, and introverted.

A mental status examination shows Mr. Diment to be alternately irritable and excited. He is wearing a bright orange top and camouflage slacks and is carrying a soft green cap. His speech is rapid and loud, and it is difficult to interrupt him. He paces the room, claims to feel "great," and is angry with his roommate for insisting that he come to the hospital. His thought processes and verbalization go off on different **tangents (tangentiality)**. He says he has no suicidal thoughts, **hallucinations**, or **delusions**.

Chapter Learning Outcomes

To be an effective member of the mental health team that will be responsible for Mr. Diment's care, you will need to be able to:

LO 18.1 Use the medical terms of psychology and psychiatry to communicate and document in writing accurately and precisely in any health care setting.

LO 18.2 Use the medical terms of psychology and psychiatry to communicate verbally with accuracy and precision in any health care setting.

LO 18.3 Recognize a uniform system for classifying and describing mental disorders.

LO 18.4 Describe the major types of anxiety disorders.

LO 18.5 Discuss psychoses and schizophrenia.

LO 18.6 Identify personality disorders.

LO 18.7 Explain the effects of common psychoactive drugs.

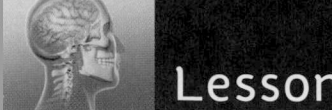
Lesson 18.1 Mental Health and Affective Disorders

Mental health is defined as emotional, behavioral, and social well-being such that an individual can cope with internal and external events. In this lesson, you will be given information about mental health disorders including affective disorders, mood disorders, schizophrenia, anxiety disorders, and psychosomatic and somatoform disorders.

This lesson and the introduction will enable you to use correct medical terminology to:

18.1.1 Distinguish between psychology and psychiatry.

18.1.2 Define mental disorder and insanity.

18.1.3 Discuss affective disorders.

18.1.4 Describe the differences between the two main types of mood disorder.

Keynotes

- Psychologists are not licensed to prescribe medications.

- As physicians, psychiatrists are licensed to prescribe medications.

- The DSM-IV classifies and describes psychiatric disorders.

- The DSM-IV contains over 200 diagnoses grouped into 17 major categories.

- The DSM-V is to be published in May 2013.

Abbreviations

DSM-IV-TR	*Diagnostic and Statistical Manual of Mental Disorders*, fourth edition, text revision; referred to as "DSM-IV"
DSM-V	*Diagnostic and Statistical Manual of Mental Disorders*, fifth edition
PhD	doctorate in philosophy
PsyD	doctorate in psychology

LO 18.3 Definitions in Mental Health

Psychology is defined as the scientific study of behavior and mental processes. **Behavior** is anything you do—talking, sleeping, reading, interacting with others. **Mental processes** are your private, internal experiences—thinking, feeling, remembering, dreaming.

A licensed specialist in psychology is called a **psychologist**. Psychologists can have a master's degree or a doctorate in philosophy **(PhD)** or a doctorate in psychology **(PsyD)**. They can practice in many different career specialties, including being a **psychotherapist** or a **psychoanalyst**.

Psychiatry is the medical specialty concerned with the origin, diagnosis, prevention, and treatment of mental, emotional, and behavioral disorders. **Psychiatrists** have an MD or DO degree and a minimum of 4 years of residency training in the specialty.

Many psychiatrists and psychologists work together in a team approach to therapy. Other health professionals in the mental health team include **clinical social workers**, **psychiatric nurses**, and **psychiatric technicians**.

Mental disorder can be defined as any behavior or emotional state that

- Causes a person to suffer emotional distress (e.g., depression, anxiety).

- Is harmful to the individual sufferer (impairs the individual's ability to work, take care of personal needs, or get along with others).

- Is self-destructive (e.g., substance abuse, gambling and other addictions, self-injury).

- Endangers others or the community (antisocial behaviors, **homicidal** intent, **pyromania** [setting fires]).

Insanity is a *legal* term for a severe mental illness, present at the time a crime was committed, that impaired the defendant's capacity to understand the moral wrong of the act. *It is not a medical diagnosis.*

Mental disorders are numerous and very diverse. A uniform system for classifying and describing them has been developed by the American Psychiatric Association. It is called the *Diagnostic and Statistical Manual of Mental Disorders*, fourth edition, text revision (**DSM-IV-TR**). The "IV" indicates that this is the fourth conceptual revision; "TR" indicates a text revision of the fourth edition. The manual is usually referred to as **DSM-IV** ("DSM-4").

The DSM-IV provides a detailed description of the symptoms seen in psychiatric disorders. These descriptions allow psychiatric disorders to be classified. It is the disorders that are classified, not the people who have the disorders. Modern mental health terminology does not use the term **schizophrenic** but uses the phrase "a person with **schizophrenia**."

WORD	PRONUNCIATION	ELEMENTS		DEFINITION
delusion	de-**LOO**-shun	S/	-ion *condition, process*	Fixed, unyielding, false belief or judgment held despite strong evidence to the contrary
		R/	**delus**- *deceive*	
delusional (adj)	de-**LOO**-shun-al	S/	-al *pertaining to*	
hallucination	hah-loo-sih-**NAY**-shun	S/	-ation *process*	Perception of an object or event when there is no such thing present
		R/	**hallucin**- *imagination*	
homicide	**HOM**-ih-side	R/CF	**hom/i**- *man*	Killing of one human by another
		R/CF	**-cid/e** *to kill*	
homicidal (adj)	hom-ih-**SIDE**-al	S/	-al *pertaining to*	Having a tendency to commit homicide
		R/	**-cid**- *to kill*	
insanity	in-**SAN**-ih-tee	S/	-ity *condition*	Nonmedical term for person unable to be responsible for actions
		P/	**in**- *not*	
		R/	**-san**- *sound, healthy*	
psychiatry	sigh-**KIGH**-ah-tree	S/	-iatry *treatment*	Diagnosis and treatment of mental disorders
		R/	**psych**- *mind*	
psychiatric (adj)	sigh-kee-**AH**-trik	S/	-ic *pertaining to*	Pertaining to psychiatry
psychiatrist	sigh-**KIGH**-ah-trist	S/	-iatrist *one who treats, practitioner*	Licensed medical specialist in psychiatry
psychology	sigh-**KOL**-oh-jee	S/	-logy *study of*	Scientific study of the human mind and behavior
		R/CF	**psych/o**- *mind*	
psychological	sigh-koh-**LOJ**-ik-al	S/	-ical *pertaining to*	Pertaining to psychology
psychologist	sigh-**KOL**-oh-jist	S/	-logist *specialist*	Licensed specialist in psychology
psychoanalysis	sigh-koh-ah-**NAL**-ih-sis	R/	-analysis *process to define*	Method of psychotherapy
psychoanalyst	sigh-koh-**AN**-ah-list	R/	-analyst *one who defines*	Practitioner of psychoanalysis
psychotherapy	sigh-koh-**THAIR**-ah-pee	S/	-therapy *treatment*	Treatment of mental disorders through communication
psychotherapist	sigh-koh-**THAIR**-ah-pist	S/	-therapist *one who treats*	Practitioner of psychotherapy
pyromania	pie-roh-**MAY**-nee-ah	S/	-mania *frenzy*	Morbid impulse to set fires
		R/CF	**pyr/o**- *fire*	
schizophrenia	skitz-oh-**FREE**-nee-ah	S/	-ia *condition*	Disorder of perception, thought, emotion, and behavior
		R/CF	**schiz/o**- *to split, cleave*	
		R/	**-phren**- *mind*	
tangentiality	tan-jen-she-**AL**-ih-tee	S/	-ity *condition, state*	Disturbance in thought processes, which move rapidly from one topic to another
		S/	-al- *pertaining to*	
tangent	**TAN**-jent	R/CF	**tangent/i**- *touch*	Sudden change of course

Exercises

A. Elements remain your best clue to the meaning of a medical term. *Match the element in the left column with its correct meaning in the right column.*   **LO 18.1, 18.3**

_____   **1.** psych/o

_____   **2.** logy

_____   **3.** mania

_____   **4.** schiz/o

_____   **5.** ity

_____   **6.** pyr/o

_____   **7.** logist

_____   **8.** in

_____   **9.** ic

_____   **10.** iatry

a. pertaining to

b. condition

c. specialist

d. not

e. fire

f. mind

g. to split

h. frenzy

i. treatment

j. study of

LO 18.3 Affective Disorders

Affective disorders are not a clearly delineated group of disorders. Included are the **mood disorders** of **unipolar** and **bipolar depression**, generalized anxiety disorder- and more specific anxiety disorders, **phobias, obsessive-compulsive disorder (OCD)**, and **posttraumatic stress disorder (PTSD)**.

Mood Disorders

You will feel sad and blue and down in the dumps from time to time and occasionally feel the grief of the death of a loved one and the tragedy of injury or severe emotional hurt. Everyone does. But people with **major depression** are so deeply sad for at least 2 weeks that they feel despairing and hopeless, see nothing but sorrow in the future, and may not want to live anymore *(Figure 18.1)*. They see themselves as worthless and unlovable. They have difficulty getting up and going to school or work. One person's depression can hurt everyone in the entire family.

Physical symptoms occur. These may include difficulty concentrating, difficulty falling asleep, feeling tired all the time, losing weight. Violent behavior or substance abuse occurs more often in depressed men than in women, though depression is more common in women.

When depression is unipolar, the episode will ease with medication. Since the 1950s, **tricyclic antidepressant (TCA) drugs** have been used for depression, but since 1990 they are being replaced by **selective serotonin reuptake inhibitors (SSRIs)** or **serotonin and norepinephrine reuptake inhibitors (SNRIs)** *(Table 18.1)*. Moderate exercise for 3 hours weekly has been shown to reduce the symptoms of depression by 47%. It is believed to alter the serotonin chemistry in the brain. In **electroconvulsive therapy (ECT)** seizures are electrically induced in anesthetized patients to treat severe depression that has not responded to other treatment.

Some people rebound to the opposite extreme of depression called **mania**, an excessive state of overexcitement and impulsive behavior. This alternation of episodes of depression with mania is called **bipolar disorder**. It used to be called **manic-depressive disorder**.

In the **manic** phase, the person is hyperactive and distractible and may not sleep for days, yet shows no fatigue. Thinking and speech are rapid and disjointed and cannot be interrupted. The person may give away possessions or go on a spending spree. Untreated pure manic episodes usually last 6 weeks. Untreated mixed (manic and depressive) episodes usually last 17 weeks.

Dysphoric mania, a form of bipolar disorder, combines the frenetic energy of mania with dark thoughts and paranoid delusions. It may be the cause of some mass shootings.

Seasonal affective disorder (SAD) is a mood disorder associated with episodes of depression during the fall and winter months, subsiding during spring and summer. It appears to be related to a lack of sunshine causing increased melatonin production by the pineal gland *(see Chapter 14)*. It can be helped by phototherapy with bright white fluorescent lights. Antidepressant drugs can also be helpful.

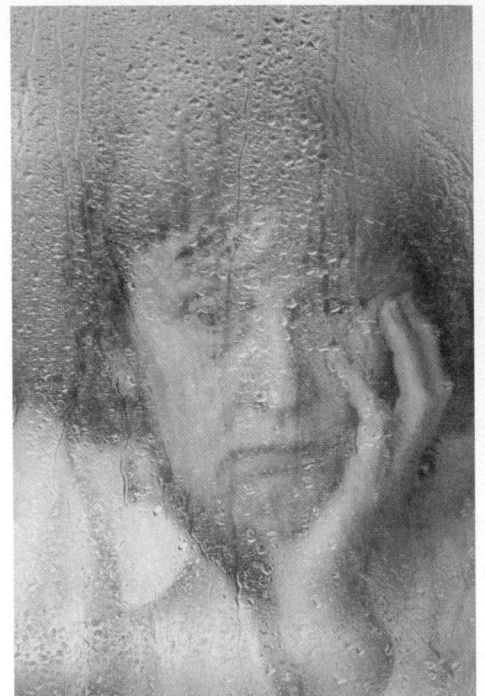

▲ **Figure 18.1** Depressed Woman at Window.

Abbreviations

ECT	electroconvulsive therapy
OCD	obsessive-compulsive disorder
PTSD	posttraumatic stress disorder
SAD	seasonal affective disorder
SNRI	serotonin and norepinephrine reuptake inhibitor
SSRI	selective serotonin reuptake inhibitor
TCA	tricyclic antidepressant

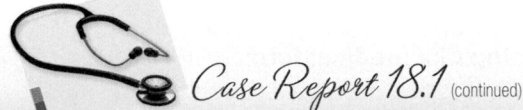

Case Report 18.1 (continued)

Mr. Harlan Diment is clearly in a manic phase. When Dr. Robert Nguyen, a psychiatrist, examined him in the Emergency Department, he believed the most likely diagnosis to be bipolar disorder. He has asked you to obtain a urine specimen to test for drugs of abuse and to do a blood test for his alcohol level, to exclude those as causes. Dr. Nguyen has ordered that Mr. Diment be admitted to the Psychiatric Unit. He will need treatment with a mood stabilizer such as lithium. If he resists admission, he can be placed on a 72-hour hold because he is a danger to himself and to others.

Table 18.1 The Depression Arsenal of Drugs

Drug Type	Generic or Brand Name
tricyclic antidepressants (TCAs)	Generic names: amitriptyline, nortriptyline, protriptyline, clomipramine, imipramine, trimipramine
selective serotonin reuptake inhibitors (SSRIs)	Generic and brand names: fluoxetine (Prozac), fluvoxamine (Luvox), paroxeline (Paxil), citalopram (Celexa), sertraline (Zoloft)
serotonin and norepinephrine reuptake inhibitors (SNRIs)	Generic and brand names: venlafaxine (Effexor), milnacipran (Dalcipran), duloxetine (Cymbalta)

WORD	PRONUNCIATION	ELEMENTS		DEFINITION
bipolar disorder	bi-**POH**-lar dis-**OR**-der	S/ P/ R/	-ar *pertaining to* bi- *two* -pol- *pole*	A mood disorder with alternating episodes of depression and mania, the two poles of the disorder
depression	de-**PRESH**-un	S/ R/	-ion *condition, process* depress- *press down*	Mental disorder with feelings of deep sadness and despair
electroconvulsive therapy	ee-**LEK**-troh-kon-**VUL**-siv **THAIR**-ah-pee	R/CF P/ R/ S/	electr/o- *electricity* -con- *with* -vuls- *tear, pull* -ive *quality of*	Passage of electric current through the brain to produce convulsions and treat persistent depression, mania, and other disorders
dysphoria	dis-**FOR**-ih-ah	S/ P/ R/	-ia *condition* dys- *bad, difficult* -phor- *carry, bear*	A condition of severe depression, agitation, and paranoid delusions
mania manic (adj) manic-depressive disorder	**MAY**-nee-ah **MAN**-ik **MAN**-ik de-**PRESS**-iv dis-**OR**-der	R/ S/ S/ R/	**Greek** *frenzy* man- *affected by frenzy* -ic *pertaining to* -ive *quality of* depress- *press down*	Mood disorder with hyperactivity, irritability, and rapid speech Pertaining to or characterized by mania An outdated name for bipolar disorder
phobia	**FOH**-bee-ah		**Greek** *fear*	Pathologic fear or dread
unipolar disorder	you-nih-**POLE**-ar dis-**OR**-der	S/ P/ R/	-ar *pertaining to* uni- *one* -pol- *pole (at the pole of depression)*	Depression

Exercises

A. Reinforce your learning of the *languages of psychology and psychiatry* by defining the difference between the following medical terms.   LO 18.1, 18.3

1. psychologist: _____

2. psychiatrist: _____

3. mental disorder: _____

4. insanity: _____

5. What is the one thing a psychiatrist can do that a psychologist cannot do? _____

_____

B. Circle the correct answer for the question.   LO 18.1, 18.3

1. Which of the following choices cannot be classified under the term *behavior*?

   a. talking

   b. sleeping

   c. reading

   d. depression

   e. interacting with others

2. Which of the following statements *best* describes a mental process?

   a. your private, internal experiences

   b. thinking

   c. feeling

   d. remembering

   e. dreaming

3. Which of the following terms contains a prefix, root, and suffix?

   a. psychology

   b. hallucination

   c. insanity

   d. homicidal

   e. psychiatry

Lesson 18.2 Anxiety Disorders

To work effectively with patients with anxiety disorders, you will need to be able to use correct medical terminology to:

18.2.1 Define the five major categories of anxiety disorders.

18.2.2 Discuss the symptoms of the five major types of anxiety disorder.

18.2.3 Specify the diagnostic criteria for posttraumatic stress disorder (PTSD).

18.2.4 Identify some of the drugs used to treat anxiety disorders.

18.2.5 Differentiate between psychosomatic and somatoform disorders.

You are

... a readjustment counseling technician in a Veterans Administration Counseling Center attached to Fulwood Medical Center.

Your patient is

... Sergeant Mike West, an Army reservist who has recently returned from his second tour of duty in Afghanistan.

Case Report 18.2

As you interview Sergeant West, you learn that he is having difficulty coping with what he experienced during wartime. The vehicle he was driving ran over an improvised explosive device (*Figure 18.2*). Two of his comrades died, and Sergeant West received shrapnel wounds in his leg and hand. He plays the tape of the incident in his mind over and over again. Loud noises, like thunderstorms, trigger paralysis. The smell of diesel brings back the memory of the vehicle on fire. Chicken on the barbecue smells like searing flesh. He can't sleep more than 3 or 4 hours a night, and then he wakes up in cold sweats. Sergeant West has become quick-tempered and doesn't like the way he is treating his wife. He is frightened to have children because of his outbursts of anger at seemingly minor upsets.

Abbreviations

CBT	cognitive behavioral therapy
CPT	cognitive processing therapy
EMDR	eye movement desensitization and reprocessing
GAD	generalized anxiety disorder
PTSD	posttraumatic stress disorder

LO 18.4 Anxiety Disorders

Anxiety disorders are the most common category of mental disorders found in the United States. They are characterized by an **unreasonable anxiety** or **fear** that is inappropriate to the circumstances and so intense and chronic that it disrupts the person's life.

There are five major categories of anxiety disorder:

1. **Generalized anxiety disorder (GAD)** consists of persistent, excessive worrying and uncontrollable anxiety that is not focused on one particular situation and has lasted for at least 6 months. People with this disorder are frightened of something but are unable to articulate a specific fear. They develop physical fear reactions including palpitations, **insomnia**, difficulty concentrating, and irritability.

2. **Posttraumatic stress disorder (PTSD)** occurs when a person who has gone through a significant trauma shows stress symptoms that last for longer than a month and impair the person's ability to function. The trauma can be a life-threatening accident, a natural disaster, loss of a loved one, torture or abuse, or combat and its related incidents.. Posttraumatic stress disorder is the diagnosis for Sergeant West.

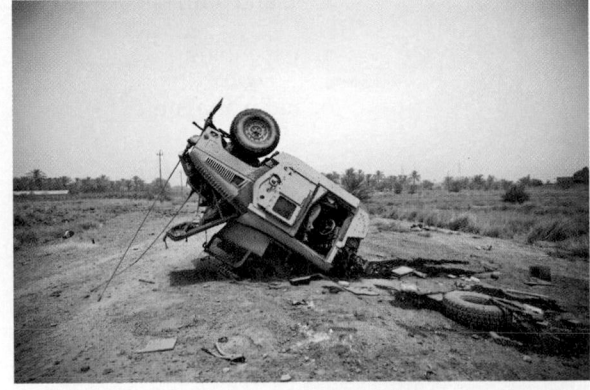

Figure 18.2 ▶ The remains of an American Humvee, one of four that were disabled by massive IEDs, lies on a dirt road on August 4, 2007, in Hawr Rajab, Iraq.

The treatment of posttraumatic stress disorder (PTSD) is **multimodal**, involving **psychopharmacotherapy**, **psychotherapy**, **social interventions**, and **patient and family education**. Forms of psychotherapy are **cognitive behavioral therapy (CBT)**, in which the traumatic experiences are relived and worked through, and **cognitive processing therapy (CPT)**, in which the thoughts and beliefs generated by the trauma are explored and reframed. **Eye movement desensitization and reprocessing (EMDR)** is also used. Social interventions to restore a sense of safety and security are a crucial element in therapy.

LO 18.1, 18.2, 18.4
Word Analysis and Definition

S = Suffix   P = Prefix   R = Root   R/CF = Combining Form

WORD	PRONUNCIATION	ELEMENTS		DEFINITION
anxiety	ang-**ZI**-eh-tee		**Greek** *distress, anxiety*	Distress caused by fear
cognitive	**KOG**-nih-tiv		**Latin** *knowledge*	Pertaining to the mental activities of thinking and learning
cognitive behavioral therapy (*Note:* Behavioral has two suffixes.)	**KOG**-nih-tiv be-**HAYV**-yur-al **THAIR**-ah-pee	S/ R/ S/ S/ R/ R/	**-ive** *quality of* **cognit-** *thinking* **-al** *pertaining to* **-ior-** *pertaining to* **behav-** *mental activity* **therapy** *medical treatment*	Psychotherapy that emphasizes thoughts and attitudes in one's behavior
cognitive processing therapy	**KOG**-nih-tiv **PROS**-es-ing **THAIR**-ah-pee	S/ R/ S/ P/ R/	**-ive** *quality of* **cognit-** *thinking* **-ing** *doing* **pro-** *before* **-cess-** *going forward*	Psychotherapy to build skills to deal with effects of the trauma in other areas of life
insomnia	in-**SOM**-nee-ah	S/ P/ R/	**-ia** *condition* **in-** *not* **-somn-** *sleep*	Inability to sleep
multimodal	mul-tee-**MOH**-dal	S/ P/ R/	**-al** *pertaining to* **multi-** *many* **-mod-** *method*	Using many methods
posttraumatic	post-traw-**MAT**-ik	S/ P/ R/	**-ic** *pertaining to* **post-** *after* **-traumat-** *wound*	Occurring after and caused by trauma
psychopharmaco-therapy	**SIGH**-koh-**FAR**-mah-koh-**THAIR**-ah-pee	S/ R/CF R/CF	**-therapy** *treatment* **psych/o-** *mind* **-pharmac/o-** *drugs*	Drug treatment of mental disorders

Exercises

A. After reading Case Report 18.2 on the opposite page, answer the following questions. *Be prepared to discuss your answers in class.* **LO 18.1, 18.4**

1. Specify the diagnostic criteria for posttraumatic stress disorder. (What can the diagnosis be based on?) _____

_____

2. What after effects of PTSD does Sergeant West now deal with on a daily basis? _____

_____

3. Is PTSD a generalized anxiety disorder? _____

4. What are some of the causes of PTSD? _____

B. Refer to the above WAD in this lesson for the answers to the following questions. *Fill in the blanks.* **LO 18.1, 18.2**

1. Which term in the WAD has an element meaning *drugs*? _____

2. Which terms in the WAD contain a prefix? _____

3. Which term in the WAD is from the Latin meaning *knowledge*? _____

4. Which term in the WAD means *inability to sleep*? _____

5. Which term in the WAD has an element meaning *many*? _____

LO 18.4 Anxiety Disorders (continued)

Keynotes

- A person called a **hypochondriac** has **hypochondriasis** and interprets some minor symptom, such as a bruise or a cough, as a sign of a serious disease and cannot believe normal physical examinations and reassurances.
- Numerous treatment options for phobias are available, including psychotherapy and the SSRIs, benzodiazepines, and **monoamine oxidase inhibitors (MAOIs)**.

Abbreviations

CBT	cognitive behavioral therapy
MAOI	monoamine oxidase inhibitor
SSRI	selective serotonin reuptake inhibitor

3. **Panic disorder** is characterized by sudden, brief attacks of **intense fear** that cause physical symptoms. The fear rises abruptly, often for no reason, and peaks in 10 minutes or less. The frequency of the attacks varies widely over many years. The disorder runs in families, but whether it is due to genetics or a shared environment is not clear. Treatment consists of medication *(Table 18.2)* and cognitive behavioral therapy (CBT).

4. **Phobias** differ from generalized anxiety and panic attacks in that a *specific* situation or object brings on the strong fear response. The danger is small, and the person realizes the fear is irrational, but there is still overwhelming anxiety. There are two categories of phobia:

   - **Situational phobias** involve a fear of specific situations. Examples include **agoraphobia** (fear of crowded places, buses, and elevators), **acrophobia** (fear of heights), fear of flying or driving in tunnels, and fear of specific animals (snakes, mice). The basic fear of being trapped in a confined space is called **claustrophobia**.
   - **Social phobias** involve fear of being embarrassed in social situations. The most common are fear of public speaking (stage fright) and of eating in public. In many, the fear is so strong that it makes normal life impossible.

5. **In obsessive-compulsive disorder (OCD)**, a majority of patients have both **obsessions** and **compulsions**. The obsessions are recurrent thoughts, fears, doubts, images, or impulses. The compulsions are recurrent, irresistible impulses to perform actions such as counting, hand washing, checking, and systematically arranging things. The recurrent actions can be violent or sexual.

Most patients recognize the senselessness of their behaviors; but if they resist doing them, the fear and anxiety become intolerable. Treatment is with CBT and one of the selective serotonin reuptake inhibitors (SSRIs) listed in *Table 18.2*.

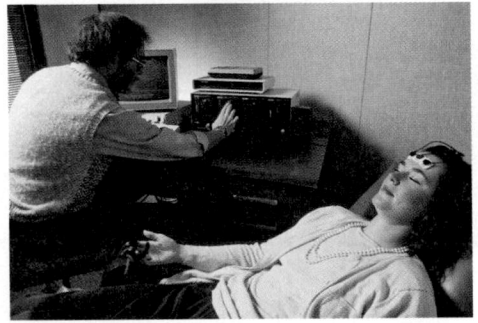

▲ **Figure 18.3**   Person Undergoing Biofeedback.

LO 18.4 Psychosomatic and Somatoform Disorders

Psychosomatic disorder is a real, physical disorder that, at least in part, has a psychologic cause. Tension headaches have real pain caused by muscle spasm, but stress and anxiety play a role in causing the symptoms. **Biofeedback** *(Figure 18.3)* and relaxation techniques can be helpful in reducing the tension and spasm.

Somatoform disorder occurs when there is no identifiable physical cause to explain physical symptoms. The symptoms are real to the patient and are not under voluntary control. In **conversion disorder**, symptoms progress to involve loss of feeling, paralysis, deafness, or blindness.

Table 18.2 Pharmacotherapy of Panic Disorder

Type of Drug	Effect
Benzodiazepines:	
alprazolam (Xanax)	Effective prophylaxis
clonazepam (Klonopin)	Reduce anticipatory anxiety
lorazepam (Ativan)	Rapid onset of action
diazepam (Valium)	
Selective Serotonin Reuptake Inhibitors (SSRIs):	
sertraline (Zoloft)	Reduce frequency of attacks
paroxetine (Paxil)	Reduce intensity of panic
fluvoxamine (Luvox)	Take 2 weeks to produce effect

WORD	PRONUNCIATION	ELEMENTS		DEFINITION
acrophobia	ak-roh-**FOH**-be-ah	S/ R/CF	-phobia *fear* **acr/o-** *peak, highest point*	Pathologic fear of heights
agoraphobia	ah-gor-ah-**FOH**-be-ah	S/ R/CF	-phobia *fear* **agor/a-** *marketplace*	Pathologic fear of being trapped in a public place
biofeedback (*Note:* This term has no prefix or suffix.)	bi-oh-**FEED**-back	R/CF R/ R/	**bi/o-** *life* -feed- *to give food, nourish* -back *back, return*	Training techniques to achieve voluntary control of responses to stimuli
claustrophobia	klaw-stroh-**FOH**-be-ah	S/ R/CF	-phobia *fear* **claustr/o-** *confined space*	Pathologic fear of being trapped in a confined space
compulsion **compulsive (adj)**	kom-**PULL**-shun kom-**PULL**-siv	S/ R/ S/	-ion *action, condition* **compuls-** *drive, compel* -ive *nature of, quality of*	Uncontrollable impulses to perform an act repetitively Possessing uncontrollable impulses to perform an act repetitively
conversion disorder	kon-**VER**-shun dis-**OR**-der		**Latin** *turn around or change*	An unconscious emotional conflict is expressed as physical symptoms with no organic basis
hypochondriac **hypochondriasis**	high-poh-**KON**-dree-ack **HIGH**-poh-kon-**DRY**-ah-sis	S/ P/ R/ S/	-iac *pertaining to* hypo- *below* -chondr- *cartilage, rib* -iasis *condition, state of*	A person who exaggerates the significance of symptoms Belief that a minor symptom indicates a severe disease
obsession **obsessive (adj)**	ob-**SESH**-un ob-**SES**-iv	S/ R/ S/	-ion *action, condition* **obsess-** *besieged by thoughts* -ive *nature of, quality of*	Persistent, recurrent, uncontrollable thoughts or impulses Possessing persistent, recurrent, uncontrollable thoughts or impulses
phobia	**FOH**-be-ah		**Greek** *fear*	Pathologic fear or dread
psychosomatic	sigh-koh-soh-**MAT**-ik	S/ R/CF R/	-tic *pertaining to* **psych/o-** *mind* -soma- *body*	Pertaining to disorders of the body usually resulting from disturbances of the mind
somatoform	so-**MAT**-oh-form	S/ R/CF	-form *appearance of* **somat/o-** *body*	Physical symptoms occurring without identifiable physical cause

Exercises

A. Meet chapter outcomes and lesson objectives by applying *the language of medical terminology* to answer the following questions. *Fill in the blanks.*   **LO 18.4**

1. What is the difference between *psychosomatic* and *somatoform* disorders?

   a. Psychosomatic disorders: _____

   b. Somatoform disorders: _____

2. What is the correct medical term for a disorder that "runs in families"? _____

3. What is the difference between *obsession* and *compulsion*?

   a. Obsession: _____

   b. Compulsion: _____

4. Explain what characterizes a *situational phobia* and a *social phobia*.

   a. Situational phobia: _____

   b. Social phobia: _____

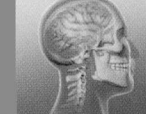

Lesson 18.3 Schizophrenia and Personality Disorders

MENTAL HEALTH

The information in this lesson will enable you to use correct medical terminology to:

18.3.1 Detail the symptoms and treatment of schizophrenia.

18.3.2 Describe the different types of personality disorders.

18.3.3 Discuss the classes of psychoactive drugs.

You are

. . . an emergency medical technician (EMT) working in the Emergency Department at Fulwood Medical Center.

Your patient is

. . . Mr. Dante Costello, a 21-year-old homeless man, brought in by the police after he was found sitting in the middle of a main street.

Case Report 18.3

Mr. Costello's explanation is "the voices told me to do it." He has heard voices telling him to do things for the past year. The voices often comment on his behavior. He has isolated himself from other people because "they are not who they say they are, and they are trying to get me." He is taking no drugs or medications and denies any **suicidal** or homicidal intent. Mr. Costello is dirty and disheveled, with poor hygiene. He can give no home or family address. His **affect** is **congruent**, though expressionless. His speech is slow, and his thoughts are disorganized and confused. The most probable diagnosis is **schizophrenia**. He needs to be admitted to the hospital because he is a danger to himself and other people.

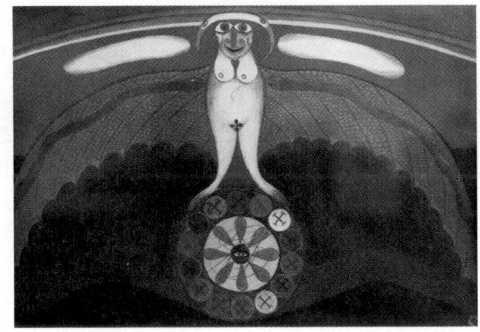

▲ **Figure 18.4** Artwork by Schizophrenic Patient.

LO 18.5 Schizophrenia

Schizophrenia is a form of **psychosis** in which there is a loss of contact with reality. People with schizophrenia do *not* have a split personality, but their words are separated from the meaning, their perceptions are separated from reality, and their behaviors are separated from their thought processes (*Figure 18.4*).

People with schizophrenia have their sensory perceptions jumbled and distorted, have difficulty concentrating, and perceive things without a stimulation—**hallucinations**. Hallucinations can occur in any of the senses but are most often auditory. These people also suffer from **delusions**, mistaken beliefs that are contrary to facts. The delusions can be **paranoid**, with pervasive distrust and suspicion of others. People with schizophrenia can withdraw from society, become homeless, and refuse to communicate (*Figure 18.5*).

Their speech is disorganized and can be incoherent. Their behaviors are often totally inappropriate. Their blunted emotions and withdrawal can progress to **catatonia**, motor immobility that can last for hours. **Mutism** is the inability or refusal to speak.

Magnetic resonance imaging (MRI) and positron emission tomography (PET) scans show brain abnormalities and changes in function.

Symptoms of schizophrenia typically come on in the late teens and twenties. Although there is no cure, it can be effectively treated with medications and programs of psychological rehabilitation (*see Chapter 18*). The goals of therapy are to reduce schizophrenic symptoms, prevent their return, and enable the patient to function in society. **Antipsychotic** medications such as olanzapine, quetiapine, and risperidone are used, either singly or in combinations if necessary, and mood stabilizers such as lithium are also used.

Case Report 18.3 (continued)

Mr. Costello stated he was hearing voices of people who were not there speaking to him (hallucination). Mr. Costello was also paranoid, believing that people were "out to get him." He withdrew from society and became homeless. His behavior of sitting immobile in the middle of the street for long periods is inappropriate and is catatonic.

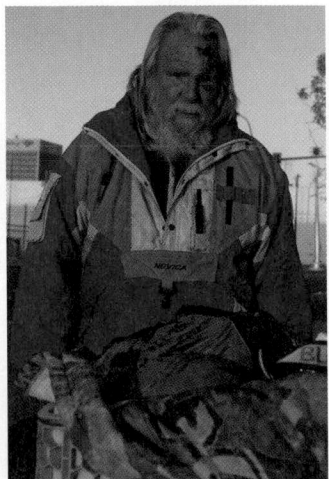

▲ **Figure 18.5** Homeless Schizophrenic Man on the Street.

WORD	PRONUNCIATION	ELEMENTS		DEFINITION
affect (noun)	**AF**-fekt		Latin *state of mind*	External display of feelings, thoughts, and emotions
catatonia	kat-ah-**TOE**-nee-ah	S/ P/ R/	**-ia** *condition* **cata-** *down* **-ton-** *pressure, tension*	Syndrome characterized by physical immobility and mental stupor
catatonic (adj)	kat-ah-**TON**-ic	S/	**-ic** *pertaining to*	Pertaining to or characterized by, catatonia
congruent	**KON**-gru-ent	S/ P/ R/	**-ent** *end result* **con-** *with* **-gru-** *to move*	Coinciding or agreeing with
mute **mutism**	MYUT **MYU**-tizm	 S/ R/	Latin *silent* **-ism** *condition, process* **mut-** *silent*	Unable or unwilling to speak Absence of speech
paranoia	par-ah-**NOY**-ah	P/ R/	**para-** *abnormal, beside* **-noia** *to think*	Mental disorder with persecutory delusions
paranoid (adj)	**PAR**-ah-noyd	S/	**-noid** *abnormal thinking*	Having delusions of persecution
psychosis	sigh-**KOH**-sis	S/ R/	**-osis** *condition* **psych-** *mind*	Disorder causing mental disruption and loss of contact with reality
psychotic (adj)	sigh-**KOT**-ik	S/ R/CF	**-tic** *pertaining to* **psych/o-** *mind*	Pertaining to or affected by psychosis
antipsychotic	**AN**-tih-sigh-**KOT**-ik	P/	**anti-** *against*	An agent helpful in the treatment of psychosis
schizophrenia	skitz-oh-**FREE**-nee-ah	S/ R/CF R/	**-ia** *condition* **schiz/o-** *to split, cleave* **-phren-** *mind*	Disorder of perception, thought, emotion, and behavior
schizophrenic (adj)	skitz-oh-**FREN**-ik	S/	**-ic** *pertaining to*	Relating to, or suffering from, schizophrenia
suicide	**SOO**-ih-side	R/CF R/CF	**su/i-** *self* **-cid/e** *kill*	The act of killing oneself Wanting to kill oneself
suicidal (adj)	**SOO**-ih-**SIGH**-dal	S/	**-al** *pertaining to*	

Exercises

A. After reading Case Report 18.3 on the opposite page, answer the following questions. *Be prepared to discuss your answers in class.*   **LO 18.1, 18.5**

1. What is the difference between *suicidal* intent and *homicidal* intent?

   a. suicidal: _____

   b. homicidal: _____

2. What is inappropriate about Mr. Costello's behavior?

   _____

   _____

3. What is amiss about his appearance?

   _____

4. Explain this sentence: "His affect is congruent, though expressionless." What does that mean?

   _____

   _____

5. Why is Mr. Costello being admitted to the hospital?

   _____

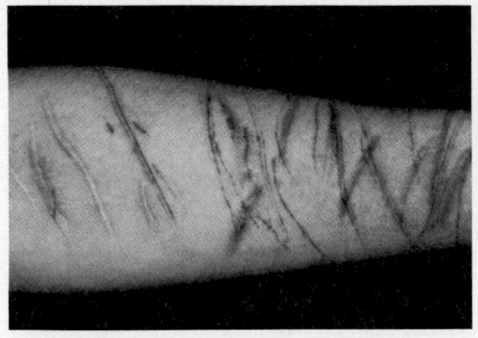

▲ **Figure 18.6**　Self-Mutilated Arm.

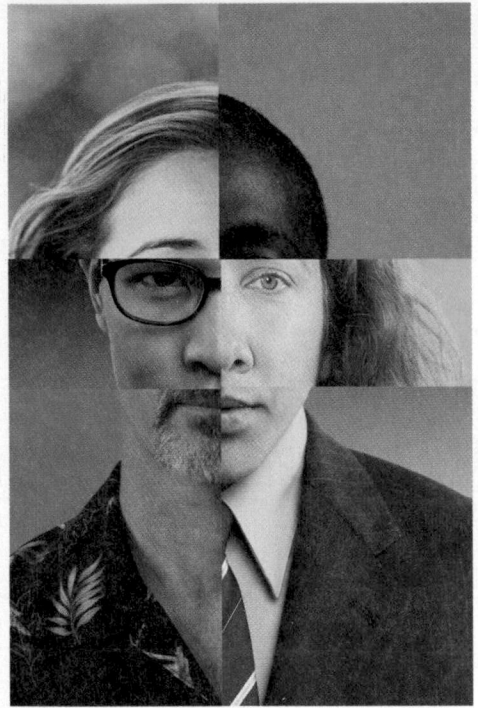

▲ **Figure 18.7**　Dissociative Identity Disorder (Multiple Personality Disorder).

Abbreviations	
BPD	borderline personality disorder
DID	dissociative identity disorder
MPD	multiple personality disorder
TTM	trichotillomania

LO 18.6　Personality Disorders

Personality is defined as an individual's unique and stable patterns of thoughts, feelings, and behaviors. When these patterns become rigid and inflexible in response to different situations, they can cause impairment of the individual's ability to deal with other people (i.e., to function socially).

Borderline personality disorder (BPD) is a frequent diagnosis in people who are impulsive, unstable in mood, and manipulative. They can be exciting, charming, and friendly one moment and angry, irritable, and sarcastic the next. Their identity is fragile and insecure, their self-worth low. They can be promiscuous and self-destructive, for example, committing **self-mutilation (self-injury)** *(Figure 18.6)* or suicide. People with **narcissistic personality disorder** have an exaggerated sense of self-importance and seek constant attention.

Antisocial personality disorder, used interchangeably with the terms **sociopath** and **psychopath**, describes people who lie, cheat, steal, make trouble for others, and have no sense of responsibility and no anxiety or guilt about their behavior. The psychopaths have these characteristics but tend to be more violent and anger more easily than sociopaths.

Schizoid and **paranoid personality disorders** describe people who are absorbed with themselves, untrusting, and fearful of closeness with others.

Treatment for personality disorders is not successful.

Dissociative Disorders

Dissociative disorders involve a disassociation (splitting apart) of past experiences from present memory or consciousness. Being unable to recall identity is called **dissociative amnesia**. The development of distinctly separate personalities is called **dissociative identity disorder (DID)**. It was formerly called **multiple personality disorder (MPD)**.

The basic origin of all these disorders is the need to escape, usually from extreme trauma, and most often from sexual, emotional, or physical abuse in childhood.

The most severe of this group of disorders is DID. Two or more distinct personalities, each with their own memories and behaviors, inhabit the same person at the same time *(Figure 18.7)*. Treatment is with psychotherapy.

Impulse Control Disorders

Impulse control disorders are an inability to resist an impulse to perform an action that is harmful to the individual or to others. These disorders include

- **Intermittent explosive disorder**, which is characterized by recurrent episodes of unrestrained aggression toward people, furniture, or property, with violent resistance to attempts to restrain. The etiology is thought to be epileptic-like activity in the brain. Medications that generate some improvement include propranolol, lithium, valproate, and phenytoin.
- **Kleptomania**, which is characterized by stealing—not for gain, but to satisfy an irresistible urge to steal. Behavioral therapy can help, and SSRIs appear to be of value.
- **Trichotillomania (TTM)**, which is characterized by the repeated urge to pull out scalp, beard, pubic, and other body hair.
- **Substance abuse** and **chemical dependence**, which involve a person's continued use of drugs or alcohol despite having had significant problems or distress related to their use. This **addiction** affects the brain and behavior and develops an increased need for the substance and an inability to stop using it.
- **Pyromania**, which is repeated fire setting with no motive other than a fascination with fire and fire engines. Some pyromaniacs end up as volunteer firefighters. Treatment with behavioral therapy is sometimes successful.

WORD	PRONUNCIATION	ELEMENTS		DEFINITION
addict addiction	ADD-ikt ah-DIK-shun	P/ R/ S/	ad- *toward* -dict *surrender* -ion *condition, action*	Person with a psychologic or physical dependence on a substance or practice Habitual psychologic and physiologic dependence on a substance or practice
amnesia	am-NEE-zee-ah		**Greek** *forgetfulness*	Total or partial inability to remember past experiences
antisocial personality disorder	AN-tee-SOH-shal per-son-AL-ih-tee dis-OR-der	S/ P/ R/ S/ S/ R/	-al *pertaining to* anti- *against* -soci- *partner, ally, community* -ity *condition, state* -al- *pertaining to* -person- *person*	Disorder of people who lie, cheat, steal, and have no guilt about their behavior
dissociative identity disorder	di-SO-see-ah-tiv eye-DEN-tih-tee dis-OR-der	P/ R/ S/	dis- *apart, away from* -soci- *partner, ally, community* -ative *quality of*	Mental disorder in which part of an individual's personality is separated from the rest, leading to multiple personalities
kleptomania	klep-toe-MAY-nee-ah	S/ R/CF	-mania *frenzy* klept/o- *to steal*	Uncontrollable need to steal
narcissism narcissistic (adj)	NAR-sih-sizm NAR-sih-SIS-tik	 S/ R/ S/	Greek mythical character, Narcissos, who was in love with his own reflection in water -ism *a process* narciss- *self-love* -istic *pertaining to*	Self-love; person interprets everything purely in relation to himself or herself Relating everything to oneself; pertaining to, or suffering from, narcissism
pathologic gambling	path-oh-LOJ-ik GAM-bling	S/ R/CF R/	-ic *pertaining to* path/o *disease* -log- *study of*	Morbid, constant, uncontrollable, destructive gambling
psychopath	SIGH-koh-path	S/ R/CF	-path *disease* psych/o- *mind*	Person with antisocial personality disorder who are prone to anger and violence
pyromania	pie-roh-MAY-nee-ah	S/ R/CF	-mania *frenzy* pyr/o- *fire*	Morbid impulse to set fires
schizoid	SKITZ-oyd	S/ R/	-oid *resemble* schiz- *split*	Withdrawn, socially isolated
self-mutilation	self-myu-tih-LAY-shun	S/ R/ R/	-ation *process* self- *own individual* -mutil- *to maim*	Injury or disfigurement made to one's own body
sociopath	SO-see-oh-path	S/ R/CF	-path *disease* soci/o- *partner, ally, community*	Person with antisocial personality disorder

Exercises

A. Use your knowledge of medical language to answer the following question.   LO 18.1, 18.6

How are psychopaths and sociopaths the same and how are they different?

1. The same: _____

2. Different: _____

LO 18.7 Psychoactive Drugs

Psychoactive drugs are chemicals that change consciousness, awareness, or perception *(Table 18.5)*. The most commonly used drugs are caffeine, tobacco, and alcohol.

Drug abuse refers to the use of drugs that cause emotional or physical harm to an individual as consumption becomes frequent and compulsive.

Addiction occurs when a person feels compelled to use a drug or perform a certain activity and cannot control the use.

Psychological dependence is the mental desire or **craving** for the effects produced by a drug.

Physical dependence is the changes in the body processes that make the drug necessary for daily functioning. If the drug is stopped, the withdrawal symptoms include physical pain, as well as intense cravings.

Tolerance occurs when the body adjusts to the effects of the drug, and higher and higher doses produce less and less effect. The brain, liver, heart, and other organs can be damaged.

Comorbidity is the presence of a combination of disorders. It is very common. Alcohol dependence and abuse overlap with almost all other mental disorders, including anxiety disorders, mood disorders, and personality disorders. In such cases, stopping drinking alcohol is only the first step in solving the problem.

Table 18.5 Psychoactive Drugs

Type/Mode of Action	Name	Common Effects	Effects of Abuse
Stimulants ("uppers") Speed up activity in the central nervous system (CNS)	caffeine	Wakefulness, shorter reaction time, alertness	Restlessness, insomnia, heartbeat irregularities
	nicotine	Varies from alertness to calmness, appetite for carbohydrates decreases	Heart disease; high blood pressure; vasoconstriction; bronchitis; emphysema; lung, throat, mouth cancer
	amphetamines	Wakefulness, alertness, increased metabolism, decreased appetite	Nervousness, high blood pressure, delusions, psychosis, convulsions, death
	cocaine	**Euphoria**, high energy, illusions of power	Excitability, paranoia, anxiety, panic, depression, heart failure, death
Depressants ("downers") Slow down activity in the CNS	alcohol	**1–2 drinks**—reduced inhibitions and anxiety	Blackouts, mental and neurologic impairment, psychosis, cirrhosis of liver, death
		Many drinks—slow reaction time, poor coordination and memory	Impaired motor and sensory functions, amnesia, loss of consciousness, death
	barbiturates and tranquilizers	Reduced anxiety and tension, sedation	
Narcotics Mimic the actions of natural **endorphins**	codeine, opium, morphine, heroin	Euphoria, pleasure, relief of pain	High tolerance of pain, nausea, vomiting, constipation, convulsions, coma, death
Psychedelics Disrupt normal thought processes	marijuana	Relaxation, euphoria, increased appetite, pain relief	Sensory distortion, hallucinations, paranoia, throat and lung damage
	LSD, mescaline, MDMA (Ecstasy)	Exhilaration, euphoria, hallucinations, insightful experiences	Panic, extreme delusions, bad trips, paranoia, psychosis

WORD	PRONUNCIATION	ELEMENTS		DEFINITION
comorbidity	koh-mor-**BID**-ih-tee	S/ P/ R/	-ity *condition, state* co- *with, together* -morbid- *disease*	Presence of two or more diseases at the same time
craving	**KRAY**-ving		Latin *desire*	Deep longing or desire
dependence	de-**PEN**-dense		Latin *to hang from*	State of needing someone or something
depressant	de-**PRESS**-ant	S/ P/ R/	-ant *agent* de- *away from* -press- *press down*	Substance that diminishes activity, sensation, or tone
endorphin	en-**DOR**-fin	P/ R/	end- *within* -orphin *morphine*	Natural substance in the brain that has same effect as opium
euphoria	yoo-**FOR**-ee-ah	S/ P/ R/	-ia *condition* eu- *normal* -phor- *bear, carry*	Exaggerated feeling of well-being
narcotic	nar-**KOT**-ik	S/ R/CF	-tic *pertaining to* narc/o- *sleep, stupor*	Drug derived from opium or a synthetic drug with similar effects
psychedelic	sigh-keh-**DEL**-ik	S/ R/CF R/	-ic *pertaining to* psych/e- *mind, soul* -del- *manifest, visible*	Agent that intensifies sensory perception
psychoactive	sigh-koh-**AK**-tiv	S/ R/CF R/	-ive *quality of, nature of* psych/o- *mind, soul* -act- *performance*	Able to alter mood, behavior, and/or cognition
stimulant	**STIM**-you-lant	S/ R/	-ant *agent* stimul- *excite*	Agent that excites or strengthens functional activity
tolerance	**TOL**-er-antz	S/ R/	-ance *condition, state of* toler- *endure*	The capacity to become accustomed to a stimulus or drug

Exercises

A. Review all the new terms you have learned on these two pages. *Choose the correct medical terminology to insert into each of the following sentences. You will use some terms twice.*   LO 18.1, 18.7

1. A diabetic with high blood pressure has a _____.

2. Caffeine and nicotine can be *both* a(n) _____ and a(n) _____.

3. Marathon runners can experience the natural stimulatory effect from _____.

4. _____ is a state that can be physical or mental.

5. The two opposite terms in the above WAD are _____ and _____.

6. An agent able to alter mood, behavior, and/or cognition is _____.

7. A natural substance in the brain that has the same effect as opium is _____.

8. A(n) _____ is an agent that excites or strengthens functional activity.

9. Deep longing or desire is a(n) _____.

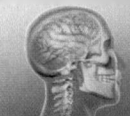

Mental Health

Challenge Your Knowledge

A. **Precision in communication requires correct spelling of the medical terms you are using.** If any of the medical terms in the following exercise are incorrectly spelled, write the correct spelling on the line next to it. Then choose one of the terms and write a sentence of clinical documentation using that term. (**LO 18.1,** *Remember, Understand, Apply*)

1. congruent   _____

2. skitzoid   _____

3. antiskiztotic   _____

4. amnessia   _____

5. cleptomania   _____

6. narcissism   _____

7. psychopath   _____

8. addiction   _____

9. piromania   _____

10. Choose any one term from 1–9 above and use it in a sentence that is not a definition.

_____

_____

B. **Elements, elements, elements.** Solid knowledge of elements will help increase your medical vocabulary. Identify the element as to type (P, R, CF, S), give the meaning of the element, and then provide a medical term containing the element. The first one is done for you. Fill in the table. (**LO 18.1, 18.2,** *Remember, Apply*)

Element	Prefix	Root/ Combining Form	Suffix	Meaning of Element	Medical Term Containing This Element
1. phobia				2.	3.
4. iatrist				5.	6.
7. phren				8.	9.
10. vuls				11.	12.
13. cognit				14.	15.
16. somn				17.	18.
19. pharmaco				20.	21.
22. acro				23.	24.
25. claustro				26.	27.
28. agora				29.	30.
31. iasis				32.	33.
34. chondr				35.	36.
37. mut				38.	39.
40. uni				41.	42.
43. sui				44.	45.

C. Terminology challenge. Once you know the meaning of an element, it always applies. First circle the prefix in each of the four terms in the left column; then write the meaning of the prefix in the middle column. Write the meaning of the term in the right column. Relate this prefix to different medical terms in other chapters. (**LO 18.1, 18.2, *Understand, Apply***)

Medical Term	Meaning of Prefix	Meaning of Medical Term
insomnia	1.	2.
multimodal	3.	4.
posttraumatic	5.	6.
bipolar	7.	8.

Terms with the same prefix from other chapters already studied:

Medical Term	Meaning of Prefix	Meaning of Medical Term
i	9.	10.
m	11.	12.
p	13.	14.
b	15.	16.

D. Abbreviations. Apply your knowledge of abbreviations to complete the following patient documentation. Choose from the following abbreviations to correctly fill in the blanks. You will have more answers than questions. (**LO 18.1, *Understand, Apply***)

ECT   CNS   PTSD   BPD   DID   CBT   SSRI   CPT   STAT

1. Patient now has developed three distinct, separate personalities. Her _____ is rapidly progressing.

2. Patient is suffering from unipolar depression, and a(n) _____ medication will be prescribed.

3. Patient's nightmares are increasing and are always the same replay of his automobile accident. I am sending him

for _____ and _____ in the hopes this can alleviate some of his _____ and help him

sleep better. Sleep medication is also prescribed.

4. Patient exhibits frequent mood changes and has become manipulative in her relationship with her parents.

Her _____ is escalating her insecurity.

5. _____ will be prescribed for this patient as a last resort for treatment of his mania.

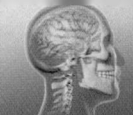

Mental Health

E. Patient education. As a health care worker, you should be prepared and equipped to explain any medical term to a patient, whether the patient requests it or you can see that the patient is not understanding what has been said by the physician. Explain to your patient the difference between the following terms. (**LO 18.2, 18.4, *Understand, Apply***)

1. a. unipolar disorder:

_____

_____

_____

b. bipolar disorder:

_____

_____

_____

2. a. psychotherapy:

_____

_____

_____

b. psychopharmacotherapy:

_____

_____

_____

3. a. addiction:

_____

_____

_____

b. abuse:

_____

_____

_____

Use any one term from questions 1–3 in a sentence of patient documentation.

4. Sentence:

_____

_____

_____

F. Prefixes. Test your recall of word element meanings by answering the following questions about prefixes. The medical term is given; on the line beside the term, write the prefix, and then circle the best answer. (**LO 18.1, 18.3, 18.4, *Understand, Apply***)

1. *bipolar:* Prefix is _____ and means

   a. one

   b. two

   c. three

   d. four

   e. five

2. *hypochondriasis:* Prefix is _____ and means

   a. after

   b. around

   c. deficient

   d. next to

   e. excessive

3. *depressant:* Prefix is _____ and means

   a. toward

   b. forming

   c. within

   d. away from

   e. around

4. *catatonia:* Prefix is _____ and means

   a. up

   b. around

   c. through

   d. down

   e. beside

5. *addiction:* Prefix is _____ and means

   a. toward

   b. from

   c. for

   d. with

   e. up

6. *euphoria:* Prefix is _____ and means

   a. marketplace

   b. mind

   c. normal

   d. madness

   e. wound

7. *paranoia:* Prefix is _____ and means

   a. above

   b. excessive

   c. abnormal

   d. condition

   e. study of

8. *unipolar:* Prefix is _____ and means

   a. one

   b. four

   c. many

   d. few

   e. none

9. *dissociative:* Prefix is _____ and means

   a. painful

   b. apart

   c. abnormal

   d. irregular

   e. together

10. *convulsive:* Prefix is _____ and means

    a. in front of

    b. with

    c. next to

    d. yellow

    e. small

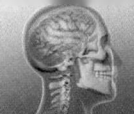

Mental Health

G. Language of psychology and psychiatry. Employ your knowledge of the *language of mental health* to match the statement in the left column with the correct medical vocabulary in the right column. Fill in the blanks. (**LO 18.1, 18.3, 18.4, 18.6,** *Understand, Apply*)

_____	1. lack of contact with reality	a. delusion
_____	2. symptoms with no physical cause	b. mutism
_____	3. refusal or inability to speak	c. dissociative amnesia
_____	4. legal term, not a diagnosis	d. personality
_____	5. motor immobility for hours	e. mental disorder
_____	6. deep sadness and despair	f. catatonia
_____	7. mistaken belief, contrary to fact	g. somatoform
_____	8. individual's unique pattern of thought	h. psychosis
_____	9. unable to recall identity	i. depression
_____	10. emotional state that is self-destructive	j. insanity

H. Deconstruct the following medical terms from this lesson into their basic elements. Then choose any four terms, and use each of them in a sentence of patient documentation. Fill in the blanks. (**LO 18.1, 18.3,** *Understand, Apply*)

Medical Term	Prefix	Root/Combining Form	Suffix
obsessive	1.	2.	3.
psychosomatic	4.	5.	6.
hypochondriac	7.	8.	9.
antipsychotic	10.	11.	12.
sociopath	13.	14.	15.
paranoia	16.	17.	18.
schizophrenia	19.	20.	21.

Sentences of patient documentation.

22. _____

_____

23. _____

_____

24. _____

_____

25. _____

_____

I. Difference between. Any health care worker in the mental health field will be interacting with psychologists and psychiatrists. Write a brief answer *in layman's terms* that explains the basic differences between the two practitioners. (**LO 18.1, 18.2, Understand, Apply**)

1. psychologist:

_____

_____

_____

2. psychiatrist:

_____

_____

_____

Meet the lesson objective by explaining the difference between

3. mental disorder:

_____

_____

_____

4. insanity:

_____

_____

_____

5. There is no listing for insanity in the DSM-IV. Why not?

_____

_____

_____

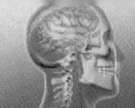

Mental Health

J. Roots/combining forms are the core foundation of every medical term. Test your knowledge of roots/combining forms in the *language of psychology and psychiatry* with this exercise. Fill in the blanks; then use any one medical term in the grid in a sentence of your choice that is not a definition. (**LO 18.2,** *Understand, Apply*)

Root/Combining Form	Element identity Meaning of Element	Medical Term with this Element	Definition of Medical Term
claustr/o	1.	2.	3.
bio	4.	5.	6.
agor/a	7.	8.	9.
somn	10.	11.	12.
acr/o	13.	14.	15.
klept/o	16.	17.	18.
cide	19.	20.	21.
schiz/o	22.	23.	24.

Sentence:

25. _____

_____

_____

K. Latin and Greek terms cannot be further deconstructed into prefix, root, or suffix. You must know them for what they are. Test your knowledge of these terms with this exercise. Match the meaning in the left column with the correct medical term in the right column. (**LO 18.2,** *Understand, Apply*)

_____ 1. turn around or change   **a.** mania

_____ 2. unable to recall identity   **b.** affect

_____ 3. knowledge   **c.** conversion

_____ 4. frenzy   **d.** phobia

_____ 5. desire   **e.** craving

_____ 6. to hang from   **f.** anxiety

_____ 7. fear   **g.** amnesia

_____ 8. distress   **h.** cognitive

_____ 9. state of mind   **i.** dependence

L. Use your knowledge of the language of psychology and psychiatry. Circle the correct answer to the following questions. *Remember:* There is only one *best* answer. (**LO 18.3, 18.4, 18.6,** *Apply*)

1. A mood disorder more common in women is

    a. PTSD

    b. SAD

    c. phobias

    d. OCD

    e. depression

2. Manic depressive disorder is now known as

    a. SAD

    b. unipolar disorder

    c. generalized anxiety disorder

    d. mania

    e. bipolar disorder

3. A TCA used to treat depression is

    a. Prozac

    b. Paxil

    c. amitriptyline

    d. Zoloft

    e. duloxetine

4. Significant trauma can lead to

    a. OCD

    b. TTM

    c. SAD

    d. DID

    e. PTSD

5. Circle the drug NOT prescribed for a panic disorder:

    a. nortriptyline

    b. Paxil

    c. Xanax

    d. Zoloft

    e. Klonopin

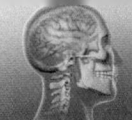

Mental Health

M. **Apply your knowledge of the language of psychology and psychiatry.** Circle the correct answer to the following questions. *Remember:* There is only one *best* answer. **(LO 18.3, 18.4, 18.6, *Apply*)**

1. A combination of CBT and EMDR would be treatment for

   a. MPD

   b. DID

   c. OCD

   d. PTSD

   e. TTM

2. No identifiable physical cause to explain physical symptoms characterizes

   a. hypochondriasis

   b. acrophobia

   c. conversion disorder

   d. agoraphobia

   e. somatoform disorder

3. Perceiving things without a stimulation is a(n)

   a. compulsion

   b. delusion

   c. hallucination

   d. obsession

   e. tangent

4. Higher doses of a drug produce less effect:

   a. psychological dependence

   b. addiction

   c. tolerance

   d. physical dependence

   e. comorbidity

5. Schizophrenia is a form of

   a. delusion

   b. phobia

   c. psychosis

   d. mood disorder

   e. obsession

N. Suffixes. Mental health practitioners can be either *psych*ologists or *psych*iatrists. The root/combining form **psych/o-** is present in all the following terms. The suffix is what makes the difference. Challenge your knowledge of the language of mental health by applying the correct term to the following statements. Fill in the blanks, using the choices below. (**LO 18.1, 18.2,** *Apply, Analyze*)

psychopath	psychiatry	psychiatric	psychotherapy
psychotic	psychopharmacotherapy	psychoanalysis	psychology
psychiatrist	psychoanalyst	psychologist	psychological
psychosomatic	psychotherapist	psychosis	psychoactive

1. An agent able to alter mood, behavior, or cognition is _____.

2. Treatment of mental disorders through communication is called _____.

3. _____ is the science concerned with the behavior of humans.

4. A licensed specialist in psychology is known as a _____.

5. The patient's _____ state was starting to affect his physical well-being.

6. A method of psychotherapy is _____.

7. What type of technician is the health care worker in the first CR at the beginning of this chapter?

    _____ technician

8. Drug treatment of mental disorders is known as _____.

9. A medical specialist in psychiatry is a _____.

10. A practitioner of psychoanalysis is called a _____.

11. Disorder causing mental disruption and loss of contact with reality is _____.

12. _____ is the medical specialty dealing with the diagnosis and treatment of mental disorders.

13. A practitioner of psychotherapy is a _____.

14. A real, physical disorder that, at least in part, has a psychological cause is _____.

15. Pertaining to or affected by psychosis is _____.

16. A serial killer can be termed a _____.

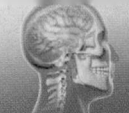

Mental Health

O. **Psychoactive drugs can be prescribed (like barbiturates and tranquilizers), or they can be self-administered (like caffeine and nicotine).** First, group the drugs from the word bank into their proper categories. Then list three bad effects resulting from abuse of each of the drug groups. Fill in the blanks. (**LO 18.7**, *Apply, Analyze*)

Word Bank:

marijuana	alcohol	nicotine	cocaine	morphine
tranquilizers	amphetamines	caffeine	heroin	barbiturates
opium	codeine	Ecstacy	LSD	mescaline

Depressants:

　1. Names of drugs in this group: _____

　2. Effects of abuse of these drugs: _____

Psychedelics:

　3. Names of drugs in this group: _____

　4. Effects of abuse of these drugs: _____

Stimulants:

　5. Names of drugs in this group: _____

　6. Effects of abuse of these drugs: _____

Narcotics:

　7. Names of drugs in this group: _____

　8. Effects of abuse of these drugs: _____

P. **Terminology in use.** Psychoactive drugs are chemicals that change consciousness, awareness, or perception. The most commonly used drugs are caffeine, tobacco, and alcohol. (**LO 18.1, 18.7**, *Apply, Analyze*)

Review Table 18.5, "Psychoactive Drugs." Then write a short paragraph using as many of the following terms as possible. For example, you can describe something you have observed in another person (say, a person who drinks too much coffee every day or someone you know who is trying to give up smoking). You might also comment on what effects on health these drugs have and how difficult it can be to give them up.

Terms to use in your short paragraph.

drug abuse	addiction	psychological dependence	tolerance	stimulant
physical dependence	comorbidity	craving	depressant	

_____

_____

_____

Q. **You will be required to document certain notes concerning Mr. Diment's behavior.** Your patient has been diagnosed with a manic episode of bipolar disorder. Reread this Case Report, and answer the following questions. (**LO 18.1, 18.5,** *Analyze*)

Case Report 18.1

Your patient is

... Mr. Harlan Diment, a 40-year-old construction worker. He was brought to the Emergency Department by his roommate, who says that Mr. Diment has slept only a couple of hours each night for the past 3 weeks. He stays up most of the night, cleaning their apartment and drinking beer. He has bought a new home entertainment set, including a big-screen plasma TV, that he cannot afford. He is very irritable and explosive when challenged about his behavior. His roommate has seen no signs of drugs and is not aware of any medical problems. Mr. Diment is usually very quiet, thoughtful, and introverted.

A mental status examination shows Mr. Diment to be alternately irritable and excited. He is wearing a bright orange top and camouflage slacks and is carrying a soft green cap. His speech is rapid and loud, and it is difficult to interrupt him. He paces the room, claims to feel "great," and is angry with his roommate for insisting that he come to the hospital. His thought processes and verbalization go off on different tangents. He says he has no suicidal thoughts, hallucinations, or delusions.

Mr. Diment is clearly in a manic phase. When Dr. Robert Nguyen, a psychiatrist, examined him in the Emergency Department, he believed the most likely diagnosis to be bipolar disorder. He has asked you to obtain a urine specimen to test for drugs of abuse and to do a blood test for his alcohol level to exclude those as causes. Dr. Nguyen has ordered that Mr. Diment be admitted to the Psychiatric Unit. He will need treatment with a mood stabilizer such as lithium. If he resists admission, he can be placed on a 72-hour hold because he is a danger to himself and to others.

1. Describe the symptoms that indicate Mr. Diment is in a manic phase of this disorder. _____

_____

_____

2. If this is a *bipolar* disorder, what is the opposite type of behavior Mr. Diment could have been exhibiting? _____

_____

_____

3. What diagnostic tests have been ordered for Mr. Diment? _____

_____

_____

4. What two factors are Dr. Nguyen looking to *exclude* as possible causes of Mr. Diment's behavior? _____

_____

_____

5. What treatment was prescribed for Mr. Diment? _____

_____

_____

6. How or why can Mr. Diment be considered a danger to himself or others? _____

_____

_____

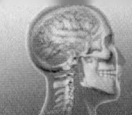

Mental Health

R. **Anxiety and impulse control disorders.** Patients with various types of anxiety and impulse control disorders are seen in the Fulwood Psychiatric Clinic. Determine the specific disorder from the description of the patient and the symptoms in the following documentation. <u>The first one is done for you</u>. Fill in the blanks. **(LO 18.4, *Analyze*)**

1. Patient suffers sudden bouts of intense fear that cause profuse sweating, nausea, and occasional vomiting.

   panic disorder
   _____

2. Patient has been arrested for shoplifting but admits to stealing many more items before she was caught today. Patient states that she steals for the "thrill of it." _____

3. Patient's house was destroyed in the flooding following Hurricane Katrina. He barely escaped with his life and now suffers from almost daily stress headaches and physical aches and pains. _____

4. Patient was locked in closets for hours at a time as a young boy. _____

5. Patient is here today by court order for psychiatric examination. Patient is suspected of setting two fires in the same neighborhood in the last 2 weeks. _____.

6. Patient is so uncomfortable on buses, subways, elevators, and crowded sidewalks that she is unable to get to work.

   _____.

7. Patient presents today with severe dermatitis on both hands. Patient states she washes her hands at least 50 times a day to be sure they are germ-free. _____

8. Patient's chief complaint today is palpitations and insomnia, which keep him awake most nights. He feels worried and anxious all the time but can give no specific reason for it. _____

S. **Differences.** Discuss and be able to explain the basic differences among the following four terms. You should be able to describe the condition and cite an example for each. Write your notes below each term. **(LO 18.7, *Analyze*)**

1. addiction:

   _____

   _____

2. tolerance:

   _____

   _____

3. physical dependence:

   _____

   _____

4. psychological dependence:

   _____

   _____

CHAPTER SUMMARY EXERCISES

A. Spelling comprehension. *Circle the correct spelling of the term.* (**LO 18.1,** *Remember*)

1. lythium	lifhium	litium	lithium	lytium
2. comorrbity	comorbidity	commorbity	comorbity	comorbity
3. paranouia	parinoia	paranoia	parenoiia	parinnoia
4. dipendance	depindince	depindance	dependence	dipendence
5. sizophrenia	schisophrenia	scizoprenia	schizophrenia	sizofrenia
6. kongruent	congruent	kongruient	congruient	congrruent
7. tolerance	tolerrence	tollerance	tolerince	tolerence
8. phobbia	pobia	fobbia	phobia	fobia
9. anesia	amisia	anmesia	amesia	amnesia
10. bipollar	bipolar	bypollar	bypolar	beipolar

B. Match the number of the correct spelling of each term in Exercise A with the following brief descriptions. (**LO 18.1,** *Understand, Apply*)

1. Pathological fear or dread
_____

2. Mood disorder with depression and mania
_____

3. Coinciding, or agreeing with
_____

4. Persecutory delusions
_____

5. Presence of two or more diseases at same time
_____

6. Inability to recall past experiences
_____

7. State of needing someone or something
_____

8. Become accustomed to a stimulus or drug
_____

9. Disorder of perception, emotion, and behavior
_____

10. Mood stabilizer
_____

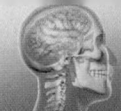
Mental Health

C. Using your knowledge of terms 1–10 in Exercises A and B and their correct spelling, write a brief sentence for each of the terms as it might appear in patient documentation. (LO 18.1, 18.3, 18.4, 18.6, *Apply*)

1. _____

2. _____

3. _____

4. _____

5. _____

6. _____

7. _____

8. _____

9. _____

10. _____

D. To meet lesson objectives and learning outcomes, be prepared to discuss the following questions in class. Be sure you can spell and pronounce each medical term correctly. (**LO 18.1, 18.2,** *Apply*)

1. List the symptoms of the five major types of anxiety disorders.

   _____

   _____

   _____

2. Detail the symptoms of schizophrenia, and explain the use of lithium in treating this condition.

   _____

   _____

   _____

3. What are the classes of psychoactive drugs? (Refer to Table 18.5.)

   _____

   _____

   _____

4. Describe the different types of personality disorders.

   _____

   _____

   _____

E. Meet the goals of each of the chapter outcomes by using the correct language of psychology and psychiatry for the answers. (**LO 18.1-18.7,** *Analyze*)

1. Use the medical language of psychology and psychiatry to communicate and document in writing accurately and precisely in any health care setting. Finish the clinical note by filling in the blank. (**LO 18.1**)

   "This patient has been hyperactive and distractible and has not slept for the past four days. He is now in the _____ phase of his condition."

2. Use the medical language of psychology and psychiatry to communicate verbally with accuracy and precision in any health care setting. Complete the sentence with the appropriate medical terms. (**LO 18.2**)

   The patient's physician has told you to administer amitriptyline to the patient today. You know this is

   a(n) _____ drug.

3. Recognize a uniform system for classifying and describing mental disorders. Fill in the blank. (**LO 18.3**)

   The _____ developed and maintains the DSM-IV-TR for classifying and describing mental disorders.

4. Describe the major types of anxiety disorders. List the five major categories of anxiety disorders. (**LO 18.4**)

   a. _____

   b. _____

   c. _____

   d. _____

   e. _____

5. Discuss *psychoses* and *schizophrenia*. Choose any *one* personality disorder and describe its symptoms and effects. (**LO 18.5**)

   Disorder: _____

   Symptoms: _____

   Effects: _____

6. Explain the effects of common psychoactive drugs. Name the effects of Klonopin. (**LO 18.6**)

   _____

Geriatrics
The Language of Gerontology

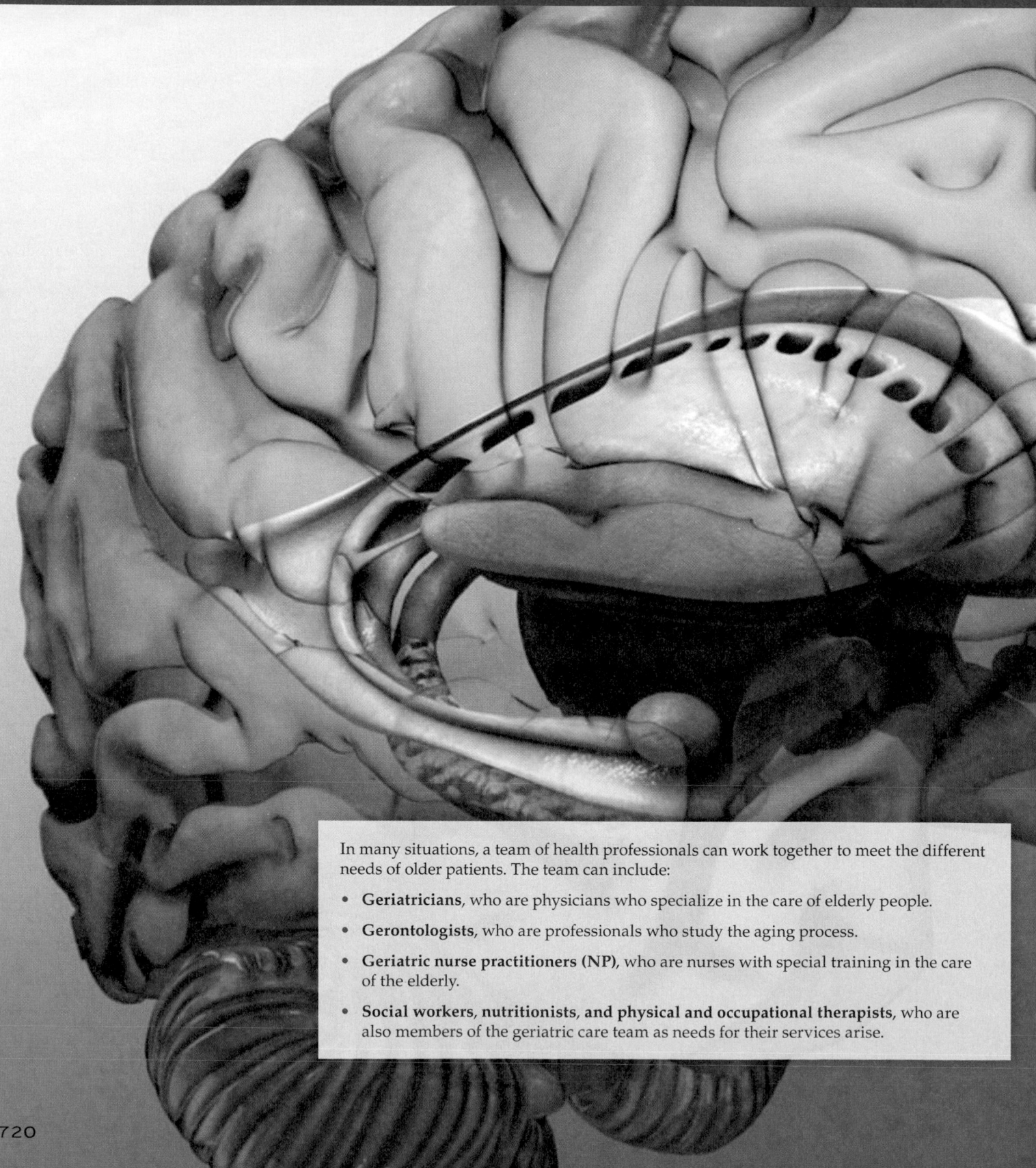

In many situations, a team of health professionals can work together to meet the different needs of older patients. The team can include:

- **Geriatricians**, who are physicians who specialize in the care of elderly people.

- **Gerontologists**, who are professionals who study the aging process.

- **Geriatric nurse practitioners (NP)**, who are nurses with special training in the care of the elderly.

- **Social workers, nutritionists, and physical and occupational therapists**, who are also members of the geriatric care team as needs for their services arise.

Case Report (CR) 19.1

You are

...a medical assistant working in the Geriatric Clinic at Fulwood Medical Center.

Your patient is

...85-year-old Mr. Mathew Hickman, who has an early dementia and a slow-growing prostate cancer for which he has opted to have no treatment.

With the help of his two daughters and day care providers, he is struggling to stay at home. His daughter, Mrs. Anna Hotteling, is with him.

Mr. Hickman:
"I'm still here, you know, somewhere inside this frail old body. I can remember yesteryear, though I'm a bit hazy about today. I can't hear you like I used to. I have difficulty starting to pee. But I can still put my socks on and tie my shoe laces. I'm not frightened of death, but the process of getting there scares the heck out of me. I've lived my life with dignity. I want to live my death the same way, you know . . . and leave with dry pants."

Chapter Learning Outcomes

To understand the changes occurring in the elderly and communicate about this with your employer, other health professionals, and patients and their families, you need to be able to:

LO 19.1 Apply the languages of geriatrics and gerontology to the anatomy, physiology, and psychology of aging in the elderly.

LO 19.2 Use the languages of geriatrics and gerontology to communicate and document in writing accurately and precisely in any health care setting.

LO 19.3 Use the languages of geriatrics and gerontology to communicate verbally with accuracy and precision in any health care setting.

LO 19.4 Compare and contrast geriatrics and gerontology.

LO 19.5 Describe the most up-to-date profile of older Americans.

LO 19.6 Discuss the terms *aging* and *senescence.*

LO 19.7 Describe the effects of senescence on the major organ systems.

LO 19.8 Explain the theories of the process of senescence.

LO 19.9 Discuss the complex effects of aging.

LO 19.10 Describe specific disorders of aging.

LO 19.11 Discuss dying and death.

LO 19.12 Identify answers to some of the important legal issues surrounding dying and death.

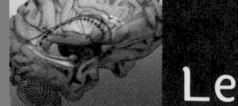

Lesson 19.1 Aging and Senescence

LESSON OBJECTIVES

The information in this lesson will enable you to:

19.1.1 Describe the links between geriatrics and gerontology.

19.1.2 Discuss the profile of the elderly population in America in 2011.

19.1.3 Discuss aging and senescence.

19.1.4 Describe changes that occur with senescence in major organ systems.

19.1.5 Outline major theories of senescence.

19.1.6 Define death and the key issues in preparing for death.

Keynotes

- **Life span** is the age to which individual humans aspire to live and the process of getting there.

- **Life expectancy** is the average length of life for any given population.

- **Longevity** is living beyond the normal life expectancy.

- **Aging** is the gradual, spontaneous change resulting in maturation through childhood, adolescence, and young adulthood. Changes then cause decline in function rather than maturation, through late adulthood and old age.

- **Senescence** is the loss over time of the ability of cells to divide, grow, and function, a process that terminates in death. It is sometimes used interchangeably with the term *aging*.

LO 19.1, 19.2, 19.4, 19.5 Aging

Gerontology is the study of the social, mental, and physical aspects of aging. Professionals from diverse fields call themselves **gerontologists**. The medical field that involves the study, care, and treatment of the elderly *(Figure 19.1)* is called **geriatrics**, and a medical specialist in geriatrics is called a **geriatrician**.

According to the statistics published by the Administration on Aging of the United States Department of Health and Human Services in 2011:

- The older population (65+) numbered 40.4 million in 2010; this is 13.1% (more than 1 in 8) of the total population of the United States.

- Older women (23.0 million) outnumber older men (17.4 million). Forty percent of older women are widows.

- Women reaching age 65 in 2010 had an average life expectancy of an additional 20.0 years; males 17.3 years.

- The older population is expected to increase to 55 million in 2020.

- The 85+ population is projected to increase from 5.5 million in 2010 to 6.6 million in 2020.

- Most older people have at least one chronic medical condition, and many have multiple conditions. The most frequently occurring chronic conditions among the elderly are diagnosed arthritis (50%), hypertension (38%), all types of heart disease (32%), any cancer (22%), and diabetes (18%). **Alzheimer** disease occurs in 13% of older people and accounts for 70% of all **dementias**.

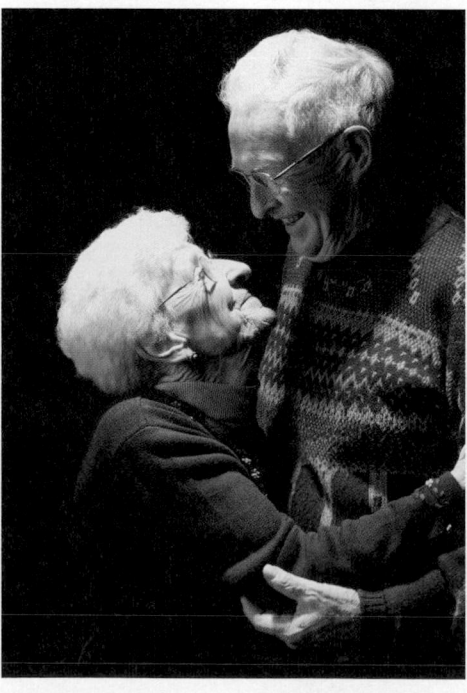

▲ **Figure 19.1** Elderly Couple.

WORD	PRONUNCIATION	ELEMENTS		DEFINITION
aging aged	**A**-jing **A**-jid		Latin *aging*	The process of human maturation and decline Having lived to an advanced age
Alzheimer disease	**AWLZ**-high-mer **DIZ**eez		Alois Alzheimer, German neurologist, 1864–1915	Common form of dementia
dementia	dee-**MEN**-she-ah	S/ P/ R/	**-ia** *condition* **de-** *without* **-ment-** *mind*	Chronic, progressive, irreversible loss of the mind's cognitive and intellectual functions
geriatrics (**Note:** This term contains two roots.) **geriatrician** **gerontology**	jer-ee-**AT**-riks jer-ee-ah-**TRISH**-an jer-on-**TOL**-oh-jee	S/ R/ R/ S/ R/CF S/	**-ics** *knowledge of* **ger-** *old age* **-iatr-** *medical treatment* **-ician** *expert* **geront/o-** *process of aging* **-logy** *study of*	Medical specialty that deals with the problems of old age Medical specialist in geriatrics Study of the process and problems of aging
life expectancy **life span**	LIFE eck-**SPEK**-tan-see LIFE SPAN	S/ R/	**-ancy** *state of* **expect-** *await* Life Old English *life* Span Old English *reach or stretch*	Statistical determination of the number of years an individual is expected to live The age that a person reaches
longevity	lon-**JEV**-ih-tee	S/ R/	**-ity** *condition, state* **longev-** *long life*	Duration of life beyond the normal expectation
senile **senescence** **senility**	**SEE**-nile seh-**NES**-ens seh-**NIL**-ih-tee	S/ R/ S/ R/ S/ R/	**-ile** *capability* **sen-** *old age* **-ence** *state of, quality of* **senesc-** *growing old* **-ity** *condition, state* **senil-** *characteristic of old age*	Characteristic of old age The state of being old Mental disorders occurring in old age

Exercises

A. Choose the correct definition for each of the following medical terms from the *languages of geriatrics and gerontology*. LO 19.1, 19.2

_____ 1. senile

_____ 2. longevity

_____ 3. senility

_____ 4. geriatrics

_____ 5. Alzheimer disease

a. mental disorders occur in old age

b. new field that involves study, care and treatment of the elderly

c. common form of dementia

d. characteristic of old age

e. duration of life beyond the normal expected time

B. Use precise medical language to answer the following questions.   LO 19.2, 19.4, 19.6

1. Differentiate between the following terms:

   a. Life span _____

   b. Life expectancy _____

   c. Geriatrics _____

   d. Gerontology _____

2. What medical term can be used interchangeably with *aging*? _____

3. Use any one term from the above WAD in a sentence of patient documentation. _____

_____

LO 19.1, 19.7 Senescence of Organ Systems

Organ systems begin to show signs of senescence at very different ages and do not degenerate at the same speed. Most physiologic studies show general peak physical performance occurs during a person's twenties, but surprisingly, **autopsies (postmortem)** in children will often reveal atherosclerosis in the arteries supplying the heart. Autopsies are usually performed by a **pathologist** or a medical examiner.

Integumentary system (see Chapter 15) changes begin in a person's forties. Melanocytes die, and hair becomes gray and thinner. The skin becomes paper thin, loses elasticity, and hangs loose, and wrinkles appear (Figure 19.2). Flat brown-black spots called **senile lentigines** (age spots) appear on the back of the hands and areas exposed to sunlight.

Special senses start to decline in the twenties. Visual acuity declines at that time. In the forties, presbyopia (see Chapter 16) begins, and many people develop cataracts later, in old age. Hearing loss occurs as the ossicles become stiffer and the number of cochlear hair cells (see Chapter 16) declines—the cause of Mr. Hickman's hearing loss in the Case Report. Taste and smell are also blunted late in life, as taste cells and olfactory buds decline in number.

Skeletal system (see Chapter 14) changes appear during a person's thirties, as osteoblasts become less active than osteoclasts. The result is osteopenia, which later develops into osteoporosis—particularly in postmenopausal women. The joints of people in their later years have less synovial fluid and thinner articular cartilage, and often, osteoarthritis results.

Muscular system (see Chapter 14) changes occur with age as muscle mass is lost **(sarcopenia)** and replaced with fat. As muscle **atrophies**, there are fewer muscle fibers to do the work; as a result, the available blood supply decreases. Tasks that used to be easy become difficult, such as buttoning shirts and tying shoelaces—one of the daily triumphs Mr. Hickman mentioned in the Case Report.

Nervous system (see Chapter 9) changes begin around age 30, when the brain weighs twice as much as it does at age 75. Motor coordination, intellectual function, and short-term memory decline more quickly than long-term memory and language skills.

Cardiovascular systems (see Chapter 10) always have coronary artery atherosclerosis, even at a very early age. As a result, when aging myocardial cells die, the heart wall gets thinner and weaker, and cardiac output declines. This causes the decline in physical capabilities with aging. Atherosclerotic plaques narrow arteries and trigger thrombosis, leading to strokes and heart attacks. In veins, valves become weaker, and blood flows back and pools in the legs, leading to poor venous return to the heart and heart failure.

Respiratory system (see Chapter 13) changes are noticeable in the thirties, as pulmonary ventilation declines. This decline is a factor in the gradual loss of stamina that occurs as people age. The rib cage becomes less flexible, and the lungs become less elastic and have fewer alveoli. Respiratory function declines. As respiratory health declines, hypoxic degenerative changes occur in all the other organ systems.

Urinary system (see Chapter 6) changes begin in a person's twenties, when the number of nephrons starts to decline. Later in life, many of the remaining glomeruli become atherosclerotic. The body's glomerular filtration rate (GFR) decreases, and the kidneys become less efficient. For example, drug doses in the elderly are generally lower than those for younger people because drugs cannot be cleared from the elderly's blood as rapidly.

Immune system (see Chapter 12) function declines in the elderly, as the amounts of lymphatic tissue and red bone marrow in their bodies decrease with age. This leads to a reduction in both cellular and humoral (antibody) immunity. As a result, the elderly have lower levels of protection against infectious diseases and cancer.

Specific **disorders of senescence** and their terminology are described in each of the body system chapters in this book.

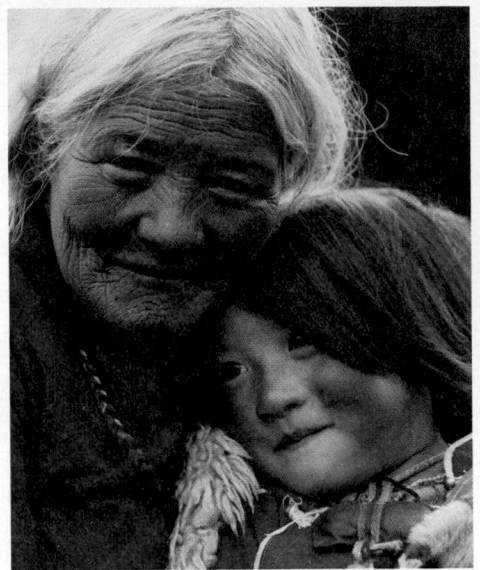

▲ **Figure 19.2** **Senescence of the Skin.** Elderly Tibetan woman with her granddaughter.

Keynotes

- Visual acuity starts to decline very early in life. Eye exercises can help prevent this normal occurrence.
- Exercise and good nutrition help prevent osteopenia.
- Exercise and good nutrition help prevent muscle degeneration.
- Exercising your brain enhances your quality of life in old age.
- Exercise and good nutrition extend **longevity** and enhance the quality of life.
- Bronchitis and emphysema, the **chronic obstructive pulmonary diseases (COPDs)**, are the cumulative effects of cigarette smoking and are a leading cause of death in old age.
- The kidneys of an 80-year-old receive only half as much blood as those of a 30-year-old because of atherosclerosis.
- Because they have lowered immunity, the elderly are advised to receive vaccinations against influenza and other infections.

Word Analysis and Definition

S = Suffix   P = Prefix   R = Root   R/CF = Combining Form

WORD	PRONUNCIATION	ELEMENTS		DEFINITION
atrophy **atrophies (verb)**	**AT**-roh-fee **AT**-roh-feez	P/ R/	a- *without* **-trophy** *development, nourishment*	Wasting or diminished volume of a tissue or organ
autopsy **postmortem (syn)**	**AWE**-top-see post-**MOR**-tem	 S/ P/ R/	Greek *see with one's own eyes* **-em** *condition* **post-** *after* **-mort-** *death*	Examination of the body and organs of a dead person to determine the cause of death
lentigo **lentigines (pl)**	len-**TIE**-go len-**TIHJ**-ih-neez		Greek *lentil*	Age spot; small, flat, brown-black spot in the skin of older people
pathologist	pa-**THOL**-oh-jist	S/ R/CF	**-logist** *one who studies, specialist* **path/o-** *disease*	A specialist in pathology (study of disease or characteristics of a particular disease)
sarcopenia	sar-koh-**PEE**-nee-ah	S/ R/CF	**-penia** *deficiency* **sarc/o-** *muscle*	Progressive loss of muscle mass and strength in aging

Exercises

A. Organ systems show various signs of senescence. *Provide one example of a sign of senescence in each organ system listed in the following table. Be sure to use correct medical terminology, and be able to explain every term you use. Fill in the blanks.*   **LO 19.7**

Organ System	Sign of Senescence
integumentary	1.
special senses (ear/eye)	2.
skeletal	3.
muscular	4.
nervous	5.
cardiovascular	6.
respiratory	7.
urinary	8.
immune	9.

Have you checked your spelling?

B. Circle the correct answer for the following questions.   **LO 19.7, 19.11**

1. What does the medical term *lentigo* identify?

   a. skin lesion

   b. skin tumor

   c. skin type

   d. skin spots

   e. skin wrinkles

2. What is the correct plural of *lentigo*?

   a. lentigos

   b. lentigoes

   c. lentigones

   d. lentigines

   e. lentigons

3. Another medical term used for *autopsy* is

   a. senescence

   b. senility

   c. geriatrics

   d. atrophy

   e. postmortem

4. What is the correct element that means *death*?

   a. post

   b. em

   c. mort

   d. auto

   e. patho

5. What is the purpose of a postmortem?

   a. to discover the patient's blood type

   b. to discover the cause of death

   c. to discover the weight of the body organs

   d. to discover the body's final blood volume

   e. to discover the presence of foreign bodies

LO 19.8 Theories of Senescence

The causes of senescence are unknown. **Heredity** plays a role because longevity or early death tends to run in families. Theories of senescence include

- **Protein abnormalities**. One-quarter of the body's protein is collagen. With age, collagen and other proteins show abnormal structures in their cells and tissues and become less soluble and more rigid. The cells accumulate more of these dysfunctional proteins as they age, and their functions are impaired, leading to **senescent** changes.

- **Free radicals**. These are chemical particles with an extra electron. For example, the stable oxygen molecule (O_2) has two atoms with many electrons. If it picks up an extra electron through some metabolic reaction, by radiation, or by chemical action, it becomes a free radical. The free radical's life is short because it combines quickly with other molecules that, in turn, become free radicals with the addition of the extra electron. A chain reaction occurs as more and more molecules become free radicals. Among the damage they cause are cancer, myocardial infarction, and perhaps senescence. They can be neutralized by **antioxidants**.

- **Autoimmune**-altered molecules *(see Chapter 12)*. These molecules may be recognized as foreign antigens, and an immune response may be generated against the body's own tissues. This theory is helped by the fact that autoimmune diseases such as rheumatoid arthritis are more common in old age.

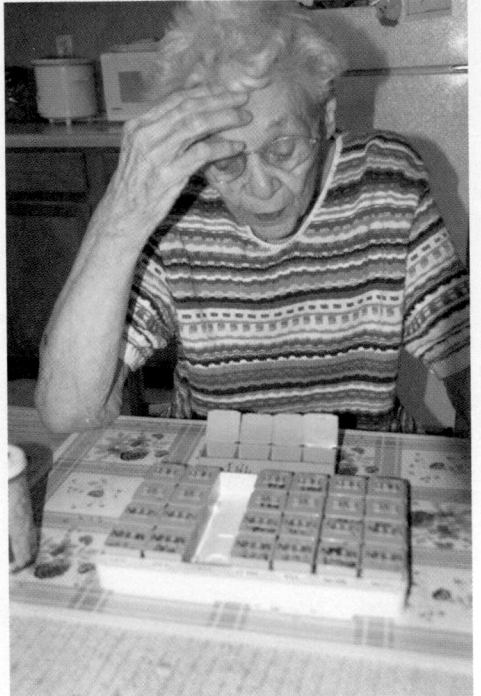

▲ **Figure 19.3** Elderly Woman Confused about Her Medications.

LO 19.9 Complex Effects of Aging

The appearance of symptoms of aging depends on the remaining healthy reserves of organs as they decline with age. For example, renal **impairment** can be part of aging, but renal **failure** is not. This decline in physiological reserve can produce complications from mild problems. For example, dehydration in mild gastroenteritis can cause confusion in the elderly, which, in turn, can lead to a fall and to a fractured femur.

Many diseases in elderly persons may present with very vague and nonspecific symptoms. For example, pneumonia can present with low-grade fever, confusion, or falls rather than with the high fever and cough seen in younger adults. **Delirium** in the elderly can be caused by something as simple as constipation. Some elderly people may have difficulty describing their symptoms, particularly if they have cognitive impairment. Therefore, time and care have to be taken to discover the root cause.

Many elderly patients take multiple **medications**, sometimes prescribed by different specialists without reference to other medications prescribed by other specialists. This **polypharmacy** can result in **adverse** drug interactions *(Figure 19.3)*. In addition, most drugs are excreted by the liver or kidneys, either of which can be impaired in the elderly. As a result, the dosage of medications may need to be adjusted to avoid excessive levels in the blood and undesirable side effects.

Aging has some benefits and advantages for many people. These include

- Increased knowledge of life (wisdom).
- Freedom from many of the day-to-day responsibilities that working adults face.
- Freedom to be gentle and grow with oneself.
- Time to enjoy family.
- Freedom to choose to participate in childrearing for grandchildren or other relatives.
- Increased participation in volunteer organizations.

Keynotes

- People older than 65 make up 13% of the population and use about 30% of all prescriptions written.

- A study of 27,600 Medicare patients documented more than 1,500 adverse drug effects (ADEs) in a single year.

- When a physician or nurse practitioner or a pharmacist oversees an elderly patient's medication regimen, drug-related problems are less likely to occur.

- The elderly patient should bring all of his/her medications to every hospital or office visit, including prescription, over-the-counter (OTC) drugs, and all supplements.

Abbreviations

ADE	adverse drug effect
OTC	over the counter

WORD	PRONUNCIATION	ELEMENTS		DEFINITION
antioxidant	an-tee-**OKS**-ih-dant	S/ P/ R/	-ant *forming* anti- *against* -oxid- *oxidize*	Substance that can prevent cell damage by neutralizing free radicals
delirium	de-**LIR**-ee-um	S/ R/	-um *structure* deliri- *confusion, disorientation*	Acute altered state of consciousness with agitation and disorientation
free radical	FREE **RAD**-ih-kal	R/ S/ R/	free *free* -al *pertaining to* radic- *root*	Short-lived product of oxidation in a cell that can damage the cell
heredity	heh-**RED**-ih-tee	S/ R/	-ity *condition, state* hered- *inherited through genes*	Transmission of characteristics from parents to offspring through genes
polypharmacy	poll-ee-**FAR**-mah-see	P/ R/	poly- *many* -pharmacy *drug*	The administration of many drugs at the same time
senescence senescent (adj)	seh-**NES**-ens	S/ R/	-ence *state of, quality of* senesc- *growing old*	The state of being old

Exercises

A. Apply the *languages of geriatrics and gerontology* to your discussions of the following questions. *Write your thoughts about the questions on the lines provided.*   **LO 19.1, 19.3, 19.9**

1. Why might Medicare patients frequently have adverse drug effects to medication?

_____

_____

_____

2. Why is it a good idea for elderly patients to bring all of their prescription medications, OTC medications, and supplements to their doctor or hospital visits?

_____

_____

_____

3. The elderly use about 30% of all prescriptions written in the United States. Why is this true?

_____

_____

_____

4. Why is it a good idea to have a doctor, nurse practitioner, or pharmacist oversee what prescriptions an elderly person is taking?

_____

_____

_____

Keynotes

The GERIATRIC GIANTS of impairment are:

- immobility
- instability
- incontinence
- impaired intellect/memory

LO 19.10 Specific Disorders of Aging

The major categories of impairment in elderly people as they begin to fail (the so-called GERIATRIC GIANTS) include

- immobility
- instability
- incontinence
- impaired intellect/memory

Immobility is a common pathway produced by many diseases and problems, particularly those that involve prolonged bed rest, immobilization, or inactivity. It can also occur when it is self-imposed, when elderly patients do not exercise to keep limbs flexible, promote circulation, and improve well-being. Many factors influencing the elderly's state of immobility are **iatrogenic**, or arising from medical regimens, institutional policies, and resident and staff characteristics in nursing homes. The negative consequences of immobility can often be avoided with careful and vigilant medical and nursing management.

Instability, or difficulty in balance *(Figure 19.4)*, is often the first problem that the elderly person encounters. The instability and associated falls can result from a single disease process or the accumulated effects of multiple diseases. It is essential to take a careful, detailed history and examination to define all the factors contributing to the instability and to develop the appropriate interventions to prevent future falls. Instability and falling are not inevitable in aging but are problems that arise from identifiable disabilities that are often treatable.

Incontinence is the inability to prevent the discharge of urine or feces. It is a common, but never normal, part of aging. In the nursing home population, some 50% of residents have urinary incontinence. There are five main types of urinary incontinence:

- **Urge incontinence**, the loss of urine before one can get to the toilet, is the most common form in the elderly. It can be caused by strokes, multiple sclerosis, dementia, and pelvic floor atrophy in women or prostate enlargement in men.
- **Stress incontinence** is caused by weak bladder muscles. It occurs when the abdominal pressure when you cough, sneeze, laugh, or climb stairs overcomes the closing pressure of the bladder.
- **Overflow incontinence** is rare. It occurs when the bladder never completely empties and leaks small amounts of urine.
- **Functional incontinence** is an inability to reach the toilet in time, for example, due to arthritis, stroke, or dementia.
- **Mixed incontinence** is usually a combination of stress and urge incontinence.

Keynotes

- **Dementia** is defined as the progressive loss, over at least six months, of cognitive and intellectual functions without impairment of consciousness or perception.
- Dementia is characterized by disorientation, impaired memory, impaired judgement, and impaired intellect.

Fecal incontinence occurs in about one-third of the elderly in institutional care, and is the second most common reason for committing the elderly to a nursing home. It can be produced by local causes such as chronic laxative abuse or muscle damage to the sphincter muscles in surgery or childbirth. It is also seen in dementia, multiple sclerosis, and diabetes.

Impaired intellect/memory that is present for at least six months is called **dementia**. The **cognitive** functions that are affected include decision making, judgment, memory, thinking, reasoning, and verbal communication. Dementia is not a normal part of aging, but advancing age is the greatest risk factor. More than 5 million people aged 65 and older have dementia and more than 500,000 people under 65 have early-onset dementia.

Alzheimer disease accounts for 70% of all dementias; it is progressive and there is no cure. Other types of dementia are vascular dementia, frontotemporal dementia, and dementia with **Lewy bodies**.

Delirium is a set of symptoms including an inability to focus attention; mental confusion; impairments in awareness, time, and space; and perhaps **hallucinations**. It often has a fluctuating course, and it can follow head trauma, stroke, drug withdrawal, hypoxia, hypoglycemia, physical illness of almost every type, and the use of opiates and benzodiazepines. Delirium is probably the single most common disorder affecting adults in hospitals and occurs in 30–40% of elderly hospitalized patients and in up to 80% of intensive care unit (ICU) patients. Treatment is to the underlying disease causing the delirium.

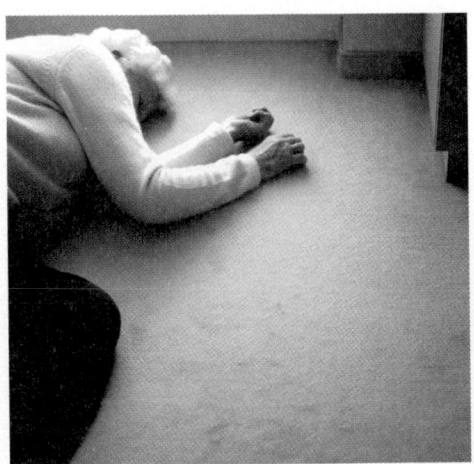

▲ **Figure 19.4** **Elderly Woman Injured in a Fall.**

WORD	PRONUNCIATION	ELEMENTS		DEFINITION
cognition	kog-**NIH**-shun		Latin *knowledge*	Process of acquiring knowledge through thinking and learning
cognitive (adj)	**KOG**-nih-tiv			Pertaining to the mental activities of thinking and learning
dementia	dee-**MEN**-she-ah	S/ P/ R/	-ia *condition* de- *without* -ment- *mind*	Chronic, progressive, and irreversible loss of the mind's cognitive and intellectual functions
hallucination	hah-loo-sih-**NAY**-shun	S/ R/	-ation *process* **hallucin-** *imagination*	Perception of an object or event when there is no such thing present
iatrogenic	ih-at-roe-**JEN**-ik	S/ R/ R/	-ic *pertaining to* **iatro-** *physician* -gen- *producing*	An unfavorable response to medical or surgical treatment, caused by the treatment itself
Lewy body	**LOO**-ih BODY		Frederic Lewy (1895–1950), German-born neurologist who became a U.S. citizen	Abnormal cells seen in a form of dementia

Exercises

A. Use the correct medical terms to answer the following questions.   LO 19.1, 19.2, 19.10

1. What are the major categories of impairment in elderly people, especially as they begin to fail?

   a. _____

   b. _____

   c. _____

   d. _____

2. Write yourself a study hint to help you remember the different categories. Share your hint with the class.

   Study hint:

   _____

   _____

   _____

   _____

3. Define the difference between

   a. immobility _____

   b. instability _____

B. Use the new medical terminology you have learned in this chapter to circle the correct answer for each question.   LO 19.10

1. What is incontinence? (Read carefully and choose the BEST answer.)

   a. inability to prevent the discharge of urine

   b. inability to prevent the discharge of feces

   c. inability to prevent the discharge of flatus

   d. inability to prevent the discharge of urine or feces

   e. inability to prevent diarrhea

2. Coughing can cause a specific type of urinary incontinence. What is the medical term for this condition?

   a. stress incontinence

   b. urge incontinence

   c. overflow incontinence

   d. functional incontinence

   e. mixed incontinence

You are
. . . a social worker in the Breast Care Clinic at Fulwood Medical Center.

Your patient is
. . . Mrs. Faye Hampson, a 42-year-old woman who has breast cancer which has metastasized to the bones in her arms and spine, generating pain for which she takes morphine orally five or six times each day. She also has metastases in her brain. She has two daughters, aged 10 and 6.

Keynotes

- Free radicals can damage cells and can be neutralized by antioxidants.
- It is highly likely that senescence has more than one etiology.
- Both PVS and MCS differ from coma, in which the individual is unresponsive and keeps his eyes closed.

Abbreviations

BD	brain death
DNR	do not resuscitate
HIPAA	Health Insurance Portability and Accountability Act
MCS	minimally conscious state
POLST	Physician's Orders for Life-Sustaining Treatment
PVS	persistent vegetative state

Case Report 19.2

Mrs. Hampson has mutation of the genes BRAC 1 and BRAC 2. She has requested that the two girls not be genetically tested until they are old enough to request the tests themselves. Mrs. Hampson is having difficulty sitting, standing, walking, and sleeping because of bone pain. She remarks, "I want to be as comfortable as possible, even if it shortens my life."

After conducting the interview with Mrs. Hampson, you decide to recommend to her and to the team caring for her that she be admitted to hospice care.

LO 19.11 Dying and Death

Death is inevitable. Just as fetal life in the womb is a preparation for birth, living and aging are a preparation for death. You can prepare for death in different ways, most of which are done with your family's involvement and many of which require legal assistance.

Medical issues are clearly significant in the process of dying. Your views on the types and extent of medical treatment you wish to have during the process of dying should be clearly stated. This is done through an **advance medical directive**, which consists of two documents:

1. **Medical (durable) power of attorney**, in which you appoint someone you know and trust as your agent and authorize that person to make medical decisions for you when you cannot.

2. **Living will**, in which you provide a set of instructions detailing what treatment you do and do not want in a terminal illness, including **hospice** treatment. If there are special instructions, such as **do not resuscitate (DNR)**, these must be stated clearly. It should also include a Health Insurance Portability and Accountability Act **(HIPAA) authorization** that enables your agent to receive the medical information about you that is necessary for making decisions about treatment. This is needed because HIPAA imposes tough privacy-of-medical-information rules on doctors and hospitals.

Your primary care doctor should have a copy of your advance medical directive and have read the document with you. This document should be part of your medical record. In some states, a document known as **Physician's Orders for Life-Sustaining Treatment (POLST)** is now available. This formal document is effectively a physician's order statement that is based on the patient's current medical condition and wishes. It has specific sections that list the patient's wishes for cardiopulmonary resuscitation (CPR), medical interventions, and artificially administered nutrition. It becomes a valid, durable component of the patient's medical record that health professionals must obey.

The process of dying, rather than death itself, is of concern to most elderly people. Dying should be dignified and free from physical and emotional pain. A **hospice** provides **palliative care** and provides for the emotional and spiritual needs of terminally ill patients and their loved ones at an inpatient facility or in the patient's home. Palliative care is designed to provide pain and symptom management to maintain the highest quality of life for as long as life remains.

Just as the moment life begins is controversial, there is no universally accepted moment of biological death.

In most states in the United States, death is now defined in terms of **brain death (BD)**, when there is no cerebral or brainstem activity and the electroencephalogram (EEG) is flat for a specific length of time *(Figure 19.5)*. Two other conditions involving brain damage and loss of brain function cause medical difficulty and should be addressed in your living will:

1. **Persistent vegetative state (PVS)** occurs in people who suffer enough brain damage that they are unaware of themselves or their surroundings, even though their eyes are open. Yet they still have certain reflexes and can breathe and pump blood because the brainstem still functions. Even reflex events like crying and smiling and the sleep–wake cycle can be seen. With medical care and artificial feeding, patients can survive for decades.

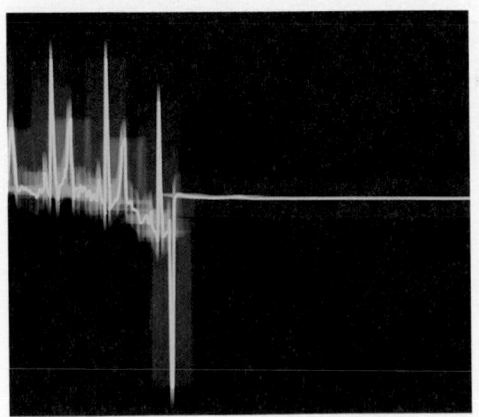

Figure 19.5 **Flat Line** ▶ **on Electroencephalogram Shows Brain Death.**

2. **Minimally conscious state (MCS)** is a condition of severely altered consciousness in which minimal evidence of awareness of self or surroundings is demonstrated. There is inconsistent communication or command following. However, positron emission tomography (PET) scans of MCS patients show cortical function when their loved ones speak to them. They are more likely to improve than are PVS patients.

WORD	PRONUNCIATION		ELEMENTS	DEFINITION
advance medical directive	ad-**VANTS MED**-ih-kal die-**REK**-tiv			Legal document signed by the patient dealing with issues of prolonging or ending life in the event of life-threatening illness
antioxidant	an-tee-**OKS**-ih-dant	S/ P/ R/	**-ant** *forming* **anti-** *against* **-oxid-** *oxidize*	Substance that can prevent cell damage by neutralizing free radicals
death	DETH		Old English *to die*	Total and permanent cessation of all vital functions
free radical	FREE **RAD**-ih-kal	R/ S/ R/	**free** *free* **-al** *pertaining to* **radic-** *root*	Short-lived product of oxidation in a cell that can be damaging to the cell
heredity	heh-**RED**-ih-tee	S/ R/	**-ity** *state, condition* **hered-** *inherited through genes*	Transmission of characteristics from parents to offspring through genes
hospice	**HOS**-pis		Latin *lodging*	Facility or program that provides care to the dying and their families
palliative care	**PAL**-ee-ah-tiv KAIR	S/ R/ R/	**-ive** *nature of, pertaining to* **palliat-** *reduce suffering* **care** *be responsible for*	Care that relieves symptoms and pain without curing
vegetative	**VEJ**-eh-tay-tiv	S/ R/	**-ive** *nature of, pertaining to* **vegetat-** *growth*	Functioning unconsciously as plant life is assumed to do

Exercises

A. Explain the difference among the following terms to a patient's relatives. *If you understand it yourself, you can explain it to someone else. Write a brief explanation for each term.* **LO 19.2, 19.3, 19.11, 19.12**

1. Persistent vegetative state:

_____

_____

2. Minimally conscious state:

_____

_____

3. Coma:

_____

_____

B. Read the following sentence from the text and be prepared to explain the medical terms to the patient's family. *Fill in the blanks in questions 1 and 2.* **LO 19.3, 19.11**

1. A hospice provides palliative care and provides for the emotional and spiritual needs of terminally ill patients and their loved ones.

_____

_____

_____

2. Hospice care can take place in an inpatient facility or in a(n) _____

_____

_____.

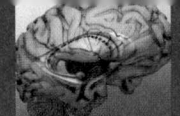
Geriatrics

Challenge Your Knowledge

A. Recall terms from previous chapters. Fill in the blank. (**LO 19.2,** *Remember*)

1. A cardiovascular surgeon will perform a _____ to open the chest for exploration or biopsy.

2. What is the important phrase (clue) in the question that will tell you the correct term to use?

_____

B. Identify the errors among the following statements the languages of geriatrics and gerontology. Circle the correct answers and then rewrite the corrections to the incorrect statements on the lines that follow. (**LO 19.2,** *Remember*)

1. *Trophy* is an element meaning *nourishment* or *development*.	T	F
2. *Post* is an element meaning *during*.	T	F
3. *Path/o* means *diagnosis*.	T	F
4. *Penia* means *deficiency*.	T	F
5. The prefix *a* means *without*.	T	F

Rewrite the incorrect statements so they are correct:

_____

_____

_____

_____

C. Abbreviations. Regardless of whether you are an administrative or clinical health care worker, you will be reading patient documentation with abbreviations, which can mean a diagnosis, procedure, disease, and so on. To interpret this documentation correctly and safely, you must know the meanings of the abbreviations. Challenge yourself to *define* each of the following abbreviations correctly. Fill in the chart, and then practice your documentation. (**LO 19.1, 19.11,** *Remember, Understand*)

Abbreviation	Meaning of Abbreviation
BD	1.
MCS	2.
PVS	3.

Choose any abbreviation from the previous table, and write one sentence of patient documentation using that abbreviation.

4. Abbreviation: _____

5. Patient documentation:

_____

_____

D. Prefixes and suffixes are good clues to the meaning of a medical term. Analyze each medical term for the meaning of its prefix and suffix. Then give the complete meaning of the medical term in the last column. Every term may not have both a prefix and a suffix. Fill in the blanks. (**LO 19.1, 19.2**, *Remember, Understand*)

Medical Term	Meaning of Prefix	Meaning of Suffix	Meaning of Medical Term
atrophy	1.	2.	3.
geriatrics	4.	5.	6.
pathologist	7.	8.	9.
antioxidant	10.	11.	12.
senile	13.	14.	15.
postmortem	16.	17.	18.
sarcopenia	19.	20.	21.
longevity	22.	23.	24.
dementia	25.	26.	27.
gerontology	28.	29.	30.

E. Elements. Even though these elements do not appear here in the context of a medical term, you should be able to recognize their meaning out of context. Match the correct element in the left column with its meaning in the right column. Fill in the blanks. (**LO 19.1, 19.2, 19.3**, *Remember, Understand*)

_____ 1. ician   a. after

_____ 2. ity   b. old age

_____ 3. trophy   c. death

_____ 4. sarco   d. against

_____ 5. ile   e. without

_____ 6. post   f. confusion

_____ 7. anti   g. expert

_____ 8. a or an   h. capability

_____ 9. deliri   i. condition, state

_____ 10. mort   j. many

_____ 11. poly   k. muscle

_____ 12. geronto   l. development

F. Latin and Greek terms cannot be further deconstructed into prefix, root, or suffix. You must know them for what they are. Test your knowledge of these terms with this exercise. Match the meaning in the left column with the correct medical term in the right column. Choose any one term and use it in a sentence that is not a definition. (**LO 19.1, 19.2**, *Remember, Understand*)

_____ 1. knowledge   a. hospice

_____ 2. to grow old   b. cognition

_____ 3. age spots   c. senescence

_____ 4. lodging   d. lentil

5. Sentence:

_____

_____

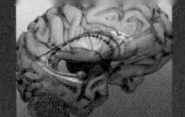
Geriatrics

G. **Medical language.** Employ the *languages of geriatrics and gerontology* to answer the following multiple-choice questions. Circle the correct answer. (**LO 19.1, 19.2, *Remember, Understand, Apply***)

1. Impaired intellect or memory that is present for at least six months is called

    a. dementia

    b. delirium

    c. hallucinations

    d. senescence

    e. cognition

2. In most U.S. states, *death* is described in terms of

    a. lack of breathing

    b. lack of blood flow to the body

    c. brain death

    d. lack of muscle response

    e. lack of speech and hearing

3. It is highly likely that senescence has more than one

    a. result

    b. free radical

    c. cause

    d. antioxidant

    e. autoimmune reaction

4. This condition is not a normal part of aging.

    a. renal failure

    b. renal impairment

    c. cataracts

    d. arthritis

    e. osteoporosis

5. A document that appoints someone you trust to make medical decisions for you is called a

    a. living will

    b. medical power of attorney

    c. DNR order

    d. consent form

    e. HIPAA authorization

6. The term meaning an unfavorable response to medical or surgical treatment, caused by the treatment itself, is

    a. polypharmacy

    b. iatrogenic

    c. senescence

    d. heredity

    e. dementia

7. Which of the following is a false statement about OTC drugs?

    a. They are available at most pharmacies.

    b. They are generally less expensive than a prescription drug.

    c. They need a prescription.

    d. They are some drugs available generically.

    e. They can save you money on medicine.

8. Free radicals can be neutralized by

    a. T lymphocytes (T cells)

    b. organ systems

    c. antioxidants

    d. enzymes

    e. hormones

9. What medical term describes an acute, altered state of consciousness with agitation and disorientation?

    a. delirium   d. persistent vegetative state

    b. dementia   e. migraine

    c. hallucination

10. Which of the following is NOT one of the so-called geriatric giants?

    a. immobility

    b. impaired intellect/memory

    c. instability

    d. incontinence

    e. loss of hearing

11. Which type of incontinence is caused by weak bladder muscles?

   a. overflow incontinence

   b. urge incontinence

   c. stress incontinence

   d. mixed incontinence

   e. functional incontinence

12. What disease accounts for 70% of all dementias?

   a. delirium

   b. Alzheimer disease

   c. fecal incontinence

   d. dementia

   e. impaired memory

13. Exercise and good nutrition are helpful in preventing

   a. wrinkles

   b. hair loss

   c. freckles

   d. osteopenia

   e. COPD

14. Which of the following statements is NOT true about hospice and the palliative care it provides?

   a. Hospice care can be provided in a hospital or in your home.

   b. Palliative care cannot cure anything.

   c. The main purpose of hospice is to alleviate pain and make you comfortable until you die.

   d. Hospice care does not charge the patient any fees.

   e. Hospice provides emotional support to the patient's family as well.

15. Which of the following statements applies to brain death?

   a. You have no cerebral or brainstem activity, and your EEG is flat for a specific length of time.

   b. You lose your sense of smell.

   c. You cannot hear anything around you.

   d. You cannot speak.

   e. You cannot walk.

H. **Terminology challenge.** Find the synonym for the medical term **autopsy**. Deconstruct each term, and provide a definition. Fill in the blanks. (**LO 19.1, 19.2,** *Remember, Understand, Apply*)

   1. A synonym for autopsy is _____.

   2. Deconstruct the synonym of autopsy into elements with meanings.

     (synonym): _____ / _____ / _____

     Elements mean P_____ /R_____ /S_____

   3. What is the definition of *autopsy*? _____

   _____

   4. What type of specialist is likely to perform an autopsy? _____

   5. What can be learned from an autopsy? _____

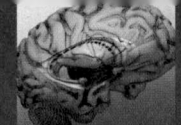
Geriatrics

I. How well do you understand what you read? Briefly explain, in your own words, each of the following statements. If there is an abbreviation, rewrite it in complete medical terms on the lines provided. (**LO 19.2, 19.9, 19.10,** *Understand*)

1. "Hospice care is palliative care."

   _____

2. "PET scans of MCS patients show corticol functions when their loved ones speak to them."

   _____

3. "The most frequently occurring chronic conditions among the elderly are: arthritis, hypertension, all types of cardiac disease, any cancer, and diabetes."

   _____

4. "Bronchitis and emphysema (the COPDs) are the cumulative effects of cigarette smoking and are a leading cause of death in old age."

   _____

J. Use one of the following words to fill in the appropriate spaces with the *language of gerontology*. Use each term only once; some terms will not be used. (**LO 19.1, 19.2,** *Understand, Apply*)

sarcopenia	pathologist	postmortem	atrophy
polypharmacy	adverse	incontinent	cognitive
dementia	iatrogenic	gastroenterologist	

1. Because she is _____, the patient needs to wear diapers.

2. The _____ will perform the autopsy tomorrow morning.

3. The patient is suffering _____ in his weakest muscles and needs physical therapy.

4. A(n) _____ drug reaction is not beneficial to the patient.

5. The (procedure) _____ will determine the cause of death.

K. Languages of geriatrics and gerontology. The following medical terms are all applicable to the *languages of geriatrics and gerontology.* Build your knowledge of their meanings by correctly using each term in a sentence of your choice that is *not a definition that appears in the text. Example:* "The life expectancy at any given age will be considerably shortened if that person smokes cigarettes." (**LO 19.1, 19.2, 19.11,** *Apply*)

| life span | life expectancy | longevity | aging | senescence |

1. _____

2. _____

3. _____

4. _____

5. Distinguish *aging* from *senescence.* Be prepared to discuss your answer in class. Write your discussion notes here:

  a. aging _____

  _____

  b. senescence _____

  _____

L. What am I? All the following statements pertain to a term that is specific to the languages of geriatrics and gerontology. Select the correct term. (**LO 19.1, 19.2,** *Apply*)

  a. I am smooth.

  b. I am brown-black.

  c. I am painless.

  d. I appear in old age.

  e. I am in a body system.

  1. Answer: I am _____.

M. The following information is for ICD codes relating to the term *senile*. Review it carefully. (**LO 19.2,** *Apply, Analyze*)

  1. *Senile* means *characteristic of old age.*

  2. *Senile* has its own listing in the Index of ICD-9 CM.

  3. Descriptive words associated with senile codes are *atrophied* (wasting away of a body part), *atrophic, degenerative,* and *failure.*

  4. *Senile cataract* is a subcategory under Cataract (366.1X).

  5. *Incipient cataract* is defined as *minor disorders of lens, not affecting vision, and due to aging.*

  6. *Senile asthenia* (797) means *lack or loss of strength* (presumably due to aging).

  7. Mental disorder codes (290–319) include *senile dementia* (290.0).

  8. The term *presenile dementia* (290.1) refers to conditions occurring *before* the patient can be deemed *senile.*

  9. The difference in one term (*senile* and *presenile*) can change the code choice.

  10. Pay attention to prefixes and adjectives in the descriptors of the code. Doing so will help you make a choice of the highest specificity of the code.

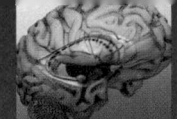

Geriatrics

N. Define the terms *agitation* and *disorientation*, and then describe the difference between the terms. (**LO 19.1, 19.10,** *Analyze*)

1. agitation

_____

_____

2. disorientation

_____

_____

3. The difference between the two is

_____

_____

O. **Why is it important to have all your legal papers in order if you become terminally ill?** Discuss what papers are necessary to have on file for the patient at the hospital. (**LO 19. 12,** *Analyze*)

_____

_____

_____

_____

_____

_____

_____

CHAPTER SUMMARY EXERCISE

A. Spelling comprehension. Circle the correct spelling of the term. (**LO 19.3,** *Remember*)

1. longivety   longevity   longevvity   lonivety   lomgevity

2. autupsy   autopsy   autopsie   atopsy   attopsy

3. jerontelogist   geronntologist   jerontologist   gerontologist   jirontologist

4. seenesence   cenescence   sinescence   ceniscence   senescence

5. integumentry   integumentery   integumentary   integomentery   integomenary

6. atrophy   atruphy   atrofi   atophy   attrophy

7 sarkopenia   sarckopenia   sarcopenia   sarcophenia   sarccopenia

8. letigenes   lettigines   letingines   letigines   lentigines

9. antioxxidents   anteoxxidints   antioxidants   antioxidints   antioxidents

10. delirium   deleriuum   dilerium   dellerium   deleriem

B. Match the number of the correct spelling of the terms in Exercise A with the following brief descriptions of the terms in this exercise. (LO 19.2, 19.3, *Apply*)

1. Examination of the deceased body organs to determine the cause of death _____

2. Duration of life beyond the normal expected _____

3. Characteristic associated with advanced age _____

4. Loss of muscle mass _____

5. Brown skin spots _____

6. Neutralize free radicals _____

7. Medical specialist for aged patient population _____

8. State of being old _____

9. The skin system covering the body _____

10. Wasting or diminished volume of a tissue or organ _____

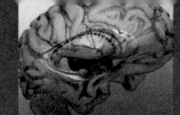

Geriatrics

C. **Using your knowledge of terms 1–10 in Exercise A and their correct spelling and definition in Exercise B, write a brief sentence for each of the terms as it might appear in patient documentation. (LO 19.2, *Apply*)**

1. _____

2. _____

3. _____

4. _____

5. _____

6. _____

7. _____

8. _____

9. _____

10. _____

D. **Each of the following surgical procedures is a removal of some body part.** Identify what is removed in each surgery. (**LO 19. 2,** *Understand*)

1. appendectomy   _____

2. lymphadenectomy   _____

3. nephrectomy   _____

4. pneumonectomy   _____

5. splenectomy   _____

6. ureterectomy   _____

7. endarterectomy   _____

8. cystectomy   _____

9. cholecystectomy   _____

10. thymectomy   _____

E. **Meet the goals of each of the chapter outcomes by using the correct languages of geriatrics and gerontology for the answers.** **(LO 19.1–19.12,** *Analyze***)**

1. Apply the language of gerontology to the anatomy, physiology, and psychology of aging in the elderly. Visual acuity declines with age. Which of the following medical terms applies to this condition? **(LO 19.1)**

   a. osteopenia

   b. presbyopia

   c. arthritic

   d. atrophy

   e. sarcopenia

2. Use the medical terms of gerontology to communicate and document in writing accurately and precisely in any health care setting. Complete the sentence appropriately. **(LO 19.2)**

   a. As muscle _____, there are fewer muscle fibers to do work.

3. Use the medical language of gerontology to communicate verbally with accuracy and precision in any health care setting. The doctor, a specialist, has told you that a patient has developed *fibromyalgia*. What type of specialist were you speaking with? Circle the correct answer. **(LO 19.3)**

   a. orthopedist

   b. podiatrist

   c. urologist

   d. hematologist

   e. pulmonologist

4. Compare and contrast *geriatrics* and *gerontology*. The medical field that involves the study, care, and treatment of the elderly is called **(LO 19.4)**

   a. gerontology

   b. geriatrics

   c. psychology

   d. neurology

   e. urologist

5. Describe the latest profile of older Americans. Circle the statement that is incorrect. **(LO 19.5)**

   a. The older population (65+) numbered 35.4 million in 2010.

   b. Older women (23.0 million) outnumber older men (17.4 million).

   c. Forty percent of older women are widows.

   d. Women reaching age 65 in 2010 had an average life expectancy of an additional 20.0 years.

   e. The older population is expected to increase to 55 million in 2020.

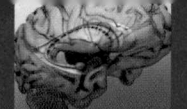

Geriatrics

6. Discuss the terms *aging* and *senescence*. Which term applies to the process, and which term applies to the state achieved by the process? (**LO 19.6**)

a. Process = _____

b. State achieved by this process = _____

7. Describe the effects of senescence on the major organ systems. Choose any one organ system and describe the effects of senescence on it. (**LO 19.7**)

Organ system _____

_____

8. Explain the theories of the process of senescence. Heredity plays a role in the cause of senescence because (**LO 19.8**)

_____

_____

9. Discuss the complex effects of aging. Decline in physiological reserve can produce complications from mild problems. Give an example of this. (**LO 19.9**)

_____

_____

10. Describe specific disorders of aging. Pick one specific disorder of aging and discuss it in class. (**LO 19.10**)

a. Disorder:

_____

_____

b. Describe the disorder:

_____

_____

11. Discuss dying and death. Which do you believe is of more concern to elderly people—dying or death? Discuss why. (**LO 19.11**)

a. More concern is for _____

b. Because

_____

_____

12. Identify answers to some of the important legal issues surrounding dying and death. Brain death, brain damage, and loss of brain function should be addressed in which legal document? (**LO 19.12**)

   a. HIPAA

   b. A will that disposes of worldly possessions

   c. DNR order

   d. Living will

   e. POA

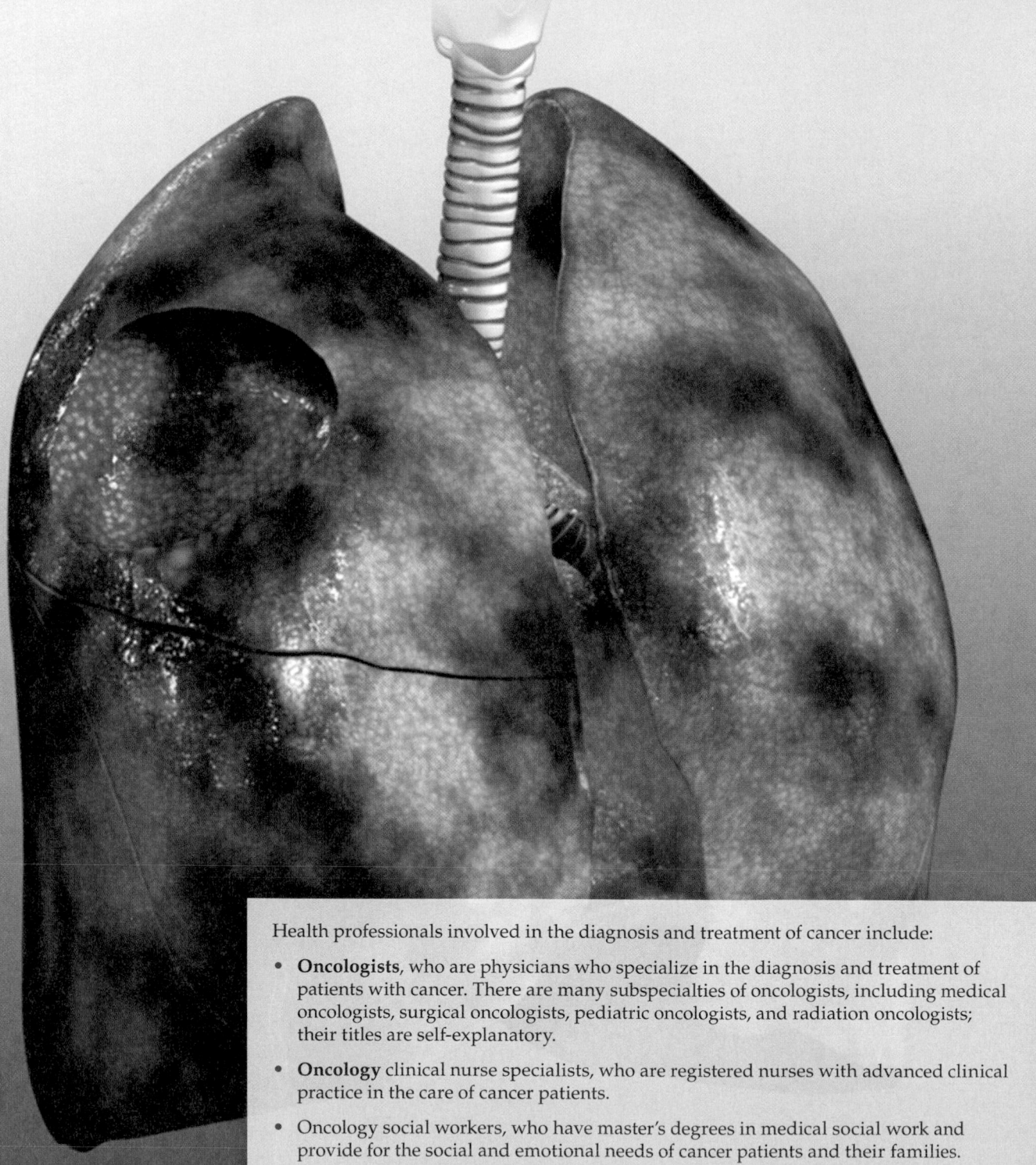

Health professionals involved in the diagnosis and treatment of cancer include:

- **Oncologists**, who are physicians who specialize in the diagnosis and treatment of patients with cancer. There are many subspecialties of oncologists, including medical oncologists, surgical oncologists, pediatric oncologists, and radiation oncologists; their titles are self-explanatory.

- **Oncology** clinical nurse specialists, who are registered nurses with advanced clinical practice in the care of cancer patients.

- Oncology social workers, who have master's degrees in medical social work and provide for the social and emotional needs of cancer patients and their families.

20

Case Report (CR) 20.1

You are

...an advanced-level respiratory therapist employed by Fulwood Medical Center, working with Tavis Senko, MD, a pulmonologist.

Your patient is

...Mrs. Raquel Sacco, a 44-year-old mother of two teenage boys, who is the owner of a quilting fabrics store. She is 2 days postop from lung surgery for non–small cell lung cancer. From her records, you see that she has two secondary (2°) metastases in her brain. She has been a nonsmoker all her life. Her 70-year-old father is a two-pack-a-day smoker, as is her husband. They both show no evidence of cancer on chest x-rays. Before Mrs. Sacco is discharged, as part of her postoperative respiratory care plan you are using incentive spirometry—also called **sustained maximal inspiration (SMI)**—to increase her inspiratory volume and improve her inspiratory muscle performance. You will also be taking an arterial blood sample to check her **arterial oxygen pressure (PaO₂)**.

Chapter Learning Outcomes

To understand the possible etiologies of cancer, its pathology and staging, and its treatment and prognosis and to communicate among the health care team as you care for Mrs. Sacco, you will need to be able to:

LO 20.1 Use the medical terms of oncology so that you communicate and document in writing accurately and precisely in any health care setting.

LO 20.2 Use the medical terms of oncology to communicate verbally with accuracy and precision in any health care setting.

LO 20.3 Discuss the different types of cancer.

LO 20.4 Describe the types of genes and their mutations that are involved in carcinogenesis.

LO 20.5 Identify environmental pollutants involved as triggers of cancer.

LO 20.6 Describe different methods of detecting cancer.

LO 20.7 Discuss different methods of treating cancer.

Note: In previous chapters on individual body systems, the terminology of cancers specific to each body system has been detailed. In this chapter, the terminology that relates to cancer in general will be explored by using lung cancer as an example.

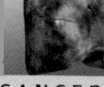

Lesson 20.1 Types of Cancer

CANCER

LESSON OBJECTIVES

Normal tissue development is a balance between cell growth and cell death. If cells multiply more quickly than cells die, tumors (neoplasms) are formed. The study of tumors is called oncology, and medical specialists in this field are called oncologists.

Neoplasms whose cells proliferate rapidly and spread to distant sites (metastasize) are called **malignant**. Neoplasms that grow slowly, stay localized, do not invade surrounding tissues, and do not metastasize are called **benign**.

The information in this lesson will enable you to use correct medical terminology to:

20.1.1 Distinguish between benign and malignant neoplasms.

20.1.2 Classify the types of cancer by the type of cell from which it originates.

20.1.3 Explain the process of carcinogenesis.

20.1.4 Discuss the roles of environmental factors in carcinogenesis.

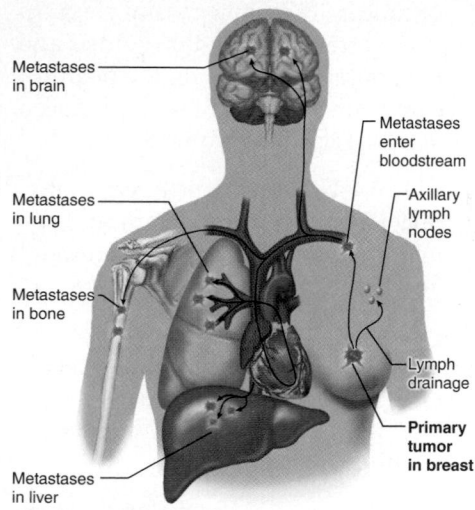

▲ **Figure 20.1** **Metastases from Primary Breast Cancer.** Metastases may be via lymph drainage to the axillary lymph nodes or via the bloodstream to the brain, lung, liver, and bone.

LO 20.3 Types of Cancer

Cancer (CA) is a class of malignant diseases characterized by uncontrolled cell division. The basic cause of this uncontrolled growth is damage to the cells' DNA. This damage produces mutations to the genes that control cell division. These mutations, which can be inherited or acquired, lead to the uncontrolled cell division and malignant tumor formation. Thus, all cancer is genetic;, that is, it develops because something in a cell's genes has changed (mutated).

Less than 10% of all cancers are inherited, that is, the genetic change is passed from parent to child. Almost 90% of cancers are acquired—something has caused the gene mutation in specific cells in a particular individual. A few genes mutated within a cell nucleus are enough to cause cancer. These gene mutations give the cells a superpower to proliferate in an uncontrolled way.

The Cells of Malignant Tumors

- Have unlimited, unregulated growth potential.
- Grow directly into adjacent tissues (invasion or **infiltration**).
- Invade the lymphatic system and are carried to local and distant lymph nodes (*Figure 20.1*).
- Invade the bloodstream and are carried to other distant organs and tissues (**metastasis**; *Figure 20.1*).

In contrast, benign tumors do not show such unregulated, invasive growth.

The Cells of Benign Tumors

- Grow slowly.
- Are surrounded by a connective tissue capsule.
- Do not invade or infiltrate adjacent tissues.
- Do not spread to other organs (metastasize) or to lymph nodes.
- Can compress surrounding tissues, causing functional problems.

Causes of Death

In the United States, the three most common causes of death are

1. Cardiovascular disease (28.5% of all deaths).
2. Cancer (22.8% of all deaths).
3. Cerebrovascular disease, primarily stroke (6.7% of all deaths).

Environmental factors, particularly cigarette smoke, are associated with many forms of cancer. In this chapter, we will use a case of lung cancer to illustrate the characteristics of an acquired cancer and to discuss methods of detection and treatment.

Keynotes

- Lung cancer causes 30.9% of all cancer cases.
- Colon cancer causes 9.6% of all cancer cases.
- Breast cancer causes 8.0% of all cancer cases.
- An estimated 1,638,910 new cancer cases and 577,190 deaths from cancer will occur in 2012.
- Between 1990 and 2007, the most recent year for which data is available, overall death rates decreased by 22% in men and 14% in women.
- The decline in cancer death rates is due to better prevention efforts, new screening methods, and more effective treatments.

Abbreviations	
CA	cancer
PaO$_2$	partial pressure of arterial oxygen
2°	secondary
SMI	sustained maximal inspiration

WORD	PRONUNCIATION		ELEMENTS	DEFINITION
benign (adj)	bee-**NINE**		Latin *kind*	Denoting the nonmalignant character of a neoplasm or illness
cancer cancerous (adj)	**KAN**-ser **KAN**-ser-ous	S/ R/	-ous *pertaining to* **cancer-** *cancer*	General term for a malignant neoplasm Pertaining to a malignant neoplasm
infiltrate infiltration	**IN**-fil-trate in-fil-**TRAY**-shun	S/ P/ R/ S/	-ate *composed of, pertaining to* in- *in* **-filtr-** *strain through* -ation *process*	To penetrate and invade a tissue or cell The invasion into a tissue or cell
malignant (adj) malignancy (noun)	mah-**LIG**-nant mah-**LIG**-nan-see	 S/ R/	Latin *hurtful* -ancy *state of* **malign-** *cancer*	Capable of invading surrounding tissues and metastasizing to distant organs Tumor that invades surrounding tissues and metastasizes to distant organs
metastasis (noun) metastases (pl) metastatic (adj)	meh-**TAS**-tah-sis meh-**TAS**-tah-seez meh-tah-**STAT**-ik	P/ R/ S/ R/	meta- *after, beyond* **-stasis** *stay in one place* -ic *pertaining to* **-stat-** *stand still*	Spread of disease from one part of the body to another Able to metastasize
neoplasm (noun) neoplastic (adj) neoplasia (*Note:* The "m" in plasm is removed to allow the elements to flow.)	**NEE**-oh-plazm **NEE**-oh-**PLAS**-tic **NEE**-oh-**PLAY**-zee-ah	P/ R/ S/ S/	neo- *new* **-plasm-** *to form* -tic *pertaining to* -ia *condition*	A new growth, either a benign or malignant tumor Pertaining to a neoplasm Process that results in formation of a tumor
oncology oncologist	on-**KOL**-oh-jee on-**KOL**-oh-jist	S/ R/CF S/	-logy *study of* **onc/o-** *tumor* -logist *one who studies, specialist*	The science dealing with cancer Medical specialist in oncology
proliferate	pro-**LIF**-eh-rate	S/ R/CF R/	-ate *composed of, pertaining to* **prol/i-** *bear offspring* **-fer-** *to bear*	To increase in number through reproduction
tumor	**TOO**-mor		Latin *swelling*	Any abnormal swelling

Exercises

A. Demonstrate that you can use various forms of the same term in correct usage. *Insert the appropriate medical term in the following blanks.* **LO 20.1, 20.3**

neoplasm   neoplastic   neoplasia

1. _____ is a process that results in the formation of a tumor, which can be either malignant or benign.

2. Another name for a tumor is a _____.

3. The tumor exhibited _____ behavior and was immediately biopsied.

metastases   metastatic   metastasis

4. A _____ carcinoma is cancer that has spread to a different site than the primary tumor.

5. The patient has _____ in his brain and kidneys.

6. Finding a primary tumor before _____ has occurred increases the chances for a cure.

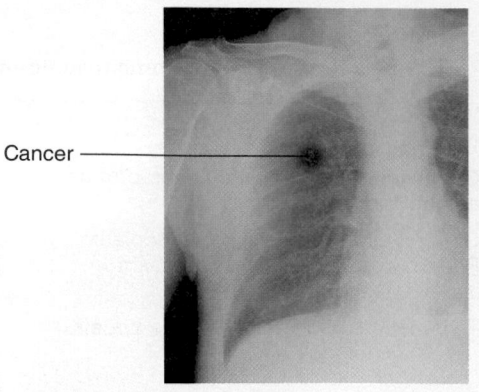

Cancer

▲ **Figure 20.2** X-ray of Small Cell Cancer of Right Upper Lung.

Abbreviations

CIS	carcinoma in situ
1°	primary

Keynote

The term **carcinoma in situ (CIS)** describes an early form of carcinoma in which there is no invasion of surrounding tissues. In many instances, it is a precursor that will transform into an invasive or malignant cancer.

- The three most common cancers in men and the three leading causes of cancer death are lung cancer, prostate cancer, and colorectal cancer.

- The three most common cancers in women are breast cancer, lung cancer, and colorectal cancer.

- The three leading causes of cancer death among women are lung cancer, breast cancer, and colorectal cancer.

LO 20.3 Types of Cancer (continued)

Within the broad classes of cancer *(Table 20.1)* are many subgroups, depending on the type of cells in the cancer.

Lung Cancer

Lung cancer has three main subgroups:

1. **Non–small cell lung cancer** accounts for 85% of cases, and 80% of patients die within 5 years of diagnosis. Included in this type are

   a. **Squamous cell carcinoma**, arising from *round cells* that have replaced damaged cells in the epithelial lining cells of a major bronchus. It accounts for 25% to 40% of lung cancers.

   b. **Adenocarcinoma**, arising from the *mucus-producing cells* in the bronchi. It accounts for between 30% and 50% of lung cancers. It is the most common lung cancer in women, and its incidence is increasing.

   c. **Large cell carcinoma**, which includes cancers that cannot be identified under the microscope as squamous cell or adenocarcinoma. It accounts for 10% to 20% of lung cancers.

Case Report 20.1 (continued)

Adenocarcinoma was found in Raquel Sacco. It was diagnosed because she had a seizure, and neurologic tests revealed the presence of two metastases in her brain. This led to a search for the primary (1°) tumor that was found in her lung *[Figure 20.2]*.

2. **Small cell lung cancer**, like squamous cell carcinoma, is derived from the epithelial cells of the bronchi but replicates at a faster rate, producing smaller cells. It accounts for 14% of all lung cancers; most patients die within 18 months of diagnosis.

3. **Mesothelioma** is a rare tumor arising from the cells lining the pleura and is associated with asbestosis.

Table 20.1 Types of Cancer

Class of Cancer	Cells of Origin	Examples
carcinoma	Epithelial	Cervical cancer, stomach cancer, squamous cell skin cancer, lung cancer
sarcoma	Connective tissue, bone cartilage, muscle	Osteosarcoma, chondrosarcoma, rhabdomyosarcoma
leukemia	Blood-forming tissues	Acute lymphocytic leukemia, chronic myelogenous leukemia
lymphoma	Lymph nodes	Hodgkin disease, non-Hodgkin lymphoma
melanoma	Melanocytes (pigment-producing skin cells)	Malignant melanoma

S = Suffix   P = Prefix   R = Root   R/CF = Combining Form

WORD	PRONUNCIATION	ELEMENTS		DEFINITION
adenocarcinoma	**AD**-eh-noh-kar-sih-**NOH**-mah	S/ R/CF R/	-oma *tumor* **aden/o-** *gland* **-carcin-** *cancer*	A cancer arising from glandular epithelial cells
asbestosis	as-bes-**TOE**-sis	S/ R/	-osis *condition* **asbest-** *asbestos*	Lung disease caused by the inhalation of asbestos particles
carcinoma	kar-sih-**NOH**-mah	S/ R/	-oma *tumor* **carcin-** *cancer*	A malignant and invasive epithelial tumor
carcinoma in situ (CIS)	kar-sih-**NOH**-mah in **SIGH**-tyu		**in situ** Latin *in its place*	Carcinoma that has not invaded surrounding tissues
chondrosarcoma	**KON**-dro-sar-**KOH**-mah	S/ R/CF R/	-oma *tumor* **chondr/o-** *cartilage* **-sarc-** *flesh*	Cancer arising from cartilage cells
mesothelioma	**MEEZ**-oh-thee-lee-**OH**-mah	S/ P/ R/	-oma *tumor* **meso-** *middle* **-theli-** *epithelium*	Cancer arising from the cells lining the pleura or peritoneum
osteosarcoma	**OS**-tee-oh-sar-**KOH**-mah	S/ R/CF R/	-oma *tumor* **oste/o-** *bone* **-sarc-** *flesh*	Cancer arising in bone-forming cells
rhabdomyosarcoma	**RAB**-doh-**MY**-oh-sar-**KOH**-mah	S/ R/CF R/CF R/	-oma *tumor* **rhabd/o-** *rod-shaped, striated* **-my/o-** *muscle* **-sarc-** *flesh*	Cancer derived from skeletal muscle
sarcoma	sar-**KOH**-mah	S/ R/	-oma *tumor* **sarc-** *flesh*	A malignant tumor originating in connective tissue

Exercises

A. Deconstruct the following *language of oncology* into elements. *These elements will form the basis for many additional oncologic terms.* Fill in the chart.   **LO 20.3**

Medical Term	Meaning of Prefix	Meaning of Root(s)/ Combining Form(s)	Meaning of Suffix	Meaning of Medical Term
sarcoma	1.	2.	3.	4.
chondrosarcoma	5.	6.	7.	8.
osteosarcoma	9.	10.	11.	12.
mesothelioma	13.	14.	15.	16.
carcinoma	17.	18.	19.	20.

21. Which of the following best describes ALL of the terms in the preceding chart? Circle the best answer.

   a. They are malignant tumors.

   b. They are noncancerous neoplasms.

   c. They are not invasive.

   d. They have no symptoms.

   e. They have no cure.

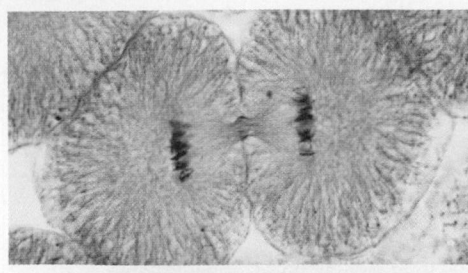

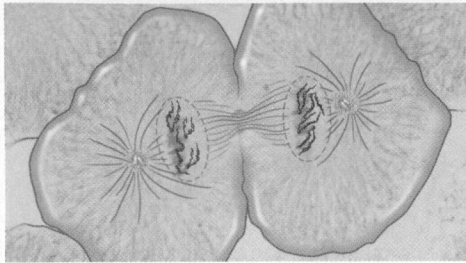

▲ **Figure 20.3** End Stage of Mitosis.
For simplicity, the schematic drawing of the cell *(bottom)* is shown with only two chromosome pairs.

Abbreviations

ETS	environmental tobacco smoke
PCD	programmed cell death
TS	tumor suppressor

Keynotes

- A pack-year equals the number of packs of cigarettes smoked per day multiplied by the number of years the person has smoked.
- Cigarette smoke contains over 60 known carcinogens.

LO 20.4 Carcinogenesis

Carcinogenesis, literally the creation of cancer, is the abnormal rate of cell division as a result of damaged DNA causing gene mutation. Normally, the balance between cell division and proliferation and cell death **(apoptosis**, or **programmed cell death [PCD])** is tightly controlled to maintain the integrity of organs and tissues. Gene mutations that cause cancer disrupt this orderly process. Mutation in a single gene is usually not enough to cause cancer, and carcinogenesis requires multiple mutations in many genes.

Most normal cells cannot divide unless a **growth factor** binds to a receptor on the cell's surface. This growth factor then stimulates the cell to undergo mitosis *(see Chapter 4)* and **differentiate** into mature, functional cells *(Figure 20.3)*.

Two types of genes have been identified that play a part in the abnormal cell division and proliferation of cancer cells:

1. **Protooncogenes** are healthy genes that promote normal cell growth. Mutated **oncogenes** cause malfunctions in the normal growth mechanisms. For example, an oncogene called *SIS* stimulates blood vessels to grow into a tumor and provide the rich blood supply it needs to proliferate rapidly. An oncogene called *RAS* generates abnormal growth-factor receptors that switch on constant cell division signals. An oncogene called *HER-2* causes many cases of breast and ovarian cancer. The drug Herceptin is an antibody that targets the HER-2 receptors on the cancer cells. This cuts off the chemical signals that the cell needs to keep proliferating. It also marks the abnormal cells for destruction by the immune system.

2. **Tumor suppressor (TS) genes** normally suppress mitosis and are activated by DNA damage. Their function is to stop cell division so that the abnormal genetic structure cannot be passed on to daughter cells. **Mutated TS genes** cannot do this, so the abnormal cells can divide and proliferate. A mutated TS gene called *p53* is present in half of all cancers and is associated with a poor prognosis and resistance to chemotherapy.

Mutations in both types of genes are usually required for cancer to develop. The oncogenes turn on the abnormal cell growth, and the mutated TS genes cannot stop it.

Cancer is due to the accumulation of genetic injury and mutations. Agents that cause these mutations are called **mutagens**, and mutagens that cause cancer are called **carcinogens**. Particular carcinogens are linked to specific types of cancer. Examples are inhalation of asbestos fibers with mesothelioma, prolonged exposure to radiation and ultraviolet radiation with melanoma and other skin malignancies, and tobacco smoking with lung cancer. Although the link between cigarette smoking and lung cancer is well established, only 15% to 20% of smokers develop lung cancer. In addition, about 10% of the population carries a gene that protects against lung cancer.

Studies in 2004 and 2005 of the epithelial cells in the large bronchi found a large number of genes altered by cigarette smoking. The studies defined genes whose alteration correlated with cumulative pack-years of smoking, and they identified 13 genes whose alterations do not return to normal after smoking is stopped. This could explain the persistent risk of lung cancer in former smokers. In addition, a subset of smokers was identified whose gene alterations have a different profile from that of other smokers. It is possible that this subset is the group who develop lung cancer.

Secondhand smoke, called **environmental tobacco smoke (ETS)**, contains the same chemicals and carcinogens as those inhaled by smokers. It is responsible for 3000 lung cancer cases each year in America. The genetic mutations caused by the carcinogens are probably similar to those in the subset of smokers discussed earlier, even though exposure to the carcinogens is much less than that for smokers.

Case Report 20.1 (continued)

Raquel Sacco probably developed her lung cancer as a result of inhaling secondhand smoke all her life (from her father and husband).

Word Analysis and Definition

WORD	PRONUNCIATION	ELEMENTS		DEFINITION
apoptosis	AP-op-TOE-sis	P/ R/	apo- *separation from* -ptosis *falling*	Programmed normal cell death
carcinogen	kar-SIN-oh-jen	S/ R/CF	-gen *produce* carcin/o- *cancer*	Cancer-producing agent
carcinogenic (adj) carcinogenesis	kar-SIN-oh-JEN-ik kar-SIN-oh-JEN-eh-sis	S/ S/	-ic *pertaining to* -genesis *source*	Causing cancer Origin and development of cancer
mutagen	MYU-tah-jen	S/ R/	-gen *produce* muta- *genetic change*	Agent that produces a mutation in a gene
oncogene	ONG-koh-jeen	S/ R/CF	-gene *producer, give birth* onc/o- *tumor*	One of a family of genes involved in cell growth that work in concert to cause cancer
oncogenic (adj) (The "e" of gene is discarded to make the word flow)	ONG-koh-JEN-ik	S/	-ic *pertaining to*	Capable of producing a neoplasm
protooncogene	pro-toe-ON-koh-jeen	S/ P/ R/CF	-gene *producer, give birth* proto- *first* -onc/o-*tumor*	A normal gene involved in normal cell growth

Exercises

A. Use the *language of oncology* to answer questions. *The following questions can be either true or false. Circle the answer, then rewrite the false statements to be true.* **LO 20.1, 20.3, 20.4**

1. Carcinogenesis is the creation of cancer. T F

2. Damaged blood cells cause gene mutation. T F

3. PCD is another term for apoptosis. T F

4. Mutagens that cause cancer are called carcinogens. T F

5. It is not possible to get cancer from secondhand smoke. T F

6. Corrections:

_____

_____

_____

B. Consult the glossary or an online medical dictionary to define the term *mutation*. *Briefly describe its role in the formation of CA.* **LO 20.1, 20.4**

1. _____

_____

_____

> ### Study Hint
> **Ptosis** is a medical term in its own right. Another example is the term **hemolysis**, in which **lysis** is also a medical term in and of itself.

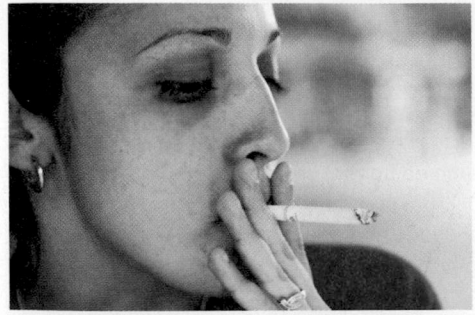

▲ **Figure 20.4** Woman Smoking.

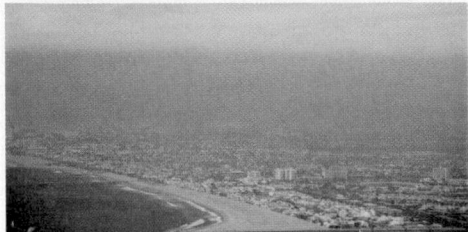

▲ **Figure 20.5** Air Pollution over a Large City.

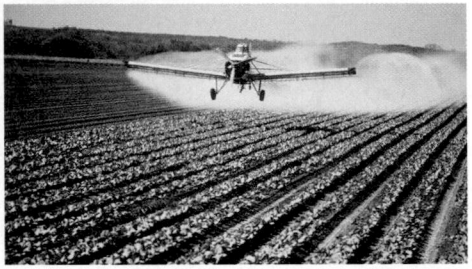

▲ **Figure 20.6** Pesticide Spraying of Field of Vegetables.

▲ **Figure 20.7** No Smoking Sign.

LO 20.5 Environmental Pollution

Pollution is a trigger of many cancers. For example, cigarette smoke *(Figure 20.4)* causes 87% of all lung cancers and acts in the following way: In the smoke are approximately 4000 chemicals, some 60 of which are known to be carcinogenic and trigger genetic mutations that lead to cancer. Among the inhaled chemicals are cyanide, benzene, formaldehyde, acetylene, tar, arsenic, and ammonia, all of which can increase the risk for cancer.

Radon, a radioactive gas that you cannot see or smell, is the second leading cause of lung cancer (after smoking). It is produced by decaying **uranium** and is found in nearly all soils. In underground miners, it increases the risk of cancer to 40%. It gets into homes through cracks in the foundations or construction joints and is a problem in 1 out of 15 homes. Cigarette smoking on top of radon significantly increases the risk of lung cancer. Testing for radon is cheap and easy.

Air pollution may be the cause of the 10% to 40% increase in lung cancer mortality between urban and rural areas *(Figure 20.5)*. **Particulate matter**, especially very small particles, includes soot; organic material such as hydrocarbons; and metals such as arsenic, chromium, and nickel—all of which are known mutagens and carcinogens. A new analysis shows that premature death from cardiovascular ailments is increased by 24% among people exposed to tiny soot particles.

Chemical toxins are estimated to cause more than 75% of all cancers. Some 77,000 chemicals are used in this country. Over 3000 are added to our food, and most Americans have between 400 and 800 chemicals stored in their bodies, mostly in fat cells. The toxins known to cause cancer include

- **Chlorine**. Used in drinking water, chlorine produces carcinogenic compounds. Cancer risk among people drinking chlorinated water is 93% higher than that of people not drinking chlorinated water.
- **Polychlorinated biphenyls (PCBs)**. These were banned years ago but still persist in the environment and are found in farmed salmon.
- **Pesticides**. According to the **Environmental Protection Agency (EPA)**, 60% of herbicides, 90% of fungicides, and 30% of insecticides are known to be carcinogenic *(Figure 20.6)*. Farmers using pesticides have a 14% greater risk for developing prostate cancer than do organic farmers.
- **Dioxins**. These are chemical compounds produced by combustion processes from waste incineration and from burning fuels like wood, coal, and oil.
- **Asbestos**. This insulating material was used in the 1950s to 1970s on floors, ceilings, water pipes, and heating ducts. When the material becomes old and crumbly, it releases fibers into the air. Inhalation of the fibers is the cause of mesothelioma.
- **Arsenic**. This is used by insecticide and herbicide sprayers and oil refinery workers.

Occupational Safety and Health Administration **(OSHA)** regulations are designed to protect workers from these environmental hazards.

Prevention of Cancer

More than 50% of cancers could be prevented by **changes in lifestyle and environment**. The same carcinogens that affect the lining of the respiratory tract cause cancer of the oral cavity, pharynx, larynx, and esophagus. They are also absorbed into the bloodstream and disseminated, thereby becoming factors that can cause cancer in the pancreas, stomach, kidney, bladder, prostate, and cervix. **Stopping smoking** alone would reduce most of the 30% of all deaths due to lung cancer and reduce the incidence of many of the other cancers related to smoking *(Figure 20.7)*.

Clean air measures that are being implemented to reduce the more than 2 billion pounds of toxic air pollutants emitted into the atmosphere annually in this country can reduce the incidence of cancer.

Obesity is said to be linked to about 10% of breast and colorectal cancers and up to 40% of kidney, esophageal, and endometrial cancers. The mechanisms of obesity linked to these cancers are not understood.

WORD	PRONUNCIATION	ELEMENTS		DEFINITION
chlorine	KLOR-een		Greek *greenish-yellow*	A toxic agent used as a disinfectant and bleaching agent
dioxin	die-OK-sin	P/ R/	di- *two* -oxin *oxygen atom*	Carcinogenic contaminant in pesticides
environment	en-VI-ron-ment	S/ R/	-ment *resulting state* environ- *surroundings*	All the external conditions affecting the life of an organism
environmental (adj)	en-VI-ron-ment-al	S/	-al *pertaining to*	Pertaining to the environment
flavonoid (alternative spelling: flavinoid)	FLAY-vih-noid	S/ R/	-oid *resembling* flavon- *yellow*	A pigment found in fruit, wine, and tea
particle	PAR-tih-kul		Latin *little piece*	A small piece of matter
particulate (adj)	par-TIK-you-late	S/ R/	-ate *composed of, pertaining to* particul- *little piece*	Relating to a fine particle
pesticide	PES-tih-side	R/CF R/CF	-cid/e *to kill* pest/i- *pest*	Agent for destroying flies, mosquitoes, and other pests
pollution	poh-LOO-shun		Latin *dirty*	Condition that is unclean, impure, and a danger to health
uranium	you-RAY-nee-um		Greek mythological character, Uranus	Radioactive metallic element

Exercises

A. Demonstrate your knowledge of the following terminology by deconstructing the terms into their elements and then using any one term in a sentence of your own choice (not directly from the text). *Fill in the blanks.*   **LO 20.1, 20.5**

1. phytochemical _____/_____/_____

    P   R/CF   S

2. environment _____/_____/_____

    P   R/CF   S

3. pesticide _____/_____/_____

    P   R/CF   S

4. dioxin _____/_____/_____

    P   R/CF   S

5. *Pick any one of these terms, and use it in a sentence.*

_____

_____

B. Name the six chemical toxins that are known to cause more than 75% of all cancers.   LO 20.1, 20.5

1. _____

2. _____

3. _____

4. _____

5. _____

6. _____

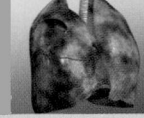

Lesson 20.2 Detecting and Treating Cancer

All that is required for cancer to develop are genetic mutations in one cell, the mother or progenitor cell. The daughter cells can reproduce rapidly, but clinical detection by physical or radiographic means is rare for a tumor mass lower than 1 billion cancer cells (about 1 cm in diameter). The earlier the tumor is detected, the better the chance of cure.

The information in this lesson will enable you to use correct medical terminology to:

20.2.1 List methods of cancer prevention.

20.2.2 Discuss methods of self-examination to detect cancer.

20.2.3 Describe methods of screening for cancer.

20.2.4 Explain therapies for treating cancer.

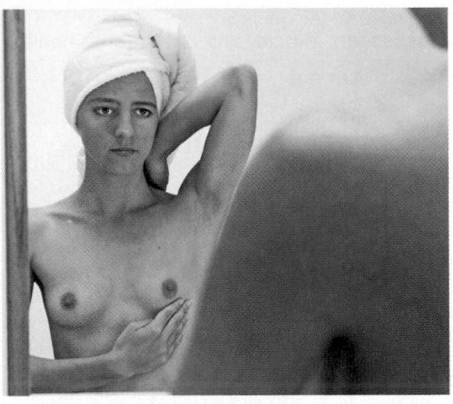

▲ **Figure 20.8** Breast Self-Examination.

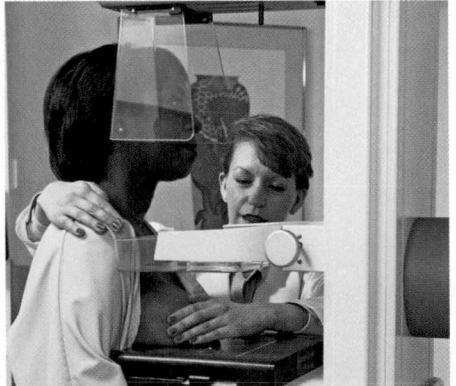

▲ **Figure 20.9** Mammography.

Abbreviations

DRE	digital rectal examination
FOBT	fecal occult blood test
MRI	magnetic resonance imaging
Pap	Papanicolaou cervical smear test
PSA	prostate-specific antigen
USPSTF	U.S. Preventive Services Task Force

LO 20.6 Detecting Cancer

Breast, testicular, and prostate cancers are often detected by **palpation**. This is why some advocacy organizations recommend monthly breast and testicular **self-examination** *(Figure 20.8)*. For prostate cancer, men aged 50 and over should be offered an annual **digital rectal examination (DRE)** and **prostate-specific antigen (PSA)** blood test periodically, although the value of the PSA test is controversial.

Melanoma of the skin is a visible cancer and **self-examination of the skin** in front of a full-length mirror should also be performed monthly by adults.

All self-examinations should be performed in conjunction with health care provider examinations. For example, a **cancer-related clinical examination** should be performed every year for those over age 40. Beginning at age 50, men and women should have a digital rectal examination annually, together with a **fecal occult blood test (FOBT)** as a screening for colon and rectal cancer. Every 10 years a colonoscopy should be performed. For most women, a **PAP test** should be performed every three to five years to detect pre-cancerous cells in the cervix *(see Chapter 8)*.

Screening for Breast Cancer

Mammograms *(Figure 20.9)* are recommended by the U.S. Preventive Services Task Force to be performed every two years between the ages 50 and 74. However, many providers and women prefer to begin screening aged 40 and to screen every 1 to 2 years.

Digital mammography records x-ray images in computer code instead of on x-ray film. This technique allows the images to be manipulated to enhance subtle changes in tissue density. Studies are being performed to see if digital mammography is more effective than conventional mammography at finding cancer.

Computer-aided detection scans a mammogram with a laser beam and converts it into a digital signal that can be processed by a computer to highlight suspicious areas. The effectiveness of this technique is also being evaluated.

Magnetic resonance imaging (MRI) creates detailed images of the breast in different planes. This technique is being evaluated for screening women at high risk for breast cancer. MRI is also being used to screen for lung cancer in high-risk patients.

Image-guided breast biopsy techniques are important in helping doctors obtain biopsies from tumors that cannot be felt but are seen on conventional mammogram. **Stereotactic-guided biopsy** is the use of a computer and scanning devices to create three-dimensional images of lesions seen on a mammogram so that a needle can be inserted accurately into the lesion. Another type of needle biopsy uses a device called a *mammatome* to gently vacuum out suspicious tissue through a needle.

Ductal lavage collects samples of cells from breast ducts for microscopic analysis. Saline solution is introduced into a milk duct through a fine catheter inserted into the opening of the duct on the surface of the nipple. The solution is then aspirated out through the catheter, and cells in it are analyzed under the microscope to check for evidence of abnormal cells.

WORD	PRONUNCIATION	ELEMENTS		DEFINITION
digital	**DIJ**-ih-tal	S/ R/	**-al** *pertaining to* **digit-** *finger or toe*	Pertaining to a finger or toe
lavage	lah-**VAHZH**		Latin *to wash*	Washing out of a hollow cavity, tube, or organ
mammogram	**MAM**-oh-gram	S/ R/CF	**-gram** *a record* **mamm/o-** *breast*	The record produced by x-ray imaging of the breast
mammography	mah-**MOG**-rah-fee	S/	**-graphy** *process of recording*	Process of x-ray examination of the breast
progenitor	pro-**JEN**-it-or	P/ R/	**pro-** *before* **-genitor** *offspring*	Founder; beginning of an ancestry
radioactive	**RAY**-dee-oh-**AK**-tiv	R/CF R/CF	**radi/o-** *radiation* **-activ/e** *movement*	Spontaneously emitting alpha, beta, or gamma rays
self-examination	**SELF**-ek-zam-ih-**NAY**-shun	S/ R/ R/	**-ation** *process* **examin-** *test, examine* **self-** *me*	The examination of part of one's own body

Exercises

A. Circle the incorrect statement and then rewrite it correctly on the following lines.   LO 20.1, 20.2, 20.3, 20.4, 20.5

1. Protooncogenes are healthy genes that promote normal cell growth.   T   F

2. Tumor suppressor (TS) genes normally suppress mitosis and are activated by DNA damage.   T   F

3. Cancer is due to the accumulation of genetic injury and mutations.   T   F

4. The oncogenes turn on the abnormal cell growth, and the mutated TS genes cannot stop it.   T   F

5. Secondhand smoke does not contain the same chemicals and carcinogens as those inhaled by smokers.   T   F

6. Corrected statement:

_____

_____

_____

_____

B. Abbreviations must be used correctly for patient safety. *Use the abbreviations in bold to identify the statements given.*   **LO 20.6**

DRE   FOBT   MRI   Pap   PET

1. diagnostic test to examine soft tissue.   Abbreviation: _____

2. gynecologic test   Abbreviation: _____

3. test for blood in the bowels   Abbreviation: _____

4. probing with a gloved finger   Abbreviation: _____

5. sectional view of the body   Abbreviation: _____

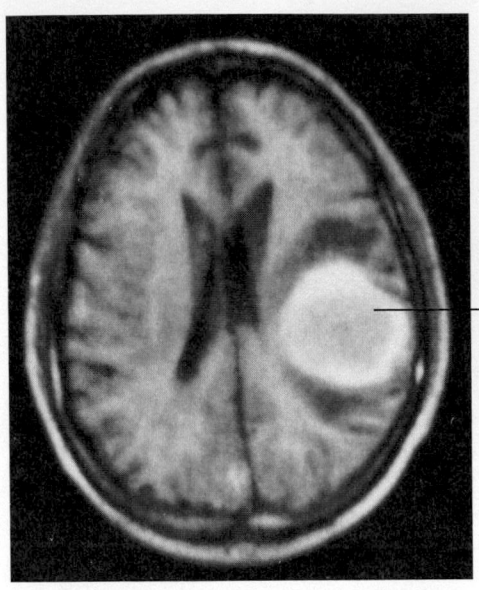

white ball "metastasis"

▲ **Figure 20.10** MRI Showing Brain Metastasis from a Lung Cancer.

LO 20.6 Detecting Lung Cancer

Chest x-rays, as a screening tool, rarely provide the first indication of lung cancer. By the time lung cancer is diagnosed by chest x-ray, it often has spread beyond the lungs.

Computed tomography (CT) scans are more effective at identifying early tumors than are chest x-rays.

Positron emission tomography (PET) scans are expensive and not widely available, but they are the most accurate noninvasive test for identifying if the cancer has spread outside lung tissue. PET use may prevent unnecessary surgeries by identifying patients whose cancer has progressed beyond the stage at which surgery is beneficial.

Magnetic resonance imaging (MRI) can locate brain and bone metastases from lung cancer *(Figure 20.10)*.

Scintigraphy utilizes low-level radioactive agents that bind to cancer cells and can be tracked by special cameras to reveal the locations of cancer cells.

Bronchoscopy can locate cancers in the major airways of the lung. Specimens are obtained for biopsy by cutting tissue, using brushings, and using a washing process called **bronchoalveolar lavage (BAL).**

Needle biopsy of tumors in the **periphery** of the lungs is performed by inserting a needle between the ribs and guiding it to the tumor by **fluoroscopy** or CT scan. The biopsy can also be performed by using **thoracoscopy,** in which a fiber-optic tube with a camera is inserted between the ribs into the pleural space to view the lungs and take a biopsy.

Mediastinoscopy uses a fiber-optic tube with a camera inserted into the mediastinum via the suprasternal notch to locate appropriate areas for biopsy if the cancer has spread to mediastinal lymph nodes.

Sputum analysis of coughed-up sputum can be a useful and cost-effective method of identifying cancer cells arising from the lining of the airways.

Biomarkers are substances that are released by specific cancers. They can be found in blood, sputum, and tissue samples. Biomarkers under investigation include **carcinoembryonic antigen (CEA),** which is found in 50% of cases of non–small cell lung cancer but is also found in colorectal, pancreatic, and breast cancer.

The blood test **anti-malignin antibody screen (AMAS)** is a general test for detecting any kind of cancer. Most cancers in their early stages secrete the antigen malignin; by using an antibody against malignin, the presence of the biomarker can be detected in the laboratory.

Alpha-fetoprotein levels may be elevated as a biomarker in cancer patients because cancer cells tend to revert to fetal characteristics.

Staging Lung Cancer

Staging defines how localized or how widespread the cancer is. Treatment and prognosis depend on the cancer's stage. The diagnostic tests described earlier are used to stage the cancer. In addition, brain metastases are identified by MRI and bone metastases by **technetium-99m (^{99m}Tc) radionuclide** bone scans.

The **tumor-node-metastasis (TNM) staging system** is used to stage cancer:

- "T" stands for *tumor* and describes its size and how far it has spread within the lung and to nearby tissues such as the pleura, diaphragm, and pericardium.
- "N" stands for spread to lymph *nodes* around the affected lung or around the other lung.
- "M" stands for *metastasis* to distant sites such as brain, liver, and bones.

Once the T, N, and M categories have been assigned, the information is combined (stage grouping) and given an overall stage of 0, I, II, III, or IV.

In many cancers, another measure of staging, called **grade,** is used. This depends on an assessment by a **pathologist** of the rate of growth of the cancer cells and how likely the cancer is to spread. The most **virulent** cancers are given a grade of 4.

Abbreviations

AMAS	anti-malignin antibody screen
BAL	bronchoalveolar lavage
CEA	carcinoembryonic antigen
CT	computed tomography
PET	positron emission tomography
^{99m}Tc	technetium 99m, a radionuclide
TNM	tumor-node-metastasis staging system for cancers

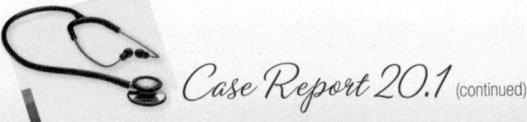

Case Report 20.1 (continued)

Because Mrs. Raquel Sacco's cancer has metastasized to her brain, she is placed in stage IV, which has only a 2% 5-year survival rate.

WORD	PRONUNCIATION	ELEMENTS		DEFINITION
biomarker	BI-oh-MARK-er	P/ R/	bio- *life* -marker *sign*	A biological marker or product by which a cell can be identified
bronchoalveolar	BRONG-koh-al-VEE-oh-lar	S/ R/CF R/	-ar *pertaining to* bronch/o- *bronchus* -alveol- *alveolus*	Pertaining to the bronchi and alveoli
fluoroscopy	flor-OS-koh-pee	S/ R/CF	-scopy *to examine* fluor/o- *x-ray beam*	Examination of the structures of the body by x-rays
grade	GRAYD		Latin *step*	In cancer pathology, a classification of the rate of growth of cancer cells
mediastinoscopy	ME-dee-ass-tih-NOS-koh-pee	S/ R/CF	-scopy *to examine* mediastin/o- *mediastinum*	Examination of the mediastinum using an endoscope
pathology	pa-THOL-oh-jee	S/ R/CF	-logy *study of* path/o- *disease*	Medical specialty dealing with the structural and functional changes of a disease process
pathologist	pa-THOL-oh-jist	S/	-logist *one who studies, specialist*	A specialist in pathology
periphery peripheral (adj)	peh-RIF-eh-ree peh-RIF-eh-ral	P/ R/	peri- *around* -phery *outer edge*	Outer part of a structure away from the center
radionuclide	RAY-dee-oh-NYU-klide	S/ R/CF R/	-ide *having a particular quality* radi/o- *radiation* -nucl- *nucleus*	Radioactive agent used in diagnostic imaging
scintigraphy	sin-TIG-rah-fee	S/ R/	-graphy *process of recording* scinti- *spark*	Recording of radioactivity with a special camera
stage	STAYJ		Latin *to stand*	Definition of extent and dissemination of a malignant neoplasm
staging	STAY-jing			Process of determination of the extent of the distribution of a neoplasm
thoracoscopy	thor-ah-KOS-koh-pee	S/ R/CF	-scopy *to examine* thorac/o- *chest*	Examination of the pleural cavity with an endoscope
virulent	VIR-you-lent		Latin *poisonous*	Extremely toxic or pathogenic

Exercises

A. Language of Oncology: Test your knowledge of the *language of oncology* with this exercise. *Circle the best answer(s). Some questions may have more than one correct answer.* **LO 20.1, 20.6**

1. Which of the following terms contains a prefix?

   periphery   thoracoscopy   virulent   pathology

2. Which term contains the suffix meaning *specialist*?

   nephrology   pathologist   pathology   fluoroscopy

3. Which term would mean a recording with a special camera?

   biomarker   thoracoscopy   scintigraphy   mediastinoscopy

4. Which is the term for something extremely toxic or poisonous?

   virulent   scintigraphy   bronchoalveolar   peripheral

5. Which of the following terms means *to examine*?

   cystoscopy   lavage   abdominocentesis   colpopexy

6. Which of the following terms is a procedure on the chest?

   cystoscopy   bronchoalveolar   bronchoscope   thoracoscopy

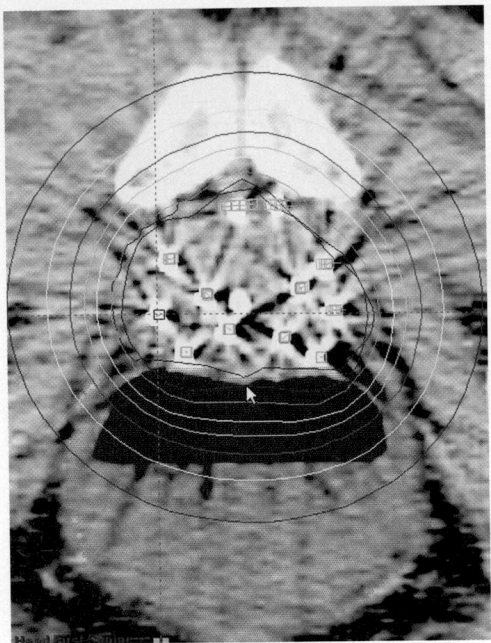

▲ **Figure 20.11** Radioactive Seeds Implanted in a Tumor.

LO 20.7 Treating Cancer

Treatment of any cancer depends on its location, its size, its localization or spread to surrounding tissues and lymph nodes, the presence of metastases, and the cancer's aggressiveness (as determined by pathologic findings on biopsy or surgical removal).

If the cancer is still localized, it can be removed and cure is possible. Unfortunately, few patients are diagnosed at such an early stage, particularly with lung cancer. Even if the original tumor is removed, cancer recurrence rates are high. Additional treatments with **radiation** and **chemotherapy** are used and can produce unpleasant side effects. A patient will have to balance a diminished quality of life against a chance for a modestly prolonged survival.

In the elderly, studies have shown that survival rates are the same for therapies aimed at relieving pain as they are for aggressive, unpleasant treatment **regimens** with their diminished quality of life.

Surgical Procedures

Surgical procedures for specific body system cancers are discussed in the relevant chapters. For example, surgery for breast cancer is covered in *Chapter 8* and for prostate cancer in *Chapter 7.*

The type of surgery for lung cancer depends on the amount of lung tissue that has to be removed.

Wedge resection (segmentectomy) removes only a small part of the lung. It is used for carcinoma in situ, small tumors, frailer patients who cannot tolerate lobectomy, or patients with lung disease.

Lobectomy is removal of one lobe of the lung and is used if the cancer has not spread beyond the lobe or into lymph nodes.

Pneumonectomy removes an entire lung and has a mortality of 5% to 8%.

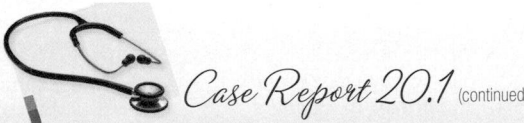

Case Report 20.1 (continued)

Lobectomy was the procedure performed on Mrs. Raquel Sacco. The respiratory therapy she is having is designed to enhance the function of her residual lung tissue.

Radiation Procedures (Radiotherapy)

Radiotherapy does not remove the lesion but distorts the DNA of the cancer cells so that they lose their ability to reproduce and to retain fluids; the cells shrink over time. Side effects of radiotherapy depend on the type of therapy used and occur when healthy cells are damaged during the treatment. Tiredness, nausea and loss of appetite, and sore skin in the treatment area can be short-term effects.

External-beam radiation focuses a beam of radiation directly on the tumor. It is generally used for metastasized cancer.

Brachytherapy implants radioactive seeds through thin tubes directly into the tumor to give high doses of radiation to the tumor while reducing radiation exposure to the surrounding tissues *(Figure 20.11)*. It can be used for inoperable cancers.

Continuous hyperfractionated accelerated radiotherapy (CHART) administers standard doses of radiation multiple times per day. It allows the total dose of radiation to be administered in a shorter period of time than the standard 6 weeks.

Stereotactic radiosurgery (SRS) uses three-dimensional computer programming to deliver a precise, single high dose of radiation in a 1-day session. The most common form of SRS used in the United States is a cobalt-60–based machine called the gamma knife. Though this technique is labeled and implied as "surgery," there is no actual surgery involved.

S = Suffix   P = Prefix   R = Root   R/CF = Combining Form

WORD	PRONUNCIATION	ELEMENTS		DEFINITION
brachytherapy	brah-kee-**THAIR**-ah-pee	R/ P/	-therapy *medical treatment* brachy- *short*	Radiation therapy in which the source of irradiation is implanted in the tissue to be treated
chemotherapy	**KEY**-moh-**THAIR**-ah-pee	R/ R/CF	-therapy *medical treatment* chem/o- *chemical*	Treatment using chemical agents
hyperfractionated (adj)	high-per-**FRAK**-shun-ay-ted	S/ P/ R/	-ated *process* hyper- *excessive* -fraction- *small amount*	Given in smaller amounts and more frequently
lobectomy	low-**BECK**-toe-me	S/ R/	-ectomy *surgical excision* lob- *lobe*	Surgical removal of a lobe of the lungs
photodynamic	foh-toe-die-**NAM**-ik	S/ R/CF R/	-ic *pertaining to* phot/o- *light* -dynam- *power*	Use of a light-sensitive drug with a laser beam to destroy cells
pneumonectomy	**NEW**-moh-**NEK**-toe-me	S/ R/	-ectomy *surgical excision* pneumon- *lung*	Surgical removal of a whole lung
radiation	ray-dee-**AY**-shun	S/ R/	-ation *process* radi- *x-ray, radiation*	Treatment with x-rays
radiotherapy	**RAY**-dee-oh-**THAIR**-ah-pee	R/CF R/	radi/o- *x-ray, radiation* -therapy *medical treatment*	Treatment using radiation
regimen	**REJ**-ih-men		Latin *direction*	Program of treatment
segmentectomy	seg-men-**TEK**-toe-me	S/ R/	-ectomy *surgical excision* segment- *section*	Surgical excision of a segment of a tissue or organ

Exercises

A. Match the element in the left column with its correct meaning in the right column. *Some of these elements have appeared in earlier chapters as well.* **LO 20.7**

_____ 1. phot/o

a. condition

_____ 6. lob

f. light

_____ 2. pneumon

b. lobe

_____ 7. therapy

g. chemical

_____ 3. brachy

c. excessive

_____ 8. osis

h. surgical excision

_____ 4. hyper

d. incision

_____ 9. chemo

i. treatment

_____ 5. ectomy

e. lung

_____ 10. otomy

j. short

B. Lung cancer usually involves surgical procedures. *Use the* language of oncology *to determine the correct answers.* **LO 20.1, 20.7**

1. The type of surgery for lung cancer depends on the amount of _____

2. What is the surgery called that removes only a small part of the lung? _____

3. Another name for the surgery in question 2 is _____

4. What surgery removes only one lobe of the lung? _____

5. What surgery removes the entire lung? _____

6. Critical thinking: Before going to surgery to remove the cancer, what should be the first step in this whole process?

    a. First step: _____

    b. Why is this done? _____

LO 20.7 Treating Cancer (continued)

Chemotherapy

(see Chapter 21)

- As well as affecting cancer cells, chemotherapy alters the function of normal cells, causing side effects.
- Gene therapy is an experimental treatment that can target healthy cells to enhance their ability to fight cancer or can target cancer cells to destroy them.

Abbreviations

FDA	Federal Drug Administration
MOAB	monoclonal antibody
NCI	National Cancer Institute
NHGRI	National Human Genome Research Institute

Chemotherapy is the use of chemical agents, the majority of which exert their effect by DNA damage that causes the cancer cells to be unable to reproduce and function, and thus they die. Unfortunately, these agents can also harm healthy cells, and that is what causes side effects. The kinds of side effects and their severity depend on the type and dose of chemotherapy. Fatigue, nausea, vomiting, and hair loss are common. Anemia and blood clotting problems can arise from the effects of the chemotherapy on the bone marrow.

Chemotherapy is usually given in regular cycles over several months. Platinum compounds, either cisplatin (Platinol) or carboplatin (Paraplatin) are used in many treatment regimens. They are mostly used with other types of **cytotoxic** drugs in two-drug or three-drug combinations. Side effects are common and vary in severity.

For some cases, chemotherapy alone can be the treatment of choice; for others, a combination of chemotherapy and radiation is used. In many cases, surgery is performed prior to or following these forms of treatment.

Biologic Therapies

Biologic therapies use the body's immune system, directly or indirectly, to attack cancer cells or to lessen the side effects that can be caused by radiation and chemotherapy. **Biologic response modifiers** alter the immune system's response to cancer cells and include interferons, interleukins, monoclonal antibodies, vaccines, and gene therapy.

Monoclonal antibodies (MOABs) are antibodies produced by a single type of cell and are specific for a single antigen. Examples of MOABs are rituximab (Rituxan), used for non-Hodgkin lymphoma, and trastuzumab (Herceptin), used in breast cancer for tumors that produce a protein called HER-2.

Antiangiogenesis therapy interferes with the genetic mechanisms that increase blood supply for the active growth of cancer cells. The drug Avastin has led to a great increase in the survival of patients with colon cancer and is also being used in lung and breast cancer.

Gene therapy is now a focus of cancer therapy. In 2005, the **National Cancer Institute (NCI)** and the **National Human Genome Research Institute (NHGRI)** announced a 3-year pilot project to map the genetic alterations in cancer cells. New technologies called **microarrays** or **gene chips** (small slivers of glass or nylon that can be coated with genes) enable every gene that is active in a cancer cell to be identified.

Gene therapy involves introducing a normal gene into a person's cells to replace an abnormal disease-producing gene *(see Chapter 21)*. Numerous trials are under way to define gene therapy's applications in the biologic treatment of cancer.

Immune therapy is a recent focus of cancer therapy research. **Vaccines** against lymphoma, prostate cancer, breast cancer, and pancreatic cancer have shown promise in stimulating the immune system to attack cancer cells and extend survival rates. In 2010, the **FDA** approved the first ever tumor vaccine, called Provenge, to treat prostate cancer. Another FDA-approved immunotherapy, Yervoy, is used in metastatic melanoma, but only extends average survival by a few months.

WORD	PRONUNCIATION	ELEMENTS		DEFINITION
angiogenesis	**AN**-jee-oh-**JEN**-eh-sis	S/ R/CF	**-genesis** *formation* **angi/o-** *blood vessel*	New formation of blood vessels
antiangiogenesis	anti-**AN**-jee-oh-**JEN**-eh-sis	P/	**anti-** *against*	The prevention of growth of new blood vessels
biology biologic (adj)	bi-**OL**-oh-jee **BI**-oh-**LOJ**-ik	S/ R/CF	**-logy** *study of* **bi/o-** *life*	Science concerned with life and living organisms
clone	KLOHN		Greek *cutting used for propagation*	A colony of organisms or cells all having identical genetic constitutions
cytotoxic (adj)	sigh-toh-**TOX**-ik	S/ R/CF	**-toxic** *able to kill* **cyt/o-** *cell*	Destructive to cells
microarray (also called gene chips)	**MY**-kroh-ah-**RAY**	P/ R/	**micro-** *small* **-array** *place in order*	Technique for studying one gene in one experiment
monoclonal (adj)	**MON**-oh-**KLO**-nal	S/ P/ R/	**-al** *pertaining to* **mono-** *one* **-clon-** *cutting used for propagation*	Derived from a protein from a single clone of cells, all molecules of which are the same

Exercises

A. Review the above WAD to find the answers to the following questions. *Circle the best answer, and then fill in the blanks.*   **LO 20.7**

1. The term containing a combining form that means *blood vessel* is

   hemolysis   angiogenesis   environmental

2. The prefix in this term means *one*:

   biologic   dioxin   monoclonal

3. The suffix in this term means *study of*:

   microarray   biology   brachytherapy

4. The suffix in this term means *able to kill*:

   cytotoxic   pnemonectomy   biologic

5. The term containing a word element that means *small* is

   lobectomy   stereotactic   microarray

6. The term that does NOT contain a prefix is

   biology   monoclonal   microarray

B. Test your recall of terms from previous chapters. *List as many terms as you can that have the suffix **-logy**, and give a brief definition of each term.*   **LO 20.1**

1. _____ means _____.

2. _____ means _____.

3. _____ means _____.

4. _____ means _____.

5. _____ means _____.

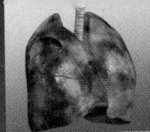

Cancer

Challenge Your Knowledge

A. **Prefixes.** Not every medical term will have a prefix; but when they do, it is an extra clue for you in determining the meaning of the term. Fill in the meaning of the prefix; then give an example of a medical term with that prefix and write the meaning of the term. (You may also use terms from previous chapters, but be prepared to define them.) (**LO 20.1,** *Remember*)

Prefix	Meaning of Prefix	Medical Term with This Prefix	Meaning of Term
apo	1.	2.	3.
di	4.	5.	6.
hyper	7.	8.	9.
meso	10.	11.	12.
meta	13.	14.	15.
micro	16.	17.	18.
mono	19.	20.	21.
neo	22.	23.	24.
peri	25.	26.	27.
pro	28.	29.	30.
proto	31.	32.	33.

B. **Roots.** Deconstruct the following medical terms by slashing (/) the elements. Define only the roots/combining forms in every term. <u>The first one is done for you.</u> Fill in the blanks. (**LO 20.1,** *Remember, Understand*)

Medical Term	Root(s)/Combining Form	Meaning of Root(s)/Combining Form
adeno/carcin/oma	*aden/o; carcin*	*gland; cancer*
mediastinoscopy	1.	2.
neoplastic	3.	4.
cytotoxic	5.	6.
bronchoalveolar	7.	8.
chondrosarcoma	9.	10.
digital	11.	12.
monoclonal	13.	14.
apoptosis	15.	16.
lobectomy	17.	18.
progenitor	19.	20.

C. Deconstruct the following medical terms into basic elements. These elements will be the basis for multiple terms in medical vocabulary. Fill in the chart. Complete the exercise by using any two terms from the chart in sentences of patient documentation. (**LO 20.1,** *Remember, Understand*)

Medical Term	Meaning of Prefix	Meaning of Root/ Combining Form	Meaning of Suffix	Meaning of Medical Term
pathology	1.	2.	3.	4.
neoplasm	5.	6.	7.	8.
infiltrate	9.	10.	11.	12.
carcinogen	13.	14.	15.	16.
metastasis	17.	18.	19.	20.
pneumonectomy	21.	22.	23.	24.
digital	25.	26.	27.	28.
fluoroscopy	29.	30.	31.	32.
oncology	33.	34.	35.	36.

37. Sentence: _____

_____

_____

38. Sentence: _____

_____

_____

D. Suffixes can provide additional information about a medical term. Analyze the suffix in each of the following terms, and use it to provide a clue about the term. Fill in the blanks. (**LO 20.1, 20.6, 20.7,** *Remember, Understand, Apply*)

1. angiogenesis: The suffix is _____ and means _____.

2. neoplasia: The suffix is _____ and means _____.

3. neoplastic: The suffix is _____ and means _____.

4. oncology: The suffix is _____ and means _____.

5. oncologist: The suffix is _____ and means _____.

6. pneumonectomy: The suffix is _____ and means _____.

7. chondrosarcoma: The suffix is _____ and means _____.

8. mediastinoscopy: The suffix is _____ and means _____.

9. scintigraphy: The suffix is _____ and means _____.

E. Study review. Cancer is a class of diseases characterized by uncontrolled cell division. Using the *language of oncology,* fill in this mini-outline and use it for study review. Fill in the blanks. (**LO 20.1, 20.4,** *Understand*)

1. Uncontrolled cell division is caused by damage to a cell's _____.

2. This damage produces _____ to the genes that cause cell division.

3. Damaged genes can be either _____ or _____.

4. Proliferation of damaged cells leads to _____ formation.

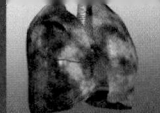

Cancer

F. Compare and contrast benign and malignant tumors to meet a lesson objective. You are given a statement about a tumor. Indicate whether it refers to a benign or malignant tumor by placing a checkmark (√) in the appropriate column. When you have finished the chart, highlight all the statements that pertain to malignant tumors *only*. (**LO 20.3,** *Understand*)

Description of Tumor	Benign	Malignant
1. Grows slowly		
2. Invades the lymph system		
3. Does not metastasize to other organs		
4. Invades the bloodstream and travels to other organs		
5. Lipoma		
6. Surrounded by connective tissue capsule		
7. Can compress surrounding tissues and cause functional problems		
8. Does not invade or infiltrate adjacent tissues		
9. Unlimited, unregulated growth potential		
10. Invades or infiltrates adjacent tissues		
11. Does not spread to lymph nodes		
12. Mesothelioma		

G. Correct usage. Demonstrate your knowledge of the *language of oncology*. These are similar medical terms, but each has only one correct use in the paragraph. Fill in the blanks. (**LO 20.1, 20.3,** *Understand, Apply*)

carcinogen   **carcinoma**   **carcinogenic**   **carcinogenesis**

1. Raquel Sacco was unknowingly exposed to a _____ in the form of secondhand smoke. This

   _____ substance brought about the _____ of her tumors. Her primary

   _____ has already metastasized; her prognosis is poor.

metastasis   **metastasized**   **metastases**   **metastatic**

2. The _____ of Raquel's primary cancer to a secondary site was discovered after diagnostic study.

   The _____ in her brain were not the site of her current surgery. Her _____

   lesions may require radiation therapy if they are inoperable. Since her cancer has already _____,

   her chances of survival are poor.

H. Cancer quiz. Assess your knowledge of this chapter by correctly answering the following questions on cancer. The *language of oncology* will aid your understanding of the questions and possible answers. Circle the correct choice, and remember there is only one *best* answer. (**LO 20.1, 20.3, 20.6,** *Understand, Apply*)

1. Second leading cause of lung cancer (after smoking):

   a. air pollution

   b. radon

   c. chemical toxins

   d. PCBs

   e. particulate matter

2. Used to vacuum out suspicious breast tissue through a needle:

   a. gamma knife

   b. lavage

   c. bronchoscopy

   d. mammatome

   e. mammogram

3. In the TNM staging system for cancer, the "N" stands for

   a. nothing

   b. normal

   c. neoplasm

   d. node

   e. noninvasive

4. SMI treatment will improve

   a. heart rate

   b. blood pressure

   c. inspiratory volume

   d. blood volume

   e. pulse rate

5. Tumor that has invaded or infiltrated has

   a. grown into adjacent tissue

   b. died

   c. become weaker

   d. mutated

   e. necrotized

6. Healthy genes that promote normal cell growth are called

   a. TS genes

   b. mutated TS genes

   c. protooncogenes

   d. mutated genes

   e. receptor genes

7. A benign tumor is

   a. not harmful

   b. cytotoxic

   c. metastatic

   d. necrotic

   e. harmful

8. An early form of carcinoma in which there is no invasion of surrounding tissues is

   a. large cell carcinoma

   b. small cell carcinoma

   c. adenocarcinoma

   d. carcinoma in situ

   e. squamous cell carcinoma

9. The abbreviation PCD means the same as

   a. protooncogene

   b. apoptosis

   c. oncogene

   d. polychlorinated biphenyls

   e. progenitor

10. Washing out of a hollow duct or cavity is

   a. stereotactic biopsy

   b. lavage

   c. curettage

   d. aspiration

   e. gavage

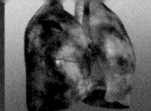

Cancer

I. Abbreviations. Use with care to ensure you are conveying precise information. Demonstrate your knowledge of this chapter's abbreviations by matching them correctly. (**LO 20.1, 20.6,** *Understand, Apply*)

_____ 1. genes normally suppress mitosis   **a.** PCD

_____ 2. injection of radioactive sugar   **b.** SMI

_____ 3. chemical toxin banned years ago   **c.** FOBT

_____ 4. general test for detecting cancer   **d.** PET

_____ 5. performed by respiratory therapist   **e.** AMAS

_____ 6. blood in stool   **f.** MRI

_____ 7. washing process with a scope   **g.** TS

_____ 8. apoptosis   **h.** PCB

_____ 9. detailed images in planes   **i.** BAL

J. Procedures. There are many different procedures associated with cancer diagnosis and treatment. Can you correctly identify these procedures used for cancer patients? Circle the best choice. (**LO 20.1, 20.7,** *Understand, Apply*)

1. The surgery Mrs. Sacco had at the site of her primary cancer:

     pneumonectomy   bronchoscopy   lobectomy

2. Examination of the pleural cavity with an endoscope:

     thoracoscopy   cystoscopy   bronchoscopy

3. Use of a chilled probe to destroy early cancer cells:

     brachytherapy   chemotherapy   cryosurgery

4. Fiber-optic tube with a camera is inserted into the chest:

     computed tomography   mediastinoscopy   fluoroscopy

5. Implants radioactive seeds into the tumor for direct radiation:

     brachytherapy   CHART   scintigraphy

6. Removal of only a small part of the lung; used for carcinoma in situ:

     SRS   segmentectomy   pneumonectomy

7. Creates three-dimensional images of a lesion for accurate insertion of a needle:

     PET scan   stereotactic guided biopsy   ductal lavage

8. Removal of an entire lung:

     lobectomy   segmentectomy   pneumonectomy

9. Employed for cutting tissue, collecting brushings, and washings in the lung:

     bronchoscopy   scintigraphy   chest x-ray

10. More effective than chest x-rays at identifying early tumors:

     CT   PET   MRI

K. Build your knowledge of elements with this exercise in the language of oncology. The element is given to you in the left column; fill in the meaning of the element in the middle column, and identify the type of element (prefix, root, combining form, or suffix) in the right column. Then combine the correct elements to form one medical term , and write a definition for that term. Fill in the blanks. (**LO 20.4, *Understand, Apply***)

Element	Meaning of Element	Type of Element (P, R, CF, S)
proto	1. _____	2. _____
apo	3. _____	4. _____
muta	5. _____	6. _____
genesis	7. _____	8. _____
gen	9. _____	10. _____
onco	11. _____	12. _____
carcino	13. _____	14. _____
ptosis	15. _____	16. _____
gene	17. _____	18. _____

19. Term: _____

20. Definition: _____

L. Patient education. Explain to your patient the difference between a benign and a malignant neoplasm. (**LO 20.3, *Apply***)

1. benign:

_____

_____

2. malignant:

_____

_____

Write a sentence of patient documentation using either the term benign or the term malignant.

3. Sentence: _____

_____

_____

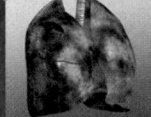
Cancer

M. **Elements.** You are given the meaning of the element. Circle the correct term in which it appears. **(LO 20.1, 20.2, *Apply, Analyze*)**

1. The root meaning *surroundings* is in the term

    environment   dioxin   pollution

2. The suffix meaning *produce* is in the term

    carcinogen   pesticide   particle

3. The prefix meaning *new* is in the term

    proliferate   neoplastic   dioxin

4. The suffix meaning *to kill* is in the term

    aminoketone   pollution   pesticide

5. The suffix meaning *pertaining to* is in the term

    pollution   environmental   hemostasis

6. The prefix meaning *two* is in the term

    pesticide   dioxin   monoclonal

7. The combining form meaning *chest* is in the term

    fluoroscopy   thoracoscopy   endoscopy

8. The root meaning *flesh* is in the term

    sarcoma   hematoma   carcinoma

N. **Elements can provide a clue to the origin of a tumor.** Analyze the medical terms in the left column, and match them to the cancer source in the right column. **(LO 20.3, 20.4, *Apply, Analyze*)**

Medical Term	Cancer Arises From
_____ 1. mesothelioma	a. epithelial cells
_____ 2. sarcoma	b. lymph nodes
_____ 3. adenocarcinoma	c. cells lining pleural cavity
_____ 4. osteosarcoma	d. connective tissue cells
_____ 5. melanoma	e. glandular epithelial cells
_____ 6. chondrosarcoma	f. skeletal muscle
_____ 7. carcinoma	g. bone-forming cells
_____ 8. lymphoma	h. pigment-producing skin cells
_____ 9. rhabdomyosarcoma	i. cartilage cells

O. Terminology challenge. All of the following medical terms have the same ending, but one term is slightly different in meaning from the others. Find the term, and explain why it is different, even though it appears the same. (**LO 20.1, 20.2, 20.3,** *Analyze*)

lymphoma   **melanoma**   **hematoma**   **carcinoma**   **sarcoma**

1. The term is _____.

2. It is different because:

_____

_____.

P. Commonalities. Analyze the following medical terms, and discover what they all have in common. Circle the correct answer. (**LO 20.6, 20.7,** *Analyze*)

1. Lobectomy, segmentectomy, and mastectomy are all

   diagnoses   procedures   diagnostic tests

2. Chondrosarcoma, adenocarcinoma, and osteosarcoma are all

   neoplasms   genes   flavonoids

3. PET, MRI, and CT are all

   blood tests   diagnostic tests   surgeries

4. Thoracoscopy, bronchoscopy, and mediastinoscopy are all

   chest procedures   pelvic procedures   abdominal procedures

5. Pathologist, oncologist, and histologist are all

   diseases   specialists   conditions

Q. Procedures. An important distinction to learn about procedures is understanding which ones are diagnostic (used to determine a diagnosis) and which ones are therapeutic (carry out treatment). Analyze the following list of medical terms and abbreviations to determine whether they are diagnostic or therapeutic procedures. Place a checkmark (√) in the appropriate column of the chart. (**LO 20.7,** *Analyze*)

Procedure	Diagnostic	Therapeutic
1. segmentectomy		
2. BAL		
3. brachytherapy		
4. DRE		
5. stereotactic biopsy		
6. pneumonectomy		
7. ductal lavage		
8. mediastinoscopy		
9. CHART		

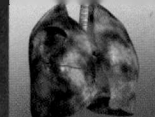

Cancer

R. Abbreviations. Transcribe into plain English the following physician orders with abbreviations. Patient safety depends on your precise interpretation of these orders. Fill in the blanks. (**LO 20.1, 20.2, _Analyze_**)

1. Patient's next yearly physical should include DRE and FOBT.

   _____

   _____

   _____

   _____

2. Schedule patient for a bronchoscopy with BAL.

   _____

   _____

   _____

   _____

3. Patient's blood work should include CEA and AMAS analysis.

   _____

   _____

   _____

   _____

4. Treatment plan includes eventual CHART or SRS after conclusion of chemotherapy.

   _____

   _____

   _____

   _____

5. I am referring this patient to the NCI for a clinical trial using MOABs for her CA.

   _____

   _____

   _____

   _____

S. Case Report. The following exercise is based entirely on the Case Report of Raquel Sacco, which was presented in this chapter. (**LO 20.1, 20.7, *Analyze***)

1. Reread this entire Case Report out loud to yourself for pronunciation practice. The medical terms you should pay particular attention to have been underlined.

2. Utilize your knowledge of the *language of oncology* (and previous chapters) to answer the following questions based on the Case Report. Fill in the blanks.

Case Report 20.1

You are

... an advanced-level <u>respiratory</u> <u>therapist</u> employed by Fulwood Medical Center, working with Tavis Senko, MD, a <u>pulmonologist.</u>

Your patient is

... Raquel Sacco, a 44-year-old mother of two teenage boys, who is the owner of a quilting fabrics store. She is 2 days postop from a lung surgery for non-small cell lung cancer. From her records, you see that she has two <u>secondary</u> <u>metastases</u> in her brain. She has been a nonsmoker all her life. Her 70-year-old father is a two-pack-a-day smoker, as is her husband. They both show no evidence of cancer on chest x-rays. Before Raquel is discharged, as part of her <u>postoperative</u> respiratory care plan you are using <u>incentive spirometry</u>—also called <u>sustained maximal inspiration</u> (SMI)—to increase her <u>inspiratory</u> volume and improve her inspiratory muscle performance. You will also be taking an <u>arterial</u> blood sample to check her arterial oxygen pressure (PaO_2).

<u>Adenocarcinoma</u> was found in Raquel Sacco. It was <u>diagnosed</u> because she had a <u>seizure,</u> and <u>neurologic</u> tests revealed the presence of two metastases in her brain, leading to a search for the <u>primary</u> tumor that was found in her lung. Raquel Sacco probably developed her lung cancer as a result of inhaling <u>secondhand</u> smoke all her life (from her father and husband). Because Raquel Sacco's cancer has <u>metastasized</u> to her brain, she is placed in stage IV. The outlook for Mrs. Sacco is bleak.

Non-Small Cell Lung Cancer Survival

Stage	5-Year Relative Survival Rate
I	47%
II	26%
III	8%
IV	2%

1. What is the meaning of the term *postoperative*? _____

_____

2. Does Mrs. Sacco have a personal history of smoking? _____

3. Is there anyone in her immediate family with a history of cancer? _____

_____

4. Define *metastases*. _____

5. Where did the metastases appear? _____

_____

6. Are the metastases the 1° or 2° cancer? _____

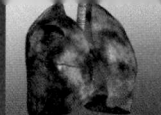

Cancer

7. Where does her 1° cancer originate? _____

8. What specific type of cancer is the 1° cancer? _____

9. What problem first brought Mrs. Sacco to the doctor? _____

10. What stage of cancer has Mrs. Sacco been diagnosed with? _____

11. Why is her prognosis bleak? _____

T. Short answers based on Case Report 20.1. (LO 20.1, 20.7, *Analyze*)

1. What is the purpose of the SMI spirometry?

   _____

   _____

   _____

2. Explain the phrase "secondhand smoke."

   _____

   _____

   _____

3. Explain the phrase "two-pack-a-day smoker."

   _____

   _____

   _____

4. How can a nonsmoker get lung cancer?

   _____

   _____

   _____

5. Record your thoughts or comments about this patient's case.

   _____

   _____

   _____

CHAPTER SUMMARY EXERCISE

A. Spelling comprehension. Circle the correct spelling of the term. (**LO 20.1,** *Remember*)

1. fluoroscopy	flueroscopy	fluorroscopy	foroscopy	floroscopy
2. apotosis	apoptosis	apoptossis	apotosus	apoptossus
3. regiment	regimen	regeemen	regimin	regimine
4. radionuclede	radionuklide	radeonuclide	rodeonuclide	radionuclide
5. levage	leevage	lavage	levege	laevage
6. porliferate	porlifferate	proliferate	proleferate	porleferate
7. metastasis	metassasis	mettasasis	meatus	metasasis
8. neoplasea	nioplasia	neoplasis	neoplasia	nioplassia
9. cytotoxic	sytotoxic	cyttotoxic	cytotoxsic	cytoxic
10. steeriotactic	stereotactic	steeriotaxic	steriotaxic	stereotaxic

B. Match the number of the correct terms in Exercise A with the following brief descriptions. (LO 20.1, 20.2, *Understand, Apply*)

a. Radioactive agent used in diagnostic imaging _____

b. Examination of the body with x-rays _____

c. Destructive to cells _____

d. Program of treatment _____

e. Process and growth of a tumor _____

f. To wash _____

g. Spread of cancer cells _____

h. Increase in number by reproducing _____

i. PCD _____

j. Three-dimensional method of locating lesions _____

C. Using your knowledge of terms 1–10 in Exercise A and their correct spelling, write a brief sentence for each of the terms as it might appear in patient documentation. (LO 20.1, *Apply*)

1. _____

2. _____

3. _____

4. _____

5. _____

6. _____

7. _____

8. _____

9. _____

10. _____

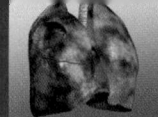

Cancer

D. **To meet learning outcomes, be prepared to discuss the following questions in class.** Be sure you can spell and pronounce each medical term correctly. (**LO 20.1, 20.2,** *Apply*)

1. Explain the role of environmental factors in carcinogenesis.

_____

_____

2. Classify the type of cancer by the type of cell from which it originates.

_____

_____

3. List methods of cancer prevention.

_____

_____

4. What types of self-examination should be employed to detect cancer?

_____

_____

5. Describe some methods of screening for cancer. _____

_____

6. What therapies are currently available for treating cancer?

_____

E. **Meet the goals of each of the chapter outcomes by using the correct language of oncology for the answers.** (**LO 20.1–20.7,** *Analyze*)

1. Use the medical terms of oncology so that you communicate and document in writing accurately and precisely in any health care setting. Finish the clinical note by filling in the blank. Proofread the following sentence for errors in fact and/or spelling. Rewrite the sentence with corrections. (**LO 20.1**)

   Mesothilioma is a rare tumor of the cells lining the plura. It is associated with asbesstosis and accounts for 10% of lung cancers.

   Corrected sentence: _____

   _____

2. Use the medical terms of oncology to communicate verbally with accuracy and precision in any health care setting. Your patient has asked you how pollution can trigger cancer. Explain that to him in layman's language. (**LO 20.2**)

   _____

   _____

   _____

   _____

3. Discuss the different types of cancer. Compare and contrast *osteosarcoma* and *mesothelioma*. (**LO 20.3**)

   a. osteosarcoma: _____

   _____

   b. mesothelioma: _____

   _____

4. Describe the types of genes and their mutations that are involved in carcinogenesis. Two types of genes have been identified that play a part in abnormal cell development. Name those genes and discuss how they operate in the cancer process. (**LO 20.4**)

   a. Genes: _____

   _____

   b. How they operate in the cancer process: _____

   _____

5. Identify environmental pollutants involved as triggers of cancer. Choose any two environmental pollutants involved as triggers of cancer and briefly discuss/describe them. (**LO 20.5**)

   a. _____

   _____

   b. _____

   _____

6. Describe different methods of detecting cancer. Which of the following is NOT a method of detecting cancer? Circle the correct answer. (**LO 20.6**)

   a. palpation

   b. DRE

   c. PSA

   d. mammogram

   e. amniocentesis

7. Discuss different methods of treating cancer. What type of radiotherapy can be considered "bloodless surgery," and why? (**LO 20.7**)

   _____

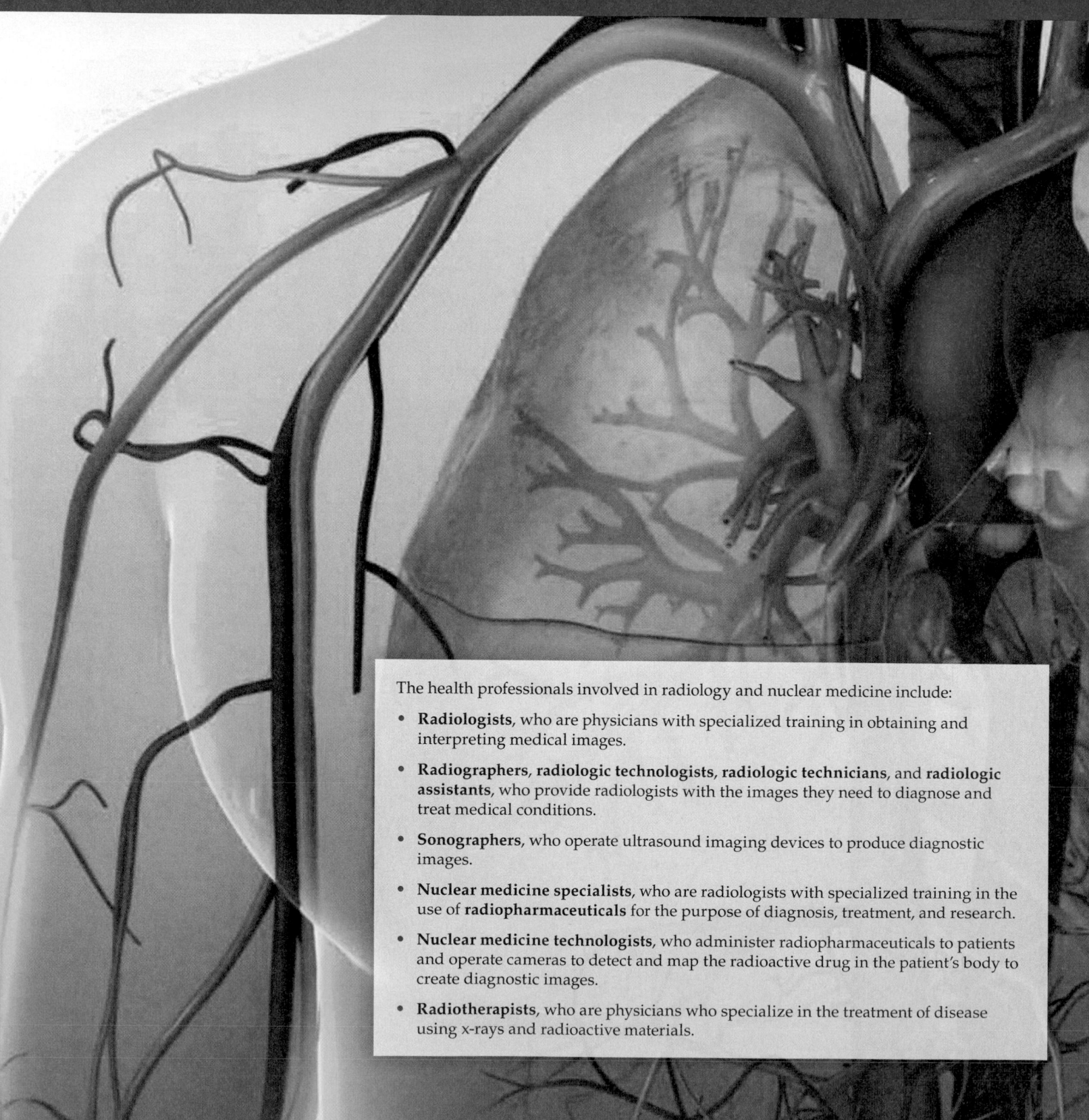

Radiology and Nuclear Medicine
The Language of Medical Imaging

The health professionals involved in radiology and nuclear medicine include:

- **Radiologists**, who are physicians with specialized training in obtaining and interpreting medical images.

- **Radiographers**, **radiologic technologists**, **radiologic technicians**, and **radiologic assistants**, who provide radiologists with the images they need to diagnose and treat medical conditions.

- **Sonographers**, who operate ultrasound imaging devices to produce diagnostic images.

- **Nuclear medicine specialists**, who are radiologists with specialized training in the use of **radiopharmaceuticals** for the purpose of diagnosis, treatment, and research.

- **Nuclear medicine technologists**, who administer radiopharmaceuticals to patients and operate cameras to detect and map the radioactive drug in the patient's body to create diagnostic images.

- **Radiotherapists**, who are physicians who specialize in the treatment of disease using x-rays and radioactive materials.

21

Case Report (CR) 21.1

You are

... Anita Scherraga, a radiologic technologist working in the radiology department at Fulwood Medical Center.

Your patient is

... Mrs. Carole Coffrey, a 46-year-old health information technologist with two children who is complaining of pain in her breasts. You are to perform a **mammogram** on Mrs. Coffrey using parallel-plate compression in a full-field digital **mammography (FFDM)** unit. You will be taking two views of Mrs. Coffrey's breasts, a head-to-foot (**craniocaudal [CC]**) and an angled side view (**mediolateral oblique [MLO]**).

Chapter Learning Outcomes

Radiology is a medical specialty that uses imaging techniques to diagnose and treat disease that can be visualized within the human body. **Nuclear medicine** is a branch of medical imaging that uses **radioactive** material to pinpoint **molecular** activity within the body in order to diagnose and treat a variety of diseases. The information in this chapter will enable you to:

LO 21.1 Use the medical terms of radiology to communicate and document in writing accurately and precisely in any health care setting.

LO 21.2 Use the medical terms of radiology to communicate verbally with accuracy and precision in any health care setting.

LO 21.3 Describe the nature and characteristics of x-rays.

LO 21.4 Identify the positions and views of the patient's body used in x-ray examinations.

LO 21.5 Discuss the different techniques for acquiring radiologic diagnostic images.

LO 21.6 Describe the nature and characteristics of radioactive materials used in medical imaging.

LO 21.7 Discuss the nuclear imaging procedures used in the diagnosis of disease.

LO 21.8 Explain the different radiologic techniques used in the treatment of disease.

LO 21.9 Describe the different nuclear medicine therapies and their effectiveness.

LESSON OBJECTIVES

X-rays were first discovered in 1895 by Wilhelm Conrad Röntgen. These x-rays, like light and radio waves, are a form of electromagnetic radiation. The information in this lesson will enable you to:

21.1.1 Discuss the wavelength characteristics of x-rays.

21.1.2 Describe how x-rays interact with and affect matter.

21.1.3 Explain how x-ray images are recorded.

21.1.4 Describe the different alignments of the body in order to produce the most informative x-ray image.

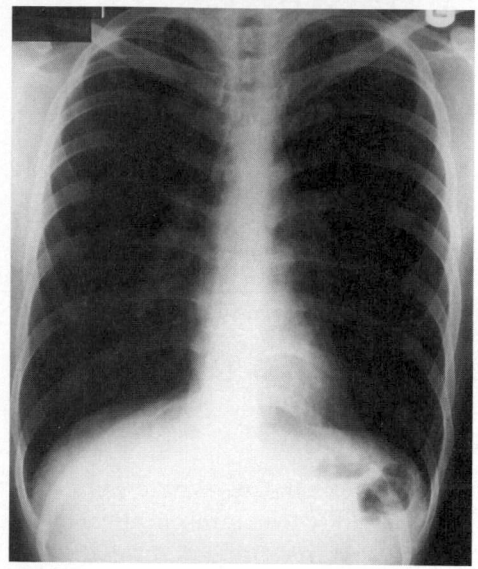

▲ **Figure 21.1** X-ray Image of a Female Chest.

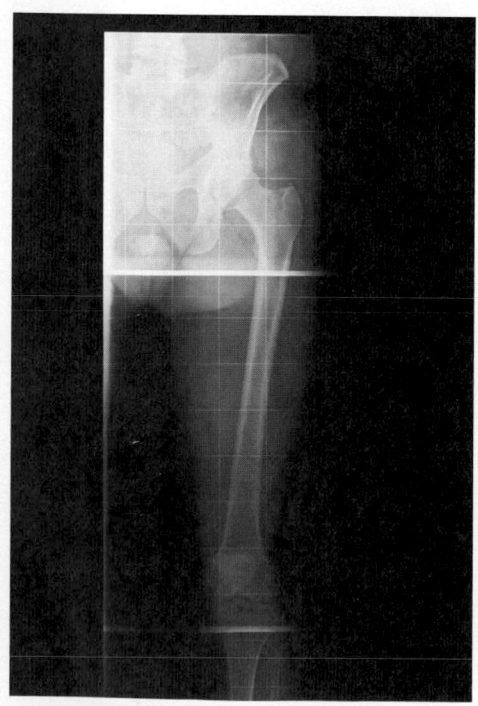

▲ **Figure 21.2** X-ray Image of Femur.

LO 21.3 X-ray Characteristics and Effects

The characteristics of x-rays include

- **Velocity.** Because they are electromagnetic, x-rays in a vacuum travel at the speed of light, 186,000 miles per second. This velocity is reduced as x-rays penetrate the different substances of the body according to their density.

- **Wavelength.** X-rays have a very short wavelength compared with other electromagnetic waveforms. Only gamma rays from an atomic explosion have a shorter wavelength. This short wavelength is a major factor in enabling x-rays to pass through many materials and tissues to different degrees. Air is the most **radiolucent** and allows the greatest penetration (photographic plates show black, *Figure 21.1*). Fat is denser than air, water is more dense, and bone is the most dense (**radiopaque**) (photographic plates show white, *Figure 21.2*).

- **Invisibility.** X-rays cannot be detected by sight, sound, or touch, so health professionals working in radiology wear a film badge to detect and record radiation to which they are exposed *(Figure 21.3)*.

- **Ionization.** An **ion** is an atom or group of atoms carrying an electric charge by having gained or lost one or more electrons. When x-rays **ionize** matter, they can both kill cancerous cells and damage normal cells to produce the side effects of radiation as well as genetic mutations that cause malignant changes. Radiation can also cause damage to a fetus, so the use of x-rays in pregnancy is kept to a minimum.

Recording of X-ray Images

A special type of photographic film is used to record x-ray pictures. The x-rays are converted into light, and the more energy that passes through body tissues to reach the photographic film or plate, the darker that region of film will be. Lungs will be dark; bones that prevent the passage of energy will be white. X-rays can now also be detected electronically using a recorder similar to that used in a digital camera. This means that they can be read immediately and stored more easily.

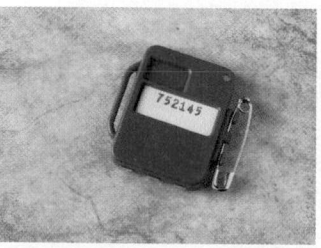

▲ **Figure 21.3** Radiation Monitor. Film badge used to determine a person's exposure to radiation. The badge is worn on a person's clothing and contains a piece of photographic film. Radiation affects the film in a similar way to light.

Abbreviations	
CC	craniocaudal
FFDM	full-field digital mammography
MLO	mediolateral oblique

Word Analysis and Definition

S = Suffix   P = Prefix   R = Root   R/CF = Combining Form

WORD	PRONUNCIATION	ELEMENTS		DEFINITION
craniocaudal	KRAY-nee-oh-KAW-dal	S/ R/ R/CF	-al *pertaining to* -caud- *tail* crani/o *skull*	A view of a structure from head to foot
electromagnetic	ee-LEK-troh-mag-NET-ik	S/ R/CF R/	-ic *pertaining to* electr/o- *electricity* -magnet- *magnet*	Pertaining to energy propagated through matter and space
ion	EYE-on		Greek *going*	An atom or group of atoms having gained or lost one or more electrons
ionization (noun)		S/ R/	-ization *process of affecting in a specific way* ion- *atom or group of atoms carrying an electric charge*	The process of causing an atom or group of atoms to gain or lose one or more electrons
ionize (verb)		S/	-ize *to affect in a specific way*	To cause the process of ionization
mammogram	MAM-oh gram	S/ R/CF	-gram *a record* mamm/o *breast*	The x-ray record produced by mammography
mammography	mah-MOG-rah-fee	S/	-graphy *process of recording*	X-ray imaging of the breast
mediolateral oblique	MEE-dee-oh-LAT-er-al oh-BLEEK	S/ R/ P/	-al *pertaining to* -later- *side* medio- *middle* oblique Latin *slanting*	An angled side view of a structure
radioactive	RAY-dee-oh-AK-tiv	R/CF R/CF	radi/o- *radiation* -active *movement*	Spontaneously emitting alpha, beta, or gamma rays
radiograph	RAY-dee-oh-graf	S/ R/CF	-graph *record* radi/o- *radiation*	Image made by exposure to x-rays
radiographer radiographic	ray-dee-OG-rah-fer ray-dee-oh-GRAF-ik	S/ S/	-er *one who records* -ic *pertaining to*	Technologist who performs x-ray procedures Pertaining to x-rays
radiology	ray-dee-OLL-oh-jee	S/ R/CF	-logy *study of* radi/o- *radiation*	The study of medical imaging
radiologic radiologist	ray-dee-oh-LOJ-ik ray-dee-OL-oh jist	S/ S/	-ic *pertaining to* -logist *specialist*	Pertaining to radiology Specialist in radiology
radiolucent	ray-dee-oh-LOO-sent	S/ R/CF	-lucent *open* radi/o- *radiation*	Penetrable by x-rays or other forms of radiation
radiopaque	ray-dee-oh-PAKE	S/	-paque *shady*	Impenetrable to x-rays or other forms of radiation
radiopharmaceutical	RAY-dee-oh-far-mah-SOO-tik-al	S/ S/ R/CF R/CF	-ical *pertaining to* -ceut- *relating to* radi/o *radiation* -pharm/a- *drug industry*	Relating to a product produced by the drug industry that is radioactive
radiotherapist	RAY-dee-oh-THER-ah-pist	S/ R/CF	-ist *specialist* radi/o- *radiation*	Specialist in the use of radiation in the treatment of patients
radiotherapy	RAY-dee-oh-THER-ah-pee	R/	-therap- *treatment*	Treatment using radiation

Exercises

A. Answer the following questions about the characteristics of x-rays. *Circle the correct answer.*   **LO 21.1, 21.3**

1. Which of the following is not a characteristic of an x-ray?

   a. velocity

   b. wavelength

   c. ionization

   d. invisibility

   e. weight

2. Which of the following characteristics of x-rays is most damaging to a fetus?

   a. velocity

   b. radiation

   c. wavelength

   d. ionization

   e. speed

3. X-rays in a vacuum travel at the speed of light. This is called

   a. wavelength

   b. radiolucent

   c. velocity

   d. radiopaque

   e. invisibility

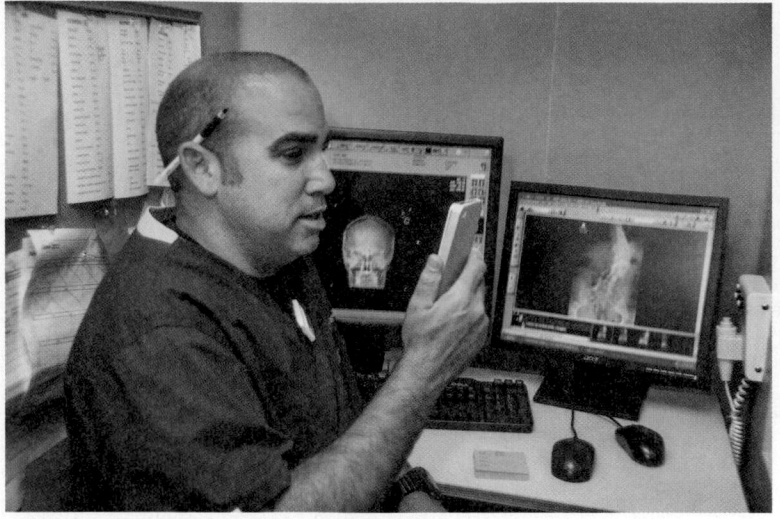

▲ **Figure 21.4** Radiologist Dictates a Report.

LO 21.4 Alignment

In many situations where x-ray images are taken, the x-ray tube that produces the radiation, the patient, and the photographic film must be aligned to direct the x-ray beam to the lesion being examined in the best possible way. Terms describing the direction of the projection of x-ray beams are of importance in chest x-rays and are

- **Posteroanterior (PA)** in which x-rays travel from a posterior source to an anteriorly placed image receiver. This is the most common chest x-ray view.

- **Anteroposterior (AP)** in which x-rays travel from an anterior source to a posteriorly placed image receiver.

- **Lateral view.** In a left lateral view, x-rays travel from a source located to the right of a patient and travel to an image recorder to the left of the patient. This is reversed in a right lateral view.

- **Oblique view in which** x-rays travel at an angle from the perpendicular plane and pass behind the heart and lung hilum to show structures normally hidden in PA and AP views.

The terms *anterior* and *posterior* and other directional terms are described in *Chapter 4*.

LO 21.5 Acquisition of Radiologic Images

Plain (Projectional) Radiography

Plain radiography was the only modality available in the first 50 years of radiology. The x-rays that pass through a patient strike an undeveloped film held in a light-tight cassette. The film is then developed chemically to produce an image on the film. Now, **digital radiography (DR)** is replacing film screen radiography; x-rays strike a plate of sensors which converts the signals generated into digital information and an image on a computer screen. Because of its lower cost and availability, plain radiography is the first-line examination of choice in radiologic diagnosis *(Figure 21.4)*. Lead aprons can be used to protect patients and technicians from receiving unwanted radiation.

Fluoroscopy

In **fluoroscopy** a continuous x-ray image is shown on a monitor like an x-ray movie. This allows real-time imaging of structures in motion, for example, blood vessels or the gastrointestinal (**GI**) tract. **Radiocontrast** agents, such as barium sulfate and iodine, are administered orally, rectally, intravenously, or into an artery and enhance the real-time imaging of dynamic processes such as blood flow in arteries and veins (**angiography**) or peristalsis in the GI tract. Iodine contrast may also be concentrated in tumors, cysts, or inflamed areas to make them more opaque and conspicuous in imaging. A barium meal *(Figure 21.5)*, also known as an upper gastrointestinal series, enables radiographs of the esophagus, stomach, and duodenum to be taken after barium sulfate is ingested. However, the diagnostic use of a barium meal has declined with the increasing use of esophagogastroduodenoscopy, which allows direct visual inspection of suspicious areas in the esophagus, stomach, and duodenum.

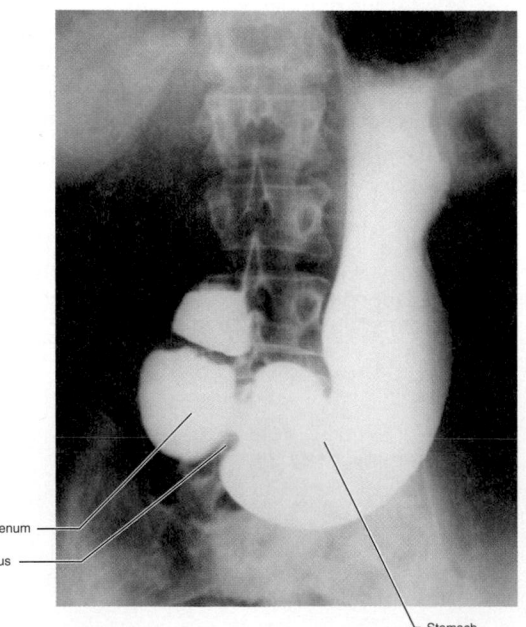

Duodenum

Pylorus

Stomach

▲ **Figure 21.5** Barium Meal Showing Stomach, Pylorus, and Duodenum.

Word Analysis and Definition

S = Suffix   P = Prefix   R = Root   R/CF = Combining Form

WORD	PRONUNCIATION	ELEMENTS		DEFINITION
angiography	an-jee-**OG**-rah-fee	S/ R/CF	**-graphy** *process of recording* **angi/o** *blood vessel*	Radiography of blood vessels after injection of contrast material
angiogram angioplasty	**AN**-jee-oh-gram **AN**-jee-oh-**PLS**-tee	S/ S/	**-gram** *a record* **-plasty** *formation*	The radiograph obtained by angiography Recanalization of a blood vessel by surgery
anteroposterior	**AN**-teh-roh-**POS**-ter-ee-or	S/ R/ R/CF	**-ior** *pertaining to* **-poster-** *coming behind* **anter/o-** *coming before*	The direction the x-ray beam passes through the patient from front to back (AP)
fluoroscopy	flor-**OS**-koh-pee	S/ R/CF	**-scopy** *to examine* **fluor/o** *x-ray beam*	Examination of the structures of the body by x-rays
oblique	ob-**LEEK**		Latin *slanting*	Slanting; in radiology, a projection that is neither frontal nor lateral
opaque	oh-**PAKE**		Latin shady	Impervious to light; impenetrable by x-rays or other forms of radiation
posteroanterior	**POS**-ter-oh-**AN**-ter-ee-or	S/ R/CF R/	**-ior** *pertaining to* **poster/o -** *coming behind* **-anter-** *coming before*	The direction the x-ray beam passes through the patient from back to front (PA)
radiocontrast	**RAY**-dee-oh-**CON**-trast	S/ S/ R/CF	**-st** *to stand* **-contra** *against* **radi/o** *radiation*	Agents that make structures stand out in x-ray imaging

Exercises

A. Use the new medical language you are learning in this chapter to answer the following questions.   LO 21.1, 21.3, 21.4, 21.5

1. What is the purpose of contrast?

_____

2. What is the difference between oblique and opaque?

   a. oblique: _____

   b. opaque: _____

3. How can these aid in diagnosis?

_____

_____

B. Using the three medical terms below, insert the appropriate medical terms into the paragraph.   LO 21.1, 21.5

   angioplasty   angiogram   angiography

1. The doctor is using _____ as a diagnostic tool. After seeing the _____, he has decided to schedule the patient for a surgical procedure. He has asked you to schedule the patient's _____ for tomorrow morning.

2. Which two terms in the above WAD box are opposites? _____ and _____ are opposites.

3. What do they describe? _____

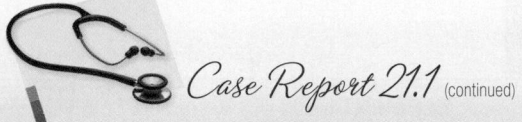
Mrs. Coffrey's mammogram report was sent to her in writing. It reads, "There are scattered **fibroglandular** densities bilaterally. There is a benign-appearing area of glandular tissue in the right lower inner breast. There are a few faint calcifications in the lower inner and central left breast. There is no associated mass or distortion."

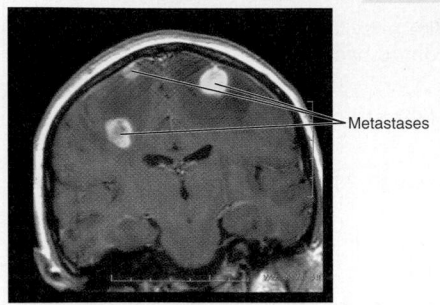

▲ **Figure 21.6** MRI of Brain Showing Metastases.

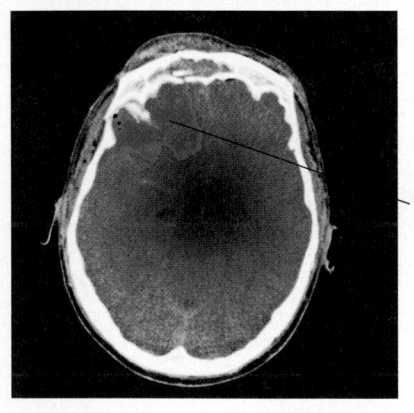

▲ **Figure 21.7** Brain Hemorrhage, Colored Computed Tomography (CT) Scan. The front of the brain is at top, and a large mass of blood (hematoma, purple) is seen at upper left in the frontal lobe. Bleeding (hemorrhage) in the brain occurs when a blood vessel, such as an artery, ruptures. It may be caused by a head injury, high blood pressure, or vascular disease. In this case a tree fell on the patient's head. The area of the brain supplied by the ruptured artery may die due to lack of oxygenated blood, leading to a stroke.

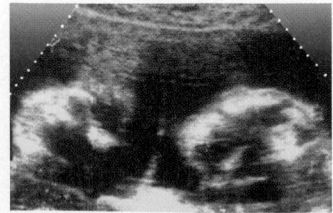

▲ **Figure 21.8** Twins, Ultrasound Biometry.

LO 21.1, 21.5 Acquisition of Radiologic Images (continued)

Interventional Radiology

Interventional radiology (**IR**) uses minimally invasive procedures both for diagnostic purposes (e.g., angiogram) and for treatment (e.g., **angioplasty**). X-ray images are used for guidance, and the basic instruments used are needles and catheters. The images provide a road map to enable the instruments to be guided to the areas containing disease for diagnosis and for treatment. Benefits from these procedures include short recovery time, shortened hospital stays, reduced infection rates, and reduced costs.

Computed Tomography

The first commercially viable computed tomography (CT) scanner was produced at EMI Labs in England in 1972. EMI owned the rights to the Beatles music, and their profits funded the research. CT scans use x-rays in conjunction with computer **algorithms** to produce a computer-generated cross-sectional image (**tomogram**) in the **axial** plane. From these images, the computer can reconstruct **coronal** and **sagittal** images. Radio-contrast agents can be used with CT to enhance the delineation of anatomy. CT scans have become the test of choice in diagnosing some emergency conditions such as cerebral hemorrhage (*Figure 21.7*), pulmonary embolism (*see Chapter 13*), aortic dissection (*see Chapter 10*), kidney stones (*see Chapter 6*) and in identifying small lung cancers (*see Chapter 13*). Unfortunately, CT scans expose the patient to much more ionizing radiation than does an x-ray.

Ultrasound

Medical **ultrasonography** uses **ultrasound** (high-frequency sound waves) functioning in real time to visualize soft tissue structures in the body No ionizing radiation is involved. Because of this, it plays a vital role in obstetrics, enabling early diagnosis of fetal abnormalities and multiple gestations (*Figure 21.8*). Ultrasound measures the severity of peripheral vascular disease and evaluates the dynamic function of the heart, heart valves, and major blood vessels. In trauma victims it can also assess the integrity of the major viscera (including liver, spleen, and kidneys) and the presence of bleeding into the peritoneum.

Magnetic Resonance Imaging

Magnetic Resonance Imaging (**MRI**) uses strong magnetic fields to align atomic nuclei in tissues, then uses a radio signal to disrupt the nuclei and observes the radio frequency signal as the nuclei return to their baseline states. MRI can produce images in axial, coronal, sagittal, and oblique planes and can also give the best soft tissue contrast of all imaging modalities. It is an important tool in musculoskeletal radiology and neuroradiology (*Figure 21.6*). Its disadvantages are that the patient has to lie in a noisy, confined space (tube) for long periods of time, and it cannot be used for patients with pacemakers or any metallic implant such as artificial joints or implanted surgical hardware (plates, rods etc.). For patients with **claustrophobia**, anti-anxiety medication can be prescribed to be taken before entering the scanner.

Teleradiology involves the transmission of radiographic digital images from one location to another for interpretation by a radiologist. It can provide real-time emergency radiology services and expert consultation round the clock.

Abbreviations	
CT	computed tomography
IR	interventional radiology
MRI	magnetic resonance imaging

Word Analysis and Definition

S = Suffix   P = Prefix   **R = Root**   **R/CF = Combining Form**

WORD	PRONUNCIATION	ELEMENTS		DEFINITION
algorithm	**AL**-go-rithm		**Greek** *number*	A process of steps to solve a problem, each depending on the outcome of the previous one
axis axial (adj)	**AXE**-is **ACK**-see-al		**Greek** *central support*	A line of central support Pertaining to an axis
claustrophobia	klaw-stroh-**FOH**-be-ah	S/ R/CF	-phobia *fear* **claustr/o** *confined space*	Pathologic fear of being trapped in a confined space
coronal	**COR**-oh-nal	S/ R/	-al *pertaining to* **coron-** *crown*	Vertical plane dividing the body into anterior and posterior portions
fibroglandular	fi-bro-**GLAN**-dyu-lar	S/ R/CF R/	-ar *pertaining to* **fibr/o-** *fiber* -glandul- *little gland*	A mixture of fibrous and glandular tissue
interventional	**IN**-ter-**VEN**-shun-al	S/ R/	-al *pertaining to* **intervention-** *to come between*	Pertaining to an overt act to change an event or outcome
sagittal	**SAJ**-ih-tal	S/ R/	-al *pertaining to* **sagitt-** *arrow*	Pertaining to the vertical plane dividing the body into right and left portions
teleradiology	**TEL**-eh-ray-dee-**OL**-oh-jee	S/ P/ R/CF	-logy *study of* tele- *distant* **radi/o** *radiation, x-ray*	The interpretation of digitized diagnostic images transmitted from a distance
tomogram tomography	**TOE**-moh-gram toe-**MOG**-rah-fee	S/ R/CF S/	-gram *writing* **tom/o-** *section* -graphy *process of recording*	Radiographic image of a selected section or slice of tissue Process of taking a tomogram
ultrasound ultrasonography	**UL**-trah-sound **ULL**-trah-soh-**NOG**-rah-fee	P/ R/ R/CF S/	ultra- *higher, beyond* -sound *noise* -son/o *sound* -graphy *process of recording*	Very high frequency sound waves Delineation of dynamic structures using sound waves

Exercises

A. Analyze the continuation of the Case Report for Mrs. Coffrey, and then answer the following questions. LO 21.1, 21.5, 21.8

1. On the lines below, write all the medical terms contained in the Case Report above.

_____

_____

2. Were there any malignancies found in Mrs. Coffrey's report?

_____

3. *Associated mass* would be another term for _____.

4. The term *bilaterally* means _____.

5. What is a *density*?

_____

B. Improve your knowledge of diagnostic procedures by matching the definition to the appropriate abbreviation. LO 21.1, 21.5

_____ **1.** This uses minimally invasive procedures for diagnosis and treatment.   **a.** MRI

_____ **2.** This is the test of choice for diagnosing some emergency conditions.   **b.** IR

_____ **3.** This uses high-frequency sound waves to visualize soft tissue.   **c.** CT

_____ **4.** Patients with pacemakers are unable to use this modality.   **d.** US

Lesson 21.2 Nuclear Medicine

Nuclear medicine imaging uses small amounts of radiopharmaceuticals that are administered to the patient and have an affinity for specific tissues to show their physiological function rather than the anatomical detail of traditional x-ray imaging. The information in this lesson will enable you to:

21.2.1 Describe characteristics and types of radiopharmaceuticals.

21.2.2 Detail imaging devices used in nuclear medicine.

21.2.3 Discuss common diagnostic uses of nuclear medicine imaging procedures.

21.2.4 Describe common nuclear medicine therapies.

Abbreviations

FDG	fludeoxyglucose
PET	positron emission tomography
SPECT	single photon emission computed tomography

LO 21.7 Radiopharmaceuticals

In nuclear medicine, **radionuclides** can be combined with pharmaceutical compounds to form radio-pharmaceuticals, which are labeled with a radioactive **tracer**. When administered to a patient orally, injected intravenously, swallowed, or inhaled as a gas, these compounds can localize to a specific organ or cells. Then, external detectors (gamma cameras) capture and form images from the radiation emitted by the tracers. This two-dimensional imaging is called **scintigraphy**. With computer processing, the information can be displayed as axial, coronal, and sagittal images *(see Chapter 4)* known as single-**photon** emission computed tomography **(SPECT)** images to produce an image of a "slice" of a patient in a particular plane. A collection of parallel slices form a slice-stack, a three-dimensional representation of how the radionuclide is distributed in the patient.

The most commonly used tracers include

- **Technetium-99m**, used in 85% of all nuclear medicine imaging including for bone scans, liver scans, renal function studies, labeling red blood cells, and use as a gaseous/aerosol.
- **Iodine-123**, used mainly for thyroid scans.
- **Iodine-131**, used mainly for the destruction of thyroid tissues.
- **Gallium-67**, used in **positron emission tomography (PET)** scans *(see the following)* and for localizing infections.
- **Indium-111**, used to label and identify the movements of white blood cells.
- **Thallium-201**, used for myocardial perfusion scans in stress tests.
- **18F-FDG** (fludeoxyglucose), used in the diagnosis and staging of cancer and most commonly in PET scans.

Positron emission tomography (PET) scanning produces two opposite travelling gamma rays to be detected concurrently to improve resolution. 18F-**FDG** is injected intravenously into the patient, and the radiation emitted is detected to produce multiplanar images of the body. Tissues, such as cancer, that are most metabolically active concentrate the 18F-FDG more than normal tissues. PET images can be fused with an anatomical CT image to improve diagnostic accuracy. In academic and research settings, PET images are now being fused with MRI images.

Radiation Dose

The radiation doses delivered to a patient in a nuclear medicine procedure present a very small risk of inducing cancer. The radiopharmaceuticals are inside the body and emit ionizing radiation that travels a short distance, thus minimizing unwanted side effects and damage to noninvolved nearby structures. The radiopharmaceuticals decay and are excreted from the body through normal bodily functions.

WORD	PRONUNCIATION	ELEMENTS		DEFINITION
photon	**FOH**-ton		Greek *light*	A particle of light or other electromagnetic radiation
positron	**POZ**-ih-tron		Greek *positive element*	A subatomic particle equal in mass to an electron but with the opposite (positive) charge
radionuclide	**RAY**-dee-oh-**NYU**-klide	S/ R/CF R/	**-ide** *having a particular quality* **radi/o-** *radiation* **-nucl-** *nucleus*	Radioactive agent used in nuclear medicine
radiopharmaceutical	**RAY**-dee-oh-far-mah-**SOO**-tik-al	S/ R/ R/CF	**-ical** *pertaining to* **-pharmaceut-** *relating to drugs* **radi/o** *radiation*	Radioactive drugs
scintigraphy	sin-**TIG**-rah-fee	S/ R/CF	**-graphy** *process of recording* **scint/i-** *spark*	Recording of radioactivity with gamma cameras
tracer	**TRAY**-ser		Latin *track*	Radioactive agent used to trace metabolic processes

Exercises

A. To improve your knowledge of radiology terms, complete the following exercises by circling the correct answer.   LO 21.6

1. Which term best describes two-dimensional imaging?

   a. ultrasound

   b. scintigraphy

   c. PET scan

   d. MRI scan

   e. interventional

2. What is a tracer?

   a. a red line that appears on the scan

   b. a radioactive agent

   c. a plastic object you swallow for the test

   d. a record produced by the test

   e. a tiny camera you swallow for the test

B. The following terms listed are all tracers. *On the line beside each tracer, write what they are doing in the body.*   **LO 21.1, 21.6, 21.7**

1. gallium-67 _____

2. thallium-201 _____

3. iodine-123 _____

4. 18F-FDG _____

5. iridium–111 _____

C. To improve your knowledge of radiology terms, complete the following exercise by writing a definition of each of the terms.   LO 21.1, 21.3

1. What is the difference between a *positron* and a *photon*?

   a. positron: _____

   b. photon: _____

Abbreviations	
3DCRT	3-dimensional conformal radiation therapy
IMRT	Intensity-modulated radiation therapy
RIT	Radioimmuno-therapy

LO 21.8, 21.9 Radiation Therapy

Radiation therapy is defined as treatment with x-rays or radionuclides.

X-ray Therapy

Ionizing radiation works by damaging the DNA of tissues exposed to it. However, the x-rays often have to pass through skin and other organs to reach a target tumor. To spare normal tissues from the harmful side effects of x-rays, narrow radiation beams are aimed from several angles to intersect at the target tumor. This provides a much larger local dose to the tumor than to the surrounding healthy tissues. It is also common to combine x-ray therapy with surgery, chemotherapy, hormone therapy, immunotherapy, or any combination.

There are five types of x-ray therapy:

- **Conventional external-beam radiation therapy** consists of a single beam of radiation delivered to the tumor from several directions. The concern is the effect of the radiation on the healthy tissues close to the tumor being irradiated. For complex reasons, large tumors respond less well to radiation than small tumors. Strategies to overcome this include surgical resection prior to chemotherapy (as in the treatment of breast cancer), chemotherapy to shrink the tumor prior to radiation therapy, and giving radiosensitizing drugs during radiation therapy. Examples are cisplatin (Platinol) and cetuximab (Erbitux).

- **Stereotactic radiation** is a specialized form of external-beam radiation therapy. It focuses radiation beams by using detailed imaging scans. In **stereotactic radiosurgery (SRS)**, radiation is applied to the tumor with multiple (as many as 200), separate narrow beams, so that the tumor receives a very high dose of radiation in one treatment, yet the surrounding tissues are minimally irradiated. In areas of the body where there is motion by breathing or blood flow, a combination of continuous imaging, motion detection, and robotic guidance enable the beams to remain focused on the tumor. **Stereotactic body radiation treatment (SBRT)** refers to the use of these techniques in such areas as the lungs. A technique called **hypofractionation** is the giving of a much higher dose of radiation per session with greater accuracy and the sparing of normal surrounding tissue. Brand names for these stereotactic radiation therapies include Gamma Knife, Cyberknife, Tomotherapy, and Truebeam.

- **3-dimensional conformal radiation therapy (3DCRT)** is the result of being able to delineate tumors and surrounding normal tissues in three dimensions using CT or MRI scanners and planning software. The profile of each radiation beam and the treatment volume conform to the shape of the tumor, allowing a higher dose of radiation to be delivered to the tumor with a reduced toxicity to the surrounding normal tissues.

- **Intensity-modulated radiation therapy (IMRT)** is the next generation of 3DCRT in which, if the tumor is wrapped around a vulnerable structure such as a blood vessel or major organ, the pattern of radiation delivery can avoid the normal structure.

- **Proton beam therapy** has the advantage that the proton only gives up its energy when it hits the tumor and does not continue on through the tumor to hit normal tissue on the far side. Very high doses of radiation can be given without adjacent normal tissue damage. Prostate cancer is the most common cancer to be treated by proton beam therapy.

Nuclear Medicine Therapy

In **radioactive iodine (I-131) therapy**, the I-131 is taken orally and absorbed into the bloodstream from the GI tract. From the blood, it is concentrated by the thyroid gland, where it destroys cells in that organ and is used to treat thyroid cancer, thyroid nodules, and hyperthyroidism. Common nuclear medicine therapies treat lymphoma, neuroendocrine tumors, and palliative bone pain. Implanted capsules of isotopes (**brachytherapy**) are used for such cancers as prostate and breast cancer.

Radioimmunotherapy (RIT) combines radiation therapy and immunotherapy. In immunotherapy, a laboratory–produced molecule called a **monoclonal antibody** is designed to recognize and bind to the surface of cancer cells; this mimics the body's naturally produced antibodies. In RIT, a monoclonal antibody is fused with a radioactive material and injected into the patient's bloodstream. The antibody travels to and binds to the cancer cells, delivering a high dose of radiation directly to the cells in the cancer.

Word Analysis and Definition

S = Suffix   P = Prefix   R = Root   R/CF = Combining Form

WORD	PRONUNCIATION	ELEMENTS		DEFINITION
brachytherapy	brak-ee-**THER**-ah-pee	P/ R/	brachy- *short* -**therapy** *medical treatment*	Internal radiation therapy delivered by placing radiation sources into the tumor
hypofractionation	hi-poh-**FRAK**-shun-a-shun	S/ P/ R/	-ination *process* hypo- *below* -**fract-** *broken*	Larger measures of a dose of radiation given less frequently
monoclonal	**MON**-oh-**KLOH**-nal	S/ P/ R/	-al *pertaining to* mono- *one, single* -**clon-** *cutting*	Pertaining to protein from a single clone of cells
photon	**FOH**-ton		Greek *light*	A particle of light or other electromagnetic radiation
proton	**PRO**-ton		Greek *first*	The positively charged unit of the nuclear mass
radioimmunotherapy	**RAY**-dee-**IMM**-you-no-**THAIR**-ah-pee	R/CF R/CF	radi/o- *radiation* -**immun/o-** *immune response* -**therapy** *Greek medical treatment*	The combination of radiotherapy and the use of antibodies, e.g., monoclonal antibodies
stereotactic	**STER**-ee-oh-**TAK**-tic	S/ R/ R/CF	-ic *-pertaining to* -**tact-** *orderly arrangement* stere/o- *three-dimensional*	Pertaining to a precise three-dimensional method to locate a lesion or a tumor

Exercises

A. Review this entire spread and WAD to find the correct answers to the following questions.   LO 21.1, 21.3, 21.8, 21.9

1. What is the difference between a *photon* and a *proton*?

   a. photon:

   _____

   b. proton:

   _____

2. Use of implanted capsules of isotopes for prostate and breast cancers is called _____.

3. Name one advantage of proton beam therapy: _____

4. Describe the technique of hypofractionation:

   _____

   _____

5. Explain the Cyberknife procedure:

   _____

   _____

B. Identify the following elements that appear in the above WAD and the text on this spread. *Match the number element to the letter definition.*   **LO 21.8, 21.9**

1. stereo   **a.** short

2. hypo   **b.** broken

3. fract   **c.** below

4. mono   **d.** three dimensional

5. clon   **e.** cutting

6. brachy   **f.** one

Radiology and Nuclear Medicine

Challenge Your Knowledge

A. The most basic element is any medical term is its root or combining form. In each of these terms, identify the root/combining form and define the meaning of the element and the term. **(LO 21.1, 21.2, *Remember*)**

Identify Root/ Combining Form	Meaning of Element	Meaning of Term
craniocaudal	1.	2.
fluoroscopy	3.	4.
anteroposterior	5.	6.
ultrasonography	7.	8.
electromagnetic	9.	10.
stereotactic	11.	12.
claustrophobia	13.	14.
radiograph	15.	16.
radiocontrast	17.	18.
angiography	19.	20.

B. Review the planes and directional terms, because they are very important in diagnostic radiology. Fill in the blanks. **(LO 21.4, *Remember, Understand, Apply*)**

1. front of the body _____

2. divides the body into upper and lower portions _____

3. side of the body _____

4. toward the midline of the body _____

5. head of the body _____

6. back of the body _____

7. divides the body into right and left portions _____

8. only horizontal plane in the body _____

9. head to foot _____

C. Circle the correct answer. (LO 21.8, 21.9, *Remember, Understand, Apply*)

1. Which x-ray characteristic is electromagnetic?

   a. speed

   b. velocity

   c. wavelength

   d. ionization

   e. invisibility

D. What am I? Think back on the medical terminology you have learned in this chapter to answer the question. Fill in the blank. (**LO 21.1, 21.3,** *Remember, Understand, Apply*)

I am impenetrable to x-rays.   I have a liquid form.   I am administered either by IV or drinking.

Answer the question, I am _____.

E. Circle the correct answer for the pronunciation; then answer question 2. (LO 21.2, 21.3, *Remember, Apply*)

1. The correct pronunciation of radiograph is

   a. ray-DE-o-graf

   b. RAY-DE-o-graf

   c. RAY-de-o-graf

   d. RAY-deo-graf

   e. RAY-dee-oh-graf

2. What is the common term for radiograph? _____

F. Each of these three medical terms has a function in radiology. Define the function on the lines provided. (**LO 21.1, 21.3,** *Understand, Apply*)

1. contrast

   _____

   _____

2. alignment

   _____

   _____

3. tracer

   _____

   _____

G. Circle the best answer. (LO 21.1, 21.2, 21.3, 21.5, *Understand, Apply*)

1. Which pair of terms could appear in a radiology report?

   a. impacted   cerumen

   b. oblique   opaque

   c. sublingual   subcutaneous

   d. tonometer   otolith

   e. cannula   catheter

Radiology and Nuclear Medicine

H.   Read the following paragraph and then circle the correct answers. (LO 21.1, 21.5, *Understand, Apply, Analyze*)

In fluoroscopy and angiography, a fluorescent screen and image intensifier tube is connected to a closed-circuit television system. This allows real-time imaging of structures in motion, for example, blood vessels or the GI tract. Radiocontrast agents, such as barium sulfate and iodine, are administered orally, rectally, intravenously, or into an artery and enhance the real-time imaging of dynamic processes such as blood flow in arteries and veins or peristalsis in the GI tract. Iodine contrast may also be concentrated in tumors, cysts, or inflamed areas to make them more opaque and conspicuous.

1. What is *real-time imaging*?

    a. You take pictures during a scan and view them later.

    b. You see images on a screen as the scan is actually happening.

    c. You take pictures before any tracer is administered.

    d. You can only take pictures at night.

    e. You can only take pictures in the morning.

2. What does *angiography* look at specifically?

    a. organs

    b. tissue

    c. blood vessels

    d. muscle

    e. tendons

3. What is the purpose of a radiocontrast agent?

    a. to enhance the image being filmed

    b. to soften the structure being filmed

    c. to block out of the picture any organs not being filmed

    d. to administer chemotherapy to a tumor being filmed

    e. to add more liquid volume to the body

4. What does radiocontrast specifically identify in the GI tract?

    a. outline of organs

    b. tumors or masses

    c. peristalsis

    d. edema

    e. clots

I. Alphabet soup. Use the correct letters to form the abbreviations necessary to match the definitions. Fill in the blanks with the correct abbreviation. (**LO 21.1, 21.2, 21.5,** *Apply*)

A B C D E F G H I J K L M N O P Q R S T U V W X Y Z

1. This term refers to the stomach and intestines. _____

2. This replaces film screen radiography. _____

3. X-rays travel from an anterior source to a posterior receiver. _____

4. This uses minimally invasive procedures. _____

5. High-frequency sound waves are used to visualize soft tissue structures. _____

6. This test gives the best soft tissue contrast of all the imaging modalities. _____

7. This scan produces a computer generated cross-sectional image in the axial plane. _____

8. This scan will produce multiplanar images of the body. _____

J. All the following terms are composed of various combinations of elements. Answer the questions, using your knowledge of the elements of the language of radiology. (**LO 21.1, 21.3, 21.4,** *Apply*)

anteroposterior   opaque   fluoroscopy   posteroanterior   oblique

claustrophobia   teleradiology   coronal   tomography

ultrasound   radiopharmaceutical

1. Which of the above terms are opposites? _____ and _____

2. Which of the above terms means *impervious to light*? _____

3. Which of the above terms means *fear of closed spaces*? _____

4. Which of the above terms has an element meaning *distant*? _____

5. Which of the above terms pertains to a *vertical plane*? _____

6. Which of the above terms has an element meaning *section*? _____

7. Which of the above terms has an element meaning *drugs*? _____

K. Build the correct medical terms by using elements from the element bank that follows (you will not use all the elements provided) to complete the terms. (**LO 21.1, 21.5, 21.6, 21.7,** *Apply*)

hypo   immune   mono   stereo   ary
brachy   fract   bi   al   mammo

1. therapy of short duration: _____/_____/therapy

2. larger measures of a dose of radiation given less frequently: _____/_____/ination

3. protein from a single clone of cells: _____/clon/_____

4. record of the breast: _____/_____/gram

5. treatment using radiation: _____/_____/_____

Radiology and Nuclear Medicine

L. **Construct medical terms with your knowledge of the language of radiology.** (LO 21.1, 21.5, 21.8, *Apply*)

1. Combine the R/CF *mamm/o* with various suffixes to complete the sentences below.

graphy   **plasty**   **gram**

The patient underwent _____ at her physician's request. After she read the _____, she recommended that the patient undergo a _____ to repair her breast.

2. Select the correct terms to complete the sentences below.

radiologist   **radiographer**   **radiographic**   **radiographs**

The chief _____ ordered various _____ studies to help determine the patient's diagnosis. The _____ performed the requested studies and after viewing the _____, the doctor was able to determine a diagnosis for the patient.

M. **Which of the following medical terms are diagnostic, and which are therapeutic?** Place a checkmark (√) in the appropriate column. (LO 21.1, 21.2, 21.7, 21.8, *Analyze*)

Medical Term	Diagnostic	Therapeutic
brachytherapy	1.	2.
radiotherapy	3.	4.
hypofractionation	5.	6.
cyberknife	7.	8.
mammogram	9.	10.
angiography	11.	12.
PET scan	13.	14.
fluoroscopy	15.	16.

17. What's the difference between *diagnostic* and *therapeutic*?

a. diagnostic:

_____

_____

b. therapeutic:

_____

_____

N. **In the following exercise, which statement is incorrect?** Identify the incorrect statement and then rewrite it correctly on the following lines. **(LO 21.1, 21.3, 21.5, *Analyze*)**

1. A tracer is a radioactive agent.   T   F

2. MRIs use gamma cameras.   T   F

3. There are five types of x-ray therapy.   T   F

4. Ionizing radiation works by damaging the DNA of tissues exposed to it.   T   F

5. *Hypofractionation* refers to the dosage of radiation.   T   F

6. Corrected statement:

_____

_____

O. **Circle the correct answer. (LO 21.1, 21.3, 21.5, *Analyze*)**

1. Which of the following pair of terms would *not* appear in a radiology report?

   a. anterior   posterior

   b. medial   lateral

   c. coronal   caudal

   d. platelet   capillary

   e. tarsus   malleolus

P. **Critical thinking.** Read the question, and then outline your thoughts. Be prepared to discuss your answer in class. **(LO 21.2, 21.6, *Analyze*)**

1. Scans can be ordered *with* contrast, *without* contrast, or *with and without* (W/WO) contrast. In what sequence would the contrast be administered if the order was for W/WO contrast?

_____

_____

_____

Radiology and Nuclear Medicine

**Q. Assign the correct term from the word bank (you will have more choices than you will need) to complete the statements.
(LO 21.1, 21.2, 21.3, 21.4, *Analyze*)**

Word Bank:

intravenously	back	teleradiology	CT scan
radiocontrast agents	ultrasonography	tomogram	concurrently
sagittal	interventional	scintigraphy	front

1. Barium sulfate and iodine are _____.

2. Delineation of dynamic structures using sound waves is _____.

3. Radiocontrast agents are administered orally, rectally, and _____.

4. A radiographic image of a selected section or slice of tissue is _____.

5. Anteroposterior x-ray beams pass through the patient from _____ to _____.

6. Digitized diagnostic images transmitted from a distance are called _____.

7. _____ is two-dimensional imaging.

8. _____ means *happening together or at the same time.*

R. Circle the correct answer. (LO 21.8, 21.9, *Analyze*)

1. Which of the following is *not* a type of x-ray therapy?

   a. stereotactic radiation

   b. conventional external-beam radiation therapy

   c. 3DCRT

   d. ultrasonography

   e. proton beam therapy

CHAPTER SUMMARY EXERCISES

A. Spelling comprehension. Circle the correct spelling of the term. (**LO 21.1,** *Remember*)

1. velocity	vellosity	veloosity	velocity	vilocity
2. radiolusent	radiolucent	radioloosent	radiolussent	radeolusent
3. opack	opaqe	opaque	opague	oppaque
4. fluoroscopy	flooroscopy	floroscopy	fluoscopy	fluosscopy
5. sintigraphy	sentigraphy	scintigraphy	sinntigraphy	scintiggraphy

B. Match the number of the correct term in Exercise A with the following brief descriptions. (**LO 21.1,** *Understand, Apply*)

1. penetrable by x-rays   _____

2. recording of radioactivity with gamma cameras   _____

3. impenetrable to x-rays   _____

4. examination of body structures by x-ray   _____

5. speed   _____

C. Using your knowledge of terms 1–5 in Exercise A and their correct spelling, write a brief sentence for each of the terms as it might appear in patient documentation. (**LO 21.1, 21.2, 21.6,** *Apply*)

1. _____

2. _____

3. _____

4. _____

5. _____

D. Alphabet soup. Listed as follows are all the letters you need to form the correct abbreviations for the statements. Some letters you will use more than once; some letters you will not use at all. (**LO 21.1, 21.6,** *Apply*)

C   A   R   F   M   P   I   L   T   E   D   G   O   N   S

1. a view of a structure from head to foot   _____

2. an angled side view of a structure   _____

3. x-ray beam that travels front to back   _____

4. stomach and intestines   _____

5. x-ray beam that travels back to front   _____

6. use of minimally invasive procedures for diagnostic and treatment purposes   _____

7. radiographic image of a selected slice of tissue   _____

8. the use of gallium in scans   _____

9. radiation-emitting IV drug used in PET scans   _____

10. combination of radiation therapy and immunotherapy   _____

Radiology and Nuclear Medicine

E. Match the correct medical term to the statement. Fill in the blanks. (**LO 21.1, 21.5,** *Analyze*)

_____ 1. can cause damage to a fetus   **a.** craniocaudal

_____ 2. a particle of light   **b.** hypofractionation

_____ 3. larger dose of radiation given less frequently   **c.** radiation

_____ 4. head to foot   **d.** stereotactic

_____ 5. special form of external-beam radiation therapy   **e.** photon

F. Circle the only false statement in the exercise, and then rewrite it correctly on the following lines. (**LO 21.5, 21.7, 21.8,** *Analyze*)

1. The advantage of proton beam therapy is that the proton only gives up its energy when it hits the tumor.   T   F

2. Conventional external beam radiation therapy consists of a single beam of radiation delivered to the tumor from several directions.   T   F

3. Cyberknife is a brand name for stereotactic radiation therapy.   T   F

4. Implanted capsules of isotopes are used in radioimmunotherapy.   T   F

5. An ion is an atom or group of atoms carrying an electrical charge.   T   F

6. Corrected statement:

_____

G. Following are actual radiology reports. Answer the questions pertaining to each report. (**LO 21.1, 21.3, 21.4, 21.5,** *Analyze*)

NM: 3-phase <u>bone scan of the lumbar spine</u>

Technique: 26.2 MCi of technetium 99-m HDP were injected intravenously with blood flow; immediate and delayed phases images of the lumbar spine were obtained.

Findings: Normal uptake is visualized in both kidneys and urinary bladder. Mild increased uptake of L3 and L4 vertebral bodies on blood flow images. There is diffuse uptake of the L3 and L4 vertebral bodies on the immediate phase and the delayed phase. Increased uptake on all 3 phases of bone scan involving the L3 and L4 vertebral bodies compatible with osteomyelitis. The patient has been scheduled for WBC tagged scan for further evaluation.

Impression: Findings compatible with L3 and L4 vertebral body osteomyelitis.

Thank you for allowing us to participate in the care of your patient.

Dictated and electronically signed by: Tuan Duc, M.D.

Review the report and answer the following questions.

1. What makes this *nuclear* medicine?_____

_____

2. What specific portion of the body was scanned? _____

3. What is the current diagnosis? _____

4. What is being tagged for the next scan?_____

<u>MRI of the brain w/wo contrast</u>

Clinical history: Breast cancer

Technique: Sagittal and axial T-1 weighted imaging, sagittal, axial and coronal, axial diffusion, axial flair and axial dual echo T2-weighted images using a 1.5 TESLA MRI system.

Comparison: This exam is compared with prior studies, most recently from June and August of this year.

Findings: The marrow signal of the skull is somewhat heterogeneous, and there is indication of a suspected metastatic lesion along the right convexity to the skeleton. There is no restricted diffusion in the brain. Small vessel white matter hyperintense changes with the hemispheric white matter in the subcortical and associated tracts have a similar pattern to the prior exams and may reflect concomitant small-vessel angiopathy. A craniotomy has been performed on the right side, and there is considerable enhancement along the craniotomy site and in the adjacent extraaxial tissue and along the lateral temporal lobe near the surgical site. There is enhancement within the surgical bed, and somewhat nodular enhancement is present within the lateral aspect of the inferior temporal gyrus. There is modest dilatation of the temporal horn of the lateral ventricle on the right in keeping with atrophy.

The degree of enhancement within the surgical bed on this exam is less avid, and there is less localized mass effect. Currently, the enhancing margin measures 1.2 cm × 1.3 cm, compared to 0.5/1.5 cm on the previous study. There are no additional new or important intracranial lesions evident on this study.

Impression: There are no new or important findings or developing area of abnormal enhancement.

Use the *language of radiology* to explain your answers.

5. What is the meaning of the following terms?

   a. sagittal _____

   b. coronal _____

6. Is a *metastatic* lesion a good or bad indication of the patient's condition, and why?_____
_____

7. What is a *convexity* to the skeleton?_____
_____

8. What part of the brain was affected by the craniotomy? _____

9. What is shrinking, once these results are compared with the previous brain study?_____
_____

10. *Lateral* means _____.

11. No *abnormal enhancement* was seen on the scan. Was this a good or bad result of the test, and why?_____
_____

Radiology and Nuclear Medicine

CT scans of the soft tissue of the head and neck with contrast

Findings: Previous right temporoparietal craniotomy. Beneath the craniotomy flap on image 7 is a vague area of enhancement coincident with encephalomalacia and the presumed surgical cavity.

No space-occupying orbital lesions. No apparent mass within the upper aerodigestive tract. No specific imaging abnormality of the submandibular or parotid glands. No mass within the thyroid gland. The right thyroid lobe is asymmetrically smaller than the contralateral side.

Scattered lymph nodes in the neck—none specifically pathologic, based on size or enhancement characteristics.

Multilevel cervical spondylosis. No definite aggressive or destructive skeletal lesion. The uppermost lungs included on this examination show no atypical mass.

Impression: Scattered small lymph nodes within the neck, none specifically pathologic.

12. *Temporoparietal craniotomy* describes what type of surgery?_____

_____

13. *Encephalomalacia* means_____

_____

14. Where is *submandibular* located? _____

15. Where is the *contralateral* side? _____

16. Scattered small lymph nodes in the neck are not *specifically pathologic.* What does this mean?_____

_____

H. Meet the goals of each of the chapter outcomes by using the correct language of radiology for the answers. (LO 21.1–21.9, *Analyze*)

1. Use the medical terms of radiology to communicate and document in writing accurately and precisely in any health care setting. **(LO 21.1)**

   Because they are electromagnetic, x-rays in a vacuum travel at the speed of light. This is known as _____.

2. Use the medical terms of radiology to communicate verbally with accuracy and precision in any health care setting.

   The radiologist has asked you to schedule the patient for an angiogram. What is an angiogram? **(LO 21.2)**

   _____

3. Describe the nature and characteristics of x-rays.

   Circle the only medical term that is a characteristic of x-rays. **(LO 21.3)**

   a. electromagnetic

   b. interventional

   c. amplitude

   d. positron

   e. radionuclide

4. Identify the positions and views of the patient's body used in x-ray examinations. List the various positions and views of the body used in x-ray examinations. (**LO 21.4**)

_____

_____

5. Discuss the different techniques for acquiring radiologic diagnostic images. Pick one technique for acquiring radiologic diagnostic images and describe it. (**LO 21.5**)

_____

_____

6. Describe the nature and characteristics of radioactive materials used in medical imaging. Pick any one radionuclide and describe its major use. (**LO 21.6**)

_____

_____

7. Discuss the nuclear imaging procedures used in the diagnosis of disease. Describe how a PET scan works and what is injected into the body to aid this process. (**LO 21.7**)

_____

_____

8. Explain the different radiologic techniques used in the treatment of disease. Explain teleradiology and how it can benefit a patient. (**LO 21.8**)

_____

_____

9. Describe the different nuclear medicine therapies and their effectiveness. What conditions do common nuclear medicine therapies treat? (**LO 21.9**)

_____

_____

Pharmacology
The Language of Pharmacology

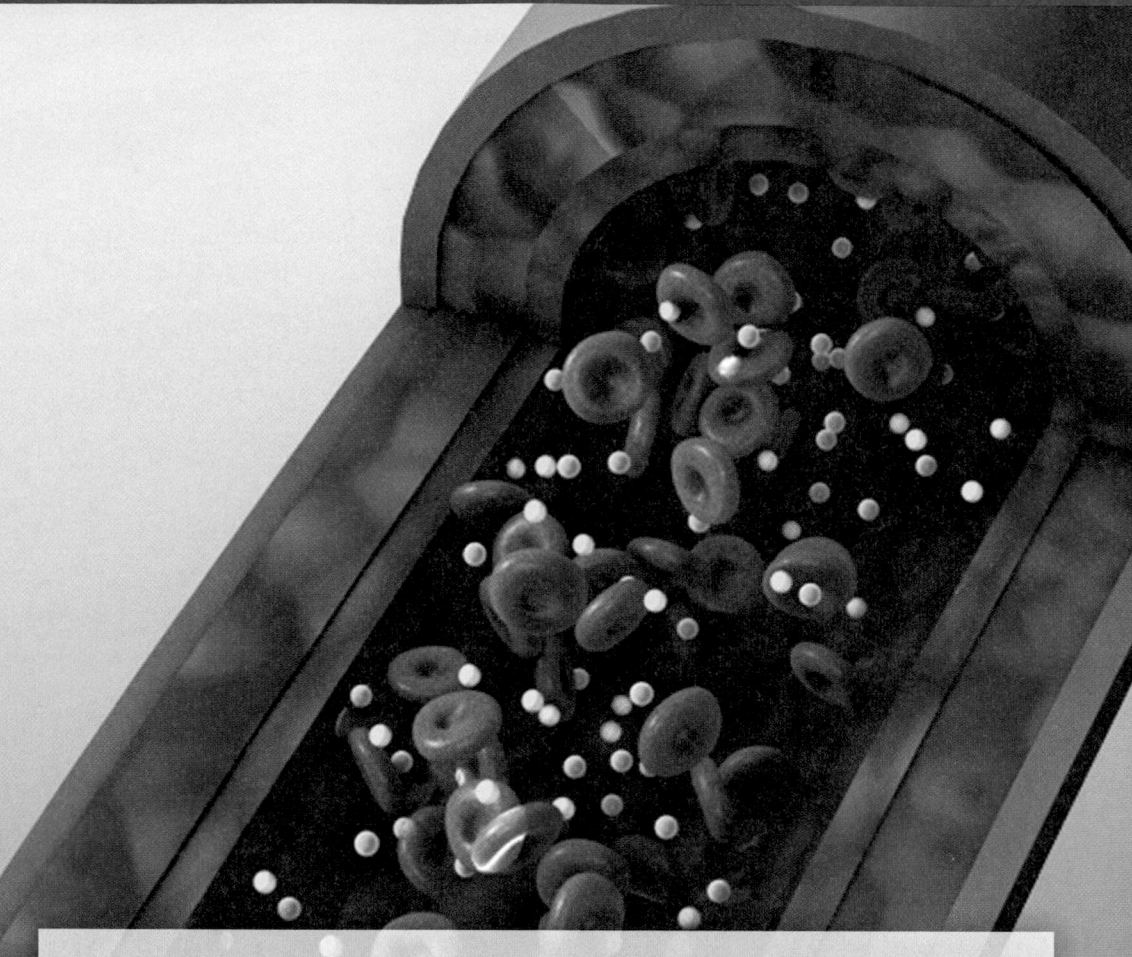

No matter in which health profession you are working, the following medical terms will be used frequently:

- **Pharmacology** is the study of drugs (**medications**) and their sources, preparation, chemistry, actions, and uses.

- A **pharmacologist**, usually a medical professional with an additional PhD, is a specialist who develops and tests drugs for medicinal use.

- A **pharmacist** is licensed to prepare and dispense drugs and compounds when given written orders from a physician. Pharmacists are knowledgeable about drugs' properties and are able to advise patients and practitioners about their effects and interactions.

- A **pharmacy** is a facility licensed to prepare and dispense drugs (medications) to the public.

- A **pharmacy technician** is trained to work under the supervision of a pharmacist to provide medications to patients.

- A **medication aide** is licensed by the state to assist competent individuals, caretakers, and licensed health care professionals to administer medications. They work mostly in nursing homes and assisted living facilities.

Case Report (CR) 22.1

You are

... a pharmacist in the pharmacy at Fulwood Medical Center. Your patient has been sent to you by Susan Lee, MD, a primary care physician at Fulwood Medical Center.

Your patient is

... Mrs. Rebecca Borodin, a frail 80-year-old widow living in an assisted living facility. She has recently begun to complain that she has difficulty recognizing and naming her fellow residents and knowing when to go to the facility's dining room for meals. In addition, it has been hard for her to eat because she suffers from dry mouth and difficulty in swallowing. She has also complained of dizziness and problems with balance; recently, she fell as a result of these problems. Her past medical history includes osteoarthritis, osteopenia, hypertension, congestive heart failure, persistent pain following herpes zoster, and stress incontinence.

Mrs. Borodin has brought in a bag containing all her medications, which include: cimetidine, acetaminophen with codeine (Tylenol #2), oxybutynin, digoxin, atenolol, alprazolam, zolpidem (Ambien), and naproxen. In addition, she takes an over-the-counter (OTC) multivitamin and melatonin.

Dr. Lee has asked you to make sure that Mrs. Borodin knows what each of the medications is for and when to take it. She has also asked you to review the drugs themselves to see if any of them could be causing her recent symptoms.

Chapter Learning Outcomes

Pharmacology is a branch of medicine concerned with the action of drugs. A drug is defined as a man-made chemical or natural substance which exerts a physiologic effect on a cell, tissue, organ, and organism. If the substance has a medicinal effect, it is called a pharmaceutical. In direct patient care pharmaceuticals are used frequently and you need to be able to:

LO 22.1 Use the medical terms of pharmacology to communicate and document in writing accurately and precisely in any health care setting.

LO 22.2 Use the medical terms of pharmacology to communicate verbally with accuracy and precision in any health care setting.

LO 22.3 Discuss the differences between the chemical name, generic name, and brand name of a drug.

LO 22.4 Define the methods used for setting and referencing the standards for the effectiveness and purity of drugs for sale in the United States.

LO 22.5 Describe controlled substance schedules.

LO 22.6 Differentiate the different routes of drug administration.

LO 22.7 Identify abbreviations used to describe drugs, their routes of administration, and their timing.

LO 22.8 Discuss methods to ensure accuracy and safety in the administration of medications.

LO 22.9 Describe the different classes of drugs, their generic and brand names, and their methods of action.

LO 22.10 Identify health professionals involved in pharmacology.

The language of pharmacology is very complex. Each drug has at least three names and is controlled by the Food and Drug Administration (**FDA**) which determines if it can be disseminated and sold. The drugs are reviewed for effectiveness and safety and are referenced for use by groups of hospitals and physicians in **formularies**. Every physician and facility has a **DEA** license number. Doctors must have this number printed or written on their prescriptions. The information in this lesson will:

22.1.1 Describe drug nomenclature.

22.1.2 Differentiate between controlled and noncontrolled drugs.

22.1.3 Discuss how standards for the quality, purity, and strength of medications are set and enforced.

22.1.4 Describe how hospitals and physicians determine which drugs they will prescribe.

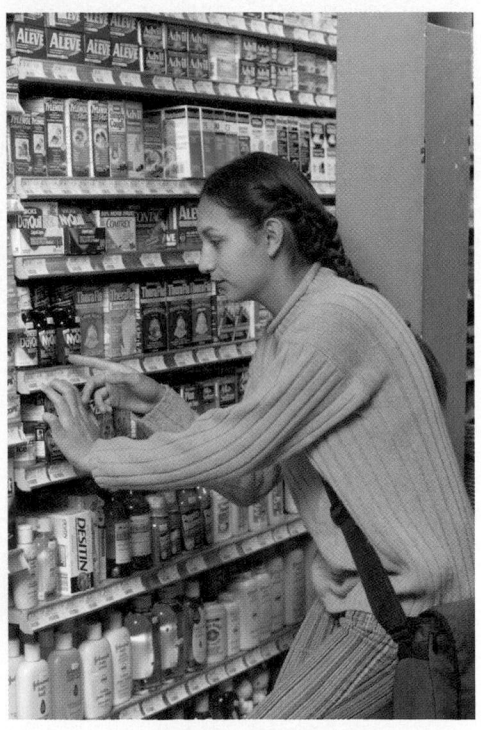

▲ **Figure 22.1** Shopping in a Pharmacy for Over the Counter (OTC) Medicines.

Abbreviation	
DEA	U.S. Drug Enforcement Agency
FDA	U.S. Food and Drug Administration
OTC	over-the-counter

LO 22.3 Drug Names

There are more than 2,400 drugs that can be **prescribed** by licensed practitioners. Each drug has three different names:

- The drug's **chemical** name (for example, 8-chloro-1-methyl-6-phenyl4H-s-triazolo-benzodiazepine), which specifies the chemical makeup of the drug, is often long and complicated.
- The drug's **generic** name (for example, alprazolam), which identifies the drug legally and scientifically; there is only one generic name for each drug.
- The drug's **brand (trade)** name (for example, Xanax), which each manufacturer gives to the drug. These names are the manufacturer's private property. There can be several brand names of a particular drug, depending on how many different companies are manufacturing the drug. The brand names are always capitalized (e.g. Xanax).

When a drug manufacturer receives U.S. **Food and Drug Administration (FDA)** approval to sell a particular drug, it is allowed to have 20 years of protected proprietary manufacture of the drug (patent) from the date of invention, which means that no other company can manufacture and sell the same drug during that period of time. After that period of time, however, the generic name of the drug becomes public property, and any drug manufacturer can manufacture and sell the drug under that generic name.

However, if a specific brand name is ordered on a **prescription** by a physician and is designated "dispense as written," no generic or other brand name may be substituted. Generic drugs are usually cheaper than brand name drugs, because several companies are competing with one another to sell them and the generic companies have not had the initial research and development costs.

LO 22.4 Drug Standards

Over the *Counter (OTC)* Drugs

Over-the-counter (OTC) drugs *(Figure 22.1)*, which are also called nonprescription drugs, are used to treat conditions that do not generally require care or a prescription from a health professional. Examples of these drugs include **analgesics**, such as aspirin or acetaminophen; **antihistamines**, such as Chlor-Trimeton and Dramamine; and some sleeping aids, such as doxylamine (an antihistamine) and melatonin. In addition, herbal preparations, vitamins, minerals, and food supplements are available without a prescription.

WORD	PRONUNCIATION	ELEMENTS		DEFINITION
analgesic	an-al-**JEE**-zic	S/ P/ R/	**-ic** *pertaining to* **an-** *without* **-alges-** *sensation of pain*	Substance that produces a reduction in the sensation of pain
antihistamine histamine	an-tee-**HISS**-tah-mean	P/ R/ R/CF	**anti-** *against* **-hist-** *derived from histidine* **-amin/e** *nitrogen compound*	Drug used to treat allergic symptoms because of its action antagonistic to histamine Compound liberated in tissues as a result of injury or an allergic response
drug	DRUG		Old English *drug*	A therapeutic agent or an addictive substance
formulary	**FORM**-you-lair-ee	S/ R/	**-ary** *pertaining to* **formul-** *form*	An official list of drugs approved for use by a hospital or group of physicians
generic	je-**NER**-ik	S/ R/	**-ic** *pertaining to* **gener-** *birth*	A non-proprietary name for a drug
medication	med-ih-**KAY**-shun	R/ R/	**medic-** *physician* **-ation** *healing*	A substance having curative properties
pharmacist pharmacy	**FAR**-mah-sist **FAR**-mah-see	S/ R/	**-ist** *specialist* **pharmac-** *drug*	Person licensed by the state to prepare and dispense drugs Facility licensed to prepare and dispense drugs
pharmacology pharmacologist	far-mah-**KOLL**-oh-jee far-mah-**KOLL**-oh jist	S/ R/CF S/	**-logy** *study* **pharmac/o** *drug* **-ist** *specialist*	Science of the preparation, uses, and effects of drugs A medical specialist in pharmacology
prescribe prescription	pre-**SKRIBE** pre-**SKRIP**-shun	P/ R/ R/ S/	**pre-** *before* **-scribe** *write* **-script** *writing* **-ion** *process, action*	To give directions in writing for the preparation and administration of a remedy A written direction for the preparation and administration of a remedy

Exercises

A. Review the Case Report and the text and use the *language of pharmacology* to answer the following questions. LO 22.1, 22.3

1. List Mrs. Borodin's symptoms and signs.

_____

_____

2. What diagnoses are in Mrs. Borodin's medical history?

_____

_____

3. Of the medications that Mrs. Borodin takes, which are OTC?

_____

_____

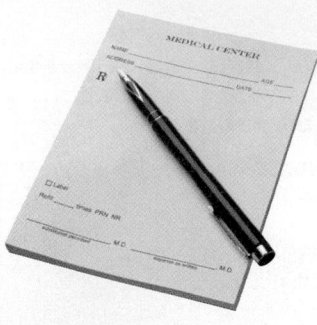

▲ Figure 22.2 Paper Prescription Pad.

LO 22.4 Drug Standards (continued)

Prescription Drugs

A prescription **medication** is legally regulated, which means that a person needs a medical prescription to purchase it *(Figure 22.2)*. Prescriptions can only be written by physicians, licensed medical practitioners, dentists, optometrists, veterinarians, and advanced nurse practitioners. Prescribed drugs must have a package insert detailing the intended effects of the drug and its **side effects**.

Regulating the safety and effectiveness of prescription drugs in the United States is the responsibility of the FDA. Another agency, the **United States Pharmacopeia (USP)**, sets the standards for the quality, purity, and safety of the medications to be enforced by the FDA to protect the public health.

Certain groups of prescription drugs that are considered to have a potential for abuse are called **controlled drugs**. Regulation of these drugs is the responsibility of the U.S. Department of Justice **Drug Enforcement Administration (DEA)**. These controlled substances are divided into five schedules, depending on their currently accepted medical use in treatment, their potential for abuse, and likelihood of causing dependence.

- **Schedule I**—controlled substances have a high potential for abuse and have no accepted medical use in treatment in the United States. Examples include heroin, marijuana, and LSD. Drugs listed in Schedule I cannot be prescribed, administered, or dispensed, but marijuana is legal for medical use in some states.

- **Schedule II**—controlled substances have a high potential for abuse. Abuse of these substances may lead to severe psychological or physical dependence. Examples include some **narcotics**, such as morphine, methadone, meperidine (Demerol), and oxycodone (OxyContin); **stimulants**, such as amphetamine, methamphetamine, and methylphenidate (Ritalin); cocaine; and barbiturates, such as pentobarbital.

- **Schedule III**—controlled substances have less potential for abuse than substances in Schedules I and II. Abuse of these substances may lead to moderate or low physical dependence or high psychological dependence. Examples include certain narcotics, including combination products with less than 15 milligrams of hydrocodone per dose (for example, Vicodin) and combination products with less than 90 milligrams of codeine per dose (for example, acetaminophen [Tylenol] with codeine). Other Schedule III nonnarcotics include **anabolic steroids**, such as oxandrolone.

- **Schedule IV**—controlled substances have a lower potential for abuse than Schedule III drugs. Schedule IV substances include benzodiazepines (for example, alprazolam [Zanax] and diazepam [Valium]).

- **Schedule V**—controlled substances have a lower potential for abuse compared to Schedule IV substances and consist primarily of preparations containing limited quantities of certain narcotics. These are generally used for **antitussive**, **antidiarrheal**, and analgesic purposes. Examples include Robitussin AC and Phenergan with codeine.

Drugs listed in Schedules II through V have accepted medical uses and therefore may be prescribed, administered, or dispensed for medical use.

Keynotes

- The **Physicians' Desk Reference (PDR)** contains detailed information on individual drugs, including their intended effects, side effects, interactions, dosage and administration. The information is provided by the manufacturers and is updated yearly.

- A **hospital formulary** provides similar information about the medications the hospital's physicians can prescribe.

- An **insurance company's formulary** provides similar information about the medications it will pay for.

Abbreviations

LSD	lysergic acid diethylamide
PDR	Physicians' Desk Reference
USP	United States Pharmacopeia

WORD	PRONUNCIATION	ELEMENTS		DEFINITION
anabolic steroid	an-a-**BOL**-ik **STER**-oyd	S/ R/ S/ R/	-ic *pertaining to* anabol- *to raise up* -oid *resemble* ster- *solid*	Prescription drug abused by some athletes to increase muscle mass
antitussive	an-the-**TUSS**-iv	S/ P/ R/	-ive *nature of, quality of* anti- *against, against* -tuss- *cough*	A cough remedy
control	kon-**TROLL**		Latin *to check an account*	To regulate, correct
generic	je-**NER**-ik	S/ R/	-ic *pertaining to* gener- *birth*	A non-proprietary name for a drug
narcotic	nar-**KOT**-ik	S/ R/CF	-tic *pertaining to* narc/o *sleep, stupor*	Drug derived from opium, or a Synthetic drug with similar effects
side effect	SIDE e-**fekt**		Old English *side* Old English *result*	An undesirable result of drug or other therapy
stimulant	**STIM**-you-lant	S/ R/	-ant *agent* stimul- *excite*	Agent that excites or strengthens functional activity

Exercises

A. Fill in the blank.   LO 22.3, 22.4

1. Which of Mrs. Borodin's medications are prescription drugs?

_____

_____

B. Circle your answer.   LO 22.3, 22.4

1. How long would a drug patent last on a brand name drug?

   a. 10 years

   b. 8 years

   c. 12 years

   d. 20 years

   e. 15 years

2. What government agency is responsible for regulating the safety and effectiveness of prescription drugs?

   a. FDIC

   b. DEA

   c. USP

   d. PDR

   e. HPV

3. Give an example of a schedule I drug with a high potential for abuse and no accepted medical use in treatment in the United States.

_____

Lesson 22.2 The Administration of Drugs

A route of administration in pharmacology and toxicology is the path by which a drug or other substance is taken into the body. Routes of administration are usually classified according to the location on the body to which the drug is applied. The routes of administration distinguish whether a drug's effect is local (as in topical) or systemic (as in enteral or parenteral administration).

The bioavailability of a drug reveals what proportion of the drug reaches the systemic blood circulation and is available to reach the intended site(s) of action. A drug's route of administration (for example, oral or intravenous [IV]) and its formulation (for example, tablet, capsule, or liquid) clearly influence its bioavailability.

The path that a drug takes from the point of its application to reach the tissue where its effect is targeted is part of pharmacokinetics—the absorption, distribution, metabolism, and elimination of drugs. A drug's interaction at its target site(s) of action is called **pharmacodynamics**. The information in this lesson will enable you to:

22.2.1 Define terms relating to a drug's ability to reach and affect a particular tissue.

22.2.2 Discuss the different routes for administering drugs.

22.2.3 Identify abbreviations used in writing medication orders.

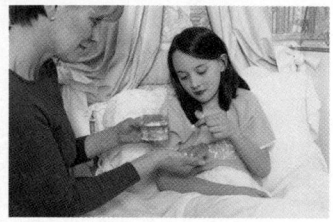

▲ **Figure 22.3** Mother Gives Medication.

Abbreviations

a.c.	before meals
b.i.d.	twice each day
GI	gastrointestinal
IV	intravenous injection
o.n.	at night
p.c.	after meals
p.o.	by mouth
PR	per rectum
p.r.n.	when necessary
q.d.	every day
q.i.d.	four times each day
Rx	prescribe
STAT	immediately
t.i.d.	three times each day

LO 22.6 Routes of Administration

Enteral Administration

Enteral administration is through the gastrointestinal (GI) tract. **Oral** is the most frequently used, convenient, and economical method of drug administration *(Figure 22.3)*. However, absorption of a drug by this route is affected by the unpredictable nature of the GI tract. For example, by affecting the gastric motility and emptying time the presence of food influences the rate and extent of drug absorption. Solid-dose forms such as tablets and capsules have a high degree of drug stability and provide accurate dosage. The use of liquids and soluble preparations is less reliable. Modified-release preparations aim to maintain plasma drug concentrations for extended periods. If they are chewed or crushed, the full dose is released immediately, leading to **toxicity**.

The **sublingual** route and the **buccal** routes provide a rich supply of blood vessels through which drugs can be directly absorbed into the systemic circulation. Wafer-based versions of drugs, such as glyceryl trinitrate in the treatment of acute angina pectoris *(see Chapter 10)*, placed under the tongue, give rapid responses to their effects.

Rectal administration in the form of **suppositories** or **enemas** is popular in some European countries, but is not easily accepted by patients in America. **Antiemetics** can be administered rectally for nausea and vomiting.

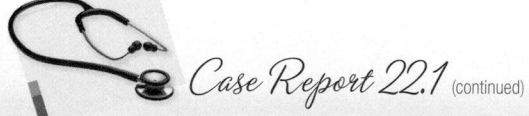

Case Report 22.1 (continued)

All the drugs that Mrs. Borodin has brought in for your inspection are administered orally.

Her medications, and their times of administration, include cimetidine 300 mg four times each day (**q.i.d.**); Tylenol #2 when necessary (**p.r.n.**) for pain; oxybutinin 5 mg three times each day (**t.i.d.**); digoxin 0.25 mg twice each day (**b.i.d.**); atenolol 100 mg at night (**o.n.**); alprazolam 0.5 mg, b.i.d.; Ambien 5 mg o.n.; and naproxen 500 mg b.i.d. In addition she takes an OTC multivitamin **q.d.** and melatonin 1 mg **o.n.**

Topical Administration

Topical administration allows a drug to be available directly at the site of action without going through the systemic circulation. For example, topical applications include steroid ointments for treating dermatitis *(Chapter 15)*, beta blocker eye drops for treating glaucoma *(Chapter 16)*, nasal medications instilled via drops or a spray, bronchodilators that are inhaled to treat asthma *(Chapter 13)*, and **pessaries** or creams containing clotrimazole (Lotrimin, Mycelex) that are inserted to treat vaginal candidiasis *(Chapter 8)*. Thus, *topical* refers to more than just application on the skin.

Drugs can also be administered into the systemic circulation through the skin. Adhesive **transdermal** patches can contain drugs that migrate across the epidermis into the blood vessel–rich dermis, where they are absorbed into the systemic circulation. Medications for motion sickness, cardiac problems, birth control, and the chemicals testosterone and nicotine are administered by transdermal patches.

WORD	PRONUNCIATION	ELEMENTS		DEFINITION
antiemetic	**AN**-tee-eh-**MET**-ik	S/ P/ R/	-tic *pertaining to* anti- *against* -eme- *to vomit*	A medication that helps to control nausea and vomiting
bioavailability	**BI**-oh-ah-**VALE**-ah-bill-ih-tee	S/ R/ R/	-ity *condition, state* bio- *life* -availabil- *to be worth*	The amount of a drug that reaches the systemic circulation and is available to reach the intended site of action
buccal	**BUCK**-al	S/ R/	-al *pertaining to* bucc- *cheek*	Inside the cheek—a site for the administration of certain medications
enema	**EN**-eh-mah		Greek *injection*	An injection of fluid into the rectum
enteral	**EN**-ter-al	S/ R/	-al *pertaining to* enter- *intestine*	Administration of medications by way of the GI tract
formulation	**FORM**-you-**LAY**-shun	S/ R/	-ation *process* formul- *form*	The form in which a drug is presented—tablet, capsule, liquid, etc.
oral	**OR**-al	S/ R/	-al *pertaining to* or- *mouth*	Pertaining to the mouth
parenteral	pah-**REN**-ter-al	S/ P/ R/	-al *pertaining to* par- *abnormal, beside* -enter- *intestine*	Administering medication by any means other than the GI tract
pessary	**PES**-ah-ree		Greek *an oval stone*	Appliance inserted into the vagina
pharmacodynamics	**FAR**-mah-co-die-**NAM**-iks	S/ R/CF R/	-ics *pertaining to* pharmac/o- *drug* -dynam- *force*	The uptake and action of drugs at their tissue site(s) of action
pharmacokinetics	**FAR**-mah-co-ki-**NET**-iks	S/ R/CF R/	-ics *pertaining to* pharmac/o- *drug* -kinet- *moving*	The movement of drugs within the body affecting absorption distribution, metabolism, and excretion
rectal	**RECK**-tal	S/ R/	-al *pertaining to* rect- *rectum*	Pertaining to the rectum
sublingual	sub-**LING**-wal	S/ P/ R/	-al *pertaining to* sub- *underneath* -lingu- *tongue*	Underneath the tongue
suppository	suh-**POS**-ih-tor-ee		Latin *placed underneath*	A small solid body containing medication that is placed in a body orifice other than the mouth to release the medication
topical	**TOP**-ih-kal	S/ R/	-al *pertaining to* topic- *local*	Medication applied to a local area
toxin	**TOK**-sin		Greek *poison*	Poisonous substance formed by a cell or organism
toxicity	toks-**ISS**-ih-tee	S/ S/ R/	-ity *state, condition* -ic- *pertaining to* tox- *poison*	The state of being poisonous
toxicology	toks-ih-**KOL**-oh-jee	R/CF S/	toxic/o *poison* -logy *study of*	The science of poisons, including their source, chemistry, actions, and antidotes
transdermal	trans-**DER**-mal	S/ P/ R/	-al *pertaining to* trans- *across, through* -derm- *skin*	Going across or through the skin

Exercises

A. Answer the questions using the *language of pharmacology*. *Controlled prescription drugs are separated into five different schedules, based on the potential for their abuse. Give one example for a drug in each Schedule. Fill in the blanks.* **LO 22.5**

1. Schedule I: _____

2. Schedule II: _____

3. Schedule III: _____

4. Schedule IV: _____

5. Schedule V: _____

LO 22.6 Routes of Administration (continued)

Parenteral Administration

Parenteral administration, which literally means *not through the GI tract*, is the injection of a drug directly into the body that bypasses the skin and mucous membranes.

The common routes of parenteral administration are

- **intramuscular (IM)** *(Figure 22.4a)*
- **intravenous (IV)** *(Figure 22.4b)*
- **subcutaneous (SC)**

Less common routes include

- **intradermal**
- **intrathecal** *(Figure 22.4c)*

Intramuscular and **subcutaneous injections** establish a "depot" for a drug that is released gradually, depending on the drug's formulation, into the systemic circulation. For example, oil-based medications are released more slowly than water-based. An IM injection of Depo-Provera, a birth control drug, works steadily for a three-month period. An **intradermal** route for medications is rarely used, except in allergy testing.

Intravenous injections enable a drug to reach its sites of action within seconds. An IV **infusion** can also deliver continuous medication—for example, morphine to patients in continuous pain or a saline drip for people needing fluids. The medications can also be given in a small solution through a **port** in intravenous tubing (**bolus**), or attached in smaller infusion containers to a larger infusion (piggyback).

Disadvantages of IV injections or infusions include the fact that patients are not typically able to self-administer them and the fact that, because it bypasses most of the body's natural defenses, IV is the most dangerous route of administration. Also, the preparation and administration of IV drugs requires the use of **aseptic** techniques. Careful training is necessary to achieve competence in the administration of IV medications.

Intrathecal injections are given into the subarachnoid space surrounding the spinal cord in the spinal canal *(see Chapter 9)*. An epidural block, which is an injection of a local anesthetic agent into the epidural space *(Figure 22.4c)*, is used often for pain management during labor *(see Chapter 8)* and occasionally for chemotherapy. An intrathecal injection's primary advantage is that the drug avoids the blood–brain barrier (BBB; *see Chapter 9*).

Methods to ensure accuracy and safety in the administration of drugs are described in the next lesson of this chapter.

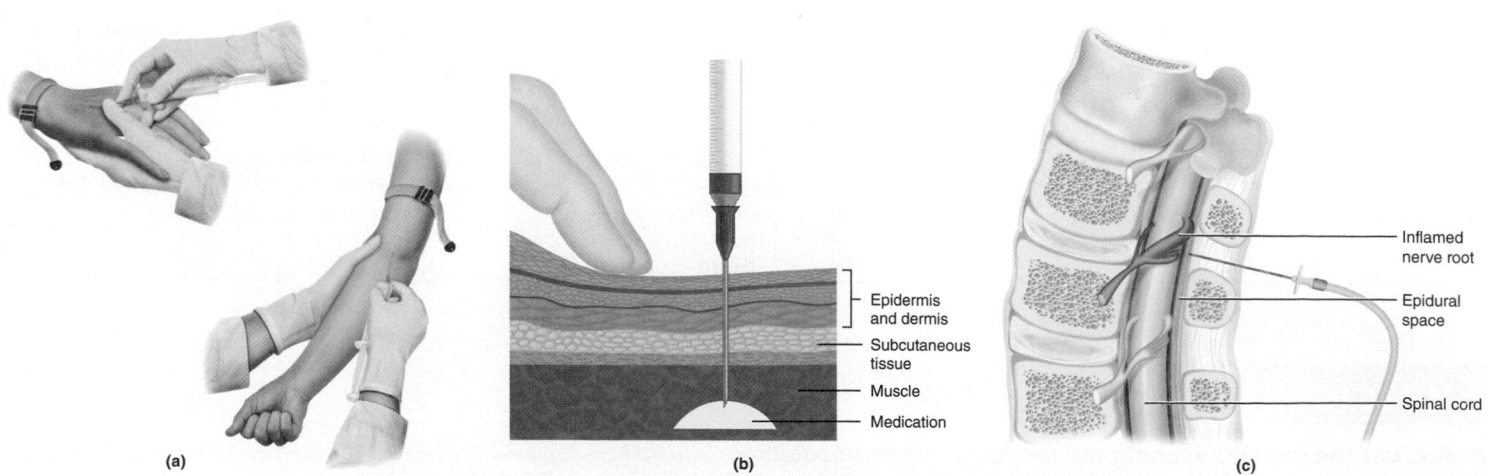

(a)   (b)   (c)

▲ **Figure 22.4**   *(a)* Inserting an Intravenous (IV) Cannula, *(b)* IM Injection, *(c)* Intrathecal Injection.

S = Suffix   P = Prefix   R = Root   R/CF = Combining Form

WORD	PRONUNCIATION	ELEMENTS		DEFINITION
aseptic (adj) (*Note:* The final "s" of the root is not used to allow the pronunciation to flow)	a-**SEP**-tik	S/ P/ R/	-tic *pertaining to* a- *without* -seps- *decay*	Pertaining to the absence of living organisms
bolus	**BOH**-lus		Greek *a lump*	Single mass of a substance
infusion	in-**FYU**-shun	P/ R/	in- *in* -fusion *to pour*	Introduction intravenously of a substance other than blood
injection	in-**JEK**-shun	R/	-jection *to throw*	Introduction of a medical substance parenterally
intradermal	in-trah-**DER**-mal	S/ P/ R/	-al *pertaining to* intra- *within* -derm- *skin*	Within the dermis
intramuscular **intrathecal** **intravenous**	in-trah-**MUSS**-kew-lar in-trah-**THEE**-kal in-trah-**VEE**-nuss	R/ R/ S/ R/	-muscul- *muscle* -thec- *sheath* -ous *pertaining to* -ven- *vein*	Within the muscle Within the subarachnoid or subdural space Inside a vein
port	PORT		Latin *gate*	A point of entry into an IV system
subcutaneous **hypodermic (syn)**	sub-kew-**TAY**-nee-us	S/ P/ R/CF	-ous *pertaining to* sub- *below* -cutan/e *skin*	Below the skin

Exercises

A. Using the specific medical language learned in this chapter, answer the following questions.   LO 22.1, 22.4, 22.6

1. Describe the difference between *pharmacokinetics* and *pharmacodynamics*.

   a. Pharmacokinetics:

   _____

   _____

   b. Pharmacodynamics:

   _____

   _____

2. Describe the difference between *intradermal* and *intrathecal* injections.

   a. Intradermal:

   _____

   _____

   b. Intrathecal:

   _____

   _____

B. The definitions of the terms are given to you. *Write the correct terms on the lines.*   **LO 22.1, 22.6**

1. absence of living organisms: _____

2. within the dermis: _____

3. point of entry into an IV system: _____

4. same as hypodermic: _____

5. single mass of a substance: _____

Lesson 22.3 Accuracy and Safety in Drug Administration

LESSON OBJECTIVES

The Centers for Disease Control and Prevention (CDC) report that in 2009, the latest year for which statistics are available, 37,485 patients in the United States died from improperly prescribed, overprescribed, or unmonitored use of tranquilizers, painkillers, and stimulant drugs. This total exceeds the number of deaths from motor vehicle accidents (36,284) and firearms (31,228). Every 14 minutes, one U.S. citizen is killed by prescribed painkillers and psychiatric drugs. Vicodin, the most prescribed medicine nationwide, kills the most pain and the most people.

The information in this lesson will enable you to:

22.3.1 **Understand that every drug has side effects that can be harmful.**

22.3.2 **Describe patterns of taking multiple self-administered drugs.**

22.3.3 **Identify the five "rights" to be addressed by patients and caregivers in administering drugs.**

22.3.4 **Discuss the importance for accurate documentation of each administration of a drug and of any error in its administration.**

Abbreviations

ADR	adverse drug reaction
AE	adverse effect
BBB	blood–brain barrier
CDC	Centers for Disease Control and Prevention
CNS	central nervous system
PCP	primary care physician

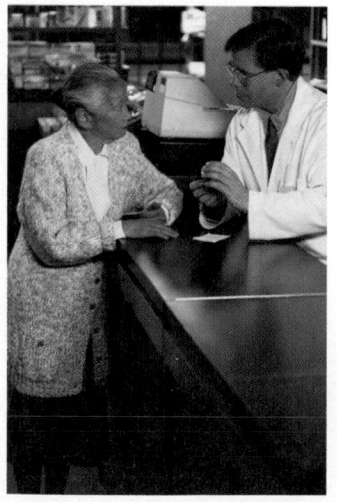

▲ **Figure 22.5**
Pharmacist Consults with Elderly Patient.

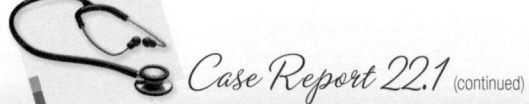

Case Report 22.1 (continued)

After reviewing Mrs. Borodin's medications with her (*Figure 22.5*), you found that she had a poor grasp of the indications for several of her medications. In addition, you found that side effects and **interactions** of several of her medications could be causing her recent symptoms of confusion, dry mouth, difficulty in swallowing, dizziness, difficulty with her balance, and falling.

For example, the benzodiazepine alprazolam (Xanax) has the side effects of fainting and dizziness, and accidental falls are common. In addition, zolpidem (Ambien), a sedative and hypnotic, interacts with Xanax and **synergistically** increases these central nervous system (**CNS**) side effects of Xanax. In addition, Mrs. Borodin is taking over-the-counter melatonin at night. You doubt that it is necessary for her to take both Ambien and melatonin. Ambien and oxybutynin list confusion, dry mouth, and dizziness among their side effects.

You ask for a conference with Dr. Lee, Mrs. Borodin's primary care physician (**PCP**), to review and possibly change her medications. Following that, you will set up a meeting with Mrs. Borodin and medication aides from the assisted living facility where she lives in order to ensure that her new medication regimen is understood and can be implemented safely and accurately.

LO 22.8 Self-Administration of Medications

The most common route of administration of medications is the self-administered oral route. Seventy-nine percent of adults older than 65 are on medications, with 39% of them taking five or more prescription drugs and 90% of them also taking over the counter (OTC) drugs. In a 2002 large study of women older than 65, 12% took 10 or more medications and 35% experienced an **adverse effect** (**AE**) from a drug. Adverse effects are harmful and undesired effects secondary to the main or therapeutic effect of the medication. Research has also found that **adverse drug reactions** (**ADR**) caused by intolerance, susceptibility, or interaction with another drug occurred in the hospitalization of some 35% of patients. In addition to hospitalization, severe adverse drug reactions can result in death or permanent **impairment** of physical activities and/or quality of life.

WORD	PRONUNCIATION	ELEMENTS		DEFINITION
adverse	**AD**-vers	P/ R/	ad- *to, into* **-verse** *turned*	Noxious, unintended, undesired
impairment	im-**PAIR**-ment	S/ R/	-ment *action, state* **impair-** *worsen*	Diminishing of normal function
interaction	in-ter-**ACK**-shun	P/ R/	inter- *between* **-action** *to do*	The action between two entities to produce or prevent an effect
reaction	ree-**ACK**-shun	P/ R/	re- *again, backward* **-action** *to do*	The response of a living tissue or organism to a stimulus
synergist	**SIN**-er-jist	S/ P/ R/	-ist *specialist* syn- *together* **erg-** *work*	Agent or process that aids the actions of another
synergism	**SIN**-er-jism	S/	-ism *condition, process*	Coordinated action of two or more agents or processes so that the combined action is greater than that of each acting separately
synergistic (adj)	sin-er-**JIST**-ic	S/	-ic *pertaining to*	Pertaining to synergism
tranquilizer	**TRANG**-kwih-lie-zer	S/ R/	-izer *affects in a particular way* **tranquil-** *calm, serene*	Agent that calms without sedating or depressing

Exercises

A. WAD search and find. *Review the above WAD before doing this exercise. The elements are given in the first column. Fill in the answers to the element questions in columns 2, 3, and 4.* **LO 22.1, 22.2**

Name of Element	Identity of Element (Prefixes, Roots, Combining Forms, Suffixes)	Meaning of Element	Word Using This Element
syn	1.	2.	3.
ad	4.	5.	6.
erg	7.	8.	9.
re	10.	11.	12.
ist	13.	14.	15.

B. Which of the following statements is the only one that is true? **LO 22.1, 22.2, 22.9**

1. A synergist is a medical professional.   T   F

2. A tranquilizer will make you sleep.   T   F

3. A reaction is a response to a stimulus.   T   F

4. An impairment is the inability to sleep.   T   F

5. An interaction involves at least five entities.   T   F

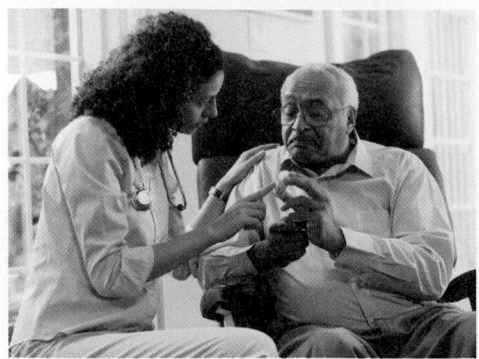

▲ **Figure 22.6** Patient Is Shown How to Check a Medication Label.

LO 22.8 Caregiver Administration of Medications

Five Rights

Before a caregiver administers a drug (medication) to a patient by any route, five factors should be addressed by the caregiver *(Figure 22.6)*.

- **Right patient**
  - Identify the patient by a bracelet or name badge. Asking the patient's name can lead to confusion, particularly in the assisted living environment.
- **Right drug**
  - Check the medication record for the name of the drug and compare with the drug in hand at three points:
    1. When taking hold of the package that contains the drug.
    2. When opening the package.
    3. When returning the package to storage.
  - **Right route**
    - Check the medication record for how to administer the drug and check the labeling of the drug to make sure it matches the prescribed route.
  - **Right dose**
    - Check that the medication record orders the same dose as that in hand.
  - **Right time**
    - Check that the time ordered or the frequency matches the current time.

In addition, the caregiver must actually watch the patient take the medication. Caregivers should not leave medications unattended and should ensure that the medication does not come into contact with any potentially **contaminated** surface or object.

Documentation of having given medication is a vital responsibility of the caregiver. Medication errors must be documented and should clearly state if it was one or more of the **Five Wrongs**—namely: the **wrong patient**, the **wrong drug**, the **wrong route**, the **wrong dose**, or the **wrong time**.

LO 22.8 Self-Administration of Drugs

For a patient at home administering his/her own medications, usually orally, the Five Rights also apply at the time of administration:

- **Right Patient**: The patient should make sure that the container or package holding the medication has his or her name on it.
- **Right Drug**: The patient should check his or her own medication record to ensure that the medication has been prescribed and stored correctly.
  - **Right Route**: The patient should check whether the medication should be swallowed whole as a capsule or tablet or taken as directed if a liquid.
  - **Right Dose**: The patient should check with his or her medication record and the label on the package that the number of tablets or capsules or the amount of liquid is correct.
  - **Right Time**: The patient should check his or her medication record and the label on the package to ensure that the medication is being taken at the right time.

Documentation of the administration of all drugs as part of the patient's medical record should be encouraged, particularly among the elderly.

Self-Administration of Insulin

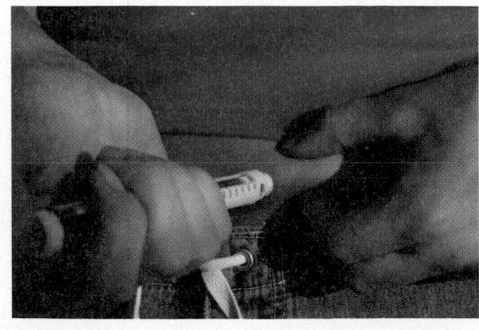

▲ **Figure 22.7** Injecting Insulin Using a Pen Device. Insulin pens are pen-like devices that allow diabetics to give themselves insulin injections without using vials and syringes.

Some 19 million people in the U.S. have been diagnosed with **diabetes**. Five million of them self-administer insulin into their subcutaneous tissue either by **syringe**, **pen injection**, high-pressure jet injection, or subcutaneous infusion pumps *(Figure 22.7)*. Inhalation of an insulin solution is also available. It is essential that the right dose of the right drug (i.e., the right type of insulin [*see next lesson*]) is given in response to the patient's blood sugar level.

WORD	PRONUNCIATION	ELEMENTS		DEFINITION
aide	ADE		Latin *to help*	An official, confidential assistant
cognitive	**KOG**-nih-tiv	S/ R/	-ive *nature of, pertaining to* cognit- *acquire knowledge*	Pertaining to the process of acquiring knowledge
capsule	**KAP**-syul	S/ R/	-ule *little* caps- *box*	A solid dosage form in which a drug is enclosed in a hard or soft shell
document (verb)	**DOK**-you-ment	S/ R/	-ment *resulting state, action* docu- *to teach*	To provide written proof
documentation (noun)	**DOK**-you-men-**TAY**-shun	S/	-ation *process*	The process of providing written proof
dose	DOS		Greek *a giving*	The quantity of a drug to be taken at one time
syringe	si-**RINJ**		Greek *pipe or tube*	An instrument used for injecting or withdrawing fluids
tablet	**TAB**-let		Latin *small table*	A solid, flattish dosage form containing medication

Exercises

A. Use your new knowledge of the *language of pharmacology* to answer the following questions. *Fill in the blanks.*   **LO 22.1, 22.6, 22.8**

1. What circumstances does a caregiver need to have correct before administering a drug to a patient?

   a. _____

   b. _____

   c. _____

   d. _____

   e. _____

2. Write a brief statement describing what can happen if any of the above criteria are not met. Be prepared to discuss this in class.

   _____

   _____

   _____

   _____

The following classification of drugs is based on that used by the Drug Effectiveness Review Project (DERP), a collaboration of public entities including Oregon Health and Science University. DERP reported on the effectiveness of the most widely used drugs. The classification meshes with the body system chapters used in this book. Each drug is listed first by its generic name and then its capitalized brand name(s). In addition, pharmacology targeted at specific problems can be found in each body system chapter. The following information will enable you to:

22.4.1 Describe different classes of drugs used for specific purposes.

22.4.2 Identify different drugs by their generic and brand names.

22.4.3 Describe the effects of drugs on their targeted tissues.

22.4.4 Discuss the route of administration for different drugs.

LO 22.9 Allergy Drugs

Nasal Corticosteroids

Nasal **corticosteroids** are a safe and effective treatment for both allergic and nonallergic rhinitis in adults and children. Eight preparations are on the market in the United States, each differing in chemistry, delivery device, propellant, potency, and dosing frequency. They include beclomethasone (Qvar, Beconase), budesonide (Rhinocort), fluticasone (Flonase, Flovent), mometasone (Nasonex), triamcinolone (Azmacort), and a combination of budesonide and formoterol (Symbicort). These drugs cause few side effects in adults, but among children their use slightly increases the risk of stunted growth.

Antihistamines

Antihistamines inhibit the effects of **histamine** at specific cell receptors. They have a number of clinical indications, including allergic conditions (for example, rhinitis, dermatoses, atopic dermatitis, contact dermatitis, allergic conjunctivitis, hypersensitivity reactions to drugs, mild transfusion reactions, and urticaria), chronic idiopathic urticaria (CIU), motion sickness, **vertigo**, and **insomnia**.

The first antihistamines to be developed readily crossed the blood–brain barrier *(see Chapter 9)*, where they could cause adverse central nervous system effects, including sedation, drowsiness, and decreased cognitive processing.

More recently developed antihistamines have higher specificity for binding to histamine receptors. Thus, they do not penetrate the blood–brain barrier well and are less likely to cause the adverse effects of the earlier antihistamines.

Antihistamines currently being developed by drug companies are intended to be natural metabolites of first-generation drugs, so they are designed to improve clinical efficacy and minimize side effects.

Many antihistamine drugs are available without a prescription. Examples include early antihistamines like brompheniramine (Dimetapp, Bromphen, Dimetane, Nasahist), chlorpheniramine (Chlor-Trimeton), clemastine (Allerhist, Tavist), and diphenhydramine (Benadryl). A newer OTC antihistamine called loratadine (Claritin), does not cause drowsiness.

More recent prescription antihistamines include cetirizine (Zyrtec), desloratadine (Clarinex), fexofenadine (Allegra), and levocetirizine (Xyzal). These antihistamines, like loratadine, are less likely to cause adverse effects like drowsiness or dry mouth. In 2011, Zyrtec and Allegra became OTC drugs.

Several antihistamine nasal sprays (for example, azelastine [Astelin]) are also available OTC. They can be effective for the treatment of such symptoms as runny nose, sneezing, and itchy nose.

WORD	PRONUNCIATION	ELEMENTS		DEFINITION
allergy	**AL**-er-jee	P/	all- *other*	State of hypersensitivity
		R/	**-ergy** *work*	
allergic (adj)	Ah-**LER**-jik	S/	-ic *pertaining to*	Pertaining to an allergy
corticosteroid	**KOR**-tih-koh-**STEHR**-oyd	S/	-steroid *steroid*	A hormone produced by the adrenal cortex
		R/CF	**cortic/o** *cortex, cortisone*	
histamine	**HISS**-tah-mean	R/	**hist-** *derived from histidine*	Compound liberated in tissues as a result of injury or an allergic response
		R/CF	**-amine** *nitrogen compound*	
antihistamine	an-tee-**HISS**-tah-mean	P/	anti- *against*	Drug used to treat allergic symptoms because of its action antagonistic to histamine
insomnia	in-**SOM**-nee-ah	S/	-ia *condition*	Inability to sleep
		P/	in- *not*	
		R/	**-somn-** *sleep*	
vertigo	**VER**-tih-go		Latin *dizziness*	Sensation of spinning or whirling

Exercises

A. Analyze the following questions and write the best answer, using the *language of pharmacology*.   LO 22.1, 22.9

1. Critical thinking: Think back to the integumentary system. What is the difference between *atopic dermatitis* and *contact dermatitis?*

   a. atopic dermatitis:

   _____

   _____

   b. contact dermititis:

   _____

   _____

2. What type of drug is prescribed for these two conditions (see question 1)?

   _____

   _____

3. Which generation of this drug (see question 2) can readily cross the blood–brain barrier?

   _____

   _____

4. What types of adverse effects will occur if the BBB is crossed?

   _____

   _____

5. What does the BBB protect?

   _____

   _____

Abbreviations	
ACE	angiotensin converting enzyme
ARB	angiotensin receptor blocker
AV	atrioventricular
CCB	calcium channel blocker
DERP	Drug Effectiveness Review Project
FDA	Food and Drug Administration
tPA	issue plasminogen activator

Keynote

Diuretics indirectly affect the heart by acting on the kidneys to stimulate urinary fluid loss, thus lessening the amount of fluid the heart must cope with; chlorothiazide (Diuril), furosemide (Lasix), and spironolactone (Aldactone) are examples of diuretics.

LO 22.9 Cardiovascular Drugs

Beta Blockers

Beta blockers diminish the effects of **epinephrine** and other stress hormones *(see Chapter 17)*. All beta blockers are approved for the treatment of hypertension. Specific beta blockers are approved for treatment of

- angina
- atrial arrhythmias *(see Chapter 10)*
- coronary artery disease
- heart failure
- hypertension
- early posttraumatic stress disorder *(see Chapter 9)*

Beta blockers are also sometimes used in the prevention of migraines. There are some 20 different beta blocking agents altogether, including propanolol (Inderal), atenolol (Tenormin), metoprolol (Lopressor), pinidolol (Visken), labetalol (Normodyne), and carvedilol (Coreg).

The **renin-angiotensin** system is a complex biological system between the heart, brain, blood vessels, and kidneys. It plays an important role in the pathology of hypertension, cardiovascular disease, chronic kidney disease, and diabetic nephropathy *(see Chapter 17)*. The potent chemical angiotensin II is formed in the blood from angiotensin I by the angiotensin converting enzyme (**ACE**). Angiotensin II causes blood vessels to contract and narrow, leading to hypertension.

ACE inhibitors inhibit, or slow, the activity of the angiotensin converting enzyme (ACE). This action decreases the formation of angiotensin II, so blood vessels dilate more and blood pressure falls. Some 10 different ACE inhibitors have been approved to control hypertension, treat heart failure, prevent strokes, and improve survival rates after heart attacks.

Angiotensin-receptor blockers (**ARBs**) block the interaction between angiotensin and the angiotensin receptors on the muscles in the wall of blood vessels, allowing blood vessels to dilate. They are used when patients are unable to tolerate ACE inhibitors because of persistent cough or, more rarely, **angioedema**.

Calcium-channel blockers (**CCBs**) inhibit the flow of calcium through channels in cardiac muscles and in the muscles in the walls of blood vessels. This leads to a decrease in muscle contraction and dilation of the blood vessels. More than 20 CCBs have been approved to treat hypertension (particularly in elderly patients), angina, arrhythmias, and Raynaud disease *(see Chapter 10)*. A high mortality rate has been reported among people who take the drugs over an extended dosage period.

Statins

Statins are a class of drugs that block the enzyme in the liver that is responsible for making **cholesterol**, an essential component in all cell membranes that is necessary for the production of bile acids, steroid hormones, and Vitamin D. However, the body's production of cholesterol also contributes to the development of atherosclerosis *(see Chapter 10)*. Seven statins are approved by the **FDA** for use; they vary in their potency to decrease cholesterol levels. Examples include atorvastatin (Lipitor), lovastatin (Mevacor), rosuvastatin (Crestor), simvastatin (Zocor), and pravastatin (Pravachol). One new drug, omega-3-acid esters (Lovaza), lowers very high triglyceride levels *(see Chapter 10)*.

Other Cardiovascular Drugs

Chronotropic drugs alter the heart rate. Epinephrine (adrenaline), norepinephrine (noradrenaline), and atropine increase the heart rate. Quinidine (Quinidex), procainamide (Pronestyl), lidocaine (Xylocaine), and propranolol (Propanolol) slow the heart.

Inotropic drugs alter the contractions of the myocardium. Digitalis and its derivatives, digoxin and digitoxin, increase the strength of contractions of the myocardium, thus leading to increased cardiac output.

Dromotropic drugs affect the conduction speed in the atrioventricular (AV) node and subsequently the rate of conduction of electrical impulses in the heart. A calcium channel blocker, such as verapamil, slows the speed of conduction through the cardiac neural system and has a negative dromotropic effect.

Anticoagulants reduce susceptibility to thrombus formation. These include aspirin, warfarin (Coumadin), heparin and a low molecular weight heparin named dalteparin (Fragmin), and new thrombin inhibitors *(see Chapter 11)* such as dabigatran etexilate (Pradaxa) and rivaroxaban (Xarelto).

- **Streptokinase**, which is derived from hemolytic streptococci, dissolves the fibrin in blood clots. If administered intravenously within 3 to 4 hours of a heart attack caused by a clot, it can be effective in dissolving the clot.

- **Tissue plasminogen activator (tPA)** binds strongly to fibrin and dissolves clots that have caused heart attacks. It is similar in effect and use to streptokinase. Reteplase (Retavase) and urokinase (Abbokinase) are forms of tPA.

Word Analysis and Definition

S = Suffix   P = Prefix   R = Root   R/CF = Combining Form

WORD	PRONUNCIATION	ELEMENTS		DEFINITION
betablocker	**BAY**-tah-**BLOCK**-er	S/ R/	beta second letter in Greek alphabet -er *agent* -block- *to obstruct*	A beta-adrenergic blocking agent used in the treatment of cardiac arrhythmias, hypertension and other diseases
chronotropic	**KRONE**-oh-**TROH**-pic	S/ R/	-tropic *change* chrono- *time*	Affecting the heart rate
dromotropic	**DROH**-moh-**TROH**-pic	R/	dromo- *race, a running*	Affecting the rate of conduction in the AV node, and subsequently the heart rate
diuretic	die-you-**RET**-ik	S/ P/ R/	-ic *pertaining to* di- *from dia- throughout* -uret- *urine, urination*	Agent that acts on the kidney to increase urine output
inhibit	in-**HIB**-it		Latin *to keep back*	To curb or restrain
inotropic	**IN**-oh-**TROH**-pic	S/ R/	-tropic *change* ino- *sinew*	Affecting the contractility of cardiac muscle
statin	**STAT**-in		Latin *condition, state*	A drug used to lower cholesterol in the bloodstream

Exercises

A. Read the following paragraphs and use the *language of pharmacology* to answer the questions.   LO 22.1, 22.9

Chronotropic drugs alter the heart rate. Epinephrine (adrenaline), norepinephrine (noradrenaline), and atropine increase the heart rate. Quinidine (Quinidex), procainamide (Pronestyl), lidocaine (Xylocaine), and propranolol (Propanolol) slow the heart.

Inotropic drugs alter the contractions of the myocardium. Digitalis and its derivatives, digoxin and digitoxin, increase the strength of contractions of the myocardium, thus leading to increased cardiac output.

1. One term in the preceding paragraphs has an element meaning *time*. That term is _____.

2. Insert that element into an English word with the same type of meaning. _____

3. Name one of the drugs in these paragraphs that is involved in the *fight-or-flight response.* _____

4. These similar terms in the paragraphs alter something in the heart:

Chronotropic drugs alter _____.

Inotropic drugs alter _____.

5. Identify the structure involved in the alterations in question 4. _____

B. Use the *language of pharmacology* to answer the questions and create a sentence.   LO 22.1, 22.3, 22.9

1. What is the function of a

a. statin: _____

b. diuretic: _____

c. betablocker: _____

2. Use any one of the above terms in a sentence of clinical documentation.

_____

_____

_____

LO 22.9 Dermatologic Drugs

No matter what the cause of skin lesions, a wide range of **topical pharmacologic agents** of different types can be used in their treatment, either to relieve symptoms or to cure the disease.

- **Antipruritics**—topical **lotions**, **ointments**, **creams**, or **sprays** that relieve itching. Corticosteroids, such as hydrocortisone, are used most frequently.

- **Antibacterials**—topical agents that eliminate the bacteria that cause epidermal infections. The antibiotic neomycin is frequently used in ointments for this purpose.

- **Antifungals**—topical agents that eliminate or inhibit the growth of fungi. Terbinafine (Lamisil) is used as a cream, gel, spray, or tablet; nystatin (Mycostatin, Nilstat) is used as a cream or ointment or as oral drops for oral candidiasis *(see Chapter 15).* A class of drugs called *imidazoles* is available in many forms, including creams, sprays, lotions, and shampoos. They include clotrimazole (Canesten, Clomazol) and ketoconazole (Ketopine, Daktagold). In oral preparations, amphotericin B (Fungizone) is used to treat oral candidiasis (thrush), and in IV therapy, it is used for systemic fungal infections. A recent study has shown that OTC mentholated ointments, such as Vicks VapoRub, can be effective in treating toenail fungus infections.

- **Parasiticides**—topical agents that kill parasites living on the skin. Hexachlorocyclohexane (Lindane 1%) is used in lotion or shampoo form to kill lice if other methods have failed.

- **Keratolytics**—topical agents that peel the skin's stratum corneum away from the other epidermal layers. Salicylic acid is used for this purpose as a **keratolytic** or **exfoliating** agent. It is used in the treatment of **acne**, **psoriasis**, **ichthyoses**, and **dandruff**. It is available in the form of wipes, creams, lotions, gels, ointments, shampoos, and patches in strengths varying from 3% to 20%.

- **Anesthetics**—topical agents that relieve pain or itching on the skin's surface. Benzocaine (ethyl ester of para-aminobenzoic acid) is used for this purpose as a numbing cream. It is given prior to injections, for infant teething, for oral ulcers, and for hemorrhoids.

- **Retinoids**—derivatives of **retinoic acid** (Vitamin A) that are used in the treatment of acne, sun spots, and psoriasis. Retinoids are powerful drugs that are used only under the strict supervision of a physician. Tretinoin (Retin-A) is used topically for the treatment of acne; isotretinoin (Accutane) is taken orally for the treatment of severe acne; etretinate (Tegison) is taken orally for the treatment of severe psoriasis, and adapalene (Differin) is used topically for the treatment of psoriasis.

S = Suffix   P = Prefix   R = Root   R/CF = Combining Form

WORD	PRONUNCIATION	ELEMENTS		DEFINITION
cream	KREEM		Latin *thick juice*	A semisolid emulsion for topical use
exfoliation	eks-**FOH**-lee-**A**-shun	S/ P/ R/	**-ion** *action, process* **ex-** *away from, out of* **-foliat-** *leaf*	Detachment and shedding of superficial cells from any tissue surface
exfoliating (adj)	eks-**FOH**-lee-**A**-ting	S/	**-ing** *quality of, doing*	The quality of exfoliation
ichthyosis	ik-thee-**OH**-sis	S/ R/	**-osis** *condition* **ichthy** *fish*	Scaling and dryness of the skin
keratolytic	**KER**-ah-toe-**LIT**-ik	S/ R/CF R/	**-ic** *pertaining to* **kerat/o-** *horn* **-lyt-** *loosening*	Causing separation or loosening of the horny layer (stratum corneum) of the epidermis
lotion	**LOW**-shun		Latin *a washing*	Liquid suspension for topical use
ointment	**OYNT**-ment		French *a smearing*	A semisolid preparation for topical use

Exercises

A. Practice your *language of pharmacology* by correctly filling in the blanks of patient documentation.   LO 22.1, 22.2, 22.9

1. What three terms describe topical medications?

   a. _____

   b. _____

   c. _____

2. Antipruritics, antibacterials, and antifungals have some things in common.

   What are they? _____

3. What type of dermatologic drug can be used to kill lice?

   _____

4. What drug is popular for treating acne? _____

5. Psoriasis and dandruff can be treated with the same kind of drug. What is it?

   _____

6. What category of drug can be given for infant teething and hemorrhoids?

   _____

B. Write one sentence of patient documentation that contains at least two terms from this lesson or the above WAD.   LO 22.1, 22.2, 22.9

1. Sentence:

   _____

   _____

   _____

LO 22.9 Endocrine Drugs

Diabetes Drugs

Antidiabetic drugs treat diabetes mellitus by lowering blood glucose levels.

Diabetes mellitus type 1 is caused by lack of **insulin** and is treated predominantly by subcutaneous injections *(see Chapter 15)* of insulin. All insulin is sold in liquid form, but in different strengths. The most common strength prescribed in the United States is U-100, which is 100 units of insulin per milliliter of liquid. The four synthetic types of insulin are

- **Rapid-acting insulin**, which begins to work after 5 to 10 minutes, peaks in about an hour, and lasts for 2 to 4 hours. Examples include insulin lispro (Humalog) and insulin aspart (NovoLog).

- **Regular-acting insulin**, which reaches the bloodstream within 30 minutes, peaks after 2 to 3 hours, and is effective for 2 to 3 hours. Examples include insulin isophane (Humulin-R and Novolin-R).

- **Intermediate-acting insulin**, which reaches the bloodstream after 2 to 4 hours, peaks 4 to 12 hours later, and is effective for 12 to 18 hours. Examples include insulin isophane (Humulin-N and Novolin-N).

- **Long-acting insulin**, which reaches the bloodstream after 6 to 10 hours and is effective for 20 to 24 hours. Examples include insulin glargine (Lantus) and insulin detemir (Levemir).

Insulin pumps deliver rapid- or regular-acting insulin continuously over a 24-hour period through a subcutaneous catheter. Buttons on the pump allow an additional bolus of insulin to be given if blood sugar levels become too high.

Diabetes mellitus type 2 is caused by resistance of the body's cells to insulin. Several types of drugs, mostly given orally, can be effective in its treatment. They are often given in combination.

- **Biguanides** increase the uptake of glucose by body cells. Metformin (Glucophage) is a first-line medication for type 2; it can be used in combination with other oral diabetic medications, particularly rosiglitazone *(see below)*. It is the most widely prescribed antidiabetic drug in the world: in the United States, more than 50 million prescriptions are written annually for its generic formulations.

- **Thiazolidinediones**, also known as glitazones, enhance use of glucose by the body's cells. The two that have FDA approval are rosiglitazone (Avandia) and pioglitazone (Actos); however, rosiglitazone is currently being evaluated for potential adverse cardiac effects.

- **Sulfonylureas** stimulate insulin release from the pancreatic beta cells. Only effective in the treatment of type 2 diabetes, they can be used in combination with metformin or thiazolidinediones. First-generation agents included tolbutamide (Orinase) and chlorpropamide (Diabinese). More effective second-generation agents include glipizide (Glucotrol) and glyburide (Micronase).

- **Exenatide** (Byetta) is the first injectable, or subcutaneous, drug approved for type 2 diabetes. It is injected subcutaneously 60 minutes before the first and last meals of the day. It stimulates insulin production from the pancreatic beta cells.

- Three oral drugs that stimulate insulin production have been approved for type 2 diabetes: sitagliptin (Januvia, approved 2006), saxagliptin (Onglyza, 2009), and linagliptin (Tradjenta, 2011). These drugs are often used in combination with metformin.

Word Analysis and Definition

S = Suffix   P = Prefix   R = Root   R/CF = Combining Form

WORD	PRONUNCIATION		ELEMENTS	DEFINITION
biguanides	bih-**GWAN**-ides		derived from chemical name 2-carbamimidoylguanidine	Class of drugs based upon this molecule used for the treatment of diabetes
diabetes mellitus	dye-ah-**BEE**-teez **MEL**-ih-tus		**diabetes** Greek *a siphon* **mellitus** Latin *sweetened with honey*	Metabolic syndrome caused by insulin deficiency and/or insulin ineffectiveness
insulin	**IN**-syu-lin	S/ R/	**in-** *chemical compound* **insul-** *island*	A hormone secreted by the islet cells of the pancreas
sulfonylureas	**SUL**-foh-nil-you-**RE**-az	P/ R/ R/	**sulf-** *contains sulfur atom* **-onyl-** *nail* **-urea** *urine*	Group of chemicals related to sulfonamides that possess hypoglycemic action
thiazolidinediones	**THIGH**-ah-**ZOL**-ih-deen-**DIE**-owns		derived from the chemical names of the class member drugs	A class of antidiabetic drugs that diminish peripheral insulin resistance

Exercises

A. Translate the following sentences into language your patient can understand.   LO 22.1, 22.2, 22.9

1. "Insulin pumps deliver rapid- or regular-acting insulin continuously over a 24 hour period through a subcutaneous catheter."
Translation:

_____

_____

_____

2. "Buttons on the pump allow an additional bolus of insulin to be given if glucose levels become too high." Translation:

_____

_____

_____

B. Write a multiple-choice test question from this spread and the above WAD. *You must give 5 possible answer choices.*   **LO 22.1, 22.2, 22.9**

1. Question:

_____

_____

_____

a. _____

b. _____

c. _____

d. _____

e. _____

Abbreviations

AI	aromatase inhibitor
ERD	estrogen-receptor downregulator
HRT	hormone replacement therapy
HT	hormone therapy
PTU	propylthiouracil
SERM	selective estrogen receptor modulator

LO 22.9 Hormone Replacement Therapy

Hormone replacement therapy (HRT) uses estrogen and progestin to treat symptoms of menopause (*see Chapter 8*). The **hormone therapy (HT)** comes as a tablet, patch, injection, vaginal cream, or vaginal ring. HRT protects against osteoporosis (*see Chapter 14*) and reduces the risk for uterine cancer, but it may increase the risk for blood clots, breast cancer, heart disease, stroke, and gallstones. At this time, short-term (up to 5 years) use of HRT given in the lowest possible dose to treat the symptoms of menopause appears to be safe for many women.

LO 22.9 Hormone Therapy

Estrogen makes hormone-receptor-positive breast cancers (*see Chapter 8*) grow. Hormone therapy (HT) medications treat hormone-receptor-positive breast cancers by lowering the amount of estrogen in the body and/or blocking the action of estrogen on breast cancer cells. They are used after surgery to help slow the growth of advanced-stage or metastatic hormone-receptor-positive breast cancers. There are three main types of HT agents:

- **Aromatase inhibitors (AIs)**, which stop the production of estrogen from androgen in post-menopausal women. These medications are anastrozole (Arimidex), exemestane (Aromasin), and letrozole (Femara). Each is given in a pill form taken once a day. Anastrozole and letrozole are available in generic form.

- **Selective estrogen receptor modulators (SERMs)**, which block estrogen in the estrogen receptors of breast cells so that the cells can't grow and multiply. The SERMs are tamoxifen (Nolvadex), raloxifene (Evista), and toremifene (Fareston).

- **Estrogen-receptor downregulators (ERDs)** act just like SERMs, sitting in the receptors of breast cells to block estrogen; fulvestrant (Faslodex) is the only approved ERD at this time.

LO 22.9 Thyroid Drugs

Thyroid hormone replacement is used to treat hypothyroidism (*see Chapter 17*) and to suppress further growth of thyroid tissue in people with thyroid cancer. Levothyroxine (Levoxyl, Synthroid, Unithroid), which is identical to the thyroid hormone T4, is the most commonly prescribed form of thyroid replacement. It is taken orally once a day.

Anti-thyroid drugs treat an overactive thyroid gland (hyperthyroidism) by decreasing its output of thyroid hormone; propylthiouracil (**PTU**) blocks the production of thyroid hormone inside the gland; methimazole (Tapazole) acts the same as PTU. Both drugs may take 1 to 4 months to normalize thyroid levels. Beta-blockers can help block the body's cells reaction to excess thyroid hormone, and iodide solutions (Lugol's solution) can prevent the release of thyroid hormone from an overactive thyroid gland.

Radioactive iodine (131-iodine, I-131), a radioactive **isotope**, is used to kill both normal and cancerous thyroid cells in hyperthyroidism and thyroid cancer.

LO 22.9 Adrenal Drugs

People with adrenal insufficiency (*see Chapter 17*) have a shortage of the hormones cortisol and aldosterone. To treat the condition, cortisol is replaced with a synthetic glucocorticoid, such as hydrocortisone (Hydrocortone, Cortef), prednisone (generic), or dexamethasone (Decadron). Aldosterone is replaced with a synthetic mineralocorticoid fludrocortisone acetate (Florinef).

Overproduction of the two hormones is usually caused by tumors of different types that are removed surgically.

WORD	PRONUNCIATION	ELEMENTS		DEFINITION
glucocorticoid	glu-coh-**KOR**-tih-koyd	S/ R/ R/CF	-oid *resemble* -cortic- *cortex, cortisone* gluc/o- *glucose*	Hormone of the adrenal cortex that helps regulate glucose metabolism
isotope	**EYE**-so-tope	P/ R/	iso- *equal* -tope *part*	Radioactive element used in diagnostic procedures
mineralocorticoid	**MIN**-er-al-oh-**KOR**-tih-koyd	S/ R/ R/CF	-oid *resemble* -cortic- *cortex, cortisone* mineral/o- *inorganic materials*	Hormone of the adrenal cortex that influences sodium and potassium metabolism
radioactive	**RAY**-dee-oh-**AK**-tiv	S/ R/CF R/	-ive *pertaining to* radi/o- *radiation* -act- *performance*	The property of emitting alpha, beta, or gamma rays

Exercises

A. Answer the questions employing the medical *language of pharmacology*.   LO 22.1, 22.2, 22.9

HORMONE-REPLACEMENT THERAPY (HRT)

Hormone replacement therapy (HRT) uses estrogen and progestin to treat symptoms of menopause. The hormone therapy (HT) comes as a tablet, patch, injection, vaginal cream, or vaginal ring. HRT protects against osteoporosis and reduces the risk for uterine cancer, but it may increase the risk for blood clots, breast cancer, heart disease, stroke, and gallstones. At this time, short-term (up to 5 years) use of HRT given in the lowest possible dose to treat the symptoms of menopause appears to be safe for many women.

1. Write on the following lines all the medical terms in this paragraph from the text. *Hint:* It will help you if you circle or highlight them first.

_____

_____

_____

_____

_____

_____

2. Write on the following lines all the good things (pros) about using HRT.

_____

_____

_____

3. Write on the following lines follows all the bad things (cons) about using HRT.

_____

_____

_____

4. Critical Thinking: If faced with these choices, what would you do, or advise someone else to do, and why?

_____

_____

_____

LO 22.9 Gastrointestinal Drugs

Antacids, which are taken orally, neutralize gastric acid and relieve heartburn and acid indigestion. Examples of antacids include

- aluminum hydroxide and magnesium hydroxide (Maalox, Mylanta)
- magnesium hydroxide (Milk of Magnesia)
- calcium carbonate (Tums, Rolaids)

Histamine-2 receptor antagonists (H$_2$-blockers) block signals that tell the stomach cells to produce acid. They are used to treat gastroesophageal reflux (GERD) and esophagitis *(see Chapter 5)*. Examples include

- cimetidine (Tagamet)
- famotidine (Pepcid)
- ranitidine (Zantac)
- nizatidine (Axid)

Less potent OTC variants of these drugs are also available.

Proton pump inhibitors (PPIs) suppress gastric acid secretion in the lining of the stomach by blocking the secretion of gastric acid from the cells into the lumen of the stomach. Examples include

- omeprazole (Prilosec)
- lansoprazole (Prevacid)
- esomeprazole (Nexium)

A new form of PPI called imidazopyridine (Tenatoprazole) appears to be extremely effective in reducing gastric acid.

Misoprostol (Cytotec) inhibits the secretion of gastric acid and is approved for the prevention of **nonsteroidal anti-inflammatory drug (NSAID)** induced gastric acid.

Sucralfate (Carafate) reacts with gastric acid (hydrogen chloride (**HCl**)) to form a paste that binds to stomach mucosal cells and inhibits the **diffusion** of acid into the stomach lumen. It also forms a protective barrier on the surface of an ulcer. Its main use is in the **prophylaxis** of stress ulcers.

Anti–H. pylori therapy *(see Chapter 5)* for the treatment of peptic ulcer and chronic gastritis is given with a combination of two antibiotics (for example, amoxicillin [generic] and clarithromycin [generic]) and a proton pump inhibitor.

Antiemetics, drugs that are effective against vomiting and nausea, are used to treat motion sickness and the side effects of opioid analgesics, general anesthetics, and chemotherapy. The types of antiemetics include

- **Serotonin antagonists**, which block serotonin receptors in the CNS and GI tract. They are used to treat postoperative and chemotherapy nausea and vomiting. Examples include dolasetron (Anzemet), granisetron (Kytril), and ondansetron (Zofran).

- **Dopamine antagonists**, which act in the brain. They are inexpensive, but have an extensive side effect profile and have been replaced by serotonin antagonists. Examples include chlorpromazine (Thorazine) and prochlorperazine (Compazine).

- **Antihistamines**, which are used to treat motion sickness, morning sickness in pregnancy, and opioid nausea. Examples include diphenhydramine (Benadryl) and promethazine (Phenergan).

- **Cannabinoids**, which are used in patients with **cachexia** or who are unresponsive to other antiemetics. Examples include cannabis (medical marijuana) and dronabinol (Marinol).

Laxative drugs are used to treat chronic constipation *(see Chapter 5)*:

- If increased water and fiber is unsuccessful, OTC forms of magnesium hydroxide are the first-line agents to be used.

- Lubiprostone (Resolor) has received FDA approval; it acts on the epithelial cells of the GI tract to produce a chloride-rich fluid that softens the **stool** and increases bowel **motility**.

Antidiarrheal drugs are widely available OTC. Examples include loperamide (Imodium A-D, Maalox), which reduces bowel motility; bismuth subsalicylate (Pepto-Bismol), which decreases the secretion of fluid into the intestine; and attapulgite (Kaopectate), which pulls diarrhea-causing substances away from the GI tract; as well as enzymes and nutrients. A combination of diphenyloxylate and atropine (Lomotil), a Schedule V drug, reduces bowel motility.

Word Analysis and Definition

S = Suffix   P = Prefix   **R** = Root   **R/CF** = Combining Form

WORD	PRONUNCIATION	ELEMENTS		DEFINITION
cachexia	kah-**KEK**-see-ah	P/ R/	cach- *bad* -exia *condition of body*	A general weight loss and wasting of the body
diffusion	dih-**FYU**-shun	S/ R/	-ion *process, action* **diffus-** *movement*	The process by which small particles move between tissues
laxative	**LAK**-sah-tiv	S/ R/CF	-tive *pertaining to* **lax/a-** *looseness*	An oral agent that promotes the expulsion of feces
motility	moh-**TILL**-ih-tee	S/ R/	-ility *condition, state of* **mot-** *to move*	The ability for spontaneous movement
stool	STOOL		Old English *a seat*	The matter discharged in one movement of the bowels

Exercises

A. Which of the following statements is NOT true? *Circle the answer and then write the corrected statement on the following lines.*
LO 22.1, 22.2, 22.9

1. Laxative drugs are used to treat chronic constipation.   T   F

2. Antihistamines treat motion sickness.   T   F

3. Antidiarrheal drugs all require prescriptions.   T   F

4. Antihistamines are used to treat morning sickness.   T   F

5. Cannabinoids are antiemetics.   T   F

6. Corrected statement:

_____

_____

_____

B. Read the statements carefully and match them with the right drugs.   LO 22.1, 22.2, 22.9

1. used to suppress gastric acid secretions   **a.** Maalox

2. used to treat opioid nausea   **b.** Imodium

3. neutralizes gastric acid and relieves heartburn   **c.** Tagamet

4. used for treatment of postoperative nausea   **d.** Nexium

5. antidiarrheal drug   **e.** Benadryl

6. blocks production of stomach acid   **f.** Zofran

LO 22.9 Musculoskeletal Drugs

NSAIDs inhibit the two cyclooxygenase (COX) enzymes that are involved in producing the inflammatory process. They have **analgesic** and **antipyretic** effects and are used for treatment of tissue injury, pyrexia, rheumatoid arthritis, osteoarthritis, gout, and nonspecific joint and tissue pains. The three major NSAIDs, each of which is available OTC, are

1. **Acetylsalicylic acid** (aspirin), which in addition to the above effects and uses also has an antiplatelet effect due to its inhibition of one of the COX enzymes; thus, it is often used in the prevention of heart attacks.

2. **Ibuprofen** (Advil, Motrin, and several other trade names), which acts by inhibiting both the COX enzymes, essential elements in the enzyme pathways involved in pain, inflammation, and fever. It is taken orally, but in 2009 an injectable form of ibuprofen (Caldolor) was approved for use. In some studies, ibuprofen has been associated with the prevention of Alzheimer and Parkinson diseases, but further studies are needed.

3. **Naproxen** (Aleve and many other trade names), which is taken orally once a day and also inhibits both the COX enzymes.

Indomethacin, an NSAID that inhibits both cyclooxygenase (COX) enzymes, is a potent drug with many serious side effects. It is not used as an analgesic for minor aches and pains or for fever.

Paracetamol (acetaminophen), an active **metabolite** of phenacetin (not an NSAID), is a widely used OTC analgesic and antipyretic. It is used for the relief of minor aches and pains and is an **ingredient** in many cold and flu remedies.

Skeletal muscle relaxants are FDA-approved for spasticity (baclofen, dantrolene, tizanidine) or for musculoskeletal conditions like multiple sclerosis (carisoprodol, chlorzoxazone, cyclobenzaprine, metaxalone, methocarbamol, orphenadrine). The only drug with available evidence of efficacy in spasticity is tizanidine (Zanaflex, Sirdalud), but cyclobenzaprine (Amrix) appears to be somewhat effective.

Keynote
___

Spasticity is a state of increased muscular tone with exaggeration of the tendon reflexes.

WORD	PRONUNCIATION	ELEMENTS		DEFINITION
analgesia	an-al-**JEE**-zee-ah	S/ P/ R/	-ia *condition* an- *without* -alges- *sensation of pain*	State in which pain is reduced
analgesic		S/	-ic *pertaining to*	Agent that produces analgesia
antipyretic	**AN**-tee-pie-**RET**-ik	S/ P/ R/	-ic *pertaining to* anti- *against* -pyret- *fever*	Agent that reduces fever
ingredient	in-**GREE**-dee-ent	P/ R/	in- *in, into* -gredient *going*	An element in a mixture
metabolism	meh-**TAB**-oh-lizm	S/ R/	-ism *condition* metabol- *change*	The constantly changing physical and chemical processes in the cell
metabolite		S/	-ite *associated with*	Any product of metabolism

Exercises

A. Employ *medical language* that you should know by now to answer the questions about the following paragraph.
   LO 22.1, 22.2, 22.9

Nonsteroidal anti-inflammatory drugs (NSAIDs) inhibit enzymes that are involved in the inflammatory process. They have **analgesic** and **antipyretic** effects and are used for treatment of tissue injury, pyrexia, rheumatoid arthritis, osteoarthritis, gout, and nonspecific joint and tissue pains.

1. Analyze the two terms in the word *anti-inflammatory* and give their meanings.

   anti:

   _____

   inflammatory:

   _____

2. *Analgesics* and *antipyretics* relieve which two symptoms?

   _____ and _____

3. What is *osteoarthritis*? _____

4. *Gout* affects which body system? _____

5. What is the main function of an NSAID?

   _____

   _____

B. Select the correct medical term to complete the following questions. *Circle the correct answer and then fill in the blanks.*   **LO 22.1, 22.2, 22.9**

1. NSAIDS inhibit enzymes that are involved in the _____ process.

   a. respiratory

   b. digestive

   c. urinary

   d. pulmonary

   e. inflammatory

2. The three major groups of NSAIDS available OTC are

   a. _____

   b. _____

   c. _____

LO 22.9 Neurologic Drugs

The transmission of impulses from one neuron to another and from a neuron to a cell is achieved by neurotransmitters at synaptic connections (*see Chapter 9*). Drugs that affect the nervous system, include

1. **Opioids**, which depress nerve transmission in the synapses of sensory pathways of the brain and spinal cord. They also bind to opioid receptors found principally in the central and peripheral nervous systems (*see Chapter 9*) and the GI tract. There are a number of broad classes of opioids:

   - **Natural opiates** are alkaloids contained in the resin of the opium poppy—primarily morphine and codeine.

   - **Semi synthetic opioids**, which are created from the natural opiates, include heroin, hydromorphone (Dilaudid), hydrocodone (Vicodin), oxycodone (Dinarkon), and buprenorphine (Subutex).

   - **Fully synthetic opioids** include fentanyl (Sublimage), pethidine (Demerol), and methadone (Symoron).

   - **Natural opioid peptides** are produced naturally in the body; they include endorphins, enkephalins, and endomorphins.

   Indications for opioids are moderate to severe pain, cough, severe diarrhea, anxiety due to shortness of breath (SOB), and opioid dependence (in which case methadone and buprenorphine are used). Opiates are addictive because they produce tolerance and physical dependence.

2. **Opiate antagonists**, such as naloxone (Narcan) and naltrexone (Revia, Depade), which prevent opiates from acting in the synapses. They can be used in cases of drug overdose and to help recovering heroin addicts stay drug-free.

3. **Analgesics**, which are drugs used to relieve pain. The major classes are

   - NSAIDs and Paracetamol (acetaminophen) (see the previous text concerning musculoskeletal drugs).

   - Opiates (see previous entry 1).

   - Combinations of the two previous classes. Examples of these prescription drugs include acetaminophen with hydrocodone (Anexsia) and acetaminophen with oxycodone (Percocet).

   - Triptans, which are effective serotonin receptor **agonists** in the treatment of migraines and cluster headaches (*see Chapter 9*) that do not respond to NSAIDs. They do not provide preventive treatment and are not a cure. Some 17 brand names of triptans are available.

4. **Inhaled anesthetics**, such as isoflurane, which act similarly to but are more powerful than sedatives; however, they are being replaced by IV agents such as propofol (Diprivan).

5. **Antiepileptics**, which act in different ways on the synaptic junctions to keep stimuli from passing across the synapse; phenobarbital, phenytoin (Dilantin), and carbamazepine (Calepsin) are examples.

6. **Alzheimer drugs**, which cannot reverse the disease process nor stop the underlying destruction of nerve cells. Only two types of drugs are FDA-approved:

   - Cholinesterase inhibitors boost the amount of **acetylcholine** available at synapses. Three cholinesterase inhibitors are available:

     – Donepezil (Aricept) is approved for all stages of Alzheimer disease.

     – Galantamine (Razadyne) is approved for mild to moderate Alzheimer disease.

     – Rivastigmine (Exelon) is approved for mild to moderate Alzheimer disease.

   - Memantine (Namenda), which regulates a different messenger chemical at the synapses, is approved for moderate to severe Alzheimer disease.
     All of these drugs are only modestly effective in reducing the rate of cognitive decline.

7. **Multiple sclerosis (MS)** (*see Chapter 9*) **drugs** used to treat **remissions** are restricted to **corticosteroids**, which reduce the inflammation that occurs during a **relapse**.

   Drugs that attempt to modify the course of the disease include beta interferons (Avonex, Betaseron, Extavia, Rebif), glatiramer (Copaxone), fingolimod (Gilenya), and natalizumab (Tysabri). Of the four types, beta interferons are used most frequently.

WORD	PRONUNCIATION	ELEMENTS		DEFINITION
narcotic	nar-**KOT**-ik	S/ R/CF	**-tic** *pertaining to* **narc/o-** *sleep, stupor*	Drug derived from opium or opium-like compounds having similar effects
opiate opioid	**OH**-pee-ate **OH**-pee-oyd		Latin *bringing sleep*	A drug derived from opium A narcotic substance, either natural or synthetic
relapse	**REE**-laps	P/ R/	**re-** *again, back* **-lapse** *to slide back*	Return of the disease manifestations after an interval of improvement
remission	ree-**MISH**-un	S/ P/ R/	**-ion** *action, condition* **re-** *again, back* **-miss-** *send*	Period when there is lessening of the manifestations of a disease

Exercises

A. Every body system has its own specific classes of drugs. *Use the* language of neurology and pharmacology *to answer the following questions.* **LO 22.1, 22.2, 22.3, 22.9**

1. Opioids depress nerve transmission in the _____ and _____.

2. Define a *semisynthetic opioid.* _____

3. Name the brands in question 2.

   _____

4. Where are natural opiates found? _____

5. Demerol, methadone, and fentanyl are what type of opioids?

   _____

B. Match the correct drugs with the following statements. **LO 22.1, 22.2, 22.3, 22.9**

1. What opiates are contained in the resin of the opium flower?

   _____ and _____

2. Opium dependence is treated with the drug _____.

3. Only one of the following conditions would require an opioid:

   a. ankylosing spondilitis

   b. Asperger's syndrome

   c. moderate to severe pain

   d. osteoarthritis

   e. hematemesis

4. A drug overdose should be treated with this opiate: _____

5. Opiate analgesics are used to relieve _____.

6. What type of flower produces opium? _____

LO 22.9 Psychiatric Drugs

1. **Antidepressants** all increase the amount of serotonin at the synapses where serotonin is a neurotransmitter *(see Chapter 9)*. Sertraline HCl (Zoloft), paroxetine (Paxil), and fluoxetine (Prozac) are examples.

2. **Stimulants**, such as caffeine, nicotine, amphetamines (Dexedrine, Adderall, Ritalin), and cocaine, enhance stimulation provided by the sympathetic nervous system. They cause the level of dopamine to rise in the synapses, leading to the pleasurable effects associated with these drugs.

3. **Sedatives**, such as barbiturates and benzodiazepines, decrease the sensitivity of the postsynaptic neurons and quiet nervous excitement. They also act on the sleep centers to induce sleep and treat **insomnia**. Newer sedative **hypnotics**, such as zolpidem (Ambien), zaleplon (Sonata), and eszopiclone (Lunesta), act on gamma-aminobutyric acid receptors. Ramelteon (Rozerem) is a selective melatonin receptor agonist.

4. **Tranquilizers**, such as chlorpromazine (Thorazine), haloperidol (Aloperidin), and the benzodiazepines (Librium, Valium, Xanax), calm like sedatives but without including a sleep-inducing effect.

5. **Mood stabilizers**, which focus on diminishing **manic** episodes, include lithium carbonate (Carbolith) and carbamazepine (Tegretol).

6. **Antipsychotics** are used to treat symptoms of **psychosis**, including schizophrenia. Chlorpromazine (Thorazine), haloperidol (Haldol), and trifluoperazine (Stelazine) are examples.

7. **Psychedelics** distort sensory perceptions—particularly sight and sound. They can be natural plant products, such as mescaline, psilocybin, and dimethyltryptamine, or they can be synthetic, such as lysergic acid diethylamide (**LSD**), methylenedioxymethamphetamine (**MDMA** or "ecstasy"), and phencyclidine (**PCP** or "angel dust"). They increase the amount of serotonin in the synaptic junctions, and some deliver additional amphetamine stimulation.

8. **Marijuana** has the active ingredient tetrahydrocannabinol (**THC**). It produces sedative-like drowsiness, like alcohol; dulls pain, like opiates; and, in high doses, distorts perception, like psychedelics. Unlike opiates or sedatives, tolerance does not occur.

Keynote

Drugs in Categories 7 and 8 are "street drugs" and it is illegal to manufacture or purchase them.

S = Suffix   P = Prefix   R = Root   R/CF = Combining Form

WORD	PRONUNCIATION	ELEMENTS		DEFINITION
sedative	SED-ah-tiv	S/ R/	-tive *quality of* sedat- *to calm*	Agent that calms nervous excitement
stabilize	STAY-bil-ize	S/ R/	-ize *action* stabil- *steady, fixed*	To make or hold firm and steady
stabilizer	STAY-bil-ize-er	S/	-er *agent*	An agent that stabilizes
stimulant	STIM-you-lant	S/ R/	-ant *forming* stimul- *excite, strengthen*	Agent that excites or strengthens functional activity
tranquilizer	TRANG-kwih-lie-zer	S/ R/	-izer *affects in a particular way* tranquil- *calm, serene*	Agent that calms without sedating or depressing

Exercises

A. Analyze the terminology in the questions and use the correct medical terminology to provide the answers.   LO 22.1, 22.2, 22.9

1. What two senses do psychedelics distort?

   a. taste and smell

   b. hearing and taste

   c. sight and sound

   d. feeling and hearing

   e. sound and smell

2. The doctor is trying to calm his patient down. He will order

   a. an antihistamine

   b. a tranquilizer

   c. an antiemetic

   d. an analgesic

   e. an antipyretic

3. What drug will produce sedative-like drowsiness, dull pain, and distort perception?

   a. marijuana

   b. Xanax

   c. Prozac

   d. Adderall

   e. Haldol

B. Interpret these statements correctly and answer the questions.   LO 22.1, 22.2, 22.9

1. Symptoms of psychosis will be treated with

   a. Keflex

   b. Demerol

   c. Thorazine

   d. Tegretol

   e. Methotrexate

2. Which is NOT a function of a sedative?

   a. quieting nervous excitement

   b. acting on sleep centers

   c. decreasing the sensitivity of postsynaptic neurons

   d. treating insomnia

   e. diminishing manic episodes

LO 22.9 Immunosuppressive Drugs

Immunosuppressive drugs are agents that inhibit or prevent activity of the immune system. They are used to

- Prevent the rejection of transplanted organs and tissues.

- Treat autoimmune diseases, such as rheumatoid arthritis, multiple sclerosis (MS), systemic lupus erythematosus (SLE), and ulcerative colitis.

- Attempt to control nonimmune diseases, such as long-term asthma.

They are classified into four groups:

1. **Glucocorticoids** influence all types of immunological and inflammatory responses, no matter what their cause. Examples include hydrocortisone and prednisone.

2. **Cytostatics** inhibit cell division. Examples include cyclophosphamide (Cytoxan), which is probably the most potent immunosuppressive agent; methotrexate (Amethopterin); azathioprine (generic); cyclosporine (Cyclosporin A); mechlorethamine (nitrogen mustard); and the antibiotic dactinomycin (Actinomycin D), which is used in kidney transplantations.

3. **Antibodies** are used as early immunosuppressive therapy to prevent acute rejection of transplants. **Monoclonal** antibodies are directed toward specific **antigens** and are used to prevent the rejection of transplanted organs. Examples include bevacizumab and panitumumab for cancer, infliximab and adalimamab for autoimmune diseases such as rheumatoid arthritis, and basiliximab and daclizumab for preventing the rejection of kidney transplants.

4. **Targeted immune modulators** are a new category of drugs used for such diseases as rheumatoid arthritis, ankylosing spondylitis, and psoriatic arthritis. Evidence of their effectiveness is evolving but is not yet conclusive.

LO 22.9 Chemotherapy Drugs

Chemotherapy is the treatment of cancer with **antineoplastic** drugs, which kill the rapidly dividing cancer cells. Unfortunately, this means that chemotherapy also harms normal cells that divide rapidly, such as those in the bone marrow, digestive tract, and hair follicles. As a result, chemotherapy commonly has side effects, such as decreased production of blood cells, nausea and vomiting, and **alopecia** (hair loss). Chemotherapy is often combined with other treatments, such as surgery and radiation *(see Chapter 21)*. The types of **chemotherapeutic** agents include **alkaloids**, such as vincristine (Oncovin) and vinblastine; **DNA modifiers**, such as cyclophosphamide (Cytoxan) and chlorambucil (Leukeran); and **cytotoxic** antibiotics, such as actinomycin (generic).

WORD	PRONUNCIATION	ELEMENTS		DEFINITION
antineoplastic (this word has two prefixes)	**ANTEE**-nee-oh-**PLAS**-tik	S/ P/ P/ R/	-ic *pertaining to* **anti-** *against* **-neo-** *new* **-plast-** *to form*	Pertaining to preventing the forming or spread of cancer cells
cytostatic (adj)	sigh-toe-**STAT**-ik	S/ R/CF R/	-ic *pertaining to* **cyt/o-** *cell* **-stat-** *standing still*	Inhibiting cell division
cytotoxic (adj)	sigh-toe-**TOX**-ik	S/	-toxic *able to kill*	Destructive to cells
modulator	mod-you-**LAY**-tor	S/ R/	-ator *agent, instrument* **modul-** *measure properly*	Agent that regulates or adjusts
monoclonal (adj)	**MON**-oh-**KLOH**-nal	S/ P/ R/	-al *pertaining to* **mono-** *one* **-clon-** *cutting used for propagation*	Derived from a single clone of cells, all molecules of which are the same in each cell

Exercises

A. Use your knowledge of *medical terminology* gained in this chapter to answer the following questions.   LO 22.1, 22.2, 22.9

1. Immunosuppressive drugs are agents that inhibit or prevent activity of the immune system.

   a. What is the main function of the immune system?

   _____

   _____

   b. Give an example of when and why you would want to suppress that function.

   _____

   _____

2. Name the autoimmune diseases that could be treated with immunosuppressive drugs.

   a. _____

   b. _____

   c. _____

   d. _____

   e. _____

B. Use the *language of pharmacology* to answer the following questions.   LO 22.1, 22.2, 22.9

1. What is a *neoplasm?*

   _____

   _____

2. Are neoplasms benign or malignant?

   _____

3. How do you know this?

   _____

   _____

LO 22.9 Respiratory Drugs

Bronchodilators relax the smooth muscles of the bronchioles—bronchodilation. Examples are theophylline and aminophylline (theophylline + ethylene diamine) taken orally but used rarely these days; **beta$_2$-agonists**, such as albuterol (Proventil), metaproterenol (Alupent), formoterol (Foradil), and salmeterol (Serevent) which are inhaled; and anticholinergics, such as ipratropium (Atrovent) which is inhaled, and tiotropium (Spiriva) which is taken orally. Newer groups of bronchodilators are **leukotriene inhibitors**, montelukast (Singulair), zafirlukast (Accolate), and zileuton (Zyflo), which are taken orally, and **mast cell stabilizers**, cromolyn sodium (Intal) and nedocromil (Tilade), which are inhaled.

Anti-inflammatory drugs, such as corticosteroids, are given by inhalation (for example, beclomethasone [Vanceril, Beclovent], budesonide [Pulmicort], fluticasone [Flovent], and triamcinolone [Azmacort]). They can also be used orally or intravenously in acute episodes of asthma or chronic obstructive pulmonary disease (COPD).

Combinations of drugs are frequently used (for example, beta$_2$-agonist + anticholinergic, albuterol + ipratropium [Combivent], inhaled corticosteroid + beta$_2$-agonist budesonide + formoterol [Symbicort], and fluticasone + salmeterol [Advair]). An oral leukotriene inhibitor is often taken in association with an inhaled corticosteroid to reduce the dose of corticosteroid.

Mucolytics are agents that break up mucus to allow it to be cleared more effectively from the airways. Examples are guaifenesin (common in OTC cough medications) and *N*-acetylcysteine (Mucomyst), taken through a **nebulizer**.

Antibiotics are used when a bacterial infection is present in COPD. Penicillin, erythromycin, cefotaxime (Claforan), and flucloxacillin (Floxapen) are frequently used.

Oxygen is used in hypoxia and can be given by nasal **cannula** or by mask and intubation. Patients with severe, chronic COPD can be attached to a portable cylinder of oxygen.

Word Analysis and Definition

S = Suffix   P = Prefix   **R = Root**   **R/CF = Combining Form**

WORD	PRONUNCIATION	ELEMENTS		DEFINITION
cannula	**KAN**-you-lah		Latin *reed*	Tube inserted into a blood vessel or cavity as a channel for fluid or gas
inhalation	in-hay-**LAY**-shun	S/ P/ R/	-ation *process* in- *in* **-hale-** *breathe*	The act of inspiration
inhaler	**IN**-hail-er	S/	-er *agent*	Instrument for administering medications by inhalation
mucolytic	**MY**-koh-**LIT**-ik	S/ R/CF R/	-ic *pertaining to* **muc/o-** *mucus* **-lyt-** *dissolve*	Agent capable of dissolving or liquefying mucus
nebulizer	**NEB**-you-lize-er	S/ R/	-izer *line of action* **nebul-** *cloud*	Device used to deliver liquid medicine in a fine mist for inhalation

Exercises

A. The following exercises require critical thinking. *Use* medical language *for the answers.*   **LO 22.1, 22.2, 22.6**

1. A nebulizer is a device used to deliver liquid medicine in a fine mist for inhalation. Is this a good or bad idea, and why? Write your thoughts on the following lines. Be prepared to discuss in class.

   a. good idea:

   _____

   _____

   b. bad idea:

   _____

   _____

2. A nebulizer and an inhaler can both deliver respiratory medicines. What is the major point of body entry for each of them?

   a. nebulizer:

   _____

   _____

   b. inhaler:

   _____

   _____

B. Circle the best answer for the following questions.   **LO 22.1, 22.2, 22.6**

1. What is a probable diagnosis for someone you see carrying around a portable oxygen tank, with a nasal cannula in place?

   a. hyperemesis   d. hematuria

   b. hypoxia   e. hypercondria

   c. hypotension

2. The purpose of a mucolytic drug is to

   a. stop nosebleeds   d. moisturize the nasal passage

   b. break up mucus   e. stop inflammation

   c. cleanse the nasal passage

3. What types of drugs are used when a bacterial infection is present in COPD?

   a. steroids   d. opioids

   b. narcotics   e. antibiotics

   c. mucolytics

LO 22.9 Urologic Drugs

Renal Drugs

Pyelonephritis, which is inflammation of the pelvis of the kidney usually spreading from a **urinary tract infection (UTI)**, is treated aggressively with antibiotics, such as an aminoglycoside (Gentamycin) together with ampicillin or ceftriaxone (Rocephin).

Nephrotic syndrome is treated initially with corticosteroids (Prednisolone), and cytostatic drugs, such as cyclophosphamide (Cytoxan) and cyclosporine (Cyclosporin A), are used for relapses.

Renal cell carcinoma is treated surgically with radical nephrectomy. As renal cell carcinoma is resistant to both radiation and chemotherapy, metastases are treated with targeted therapies using drugs such as temsirolimus (Torisel) and bevacizumab (Avastin). Despite these drugs, the overall survival rate has not improved much.

Renal stones can be prevented by alkalinization of the urine with acetazolamide (Diamox) and with dyazide diuretics, such as chlorthalidone (Thalitone).

Renal transplant patients receive a regimen of drugs to prevent rejection. The most common regimen is a cocktail of tacrolimus (Prograf), mycophenolate (Cellcept), and prednisone (generic).

In patients with chronic renal disease and diminished renal function, dosing of renally excreted drugs should be adjusted by reducing the dose, increasing the dosing interval, or both. Drugs that have to be adjusted include antihypertensive agents, hypoglycemic agents, antimicrobials, analgesics, NSAIDs, and many herbal products.

Non-Renal Urinary Tract Infection Drugs

UTIs, including **cystitis**, are treated with antibiotics, such as trimethoprim (Trimpex, Primsol), nitrofurantoin (Furadantin, Macrobid), or one of the many cephalosporins. Infections that spread from the urinary tract to the epididymis (epididymitis) and the testes (orchitis) are treated with cefalexin or ciprofloxacin.

Sexually transmitted diseases (STDs) are caused by a variety of organisms in both men and women. They require different treatments, depending on the organism.

- **Chlamydia** is treated with a single dose of azithromycin (Zithromax and others) or a week of doxycycline (Vibramycin and others) in both sexes.

- **Trichomoniasis** is treated with metronidazole (Flagyl) or tinidazole (Tindamax).

- **Gonorrhea** has become resistant to most classes of antibiotics except cephalosporins, such as ceftriaxone (Rocephin) and cefixime (Suprax).

- **Bacterial vaginosis** is treated with metronidazole (Flagyl) or clindamycin (Cleocin).

- **Pelvic inflammatory disease (PID)**, which is usually a complication of chlamydia or gonorrhea, is treated with antibiotic combinations of two drugs—for example, cefotetan (Cefotan) and doxycycline (Vibramycin); clindamycin (Cleocin) and gentamicin (Garamycin); or cefoxitin (Cefotan) and doxycycline (Vibramycin).

- **Genital herpes infections** have no cure, but antiviral medications, such as acyclovir (Zovirax), famaciclovir (Famvir), and valacyclovir (Valtrex), can prevent or cut short outbreaks.

- **Syphilis** in its early stages requires a single dose of IM penicillin. If the infection has been present for more than a year, additional doses are required.

- **Human papilloma virus (HPV)** has 40 different types that infect the genital area. HPV can cause cervical cancer. There is no known treatment, but two vaccines are approved by the FDA. Cervarix protects against HPV types 16 and 18. Gardasil protects against types 6, 11, 16, and 18. Both protect against HPV types that cause 70% of cervical cancers, and Gardasil protects against HPV types that cause 90% of genital warts.

- **Human immunodeficiency virus (HIV) infections** have no cure. The aim of treatment is to maintain a good quality of life and prevent the development of **acquired immunodeficiency syndrome (AIDS)**. Highly active antiretroviral therapy (**HAART**) is a combination of at least three drugs belonging to at least two types of **antiretroviral** agents. Without HAART, HIV infection progresses to AIDS in approximately 9 to 10 years.

WORD	PRONUNCIATION	ELEMENTS		DEFINITION
antiretroviral	AN-tee-RET-roh-vi-ral	S/	-al *pertaining to*	An agent that inhibits or kills any virus of the family
		P/	anti- *against*	
retrovirus	RET-roh-vi-rus	P/	-retro- *back, backward*	A virus with RNA core genetic material
		R/	-vir- *virus*	
genital	JEN-it-al	S/	-al *pertaining to*	Relating to the male or female sex organs
		R/	genit- *primary male or female sex organs*	
genitalia	JEN-ih-TAY-lee-ah	S/	-ia *condition*	External and internal organs of reproduction
vaginosis	vah-jih-NOH-sis	S/	-osis *condition*	Any disease of the vagina
		R/	vagin- *vagina*	
vaginitis	vah-jih-NIE-tis	S/	-itis *inflammation*	Inflammation of the vagina

Exercises

A. Review what you learned in the earlier chapters about word elements. *Fill in the answers on the following lines.*   **LO 22.1, 22.2, 22.9**

1. What is most unusual about the term *antiretroviral*?

_____

_____

2. Vaginosis would be found in which body system?

_____

_____

3. What is the only term in the above WAD that can apply to both males and females?

_____

B. Match the condition with the drug(s) used to treat it. *Choose the correct term in the second column.*   **LO 22.1, 22.2, 22.9**

1. syphilis   **a.** antibiotic combination of two drugs

2. used to treat pyelonephritis   **b.** HAART

3. PID   **c.** IM penicillin

4. bacterial vaginosis   **d.** antibiotics

5. HIV   **e.** Flagyl

LO 22.9 Urologic Drugs (continued)

Prostate Drugs

Prostatitis is usually an extension of an *E. coli* UTI. In the acute phase, antibiotics such as trimethoprim-sulfamethoxazole (Bactrim, Septa), fluoroquinolones (Floxin, Cipro), or doxycycline (Vibramycin) are given for 14 days. If the disease is chronic, the regimen is continued for 4 to 12 weeks.

Benign prostatic hypertrophy (BPH) can be treated with two main types of medication. **Alpha blockers**, such as doxazosin (Cardura) or alfuzosin (Uroxatral), relax smooth muscle at the bladder neck to allow a freer flow of urine. **5-alpha-reductase inhibitors**, such as finasteride (Proscar, Propecia) and dutasteride (Avodart), inhibit the production of dihydrotestosterone, which is believed to stimulate the prostate cells to grow.

Prostate cancer is treated primarily with surgery or radiation therapy. Other treatments such as hormonal or chemotherapy are not approved by the Federal Drug Administration (FDA).

Other Nonrenal Urinary Tract Drugs

Erectile dysfunction can be treated with drugs designed to improve the flow of blood to the penis. Examples include sildenafil (Viagra), tadalafil (Cialis), vardenafil (Levitra), and alprostadil (Edex, Caverject), which is injected into one of the corpus cavernosa of the penis. The latter drug is sometimes used for the treatment of **impotence**.

Urinary incontinence, which is any involuntary leakage of urine, almost always results from an underlying treatable medical condition. In an **overactive bladder**, which causes incontinence, drugs that relax the bladder muscle wall can alleviate the symptoms. They include tolterodine (Detrol), oxybutynin (Ditropan), trospium (Sanctura), solifenacin (Vesicare), darifenacin (Enablex), and an oxybutynin skin patch (Oxytrol).

WORD	PRONUNCIATION	ELEMENTS		DEFINITION
dysfunction	dis-**FUNK**-shun	P/	dys- *difficult, painful*	Difficulty in performing
		R/	**-function** *perform*	
dysfunctional (adj)	dis-**FUNK**-shun-al	S/	-al *pertaining to*	Having difficulty in performing
impotence	**IM**-poh-tence		Latin *inability*	Inability to achieve an erection
overactive	**OH**-ver-**ACK**-tiv	S/	-ive *function, connection*	An exaggerated response
		P/	over- *above*	
		R/	-act- *process of doing*	

Exercises

A. Use the *language of the urinary system* and the *language of pharmacology* to answer the questions. *Fill in the blanks.*
   LO 22.1, 22.2, 22.9

1. What is urinary incontinence?

   _____

2. What can cause this incontinence?

   _____

3. What type of drugs can alleviate the symptoms of urinary incontinence?

   _____

4. What usual types of delivery methods do the drugs in question 3 have?

   a. _____

   b. _____

B. Precision in communication involves correct spelling. *Circle the pair of terms that is spelled incorrectly. Rewrite them as correct on the following lines.*   **LO 22.1, 22.2, 22.9**

1. dysfunction   overactive

2. inhibbitors   impotance

3. erectile   cavernosums

4. prostatitis   genital

5. genitalia   pelvic

6. Corrected terms: _____ and _____

C. In the following group of terms, circle any that are NOT a diagnosis. *Take any one term that is not a diagnosis and write a sentence containing that term. The sentence cannot be from the text or the above WAD.*   **LO 22.1, 22.2, 22.9**

vaginitis	genitalia	PID	HIV	genital herpes
analgesic	antitussive	formulary	anabolic	narcotic

1. Appropriate use of a term that is not a diagnosis:

   Term: _____

   _____

   _____

Pharmacology

Challenge Your Knowledge

A. Abbreviations are an important part of clinical documentation. Make sure you know what they mean. Insert the correct abbreviation in the appropriate space. (**LO 22.1, 22.2, 22.7,** *Remember, Understand, Apply*)

ac   b.i.d.   t.i.d   q.i.d.   o.n.   p.o.   p.r.n.   GI   IM   p.c.

1. Mr. Baker's doctor has told you to administer his medication _____ (before meals).

2. The medicine prescribed by the doctor will help Mr. Baker's (gastrointestinal) _____ problem.

3. This medication is to be given to the patient _____ (at night).

4. The patient needs the medication _____ (three times each day).

5. Since her coughing is improving, the patient only needs the medication _____ (when necessary).

6. This medicine should be given _____ (after meals); otherwise, it will upset the patient's stomach.

7. Administer this medication for the patient by _____ (intramuscular) injection.

8. The prescription was written to be taken _____ (four times each day) _____ (by mouth).

9. Do not confuse _____ (twice each day) with _____ (three times each day).

B. Who are the only healthcare personnel licensed to write prescriptions? (**LO 22.2, 22.10,** *Remember, Understand*)

1. _____

C. How do physicians determine which drugs they will prescribe? (**LO 22.2, 22.8,** *Analyze, Apply*)

_____

_____

D. What is the purpose of a port? Circle the correct answer. (**LO 22.2, 22.6, 22.7,** *Remember*)

1. to divert fluids away from the site

2. to provide an entry site for IV fluids

3. to separate veins and arteries

4. to speed the process of blood circulation

5. to help prevent clots

E. To meet lesson objectives and learning outcomes, be prepared to discuss the following questions in class. Be sure you can spell and pronounce each medical term correctly. **(LO 22.1, 22.2, 22.6, *Apply*)**

1. **Enteral** delivery of medications is through the:

   a. mouth   **d.** GI tract

   b. rectum   **e.** pulmonary vein

   c. anus

2. Why do doctors use the enteral delivery route of medication?

   _____

   _____

   _____

3. What does *paraenteral* mean?

   _____

   _____

   _____

F. Analyze the following paragraph and use the correct medical language to answer the questions. (LO 22.1, 22.2. 22.8, *Apply, Analyze*)

Mrs. Edna Whitman, a 78-year-old woman, was brought to the ER by ambulance early Sunday morning bleeding profusely from a long laceration on her leg. She had tripped over a raised crack in the sidewalk and fell, cutting her leg. After examining her and taking her medical history the ER doctor determined she was taking aspirin every day to thin her blood.

   Mrs. Whitman was confused and unable to tell the doctor how much aspirin she had taken during the prior week. The doctor sutured her laceration and tested her blood for the amount of anticoagulant she had. Anticoagulants reduce susceptibility to thrombus formation. Mrs. Whitman had overdosed on aspirin and needs someone to carefully oversee her drug regimen.

1. What is the purpose of taking aspirin every day?

   _____

2. What is a thrombus?

   _____

3. What can be caused by a thrombus? _____ and _____

4. What is another term for *sutured*? _____

5. Anticoagulants act on which component of blood?

   a. red blood cell   **d.** serum

   b. white blood cell   **e.** platelets

   c. plasma

Pharmacology

G. Reread the Case Report and use your knowledge of medical language to create your answers to the following questions. (LO 22.1, 22.3, 22.9, *Analyze*)

Case Report 22.1

You are

...a pharmacist in the pharmacy at Fulwood Medical Center. Your patient has been sent to you by Susan Lee, MD, a primary care physician at Fulwood Medical Center.

Your patient is

...Mrs. Rebecca Borodin, a frail 80-year-old widow living in an assisted living facility. She has recently begun to complain that she has difficulty recognizing and naming her fellow residents and knowing when to go to the facility's dining room for meals. In addition, it has been hard for her to eat because she suffers from dry mouth and difficulty in swallowing. She has also complained of dizziness and problems with balance; recently, she fell as a result of these problems. Her past medical history includes osteoarthritis, osteopenia, hypertension, congestive heart failure, persistent pain following herpes zoster, and stress incontinence.

Mrs. Borodin has brought in a bag containing all her medications, which include: cimetidine, acetaminophen with codeine (Tylenol #2), oxybutynin, digoxin, atenolol, alprazolam, zolpidem (Ambien), and naproxen. In addition, she takes an OTC multivitamin and melatonin.

Dr. Lee has asked you to make sure that Mrs. Borodin knows what each of the medications is for and when to take it. She has also asked you to review the drugs themselves to see if any of them could be causing her recent symptoms.

1. What health professionals in this case report are involved in Mrs. Borodin's care?

   _____

2. What are Mrs. Borodin's chief complaints?

   _____

   _____

3. Does Mrs. Borodin have a chronic history of falling?

   _____

   _____

4. What body systems are represented in Mrs. Borodin's diagnoses from her past medical history?

   _____

   _____

   _____

   _____

5. What OTC medications does Mrs. Borodin use?

   _____

6. Digoxin is taken for _____ .

   Ambien is taken for _____ .

   Naproxen is taken for _____ .

H. **What am I?** Fill in the blank with the correct answer. (**LO 22.2, 22.3, 22.8, 22.9,** *Remember, Apply, Analyze*)

1. I do not need a prescription

2. I can treat minor aches and pains

3. I am usually cheaper than a prescription drug

4. I can be used to help you sleep

5. I can boost your health.

6. I am _____.

I. **What is the difference between an *infusion* and an *injection?*** Fill in the blanks. (**LO 22.2,** *Understand, Apply*)

a. Infusion: _____

_____

b. Injection: _____

_____

J. **Translate this sentence into layman's language.** (**LO 22.2, 22.6,** *Understand, Apply*)

"The sublingual route and the buccal routes provide a rich supply of blood vessels through which drugs can be directly absorbed into the systemic circulation."

_____

_____

_____

_____

K. **Fill in the blanks with the correct abbreviations.** (**LO 22.2, 22.7,** *Remember, Understand*)

1. by mouth _____

2. doctors check drugs in this book _____

3. federal government agency _____

4. when necessary _____

5. does not need a prescription _____

L. All of these drugs have the prefix "anti-." Define what they work against. (**LO 22.2, 22.9,** *Remember, Apply*)

1. antiduretic: _____

2. antidepressant: _____

3. antihistamine: _____

4. anticoagulant: _____

5. antibiotic: _____

Pharmacology

CHAPTER SUMMARY EXERCISES

A. Spelling comprehension. Circle the correct spelling of the term. (**LO 22.1,** *Remember*)

1. pharmasist	pharmocist	pharmycyst	pharmacist	pharmmocist
2. antetussive	antitusive	antitussive	antetusive	antretusive
3. formularly	formulary	formularrly	formullary	formmularly
4. anabolic	annabolic	anebolic	anabollic	annebolic
5. parenterral	parentteral	parrental	parenteral	parenterall

B. Match the number of the correct term in Exercise A with the following brief description of the term. (**LO 22.1,** *Understand, Apply*)

1. Official list of drugs approved for use by a hospital or group of physicians _____

2. Person licensed by the state to prepare and dispense drugs _____

3. Pertaining to "raising up"—used by athletes to increase muscle mass _____

4. Administering medication by any means other than the GI tract _____

5. A cough remedy _____

C. Using your knowledge of terms 1–10 in Exercise A and their correct spelling, write a brief sentence for each of the terms as it might appear in patient documentation. (**LO 22.1, 22.2, 22.6,** *Apply*)

1. _____

2. _____

3. _____

4. _____

5. _____

D. Circle the correct answer. The path by which a drug or other substance is taken into the body is called: (**LO 22.2, 22.6,** *Remember, Apply*)

1. bioavailability

2. digestion

3. absorption

4. a route of administration

5. biokinetics

E. What do psychedelics distort? Circle the best answer. (**LO 22.2, 22.5, 22.9,** *Remember, Apply*)

1. balance

2. sight and sound

3. smell

4. smell and taste

5. light

F. **What would an ENT physician prescribe for a patient with a heavy cough?** Circle the correct answer. (**LO 22.2, 22.3, 22.9,** *Understand, Apply*)

1. antiemetic

2. antihistamine

3. antitussive

4. anticoagulant

5. antidepressant

G. **Circle the incorrect statement about beta blockers.** (**LO 22.2, 22.3, 22.9,** *Remember, Understand*)

1. Beta blockers diminish the effects of epinephrine. T   F

2. Beta blockers diminish the effects of stress hormones. T   F

3. All beta blockers are approved for the treatment of HBP. T   F

4. Beta blockers have to be administered intravenously. T   F

5. Beta blockers can treat angina. T   F

H. **Circle the correct answer.** (**LO 22.1, 22.7, 22.8, 22.10,** *Remember, Understand, Apply*)

1. The MOST important job of the pharmacist is:

   a. to count pills.

   b. to make sure you are getting the right prescription.

   c. to make sure he is giving the right prescription to the right person.

   d. to make sure any drug he is giving you will not interact with the other drugs you are taking.

   e. to make sure your prescription has not expired.

2. Circle the correct pair of abbreviations that are both government agencies controlling drugs.

   a. HIV   HPV

   b. MRI   STAT

   c. FDA   DEA

   d. BPH   OTC

   e. DVT   CRF

3. Which of the following does not refer to a drug name?

   a. chemical

   b. generic

   c. brand

   d. trade

   e. popular

Chapter 22 Review

Pharmacology

I. Write a brief answer for each of the questions below. (**LO 22.1, 22.4,** *Apply, Analyze*)

   1. What is the purpose of a patent on a drug?

   _____

   2. How many years can a patent be enforced?

   _____

   3. What does "proprietary" mean?

   _____

J. Give an example of five products that are health aids available OTC and are not prescription drugs. (**LO 22.1, 22.2,** *Understand, Apply*)

   1. _____

   2. _____

   3. _____

   4. _____

   5. _____

K. Which of the following is NOT a possible side effect from a drug: (**LO 22.1, 22.2, 22.8,** *Understand, Apply*)

   1. nausea

   2. dizziness

   3. blurred vision

   4. hemorrhage

   5. headache

L. Which U.S. agency sets the standards for the quality, purity, and safety of medications? (**LO 22.4, 22.8,** *Remember, Apply*)

   1. USP

   2. USPS

   3. CDC

   4. BATF

   5. AAP

M. Think about the question, then write your answers on the lines below. Controlled substances are divided into five schedules, depending on: (**LO 22.1, 22.2, 22.5,** *Remember, Apply*)

   1. _____

   2. _____

   3. _____

N. Which of the following terms would a pharmacist NOT use? **(LO 22.2, 22.3,** *Remember, Understand*)

1. beta blocker

2. antihistamine

3. anticoagulant

4. synthyroid

5. cadaver

O. Translate the following sentence into words your patient can understand. **(LO 22.1, 22.2, 22.6,** *Remember, Understand*)

1. "Five million people self-administer insulin into their subcutaneous tissue either by syringe, pen injection, high-pressure jet injection, or subcutaneous infusion pumps. Inhalation of an insulin solution is also available." (*HINT:* underline or highlight all the medical terms in the sentence, then translate them.)

2. Translation: _____

_____

_____

_____

P. Match the correct medical term to the brief definition given below. **(LO 22.2, 22.3,** *Remember, Apply*)

1. dissolves clots that have caused heart attacks   a. anticoagulents

2. warfarin   b. streptokinase

3. derived from hemolytic streptococci   c. Abbokinase

4. urokinase   d. Coumadin

5. reduce thrombus formation   e. tPA

Q. Meet the goals of each of the chapter outcomes by using the correct language of pharmacology for the answers. **(LO 22.1–22.10,** *Analyze*)

1. Use the medical terms of pharmacology to communicate and document in writing accurately and precisely in any health care setting. Circle the statement that is incorrect. **(LO 22.1)**

   a. Marijuana dulls pain.

   b. Psychedelics can be natural plant products.

   c. Antipsychotics treat symptoms of psychosis.

   d. Tranquilizers can calm you and put you to sleep.

   e. Tegretol and lithium are mood stabilizers.

2. Use the medical *terms of pharmacology* to communicate verbally with accuracy and precision in any health care setting. **(LO 22.2)**

   a. The doctor has told you she is ordering Mucomyst for her patient. You will need to administer this medication through a

   _____.

Pharmacology

3. Discuss the differences between the chemical name, generic name, and brand name of a drug. List the chemical name, generic name, and brand name for a drug that clears mucus. **(LO 22.3)**

   a. chemical name _____

   b. generic name _____

   c. brand name _____

4. Define the methods used for setting and referencing the standards for the effectiveness and purity of drugs for sale in the United States. Regulation of controlled drugs is the responsibility of which federal agency? **(LO 22.4)**

   _____

5. Describe controlled substance schedules. The drugs in which drug schedule cannot be prescribed, dispensed, or administered? **(LO 22.5)**

   Drug Schedule _____ prohibits dispensing drugs that cannot be prescribed, dispensed

   or administered.

6. Identify the different routes of drug administration. Choose from the following terms the correct route of administration. Fill in the blanks. You will not use all the choices. **(LO 22.6)**

   enteral   oral   rectal   buccal   sublingual   transdermal   intravenous

   a. You have placed a patch containing pain medicine on your patient's back. Which route of administration

   is that? _____

   b. Mr. Matthews has to put his medicine under his tongue. Which route of administration is that? _____

   c. Dr. Philips has ordered a suppository for Mrs. Johnson. Which route of administration is that? _____

   d. Dr. Mallard prescribed pain pills for Mr. Cosmos. Which route of administration is that? _____

7. Identify abbreviations used to describe drugs, their routes of administration, and their timing. Match the abbreviation to the correct statement. **(LO 22.7)**

   _____   **a.** p.r.n.   **i.** intramuscular

   _____   **b.** t.i.d.   **ii.** by mouth

   _____   **c.** b.i.d.   **iii.** when necessary

   _____   **d.** IM   **iv.** twice each day

   _____   **e.** p.o.   **v.** three times each day

8. Discuss methods to ensure accuracy and safety in the administration of medications. What are the five rights of medicine administration? **(LO 22.8)**

   a. _____

   b. _____

   c. _____

   d. _____

   e. _____

9. Describe the different classes of drugs, their generic and brand names, and their methods of action. Pick any class of drugs and describe its generic and brand names and what they act on in the body. (**LO 22.9**)

a. Class of drugs: _____

b. Generic names: _____

c. Brand names: _____

d. What they act on in the body: _____

10. Identify health professionals involved in pharmacology. What is the difference between a pharmacist and a pharmacologist? (**LO 22.10**)

a. Pharmacist: _____

b. Pharmacologist: _____

Coder's Tip:

The documentation offered in the patient's chart contains many important terms for correct code choice of adverse effects of drug administration. Pay careful attention to key words such as *right, wrong, correct, incorrect,* etc. Read the code descriptors carefully to match them up with your documentation.

Ask these questions to determine what you are looking for.

1. Right or wrong patient?

2. Right or wrong drug?

3. Right or wrong route (properly administered)?

4. Right or wrong dose?

5. Right or wrong time?

Note the defining terms that are helpful in code selection.

6. *Accidental* overdose of drug and *wrong drug given* or taken in error—E850.0–E 858.9.

7. *Correct drug properly administered* in therapeutic or prophylactic dosage, as the cause of an adverse effect—E930.0–E949.9.

8. Wrong drug given in error—NEC 977.9.

9. Consult the table of drugs and chemicals to code the drug involved in the adverse effect.

Appendices

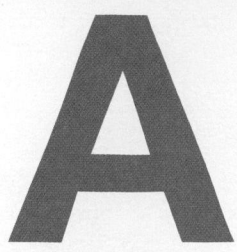

End-of-Book Exercises

The following additional exercises draw from all the previous chapters in the text and will help you review some of the basic elements of medical terminology.

Use These Exercises to Prepare for Cumulative Exams

A. Elements associated with body systems. The body systems are listed for you in the left column. Choose one root/combining form for each body system; define the meaning of the element, and find an example of a medical term using that element. Fill in the table. (**LO 1.2, 1.5, 2.8, 3.2,** *Remember, Understand, Apply*)

	Body System	Root/Combining Form	Meaning of Element	Medical Term Using This Element
1.	integumentary	1.	1.	1.
2.	musculoskeletal	2.	2.	2.
3.	nervous	3.	3.	3.
4.	endocrine	4.	4.	4.
5.	cardiovascular	5.	5.	5.
6.	lymphatic	6.	6.	6.
7.	digestive	7.	7.	7.
8.	respiratory	8.	8.	8.
9.	urinary	9.	9.	9.
10.	reproductive	10.	10.	10.

B. Elements by grouping. List all the elements that denote a color. <u>The first one is done for you.</u> (**LO 2.5, 2.6,** *Understand, Analyze*)

	Element	Color
1.	*leuk/o*	*white*
2.		
3.		
4.		
5.		
6.		
7.		
8.		

C. List all the elements that denote a location or direction (above, below, etc.). <u>The first one is done for you.</u>
(**LO 2.5, 2.6,** *Understand, Analyze*)

	Element	Location
1.	*epi*	*above*
2.		
3.		
4.		
5.		
6.		
7.		
8.		
9.		
10.		
11.		
12.		

D. List all the elements that denote a number. <u>The first one is done for you.</u> (**LO 2.5, 2.6,** *Understand, Analyze*)

	Element	Number
1.	*mono*	*one*
2.		
3.		
4.		
5.		
6.		
7.		
8.		

E. Difference between elements. Many elements sound and look similar but have very different meanings. Be precise in your communication—patient safety depends on you! (**LO 1.5, 1.8, *Apply, Analyze***)

	Element	Type of Element (P/R/CF/S)	Meaning of Element	Medical Term Containing this Element from Any Chapter
1.	pheresis			
2.	phoresis			
3.	colo			
4.	colpo			
5.	echo			
6.	ectop			
7.	radiculo			
8.	reticulo			
9.	metacarpo			
10.	metatarso			
11.	vaso			
12.	veno			
13.	photon			
14.	proton			
15.	enteral			
16.	paraenteral			
17.	necro			
18.	narco			
19.	sacro			
20.	sarco			

F. Elements. Reinforce your knowledge of elements with this comprehensive list. Identify the element as to type, give its meaning, and then use it in an appropriate medical term. Fill in the chart. <u>The first one is done for you.</u> (**LO 1.5, 1.6, 2.7, 3.2, 3.6,** *Understand, Apply, Analyze*)

	Element	Type of Element (P/R/CF/S)	Meaning of Element	Medical Term Containing This Element
1.	*a, an*	*P*	*without*	*anencephaly*
2.	ger			
3.	mort			
4.	angio			
5.	patho			
6.	sarco			
7.	bucc			
8.	chole			
9.	claustro			
10.	tele			
11.	radio			
12.	fract			
13.	stero			
14.	contro			
15.	fluoro			
16.	ment			
17.	histo			
18.	hydro			
19.	pharmaco			
20.	tuss			
21.	mania			
22.	lingu			
23.	toxico			
24.	neo			
25.	psycho			
26.	toxico			
27.	rrhea			
28.	stomy			
29.	terato			
30.	thrombo			
31.	viscer			
32.	xeno			

G. Spelling demons. Precision in communication and professionalism require correct spelling of all medical terms. Circle the correct spelling of each term; then on the line below, deconstruct the correct spelling of the term with slashes, and write a brief explanation of the medical term. (**LO 3.6,** *Understand, Apply, Analyze*)

1. acondroplasia   achondroplasia   acondroplesia

___

2. hemorrhage   hemmorrhage   hemorhage

___

3. cirrosis   sirosis   cirrhosis

___

4. cenessance   senescence   senescience

___

5. antiarrythmics   antiarrhthmics   antiarrhythmics

___

6. intratecal   interthecal   intrathecal

___

7. parmacist   pharmasist   pharmacist

___

8. diverticulosis   deverticulosis   diverticculosis

___

9. cholecystectomy   colecystectomy   collecystectomy

___

10. algorithim   allgorithem   algoreithim

___

11. sintigraphy   scintigraphy   cintigraphy

___

12. exophthalmos   exopthalamos   exophtalamos

___

13. nosocomial   nosoccomial   nossocomial

___

14. parmacy   pharmacy   farmacy

___

15. fluoroscopy   fluoroscopy   fouroscopy

___

16. gastroesophageal   gastroesopageal   gastroesophagial

17. pneumonitis   penummonitis   pneumonnitis

18. oophorectomy   ophorectomy   ooporectomy

19. parenteral   parrentiral   perenteral

20. tonsillectomy   tonsilectomy   tonssilectomy

21. thyrotoxicosis   thyroidtoxicosis   thyrotoxicossis

H. Review of latin/greek terms that do not deconstruct into elements. You must know these terms for what they are. Fill in the table. <u>A sample is shown on the first line.</u> (**LO 1.7, 3.6, *Understand, Apply, Analyze***)

	Medical Term	**Meaning of Term in Latin/ Greek**	**Application to Medical Terminology**
	cruciate	*cross*	*anterior cruciate ligament*
1.	ion		
2.	viscous		
3.	oblique		
4.	calculus		
5.	patent		
6.	opaque		
7.	axis		
8.	autopsy		
9.	lymph		
10.	lentigo		
11.	lavage		
12.	ptosis		
13.	enema		
14.	bolus		
15.	tracer		
16.	ganglion		
17.	cartilage		

I. Body systems. Use your knowledge of medical terminology to fill in the following chart with terms applicable to each specific body system. There may not be an appropriate answer for every blank. The first one is done for you. (**LO 1.1, 2.2, 3.1, 3.5,** *Remember, Apply*)

	Body System	Study Of (practice)	One Who Studies (practitioner)	Disease	Procedure
1.	*integumentary*	*dermatology*	*dermatologist*	*eczema*	*excisional biopsy*
2.	musculoskeletal				
3.	nervous				
4.	endocrine				
5.	cardiovascular				
6.	special senses/eye				
7.	digestive				
8.	respiratory				
9.	urinary				
10.	reproductive				

J. Symptoms/chief complaint. The patients of Fulwood Medical Center have come into the various clinics with the following complaints. Use the correct medical terminology to enter the chief complaint in the patient's chart. (**LO 1.1, 1.6, 2.7, 3.6,** *Understand, Apply, Analyze*)

	Patient Complaint	Correct Medical Terminology for Chart
1.	double vision	
2.	blood in urine	
3.	ringing in ears	
4.	painful breathing	
5.	pus in gums	
6.	sore throat	
7.	loss of cognitive and intellectual function	
8.	pink eye	
9.	fear of heights	
10.	low blood pressure	
11.	bad headaches	
12.	inability to urinate	
13.	dizziness	
14.	lack of bowel movements	
15.	broken wrist	
16.	nosebleeds	
17.	impacted earwax	
18.	bed-wetting	
19.	heavy menstrual bleeding	
20.	stomachache	

K. Transcription exercise. The following paragraphs from patient documentation and office forms contain errors. Locate the errors in the paragraph, circle them, then rewrite the correct medical terminology on the line below. (**LO 1.8, 2.7, 3.6,** *Remember, Apply, Analyze*)

1. Hemmostasis was accomplished using electrocogulation. The patient had a slight commuted fracture of the medial maleolus. The wound was irrigated and debris was removed.

   _____

2. The patient is a 58-year-old black female with an osteosarcoma of the pelvis who underwent successful wide resuction and reconstruction; however, 2 weeks later her wound became infected and perforated the rectim, which resulted in gross contammination.

   _____

3. Under general anesthesia it was clear that the patient had a grade II tear of the latteral colateral ligament as well as an anterior and posterior cruxiate ligament tear.

   _____

4. PA/lateral CXR: The heart size is normal. There is bilateral atellectasis noted. There is density within the overlying soft tissues of the right chest consistent with recent right-sided breast biopsie. There is no evidence of plural efusion or pneumothorax.

   _____

5. CT scan: Numerous enlarged, abnormal-appearing limph nodes in the right axila, with markedly thickened cortices and hillar effacement. Concerning for lympoma or metastaic disease. Further follow-up is recommended.

   _____

6. MRI scan: There is diffuse fatty infiltration of the liver. The spleen is unremarkable as well as kidneys and adrennal glands. There is no retroperitonial adenopathy or abdominal aortic aneursm. There are multiple calcifications within the galbladder consistent with choleithiasis.

   _____

7. Increased activity at the ankles and feet is seen bilateraly, likely related to degenerative/hypertopic changes. There is minimal increased activity at both shoulders and at the right sternocavicular joint, likely related to arthritic changes. No other significant abnormality is identified.

   _____

8. Past medical history of childhood diseases:

diphtheria	smallpox	scarlet fever	rhumatic fever
chorea	tyhphoid	whoping cough	chickenbox
mumps	meseles	tonsilitis	rubela

9. Past medical illness occurring within the last 3 years:

punmonia	plurisy	arthralgia	migrain headaches
malaria	sleep apnia	broncitis	cardiomyopathy
conjunctivetis	gout	otitus media	anemmia

10. The gastriscope was advanced into the distal esopagus, which was essentially normal. Advancement of the scope into the stomach showed evidence of erytema and gasritis. The pylorus was intubated, and the duodenal bulb was visualized.

   _____

L. Coding exercise. Solid knowledge of medical terminology will help you to better understand the coding systems. Volumes I and II of ICD-9-CM contain diagnosis codes. CPT codes are used to bill physician fees for procedures and services. In the following chart, choose whether each medical term requires an ICD-9-CM code or a CPT code (put a checkmark √ in the appropriate column), and identify the specialist associated with the medical term. (**LO 1.6, 2.7, 3.5,** *Remember, Understand, Apply*)

	Medical Term	Diagnosis (ICD-9 CM)	Procedures/Services (CPT)	Specialist Consulted
1.	otitis media			
2.	SAD			
3.	blepharoplasty			
4.	thoracotomy			
5.	neuralgia			
6.	nephrosis			
7.	herniorrhaphy			
8.	depression			
9.	osteoporosis			
10.	lithotripsy			
11.	senility			
12.	osteotomy			
13.	amniocentesis			
14.	jejunostomy			
15.	hemoptysis			
16.	rhinitis			
17.	gastroscopy			
18.	anorexia			
19.	anal fistula			
20.	MRI			
21.	hematuria			
22.	hysteroscopy			
23.	neoplasm			
24.	PET			
25.	CF			
26.	venogram			

M. Definitions. Write a brief definition for each of the following signs and symptoms a patient may experience. (**LO 3.5, 3.6,** *Remember, Understand, Apply*)

1. claustrophobia   _____

2. pallor   _____

3. cyanosis   _____

4. mania   _____

5. edema   _____

6. epistaxis   _____

7. febrile   _____

8. delete   _____

9. jaundice   _____

10. hypertension   _____

11. hyperpnea   _____

12. polydipsia   _____

13. petechia   _____

14. pes planus   _____

15. dementia   _____

16. palpitation   _____

17. malunion   _____

18. tetany   _____

19. contracture   _____

20. wheals   _____

N. Surgical suffixes. The following suffixes are all associated with surgical procedures. CPT codes are specific as to type of procedure—you can't code and bill a nephrotomy if the patient actually had a nephrectomy. You must code what is documented in the medical record. Know your suffixes! This chart contains surgical suffixes. Give the meaning of the suffix, an example of the suffix in a term, and the definition of the term. The first one is done for you. (**LO 2.2, 2.3, 2.7,** *Understand, Apply, Analyze*)

	Suffix	Suffix Meaning	Example of Term	Meaning of the Term
1.	*ectomy*	*removal of*	*nephrectomy*	*removal of the kidney*
2.	centesis			
3.	cision			
4.	desis			
5.	ostomy			
6.	pexy			
7.	plasty			
8.	rrhaphy			
9.	tomy			
10.	tripsy			

O. Work with more surgical terms. Write a brief description of the procedure each term represents. Fill in the blanks. (**LO 2.2, 2.5, 2.8,** *Understand, Apply, Analyze*)

1. abdominocentesis _____
   _____

2. catheterization _____
   _____

3. ligation _____
   _____

4. amputation _____
   _____

5. incision _____
   _____

6. curettage _____
   _____

7. aspiration _____
   _____

8. debridement _____
   _____

9. cauterization _____
   _____

10. ablation _____
    _____

11. resection _____
    _____

12. dilation _____
    _____

13. manipulation _____
    _____

14. allograft _____
    _____

15. excision _____
    _____

16. suture _____
    _____

P. Abbreviations. Reading patient documentation to extract/abstract information for coding purposes requires that you understand what you are reading. Identify the abbreviations in the following chart. Check (√) whether the abbreviation is a diagnosis, a procedure, or something else. In the right column, write the meaning of the abbreviation. (**LO 2.2, 2.5, 2.8**, *Remember, Understand, Apply, Analyze*)

	Abbreviation	Diagnosis	Procedure	Other	Meaning of Abbreviation
1.	DNR				
2.	q.i.d.				
3.	SOB				
4.	CPR				
5.	UTI				
6.	BD				
7.	CSF				
8.	ABG				
9.	CXR				
10.	DJD				
11.	p.r.n.				
12.	CBC				
13.	ARDS				
14.	AKA				
15.	CAD				
16.	AU				
17.	COPD				
18.	DEXA				
19.	WBC				
20.	EEG				
21.	ROM				
22.	STAT				
23.	CXR				
24.	AP				
25.	GYN				

Q. Use your knowledge of medical language and abbreviations to analyze the following groups of terms and determine what they have in common. (**LO 2.8,** *Understand, Apply, Analyze, Evaluate*)

1. *comminuted, pathologic, displaced*

   All relate to _____.

2. *onychomycosis, matrix, paronychia*

   All relate to _____.

3. *erythrocyte, thrombocyte, leukocyte*

   All relate to _____.

4. *biceps, deltoid, brachioradialis*

   All relate to _____.

5. *antibiotic, antitussive, antihistamine*

   All relate to _____.

6. *zygote, embryo, fetus*

   All relate to _____.

7. *interventional, scintigraphy, stereotactic*

   All relate to _____.

8. *thelarche, pubarche, menarche*

   All relate to _____.

9. *phobia, mania, psychosis*

   All relate to _____.

10. *cholesteatoma, tympanostomy, auricle*

    All relate to _____.

11. *FDA, OTC, DEA*

    All relate to _____.

12. *surfactant, inflate, hilum*

    All relate to _____.

13. *oblique, opaque, contrast*

    All relate to _____.

14. *enuresis, polyuria, glycosuria*

    All relate to _____.

15. *lymphadenectomy, lymphadenitis, lymphadenopathy*

    All relate to _____.

16. *senescence, longevity, senility*

    All relate to _____.

Congratulations on a job well done!

Word Parts

B

Note: For easy identification, the word parts in this appendix appear in the same colors as they do in the Word Analysis and Definition boxes: suffix, prefix, root, root/combining form. Any term that is used in the text in both root and combining form is shown in this appendix only as a combining form. Sometimes the same element (for example, "ac") can function in different parts of the medical term.

WORD PART	DEFINITION
-ac	pertaining to
-al	pertaining to
-ar	pertaining to
-ary	pertaining to
a-	not, without, into
ab-	away from
abdomin/o	abdomen
ability	competence
ablat	take away
-able	capable of
abort	fail at onset
absorpt	to swallow, take in
ac-	toward
-acea	condition, remedy
acetyl	acetyl
acid/o	acid, low pH
acin	grape
acous	hearing
acr/o	peak, extremity, highest point
acro-	peak, highest point, extremity
acromi/o	acromion
act	to do, perform, performance

WORD PART	DEFINITION
activ/e	movement
acu-	sharp
acu	needle, sharp
acumin	to sharpen
ad-	to, toward, near, into
adapt	to adjust
-ade	process
aden/o	gland
adenoid	adenoid
adipos/e	fat
adjust	alter
adjuv	give help
adnex	connected parts
adolesc	beginning of adulthood
adren/o	adrenal gland
aer/o	air, gas
ag-	to
-age	related to
agglutin	sticking together, clumping
-ago	disease
agon	contest against, fight against
-agon	contest

S = Suffix   P = Prefix   **R = Root**   **R/CF = Combining Form**

WORD PART	DEFINITION
agor/a	marketplace
-agra	rough
-al	pertaining to
alanine	an amino acid, protein synthesized in muscle
albin/o	white
albumin	albumin
ald/o	organic compound
-ale	pertaining to
alges	sensation of pain
-algia	pain, painful condition
aliment	nourishment
-alis	pertaining to
alkal	base
all/o	strange, other, different
aller	allergy
allo-	other, different, strange
alopec-	baldness, mange
alpha-	first letter in Greek alphabet
alveol	alveolus, air sac
-aly	condition
ambly-	dull
ambulat	to walk, walking
amin/o	nitrogen compound
-amine	nitrogen-containing
ammon	ammonia
amni/o	amnion, fetal membrane
amnios	amnion, fetal membrane
amoeb	amoeba
amph-	around
ampull	bottle-shaped
amput	to prune, lop off
amyl	starch
an-	not, lack of, without
-an	pertaining to
an/o	anus
ana-	away from, excessive

WORD PART	DEFINITION
ana	apart from
anabol	build up
analysis	process to define
analyst	one who defines
anastom	join together
-ance	condition, state of
-ancy	state of
andr/o	male, masculine
aneurysm	dilation
angi/o	blood vessel, lymph vessel
angina	sore throat, chest pain radiating to throat
ankyl	stiff
ant-	against
-ant	forming, pertaining to, agent
ante-	before, forward
anter	before, front part
anthrac	coal
anti-	against
aort	aorta
apo-	different from, separation from, off
append	appendix
apse	clasp
aqu/a	watery
-ar	pertaining to
arachn	cobweb, spider
-arche	beginning
aria	air
-arian	one who is
-aris	pertaining to
aroma	smell, sweet herb
array	place in order
arteri/o	artery
arteriosus	like an artery
arthr/o	joint
articul	joint

S = Suffix   P = Prefix   **R = Root   R/CF = Combining Form**

WORD PART	DEFINITION
-ary	pertaining to
asbest	asbestos
asc	belly
ascit	fluid in the belly
-ase	enzyme
aspartate	an amino acid
aspergill	*Aspergillus*
aspirat	to breathe in, remove by suction
assay	evaluate
assist	aid, help
astr/o	star
-ata	action, place, use
-ate	composed of, pertaining to, process
-ated	process, composed of
atel	incomplete
ather/o	porridge, gruel, fatty substance
athet	without position, uncontrolled
-atic	pertaining to
-ation	process
-ative	pertaining to, quality of
-ator	agent, instrument, person or thing that does something
atri/o	entrance, atrium
-atric	treatment
attent	awareness
attenu	to weaken
audi/o	hearing
audit	hearing
aur-	ear
auscult	listen to
auto-	self, same
avail	useful
axill	armpit
ayur-	life
azot	nitrogen
back	back, return

WORD PART	DEFINITION
-back	back, toward the starting point
bacter	bacterium
bacteri/o	bacteria
balan	glans penis
bar	pressure
bari	weight
bas/o	base, opposite of acid
basal/e	deepest part
basil	base, support
be	life
behav	mental activity
beta	second letter of Greek alphabet
bi-	two, twice, double
bi/o	life
-bic	life
-bil	able
bil/i	bile
bio-	life
bio	life
biot	life
-blast	embryo, germ cell, immature cell
blast/o	immature cell, germ cell
blephar/o	eyelid
body	body, mass, substance
bov	cattle
brachi/o	arm
brachii	of the arm
brachy-	short
brady-	slow
bride	rubbish, rubble
bronch/o	bronchus
brucell	from pathologist David Bruce
bucc	cheek
buccin	cheek

S = Suffix   P = Prefix   **R = Root**   R/CF = Combining Form

WORD PART	DEFINITION
bulb/o	bulb
burs	bursa
calc/i	calcium
calcul	stone, little stone
callos	thickening
calor	heat
cancer	cancer
candid	*Candida,* a yeast
capill	hairlike structure, capillary
capit	head
capn	carbon dioxide
caps	box, cover, shell
capsul	little box
carb/o	carbon
carboxy	group of organic compounds
carcin/o	cancerous, cancer
card	heart
cardi/o	heart
cardia	heart
care	be responsible for
caroten/e	yellow-red pigment
carotid	large neck artery
carp/o	bones of the wrist
cartilag/e	cartilage
cata-	down
catabol	break down
catechol	benzene derivative
cathet	insert, catheter
caud/a	tail
cava	cave
cavern	cave
cec	cecum
-cele	cave, hernia, swelling
celi	abdomen
cellul	small cell
cent-	hundred

WORD PART	DEFINITION
cent	hundred
-centesis	to puncture
centr/o	central
cephal/o	head
cephalus	head
-cephalus	head
cephaly	condition of the head
ceps	head
-ceps	head
cept	to receive
cerebell	little brain, cerebellum
cerebr/o	brain
cervic	neck, cervix
cess	going forward
chancr	chancre
chem/o	chemical
chemic	chemical
chete	hair
-chezia	pass a stool
chir/o	hand
chlor/o	green
chol/e	bile
cholangi	bile duct
cholecyst	gallbladder
choledoch/o	common bile duct
choline	choline
chondr/o	cartilage, rib
chori/o	chorion, membrane
chorion	chorion
chrom/o	color
chromat	color
chron/o	time
chym/o	chyme
cid/e	to kill
-cidal	pertaining to killing
-cide	to kill

S = Suffix   P = Prefix   R = Root   R/CF = Combining Form

WORD PART	DEFINITION
cili	hairlike structure, eyelid
circum-	around
cirrh	yellow
cis	to cut
cit/i	cell
-clast	break, break down
claudic	limp
claustr/o	confined space
clav	clavicle
clave	lock
clavicul	clavicle
-cle	small
clitor	clitoris
clon	cutting used for propagation
-clonus	violent action
co-	with, together
coagul/o	clotting, clump
coarct	press together, narrow
cobal	cobalt
cocc	spherical bacterium, berry
cochle	cochlea
code	information system
cognit	thinking
coit	sexual intercourse
col-	before
col	colon
coll/a	glue
colon	colony
colon/o	colon
coloniz	form a colony
colp/o	vagina
com-	with, together
com	take care of
combin	combine
comminut	break into small pieces
commodat	adjust

WORD PART	DEFINITION
compat	tolerate
compet	strive together
complete	fill in
complex	woven together
compli	fulfill
compress	press together
compuls	drive, compel
con-	with, together
concav	arched, hollow
concept	become pregnant
concuss	shake violently
condyl	knuckle
confus	bewildered
congest	accumulation of fluid
coni	dust
coniz	cone
conjunctiv	conjunctiva
conscious	aware
constip	press together
constrict	narrow, to narrow
contagi/o	transmissible by contact
contamin	to corrupt, make unclean
contin	hold together
contra-	against
contract	draw together, pull together
contus	bruise
convalesc	recover
cor	heart, pupil
cori	skin
corne/o	cornea
coron	crown, coronary
corpor/e	body
corpus	body
cort	cortex
cortic/o	cortex, cortisone
cortis	cortisone

WORD PART	DEFINITION
cost	rib
crani/o	cranium, skull
cre	separation
crease	groove
creat	flesh
creatin	creatine
cret	to separate
cretin	cretin
crimin	distinguish
crine	secrete
-crine	secrete
crista	crest
-crit	to separate
crown	crown
cry/o	icy cold
crypt-	hidden
cub	cube
cubit	elbow
cubitus	lying down
cune/i	wedge
cur	cleanse, cure
curat	to care for
curett	to cleanse
curr	to run
cursor	run
cusp	point
cutan/e	skin
cyan/o	dark blue
-cyst	cyst, sac, bladder
cyst/o	bladder, sac, cyst
cysteine	an amino acid
cyt/o	cell
-cyte	cell
cyth	cell
dacry/o	tears, lacrimal duct
dai	day

WORD PART	DEFINITION
de-	from, take away, out of, without
defec	clear out waste
deferens	carry away
defici	failure, lacking, inadequate
degenerat	deteriorate
deglutit	to swallow
del	visible, manifest
deliri	confusion, disorientation
delt	Greek letter delta
delus	deceive
dem	the people
demi-	half
dendr/o	treelike, branching structure
dent	tooth
depend	relying on
depress	press down
derm/a	skin
dermat/o	skin
dermis	skin
-desis	bind together, fixation of bone or joint
di-	two, complete
dia-	complete, through
diabet	diabetes
diagnost	decision
dialectic	argument
dialy	separate
diaphor	sweat
diaphragm/a	diaphragm
dict	consent, surrender
didym/o	testis
didymis	testis
diet	a way of life
different	not identical
digest	to break down, break up
digit	finger or toe
dilat	open up, expand, open out

WORD PART	DEFINITION
dips	thirst
dis-	apart, away from
discipl	understand
disciplin	disciple, instruction
dist	away from the center
-dium	appearance
diuret	increase urine output
diverticul	by-road
dorm	sleep
dors/i	back
drome	running
drop	liquid globule
duce	to lead
ducer	to lead, leader
duct	to lead
ductus	leading
duoden	twelve, duodenum
dur/a	hard, dura mater
dwarf	miniature
dynam/o	power
-dynia	pain
dys-	bad, difficult, painful
e-	out of, from
-eal	pertaining to
ease	normal function, freedom from pain
ec-	out, outside
ech/o	sound wave
echin	hedgehog
eclamps	shining forth
eco-	environment
-ectasis	dilation
-ectomy	excision, surgical excision
ectop	on the outside, displaced
eczema	eczema
-ed	pertaining to
edema	edema, swelling

WORD PART	DEFINITION
efface	wipe out
effus	pour out
ejacul	shoot out
el	wart, nail
elasma	plate
elect	choice
electr/o	electric, electricity
elimin	throw away, expel
-elle	small
em-	in, into
-em	condition
-ema	result
emac/i	make thin
embol	plug
embry/o	embryo, fertilized egg
eme	to vomit
emesis	vomiting
-emesis	to vomit, vomiting
emia	blood
-emia	blood, blood condition
-emic	in the blood
emmetr-	measure
emuls	suspend in a liquid
emulsific	to milk out, to drain out
en-	in
-ence	forming, quality of, state of
encephal/o	brain
encephaly	condition of the brain
-ency	condition, state of, quality, quality of
end-	inside, within
endo-	inner, inside, within
-ent	end result, pertaining to, state of, end, forming
enter/o	intestine
entery	intestine
enur	urinate
environ	surroundings

S = Suffix   P = Prefix   R = Root   R/CF = Combining Form

WORD PART	DEFINITION
-eon	one who does
eosin/o	dawn
ependym	lining membrane
epi-	above, upon, over
epilep	seizure
epiphys/e	growth
episi/o	vulva
equi-	equal
equin/a	horse
equip	to fit out
-er	agent, one who does
erect	straight, to set up
erg/o	work
-ergy	process of working
-ery	condition, process of
erysi-	red
erythemat	redness
erythr/o	red
-escent	process
-esis	abnormal condition
eso-	inward
esophag/e	esophagus
essent	existence
esthes	sensation
esthet	sensation, perception
estr/o	woman
ethm	sieve
eti/o	cause
-etic	pertaining to
-etics	pertaining to
-ette	little
eu-	good, normal
ex-	away from, out, out of
exacerb	increase, aggravate
examin	test, examine
excret	separate, discharge

WORD PART	DEFINITION
exo-	outside, outward
expect	await
expir	breathe out
extra-	out of, outside
fac/i	face
factor	maker
farct	stuff
fasc/i	fascia
febr	fever
fec	feces
feed	to give food, nourish
femor	femur
fer	to bear, carry
ferrit	iron
fertil	able to conceive
fertiliz	to bear, make fruitful
fet/o	fetus
fibr/o	fiber, fibrous
fibril	small fiber
fibrin/o	fibrin
-fication	remove
fida	split
field	definite area
filar	roundworm
filtr	strain through
fiss	split
fistul	tube, pipe
flat	flatus
flate	blow into
flatul	excessive gas
flavon	yellow
flex	bend
fluid/o	to flow
fluo-	fluorine
fluor/o	flux, flow, x-ray beam
flux	flow

S = Suffix   P = Prefix   R = Root   R/CF = Combining Form

WORD PART	DEFINITION
foc	center, focus
follicul	follicle
foramin	opening, foramen
fore-	in front
-form	appearance of, resembling
form	shape, appearance of
format	to form
fract	break
fraction	small amount
free	free
frequ	repeated, often
front	front, forehead
fruct	fruit
funct	perform
fund/o	fundus
fung/i	fungus
fusion	to pour
galact/o	milk
gall	bile
galvan	low-voltage current
gastr/o	stomach
gastrin	stomach hormone
gastrocnem	calf of leg
gemin	twin, double
gen-	birth, origin
-gen	create, produce, form
gen/o	to create, to produce
-gene	producer, give birth
gener	produce
-genes	producing
genesis	origin, creation, production
-genesis	creation, origin, formation, source
genet	origin
-genic	creation, producing
genit	bring forth, birth, primary male or female sex organ

WORD PART	DEFINITION
genitor	offspring
ger	old age
geront/o	process of aging
gest	gestation, pregnancy, produce
gestat	gestation, pregnancy, to bear
gigant	giant
gingiv	gums
gland	gland
glauc	lens opacity, gray
gli/o	glue, supportive tissue of nervous system
glia	glue, supportive tissue of nervous system
-glia	glue, supportive tissue of nervous system
glob	globe
globin/o	protein
globul	globular, protein
glomerul/o	glomerulus
gloss/o	tongue
glott	mouth of windpipe
glottis	windpipe
gluc/o	glucose, sugar
glut/e	buttocks
glutin	glue, stick together
glyc/o	glycogen, glucose, sugar
glycer	glycerol, sweet
gnath	jaw
gnose	recognize an abnormal condition
gnosis	knowledge
gomph	bolt, nail
gon/o	seed
gonad/o	gonads, testes or ovaries
gong	daily practice
-grade	going, level
graft	splice, transplant
-graft	tissue for transplant
graine	head pain

WORD PART	DEFINITION
-gram	a record, drawing, recording
grand-	big
granul/o	granule, small grain
-graph	to record, write
-grapher	one who records
-graphy	process of recording
gravid	pregnant
gravida	pregnant woman
gravis	serious
green	green
gru	to move
guan	dung
gurgit	flood
gynec/o	woman, female
habilitat	restore
hale	breathe
halit	breath
hallucin	imagination
hallux	big toe
hem/o	blood
hemangi/o	blood vessel
hemat/o	blood
heme	red iron-containing pigment
hemi-	half
hepar	liver
hepat/o	liver
herb/i	plant
hered	inherited through genes
herni/o	hernia, rupture
herp	blister
heter/o	different
hetero-	different
hist	derived from histidine
hist/o	tissue
holist	entire, whole
hom/i	man

WORD PART	DEFINITION
home/o	the same
homo-	same, alike
hormon/e	chemical messenger
humor	fluid
hyal	glass
hydr/o	water
hyp-	below
hyper-	above, beyond, excess, excessive
hypn/o	sleep
hypo-	below, deficient, smaller, low, under
hyster/o	uterus
-ia	condition
-iac	pertaining to
-ial	pertaining to
-ian	one who does, specialist
-ias	condition
-iasis	condition, state of
iatr	medical treatment, treatment
-iatric	relating to medicine, medical knowledge
iatrics	field of medicine, healing
-iatrist	practitioner, one who treats
-iatry	treatment, field of medicine
-ible	can do, able to
-ic	pertaining to
-ica	pertaining to
-ical	pertaining to
-ician	expert, specialist
-ics	knowledge of
ict	seizure
icterus	jaundice
-id	having a particular quality, pertaining to
-ide	having a particular quality
idi/o	personal, distinct
ifer	to bear, carry
-ify	to become
-il	capability

S = Suffix   P = Prefix   R = Root   R/CF = Combining Form

WORD PART	DEFINITION
-ile	capable, capability, pertaining to
ile/o	ileum
ili	ilium
-ility	having the quality of, state of
im-	not, in
imag	likeness
immun/o	immune, immune response, immunity
immuniz	make immune
impair	worsen
imped/e	obstruct
imperfecta	unfinished
-imus	most
in-	not, into, in, without
-in	chemical, chemical compound, substance
incis	cut into
incub	sit on, lie on, hatch
index	to declare
-ine	pertaining to, substance
infant	infant
infect/i	tainted, internal invasion
infer	below, beneath
infest	invade, attack
inflammat	set on fire
inflat	blow up
infra-	below, beneath
-ing	quality of, doing
ingest	carry in
inguin	groin
inhal	breathe in
inhibit	repress
inject	force in
ino	sinew
insect/i	insect
insert	put together
inspir	breathe in

WORD PART	DEFINITION
insul	island
integr	whole
integ/u	covering of the body
intellect/u	perception, discernment
inter-	between
interstit	spaces within tissues
intestin	gut, intestine
intra-	inside, within
intrins	on the inside
intus-	within
iod/o	violet, iodine
-ion	action, condition, process
-ior	pertaining to, suffix for comparatives
-iosum	pertaining to
-ious	pertaining to
ir-	in
-is	belonging to, pertaining to, condition
isch	to keep back
-ism	action, condition, process
-ismus	take action
iso-	equal
-isone	cortisone
-ist	agent, specialist
-istic	pertaining to
-istry	specialty
-isy	inflammation
-ites	associated with
-itic	pertaining to
-ition	process
-itis	inflammation, infection
-ity	condition, state
-ium	structure
-ius	pertaining to
-ive	nature of, quality of, pertaining to
-iz	subject to

S = Suffix   P = Prefix   R = Root   R/CF = Combining Form

WORD PART	DEFINITION
-ization	process of creating, process of affecting in a specific way
-ize	action, affect in a specific way, policy
-ized	affected in a specific way
-izer	affects in a particular way, line of action
jejun	jejunum
jugul	throat
junct	joining together
juxta-	beside, near, close to
kal	potassium
kary/o	nucleus
kel/o	tumor
kerat/o	cornea
keratin/o	keratin
kern	nucleus
ket/o	ketone
keton	ketone
ketone	organic compound, ketone
kin	motion
kinase	enzyme
-kine	movement
kines/i	movement
kinet	motion
-kinin	move in
klept/o	to steal
kyph/o	bent
labi	lip
labyrinth	inner ear
lacer	to tear
lacrim	tears, tear duct
lact/e	milk
lactat	secrete milk
lapar/o	abdomen in general
lapse	clasp, fall together
-lapse	fall together, slide
laryng/o	larynx

WORD PART	DEFINITION
laser	acronym for *l*ight *a*mplification by *s*timulated *e*mission of *r*adiation
lash	end of whip
lat	to take
later	side, at the side
latiss	wide
-le	small
lei/o	smooth
-lemma	covering
-lepsy	seizure
lept	thin, small
-let	small
leuk/o	white
lex	word
librium	balance
ligament	ligament
ligat	tie up, tie off
lign	line
line	a mark
-ling	small
lingu	tongue
lip/o	fat, fatty tissue
lipid	fat
-lith	stone
lith/o	stone
liv	life
load	to carry
lob	lobe
locat	a place
log	to study, study of
-logist	one who studies, specialist
logous	relation
logy	study of
-logy	to study, study of
longev	long life
lord	curve, swayback

S = Suffix   P = Prefix   R = Root   R/CF = Combining Form

WORD PART	DEFINITION
lubric	make slippery
lucid	bright, clear
lumb	lower back, loin
lump	piece
lun	moon
-lus	small
lute	yellow
luxat	dislocate
ly	break down, separate
-ly	going toward, every
lymph/o	lymph
lymphaden/o	lymph node
lymphangi/o	lymphatic vessels
lys/o	decompose, decomposition, dissolve
lysis	destruction, to separate
-lysis	destroy, destruction, dissolve, separate, break down
lyt	dissolve
-lyte	soluble
-lytic	relating to destruction
lyze	destruct, dissolve, destroy
macro-	large
macul	spot
magnet	magnet
mak	makes
-maker	one who makes
mal-	bad, inadequate
mal	bad
-malacia	abnormal softness
malign	harmful, bad, cancer
malleol	small hammer, malleolus
mamm/o	breast
man/o	pressure
mandibul	the jaw
mania	frenzy
-mania	frenzy, madness

WORD PART	DEFINITION
manic	affected by frenzy
manipul	handful, use of hands
marker	sign
mast	breast
mastic	chew
mastoid	mastoid process
mater	mother
matern	mother
matur	ripe, ready
mature	ripe, ready, fully developed
medi	middle
media-	middle
mediastin/o	mediastinum, middle septum
medic	medicine
medulla	middle
mega-	enormous
megaly	enlargement
-megaly	enlargement
mei	lessening
mela	black
melan/o	melanin, black pigment, black
mellit	sweetened with honey
membran/o	cover, skin
men/o	menses, monthly, month
mening/o	meninges, membranes
menisc	crescent, meniscus
menstru	menses, occurring monthly
ment	mind, chin
-ment	action, state, resulting state
mere	part
mero-	partial
mes-	middle
meso-	middle
meta-	after, subsequent to, beyond
metabol	change
metacarp	bones of the hand

S = Suffix   P = Prefix   **R = Root**   **R/CF = Combining Form**

WORD PART	DEFINITION
metatars	bones of the foot
meter	measure
-meter	measure, instrument to measure
metr/o	uterus
-metrist	skilled in measurement
-metry	process of measuring
mi-	derived from hemi, half
micr/o	small
micro-	small
mictur	make urine, pass urine
mid-	middle
mileusis	lathe
milli	one-thousandth
min	amine
miner	mines
mineral/o	inorganic materials
miss	send
mit/o	thread, threadlike structure
mitr-	having two points
mitt	to send
mod	nature, form, method
molec	mass
mollusc	soft
mon	single
monas	unit
monil	type of fungus
mono-	one, single
morbid	disease
morph/o	shape
morphin	morphine
mort	death
mot	move
motiv	move
muc/o	mucous membrane, mucus
mucos/a	lining of a cavity

WORD PART	DEFINITION
multi-	many
mune	in service
muscul/o	muscle
mut	silent
muta	genetic change
mutil	to maim
my/o	muscle
myc/o	fungus
myel/o	spinal cord, bone marrow
myelin	in the spinal cord, myelin
myo-	to blink
my/o	muscle
myring/o	tympanic membrane, eardrum
myx-	mucus
narc/o	stupor, sleep
narciss	self-love
nas/o	nose
nat/e	birth, born
natr/i	sodium
natur/o	nature
nebul	cloud
necr/o	death
neo-	new
nephr/o	kidney
nerv	nerve
-ness	quality, state
neur/o	nerve, nervous tissue, nerve tissue
neutr/o	neutral
-nic	pertaining to
nitr/o	nitrogen
noct-	night
noia	to think
nom	law
non-	no
nor-	normal

S = Suffix   P = Prefix   R = Root   R/CF = Combining Form

WORD PART	DEFINITION
norm-	normal
nos/o	disease
nucl	nucleus
nucle/o	nucleus
nucleol	small nucleus
nutri	nourish
nutrit	nourishment
o/o	egg
oblong	elongated
obsess	besieged by thoughts
obstetr	midwifery
occipit	back of head
occult/a	hidden
occupation	work
ocul/o	eye
ode	way, road, path
odont	tooth
odyn/o	pain
-oid	appearance of, resemble, resembling
-ol	alcohol, chemical substance
-ola	small
-ole	small
olfact	smell
olig/o-	scanty, too little
olig-	too little, scanty
om/o	body, tumor
-oma	tumor, mass
omone	excite, stimulate
onc/o	tumor
-one	chemical substance, hormone
onych/o	nail
opheles	be of service
ophthalm/o	eye
opia	sight
opportun	take advantage of

WORD PART	DEFINITION
-opsis	vision
-opsy	to view
opt/o	vision
-or	a doer, one who does, that which does something
or/o	mouth
orbit	orbit
orch/o	testicle
ordin	arrange
orex	appetite
organ	organ, tool, instrument, organic
orth/o	straight
orthot	correct
-orum	function of
-ory	having the function of
os	mouth
-osa	like
-ose	full of, condition
-osis	condition
osmo	push
osmol	concentration
oss/i	bone
oste/o	bone
-osus	condition
ot/o	ear
-otomy	incision
-ous	pertaining to
ov/i	egg
ovari	ovary
ovul	ovum, egg
ox/y	oxygen
-oxia	oxygen condition
oxid	oxidize
oxin	oxygen atom
oxytoc	swift birth

S = Suffix   P = Prefix   **R = Root**   **R/CF = Combining Form**

WORD PART	DEFINITION
pace	step, pace
pact	driven in
palat	palate
palliat	reduce suffering
palpat	touch, stroke
palpit	throb
pan-	all
pancreat	pancreas
pant/o	entire
panto-	entire
papill/o	pimple
par-	abnormal, beside
para-	adjacent to, alongside, beside, abnormal
para	to bring forth
parasit	parasite
paresis	weakness
pareun	lying beside, sexual intercourse
pariet	wall
paroxysm	irritation
particul	little piece
partum	childbirth, to bring forth
pat	lie open
patell	patella
patent	lie open
-path	disease
path/o	disease
pathet	suffering
-pathic	pertaining to a disease
pathy	emotion, disease
-pathy	disease
paus/e	cessation
-pause	cessation
pector	chest
ped	child, foot
pedicul	louse
pelas	skin

WORD PART	DEFINITION
pell	skin
pelv	pelvis
pen	penis
-penia	deficient, deficiency
peps	digestion
pepsin/o	pepsin
pept/i	digest, digestion, amino acid
per-	intense, through
perforat	bore through
perfus/e	to pour
peri-	around
perin/e	perineum
peripher	external boundary, outer part, outer edge
periton/e	stretch over, peritoneum
perium	bringing forth
perm/e	pass through
person	person
pes	foot
pest/i	pest, nuisance
petit-	small
-pexy	fixation, surgical fixation
phaco-	lens
phag/e	to eat
-phage	to eat
-phagia	swallowing, eating
phalang/e	phalanx
pharmac/o	drug
pharyng/e	pharynx
pharynx	throat, pharynx
phen/o	to display
phenol	benzene derivative
phenyl	chemical group
pheo-	gray
pher-	carrying
pher/o	to carry

S = Suffix   P = Prefix   **R = Root**   **R/CF = Combining Form**

WORD PART	DEFINITION
-pheresis	removal
phery	outer edge
-phil	attraction
-phile	attraction
-philia	attraction
phim	muzzle
phleb/o	vein
phob	fear
-phobia	fear
phon/o	sound, voice
phor/e	bear, carry
phosph	phosphorus
phot/o	light
phren	mind
phylac	protect
phylaxis	protection
-phyll	leaf
phys	nature
physema	blowing
physi/o	body
physic	body
physis	growth
phyt/o	plant
pia	delicate
pituit	pituitary
placed	in an area
plak	plate, plaque
plant	insert, plant
planus	flat surface
plas	molding, formation
-plasia	formation
-plasm	something formed
plasm/o	to form
-plasty	formation, repair, surgical repair
plate	flat

WORD PART	DEFINITION
pleg	paralysis
plete	filled
pleur	pleura
plexy	stroke
pnea	to breathe
pneum/o	air, lung
pneumat	structure filled with air
pneumon	air, lung
pod	foot
-poiesis	to make
-poiet	the making
-poietin	the maker
poikilo-	irregular
point	to pierce
pol	pole
polio-	gray matter
pollut	to defile
poly-	excessive, many, much
polyp	polyp
poplit/e	ham, back of knee
por/o	opening
post-	after
poster	coming behind
pract	efficient, practical
prand/i	breakfast
pre-	before, in front of
precis	accurate
predn	a derivative of cholesterol
pregn	with child, pregnant
presby	old person
press	press close, press down, squeeze
prevent	prevent
primi-	first
pro-	before, in front, projecting forward
proct/o	anus and rectum

S = Suffix   P = Prefix   **R = Root**   **R/CF = Combining Form**

WORD PART	DEFINITION	WORD PART	DEFINITION
product	lead forth	pyrid	heat
prol/i	bear offspring	qi	vital force
prolifer	bear offspring	quadr	four
pronat	bend down	quadrant	quarter
prost/a	prostate	quadri-	four
prot/e	protein	radi/o	x-ray, radiation, radius
protein	protein	radial	radius
proto-	first	radic	root
proton	first	re-	again, back, backward
provis	provide	recept	receive
proxim	nearest	rect/o	rectum
prurit	itch	reflex/o	to reflect, bend back
pseudo-	false	regul	to rule
psych/o	mind, soul	remiss	send back, give up
pteryg	wing	ren	kidney
ptosis	drooping, falling	replic	reply
-ptosis	drooping	rescein	resin
ptysis	spit	resect/o	cut off
pub	pubis	resid/u	left over, what is left over
puber	growing up	resist	to withstand
pubesc	to reach puberty	restor	renew
puer	child	resuscit	revival from apparent death
pulmon/o	lung	reticul	fine net, network
puls	to drive	retin/o	retina
pump	pump	retinacul	hold back
punct	puncture	retro-	backward
pur	pus	rhabd/o	rod-shaped, striated
purg	cleanse, evacuate, throw up	rheumat	a flow, rheumatism
purif	make pure	rhin/o	nose
purul	pus	rhythm	rhythm
py/o	pus	rib/o	like a rib
pyel/o	renal pelvis	ribo-	from gum Arabic
pylor	gate, pylorus	ribo	pentose, a sugar
pyr/o	fire, heat, fever	rig	water
pyret	fever	rigid	stiff
pyrex	fever, heat	rit/u	right

S = Suffix   P = Prefix   **R = Root**   **R/CF = Combining Form**

WORD PART	DEFINITION
rose	rose
rotat	rotate
-rrhage	to flow profusely
-rrhagia	excessive flow, discharge
-rrhaphy	suture
rrhea	flow, discharge
-rrhea	flow, discharge
-rrhoid	flow
rrythm	rhythm
-rubin	rust colored
rumin	throat
-ry	occupation
sacchar	sugar
sacr/o	sacrum
sagitt	arrow
saliv	saliva
salping/o	fallopian tube, uterine tube
salpinx	trumpet
san	sound, healthy
sanit	health
sanitiz	make healthy
sapon	soap
sarc/o	flesh, sarcoma, muscle
satur	to fill
scapul	scapula
schiz/o	to split, cleave
scinti	spark
scintill	spark
scler/o	hard, white of eye, hardness
scope	instrument for viewing
-scope	instrument for viewing, instrument
-scopy	to examine, to view, visual examination
scorb	scurvy
script	writing, thing copied
scrot	scrotum
seb/o	sebum

WORD PART	DEFINITION
sebac/e	wax
secret	secrete, produce, separate
sect	cut off
sedat	to calm
sedent	sitting
segment	section
seiz	to grab, convulse
self	me, own individual
semi-	half
semin	scatter seed
semin/i	semen
sen	old age
senesc	growing old
senil	characteristic of old age
sens	feel
sensitiv	sensitive, feeling, sensitivity
sensor/i	sensation, sensory
separat	move apart
seps	decay, infection
sept/o	septum, partition
septic	infected
ser/o	serum, serous
sib	relative
-side	glycoside
sigm	Greek letter "S"
sigmoid/o	sigmoid colon
silic	silicon, glass
simi	ape, monkey
simul	imitate
sin/o	sinus
-sine	fold, pocket
sinus	sinus
sipid	flavor
-sis	abnormal condition, process
sit/u	place
skelet	skeleton

S = Suffix   P = Prefix   R = Root   R/CF = Combining Form

WORD PART	DEFINITION
skin	skin
smear	spread
soc	partner
soci/o	partner, ally, community
soma	body
somat/o	body
some	body
somn/o	sleep
somy	chromosome
son/o	sound
sorbit	fruit of a tree
sorpt	swallow
sound	noise
spad	tear or cut
spasm	spasm, sudden involuntary tightening
spast	tight
specif	species
sperm/i	sperm
spermat/o	sperm
sphen	wedge
spher/o	sphere
sphygm/o	pulse
spin/o	spine, spinal cord
spir/o	spiral, coil
spirat	breathe
spirit/u	spirit
spiro-	spiral, coil
splen/o	spleen
spondyl	vertebra
spong/i	sponge
spongios	sponge
spor/e	spore
stabil	stand firm
stable	steady
stag	standing place
stalsis	to constrict

WORD PART	DEFINITION
-stalsis	constrict, constriction
staphyl/o	bunch of grapes
stasis	stagnate, stay in one place, placement
-stasis	control, stop, stand still
stat	stand still
-static	to make stand, stop
-statin	inhibit
stax	fall in drops
steat	fat
stein	stone
sten/o	narrow, contract
ster	solid, steroid
stere/o	three-dimensional
steril	barren
stern	chest, breastbone
-steroid	steroid
-sterol	steroid
steron	steroid
-sterone	sterol
steth/o	chest
sthen	strength
stick	branch, twig
stigmat	focus
stimul	excite, strengthen
stin	partition
stip	press
stit/i	space
stoma	mouth
-stomy	new opening
stone	stone, pebble
storm	crisis
strab	squint
strat	layer
strept/o	twisted
strepto-	curved
study	inquiry

S = Suffix   P = Prefix   R = Root   R/CF = Combining Form

WORD PART	DEFINITION
su/i	self
sub-	below, under, slightly, underneath
sucr	sucrose, table sugar
suffic/i	enough
sulf	sulfur
super-	above, excessive
super	above
supinat	bend backward
supplement	supply to remedy a deficiency
suppress	pressed under, push under
supra-	above, excessive
surf	surface
surfact	surface
surg	operate
suscept	to take up
-sylated	linked
sym-	together
symptomat	symptom
syn-	together
syn/o	synovial membrane
syndesm	bind together
synov	synovial membrane
syring/o	tube, pipe
system	body system
systol/e	contraction
tachy-	rapid
tact	orderly arrangement
tag	touch
tain	hold
tali	ankle bone
tamin	touch
tampon	plug
tangent/i	touch
tarsus	flat surface
tax	coordination
tect/o	to shelter

WORD PART	DEFINITION
tempor/o	time, temple, side of head
ten/o	tendon
tendin	tendon
tens	pressure
-tensin	tense, taut
terat/o	monster, malformed fetus
term	normal gestation
test/o	testis, testicle
testicul	testicle, testis
tetra-	four
thalam	thalamus
thalass	sea
thec	sheath
thel	breast, nipple
thel/i	lining
then	motion
thenar	palm
therap/o	healing, treatment
therapeut	healing, treatment
therapy	medical treatment
-therapy	treatment
therm/o	heat
thesis	to arrange, place
thet	place, arrange
thi	sulfur
thora	chest
thorac/o	chest
thorax	chest
thromb/o	blood clot, clot
thrombin	clot
thym	thymus gland, the mind
thyr/o	thyroid
thyroid	thyroid
-tic	pertaining to
-tion	process, being
-tiz	pertaining to

S = Suffix   P = Prefix   R = Root   R/CF = Combining Form

WORD PART	DEFINITION
toc	labor, birth
toler	endure
tom/o	section, incise, cut
-tome	instrument to cut
-tomy	surgical incision
ton/o	pressure, tension
tonsil	tonsil
tonsill/o	tonsil
tope	part, location
topic	local
-tous	pertaining to
tox/o	poison
-toxic	able to kill
toxic/o	poison
toxin	poison
trache/o	trachea, windpipe
tract	draw, pull
tranquil	calm
trans-	across, through
trauma	wound, injury
tresia	a hole
tri-	three
trich/o	hair, flagellum
trichin/o	hair
-tripsy	to crush
-tripter	crusher
trochle	pulley
trop	turn, turning
troph	development, nourishment
trophy	development, nourishment
-tropic	stimulator, change
-tropin	nourishing, stimulation
tryps	friction
tub/a	tube
tubercul	swelling, tuberculosis, nodule
tubul	small tube

WORD PART	DEFINITION
tuss/i	cough
tussis	cough
-ty	quality, state
tympan/o	eardrum, tympanic membrane
-type	model, particular kind, group
typh	typhus
-ula	small thing
ulcer	a sore
-ule	little, small
-ulent	abounding in
uln/a	forearm bone
ultra-	higher, beyond
-um	tissue, structure
umbilic	belly button, navel, umbilicus
un-	not
un	one
uni-	one
ur/o	urinary system
urac	urinary bladder
-ure	process, result of
uresis	to urinate
uret	ureter, urine, urination
ureter/o	ureter
urethr/o	urethra
uria	urine
-uria	urine
urin/a	urine
-us	pertaining to
uter/o	uterus
uve	uvea
uvul	uvula
vaccin	vaccine, giving a vaccine
vag	vagus nerve
vagin	sheath, vagina
valgus	turn out
valv	valve

S = Suffix   P = Prefix   **R = Root**   **R/CF = Combining Form**

WORD PART	DEFINITION
varic/o	varicosity; dilated, tortuous vein
vas/o	blood vessel, duct
vascul	blood vessel
ved	knowledge
veget	plants
vegetat	growth
ven/o	vein
ventil	wind
ventr	belly
ventricul	ventricle
vers	turned
verse	travel
-version	change
vert	to turn
vertebr/a	vertebra
vesic	sac containing fluid
vestibul/o	vestibule of inner ear
via	the way
violet	bluish purple
vir	virus
viril	masculine
virus	poison
visc/o	sticky

WORD PART	DEFINITION
viscer	an internal organ
visu	sight
vit/a	life
voc	voice
vol	volume
volunt	free will
-volut	rolled up
volut/e	shrink, roll up
vuls	tear, pull
vulv/o	vulva
whip	to swing
xanth	yellow
xen/o	foreign material
xeno-	foreign
-xis	condition
-yl	substance
zea-	to live
-zoa	animal
zyg	zygote
zygot	yoked together
zyme	fermenting, enzyme, transform
-zyme	enzyme

Abbreviations

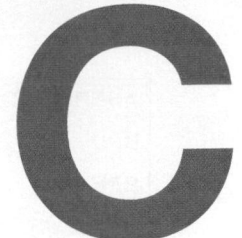

ABBREVIATION	DEFINITION
μg	microgram; one-millionth of a gram
↑	increase/ above
↓	decrease/ below
1°	primary
2°	secondary
99mTc	technetium 99m, a radionuclide
ABG	arterial blood gas
ABI	ankle/brachial index
ABO	a blood group system
AC	acromioclavicular
ACE	angiotensin-converting enzyme
ACEP	American College of Emergency Physicians
ACL	anterior cruciate ligament
ACTH	adrenocorticotropic hormone
AD	right ear
ADD	attention deficit disorder
ADH	antidiuretic hormone
ADHD	attention deficit hyperactivity disorder
ADLs	activities of daily living
AED	automatic external defibrillator
AFP	alpha-fetoprotein
AI	adequate intake
AIDS	acquired immunodeficiency syndrome
ALL	acute lymphoblastic leukemia
ALP	alkaline phosphatase
ALS	amyotrophic lateral sclerosis
ALT	alanine aminotransferase
AMAS	anti-malignin antibody screen

ABBREVIATION	DEFINITION
ANS	autonomic nervous system
AOM	acute otitis media
AP	anteroposterior
aPTT	activated partial thromboplastin time
ARDS	acute respiratory distress syndrome
ARF	acute respiratory failure
ARF	acute renal failure
AROM	active range of motion
AS	left ear
ASD	atrial septal defect
ASD	autism spectrum disorder
ASHD	arteriosclerotic heart disease
AST	aspartate aminotransferase
AU	both ears
AV	atrioventricular
AVM	arteriovenous malformation
BAL	bronchoalveolar lavage
BBB	blood–brain barrier
BCIA	Biofeedback Certification Institute of America
BD	brain death
BKA	below-the-knee amputation
BM	bowel movement
BMD	bone mineral density
BMR	basal metabolic rate
BNP	B-type natriuretic peptide
BOM	bilateral otitis media
BP	blood pressure

ABBREVIATION	DEFINITION
BPD	borderline personality disorder
BPH	benign prostatic hyperplasia
BPPV	benign paroxysmal positional vertigo
BRCA1	a gene, which when mutated, increases risk for breast and ovarian cancer
BRCA2	a gene, which when mutated, increases risk for breast cancer (BReast CAncer 2)
BSE	bovine spongiform encephalopathy
BSE	breast self-examination
BSI	Body Substance Isolation
BUN	blood urea nitrogen
C1–C8	cervical spinal nerves
C5	fifth cervical vertebra or nerve
CA	cancer
CABG	coronary artery bypass graft
CAD	coronary artery disease
CAM	complementary and alternative medicine
CAO	chronic airway obstruction
CAPD	continuous ambulatory peritoneal dialysis
CBC	complete blood count
CBT	cognitive behavioral therapy
CD	cluster of differentiation; coreceptors of cell membranes to recognize specific antigens
CD	conduct disorder
CD8	helper T cell
CDC	Centers for Disease Control and Prevention
CEA	carcinoembryonic antigen
CF	cystic fibrosis
CHART	continuous hyperfractionated accelerated radiotherapy
CHD	congenital heart disease
CHES	Certified Health Education Specialist
CHF	congestive heart failure
CIS	carcinoma in situ
CJD	Creutzfeldt-Jakob disease
CK	creatine kinase

ABBREVIATION	DEFINITION
CKD	chronic kidney disease
CMA	Certified Medical Assistant
CMV	cytomegalovirus
CNA	Certified Nurse Assistant
CNS	central nervous system
c/o	complains of
CO_2	carbon dioxide
COPD	chronic obstructive pulmonary disease
COT	Certified Occupational Therapist
COTA	Certified Occupational Therapist Assistant
CP	cerebral palsy
CPAP	continuous positive airway pressure
CPR	cardiopulmonary resuscitation
CPT	cognitive processing therapy
CRF	chronic renal failure
CRP	C-reactive protein
C-section	cesarean section
CSF	cerebrospinal fluid
CT	computed tomography
CVA	cerebrovascular accident
CVP	central venous pressure
CVS	cardiovascular system
CVT	cardiovascular technician
CXR	chest x-ray
D&C	dilation and curettage
DASH	Dietary Approaches to Stop Hypertension
DDAVP	synthetic ADH
DEXA	dual-energy x-ray absorptiometry
DHEA	dehydroepiandrosterone
DI	diabetes insipidus
DIC	disseminated intravascular coagulation
DID	dissociative identity disorder
DIFF	differential white blood cell count
DJD	degenerative joint disease
DKA	diabetic ketoacidosis

ABBREVIATION	DEFINITION
dL	deciliter; one-tenth of a liter
DM	diabetes mellitus
DMD	Duchenne muscular dystrophy
DNA	deoxyribonucleic acid
DNR	do not resuscitate
DO	doctor of osteopathy
DRE	digital rectal examination
DSHEA	Dietary Supplements Health and Education Act
DSM-IV	*Diagnostic and Statistical Manual of Mental Disorders,* fourth edition
DUB	dysfunctional uterine bleeding
DVT	deep vein thrombosis
Dx	diagnosis
EBT	electron beam tomography
EBV	Epstein-Barr virus
ECG	electrocardiogram
E. coli	*Escherichia coli*
ECT	electroconvulsive therapy
ED	erectile dysfunction
EEG	electroencephalogram
EFA	essential fatty acid
EKG	electrocardiogram
ELISA	enzyme-linked immunosorbent assay
EMDR	eye movement desensitization and reprocessing
EMF	electromagnetic field
EMG	electromyogram
EMT	emergency medical technician
EMT-1	emergency medical technician–first responder
EMT-P	emergency medical technician–paramedic
EP	evoked potential
EPA	U. S. Environmental Protection Agency
ER	Emergency Room
ERCP	endoscopic retrograde cholangiopancreatography
ESR	erythrocyte sedimentation rate

ABBREVIATION	DEFINITION
ESRD	end-stage renal disease
ESWL	extracorporeal shock wave lithotripsy
ETS	environmental tobacco smoke
FAS	fetal alcohol syndrome
FDA	U.S. Food and Drug Administration
FEV1	forced expiratory volume in 1 second
fL	femtoliter; one-quadrillionth of a liter
FOBT	fecal occult blood test
FSH	follicle-stimulating hormone
FTT	failure to thrive
FUS	focused ultrasound surgery
FVC	forced vital capacity
Fx	fracture
g	gram
GAD	generalized anxiety disorder
GDM	gestational diabetes mellitus
GERD	gastroesophageal reflux disease
GFR	glomerular filtration rate
GGT	gamma-glutamyl transpeptidase
GH	growth hormone, somatotropin
GI	gastrointestinal
GI	glycemic index
GL	glycemic load
GMP	good manufacturing practice
GnRH	gonadotropin-releasing hormone
GSR	galvanic skin response
GTT	glucose tolerance test
GYN	gynecology
H1N1	swine flu virus
H_2-blocker	histamine-2 receptor antagonist
H5N1	subtype of avian influenza virus
HAV	hepatitis A virus
Hb	hemoglobin
Hb A1c	glycosylated hemoglobin A1c
HBOT	hyperbaric oxygen therapy
HBV	hepatitis B virus
HCG	human chorionic gonadotropin

ABBREVIATION	DEFINITION
HCL	hydrochloric acid
Hct	hematocrit
HCV	hepatitis C virus
HDL	high-density lipoprotein
HDN	hemolytic disease of the newborn
Hg	mercury
Hgb	hemoglobin
HIPAA	Health Insurance Portability and Accountability Act
HIV	human immunodeficiency virus
HLA	human leukocyte antigen
HLD	high-level disinfection
HMD	hyaline membrane disease
H/O	history of
HPI	history of present illness
HPV	human papillomavirus
HRT	hormone replacement therapy
HSV	herpes simplex virus
HSV-1	herpes simplex virus, type 1
HUS	hemolytic uremic syndrome
IADLs	instrumental activities of daily living
IBS	irritable bowel syndrome
ICD	implantable cardioverter/defibrillator
IDDM	insulin-dependent diabetes mellitus
Ig	immunoglobulin
IgA	immunoglobulin A
IgD	immunoglobulin D
IgE	immunoglobulin E
IgF	insulinlike growth factor
IgG	immunoglobulin G
IgM	immunoglobulin M
IM	intramuscular
INR	international normalized ratio
ITP	idiopathic (or immunologic) thrombocytopenic purpura
IU	international unit(s)
IUD	intrauterine device

ABBREVIATION	DEFINITION
IV	intravenous
IVC	inferior vena cava
IVF	in vitro fertilization
IVP	intravenous pyelogram
JC	Joint Commission
JRA	juvenile rheumatoid arthritis
KUB	x-ray of abdomen to show kidneys, ureters, and bladder
L	liter
L1–L5	lumbar nerves spine or vertebrae
LASER	light amplification by stimulated emission of radiation
LCC-ST	Liaison Council on Certification for the Surgical Technologist
LD	learning disability
LDL	low-density lipoprotein
LED	light emission diode
LEEP	loop electrosurgical excision procedure
LFT	liver function test
LH	luteinizing hormone
LLQ	left lower quadrant
LOC	loss of consciousness
LPN	licensed practical nurse
LSD	lysergic acid diethylamide (acid)
LUQ	left upper quadrant
LVN	licensed vocational nurse
MAOI	monoamine oxidase inhibitor
mcg	microgram; one-millionth of a gram
MCH	mean corpuscular hemoglobin (the average amount of hemoglobin in the average red blood cell)
MCHC	mean corpuscular hemoglobin concentration (the average concentration of hemoglobin in a given volume of red blood cells)
MCP	metacarpophalangeal
MCS	minimally conscious state
MCV	mean corpuscular volume (the average volume of a red blood cell)

ABBREVIATION	DEFINITION
MD	doctor of medicine
MDMA	methylenedioxymethamphetamine (ecstasy)
mg	milligram
MHC	major histocompatibility complex
MI	myocardial infarction
mL	milliliter
mm³	cubic millimeter
MOAB	monoclonal antibody
MODY	mature-onset diabetes of youth
MPD	multiple personality disorder
MRA	magnetic resonance angiography
MRI	magnetic resonance imaging
mRNA	messenger RNA
MRSA	methicillin-resistant Staphylococcus aureus
MS	multiple sclerosis
NCBTMB	National Certification Board for Therapeutic Massage and Bodywork
NCCAM	National Center for Complementary and Alternative Medicine
NCCAOM	National Certifying Commission for Acupuncture and Oriental Medicine
NCI	National Cancer Institute
NCTMB	National Certificate for Therapeutic Massage and Bodywork
NHGRI	National Human Genome Research Institute
NHLBI	National Heart, Lung, and Blood Institute
NIDDM	non-insulin-dependent diabetes mellitus
NIH	National Institutes of Health
NKA	no known allergies
NMS	neurally mediated syncope
NO	nitric oxide
NPH	neutral protamine Hagedorn insulin
NRDS	neonatal respiratory distress syndrome
NSAID	nonsteroidal anti-inflammatory drug
O₂	oxygen
OA	osteoarthritis

ABBREVIATION	DEFINITION
OB	obstetrics
OCD	obsessive-compulsive disorder
OD	doctor of osteopathy
OD	right eye
ODD	oppositional defiant disorder
OGTT	oral glucose tolerance test
OME	otitis media with effusion
omega-3	alpha-linolenic acid
omega-6	linolenic acid
OR	operating room
OS	left eye
OSHA	Occupational Safety and Health Administration
OT	ophthalmic technician
OT	oxytocin
OT	occupational therapist
OTC	over-the-counter
OU	both eyes
P	pulse (rate)
PA	posteroanterior
PaO₂	partial pressure of arterial oxygen
Pap	Papanicolaou (Pap test, Pap smear)
PAT	paroxysmal atrial tachycardia
PCBs	polychlorinated biphenyls
PCD	programmed cell death
PCL	posterior cruciate ligament
PCOS	polycystic ovarian syndrome
PCP	phencyclidine (angel dust)
PDA	patent ductus arteriosus
PDD-NOS	pervasive developmental disorder–not otherwise specified
PDT	postural drainage therapy
PE	pressure equalization (tube)
PEEP	positive end-expiratory pressure
PEFR	peak expiratory flow rate
PET	positron emission tomography

ABBREVIATION	DEFINITION
PFT	pulmonary function test
pg	picogram; one-trillionth of a gram
PGY	pregnancy
pH	hydrogen ion concentration
PhD	doctor of philosophy
PID	pelvic inflammatory disease
PIP	proximal interphalangeal
PKD	polycystic kidney disease
PKU	phenylketonuria
PMDD	premenstrual dysphoric disorder
PMNL	polymorphonuclear leukocyte
PMS	premenstrual syndrome
PNS	peripheral nervous system
p.o.	by mouth
polio	poliomyelitis
PPH	postpartum hemorrhage
PPI	proton pump inhibitor
PPS	postpolio syndrome
PRL	prolactin
p.r.n.	when necessary
PSA	prostate-specific antigen
PsyD	doctor of psychology
PT	physiotherapy
PT	prothrombin time
PT	physical therapy, physical therapist
PTA	physical therapy assistant
PTCA	percutaneous transluminal coronary angioplasty
PTH	parathyroid hormone
PTSD	posttraumatic stress disorder
PVC	premature ventricular contraction
PVD	peripheral vascular disease
PVS	persistent vegetative state
q.4.h.	every 4 hours
q.i.d.	four times a day
R	respiration (rate)

ABBREVIATION	DEFINITION
RA	rheumatoid arthritis
RBC	red blood cell
RDA	recommended dietary allowance
RDS	respiratory distress syndrome
RF	radiofrequency
Rh	Rhesus
RhoGAM	Rhesus immune globulin
RICE	rest, ice, compression, elevation
RLQ	right lower quadrant
RN	registered nurse
RNA	ribonucleic acid
ROM	range of motion
RSV	respiratory syncytial virus
RT	radiology technician
RU-486	mifepristone
RUQ	right upper quadrant
S1–S5	sacral nerves or vertebrae
SA	sinoatrial
SAD	seasonal affective disorder
SARS	severe acute respiratory syndrome
SBS	shaken baby syndrome
SC	subcutaneous
SCI	spinal cord injury
SET	self-examination of the testes
SFD	small for date
SG	specific gravity
SGA	small for gestational age
SGOT	serum glutamic-oxaloacetic acid transaminase (AST)
SGPT	serum glutamic-pyruvic transaminase (ALT)
SI	sacroiliac
SIDS	sudden infant death syndrome
SLE	systemic lupus erythematosus
SMI	sustained maximal inspiration
SNRI	serotonin and norepinephrine reuptake inhibitor
SOB	short(ness) of breath

ABBREVIATION	DEFINITION
SP	Standard Precautions
SRS	stereotactic radiosurgery
SSA	Sjögren syndrome antibodies A
SSB	Sjögren syndrome antibodies B
SSRI	selective serotonin reuptake inhibitor
STAT	immediately
STD	sexually transmitted disease
SVC	superior vena cava
T	temperature
T1	first thoracic vertebra or nerve
T1–T12	thoracic spinal nerves or vertebrae
T_3	triiodothyronine
T_4	tetraiodothyronine (thyroxine)
TB	tuberculosis
TBI	traumatic brain injury
TCA	tricyclic antidepressant
TED	thromboembolic deterrent
TEE	transesophageal echocardiography
TENS	transcutaneous electrical nerve stimulation
THC	tetrahydrocannabinol (marijuana)
THR	total hip replacement
TIA	transient ischemic attack
TIBC	total iron-binding capacity
t.i.d.	(Latin *ter in die*) three times a day
TMJ	temporomandibular joint
TNM	tumor-node-metastasis (staging system for cancer)
TOF	tetralogy of Fallot

ABBREVIATION	DEFINITION
tPA	tissue plasminogen activator
TPN	total parenteral nutrition
TS	tumor suppressor
TSH	thyroid-stimulating hormone
TTM	trichotillomania
TTN	transient tachypnea of the newborn
TTP	thrombotic thrombocytopenic purpura
TURP	transurethral resection of the prostate
U	unit
UA	urinalysis
μg	microgram; one-millionth of a gram
UP	Universal Precautions
URI	upper respiratory infection
USDA	U.S. Department of Agriculture
UTI	urinary tract infection
UV	ultraviolet
VCUG	voiding cystourethrogram
VEP	visual evoked potential
V-fib	ventricular fibrillation
VS	vital signs
VSD	ventricular septal defect
vWD	von Willebrand disease
vWF	von Willebrand factor
WAD	Word Analysis and Definition (box)
WBC	white blood cell; white blood (cell) count
WNL	within normal limits
WNV	West Nile virus

A

abdomen (**AB**-doh-men) Part of the trunk between the thorax and the pelvis.

abdominal (ab-**DOM**-in-al) Pertaining to the abdomen.

abdominopelvic (ab-**DOM**-ih-no-**PEL**-vik) Pertaining to the abdomen and pelvis.

abducens (ab-**DYU**-senz) Sixth (VI) cranial nerve; responsible for eye movement.

abduction (ab-**DUCK**-shun) Action of moving away from the midline.

ablation (ab-**LAY**-shun) Removal of tissue to destroy its function.

abortion (ah-**BOR**-shun) Spontaneous or induced expulsion of an embryo or fetus from the uterus.

abortus (ah-**BOR**-tus) Product of abortion.

abrasion (ah-**BRAY**-shun) Area of skin or mucous membrane that has been scraped off.

abruptio (ab-**RUP**-she-oh) Placenta abruptio is the premature detachment of the placenta.

absorption (ab-**SORP**-shun) Uptake of nutrients and water by cells in the GI tract.

accessory (ack-**SESS**-oh-ree) Eleventh (XI) cranial nerve; supplying neck muscles, pharynx, and larynx.

accommodation (ah-kom-oh-**DAY**-shun) The act of adjusting something to make it fit the needs; in the case of the eye, the lens adjusts itself.

acetabulum (as-eh-**TAB**-you-lum) The cup-shaped cavity of the hip bone that receives the head of the femur to form the hip joint.

acetaminophen (ah-seat-ah-**MIN**-oh-fen) Medication that is an analgesic and an antipyretic.

acetone (**ASS**-eh-tone) Ketone that is found in blood, urine, and breath when diabetes mellitus is out of control.

acetylcholine (**AS**-eh-til-**KOH**-leen) Parasympathetic neurotransmitter.

Achilles tendon (ah-**KILL**-eeze) A tendon formed from the gastrocnemius and soleus muscles and inserted into the calcaneus. Also called *calcaneal tendon*.

achondroplasia (a-kon-droh-**PLAY**-ze-ah) Condition with abnormal conversion of cartilage into bone, leading to dwarfism.

acid (**ASS**-id) Substance with a pH below 7.0.

acinar cells (**ASS**-in-ar **SELLS**) Enzyme-secreting cells of the pancreas.

acne (**AK**-nee) Inflammatory disease of sebaceous glands and hair follicles.

acoustic (ah-**KOOS**-tik) Pertaining to hearing.

acquired (ah-**KWIRED**) A condition that is not inherited.

acquired immunodeficiency syndrome (AIDS) (ah-**KWIRED** **IM**-you-noh-de-**FISH**-en-see **SIN**-drome) Infection with the HIV virus.

acromegaly (ak-roe-**MEG**-ah-lee) Enlargement of the head, face, hands, and feet due to excess growth hormone in an adult.

acromioclavicular (AC) (ah-**CROW**-mee-oh-klah-**VICK**-you-lar) The joint between the acromion and the clavicle.

acromion (ah-**CROW**-mee-on) Lateral end of the scapula, extending over the shoulder joint.

acrophobia (ak-roh-**FOH**-be-ah) Pathologic fear of heights.

activities of daily living (ADLs) (ak-**TIV**-ih-tees of **DAY**-lee **LIV**-ing) Daily routines for mobility and personal care: bathing, dressing, eating, and moving.

acuminata (a-**KYU**-min-ah-ta) Tapering to a point.

acupoint (**AK**-you-point) Point of entry in the skin to a meridian.

acupressure (**AK**-you-presh-ur) Application of pressure to acupoints.

acupuncture (ak-you-**PUNK**-chur) Use of sterile, hair-thin needles to stimulate the energy pathways known as meridians.

acute (ah-**KYUT**) Describes a disease of sudden onset that is usually severe and of short duration.

adapt (ad-**APT**) To adjust to different conditions.

adaptation (ad-ap-**TAY**-shun) Change in function or structure of an organ to meet new conditions.

adaptive equipment (a-**DAP**-tiv ee-**KWIP**-ment) Devices and supplies that enable a disabled individual to perform specific functions.

addict (**ADD**-ikt) Person with a psychologic or physical dependence on a substance or practice.

addiction (ah-**DIK**-shun) Habitual psychological and physiologic dependence on a substance or practice.

addictive (ah-**DIK**-tiv) Pertaining to or causing addiction.

Addison disease (**ADD**-ih-son **DIZ**-eez) An autoimmune disease leading to decreased production of adrenocortical steroids.

adduction (ah-**DUCK**-shun) Action of moving toward the midline.

adenine (**AD**-eh-neen) One of the chemical bases found in, and comprising the sequence of, both DNA and RNA.

adenocarcinoma (**AD**-eh-noh-kar-sih-**NOH**-mah) A cancer arising from glandular epithelial cells.

adenohypophysis (**AD**-en-oh-hi-**POF**-ih-sis) Anterior lobe of the pituitary gland.

adenoid (**ADD**-eh-noyd) Single mass of lymphoid tissue in the midline at the back of the throat.

adenomyosis (**AD**-en-oh-my-**OH**-sis) The implantation of endometrial glandular tissue in the myometrium.

adherence (ad-**HERE**-ents) The act of sticking to something.

adipose (**ADD**-i-pose) Containing fat.

adiposity (ad-ih-**POSS**-ih-tee) Excessive accumulation of fat in a site, organ, or body.

adjunct (**AJ**-ungkt) Something that is joined to another but is not an essential part.

adjustment (ah-**JUST**-ment) The action of bringing a body part into alignment with the others. Also called *manipulation.*

adjuvant (**AD**-joo-vant) Additional treatment after a primary treatment has been used.

adnexa (ad-**NEK**-sa) Parts accessory to an organ or structure. Singular *adnexum.*

adnexal (ad-**NEK**-sal) Pertaining to accessory structures; for example, structures alongside the uterus.

adolescence (ad-oh-**LESS**-ents) Stage that begins with puberty and ends with physical maturity.

adolescent (ad-oh-**LESS**-ent) Pertaining to adolescence or a person in that stage.

adrenal gland (ah-**DREE**-nal GLAND) The suprarenal, or adrenal, gland on the upper pole of each kidney.

adrenalectomy (ah-dree-nal-**ECK**-to-me) Removal of part or all of an adrenal gland.

adrenaline (ah-**DREN**-ah-lin) One of the catecholamines. Also called *epinephrine.*

adrenergic (ad-re-**NER**-jik) Relating to the autonomic nervous system.

adrenocortical (ah-dree-noh-**KOR**-tih-kal) Pertaining to the cortex of the adrenal gland.

adrenocorticotropic hormone (ah-**DREE**-noh-**KOR**-tih-koh-**TROH**-pik HOR-mohn) Hormone of the anterior pituitary that stimulates the cortex of the adrenal gland to produce its own hormones.

adrenogenital syndrome (ah-**DREE**-no-**JEN**-it-al **SIN**-drome) Hypersecretion of androgens from the adrenal gland.

advance medical directive (ad-**VANTS** MED-ih-kal die-**REK**-tiv) Legal document signed by the patient dealing with issues of prolonging or ending life in the event of life-threatening illness.

adventitia (ad-ven-**TISH**-ah) Outer layer of connective tissue covering blood vessels or organs.

aerobic (air-**OH**-bik) An organism capable of living in the presence of oxygen.

affect (**AF**-fekt) External display of feelings, thoughts, and emotions.

afferent (**AF**-eh-rent) Conducting impulses inward *toward* the spinal cord or brain.

agar (**AH**-gar) A derivative of seaweed used as a culture medium.

aged (**A**-jid) Having lived to an advanced age.

agenesis (a-**JEN**-eh-sis) Failure to develop any organ or any part.

agglutinate (ah-**GLUE**-tin-ate) Stick together to form clumps.

agglutination (ah-glue-tih-**NAY**-shun) Process by which cells or other particles adhere to each other to form clumps.

aging (**A**-jing) The process of human maturation and decline.

agonist (**AG**-on-ist) Agent combines with receptors to initiate drug actions.

agoraphobia (ah-gor-ah-**FOH**-be-ah) Pathologic fear of being trapped in a public place.

agranulocyte (a-**GRAN**-you-lo-site) A white blood cell without any granules in its cytoplasm.

alanine aminotransferase (**ALT**) (**AL**-ah-neen ah-**ME**-no-**TRANS**-fer-aze) Enzyme that is found in liver cells and leaks out into the bloodstream when the cells are damaged, enabling liver damage to be diagnosed.

albinism (**AL**-bih-nizm) Genetic disorder with lack of melanin.

albino (al-**BY**-no) Person with albinism.

albumin (al-**BYU**-min) Simple, soluble protein.

aldosterone (al-**DOS**-ter-own) Mineralocorticoid hormone of the adrenal cortex.

aldosteronism (al-**DOS**-ter-on-izm) Condition caused by excessive secretion of aldosterone. Also called *Conn syndrome.*

aldosteronoma (al-**DOS**-ter-on-oma) Benign adenoma of the adrenal cortex.

Alexander technique (al-eg-**ZAN**-der tek-**NEEK**) The use of awareness and exercises to improve posture, breathing, and movement.

alignment (a-**LINE**-ment) A state of being in the correct position in relation to other structures.

alimentary (al-ih-**MEN**-tar-ee) Pertaining to the digestive tract.

alkaline (**AL**-kah-line) Substance with a pH above 7.0. Also called *basic.*

alkaloid (**AL**-ka-loyd) Alkaline substances with pharmacologic activity synthesized from plants.

allele (ah-**LEEL**) Genetic variant found on the same locus of a pair of chromosomes.

allergen (**AL**-er-jen) Substance producing a hypersensitivity (allergic) reaction.

allergic (ah-**LER**-jik) Pertaining to being hypersensitive.

allergy (**AL**-er-jee) Hypersensitivity to an allergen.

allogen (**AL**-oh-jen) Antigen from someone else in the same species.

allograft (**AL**-oh-graft) Tissue graft from another person or cadaver.

alloimmune (**AL**-oh-im-**YUNE**) Reaction directed against foreign tissue.

allopathic medicine (al-oh-**PATH**-ic MED-ih-sin) Conventional medical practice.

allyl sulfides (**AL**-il **SUL**-fides) Group of substances found in garlic and onions that can reduce blood cholesterol.

alopecia (al-oh-**PEE**-shah) Partial or complete loss of hair, naturally or from medication.

alpha-fetoprotein (**AL**-fah-fee-toe-**PRO**-teen) Protein normally produced only by the fetus.

alveolus (al-**VEE**-oh-lus) Terminal element of the respiratory tract. Plural *alveoli.*

Alzheimer disease (**AWLZ**-high-mer DIZ-eez) Common form of dementia.

amblyopia (am-blee-**OH**-pee-ah) Failure or incomplete development of the pathways of vision to the brain.

amenorrhea (a-men-oh-**REE**-ah) Absence or abnormal cessation of menstrual flow.

amino acid (ah-ME-no ASS-id) The basic building block of protein.

aminoketone (ah-ME-no-KEY-tone) By-product of nicotine.

ammonia (ah-MOAN-ih-ah) Toxic breakdown product of amino acids.

amnesia (am-NEE-zee-ah) Total or partial inability to remember past experiences.

amniocentesis (AM-nee-oh-sen-tee-sis) Removal of amniotic fluid for diagnostic purposes.

amnion (AM-nee-on) Membrane around the fetus that contains amniotic fluid.

amniotic (am-nee-OT-ic) Pertaining to the amnion.

amoeba (ah-ME-bah) Single-celled organism that changes shape as it moves.

amoebiasis (ah-me-BY-ah-sis) Infection with *Amoeba*.

ampulla (am-PULL-ah) Dilated portion of a canal or duct.

amputation (am-pyu-TAY-shun) Process of removing a limb, a part of a limb, a breast, or some other projecting part.

amputee (AM-pyu-tee) A person with an amputation.

amylase (AM-il-aze) One of a group of enzymes that break down starch.

amyotrophic (a-my-oh-TROH-fik) Pertaining to muscular atrophy.

anabolism (an-AB-oh-lizm) The buildup of complex substances in the cell from simpler ones as a part of metabolism.

anaerobic (an-air-OH-bik) An organism capable of growing in the absence of oxygen.

analgesia (an-al-JEE-ze-ah) State in which pain is reduced.

analgesic (an-al-JEE-zic) Substance that reduces the response to pain.

anaphylactic (AN-ah-fih-LAK-tik) Pertaining to anaphylaxis.

anaphylaxis (AN-ah-fih-LAK-sis) Immediate severe allergic response.

anastomosis (ah-NAS-to-MO-sis) A surgically made union between two tubular structures. Plural *anastomoses*.

anatomical (an-ah-TOM-ik-al) Pertaining to anatomy.

anatomy (ah-NAT-oh-mee) Study of the structures of the human body.

ancillary (AN-sil-air-ree) Accessory, adjunct.

androgen (AN-droh-jen) Hormone that promotes masculine characteristics.

anemia (ah-NEE-me-ah) Decreased number of red blood cells.

anemic (ah-NEE-mik) Pertaining to or suffering from anemia.

anencephaly (AN-en-SEF-ah-lee) Born without cerebral hemispheres.

anesthesia (an-es-THEE-zee-ah) Complete loss of sensation.

anesthesiologist (AN-es-thee-zee-OL-oh-jist) Medical specialist in anesthesia.

anesthesiology (AN-es-thee-zee-OL-oh-jee) Medical specialty related to anesthesia.

anesthetic (an-es-THET-ic) Substance that takes away feeling and pain.

aneurysm (AN-yur-izm) Circumscribed dilation of an artery or cardiac chamber.

angiogenesis (AN-jee-oh-JEN-eh-sis) New formation of blood vessels.

angiogram (AN-jee-oh-gram) Radiograph obtained after injection of radiopaque contrast material into blood vessels.

angiography (an-jee-OG-rah-fee) Radiography of vessels after injection of contrast material.

angioplasty (AN-jee-oh-PLAS-tee) Recanalization of a blood vessel by surgery.

angiotensin (an-jee-oh-TEN-sin) An agent that constricts blood vessels.

anomaly (ah-NOM-ah-lee) A structural abnormality.

Anopheles (ah-NOF-eh-leez) A type of mosquito.

anorchism (an-OR-kizm) Absence of testes.

anorexia (an-oh-RECK-see-ah) Severe lack of appetite; *or* an aversion to food.

anoscopy (A-nos-koh-pee) Endoscopic examination of the anus.

anoxia (an-OCK-see-ah) Without oxygen.

anoxic (an-OCK-sik) Pertaining to or suffering from a lack of oxygen.

antacid (ant-ASS-id) Agent that neutralizes acidity.

antagonism (an-TAG-oh-nizm) Situation of opposing.

antagonist (an-TAG-oh-nist) An opposing structure, agent, disease, or process.

antagonistic (an-TAG-oh-nist-ik) Having an opposite function.

anterior (an-TER-ee-or) Front surface of body; situated in front.

anteversion (an-teh-VER-shun) Forward tilting of the uterus.

antevert (an-teh-VERT) Tilted forward.

anthracosis (an-thra-KOH-sis) Lung disease caused by the inhalation of coal dust.

anthrax (AN-thraks) A severe infectious disease.

antiangiogenesis (anti-AN-jee-oh-JEN-eh-sis) The prevention of growth of new blood vessels.

antibiotic (AN-tih-bye-OT-ik) A substance that has the capacity to destroy bacteria and other microorganisms.

antibody (AN-tih-body) Protein produced in response to an antigen. Plural *antibodies*.

anticoagulant (AN-tee-ko-AG-you-lant) Substance that prevents clotting.

antidiuretic (AN-tih-die-you-RET-ik) An agent that decreases urine production.

antidiuretic hormone (ADH) (AN-tih-die-you-RET-ik HOR-mohn) Posterior pituitary hormone that decreases urine output by acting on the kidney. Also called *vasopressin*.

antiepileptic (AN-tee-epih-LEP-tik) A pharmacologic agent capable of preventing or arresting epilepsy.

antigen (AN-tee-jen) Substance capable of triggering an immune response.

antihistamine (an-tee-HISS-tah-mean) Drug used to treat allergic symptoms because of its action antagonistic to histamine.

anti-inflammatory (AN-tee-in-FLAM-ah-tor-ee) Agent that reduces inflammation by acting on the body's response mechanisms without affecting the causative agent.

antimicrobial (AN-tee-my-KROH-bee-al) Agent for destroying or preventing multiplication of organisms.

antioxidant (an-tee-OKS-ih-dant) Substance that can prevent cell damage by neutralizing free radicals.

antipruritic (AN-tee-pru-RIT-ik) Medication against itching.

antipsychotic (AN-tih-sigh-KOT-ik) An agent helpful in the treatment of psychosis.

antipyretic (AN-tee-pie-RET-ik) Agent that reduces fever.

antisepsis (an-tih-SEP-sis) Inhibiting the growth of infectious agents.

antiseptic (an-tih-SEP-tic) Pertaining to antisepsis, *or* an agent capable of producing antisepsis.

antisocial personality disorder (AN-tee-SOH-shal per-son-AL-ih-tee dis-OR-der) Disorder of people who lie, cheat, and steal and have no guilt about their behavior.

antithyroid (an-tee-THIGH-royd) A substance that inhibits production of thyroid hormones.

antrum (AN-trum) A nearly closed cavity or chamber.

anuria (an-YOU-ree-ah) Absence of urine production.

anus (A-nuss) Terminal opening of the digestive tract through which feces are discharged.

anxiety (ang-ZI-eh-tee) Distress caused by fear

aorta (a-OR-tuh) Main trunk of the systemic arterial system.

apex (A-peks) Tip or end of cone-shaped structure, such as the heart.

Apgar score (AP-gar SKOR) Evaluation of newborn status.

apheresis (a-fer-EE-sis) Extraction of one element from donated blood.

aphonia (a-FO-nee-ah) Loss of voice.

aphthous ulcer (AF-thus UL-ser) Painful small oral ulcer (canker sore).

aplastic anemia (a-PLAS-tik ah-NEE-me-ah) Condition in which the bone marrow is unable to produce sufficient red cells, white cells, and platelets.

apnea (AP-nee-ah) Absence of spontaneous respiration.

apocrine (AP-oh-krin) Apocrine sweat glands that open into the hair follicle.

apoptosis (AP-op-TOE-sis) Programmed normal cell death.

appendectomy (ah-pen-DEK-toe-me) Surgical removal of the appendix.

appendicitis (ah-pen-dih-SIGH-tis) Inflammation of the appendix.

appendix (ah-PEN-dicks) Small blind projection from the pouch of the cecum.

aqueous humor (ACHE-we-us HEW-mor) Watery liquid in the anterior and posterior chambers of the eye.

arachnoid mater (ah-RACK-noyd MAY-ter) Weblike middle layer of the three meninges.

areola (ah-REE-oh-luh) Circular reddish area surrounding the nipple.

aromatherapy (ah-ROH-mah-THAIR-ah-pee) Use of essential oils to promote well-being.

aromatic (ah-roh-MAT-ik) Having an agreeable spicy odor; *or* one of a group of vegetable drugs.

arrhythmia (a-RITH-me-ah) An abnormal heart rhythm.

arteriography (ar-teer-ee-OG-rah-fee) X-ray visualization of an artery after injection of contrast material.

arteriole (ar-TER-ee-ole) Small terminal artery leading into the capillary network

arteriosclerosis (ar-TIER-ee-oh-skler-OH-sis) Hardening of the arteries.

arteriosclerotic (ar-TIER-ee-oh-skler-OT-ik) Pertaining to or suffering from arteriosclerosis.

arteriovenous malformation (ar-TEER-e-o-VE-nus mal-for-MAY-shun) An abnormal communication between an artery and a vein.

artery (AR-ter-ee) Thick-walled blood vessel carrying blood away from the heart.

arthritis (ar-THRY-tis) Inflammation of a joint or joints.

arthrocentesis (AR-throw-sen-TEE-sis) Withdrawal of fluid from a joint through a needle.

arthrodesis (ar-THROW-dee-sis) Fixation or stiffening of a joint by surgery.

arthrography (ar-THROG-ra-fee) X-ray of a joint taken after the injection of a contrast medium into the joint.

arthroplasty (AR-throw-plas-tee) Surgery to restore as far as possible the function of a joint.

arthroscope (AR-thro-skope) Endoscope used to examine the interior of a joint.

arthroscopy (ar-THROS-koh-pee) Visual examination of the interior of a joint.

articulate (ar-TIK-you-late) To form a joint so as to allow movement.

articulation (ar-tik-you-LAY-shun) Joint formed to allow movement.

asana (ah-SAH-nah) Yoga posture or steady position of the body to open energy channels.

asbestosis (as-bes-TOE-sis) Lung disease caused by the inhalation of asbestos particles.

Ascaris lumbricoides (AS-kah-ris lum-bri-KOY-deez) Large roundworm parasite.

ascites (ah-SIGH-teez) Accumulation of fluid in the abdominal cavity.

ascorbic acid (as-KOR-bic ASS-id) Vitamin C, which prevents scurvy.

asepsis (a-SEP-sis) Absence of living pathogenic organisms.

Ashkenazi (ASH-ke-NAZ-ih) Jews of eastern European ancestry.

aspartate aminotransferase (AST) (as-PAR-tate ah-me-no-TRANS-fer-aze) Enzyme that is found in liver cells and leaks out into the bloodstream when the cells are damaged, enabling liver damage to be diagnosed.

Asperger syndrome (AHS-per-ger SIN-drome) Developmental disorder of children.

aspergilloma (AS-per-ji-LOH-mah) Infectious granuloma.

aspergillosis (AS-per-ji-LOH-sis) Presence of *Aspergillus* in the body.

Aspergillus (as-per-JILL-us) A type of fungus.

aspiration (AS-pih-RAY-shun) Removal by suction of fluid or gas from a body cavity.

assistive device (ah-SIS-tiv de-VICE) Tool, software, or hardware to assist in performing daily activities.

assistive therapy (ah-SIS-tiv THAIR-ah-pee) Use of methods, technology, and devices to help people with disabilities achieve specific functions.

asthma (AZ-mah) Episodes of breathing difficulty due to narrowed or obstructed airways.

astigmatism (ah-STIG-mah-tism) Inability to focus light rays that enter the eye in different planes.

astrocyte (ASS-troh-site) Star-shaped connective tissue cell in the nervous system.

astrocytoma (ASS-troh-sigh-TOE-mah) Brain tumor derived from astrocytes.

asystole (a-SIS-toe-lee) Absence of contractions of the heart.

ataxia (a-TAK-see-ah) Inability to coordinate muscle activity, leading to jerky movements.

atelectasis (at-el-ECK-tah-sis) Collapse of part of a lung.

atherectomy (ath-er-EK-toe-me) Surgical removal of the atheroma.

atheroma (ath-er-ROE-mah) Lipid deposit in the lining of an artery.

atherosclerosis (ATH-er-oh-skler-OH-sis) Atheroma in arteries.

athetosis (ath-eh-TOE-sis) Slow, writhing involuntary movements.

atom (AT-om) A small unit of matter.

atonic (a-TOHN-ik) Without normal muscular tone.

atopy (AY-toh-pee) State of hypersensitivity to an allergen—allergic.

atresia (a-TREE-zee-ah) Congenital absence of a normal opening or lumen.

atrioventricular (AV) (A-tree-oh-ven-TRICK-you-lar) Pertaining to both the atrium and the ventricle.

atrium (A-tree-um) Chamber where blood enters the heart on both right and left sides. Plural *atria.*

atrophy (AT-roh-fee) The wasting away or diminished volume of tissue, an organ, or a body part.

atropine (AT-ro-peen) Pharmacologic agent used to dilate pupils.

attenuate (ah-TEN-you-ate) Weaken the ability of an organism to produce disease.

attenuated (ah-TEN-you-a-ted) Weakened.

atypical (a-TIP-ih-kal) Something that does not conform to the normal type.

audiologist (aw-dee-OL-oh-jist) Specialist in evaluation of hearing function.

audiology (aw-dee-OL-oh-jee) Study of hearing disorders.

audiometer (aw-dee-OM-ee-ter) Instrument to measure hearing.

audiometric (AW-dee-oh-MET-rik) Pertaining to the measurement of hearing.

auditory (AW-dih-tor-ee) Pertaining to the sense or the organs of hearing.

aura (AWE-rah) Sensory experience preceding an epileptic seizure or a migraine headache.

auricle (AW-ri-kul) The shell-like external ear.

auscultation (aws-kul-TAY-shun) Diagnostic method of listening to body sounds with a stethoscope.

autism (AWE-tizm) Developmental disorder of children.

autoantibody (aw-toe-AN-tee-bod-ee) Antibody produced in response to an antigen from the host's own tissue.

autoclave (AW-toe-klayv) Apparatus for sterilization by steam under pressure.

autograft (AWE-toe-graft) A graft using tissue taken from the individual who is receiving the graft.

autoimmune (aw-toe-im-YUNE) Immune reaction directed against a person's own tissue.

autologous (awe-TOL-oh-gus) Blood transfusion with the same person as donor and recipient.

autolysis (awe-TOL-ih-sis) Self-destruction of cells by enzymes within the cells.

autonomic (awe-toh-NOM-ik) Not voluntary; pertaining to the self-governing visceral motor division of the peripheral nervous system.

autopsy (AWE-top-see) Examination of the body and organs of a dead person to determine the cause of death.

autosome (AWE-toe-soam) Any chromosome other than a sex chromosome.

avascular (a-VAS-cue-lar) Without a blood supply.

avian (A-vee-an) Pertaining to birds.

avulsion (a-VUL-shun) Forcible separation or tearing away, often of a tendon from bone.

axilla (AK-sill-ah) Medical name for the armpit. Plural *axillae.*

axon (ACK-son) Single process of a nerve cell carrying nervous impulses away from the cell body.

Ayurvedic (ah-yur-VED-ik) A system of medicine arising from Hindu culture.

azotemia (azo-TEE-me-ah) Excess nitrogenous waste products in the blood.

B

Babinski sign (bah-BIN-skee SINE) Abnormal neurologic response to plantar reflex that is normal in infants.

bacillus (ba-SIL-us) A rod-shaped bacterium. Plural *bacilli.*

bacterial (bak-TEER-ee-al) Pertaining to bacteria.

bacterium (bak-TEER-ee-um) A unicellular, simple, microscopic organism. Plural *bacteria.*

balanitis (bal-ah-NIE-tis) Inflammation of the glans and prepuce of the penis.

bariatric (bar-ee-AT-rik) Treatment of obesity.

basal metabolic rate (BAY-sal met-ah-BOL-ic RATE) Energy the body requires to function at rest.

basilar (BAS-ih-lar) Pertaining to the base of a structure.

basophil (BAY-so-fill) A basophil's granules attract a basic blue stain in the laboratory.

Bell palsy (BELL PAWL-ze) Paresis or paralysis of one side of the face.

benign (bee-NINE) Denoting the nonmalignant character of a neoplasm or illness

beriberi (BER-ee-BER-ee) Disease produced by thiamine deficiency.

beta (BAY-tah) Second letter in the Greek alphabet.

beta carotene (BAY-tah KAR-oh-teen) Yellow-red pigment in fruits and vegetables.

biceps brachii (BYE-sepz BRAY-key-eye) A muscle of the upper arm that has two heads or points of origin on the scapula.

biconcave (bi-KON-cave) Having a hollowed surface on both sides of a structure.

bicuspid (by-KUSS-pid) Having two points; a bicuspid heart valve has two flaps, and a bicuspid (premolar) tooth has two points.

bifid (BIH-fid) Separated into two parts.

bilateral (by-LAT-er-al) On two sides; for example, in both ears.

bile (BILE) Fluid secreted by the liver into the duodenum.

bile acids (BILE ASS-ids) Steroids synthesized from cholesterol.

biliary (BILL-ee-air-ee) Pertaining to bile or the biliary tract.

bilirubin (bill-ee-RU-bin) Bile pigment formed in the liver from hemoglobin.

binge eating (BINJ EE-ting) Eating with periods of excessive intake.

bioavailable (BI-oh-ah-VAIL-ah-bul) Capable of being absorbed into the bloodstream.

biofeedback (bi-oh-FEED-back) Training techniques to achieve voluntary control of responses to stimuli.

biofield (bi-oh-FIELD) Area of energy in and surrounding the body.

biology (bi-OL-oh-jee) Science concerned with life and living organisms.

biomarker (bi-oh-MARK-er) A biological marker or product by which a cell can be identified.

biopsy (BI-op-see) Removing tissue from a living person for laboratory examination.

biopsy removal (BI-op-see re-MUV-al) Used for small tumors when complete removal provides tissue for a biopsy and cures the lesion. Also called *excisional biopsy.*

biotin (BI-oh-tin) Vitamin B_2.

bipolar disorder (bi-POH-lar dis-OR-der) A mood disorder with alternating episodes of depression and mania

bladder (BLAD-er) Hollow sac that holds fluid; for example, urine or bile.

blastocyst (BLAS-toe-sist) The developing embryo during the first 2 weeks.

blepharitis (blef-ah-RYE-tis) Inflammation of the eyelid.

blepharoplasty (BLEF-ah-ro-plas-tee) Surgical repair of the eyelid.

blepharoptosis (BLEF-ah-ROP-toe-sis) Drooping of the upper eyelid.

blood-brain barrier (BBB) (BLUD BRAYN BAIR-ee-er) A selective mechanism that protects the brain from toxins and infections.

bolus (BOH-lus) Single mass of a substance.

bonding (BON-ding) Formation of a close and lasting emotional attachment.

Botox (BO-tox) Neurotoxin injected into the muscles of the face to prevent the muscles from contracting and causing wrinkles.

botulism (BOT-you-lizm) Food poisoning caused by the neurotoxin produced by *Clostridium botulinum.*

bovine spongiform encephalopathy (BO-vine SPON-jee-form en-sef-ah-LOP-ah-thee) Disease of cattle (mad cow disease) that can be transmitted to humans, causing Creutzfeldt-Jakob disease.

bowel (BOUGH-el) Another name for intestine.

brace (BRACE) Appliance to support a part of the body in its correct position.

brachial (BRAY-kee-al) Pertaining to the arm.

brachialis (BRAY-kee-al-is) Muscle that lies underneath the biceps and is the strongest flexor of the forearm.

brachiocephalic (BRAY-kee-oh-seh-FAL-ik) Pertaining to the head and arm, as an artery supplying blood to both.

brachioradialis (BRAY-kee-oh-RAY-dee-al-is) Muscle that helps flex the forearm.

brachytherapy (brah-kee-THAIR-ah-pee) Radiation therapy in which the source of irradiation is implanted in the tissue to be treated.

bradycardia (brad-ee-KAR-dee-ah) Slow heart rate (below 60 beats per minute).

bradypnea (brad-ip-NEE-ah) Slow breathing.

brainstem (BRAYNSTEM) Region of the brain that includes the thalamus, pineal gland, pons, fourth ventricle, and medulla oblongata.

breech (BREECH) Buttocks-first presentation of the fetus at delivery.

bronchiectasis (brong-kee-ECK-tah-sis) Chronic dilation of the bronchi following inflammatory disease and obstruction.

bronchiole (BRONG-key-ole) Increasingly smaller subdivisions of bronchi.

bronchiolitis (brong-kee-oh-LYE-tis) Inflammation of the small bronchioles.

bronchoalveolar (BRONG-koh-al-VEE-oh-lar) Pertaining to the bronchi and alveoli.

bronchoconstriction (BRONG-koh-kon-STRIK-shun) Reduction in diameter of a bronchus.

bronchodilator (BRONG-koh-die-LAY-tor) Agent that increases the diameter of a bronchus.

bronchogenic (brong-koh-JEN-ik) Arising from a bronchus.

bronchopneumonia (BRONG-koh-new-MOH-nee-ah) Acute inflammation of the walls of smaller bronchioles with spread to lung parenchyma.

bronchopulmonary dysplasia (BRONG-koh-PUL-moh-nair-ee dis-PLAY-zee-ah) Chronic lung disorder in premature infants after prolonged mechanical ventilation.

bronchoscope (BRONG-koh-skope) Endoscope used for bronchoscopy.

bronchoscopy (brong-KOS-koh-pee) Examination of the interior of the tracheobronchial tree with an endoscope.

bronchus (BRONG-kuss) One of two subdivisions of the trachea. Plural *bronchi*.

brucellosis (brew-sel-OH-sis) Undulant fever.

bruxism (BRUK-sizm) Gritting or grinding together of the teeth, often during sleep.

bubo (BYU-bo) Swollen, inflamed lymph node. Plural *buboes*.

buccal smear (BUCK-al SMEER) Use of a small brush or cotton swab to collect cells from the inside surface of the cheek.

buccinator (BUCK-sin-a-tor) Buccinator muscle is the muscle in the cheek.

buffer (BUFF-er) Substance that resists a change in pH.

bulbourethral (BUL-boh-you-REE-thral) Pertaining to the bulbous penis and urethra.

bulimia (byu-LEEM-ee-ah) Episodic bouts of excessive eating with compensatory throwing up.

bulla (BULL-ah) Bubblelike dilated structure. Plural *bullae*.

bundle of His (HISS) Pathway for electrical signals to be transmitted to the ventricles.

bunion (BUN-yun) A swelling at the base of the big toe.

bursa (BURR-sah) A closed sac containing synovial fluid.

bursitis (burr-SIGH-tis) Inflammation of a bursa.

C

café-au-lait (KAF-ay-oh-LAY) Color of skin macules in neurofibromatosis.

calcaneus (kal-KAY-knee-us) Bone of the tarsus that forms the heel.

calcitonin (kal-sih-TONE-in) Thyroid hormone that moves calcium from blood to bones.

calcitriol (KAL-sih-TRY-ol) Potent form of vitamin D that acts as a hormone.

calculus (KAL-kyu-lus) Small stone. Plural *calculi*.

callus (KAL-us) The mass of fibrous connective tissue that forms at a fracture site and becomes the foundation for the formation of new bone.

caloric (kah-LOR-ik) Pertaining to calories.

Calorie (KAL-oh-ree) An expression of the energy content of food; capitalize "C" always.

calyx (KAY-licks) Funnel-shaped structure. Plural *calyces*.

cancellous (KAN-sell-us) Bone that has a spongy or latticelike structure.

cancer (KAN-ser) General term for a malignant neoplasm.

cancerous (KAN-ser-ous) Pertaining to a malignant neoplasm.

Candida (KAN-did-ah) A yeastlike fungus.

candidiasis (can-dih-DIE-ah-sis) Infection with the yeastlike fungus *Candida*. Also called *thrush*.

canker; canker sore (KANG-ker SOAR) Nonmedical term for aphthous ulcer. Also called *mouth ulcer*.

cannula (KAN-you-lah) Tube inserted into a blood vessel or cavity as a channel for fluid.

canthus (KAN-thus) Corner of the eye where the upper and lower lids meet. Plural *canthi*.

capillary (KAP-ih-lair-ee) Minute blood vessel between the arterial and venous systems.

capsid (KAP-sid) Protein shell surrounding the nucleic acid in the core of a virus.

capsule (KAP-syul) Fibrous tissue layer surrounding a joint or some other structure.

carbohydrate (kar-boh-HIGH-drate) Group of organic food compounds that includes sugars, starch, glycogen, and cellulose.

carboxypeptidase (kar-box-ee-PEP-tide-ase) Enzyme that breaks down protein.

carbuncle (KAR-bunk-ul) Infection of many furuncles in a small area, often on the back of the neck.

carcinogen (kar-SIN-oh-jen) Cancer-producing agent.

carcinogenesis (kar-SIN-oh-JEN-eh-sis) Origin and development of cancer.

carcinoma (kar-sih-NOH-mah) A malignant and invasive epithelial tumor.

carcinoma in situ (kar-sih-NOH-mah IN SIGH-tyu) Carcinoma that has not invaded surrounding tissues.

cardiac (KAR-dee-ak) Pertaining to the heart.

cardiogenic (KAR-dee-oh-JEN-ik) Of cardiac origin.

cardiologist (kar-dee-OL-oh-jist) A medical specialist in diagnosis and treatment of the heart (cardiology).

cardiology (kar-dee-OL-oh-jee) Medical specialty of diseases of the heart.

cardiomegaly (KAR-dee-oh-MEG-ah-lee) Enlargement of the heart.

cardiomyopathy (KAR-dee-oh-my-OP-ah-thee) Disease of heart muscle, the myocardium.

cardiopulmonary resuscitation (KAR-dee-oh-PUL-mo-nary ree-sus-ih-TAY-shun) The attempt to restore cardiac and pulmonary function.

cardiovascular (KAR-dee-oh-VAS-kyu-lar) Pertaining to the heart and blood vessels.

cardioversion (KAR-dee-oh-VER-shun) Restoration of a normal heart rhythm by electrical shock. Also called *defibrillation*.

cardioverter (KAR-dee-oh-VER-ter) Device used to generate electrical shock for cardioversion.

caries (KARE-eez) Bacterial destruction of teeth.

carotenoid (kah-ROT-en-oyd) Organic pigment occurring naturally in plants.

carotid (kah-ROT-id) Main artery of the neck.

carotid endarterectomy (kah-ROT-id END-ar-ter-EK-toe-me) Surgical removal of diseased lining from the carotid artery to leave a smooth lining.

carpal (KAR-pal) Pertaining to the wrist.

carpus (KAR-pus) Collective term for the eight carpal bones of the wrist.

carrier (KAH-ree-er) A person with an autosomal recessive gene for a disease. Also called *heterozygote*.

cartilage (KAR-tih-lage) Nonvascular, firm connective tissue found mostly in joints.

cast (KAST) A cylindrical mold formed by materials in kidney tubules.

catabolism (kah-TAB-oh-lizm) Breakdown of complex substances into simpler ones as a part of metabolism.

cataplexy (KAT-ah-plek-see) Sudden loss of muscle tone with brief paralysis.

cataract (KAT-ah-ract) Complete or partial opacity of the lens.

catatonia (kat-ah-TOE-nee-ah) Syndrome characterized by physical immobility and mental stupor.

catecholamine (kat-eh-COAL-ah-meen) Any major hormones in stress response; includes epinephrine and norepinephrine.

catheter (KATH-eh-ter) Hollow tube that allows passage of fluid into or out of a body cavity, organ, or vessel.

catheterization (KATH-eh-ter-ih-ZAY-shun) Introduction of a catheter.

catheterize (KATH-eh-teh-RIZE) To introduce a catheter.

cauda equina (KAW-dah eh-KWY-nah) Bundle of spinal nerves in the vertebral canal below the ending of the spinal cord.

caudal (KAW-dal) Pertaining to or nearer to the tail.

cautery (KAW-ter-ee) Agent or device used to burn or scar a tissue.

cavernosa (kav-er-NOH-sah) Resembling a cave.

cavity (KAV-ih-tee) Hollow space or body compartment. Plural cavities.

cecum (SEE-kum) Blind pouch that is the first part of the large intestine.

celiac (SEE-lee-ack) Relating to the abdominal cavity.

celiac disease (SEE-lee-ak diz-eez) Disease caused by sensitivity to gluten.

cell (SELL) The smallest unit capable of independent existence.

cellular (SELL-you-lar) Pertaining to a cell.

cellulitis (sell-you-LIE-tis) Infection of subcutaneous connective tissue.

cellulose (SELL-you-lohse) Major constituent of cell walls of plants.

centromere (SEN-troh-mere) Junction that holds two chromatids together to form a chromosome.

cephalic (se-FAL-ik) Pertaining to or nearer to the head.

cerebellum (ser-eh-BELL-um) The most posterior area of the brain.

cerebrospinal (SER-eh-broh-SPY-nal) Pertaining to the brain and spinal cord.

cerebrospinal fluid (CSF) (SER-eh-broh-SPY-nal FLU-id) Fluid formed in the ventricles of the brain; surrounds the brain and spinal cord.

cerebrum (SER-ee-brum) The major portion of the brain divided into two hemispheres (cerebral hemispheres) separated by a fissure.

cerumen (seh-ROO-men) Waxy secretion of the ceruminous glands of the external ear.

cervical (SER-vih-kal) Pertaining to the cervix or to the neck region.

cervix (SER-viks) The lower part of the uterus.

cesarean section (seh-ZAH-ree-an SEK-shun) Extraction of the fetus through an incision in the abdomen and uterine wall. Also called C-section.

chakra (CHAK-rah) One of seven centers of energy in the body.

chalazion (kah-LAY-zee-on) Cyst on the outer edge of an eyelid.

chancre (SHAN-ker) Primary lesion of syphilis.

chancroid (SHAN-kroyd) Infectious, painful, ulcerative STD not related to syphilis.

Charcot joint (SHAR-koh JOYNT) Bone and joint destruction secondary to a neuropathy and loss of sensation.

chemoprophylaxis (KEEM-oh-PRO-fil-ak-sis) Prevent infection by use of chemicals or drugs.

chemotherapy (KEY-moh-THAIR-ah-pee) Treatment using chemical agents.

chi (CHEE) Universal life force. Also spelled qi.

chiasm (KYE-asm) X-shaped crossing of the two optic nerves at the base of the brain. Alternative term chiasma.

chickenpox (CHICK-en-pocks) Acute, contagious viral disease. Also called varicella.

chiropractic (kye-roh-PRAK-tik) Diagnosis, treatment, and prevention of mechanical disorders of the musculoskeletal system.

chiropractor (kye-roh-PRAK-tor) Practitioner of chiropractic.

chlamydia (klah-MID-ee-ah) A species of bacteria causing a sexually transmitted disease.

chlorine (KLOR-een) A toxic agent used as a disinfectant and bleaching agent.

chlorophyll (KLOR-oh-fil) Light-absorbing pigment in plants.

cholangiography (KOH-lan-jee-OG-rah-fee) X-ray of the bile ducts after injection or ingestion of a contrast medium.

cholecystectomy (KOH-leh-sis-TECK-toe-me) Surgical removal of the gallbladder.

cholecystitis (KOH-leh-sis-TIE-tis) Inflammation of the gallbladder.

cholecystokinin (KOH-leh-sis-toe-KIE-nin) Hormone secreted by the lining of the intestine that stimulates secretion of pancreatic enzymes and contraction of the gallbladder.

choledocholithiasis (koh-leh-DOH-koh-lih-THIGH-ah-sis) Presence of a gallstone in the common bile duct.

cholelithiasis (KOH-leh-lih-THIGH-ah-sis) Condition of having bile stones (gallstones).

cholelithotomy (KOH-leh-lih-THOT-oh-me) Surgical removal of a gallstone(s).

cholera (KOL-er-ah) Acute endemic infectious disease.

cholestatic (koh-les-TAT-ik) Stopping the flow of bile.

cholesteatoma (koh-less-tee-ah-TOE-mah) Yellow, waxy tumor arising in the middle ear.

cholesterol (koh-LESS-ter-ol) Steroid formed in liver cells; the most abundant steroid in tissues and circulates in the plasma attached to proteins of different densities.

choline (KOH-leen) An amine found in most tissues; a precursor for acetylcholine.

chondromalacia (KON-dro-mah-LAY-she-ah) Softening and degeneration of cartilage.

chondrosarcoma (KON-dro-sar-KOH-mah) Cancer arising from cartilage cells.

chordae tendineae (KOR-dee ten-DIN-ee) Tendinous cords attaching the bicuspid and tricuspid valves to the heart wall.

chorea (kor-EE-ah) Involuntary, irregular spasms of limb and facial muscles.

choriocarcinoma (KOH-ree-oh-kar-sih-NOH-mah) Highly malignant cancer in a testis or ovary.

chorion (KOH-ree-on) The fetal membrane that forms the placenta.

chorionic (koh-ree-ON-ick) Pertaining to the chorion.

chorionic villus (koh-ree-ON-ik VILL-us) Vascular process of the embryonic chorion to form the placenta.

choroid (KOR-oid) Region of the retina and uvea.

chromatid (KROH-ma-tid) One of the two strands of a chromosome.

chromatin (KROH-ma-tin) Substance composed of DNA that forms chromosomes during cell division.

chromosome (KROH-moh-sohm) Body in the nucleus that contains DNA and genes.

chronic (KRON-ik) Describes a persistent, long-term disease.

chronotropic (KRONE-oh-TROH-pic) Affecting the heart rate.

chyle (KYLE) A milky fluid that results from the digestion and absorption of fats in the small intestine.

chyme (KYME) Semifluid, partially digested food passed from the stomach into the duodenum.

chymotrypsin (kye-moh-TRIP-sin) Trypsin found in chyme.

ciliary body (SILL-ee-ary BOD-ee) Muscles that make the eye lens thicker and thinner.

cilium (SILL-ee-um) Hairlike motile projection from the surface of a cell. Plural *cilia*.

circulation (SER-kyu-LAY-shun) Continuous movement of blood through the heart and blood vessels.

circumcision (ser-kum-SIZH-un) To remove part or all of the prepuce.

circumduction (ser-kum-DUCK-shun) Movement of an extremity in a circular motion.

cirrhosis (sir-ROE-sis) Extensive fibrotic liver disease.

claudication (klaw-dih-KAY-shun) Intermittent leg pain and limping.

claustrophobia (klaw-stroh-FOH-be-ah) Pathologic fear of being trapped in a confined space.

clavicle (KLAV-ih-kul) Curved bone that forms the anterior part of the pectoral girdle.

clean (KLENE) Free from visible contamination.

cleft lip (KLEFT LIP) Congenital defect of the upper lip.

cleft palate (KLEFT PAL-ate) Congenital defect of the upper palate.

clitoris (KLIT-oh-ris) Erectile organ of the vulva.

clonic (KLON-ik) State of rapid successions of muscular contractions and relaxations.

closed fracture (KLOSD FRAK-chur) A bone is broken but the skin over it is intact.

Clostridium botulinum (klos-TRID-ee-um bot-you-LIE-num) Bacterium that causes food poisoning.

Clostridium difficile (klos-TRID-ee-um dif-ih-SEE-il) Gram-positive rod producing powerful exotoxins that cause colitis.

clot (KLOT) The mass of fibrin and cells that is produced in a wound.

coagulant (koh-ag-you-LANT) Substance that induces clotting.

coagulate (koh-AG-you-late) Form a clot.

coagulation (koh-ag-you-LAY-shun) The process of blood clotting.

coagulopathy (koh-ag-you-LOP-ah-thee) Disorder of blood clotting. Plural *coagulopathies.*

coarctation (koh-ark-TAY-shun) Constriction, stenosis, particularly of the aorta.

coccus (KOK-us) Round, spheroid bacterium. Plural *cocci.*

coccyx (KOK-sicks) Small tailbone at the lower end of the vertebral column.

cochlea (KOK-lee-ah) An intricate combination of passages; used to describe the part of the inner ear used in hearing.

cochlear (KOK-lee-ar) Pertaining to the cochlea.

coenzyme (koh-EN-zime) Substance required for an enzyme to function.

cognition (kog-NIH-shun) Process of acquiring knowledge through thinking, learning, and memory.

cognitive (KOG-nih-tiv) Pertaining to the mental activities of thinking and learning.

cognitive behavioral therapy (CBT) (KOG-nih-tiv be-HAYV-yur-al THAIR-ah-pee) Psychotherapy that emphasizes thoughts and attitudes in one's behavior.

cognitive processing therapy (KOG-nih-tiv PROS-es-ing THAIR-ah-pee) Psychotherapy to build skills to deal with effects of the trauma in other areas of life.

coitus (KOH-it-us) Sexual intercourse.

colic (KOL-ik) Spasmodic, crampy pains in the abdomen; in young infants, persistent crying and irritability thought to be arising from pain in the intestines.

colitis (koh-LIE-tis) Inflammation of the colon.

collagen (KOL-ah-jen) Major protein of connective tissue, cartilage, and bone.

collateral (koh-LAT-er-al) Situated at the side, often to bypass an obstruction.

Colles fracture (KOL-ez FRAK-chur) Fracture of the distal radius at the wrist.

colloid (COLL-oyd) Liquid containing suspended particles.

colon (KOH-lon) The large intestine, extending from the cecum to the rectum.

colonization (KOL-on-ih-ZAY-shun) Formation of a population of microorganisms.

colonoscopy (koh-lon-OSS-koh-pee) Examination of the inside of the colon by endoscopy.

color Doppler ultrasonography (DOP-ler UL-trah-soh-NOG-rah-fee) Computer-generated color image to show directions of blood flow.

colostomy (ko-LOSS-toe-me) Artificial opening from the colon to the outside of the body.

colostrum (koh-LOSS-trum) The first breast secretion at the end of pregnancy.

colpopexy (KOL-poh-peck-see) Surgical fixation of the vagina.

coma (KOH-mah) State of deep unconsciousness.

comatose (KOH-mah-toes) Being in a coma.

comedo (KOM-ee-doh) A whitehead or blackhead caused by too much sebum and too many keratin cells blocking the hair follicle. Plural *comedones.*

comminuted fracture (KOM-ih-nyu-ted FRAK-chur) A fracture in which the bone is broken into pieces.

comorbidity (koh-mor-BID-ih-tee) Presence of two or more diseases at the same time.

competent (KOM-peh-tent) Capable of performing a task or function.

complement (KOM-pleh-ment) Group of proteins in serum destroy bacteria and other cells.

complete (kom-PLEET) Whole, entire, total.

complete fracture (kom-PLEET FRAK-chur) A bone is fractured into two separate pieces.

compliance (kom-PLY-ance) Measure of the capacity of a chamber or hollow viscus to expand; for example, compliance of the lungs.

compression (kom-PRESH-un) A squeezing together so as to increase density and/or decrease a dimension of a structure.

compression fracture (kom-PRESH-un FRAK-chur) Fracture of a vertebra causing loss of height of the vertebra.

compulsion (kom-PULL-shun) Uncontrollable impulses to perform an act repetitively.

compulsive (kom-PULL-siv) Possessing uncontrollable impulses to perform an act repetitively.

conception (kon-SEP-shun) Fertilization of the egg by sperm to form a zygote.

concha (KON-kah) Shell-shaped bone on the medial wall of the nasal cavity. Plural *conchae.*

concussion (kon-KUSH-un) Mild head injury.

condom (KON-dom) A sheath or cover for the penis or vagina to prevent conception and infection.

conduction (kon-DUCK-shun) Process of transmitting energy.

conductive hearing loss (kon-DUK-tiv) Hearing loss caused by lesions in the outer ear or middle ear.

condyle (KON-dile) Large, smooth rounded expansion of the end of a bone that forms a joint with another bone.

condyloma (kon-dih-LOW-ma) Warty growth on external genitalia. Plural *condylomata.*

confusion (kon-FEW-zhun) Mental state in which environmental stimuli are not processed appropriately.

congenital (kon-JEN-ih-tal) Present at birth, either inherited or due to an event during gestation up to the moment of birth.

congruent (KON-gru-ent) Coinciding or agreeing with.

conization (koh-nih-ZAY-shun) Surgical excision of a cone-shaped piece of tissue.

conjunctiva (kon-junk-TIE-vah) Inner lining of the eyelids.

conjunctivitis (kon-junk-tih-VI-tis) Inflammation of the conjunctiva.

Conn syndrome (KON SIN-drom) Condition caused by excessive secretion of aldosterone. Also called *aldosteronism.*

conscious (KON-shus) Having present knowledge of oneself and one's surroundings.

consciousness (KON-shus-ness) The state of being aware of and responsive to the environment.

constipation (kon-stih-PAY-shun) Hard, infrequent bowel movements.

contagiosum (kon-TAY-jee-oh-sum) Infection spread from one person to another by direct contact.

contagious (kon-TAY-jus) Able to be transmitted, as infections transmitted from person to person or from person to air or surface to person.

contaminate (kon-TAM-in-ate) To cause the presence of an infectious agent to be on any surface.

contamination (KON-tam-ih-NAY-shun) Presence of an infectious agent on a surface or in a substance.

contraception (kon-trah-SEP-shun) Prevention of conception.

contraceptive (kon-trah-SEP-tiv) An agent that prevents conception.

contract (kon-TRAKT) Draw together or shorten.

contracture (kon-TRAK-chur) Muscle shortening due to spasm or fibrosis.

contrecoup (KON-treh-koo) Injury to the brain at a point directly opposite the point of original contact.

contusion (kon-TOO-zhun) Bruising of a tissue, including the brain.

conversion disorder (kon-VER-shun dis-OR-der) An unconscious emotional conflict is expressed as physical symptoms with no organic basis.

convulsion (kon-VUL-shun) Alternative name for seizure.

coordinate (ko-OR-din-ate) To bring together different structures into a harmonious function.

cor pulmonale (KOR pul-moh-NAH-lee) Right-sided heart failure arising from chronic lung disease.

coreceptor (koh-ree-SEP-tor) Cell surface protein that enhances the sensitivity of an antigen receptor.

cornea (KOR-nee-ah) The central, transparent part of the outer coat of the eye covering the iris and pupil.

coronal (KOR-oh-nal) Pertaining to the vertical plane dividing the body into anterior and posterior portions.

coronal plane (KOR-oh-nal PLAIN) Vertical plane dividing the body into anterior and posterior portions.

coronary circulation (KOR-oh-nair-ee SER-kyu-LAY-shun) Blood flow through the vessels supplying the heart.

corpus (KOR-pus) Major part of a structure. Plural *corpora.*

corpus albicans (KOR-pus AL-bih-kanz) An atrophied corpus luteum.

corpus callosum (KOR-pus kah-LOW-sum) Bridge of nerve fibers connecting the two cerebral hemispheres.

corpus luteum (KOR-pus LOO-teh-um) Yellow structure formed at the site of a ruptured ovarian follicle.

corpuscle (KOR-pus-ul) A blood cell.

cortex (KOR-teks) Outer portion of an organ, such as bone; *or* gray covering of cerebral hemispheres. Plural *cortices.*

corticoid (KOR-tih-koyd) One of the steroid hormones produced by the adrenal cortex. Also called *corticosteroid.*

corticosteroid (KOR-tih-koh-STEHR-oyd) A hormone produced by the adrenal cortex.

corticotropin (KOR-tih-koh-TROH-pin) Pituitary hormone that stimulates the cortex of the adrenal gland to secrete corticosteroids.

cortisol (KOR-tih-sol) One of the glucocorticoids produced by the adrenal cortex; has anti-inflammatory effects. Also called *hydrocortisone.*

coryza (ko-RYE-zah) Viral inflammation of the mucous membrane of the nose. Also called *rhinitis.*

counseling (KOWN-sel-ing) Professional relationship to transmit advice to direct the judgment of another.

coup (KOO) Injury to the brain occurring directly under the skull at the point of impact.

coxa (COCK-sah) Hip bone. Plural *coxae.*

cranial (KRAY-nee-al) Pertaining to the skull.

craniofacial (KRAY-nee-oh-FAY-shal) Pertaining to both the face and the cranium.

craniosacral (KRAY-nee-oh-SAY-kral) Referring to the cranium and sacrum.

cranium (KRAY-nee-um) The upper part of the skull that encloses and protects the brain.

craving (KRAY-ving) Deep longing or desire.

creatine kinase (KREE-ah-teen KI-naze) Enzyme elevated in plasma following heart muscle damage in myocardial infarction.

creatinine (kree-AT-ih-neen) Breakdown product of the skeletal muscle protein creatine.

cretin (KREH-tin) A person with severe congenital hypothyroidism.

cretinism (KREH-tin-izm) Condition of severe congenital hypothyroidism.

Creutzfeldt-Jakob disease (KROITS-felt-YAK-op DIZ-eez) Progressive incurable neurologic disease caused by infectious prions.

cricoid (CRY-koyd) Ring-shaped cartilage in the larynx.

crista ampullaris (KRIS-tah am-PULL-air-is) Mound of hair cells and gelatinous material in the ampulla of a semicircular canal.

criterion (kri-TEER-ee-on) Standard or rule for judging. Plural *criteria.*

Crohn disease (KRONE DIZ-eez) Inflammatory bowel disease with narrowing and thickening of the terminal small bowel. Also called *regional enteritis.*

croup (KROOP) Infection of the upper airways in children; characterized by a barking cough. Also called *laryngotracheobronchitis.*

crown (KROWN) Part of tooth above the gum.

crowning (KROWN-ing) During childbirth, when the maximum diameter of the baby's head comes through the vulvar ring.

cruciate (KRU-she-ate) Shaped like a cross.

cryokinetics (CRY-oh-kih-NET-iks) Combination of cold therapy with exercise.

cryoneurolysis (cry-oh-NYUR-oh-lie-sis) Temporary deactivation of nerve tissue using extreme cold.

cryopexy (cry-oh-PEX-ee) Repair of a detached retina by freezing it to surrounding tissue.

cryosurgery (cry-oh-SUR-jer-ee) Use of liquid nitrogen or argon gas in a probe to freeze and kill abnormal tissue.

cryotherapy (CRY-oh-THAIR-ah-pee) The use of cold in the treatment of injury.

cryptorchism (krip-TOR-kizm) Failure of one or both testes to descend into the scrotum.

curative (KYUR-ah-tiv) That which heals or cures.

curettage (kyu-reh-TAHZH) Scraping of the interior of a cavity.

curette (kyu-RET) Scoop-shaped instrument for scraping the interior of a cavity or removing new growths.

Cushing syndrome (KUSH-ing SIN-drom) Hypersecretion of cortisol (hydrocortisone) by the adrenal cortex.

cuspid (KUSS-pid) Tooth with one point.

cutaneous (kyu-TAY-nee-us) Pertaining to the skin.

cuticle (KEW-tih-cul) Nonliving epidermis at the base of the fingernails and toenails.

cyanocobalamin (SIGH-an-oh-koh-BAL-ah-min) Vitamin B_{12}.

cyanosis (sigh-ah-NO-sis) Blue discoloration of the skin, lips, and nail beds due to low levels of oxygen in the blood.

cyanotic (sigh-ah-NOT-ik) Marked by cyanosis.

cyst (SIST) An abnormal, fluid-containing sac.

cystic (SIS-tik) Relating to a cyst.

cystic fibrosis (CF) (SIS-tik fie-BRO-sis) Genetic disease in which excessive viscid mucus obstructs passages, including bronchi.

cystitis (sis-TIE-tis) Inflammation of the urinary bladder.

cystocele (SIS-toh-seal) Hernia of the bladder into the vagina.

cystopexy (SIS-toh-pek-see) Surgical procedure to support the urinary bladder.

cystoscope (SIS-toh-skope) An endoscope inserted to view the inside of the bladder.

cystoscopy (sis-TOS-koh-pee) The process of using a cystoscope.

cystourethrogram (sis-toh-you-REETH-roe-gram) X-ray image during voiding to show the structure and function of the bladder and urethra.

cytokine (SIGH-toh-kine) Proteins produced by different cells that communicate with other cells in the immune system.

cytosine (SIGH-toh-seen) One of the chemical bases found in, and comprising the sequence of, both DNA and RNA.

cytology (SIGH-tol-oh-gee) Study of the cell.

cytomegalovirus (sigh-toh-MEG-ah-loh-VIE-rus) A group of herpesviruses that can cause congenital infections.

cytoplasm (SIGH-toh-plazm) Clear, gelatinous substance that forms the substance of a cell except for the nucleus.

cytosine (**SIGH**-toh-seen) One of the chemicals found in both DNA and RNA.

cytotoxic (sigh-toh-**TOX**-ik) Destructive to cells.

D

dacryocystitis (**DAK**-re-oh-sis-**TIE**-tis) Inflammation of the lacrimal sac.

dacryostenosis (**DAK**-re-oh-ste-**NO**-sis) Narrowing of the nasolacrimal duct.

dandruff (**DAN**-druff) Seborrheic scales from the scalp.

death (**DETH**) Total and permanent cessation of all vital functions.

debridement (day-**BREED**-mon) The removal of injured or necrotic tissue.

decongestant (dee-con-**JESS**-tant) Agent that reduces the swelling and fluid in the nose and sinuses.

decubitus ulcer (de-**KYU**-bit-us **UL**-ser) Sore caused by lying down for long periods of time.

decussate (**DEE**-kuss-ate) Cross over like the arms of an "X."

defecation (def-eh-**KAY**-shun) Evacuation of feces from the rectum and anus.

defect (**DEE**-fect) An absence, malformation, or imperfection.

defective (dee-**FEK**-tiv) Imperfect.

defibrillation (dee-fib-rih-**LAY**-shun) Restoration of uncontrolled twitching of cardiac muscle fibers to normal rhythm.

defibrillator (dee-fib-rih-**LAY**-tor) Instrument for defibrillation.

deformity (de-**FOR**-mih-tee) A permanent structural deviation from the normal.

degenerative (dee-**JEN**-er-a-tiv) Relating to the deterioration of a structure.

deglutition (dee-glue-**TISH**-un) The act of swallowing.

dehydration (dee-high-**DRAY**-shun) Process of losing body water.

dehydroepiandrosterone (**DHEA**) (de-**HIGH**-droh-epee-an-**DROS**-ter-own) Precursor to testosterone; produced in the adrenal cortex.

delirium (de-**LIR**-ee-um) Acute altered state of consciousness with agitation and disorientation; condition is reversible.

deltoid (**DEL**-toyd) Large, fan-shaped muscle connecting the scapula and clavicle to the humerus.

delusion (de-**LOO**-shun) Fixed, unyielding, false belief or judgment held despite strong evidence to the contrary.

dementia (dee-**MEN**-she-ah) Chronic, progressive, irreversible loss of the mind's cognitive and intellectual functions.

demyelination (dee-**MY**-eh-lin-**A**-shun) Process of losing the myelin sheath of a nerve fiber.

dendrite (**DEN**-dright) Branched extension of the nerve cell body that receives nervous stimuli.

dental (**DEN**-tal) Pertaining to the teeth.

dentin (**DEN**-tin) Dense, ivorylike substance located under the enamel in a tooth.

dentist (**DEN**-tist) Legally qualified specialist in dentistry.

dentistry (**DEN**-tis-tree) Evaluation, diagnosis, prevention, and treatment of conditions of the oral cavity and associated structures.

deoxyribonucleic acid (**DNA**) (dee-**OCK**-see-**RYE**-boh-noo-**KLEE**-ik **ASS**-id) Source of hereditary characteristics found in chromosomes.

dependence (de-**PEN**-dense) State of needing someone or something.

dependent (de-**PEN**-dent) Having to rely on someone else.

depressant (de-**PRESS**-ant) Substance that diminishes activity, sensation, or tone.

depression (de-**PRESH**-un) Mental disorder with feelings of deep sadness and despair.

dermatitis (der-mah-**TYE**-tis) Inflammation of the skin.

dermatologist (der-mah-**TOL**-oh-jist) Medical specialist in diseases of the skin.

dermatology (der-mah-**TOL**-oh-jee) Medical specialty concerned with disorders of the skin.

dermatome (**DER**-mah-tome) The area of skin supplied by a single spinal nerve; alternatively, an instrument used for cutting thin slices.

dermatomyositis (**DER**-mah-toe-**MY**-oh-site-is) Inflammation of the skin and muscles.

dermis (**DER**-miss) Connective tissue layer of the skin beneath the epidermis.

detoxification (de-**TOKS**-ih-fi-**KAY**-shun) Removal of poison from a tissue or substance.

deviation (de-ve-**A**-shun) A turning aside from a normal course.

diabetes insipidus (dye-ah-**BEE**-teez in-**SIP**-ih-dus) Excretion of large amounts of dilute urine as a result of inadequate ADH production.

diabetes mellitus (dye-ah-**BEE**-teez **MEL**-ih-tus) Metabolic syndrome caused by absolute or relative insulin deficiency and/or insulin ineffectiveness.

diabetic (dye-ah-**BET**-ik) Pertaining to or suffering from diabetes.

diagnose (die-ag-**NOSE**) To make a diagnosis.

diagnosis (die-ag-**NO**-sis) The determination of the cause of a disease. Plural *diagnoses.*

diagnostic (die-ag-**NOS**-tik) Pertaining to or establishing a diagnosis.

dialectic (die-ah-**LEK**-tik) Logical argumentation.

dialysis (die-**AL**-ih-sis) An artificial method of filtration to remove excess waste materials and water from the body.

dialyzer (**DIE**-ah-lie-zer) Machine for dialysis.

diaphoresis (**DIE**-ah-foh-**REE**-sis) Sweat or perspiration.

diaphoretic (**DIE**-ah-foh-**RET**-ic) Pertaining to sweat or perspiration.

diaphragm (**DIE**-ah-fram) A ring and dome-shaped material inserted in the vagina to prevent pregnancy; *or* the musculomembranous partition separating the abdominal and thoracic cavities.

diaphragmatic (**DIE**-ah-frag-**MAT**-ic) Pertaining to the diaphragm.

diaphysis (die-**AF**-ih-sis) The shaft of a long bone.

diarrhea (die-ah-REE-ah) Abnormally frequent and loose stools.

diastasis (die-ASS-tah-sis) Separation of normally joined parts.

diastole (die-AS-toe-lee) Dilation of heart cavities, during which they fill with blood.

diet (DIE-et) Specific course of eating and drinking.

dietary (DIE-et-ary) Pertaining to a diet.

dietetics (die-eh-TET-iks) Application of diet to prevention and treatment of disease.

dietician (die-eh-TISH-un) Licensed professional in dietetics. Alternative spelling *dietitian*.

differential (dif-er-EN-shal) A differential white blood cell count lists percentages of the different leukocytes in a blood sample.

diffuse (dih-FUSE) To disseminate or spread out.

diffusion (dih-FYU-zhun) The means by which small particles move between tissues.

DiGeorge syndrome (dee-JORJ SIN-drome) Congenital absence of the thymus gland.

digestion (die-JEST-shun) Breakdown of food into elements suitable for cell metabolism.

digestive (die-JEST-iv) Relating to digestion.

digital (DIJ-ih-tal) Pertaining to a finger or toe.

diglyceride (die-GLISS-eh-ride) Substance with two fatty acids.

dilation (die-LAY-shun) Stretching or enlarging of an opening.

diode (DIE-ode) Allows electrical current to flow in one direction only.

dioxin (die-OK-sin) Carcinogenic contaminant in pesticides.

diphtheria (dif-THEER-ee-ah) Disease with a thick, membranous (leathery) coating of the pharynx.

diplegia (die-PLEE-jee-ah) Paralysis of all four limbs, with the two legs affected most severely.

disability (dis-ah-BILL-ih-tee) Diminished capacity to perform certain activities or functions.

disaccharide (die-SACK-ah-ride) A combination of two monosaccharides; for example, table sugar.

discipline (DIS-ih-plin) Training for proper conduct or action.

discrimination (DIS-krim-ih-NAY-shun) Ability to distinguish between different things.

disinfectant (dis-in-FEK-tant) Agent that disinfects.

disinfection (dis-in-FEK-shun) Process of destruction of microorganisms by chemical agents.

dislocation (dis-low-KAY-shun) The state of being completely out of joint.

displaced fracture (dis-PLAYSD FRAK-chur) A fracture in which the fragments are separated and are not in alignment.

disseminate (dih-SEM-in-ate) Widely scattered throughout the body or an organ.

dissociative identity disorder (di-SO-see-ah-tiv eye-DEN-tih-tee dis-OR-der) Mental disorder in which of an individual's personality is separated from the rest, leading to multiple personalities.

distal (DISS-tal) Situated away from the center of the body.

diuresis (die-you-REE-sis) Excretion of large volumes of urine.

diuretic (die-you-RET-ik) Agent that increases urine output.

diverticulitis (DIE-ver-tick-you-LIE-tis) Inflammation of the diverticula.

diverticulosis (DIE-ver-tick-you-LOW-sis) Presence of a number of small pouches in the wall of the large intestine.

diverticulum (die-ver-TICK-you-lum) A pouchlike opening or sac from a tubular structure (e.g., gut). Plural *diverticula*.

dizygotic (die-zye-GOT-ik) Twins from two separate zygotes.

dominant gene (DOM-ih-nant JEEN) Single allele that is expressed as a trait or characteristic.

dopamine (DOH-pah-meen) Neurotransmitter in some specific small areas of the brain.

Doppler (DOP-ler) Diagnostic instrument that sends an ultrasonic beam into the body.

Doppler ultrasonography (DOP-ler UL-trah-soh-NOG-rah-fee) Imaging that detects direction, velocity, and turbulence of blood flow; used in workup of stroke patients.

dormant (DOR-mant) Inactive.

dorsal (DOR-sal) Pertaining to the back or situated behind.

dorsum (DOR-sum) Upper, posterior, or back surface.

dosha (DOH-sha) Psychophysical constitution of the body in Ayurvedic medicine.

Down syndrome (DOWN SIN-drome) A syndrome with variable abnormalities associated with three chromosomes 21.

droplet (DROP-let) Globule of liquid; for example, that which is ejected from the mouth during speaking, coughing, sneezing.

Duchenne muscular dystrophy (DOO-shen MUSS-kyu-lar DISS-troh-fee) A condition with symmetrical weakness and wasting of pelvic, shoulder, and proximal limb muscles.

ductus arteriosus (DUK-tus ar-TEER-ih-OH-sus) Fetal vessel that connects the descending aorta with the left pulmonary artery.

ductus deferens (DUK-tus DEH-fuh-renz) Tube that receives sperm from the epididymis. Also known as *vas deferens*.

duodenal (du-oh-DEE-nal) Pertaining to the duodenum.

duodenum (du-oh-DEE-num) The first part of the small intestine; approximately 12 finger-breadths (9 to 10 inches) in length.

Dupuytren (du-pwe-TRAHN) Dupuytren contracture is thickening and shortening of fibrous bands in the palm of the hand.

dura mater (DYU-rah MAY-ter) Hard, fibrous outer layer of the meninges.

dwarfism (DWORF-izm) Short stature due to underproduction of growth hormone.

dysentery (DIS-en-tare-ee) Disease with diarrhea, bowel spasms, fever, and dehydration.

dysfunctional (dis-FUNK-shun-al) Having difficulty in performing.

dyslexia (dis-LEK-see-ah) Impaired reading and writing ability below the person's level of intelligence.

dyslexic (dis-LEK-sik) Pertaining to or suffering from dyslexia.

dyslipidemia (DIS-li-pi-DEE-me-ah) Abnormal (and "bad") levels of blood lipids.

dysmenorrhea (dis-men-oh-REE-ah) Painful and difficult menstruation.

dyspareunia (dis-pah-RUE-nee-ah) Pain during sexual intercourse.

dyspepsia (dis-PEP-see-ah) "Upset stomach," epigastric pain, nausea, and gas.

dysphagia (dis-FAY-jee-ah) Difficulty in swallowing.

dysplasia (dis-PLAY-zee-ah) Abnormal tissue formation.

dyspnea (disp-NEE-ah) Difficulty breathing.

dysrhythmia (dis-RITH-me-ah) An abnormal heart rhythm.

dysuria (dis-YOU-ree-ah) Difficulty or pain with urination.

E

eccrine (EK-rin) Coiled sweat gland that occurs in skin all over the body.

echinacea (ek-ih-NAY-sha) Spiky North American herb.

echocardiography (EK-oh-kar-dee-OG-rah-fee) Ultrasound recording of heart function.

echoencephalography (EK-oh-en-sef-ah-LOG-rah-fee) Use of ultrasound in the diagnosis of intracranial lesions.

eclampsia (ek-LAMP-see-uh) Convulsions in a patient with preeclampsia.

ecologic (ee-koh-LOJ-ik) Pertaining to the study of the environment.

ecology (ee-KOL-oh-jee) Interrelationship between living organisms with each other and the environment.

ectopic (ek-TOP-ik) Out of place, not in a normal position.

eczema (EK-zeh-mah) Inflammatory skin disease often with a serous discharge.

edema (ee-DEE-mah) Excessive accumulation of fluid in cells and tissues.

edematous (ee-DEM-ah-tus) Pertaining to or marked by edema.

effacement (ee-FACE-ment) Thinning of the cervix in relation to labor.

efferent (EF-eh-rent) Conducting impulses outward away from the brain or spinal cord.

effusion (eh-FYU-shun) Collection of fluid that has escaped from blood vessels into a cavity or tissues.

ejaculate (ee-JACK-you-late) To expel suddenly; *or* the semen expelled in ejaculation.

ejaculation (ee-JACK-you-LAY-shun) Process of expelling semen suddenly.

elective (e-LEK-tiv) Surgery that is not urgent or vital.

electrocardiogram (ECG or EKG) (ee-lek-troh-KAR-dee-oh-gram) Record of the electrical signals of the heart.

electrocardiograph (ee-lek-troh-KAR-dee-oh-graf) Machine that makes the electrocardiogram.

electrocardiography (ee-LEK-troh-kar-dee-OG-rah-fee) Interpretation of electrocardiograms.

electroconvulsive therapy (ee-LEK-troh-kon-VUL-siv THAIR-ah-pee) Passage of electric current through the brain to produce convulsions and treat persistent depression mania, and other disorders.

electrode (ee-LEK-trode) A device for conducting electricity.

electroencephalogram (EEG) (ee-LEK-troh-en-SEF-ah-low-gram) Record of the electrical activity of the brain.

electroencephalograph (ee-LEK-troh-en-SEF-ah-low-graf) Device used to record the electrical activity of the brain.

electroencephalography (ee-LEK-troh-en-SEF-ah-LOG-rah-fee) The process of recording the electrical activity of the brain.

electrolyte (ee-LEK-troh-lite) Substance that, when dissolved in a suitable medium, forms electrically charged particles.

electromagnetic (ee-LEK-troh-mag-NET-ik) Pertaining to energy propagated through matter and space.

electromyogram (ee-lek-troh-MY-oh-gram) Recording of electric currents associated with muscle action.

electromyography (ee-LEK-troh-my-OG-rah-fee) Recording of electrical activity in muscle.

electroneurodiagnostic (ee-LEK-troh-NYUR-oh-die-ag-NOS-tik) Pertaining to the use of electricity in the diagnosis of a neurologic disorder.

elimination (e-lim-ih-NAY-shun) Removal of waste material from the digestive tract.

emaciation (ee-may-see-AY-shun) Abnormal thinness.

embolus (EM-boh-lus) Detached piece of thrombus, mass of bacteria, quantity of air, or foreign body that blocks a vessel.

embryo (EM-bree-oh) Developing organism from conception until the end of the second month.

embryology (em-bree-OL-oh-jee) Science of the origin and early development of an organism.

embryonic (em-bree-ON-ic) Pertaining to the embryo.

emesis (EM-eh-sis) Vomit.

eminence (EM-ih-nens) A higher place or part.

emmetropia (emm-eh-TROH-pee-ah) Normal refractive condition of the eye.

empathy (EM-pah-thee) Ability to place yourself into the feelings, emotions, and reactions of another person.

emphysema (em-fih-SEE-mah) Dilation of respiratory bronchioles and alveoli.

empyema (EM-pie-EE-mah) Pus in a body cavity, particularly in the pleural cavity.

emulsify (eh-MUL-sih-fye) Break up into very small droplets to suspend in a solution (emulsion).

enamel (ee-NAM-el) Hard substance covering a tooth.

encephalitis (en-SEF-ah-LIE-tis) Inflammation of brain cells and tissues.

encephalocele (en-SEF-ah-loh-seal) Congenital defect of the cranium with herniation of brain tissue.

encephalomyelitis (en-SEF-ah-loh-MY-eh-lie-tis) Inflammation of the brain and spinal cord.

encode (en-KODE) Convert information.

encopresis (en-koh-PREE-sis) Repeated soiling with feces.

endarterectomy (END-ar-ter-EK-toe-me) Surgical removal of plaque from an artery.

endemic (en-**DEM**-ik) Disease always present in a community.

endocarditis (**EN**-doh-kar-**DIE**-tis) Inflammation of the lining of the heart.

endocardium (**EN**-doh-**KAR**-dee-um) The inside lining of the heart.

endocrine (**EN**-doh-krin) Pertaining to a gland that produces an internal or hormonal secretion and secretes it into the bloodstream.

endocrine gland (**EN**-doh-krin GLAND) A gland that produces an internal or hormonal secretion and secretes it into the bloodstream.

endocrinologist (**EN**-doh-krih-**NOL**-oh-jist) A medical specialist in endocrinology.

endocrinology (**EN**-doh-krih-**NOL**-oh-jee) Medical specialty concerned with the production and effects of hormones.

endogenous (en-**DOJ**-en-us) Produced within the organism.

endometrial (en-doh-**ME**-tree-al) Pertaining to the inner lining of the uterus.

endometriosis (**EN**-doh-me-tree-**OH**-sis) Endometrial tissue in the abdomen outside the uterus.

endometrium (en-doh-**ME**-tree-um) Inner lining of the uterus.

endoplasmic reticulum (**EN**-doh-**PLAZ**-mik reh-**TIC**-you-lum) Structure inside a cell that synthesizes steroids, detoxifies drugs, and manufactures cell membranes.

endorphin (en-**DOR**-fin) Natural substance in the brain that has the same effect as opium.

endoscope (**EN**-doh-skope) Instrument for examining the inside of a tubular or hollow organ.

endoscopy (en-**DOS**-koh-pee) The use of an endoscope.

endospore (**EN**-doh-spor) Spore produced inside a cell and capable of resisting heat, freezing, radiation, and chemicals.

endosteum (en-**DOSS**-tee-um) A membrane of tissue lining the inner (medullary) cavity of a long bone.

endotracheal (en-doh-**TRAY**-kee-al) Pertaining to being inside the trachea.

enema (**EN**-eh-mah) An injection of fluid into the rectum.

enteric (en-**TEHR**-ik) Pertaining to the intestine.

enteroscope (**EN**-ter-oh-**SKOPE**) Slender, tubular instrument with light source and camera to visualize the digestive tract.

enteroscopy (en-ter-**OSS**-koh-pee) The examination of the lining of the digestive tract.

enuresis (en-you-**REE**-sis) Bed-wetting; urinary incontinence.

environment (en-**VI**-ron-ment) All the external conditions affecting the life of an organism.

environmental (en-**VI**-ron-ment-al) Pertaining to the environment.

enzyme (**EN**-zime) Protein that induces changes in other substances.

eosinophil (ee-oh-**SIN**-oh-fill) An eosinophil's granules attract a rosy-red color on staining.

ependyma (ep-**EN**-dih-mah) Membrane lining the central canal of the spinal cord and the ventricles of the brain.

ependymoma (eh-pen-dih-**MOH**-mah) Benign tumor arising from cells lining the ventricles.

epicardium (**EP**-ih-kar-**DEE**-um) The outer layer of the heart wall.

epicondyle (ep-ih-**KON**-dile) Projection above the condyle for attachment of a ligament or tendon.

epidemic (ep-ih-**DEM**-ik) Outbreak in a community of a disease or a health-related behavior.

epidermis (ep-ih-**DER**-miss) Top layer of the skin.

epididymis (**EP**-ih-**DID**-ih-miss) Coiled tube attached to the testis.

epididymitis (**EP**-ih-did-ih-**MY**-tis) Inflammation of the epididymis.

epididymoorchitis (ep-ih-**DID**-ih-moh-or-**KIE**-tis) Inflammation of the epididymis and testicle. Also called *orchitis.*

epidural (ep-ih-**DYU**-ral) Above the dura.

epidural space (ep-ih-**DYU**-ral SPASE) Space between the dura mater and the wall of the vertebral canal or skull.

epigastric (ep-ih-**GAS**-trik) Abdominal region above the stomach.

epiglottis (ep-ih-**GLOT**-is) Leaf-shaped plate of cartilage that shuts off the larynx during swallowing.

epiglottitis (ep-ih-**GLOT**-eye-tis) Inflammation of the epiglottis.

epilepsy (**EP**-ih-**LEP**-see) Chronic brain disorder due to paroxysmal excessive neuronal discharges.

epinephrine (ep-ih-**NEF**-rin) Main catecholamine produced by the adrenal medulla. Also called *adrenaline.*

epiphyseal plate (eh-**PIF**-ih-see-al PLATE) Layer of cartilage between the epiphysis and metaphysis where bone growth occurs.

epiphysis (eh-**PIF**-ih-sis) Expanded area at the proximal and distal ends of a long bone that provides increased surface area for attachment of ligaments and tendons.

episiotomy (eh-piz-ee-**OT**-oh-me) Surgical incision of the vulva.

epispadias (ep-ih-**SPAY**-dee-as) Condition in which the urethral opening is on the dorsum of the penis.

epistaxis (ep-ih-**STAK**-sis) Nosebleed.

epithelium (ep-ih-**THEE**-lee-um) Tissue that covers surfaces or lines cavities.

equilibrium (ee-kwi-**LIB**-ree-um) Being evenly balanced.

erectile (ee-**REK**-tile) Capable of erection or being distended with blood.

erection (ee-**REK**-shun) Distended and rigid state of an organ.

ergonomic (err-go-**NOM**-ick) Term applied to a workplace tool or equipment designed to prevent worker injury and discomfort.

erosion (ee-**ROE**-shun) A shallow ulcer in the lining of a structure.

erythema infectiosum (er-ih-**THEE**-mah in-fek-she-**OH**-sum) Mild infectious disease of childhood with a flushed-cheek appearance. Also called *fifth disease.*

erythroblast (eh-**RITH**-ro-blast) Precursor to a red blood cell.

erythroblastosis fetalis (eh-**RITH**-ro-blast-oh-sis fee-**TAH**-lis) Hemolytic disease of the newborn due to Rh incompatibility.

erythrocyte (eh-**RITH**-roh-site) Another name for a red blood cell.

erythropoiesis (eh-**RITH**-ro-poy-**EE**-sis) The formation of red blood cells.

erythropoietin (eh-**RITH**-ro-**POY**-ee-tin) Protein secreted by the kidney that stimulates red blood cell production.

eschar (**ESS**-kar) The burned, dead tissue lying on top of third-degree burns.

Escherichia coli (esh-eh-**RIK**-ee-ah **KOH**-lie) Organism in the intestine; releases an exotoxin that causes diarrhea.

esophagitis (ee-**SOF**-ah-**JI**-tis) Inflammation of the lining of the esophagus.

esophagus (ee-**SOF**-ah-gus) Tube linking the pharynx and the stomach.

esotropia (es-oh-**TROH**-pee-ah) A turning of the eye inward toward the nose.

essential (eh-**SEN**-shal) Amino acids that cannot be synthesized by the body.

estrogen (**ES**-troh-jen) Generic term for hormones that stimulate female secondary sex characteristics.

ethmoid (**ETH**-moyd) Bone that forms the back of the nose and encloses numerous air cells.

eumelanin (**YOU**-mel-ah-nin) The dark form of the pigment melanin.

euphoria (yoo-**FOR**-ee-ah) Exaggerated feeling of well-being.

eupnea (yoop-**NEE**-ah) Normal breathing.

eustachian tube (you-**STAY**-shun **TYUB**) Tube that connects the middle ear to the nasopharynx. Also called *auditory tube.*

euthyroid (you-**THIGH**-royd) Normal thyroid function.

eversion (ee-**VER**-shun) A turning outward.

evolve (ee-**VOLV**) To develop gradually.

exacerbation (ek-zas-er-**BAY**-shun) Period in which there is an increase in the severity of a disease.

exanthem (ek-**ZAN**-them) Skin eruption or rash occurring as the outward sign of a viral or bacterial disease.

excoriate (eks-**KOR**-ee-ate) To scratch.

excoriation (eks-**KOR**-ee-**AY**-shun) Scratch marks.

excrement (**EKS**-kreh-ment) Waste matter such as feces.

excrete (eks-**KREET**) To pass out of the body waste products of metabolism.

excretion (eks-**KREE**-shun) Removal of waste products of metabolism out of the body.

exhale (**EKS**-hail) Breathe out.

exocrine gland (**EK**-soh-krin **GLAND**) A gland that secretes outwardly through excretory ducts.

exogenous (ex-**OJ**-en-us) Originating outside the organism.

exophthalmos (ek-sof-**THAL**-mos) Protrusion of the eyeball.

exotropia (ek-soh-**TROH**-pee-ah) A turning of the eye outward away from the nose.

expectorate (ek-**SPEC**-toh-rate) Cough up and spit out mucus from the respiratory tract.

expiration (**EKS**-pih-**RAY**-shun) Breathe out.

extension (eks-**TEN**-shun) Straighten a joint to increase its angle.

extracorporeal (**EKS**-trah-kor-**POH**-ree-al) Outside the body.

extravasate (eks-**TRAV**-ah-sate) To ooze out from a vessel into the tissues.

extrinsic (eks-**TRIN**-sik) Extrinsic eye muscles are located on the outside of the eye, as opposed to intrinsic muscles, which are located inside the eye.

F

facet (**FAS**-et) Small smooth area around a pain-producing nerve.

facial (**FAY**-shal) Seventh (VII) cranial nerve; supplying the forehead, nose, eyes, mouth, and jaws.

facies (**FASH**-eez) Facial expression and features characteristic of a specific disease.

fallopian tubes (fah-**LOW**-pee-an) Uterine tubes connected to the fundus of the uterus.

Fallot (fah-**LOW**) Person who first described the tetralogy of congenital heart defects.

fascia (**FASH**-ee-ah) Sheet of fibrous connective tissue.

fascicle (**FAS**-ih-kull) Bundle of muscle fibers.

fasciectomy (fash-ee-**EK**-toe-me) Surgical removal of fascia.

fasciitis (fash-ee-**I**-tis) Inflammation of the fascia.

fasciotomy (fash-ee-**OT**-oh-me) An incision through a band of fascia, usually to relieve pressure on underlying structures.

fat (**FAT**) Lipid that is solid at room temperature.

fatty acid (**FAT**-ee **ASS**-id) An acid obtained from the hydrolysis of fats.

febrile (**FEB**-ril or **FEB**-rile) Pertaining to or suffering from a fever.

fecal (**FEE**-kal) Pertaining to feces.

feces (**FEE**-sees) Undigested, waste material discharged from the bowel.

Feldenkrais method (**FEL**-den-kries **METH**-od) Series of exercises to discover new ways of pain-free movement.

femoral (**FEM**-oh-ral) Pertaining to the femur.

femur (**FEE**-mur) The thigh bone.

ferritin (**FER**-ih-tin) Iron-protein complex that regulates iron storage and transport.

fertilization (**FER**-til-eye-**ZAY**-shun) Union of a male sperm and a female egg.

fertilize (**FER**-til-ize) To penetrate an oocyte with a sperm so as to impregnate.

fertilizer (**FER**-tih-lie-zer) Substance used to increase the yield of crops.

festinant (**FES**-tih-nant) Shuffling, falling-forward gait.

fetal (**FEE**-tal) Pertaining to the fetus.

fetus (**FEE**-tus) Human organism from the end of the eighth week after conception to birth.

fever (**FEE**-ver) Increased body temperature that is a physiologic response to disease.

fiber (**FIE**-ber) Carbohydrate not digested by intestinal enzymes; *or* a strand or filament.

fibrillation (fi-brih-LAY-shun) Uncontrolled quivering or twitching of the heart muscle.

fibrin (FIE-brin) Stringy protein fiber that is a component of a blood clot.

fibrinogen (fie-BRIN-oh-jen) Precursor of fibrin in blood-clotting process.

fibroadenoma (FIE-broh-ad-en-OH-mah) Benign tumor containing much fibrous tissue.

fibroblast (FIE-bro-blast) Cell that forms collagen fibers.

fibrocartilage (fie-bro-KAR-til-age) Cartilage containing collagen fibers.

fibrocystic disease (fie-broh-SIS-tik DIZ-eez) Benign breast disease with multiple tiny lumps and cysts.

fibroid (FIE-broyd) Uterine tumor resembling fibrous tissue.

fibromyalgia (fie-bro-my-AL-jee-ah) Pain in the muscle fibers.

fibromyoma (FIE-bro-my-OH-mah) Benign neoplasm derived from smooth muscle containing fibrous tissue.

fibrosis (fie-BROH-sis) Repair of dead tissue cells by formation of fibrous tissue.

fibrous (FIE-brus) Tissue containing fibroblasts and fibers.

fibula (FIB-you-lah) The smaller of the two bones of the lower leg.

filter (FIL-ter) A porous substance through which a liquid or gas is passed to separate out contained particles; or to use a filter.

filtrate (FIL-trate) That which has passed through a filter.

filtration (fil-TRAY-shun) Process of passing liquid through a filter.

fimbria (FIM-bree-ah) A fringelike structure on the surface of a cell or microorganism. Plural *fimbriae*.

fissure (FISH-ur) Deep furrow or cleft. Plural *fissures*.

fistula (FIS-tyu-lah) Abnormal passage.

flagellum (fla-JELL-um) Tail of a sperm. Plural *flagella*.

flatulence (FLAT-you-lents) Excessive amount of gas in the stomach and intestines.

flatus (FLAY-tus) Gas or air expelled through the anus.

flavonoid (FLAY-vih-noid) A pigment found in fruit, wine, and tea. Also spelled *flavinoid*.

flex (FLEKS) To bend a joint so that the two parts come together.

flexion (FLEK-shun) Bend a joint to decrease its angle.

flexor (FLEK-sor) Muscle or tendon that flexes a joint.

flexure (FLEK-shur) A bend in a structure.

flora (FLO-rah) Microorganisms covering the exterior and interior of a healthy animal.

fluidized therapy (FLU-id-ized THAIR-ah-pee) Use of suspended particles in a hot air stream to apply heat.

fluidotherapy (FLU-id-oh-THAIR-ah-pee) A form of heat therapy.

fluorescein (flor-ESS-ee-in) Dye that produces a vivid green color under a blue light to diagnose corneal abrasions and foreign bodies.

fluoride (FLOR-ide) Chemical found in bones and teeth.

fluoroscopy (flor-OS-koh-pee) Examination of the structures of the body by x-rays.

folate (FO-late) Natural B$_9$ vitamin.

folic acid (FO-lik ASS-id) Synthetic B$_9$ vitamin.

follicle (FOLL-ih-kull) Spherical mass of cells containing a cavity or a small cul-de-sac, such as a hair follicle.

follicular (fo-LIK-you-lar) Pertaining to a follicle.

fomites (FO-my-teez) Bedding, clothing, towels, etc., that can harbor and transmit a disease agent.

foramen (fo-RAY-men) An opening through a structure. Plural *foramina*.

forceps extraction (FOR-seps ek-STRAK-shun) Assisted delivery of the baby by an instrument that grasps the head of the baby.

foreskin (FOR-skin) Skin that covers the glans penis.

fornix (FOR-niks) Arch-shaped, blind-ended part of the vagina behind and around the cervix. Plural *fornices*.

fovea centralis (FOH-vee-ah sen-TRAH-lis) Small pit in the center of the macula that has the highest visual acuity.

free radical (FREE RAD-ih-kal) Short-lived product of oxidation in a cell that can be damaging to the cell.

frenulum (FREN-you-lum) Fold of mucous membrane between the glans and the prepuce.

frequency (FREE-kwen-see) The number of times something happens in a given time (e.g., passing urine).

frontal (FRON-tal) Pertaining to the vertical plane dividing the body into anterior and posterior portions.

frontal lobe (FRON-tal LOBE) Area of brain behind the frontal bone.

fructosamine (FRUK-toe-sah-meen) Organic compound with fructose as its base.

fructose (FRUK-toes) Sugar found in fruits and honey.

function (FUNK-shun) The ability of an organ or tissue to perform its special work.

fundoscopy (fun-DOS-koh-pee) Examination of the fundus (retina) of the eye.

fundus (FUN-dus) Part farthest from the opening of a hollow organ.

fungicide (FUN-jee-side) Agent for destroying fungi.

fungus (FUN-gus) General term used to describe yeasts and molds. Plural *fungi*.

furuncle (FU-rung-kel) An infected hair follicle that spreads into the tissues around the follicle.

G

galactorrhea (gah-LAK-toe-REE-ah) Abnormal flow of milk from the breasts.

gallbladder (GAWL-blad-er) Receptacle on the inferior surface of the liver for storing bile.

gallstone (GAWL-stone) Hard mass of cholesterol, calcium, and bilirubin that can be formed in the gallbladder and bile duct.

galvanic (gal-VAN-ik) Pertaining to electric current.

ganglion (GANG-lee-on) Collection of nerve cell bodies outside the CNS; *or* a fluid-containing swelling attached to the synovial sheath of a tendon. Plural *ganglia*.

gastric (GAS-trik) Pertaining to the stomach.

gastrin (GAS-trin) Hormone secreted in the stomach that stimulates secretion of HCl and increases gastric motility.

gastritis (gas-TRY-tis) Inflammation of the lining of the stomach.

gastrocnemius (gas-trok-NEE-me-us) Major muscle in back of the lower leg (the calf).

gastrocolic reflex (gas-troh-KOL-ik RE-fleks) Taking food into the stomach leads to mass movement of feces in the colon and the desire to defecate.

gastroenteritis (GAS-troh-en-ter-I-tis) Inflammation of the stomach and intestines.

gastroenterologist (GAS-troh-en-ter-OL-oh-jist) Medical specialist in gastroenterology.

gastroenterology (GAS-troh-en-ter-OL-oh-gee) Medical specialty of the stomach and intestines.

gastroesophageal (GAS-troh-ee-sof-ah-JEE-al) Pertaining to the stomach and esophagus.

gastrointestinal (GI) (GAS-troh-in-TESS-tin-al) Relating to the stomach and intestines.

gastroscope (GAS-troh-skope) Endoscope for examining the inside of the stomach.

gastroscopy (gas-TROS-koh-pee) Endoscopic examination of the stomach.

Gaucher disease (go-SHAY DIZ-eez) Congenital disorder of fat metabolism.

gavage (guh-VAHZH) Forced feeding by stomach tube.

gene (JEEN) Functional segment of the DNA molecule.

genetic (jeh-NET-ik) Pertaining to a gene.

geneticist (jeh-NET-ih-sist) A specialist in genetics.

genetics (jeh-NET-iks) Science of the inheritance of characteristics.

genistein (JEN-is-tine) Flavonoid found in soy.

genital (JEN-ih-tal) Relating to reproduction or to the male or female sex organs.

genitalia (JEN-ih-TAY-lee-ah) External and internal organs of reproduction.

genome (JEE-nome) Complete set of genes.

genomics (jee-NOME-iks) Study of the structure, function, and information content of the genome.

genotype (jee-NOH-type) Specific genetic constitution of an individual.

geriatrician (jer-ee-ah-TRISH-an) Medical specialist in geriatrics.

geriatrics (jer-ee-AT-riks) Medical specialty that deals with the problems of old age.

gerontologist (jer-on-TOL-oh-jist) Medical specialist in gerontology.

gerontology (jer-on-TOL-oh-jee) Study of the process and problems of aging.

gestation (jes-TAY-shun) Period from conception to birth.

Giardia (jee-AR-dee-ah) Parasite in the small intestine.

giardiasis (jee-ar-DIE-ah-sis) Infection with *Giardia*, causing diarrhea.

gigantism (JI-gan-tizm) Abnormal height and size of the entire body.

gingiva (JIN-jih-vah) Tissue surrounding teeth and covering the jaw.

gingival (JIN-jih-vul) Pertaining to the gums.

gingivectomy (jin-jih-VEC-toe-me) Surgical removal of diseased gum tissue.

gingivitis (jin-jih-VI-tis) Inflammation of the gums.

Ginkgo **biloba** (GING-koh BIL-oh-bah) Extract of leaves used as a vasodilator.

ginseng (JIN-seng) Extract made from the root of a Chinese plant.

glans (GLANZ) Head of the penis or clitoris.

glaucoma (glau-KOH-mah) Increased intraocular pressure.

glia (GLEE-ah) Connective tissue that holds a structure together.

glioblastoma multiforme (GLIE-oh-blas-TOE-mah) A malignant form of brain cancer.

glioma (gli-OH-mah) Tumor arising in a glial cell.

globulin (GLOB-you-lin) Family of blood proteins.

glomerulonephritis (glo-MER-you-low-nef-RYE-tis) Infection of the glomeruli of the kidney.

glomerulus (glo-MER-you-lus) Plexus of capillaries; part of a nephron. Plural *glomeruli.*

glossodynia (gloss-oh-DIN-ee-ah) Painful, burning tongue.

glossopharyngeal (GLOSS-oh-fah-RIN-jee-al) Ninth (IX) cranial nerve; supplying the tongue and pharynx.

glottis (GLOT-is) Vocal apparatus of the larynx.

glucagon (GLU-kah-gon) Pancreatic hormone that supports blood glucose levels.

glucocorticoid (glu-co-KOR-tih-koyd) Hormone of the adrenal cortex that helps regulate glucose metabolism.

gluconeogenesis (GLU-ko-nee-oh-JEN-eh-sis) Formation of glucose from noncarbohydrate sources.

glucose (GLU-kose) The final product of carbohydrate digestion and the main sugar in the blood.

gluteal (GLU-tee-al) Pertaining to the buttocks.

gluten (GLU-ten) Insoluble protein found in wheat, barley, and oats.

gluteus (GLU-tee-us) Term that refers to a muscle in the buttocks.

glycemic index (glye-SEE-mic IN-deks) Measure of the rapidity in the rise of blood glucose after ingestion of carbohydrates.

glycemic load (glye-SEE-mic LOHD) Takes into account the amount of sugar available in the food to cause the rise in blood sugar.

glycogen (GLYE-koh-gen) The body's principal carbohydrate reserve, stored in the liver and skeletal muscle.

glycogenolysis (GLYE-koh-jen-oh-LYE-sis) Conversion of glycogen to glucose.

glycoprotein (GLYE-koh-PRO-teen) Combination of carbohydrate and protein.

glycosuria (GLYE-koh-SYU-ree-ah) Presence of glucose in urine.

glycosylated hemoglobin (Hb A1c) (GLYE-koh-sih-lay-ted HE-moh-GLOW-bin) Hemoglobin A fraction linked to glucose; used as an index of glucose control.

goiter (GOY-ter) Enlargement of the thyroid gland.

Golgi complex (GOAL-jee KOM-pleks) Organelle involved in synthesis of carbohydrates and glycoproteins.

gomphosis (gom-FOE-sis) Joint formed by a peg and socket. Plural *gomphoses.*

gonad (GO-nad) Testis or ovary. Plural *gonads.*

gonadotropin (GO-nad-oh-TROH-pin) Hormone capable of promoting gonad function.

gonorrhea (gon-oh-REE-ah) Specific contagious sexually transmitted infection.

gout (GOWT) Painful arthritis of the big toe and other joints.

grade (GRAYD) In cancer pathology, a classification of the rate of growth of cancer cells.

graft (GRAFT) Transplantation of living tissue.

Gram stain (GRAM STAYN) A method for differential staining of bacteria.

grand mal (GRAHN MAL) Old name for a generalized tonic-clonic seizure.

granulation (gran-you-LAY-shun) New fibrous tissue formed during wound healing.

granulocyte (GRAN-you-loh-site) A white blood cell that contains multiple small granules in its cytoplasm.

granulosa cell (gran-you-LOH-sah SELL) Cell lining the ovarian follicle.

Graves disease (GRAVZ DIZ-eez) Hyperthyroidism with toxic goiter.

gravid (GRAV-id) Pregnant.

gravida (GRAV-ih-dah) A pregnant woman.

gravidarum (gra-vih-DAR-um) Relating to pregnant women.

gray matter (GRAY MATT-er) Regions of the brain and spinal cord occupied by cell bodies and dendrites.

greenstick fracture (GREEN-stik FRAK-chur) A fracture in which one side of the bone is partially broken and the other side is bent; occurs mostly in children.

guanine (GWAH-neen) One of the chemical bases found in, and comprising the sequence of, both DNA and RNA.

Guillain-Barré syndrome (GEE-yan-bah-RAY SIN-drom) Disorder in which the body makes antibodies against myelin, disrupting nerve conduction.

gynecologist (guy-nih-KOL-oh-jist) Specialist in gynecology.

gynecology (guy-nih-KOL-oh-jee) Medical specialty for the care of the female reproductive system.

gynecomastia (GUY-nih-koh-MAS-tee-ah) Enlargement of the breast.

gyrus (JI-rus) Rounded elevation on the surface of the cerebral hemispheres. Plural *gyri.*

H

hairline fracture (HAIR-line FRAK-chur) A fracture without separation of the fragments.

halitosis (hal-ih-TOE-sis) Bad odor of the breath.

hallucination (hah-loo-sih-NAY-shun) Perception of an object or event when there is no such thing present.

hallux valgus (HAL-uks VAL-gus) Deviation of the big toe toward the lateral side of the foot.

handicap (HAND-ee-cap) Condition that interferes with a person's ability to function normally.

hapten (HAP-ten) Small molecule that has to bind to a larger molecule to form an antigen.

Hashimoto disease (hah-shee-MOH-toe DIZ-eez) Autoimmune disease of the thyroid gland. Also called *Hashimoto thyroiditis.*

haversian canals (hah-VER-shan ka-NALS) Vascular canals in bone. Also called *central canals.*

head (HED) The rounded extremity of a bone.

Heberden node (HEH-ber-den NOHD) Bony lump on the terminal phalanx of the fingers in osteoarthritis.

helix (HE-liks) A line in the shape of a coil.

helminth (HELL-minth) Any intestinal wormlike parasite.

hemangioma (he-MAN-jee-oh-mah) Abnormal mass of proliferating blood vessels.

hematemesis (he-mah-TEM-eh-sis) Vomiting of red blood.

hematochezia (he-mat-oh-KEY-zee-ah) The passage of red, bloody stools.

hematocrit (Hct) (HE-mat-oh-krit) Percentage of red blood cells in blood.

hematologist (he-mah-TOL-oh-jist) Specialist in hematology.

hematology (he-mah-TOL-oh-jee) Medical specialty of disorders of blood.

hematoma (he-mah-TOH-mah) Collection of blood that has escaped from the blood vessels into tissue. Also called *bruise.*

hematopoietic (HE-mah-toh-poy-ET-ick) Pertaining to the making of red blood cells.

hematuria (he-mah-TYU-ree-ah) Blood in the urine.

heme (HEEM) The iron-based component of hemoglobin that carries oxygen.

hemifacial (hem-ee-FAY-shal) Pertaining to one side of the face.

hemiparesis (HEM-ee-pah-REE-sis) Weakness of one side of the body.

hemiplegia (hem-ee-PLEE-jee-ah) Paralysis of one side of the body.

Hemoccult test (HEEM-oh-kult TEST) *Hemoccult* (trade name for a fecal occult blood test).

hemochromatosis (HE-mah-krom-ah-TOE-sis) Dangerously high levels of iron in the body with deposition of iron pigments in tissues.

hemodialysis (HE-moh-die-AL-ih-sis) An artificial method of filtration to remove excess waste materials and water directly from the blood.

hemodynamics (HE-moh-die-NAM-iks) The science of the blood flow through the circulation.

hemoglobin (HE-moh-GLOW-bin) Red-pigmented protein that is the main component of red blood cells.

hemoglobinopathy (HE-moh-GLOW-bih-NOP-ah-thee) Disease caused by the presence of an abnormal hemoglobin in the red blood cells.

hemolysis (he-MOL-ih-sis) Destruction of red blood cells so that hemoglobin is liberated.

hemolytic (he-moh-LIT-ik) Pertaining to the process of destruction of red blood cells.

hemophilia (he-moh-FILL-ee-ah) An inherited disease from a deficiency of clotting factor VIII.

hemoptysis (he-MOP-tih-sis) Bloody sputum.

hemorrhage (HEM-oh-raj) To bleed profusely.

hemorrhoid (HEM-oh-royd) Dilated rectal vein producing painful anal swelling. Plural *hemorrhoids.*

hemorrhoidectomy (HEM-oh-roy-DEK-toh-me) Surgical removal of hemorrhoids.

hemostasis (he-moh-STAY-sis) Controlling or stopping bleeding.

hemothorax (he-moh-THOR-ax) Blood in the pleural cavity.

heparin (HEP-ah-rin) An anticoagulant secreted particularly by liver cells.

hepatic (hep-AT-ik) Pertaining to the liver.

hepatitis (hep-ah-TIE-tis) Inflammation of the liver.

hepatocellular (HEP-ah-toe-SELL-you-lar) Pertaining to liver cells.

herbicide (ER-bih-side) Agent for destroying plants.

heredity (heh-RED-ih-tee) Transmission of characteristics from parents to offspring through genes.

hernia (HER-nee-ah) Protrusion of a structure through the tissue that normally contains it.

herniate (HER-nee-ate) To protrude.

herniation (HER-nee-ay-shun) Protrusion of an anatomical structure from its normal location.

herniorrhaphy (HER-nee-OR-ah-fee) Repair of a hernia.

herpangina (her-PAN-ji-nah) Ulcerative disease of the throat.

herpes simplex virus (HSV) (HER-peez SIM-pleks VIE-rus) Disease that manifests with painful, watery blisters on the skin and mucous membranes.

herpes zoster (HER-pees ZOS-ter) Painful eruption of vesicles that follows a dermatome or nerve root on one side of the body. Also called *shingles.*

heterograft (HET-er-oh-graft) A graft using tissue taken from another species. Also known as *xenograft.*

heterophile (HET-er-oh-file) Pertaining to antibodies present during a disease but not directed against the causative agent.

heterozygous (HET-er-oh-ZIE-gus) Carries a different version (allele) of a specific gene on each of the two corresponding chromosomes.

hiatus (high-AY-tus) An opening through a structure.

hilum (HIGH-lum) The site where the nerves and blood vessels enter and leave an organ. Plural *hila.*

hirsutism (HER-sue-tizm) Excessive body and facial hair.

histamine (HISS-tah-mean) Compound liberated in tissues as a result of injury or an allergic response.

histology (his-TOL-oh-jee) Structure and function of cells, tissues, and organs.

Hodgkin lymphoma (HOJ-kin lim-FO-muh) Disease marked by chronic enlargement of lymph nodes spreading to other nodes in an orderly way.

holistic (ho-LIS-tik) Pertaining to the care of the whole person in physical, mental, emotional, and spiritual dimensions.

homeopath (HO-mee-oh-path) Practitioner of homeopathy.

homeopathy (ho-mee-OP-ah-thee) Treatment of disease with minute doses of substances.

homeostasis (ho-mee-oh-STAY-sis) Stability or equilibrium of a system or the body's internal environment.

homicidal (hom-ih-SIDE-al) Having a tendency to commit homicide.

homicide (HOM-ih-side) Killing of one human by another.

homocysteine (ho-moh-SIS-teen) An amino acid similar to cysteine.

homograft (HOH-moh-graft) Skin graft from another person or a cadaver.

homozygous (hoh-moh-ZIE-gus) Having two identical copies of a specific gene on the two homologous chromosomes.

hordeolum (hor-DEE-oh-lum) Abscess in an eyelash follicle. Also called *stye.*

hormone (HOR-mohn) Chemical formed in one tissue or organ and carried by the blood to stimulate or inhibit a function of another tissue or organ.

Horner syndrome (HOR-ner SIN-drome) Disorder of the sympathetic nerves to the face and eye.

hospice (HOS-pis) Facility or program that provides care to the dying and their families.

host (HOST) Organism on which organisms live.

human immunodeficiency virus (HIV) (HYU-man IM-you-noh-dee-FISH-en-see VIE-rus) Etiologic agent of acquired immunodeficiency syndrome (AIDS).

human papilloma virus (HPV) (HYU-man pap-ih-LOW-mah VIE-rus) Causes warts on the skin and genitalia and can increase the risk for cervical cancer.

humerus (HYU-mer-us) Single bone of the upper arm.

humoral immunity (HYU-mor-al im-YOU-nih-tee) Defense mechanism arising from antibodies in the blood.

Huntington disease (HUN-ting-ton DIZ-eez) Progressive inherited, degenerative, incurable neurologic disease. Also called *Huntington chorea.*

hyaline (HIGH-ah-line) Cartilage that looks like frosted glass and contains fine collagen fibers.

hyaline membrane disease (HIGH-ah-line MEM-brain DIZ-eez) Respiratory distress syndrome of the newborn.

hydrocele (HIGH-droh-seal) Collection of fluid in the space of the tunica vaginalis.

hydrocephalus (high-droh-SEF-ah-lus) Enlarged head due to excess CSF in the cerebral ventricles.

hydrochloric acid (HCl) (high-droh-KLOR-ic ASS-id) The acid of gastric juice.

Hydrocollator (high-droh-KOLL-ay-tor) Synthetic hot or cold gel used to stimulate a rise or fall in tissue temperature.

hydrocortisone (high-droh-KOR-tih-sohn) Potent glucocorticoid with anti-inflammatory properties. Also called *cortisol.*

hydrogenated (HIGH-droh-jeh-NAY-ted) Addition of hydrogen to unsaturated oils to solidify them and produce trans fats.

hydronephrosis (HIGH-droh-neh-FRO-sis) Dilation of the pelvis and calyces of a kidney.

hydronephrotic (HIGH-droh-neh-FROT-ik) Pertaining to or suffering from the dilation of the pelvis and calyces of the kidney.

hymen (HIGH-men) Thin membrane partly occluding the vaginal orifice.

hyperactivity (HIGH-per-ac-TIV-ih-tee) Excessive restlessness and movement.

hyperbaric (high-per-BAR-ik) Pressure greater than atmospheric pressure.

hypercalcemia (HIGH-per-cal-SEE-me-ah) Excessive level of calcium in the blood.

hypercapnia (HIGH-per-KAP-nee-ah) Abnormal increase of carbon dioxide in the arterial bloodstream.

hypercarotenemia (HIGH-per-KAR-o-teh-NEE-me-ah) Excessive level of the yellow-red pigment carotene in the blood.

hyperemesis (high-per-EM-ee-sis) Excessive vomiting.

hyperflexion (high-per-FLEK-shun) Flexion of a limb or part beyond the normal limits.

hyperfractionated (high-per-FRAK-shun-ay-ted) Given in smaller amounts and more frequently.

hyperglycemia (HIGH-per-gly-SEE-me-ah) High level of glucose (sugar) in blood.

hyperglycemic (HIGH-per-gly-SEE-mik) Pertaining to high blood sugar.

hyperimmune globulin (HIGH-per-im-YUNE GLOB-you-lin) Immunoglobulin prepared from serum of people with a high antibody titer to a specific virus.

hyperinflation (HIGH-per-in-FLAY-shun) Overdistension of pulmonary alveoli with air resulting from airway obstruction.

hyperkalemia (HIGH-per-kah-LEE-me-ah) High level of potassium in the blood.

hypernatremia (HIGH-per-nah-TREE-me-ah) High level of sodium in the blood.

hyperopia (high-per-OH-pee-ah) Able to see distant objects but unable to see close objects.

hyperosmolar (HIGH-per-os-MOH-lar) Marked hyperglycemia without ketoacidosis.

hyperparathyroidism (HIGH-per-para-THIGH-royd-ism) Excessive levels of parathyroid hormone.

hyperplasia (high-per-PLAY-zee-ah) Increase in the *number* of the cells in a tissue or organ.

hyperpnea (high-perp-NEE-ah) Deeper and more rapid breathing than normal.

hypersecretion (HIGH-per-seh-KREE-shun) Excessive secretion of mucus (or enzymes or waste products).

hypersensitivity (HIGH-per-sen-sih-TIV-ih-tee) Exaggerated abnormal reaction to an allergen.

hypersplenism (high-per-SPLEN-izm) Condition in which the spleen removes blood components at an excessive rate.

hypertension (HIGH-per-TEN-shun) Persistent high arterial blood pressure.

hypertensive (HIGH-per-TEN-siv) Suffering from hypertension.

hyperthyroidism (high-per-THIGH-royd-ism) Excessive production of thyroid hormones.

hypertrophy (high-PER-troh-fee) Increase in size, but not in number, of an individual tissue element.

hypha (HIGH-fah) Branching tubular fungal cell. Plural *hyphae.*

hypnosis (hip-NOH-sis) Changed state of consciousness.

hypnotherapy (hip-noh-THAIR-ah-pee) Use of hypnosis in treatment of disorders.

hypochondriac (high-poh-KON-dree-ack) A person who exaggerates the significance of symptoms.

hypochondriasis (HIGH-poh-kon-DRY-ah-sis) Belief that a minor symptom indicates a severe disease.

hypochromic (high-poh-CROW-mik) Pale in color, as in RBCs when hemoglobin is deficient.

hypodermis (high-poh-DER-miss) Tissue layer below the dermis.

hypogastric (high-poh-GAS-trik) Abdominal region below the stomach.

hypoglossal (high-poh-GLOSS-al) Twelfth (XII) cranial nerve; supplying muscles of the tongue.

hypoglycemia (HIGH-poh-glie-SEE-me-ah) Low level of glucose (sugar) in the blood.

hypoglycemic (HIGH-poh-glie-SEE-mik) Pertaining to or suffering from hypoglycemia.

hypogonadism (HIGH-poh-GOH-nad-izm) Deficient gonad production of sperm or eggs or hormones.

hypokalemia (HIGH-poh-kah-LEE-me-ah) Low level of potassium in the blood.

hyponatremia (HIGH-poh-nah-TREE-me-ah) Low level of sodium in the blood.

hypoparathyroidism (HIGH-poh-para-THIGH-royd-ism) Deficient levels of parathyroid hormone.

hypophysis (high-POF-ih-sis) Another name for the pituitary gland.

hypopituitarism (HIGH-poh-pih-TYU-ih-tah-rizm) Condition of one or more deficient pituitary hormones.

hypospadias (high-poh-SPAY-dee-as) Urethral opening more proximal than normal on the ventral surface of the penis.

hypotension (HIGH-poh-TEN-shun) Persistent low arterial blood pressure.

hypothalamic (high-poh-tha-LAM-ik) Pertaining to the hypothalamus.

hypothalamus (high-poh-THAL-ah-muss) Area of gray matter forming part of the walls and floor of the third ventricle.

hypothenar (high-poh-THAY-nar) Fleshy eminence at the base of the little finger.

hypothermia (high-poh-THER-me-ah) Very low core body temperature.

hypothyroidism (high-poh-THIGH-royd-ism) Deficient production of thyroid hormones.

hypotonia (high-poh-TOE-nee-ah) Diminished muscle tone.

hypotonic (high-poh-TON-ik) Pertaining to or suffering from hypotonia.

hypovolemic (HIGH-poh-vo-LEE-mick) Having decreased blood volume in the body.

hypoxia (high-POCK-see-ah) Decrease below normal levels of oxygen in tissues, gases, or blood.

hypoxic (high-POCK-sik) Deficient in oxygen.

hysterectomy (his-ter-EK-toe-me) Surgical removal of the uterus.

hysterosalpingogram (HIS-ter-oh-sal-PING-oh-gram) Radiograph of the uterus and uterine tubes after injection of contrast material.

hysteroscopy (his-ter-OS-koh-pee) Visual inspection of the uterine cavity using an endoscope.

I

ictal (ICK-tal) Pertaining to, or condition caused by, a stroke or epilepsy.

idiopathic (ID-ih-oh-PATH-ik) Pertaining to a disease of unknown etiology.

ileocecal (ILL-ee-oh-SEE-cal) Pertaining to the junction of the ileum and cecum.

ileocecal sphincter (ILL-ee-oh-SEE-cal SFINK-ter) Band of muscle that encircles the junction of the ileum and cecum.

ileoscopy (ill-ee-OS-koh-pee) Endoscopic examination of the ileum.

ileostomy (ill-ee-OS-toe-me) Artificial opening from the ileum to the outside of the body.

ileum (ILL-ee-um) Third portion of the small intestine.

iliac (ILL-ee-ack) Pertaining to or near the ilium (pelvic bone).

ilium (ILL-ee-um) Large wing-shaped bone at the upper and posterior part of the pelvis. Plural *ilia.*

imagery (IM-aj-ree) Visualization of pleasant fantasies.

immune (im-YUNE) Protected from an infectious disease.

immune serum (im-YUNE SEER-um) Serum taken from another human or animal that has antibodies to a disease. Also called *antiserum.*

immunity (im-YOU-nih-tee) State of being protected.

immunization (im-you-nih-ZAY-shun) Administration of an agent to provide immunity.

immunize (IM-you-nize) To make resistant to an infectious disease.

immunoassay (IM-you-noh-ASS-ay) Biochemical test to measure the amount of a substance in a liquid, using the reaction of an antibody to its antigen.

immunodeficiency (IM-you-noh-dee-FISH-en-see) Failure of the immune system.

immunoglobulin (IM-you-noh-GLOB-you-lin) Specific protein evoked by an antigen. All antibodies are immunoglobulins.

immunologist (im-you-NOL-oh-jist) Medical specialist in immunology.

immunology (im-you-NOL-oh-jee) The science and practice of immunity and allergy.

immunosuppression (IM-you-noh-suh-PRESH-un) Suppression of the immune response by an outside agent, such as a drug.

impacted (im-PAK-ted) Immovably wedged, as with earwax blocking the external canal.

impacted fracture (im-PAK-ted FRAK-chur) A fracture in which one bone fragment is driven into the other.

impairment (im-PAIR-ment) Diminishing of normal function.

impedance (im-PEE-dahns) Resistance to the flow of an electric current.

impermeable (im-PER-me-ah-bull) Does not allow passage of anything.

impetigo (im-peh-TIE-go) Infection of the skin producing thick, yellow crusts.

implant (im-PLANT) To insert material into tissues; *or the* material inserted into tissues.

implantable (im-PLAN-tah-bul) Able to be inserted into tissues.

implantation (im-plan-TAY-shun) Attachment of a fertilized egg to the endometrium.

impotence (IM-poh-tence) Unable to achieve an erection.

impulsive (im-PUL-siv) Inability to resist performing inappropriate actions.

in situ (IN SIGH-tyu) In the correct place.

in utero (IN YOU-ter-oh) Within the womb; not yet born.

in vitro fertilization (IVF) (IN VEE-troh FER-til-eye-ZAY-shun) Process of combining a sperm and egg in a laboratory dish and placing the resulting embryos inside a uterus.

inattention (IN-ah-TEN-shun) Lack of concentration and direction.

incision (in-SIZH-un) A cut or surgical wound.

incisor (in-SIGH-zor) Chisel-shaped tooth.

incompatible (in-kom-PAT-ih-bul) Substances that interfere with each other physiologically.

incompetence (in-KOM-peh-tense) Failure of valves to close completely.

incomplete (in-kom-PLEET) Lacking some part.

incomplete fracture (in-kom-PLEET FRAK-chur) A fracture that does not extend across the bone, as in a hairline fracture.

incontinence (in-KON-tin-ence) Inability to prevent discharge of urine or feces.

incubation (in-kyu-BAY-shun) Process of developing an infection.

incus (IN-cuss) Middle one of the three ossicles in the middle ear; shaped like an anvil.

independence (in-de-PEN-denz) State of being independent.

independent (in-de-PEN-dent) Able to fend for oneself.

index (IN-deks) A standard indicator of measurement. Plural *indices.*

indole (IN-dole) A phytochemical that makes estrogen less effective.

infancy (IN-fan-see) The first year of life.

infant (IN-fant) Child in the first year of life.

infant formula (IN-fant FOR-myu-lah) Commercial product for infants manufactured from cows' milk or soy milk.

infarct (in-FARKT) Area of cell death resulting from an infarction.

infarction (in-**FARK**-shun) Sudden blockage of an artery.

infect (in-**FEKT**) To invade an organism with disease-producing microorganisms.

infection (in-**FEK**-shun) Invasion of the body by disease-producing microorganisms.

infectious (in-**FEK**-shus) Capable of being transmitted; *or* caused by infection by a microorganism.

inferior (in-**FEE**-ree-or) Situated below.

infertility (in-fer-**TIL**-ih-tee) Inability to conceive over a long period of time.

infestation (in-fes-**TAY**-shun) Act of being invaded on the skin by a troublesome other species, such as a parasite.

infiltrate (**IN**-fil-trate) To penetrate and invade into a tissue or cell.

infiltration (in-fil-**TRAY**-shun) The invasion into a tissue or cell.

inflate (in-**FLAYT**) Expand with air.

inflation (in-**FLAY**-shun) Process of expanding with air.

infundibulum (**IN**-fun-**DIB**-you-lum) Funnel-shaped structure. Plural *infundibula*.

infusion (in-**FYU**-zhun) Introduction intravenously of a substance other than blood.

ingestion (in-**JEST**-shun) Intake of food, either by mouth or through a nasogastric tube.

inguinal (**IN**-gwin-al) Pertaining to the groin.

inhale (**IN**-hail) Breathe in.

inherent (in-**HAIR**-ent) Occurring as a natural part of something.

inherited (in-**HAIR**-it-ed) Acquired through the genetic code.

innate (ih-**NATE**) Present at birth; arising from the intellect.

inotropic (**IN**-oh-**TROH**-pic) Affecting the contractility of cardiac muscle.

insanity (in-**SAN**-ih-tee) Nonmedical term for a person unable to be responsible for his or her actions.

insecticide (in-**SEK**-tih-side) Agent for destroying insects.

insemination (in-sem-ih-**NAY**-shun) Introduction of semen into the vagina.

insertion (in-**SIR**-shun) The insertion of a muscle is the attachment of a muscle to a more movable part of the skeleton, as distinct from the origin.

insomnia (in-**SOM**-nee-ah) Inability to sleep.

inspiration (in-spih-**RAY**-shun) Breathe in.

instability (in-stah-**BIL**-ih-tee) Abnormal tendency of a joint to partially or fully dislocate.

insufficiency (in-suh-**FISH**-en-see) Lack of completeness of function; in the heart, failure of a valve to close properly.

insulin (**IN**-syu-lin) A hormone secreted by the pancreas.

integrate (**IN**-teh-grate) To bring together into a complete and harmonious whole.

integument (in-**TEG**-you-ment) Organ system that covers the body, the skin being the main organ within the system.

integumentary (in-**TEG**-you-**MEN**-tah-ree) Pertaining to the covering of the body.

intellectual (in-teh-**LEK**-chu-al) Pertaining to the capacity for thinking and acquiring knowledge.

interatrial (**IN**-ter-**AY**-tree-al) Between the atria of the heart.

intercostal (**IN**-ter-**KOS**-tal) The space between two ribs.

intermittent (**IN**-ter-**MIT**-ent) Alternately ceasing and beginning again.

interosseous (in-ter-**OSS**-ee-us) A structure between bones, such as the muscles between the metacarpals.

interphalangeal (**IN**-ter-fay-**LAN**-jee-al) Pertaining to the joints between two phalanges.

interstitial (in-ter-**STISH**-al) Pertaining to spaces between cells in a tissue or organ.

interventricular (**IN**-ter-ven-**TRIK**-you-lar) Between the ventricles of the heart.

intervertebral (**IN**-ter-**VER**-teh-bral) The space between two vertebrae.

intestine (in-**TES**-tin) The digestive tube from stomach to anus.

intima (**IN**-tih-ma) Inner layer of a structure, particularly a blood vessel.

intolerance (in-**TOL**-er-ance) Inability of the small intestine to digest and dispose of a particular dietary constituent.

intracellular (in-trah-**SELL**-you-lar) Within the cell.

intracranial (in-trah-**KRAY**-nee-al) Within the cranium (skull).

intradermal (in-trah-**DER**-mal) Within the dermis.

intramuscular (in-trah-**MUSS**-kew-lar) Within the muscle.

intraocular (in-trah-**OCK**-you-lar) Pertaining to the inside of the eye.

intrathecal (**IN**-trah-**THEE**-kal) Within the subarachnoid or subdural space.

intrauterine (**IN**-trah-**YOU**-ter-ine) Inside the uterine cavity.

intravenous (**IN**-trah-**VEE**-nuss) Inside a vein.

intrinsic (in-**TRIN**-sik) Any muscle whose origin and insertion are entirely within the structure under consideration; for example, muscles inside the vocal cords or the eye.

intrinsic factor (in-**TRIN**-sik **FAK**-tor) Substance that makes the absorption of vitamin B_{12} happen.

intubation (**IN**-tyu-**BAY**-shun) Insertion of a tube into the trachea.

intussusception (**IN**-tuss-sus-**SEP**-shun) The slipping of one part of the bowel inside another to cause obstruction.

inversion (in-**VER**-shun) A turning inward.

involuntary (in-**VOL**-un-tah-ree) Not under control of the will.

involute (in-voh-**LUTE**) To return to a former condition; *or* decline associated with advanced age.

involution (in-voh-**LOO**-shun) A decrease in size or vigor.

iodine (**EYE**-oh-dine or **EYE**-oh-deen) Chemical element, the lack of which causes thyroid disease.

iris (**EYE**-ris) Colored portion of the eye with the pupil in its center.

irrigation (ih-rih-**GAY**-shun) Use of water to clean wax out of the external ear canal.

ischemia (is-**KEE**-me-ah) Lack of blood supply to a tissue.

ischium (**ISS**-kee-um) Lower and posterior part of the hip bone. Plural *ischia*.

Ishihara color system (ish-ee-**HAR**-ah) Test for color vision defects.

islet cells (**I**-let **SELLS**) Hormone-secreting cells of the pancreas.

islets of Langerhans (**EYE**-lets of **LAHNG**-er-hahnz) Areas of pancreatic cells that produce insulin and glucagon.

isoflavone (**I**-zo-**FLAY**-vone) Phytochemical that imitates estrogen.

isolate (**I**-so-late) To separate from others.

isotope (**I**-so-tope) Radioactive element used in diagnostic procedures.

isthmus (**IS**-mus) Part connecting two larger parts; for example, the uterus to the uterine tube.

J

Jaeger reading cards (**YA**-ger) Type in different sizes of print for testing near vision.

jaundice (**JAWN**-dis) Yellow staining of tissues with bile pigments, including bilirubin.

jejunum (je-**JEW**-num) Segment of small intestine between the duodenum and the ileum where most of the nutrients are absorbed.

jugular (**JUG**-you-lar) Pertaining to the throat.

juvenile (**JU**-ven-ile) Between the ages of 2 and 17 years.

K

Kaposi sarcoma (ka-**POH**-see sar-**KOH**-mah) A malignancy often seen in AIDS patients.

karyotype (**KAIR**-ee-oh-type) Map of chromosomes of an individual cell.

Kegel exercises (**KEG**-al **EKS**-er-size-ez) Contraction and relaxation of the pelvic floor muscles to improve urethral and rectal sphincter function.

keloid (**KEY**-loyd) Raised, irregular, lumpy, shiny scar due to excess collagen fiber production during healing of a wound.

keratin (**KER**-ah-tin) Protein found in the dead outer layer of skin and in nails and hair.

keratinocyte (ke-**RAT**-in-oh-site) Cell producing a tough, horny protein (keratin) in the process of differentiating into the dead cells of the stratum corneum.

keratomileusis (ker-ah-**TOE**-mill-oo-sis) A surgical procedure that involves cutting and shaping the cornea.

keratotomy (ker-ah-**TOT**-oh-mee) Incision in the cornea.

kernicterus (ker-**NICK**-ter-us) Bilirubin staining of the basal nuclei of the brain.

ketoacidosis (**KEY**-toe-as-ih-**DOE**-sis) Excessive production of ketones, making the blood acid.

ketone (**KEY**-tone) Chemical formed in uncontrolled diabetes or in starvation.

ketosis (key-**TOE**-sis) Excess production of ketones.

ki (**KEY**) Universal energy of life.

kidney (**KID**-nee) Organ of excretion.

kinesiology (ki-**NEE**-see-**OL**-oh-jee) Study of muscles and body parts involved in movement.

kleptomania (klep-toe-**MAY**-nee-ah) Uncontrollable need to steal

Klinefelter syndrome (**KLINE**-fel-ter **SIN**-drome) Genetic anomaly in males with XXY chromosomes.

Koplik spots (**KOP**-lik **SPOTZ**) Small red spots with a white center on the buccal mucosa early in measles.

kyphosis (ki-**FOH**-sis) A normal posterior curve of the thoracic spine that can be exaggerated in disease.

L

labium (**LAY**-bee-um) Fold of the vulva. Plural *labia*.

labor (**LAY**-bore) Process of expulsion of the fetus.

labrum (**LAY**-brum) Cartilage that forms a rim around the socket of the hip joint.

labyrinth (**LAB**-ih-rinth) The inner ear.

labyrinthitis (**LAB**-ih-rin-**THI**-tis) Inflammation of the inner ear.

laceration (lass-eh-**RAY**-shun) A tear of the skin.

lacrimal (**LAK**-rim-al) Pertaining to tears.

lactase (**LAK**-tase) Enzyme that breaks down lactose to glucose and galactose.

lactation (lak-**TAY**-shun) Production of milk.

lacteal (**LAK**-tee-al) A lymphatic vessel carrying chyle away from the intestine.

lactiferous (lak-**TIF**-er-us) Pertaining to or yielding milk.

lactose (**LAK**-toes) The disaccharide found in cow's milk.

lactovegetarian (**LAK**-toe-**VEJ**-eh-**TAR**-ee-an) Person whose diet consists of only plants and dairy products.

lacuna (la-**KOO**-nah) Small space or cavity within the matrix of bone. Plural *lacunae*.

lanugo (la-**NYU**-go) Fine, soft hair on the fetal body.

laparoscope (**LAP**-ah-roh-skope) Instrument (endoscope) used for viewing the abdominal contents.

laparoscopic (**LAP**-ah-rah-**SKOP**-ik) Pertaining to laparoscopy.

laparoscopy (lap-ah-**ROS**-koh-pee) Examination of the contents of the abdomen using an endoscope.

larva (**LAR**-vah) Stage in the development of an insect or intestinal parasite. Plural *larvae*.

laryngitis (lar-in-**JEYE**-tis) Inflammation of the larynx.

laryngopharynx (lah-**RING**-oh-**FAIR**-inks) Region of the pharynx below the epiglottis that includes the larynx.

laryngoscope (lah-**RING**-oh-skope) Hollow tube with a light and camera used to visualize or operate on the larynx.

laryngotracheobronchitis (lah-**RING**-oh-**TRAY**-kee-oh-brong-**KI**-tis) Inflammation of the larynx, trachea, and bronchi. Also called *croup*.

larynx (**LAIR**-inks) Organ of voice production.

laser (**LAY**-zer) Intense, narrow beam of monochromatic light.

laser surgery (LAY-zer SUR-jer-ee) Use of a concentrated, intense narrow beam of electromagnetic radiation for surgery.

latent (LAY-tent) Dormant, not discernible.

lateral (LAT-er-al) Situated at the side of a structure.

latex (LAY-tecks) Manufactured from the milky liquid in rubber plants; used for gloves in patient care.

latissimus dorsi (lah-TISS-ih-muss DOOR-sigh) The widest (broadest) muscle in the back.

lavage (lah-VAHZH) Washing out of a hollow cavity, tube, or organ.

legume (LEG-yoom) Family of plants including peas, beans, and lentils.

leiomyoma (LIE-oh-my-OH-mah) Benign neoplasm derived from smooth muscle.

lens (LENZ) Transparent refractive structure behind the iris.

lentigo (len-TIE-go) Age spot; small, flat, brown-black spot in the skin of older people. Plural *lentigines.*

leptin (LEP-tin) Hormone secreted by adipose tissue.

lesion (LEE-zhun) Pathologic change or injury in a tissue.

leukemia (loo-KEE-mee-ah) Disease in which the blood is taken over by white blood cells and their precursors.

leukocoria (loo-koh-KOH-ree-ah) Reflection in the pupil of a white mass in the eye.

leukocyte (LOO-koh-site) Another term for *white blood cell.* Alternative spelling *leucocyte.*

leukocytosis (LOO-koh-sigh-TOE-sis) An excessive number of white blood cells.

leukoencephalopathy (LOO-koh-en-sef-ah-LOP-ah-thee) Disease-producing destruction of white matter of the brain.

leukopenia (loo-koh-PEE-nee-ah) A deficient number of white blood cells.

leukoplakia (loo-koh-PLAY-kee-ah) White patch on the oral mucous membrane, often precancerous.

libido (li-BEE-doh) Sexual desire.

life expectancy (LIFE eck-SPEK-tan-see) Statistical determination of the number of years an individual is expected to live.

life span (LIFE SPAN) The age that a person reaches.

ligament (LIG-ah-ment) Band of fibrous tissue connecting two structures.

ligate (LIE-gate) Tie off a structure, such as a bleeding blood vessel.

ligation (lie-GAY-shun) Use of a tie to close a tube.

ligature (LIG-ah-chur) Thread or wire tied around a tubal structure to close it.

limbic (LIM-bic) Pertaining to the limbic system, an array of nerve fibers surrounding the thalamus.

linear fracture (LIN-ee-ar FRAK-chur) A fracture running parallel to the length of the bone.

lipase (LIE-paze) Enzyme that breaks down fat.

lipectomy (lip-ECK-toe-me) Surgical removal of adipose tissue.

lipid (LIP-id) General term for all types of fatty compounds; for example, cholesterol, triglycerides, and fatty acids.

lipoprotein (LIE-poh-pro-teen) Molecules made of combinations of fat and protein.

lithotripsy (LITH-oh-trip-see) Crushing stones by sound waves.

lithotripter (LITH-oh-trip-ter) Instrument that generates sound waves.

liver (LIV-er) Body's largest internal organ, located in the right upper quadrant of the abdomen.

lobe (LOBE) Subdivision of an organ or some other part.

lobectomy (low-BECK-toe-me) Surgical removal of a lobe of the lungs.

lochia (LOW-kee-uh) Vaginal discharge following childbirth.

locus (LOW-kus) A specific site; for example, the position a gene occupies on a chromosome.

longevity (lon-JEV-ih-tee) Duration of life beyond the normal expectation.

loop of Henle (LOOP of HEN-lee) Part of the renal tubule where reabsorption occurs.

lordosis (lore-DOH-sis) An exaggerated forward curvature of the lumbar spine.

louse (LOWSE) Parasitic insect. Plural *lice.*

lubricant (LOO-bri-cant) Substance for reducing friction.

lumbar (LUM-bar) Pertaining to the region in the back and sides between the ribs and pelvis.

lumen (LOO-men) The interior space of a tubelike structure.

lumpectomy (lump-ECK-toe-me) Removal of a lesion with preservation of surrounding tissue.

luteal (LOO-tee-al) Pertaining to a corpus luteum.

lutein (LOO-tee-in) Yellow pigment.

luteum (LOO-tee-um) Corpus luteum is the yellow (lutein) body formed after an ovarian follicle ruptures.

lycopene (LIE-koh-peen) Carotenoid that gives tomatoes their red color.

Lyme disease (LIME DIZ-eez) Disease transmitted by the bite of an infected deer tick.

lymph (LIMF) A clear fluid collected from tissues and transported by lymph vessels to the venous circulation.

lymphadenectomy (lim-FAD-eh-NECK-toe-me) Surgical excision of a lymph node.

lymphadenitis (lim-FAD-eh-neye-tis) Inflammation of a lymph node.

lymphadenopathy (lim-FAD-eh-NOP-ah-thee) Any disease process affecting a lymph node.

lymphangiogram (lim-FAN-jee-oh-gram) Radiographic images of lymph vessels and nodes following injection of contrast material.

lymphatic (lim-FAT-ik) Pertaining to lymph or the lymphatic system.

lymphedema (LIMF-e-dee-mah) Tissue swelling due to lymphatic obstruction.

lymphocyte (LIM-foh-site) Small white blood cell with a large nucleus.

lymphoid (LIM-foyd) Resembling lymphatic tissue.

lymphoma (lim-FO-muh) Any neoplasm of lymphatic tissue.

lysis (LIE-sis) Destruction of a cell; gradual decline of a disease (as opposed to a crisis).

lysosome (LIE-soh-sohm) Enzyme that digests foreign material and worn-out cell components.

lysozyme (LIE-soh-zime) Enzyme that dissolves the cell walls of bacteria.

M

macrocyte (MAK-roh-site) Large red blood cell.

macrocytic (mak-roh-SIT-ik) Pertaining to macrocytes.

macrophage (MAK-roh-fayj) Large white blood cell that removes bacteria, foreign particles, and dead cells.

macula (MAK-you-lah) Small area of special function; in the ear, a sensory receptor. Plural *maculae.*

macula lutea (MAK-you-lah LOO-tee-ah) Yellowish spot on the back of the retina; contains the fovea centralis.

macule (MAK-yul) Small, flat spot or patch on the skin.

majus (MAY-jus) Bigger or greater; for example, labia majora. Plural *majora.*

malabsorption (mal-ab-SORP-shun) Inadequate gastrointestinal absorption of nutrients.

malaria (mah-LAIR-ee-ah) Disease transmitted by the bite of a female *Anopheles* mosquito.

malformation (MAL-for-MAY-shun) Failure of proper or normal development.

malfunction (mal-FUNK-shun) Inadequate or abnormal function.

malignancy (mah-LIG-nan-see) Tumor that invades surrounding tissues and metastasizes to distant organs.

malignant (mah-LIG-nant) Capable of invading surrounding tissues and metastasizing to distant organs.

malleus (MAL-ee-us) Outer (lateral) one of the three ossicles in the middle ear; shaped like a hammer.

malnutrition (mal-nyu-TRISH-un) Inadequate nutrition from poor diet or inadequate absorption of nutrients.

malunion (mal-YOU-nee-un) Condition in which the two bony ends of a fracture fail to heal together correctly.

mammary (MAM-ah-ree) Relating to the lactating breast.

mammogram (MAM-oh-gram) The record produced by x-ray imaging of the breast.

mammography (mah-MOG-rah-fee) Process of x-ray examination of the breast.

mandible (MAN-di-bel) Lower jawbone.

mandibular (man-DIB-you-lar) Pertaining to the mandible.

mania (MAY-nee-ah) Mood disorder with hyperactivity, irritability, and rapid speech.

manic-depressive disorder (MAN-ik de-PRESS-iv dis-OR-der) An outdated name for bipolar disorder.

manipulation (mah-NIP-you-lay-shun) Hands-on adjustment of joints, particularly of the spine.

manipulative (mah-NIP-you-lay-tiv) Pertaining to manipulation.

Marfan syndrome (mahr-FAN SIN-drome) Genetic condition with malformation of elastic connective tissue.

marijuana (mar-ih-HWAN-ah) Dried, flowering leaves of the plant *Cannabis sativa.*

marrow (MAH-roe) Fatty, blood-forming tissue in the cavities of long bones.

massage (mah-SAHZH) Application of pressure or vibration to soft body tissues.

masseter (MASS-eh-ter) Muscle that closes the mouth.

mastalgia (mass-TAL-jee-uh) Pain in the breast.

mastectomy (mass-TECK-toe-me) Surgical excision of the breast.

masticate (MAS-tih-kate) To chew.

mastitis (mass-TIE-tis) Inflammation of the breast.

mastoid (MASS-toyd) Small bony protrusion immediately behind the ear.

maternal (mah-TER-nal) Pertaining to or derived from the mother.

matrix (MAY-triks) Substance that surrounds cells, is manufactured by the cells, and holds them together.

maturation (mat-you-RAY-shun) Process of achieving full development.

maxilla (mak-SILL-ah) Upper jawbone, containing right and left maxillary sinuses.

maximus (MAKS-ih-mus) The gluteus maximus muscle is the largest muscle in the body, covering a large part of each buttock.

McBurney point (mack-BUR-nee POYNT) One-third the distance from the anterior superior iliac spine to the umbilicus.

measles (ME-zelz) Acute, contagious disease of childhood. Also known as *rubeola.*

meatus (me-AY-tus) Passage or channel; also used to denote the external opening of a passage.

meconium (meh-KOH-nee-um) The first bowel movement of the newborn.

media (ME-dee-ah) Middle layer of a structure, particularly a blood vessel.

medial (ME-dee-al) Nearer to the middle of the body.

mediastinoscopy (ME-dee-ass-tih-NOS-koh-pee) Examination of the mediastinum using an endoscope.

mediastinum (ME-dee-ass-TIE-num) Area between the lungs containing the heart, aorta, venae cavae, esophagus, and trachea.

mediate (ME-dee-ate) Effect by means of an intermediary substance or person.

meditation (med-ih-TAY-shun) The focusing of attention or freeing the mind of thoughts as part of a formalized spiritual practice.

medius (ME-dee-us) The gluteus medius muscle is partly covered by the gluteus maximus; it originates on the ilium and is inserted into the femur.

medulla (meh-DULL-ah) Central portion of a structure surrounded by cortex.

medulla oblongata (meh-DULL-ah ob-lon-GAH-tah) Most posterior subdivision of the brainstem; continuation of the spinal cord.

megakaryocyte (MEG-ah-kair-ee-oh-site) Large cell with a large nucleus. Parts of the cytoplasm break off to form platelets.

megavitamin (meg-ah-VIE-tah-min) Large dose of a vitamin.

meiosis (my-OH-sis) Two rapid cell divisions, resulting in half the number of chromosomes.

melanin (MEL-ah-nin) Black pigment found in the skin, hair, and retina.

melanocyte (MEL-ann-oh-cyte) Cell that synthesizes (produces) melanin.

melanoma (MEL-ah-NO-mah) Malignant neoplasm formed from cells that produce melanin.

melatonin (mel-ah-TONE-in) Hormone formed by the pineal gland.

melena (mel-EN-ah) The passage of black, tarry stools.

membrane (MEM-brain) Thin layer of tissue covering a structure or cavity.

menarche (meh-NAR-key) First menstrual period.

Mendelian (men-DEE-lee-an) Described by Gregor Mendel.

Ménière disease (men-YEAR DIZ-eez) Disorder of the inner ear with a cluster of symptoms of acute attacks of tinnitus, vertigo, and hearing loss.

meninges (meh-NIN-jeez) Three-layered covering of the brain and spinal cord.

meningioma (meh-NIN-jee-OH-mah) Tumor arising from the arachnoid layer of the meninges.

meningitis (men-in-JIE-tis) Acute infectious disease of children and young adults.

meningocele (meh-NING-oh-seal) Protrusion of the meninges from the spinal cord or brain through a defect in the vertebral column or cranium.

meningococcal (meh-nin-goh-KOK-al) Pertaining to the *meningococcus* bacterium.

meningomyelocele (meh-NIN-goh-MY-el-oh-seal) Protrusion of the spinal cord and meninges through a defect in the vertebral arch of one or more vertebrae.

meniscectomy (men-ih-SEK-toh-me) Excision (cutting out) of all or part of a meniscus.

meniscus (meh-NISS-kuss) Disc of connective tissue cartilage between the bones of a joint; for example, in the knee joint. Plural *menisci.*

menopausal (MEN-oh-paws-al) Pertaining to menopause.

menopause (MEN-oh-paws) Permanent ending of menstrual periods.

menorrhagia (men-oh-RAY-jee-ah) Excessive menstrual bleeding.

menses (MEN-seez) Monthly uterine bleeding.

menstruate (MEN-stru-ate) The act of menstruation.

menstruation (men-stru-AY-shun) Synonym of *menses.*

meridian (meh-RID-ee-an) Energy line connecting different anatomical sites.

merocrine (MARE-oh-krin) Another name for *eccrine.*

mesentery (MESS-en-ter-ree) A double layer of peritoneum enclosing the abdominal viscera.

mesothelioma (MEEZ-oh-thee-lee-OH-mah) Cancer arising from the cells lining the pleura or peritoneum.

metabolic acidosis (met-ah-BOL-ik ass-ih-DOE-sis) Decreased pH in the blood and body tissues as a result of an upset in metabolism.

metabolism (meh-TAB-oh-lizm) The constantly changing physical and chemical processes occurring in the cell.

metacarpal (MET-ah-KAR-pal) The five bones between the carpus and the fingers.

metacarpophalangeal (MET-ah-KAR-poh-fay-LAN-jee-al) Pertaining to the joints between the metacarpal bones and the phalanges.

metaphysis (meh-TAF-ih-sis) Region between the diaphysis and the epiphysis where bone growth occurs.

metastasis (meh-TAS-tah-sis) Spread of a disease from one part of the body to another. Plural *metastases.*

metastasize (meh-TAS-tah-size) To spread to distant parts.

metastatic (meh-tah-STAT-ik) Pertaining to the character of cells that can metastasize.

metatarsus (MET-ah-TAR-sus) A collective term referring to the five parallel bones of the foot between the tarsus and the phalanges.

metrorrhagia (MEH-troh-RAY-jee-ah) Irregular uterine bleeding between menses.

microalbuminuria (MY-kroh-al-byu-min-YOU-ree-ah) Presence of very small quantities of albumin in urine that cannot be detected by conventional urine testing.

microaneurysm (my-kroh-AN-yu-rizm) Focal dilation of retinal capillaries.

microangiopathy (MY-kroh-an-jee-OP-ah-thee) Disease of the very small blood vessels (capillaries).

microarray (MY-kroh-ah-RAY) Technique for studying one gene in one experiment. Also called *gene chips.*

microbe (MY-krohb) Short for *microorganism.*

microcephaly (MY-kroh-SEF-ah-lee) An abnormally small head.

microcytic (my-kroh-SIT-ik) Pertaining to a small cell.

microglia (my-KROH-glee-ah) Small nervous tissue cells that are phagocytes.

microorganism (MY-kroh-OR-gan-izm) Any organism too small to be seen by the naked eye.

microscope (MY-kroh-skope) Instrument for viewing something small that cannot be seen in detail by the naked eye.

microscopic (MY-kroh-SKOP-ik) Visible only with the aid of a microscope.

micturate (MIK-choo-rate) Pass urine.

micturition (mik-choo-RISH-un) Act of passing urine.

migraine (MY-grain) Paroxysmal severe headache confined to one side of the head.

mineral (MIN-er-al) Inorganic compound usually found in earth's crust.

mineralocorticoid (MIN-er-al-oh-KOR-tih-koyd) Hormone of the adrenal cortex that influences sodium and potassium metabolism.

minimus (MIN-ih-mus) The gluteus minimus is the smallest of the gluteal muscles and lies under the gluteus medius.

minus (MY-nus) Smaller or lesser; for example, labia minora. Plural *minora*.

mitochondrion (my-toe-KON-dree-on) Organelle that generates, stores, and releases energy for cell activities. Plural *mitochondria*.

mitosis (my-TOE-sis) Cell division to create two identical cells, each with 46 chromosomes.

mitral (MY-tral) Shaped like the headdress of a Catholic bishop.

modality (moh-DAL-ih-tee) A form of therapeutic agent or regimen.

modify (MOD-ih-fie) Change the form or qualities of something.

molar (MO-lar) One of six teeth in each jaw that grind food.

molasses (mo-LASS-iz) Dark-colored syrup produced during the refining of sugar.

mold (MOLD) Filamentous fungus.

mole (MOLE) Benign localized area of melanin-producing cells.

molecule (MOLL-eh-kyul) Very small particle consisting of two or more atoms held tightly together.

molluscum (moh-LUS-kum) Soft, round tumor of the skin caused by a virus.

molluscum contagiosum (moh-LUS-kum kon-TAY-jee-oh-sum) An STD caused by a virus.

monoclonal (MON-oh-KLO-nal) Derived from a protein from a single clone of cells, all molecules of which are the same.

monocyte (MON-oh-site) Large white blood cell with a single nucleus.

monoglyceride (mon-oh-GLISS-eh-ride) A fatty substance with a single fatty acid.

mononeuropathy (MON-oh-nyu-ROP-ah-thee) Disorder affecting a single nerve.

mononucleosis (MON-oh-nyu-klee-OH-sis) Presence of large numbers of mononuclear leukocytes.

monoplegia (MON-oh-PLEE-jee-ah) Paralysis of one limb.

monosaccharide (MON-oh-SACK-ah-ride) Simplest form of sugar; for example, glucose.

Monospot test (MON-oh-spot TEST) Detects heterophile antibodies in infectious mononucleosis.

monozygotic (MON-oh-zye-GOT-ik) Twins from a single zygote.

mons pubis (MONZ PYU-bis) Fleshy pad with pubic hair, overlying the pubic bone.

Moro reflex (MOR-oh RE-fleks) Neonatal brainstem reflex. Also called *startle reflex*.

morphine (MOR-feen) Derivative of opium used as an analgesic or sedative.

mortality (mor-TAL-ih-tee) Fatal outcome or death rate.

morula (MOR-you-lah) Ball of cells formed from divisions of a zygote.

mosquito (mos-KEY-toe) Blood-sucking insect. Plural *mosquitoes*.

motile (MOH-til) Capable of spontaneous movement.

motility (moh-TILL-ih-tee) The ability for spontaneous movement.

motivation (moh-tih-VAY-shun) Force that enables a person to meet a need or achieve a goal.

motor (MOH-tor) Pertaining to nerves that send impulses out to cause muscles to contract or glands to secrete.

mouth (MOWTH) External opening of a cavity or canal.

mucin (MYU-sin) Protein element of mucus.

mucociliary (MYU-koh-SIL-ih-ah-ree) Pertaining to the ciliated epithelium lining the bronchial tree.

mucolytic (MYU-koh-LIT-ik) Agent capable of dissolving or liquefying mucus.

mucopurulent (myu-koh-PYUR-you-lent) Mixture of pus and mucus.

mucosa (myu-KOH-sah) Lining of a tubular structure. Another name for *mucous membrane*.

mucous (MYU-kus) Relating to mucus or the mucosa.

mucus (MYU-kus) Sticky secretion of cells in mucous membranes.

multidisciplinary (mul-tee-DIS-ih-plih-NAR-ee) Involving health care providers from more than one profession

multifocal (mul-tee-FOH-kal) Arising from many centers.

multimodal (mul-tee-MOH-dal) Using many methods.

multipara (mul-TIP-ah-ruh) Woman who has given birth to two or more children.

murmur (MUR-mur) Abnormal sound heard on auscultation of the heart or blood vessels.

Murphy sign (MUR-fee SINE) Tenderness in the right subcostal area on inspiration, associated with acute cholecystitis.

muscle (MUSS-el) Tissue consisting of contractile cells.

muscularis (muss-kyu-LAR-is) The muscular layer of a hollow organ or tube.

musculoskeletal (MUSS-kyu-loh-SKEL-eh-tal) Pertaining to the muscles and the bony skeleton.

mutagen (MYU-tah-jen) Agent that produces a mutation in a gene.

mutation (myu-TAY-shun) Change in the chemistry of a gene.

mute (MYUT) Unable or unwilling to speak.

mutism (MYU-tizm) Absence of speech.

myasthenia gravis (my-as-THEE-nee-ah GRA-vis) Disorder of fluctuating muscle weakness.

mycelium (my-SEE-lee-um) Mass of hyphae forming a colony of fungi.

mycologist (my-KOL-oh-jist) Specialist in mycology.

mycology (my-KOL-oh-jee) Study of fungi.

myelin (MY-eh-lin) Material of the sheath around the axon of a nerve.

myelitis (MY-eh-LIE-tis) Inflammation of the spinal cord.

myelocele (MY-eh-low-seal) Protrusion of the spinal cord through a defect in the vertebral arch.

myelography (my-eh-LOG-rah-fee) Radiography of the spinal cord and nerve roots after injection of a contrast medium into the subarachnoid space.

myeloid (MY-eh-loyd) Resembling cells derived from bone marrow.

myelomeningocele (MY-eh-low-meh-NING-oh-seal) Protrusion of the spinal cord and meninges through a defect in the vertebral arch of one or more vertebrae.

myocarditis (MY-oh-kar-DIE-tis) Inflammation of the heart muscle.

myocardium (MY-oh-KAR-dee-um) All the heart muscle.

myofascial (MY-oh-FASH-ee-al) Relating to the fascia surrounding and separating muscle tissue.

myoglobin (MY-oh-GLOW-bin) Protein of muscle that stores and transports oxygen.

myoma (my-OH-mah) Benign tumor of muscle.

myomectomy (my-oh-MEK-toe-me) Surgical removal of a myoma (fibroid).

myometrium (my-oh-ME-tree-um) Muscle wall of the uterus.

myopia (my-OH-pee-ah) Able to see close objects but unable to see distant objects.

myotherapy (MY-oh-THAIR-ah-pee) Treatment of muscles by massage.

myringotomy (mir-in-GOT-oh-me) Incision in the tympanic membrane.

myxedema (miks-eh-DEE-muh) Severe hypothyroidism.

N

narcissism (NAR-sih-sizm) Self-love; person interprets everything purely in relation to himself or herself.

narcissistic (NAR-sih-SIS-tik) Relating everything to oneself.

narcolepsy (NAR-coh-lep-see) Condition with frequent incidents of sudden, involuntary deep sleep.

narcotic (nar-KOT-ik) Drug derived from opium or a synthetic drug with similar effects.

naris (NAH-ris) Nostril. Plural *nares.*

nasal (NAY-zal) Pertaining to the nose.

nasogastric (NAY-zoh-GAS-trik) Pertaining to the nose and stomach.

nasolacrimal duct (NAY-zoh-LAK-rim-al DUKT) Passage from the lacrimal sac to the nose.

nasopharynx (NAY-zoh-FAIR-inks) Region of the pharynx at the back of the nose and above the soft palate.

natriuretic peptide (NAH-tree-you-RET-ik PEP-tide) Protein that increases the excretion of sodium.

naturopath (NAH-chur-oh-path) Practitioner of naturopathy.

naturopathic medicine (NAH-chur-oh-PATH-ik MED-ih-sin) A system of healing based on the healing power of nature.

naturopathy (nah-chur-OP-ah-thee) Holistic system of medicine with a natural approach to healing.

nebulizer (NEB-you-liz-er) Device used to deliver liquid medicine in a fine mist.

necrosis (neh-KROH-sis) Pathologic death of cells or tissue.

necrotic (neh-KROT-ik) Affected by necrosis.

necrotizing fasciitis (neh-kroh-TIZE-ing fash-eh-EYE-tis) Inflammation of fascia, producing death of the tissue.

Neisseria gonorrhoeae (ni-SEE-ree-ah gon-oh-REE-ee) Bacterium that causes gonorrhea.

neonatal (NEE-oh-NAY-tal) Pertaining to the newborn infant or the newborn period.

neonate (NEE-oh-nate) A newborn infant.

neoplasia (NEE-oh-PLAY-zee-ah) Process that results in formation of a tumor.

neoplasm (NEE-oh-plazm) A new growth, either a benign or malignant tumor.

neoplastic (NEE-oh-PLAS-tic) Pertaining to a neoplasm.

nephrectomy (neh-FREK-toe-me) Surgical removal of a kidney.

nephritis (neh-FRY-tis) Inflammation of the kidney.

nephrolithiasis (NEF-roe-lih-THIGH-ah-sis) Presence of a kidney stone.

nephrolithotomy (NEF-roe-lih-THOT-oh-me) Incision for removal of a stone.

nephrologist (neh-FROL-oh-jist) Medical specialist in disorders of the kidney.

nephrology (neh-FROL-oh-jee) Medical specialty of diseases of the kidney.

nephron (NEF-ron) Filtration unit of the kidney; glomerulus + renal tubule.

nephropathy (neh-FROP-ah-thee) Any disease of the kidney.

nephroscope (NEF-roe-skope) Endoscope used to view the inside of the kidney.

nephroscopy (neh-FROS-koh-pee) Examination of the kidney.

nephrotic syndrome (neh-FROT-ik SIN-drome) Glomerular disease with marked loss of protein. Also known as *nephrosis.*

nerve (NERV) A cord of fibers in connective tissue conduct impulses.

nerve conduction study (NERV kon-DUK-shun STUD-ee) Procedure for measuring the speed at which an electrical impulse travels along a nerve.

neural (NYU-ral) Pertaining to nervous tissue.

neural tube (NYU-ral TYUB) Embryologic tubelike structure that forms the brain and spinal cord.

neuralgia (nyu-RAL-jee-ah) Pain in the distribution of a nerve.

neurilemma (nyu-ri-LEM-ah) Covering of a nerve around the myelin sheath.

neuroglia (nyu-roh-GLEE-ah) Connective tissue holding nervous tissue together.

neurohypophysis (NYUR-oh-high-POF-ih-sis) Posterior lobe of the pituitary gland.

neurologist (nyu-ROL-oh-jist) Medical specialist in disorders of the nervous system.

neurology (nyu-ROL-oh-jee) Medical specialty of disorders of the nervous system.

neuromuscular (NYUR-oh-MUSS-kyu-lar) Pertaining to both nerves and muscles.

neuron (NYUR-on) Technical term for a nerve cell; consists of the cell body with its dendrites and axons.

neuropathy (nyu-ROP-ah-thee) Any disease of the nervous system.

neurosurgeon (NYU-roh-SUR-jun) Specialist in operating on the nervous system.

neurosurgery (NYU-roh-SUR-jer-ee) Medical specialty in surgery of the nervous system.

neurotoxin (NYUR-oh-tock-sin) Agent that poisons the nervous system.

neurotransmitter (NYUR-oh-trans-MIT-er) Chemical agent that relays messages from one nerve cell to the next.

neutropenia (NEW-troh-PEE-nee-uh) A deficiency of neutrophils.

neutrophil (NEW-troh-fill) A neutrophil's granules take up (purple) stain equally, whether the stain is acid or alkaline.

neutrophilia (NEW-troh-FILL-ee-ah) An increase in neutrophils.

nevus (NEE-vus) Congenital or acquired lesion of the skin. Plural *nevi.*

niacin (NI-ah-sin) Vitamin B_3.

nipple (NIP-el) Projection from the breast into which the lactiferous ducts open.

nitrite (NI-trite) Chemical formed in urine by *E. coli* and other microorganisms.

nitrogenous (ni-TROJ-en-us) Containing or generating nitrogen.

nocturia (nok-TYU-ree-ah) Excessive urination at night.

node (NOHD) A circumscribed mass of tissue.

nodule (NOD-yule) Small node or knotlike swelling.

nonessential (NON-ee-SEN-shal) Can be synthesized by the body.

nonunion (non-YOU-nee-un) Total failure of healing of a fracture.

norepinephrine (NOR-ep-ih-NEFF-rin) Parasympathetic neurotransmitter that is a catecholamine hormone of the adrenal gland. Also called *noradrenaline.*

nosocomial (noh-soh-KOH-mee-al) Acquired while in the hospital.

nuchal cord (NYU-kul KORD) Loop of umbilical cord around the fetal neck.

nucleolus (nyu-KLEE-oh-lus) Small mass within the nucleus.

nucleus (NYU-klee-us) Functional center of a cell or structure.

null cells (NULL SELLS) Lymphocytes with no surface markers, unlike T cells or B cells.

nutrient (NYU-tree-ent) A substance in food required for normal physiologic function.

nutrition (nyu-TRISH-un) The study of food and liquid requirements for normal function of the human body.

nutritionist (nyu-TRISH-un-ist) Certified professional in nutrition science.

nutritive (NYU-trih-tiv) Providing nourishment.

O

obesity (oh-BEE-sih-tee) Excessive amount of fat in the body.

oblique fracture (ob-LEEK FRAK-chur) A diagonal fracture across the long axis of the bone.

obsession (ob-SESH-un) Persistent, recurrent, uncontrollable thoughts or impulses.

obsessive (ob-SES-iv) Possessing persistent, recurrent, uncontrollable thoughts or impulses.

obstetrician (ob-steh-TRISH-un) Medical specialist in obstetrics.

obstetrics (OB) (ob-STET-ricks) Medical specialty for the care of women during pregnancy and the postpartum period.

occipital (ock-SIP-it-al) The back of the skull.

occipital lobe (ock-SIP-it-al LOBE) Posterior area of the cerebral hemispheres.

occlude (o-KLUDE) To close, plug, or completely obstruct.

occlusion (o-KLU-zhun) A complete obstruction.

occult (oh-KULT) Not visible on the surface.

occupational therapy (OCK-you-PAY-shun-al THAIR-ah-pee) Use of work and recreational activities to increase independent function.

ocular (OCK-you-lar) Pertaining to the eye.

oculomotor (OCK-you-loh-MOH-tor) Third (III) cranial nerve; moves the eye.

olfaction (ol-FAK-shun) Sense of smell.

olfactory (ol-FAK-toh-ree) First (I) cranial nerve; carries information related to the sense of smell.

oligodendrocyte (OL-ih-goh-DEN-droh-site) Connective tissue cell of the central nervous system that forms a myelin sheath.

oligodendroglioma (OL-ih-goh-DEN-droh-gly-OH-mah) A slow-growing tumor in the cerebral hemisphere of an adult.

oligohydramnios (OL-ih-goh-high-DRAM-nee-os) Too little amniotic fluid.

oliguria (ol-ih-GYUR-ee-ah) Scanty production of urine.

omentum (oh-MEN-tum) Membrane that encloses the bowels.

oncogene (ONG-koh-jeen) One of a family of genes involved in cell growth that work in concert to cause cancer.

oncogenic (ONG-koh-JEN-ik) Capable of producing a neoplasm.

oncologist (on-KOL-oh-jist) Medical specialist in oncology.

oncology (on-KOL-oh-jee) The science dealing with cancer.

onychomycosis (oh-ni-koh-my-KOH-sis) Condition of a fungus infection in a nail.

oocyte (OH-oh-site) Female egg cell.

oogenesis (oh-oh-JEN-eh-sis) Development of a female egg cell.

open fracture (OH-pen FRAK-chur) The skin over the fracture is broken.

ophthalmia neonatorum (off-THAL-me-ah ne-oh-nay-TOR-um) Conjunctivitis of the newborn.

ophthalmologist (off-thal-MALL-oh-jist) Medical specialist in ophthalmology.

ophthalmology (off-thal-MALL-oh-jee) Medical specialty that diagnoses and treats diseases of the eye.

ophthalmoscope (off-THAL-moh-skope) Instrument for viewing the retina.

ophthalmoscopic (OFF-thal-MOS-koh-pik) Pertaining to the use of an ophthalmoscope.

ophthalmoscopy (OFF-thal-MOS-koh-pee) The process of viewing the retina.

opiate (OH-pee-ate) A drug derived from opium.

opportunistic (OP-or-tyu-NIS-tik) An organism or a disease in a host with lowered resistance.

opportunistic infection (OP-or-tyu-NIS-tik in-FEK-shun) An infection that causes disease when the immune system is compromised for other reasons.

opposition (op-oh-SIH-shun) The movement of the thumb across the palm of the hand to touch the tips of the other fingers.

optic (OP-tick) Pertaining to the eye; *or* second (II) cranial nerve, which carries visual information.

optometrist (op-TOM-eh-trist) Someone who is skilled in the measurement of vision but cannot treat eye diseases or prescribe medication.

oral (OR-al) Pertaining to the mouth.

orbit (OR-bit) The bony socket that holds the eyeball.

orchiectomy (or-key-ECK-toe-me) Removal of one or both testes.

orchiopexy (OR-kee-oh-PEK-see) Surgical fixation of a testis in the scrotum.

orchitis (or-KIE-tis) Inflammation of the testis. Also called *epididymoorchitis.*

organ (OR-gan) Structure with specific functions in a body system.

organelle (OR-gah-nell) Part of a cell having a specialized function(s).

organic (or-GAN-ik) Compound with carbon atoms; *or* food produced without using chemicals.

organism (OR-gan-izm) Any whole, living individual whether animal or plant.

organophosphate (OR-ga-no-FOS-fate) Organic phosphorus compound used as an insecticide.

orifice (OR-ih-fis) Any opening or aperture.

origin (OR-ih-gin) Fixed source of a muscle at its attachment to bone.

oropharynx (OR-oh-FAIR-inks) Region at the back of the mouth between the soft palate and the tip of the epiglottis.

orthopedic (or-tho-PEE-dik) Pertaining to the correction and cure of deformities and diseases of the musculoskeletal system; originally, most of the deformities treated were in children. Also spelled *orthopaedic.*

orthopedist (or-tho-PEE-dist) Specialist in orthopedics.

orthopnea (or-THOP-nee-ah) Difficulty in breathing when lying flat.

orthopneic (or-THOP-nee-ik) Pertaining to or affected by orthopnea.

orthotic (or-THOT-ik) Orthopedic appliance used to correct an abnormality.

orthotist (or-THOT-ist) Maker and fitter of orthopedic appliances.

os (OS) Opening into a canal; for example, the cervix.

osmosis (oz-MO-sis) The passage of water across a cell membrane.

ossicle (OS-ih-kel) A small bone, particularly relating to the three bones in the middle ear.

osteoarthritis (OS-tee-oh-ar-THRI-tis) Chronic inflammatory disease of the joints with pain and loss of function.

osteoblast (OS-tee-oh-blast) Bone-forming cell.

osteoclast (OS-tee-oh-klast) Bone-removing cell.

osteocyte (OS-tee-oh-site) Bone-maintaining cell.

osteogenesis (OS-tee-oh-JEN-eh-sis) Creation of new bone.

osteogenesis imperfecta (OS-tee-oh-JEN-eh-sis im-per-FEK-tah) Inherited condition in which bone formation is incomplete, leading to fragile, easily broken bones.

osteogenic sarcoma (OS-tee-oh-JEN-ik sar-KOH-mah) Malignant tumor originating in bone-producing cells.

osteomalacia (OS-tee-oh-mah-LAY-she-ah) Soft, flexible bones lacking in calcium (rickets).

osteomyelitis (OS-tee-oh-my-eh-LIE-tis) Inflammation of bone tissue.

osteopath (OS-tee-oh-path) Practitioner of osteopathy.

osteopathy (OS-tee-OP-ah-thee) Medical practice based on maintaining the structural integrity of the musculoskeletal system.

osteopenia (OS-tee-oh-PEE-nee-ah) Decreased calcification of bone.

osteoporosis (OS-tee-oh-poh-ROE-sis) Condition in which the bones become more porous, brittle, and fragile and are more likely to fracture.

osteosarcoma (OS-tee-oh-sar-KOH-mah) Cancer arising in bone-forming cells.

ostomy (OS-toe-me) Surgery to create an artificial opening into a tubular structure.

otitis media (oh-TIE-tis ME-dee-ah) Inflammation of the middle ear.

otolith (OH-toe-lith) A calcium particle in the vestibule of the inner ear.

otologist (oh-TOL-oh-jist) Medical specialist in diseases of the ear.

otology (oh-TOL-oh-jee) Study of the function and diseases of the ear.

otomycosis (OH-toe-my-KOH-sis) Fungal infection of the external ear.

otorhinolaryngologist (oh-toe-rhino-lah-rin-GOL-oh-jist) Ear, nose, and throat medical specialist.

otosclerosis (oh-toe-sklair-OH-sis) Hardening at the junction of the stapes and oval window that causes loss of hearing.

otoscope (OH-toe-skope) Instrument for examining the ear.

otoscopic (oh-toe-SKOP-ik) Pertaining to examination with an otoscope.

otoscopy (oh-TOS-koh-pee) Examination of the ear.

ovarian (oh-VAIR-ee-an) Pertaining to the ovary.

ovary (OH-va-ree) One of the paired female egg-producing glands.

ovulation (OV-you-LAY-shun) Release of an oocyte from a follicle.

ovum (OH-vum) Egg. Also called *oocyte.* Plural *ova.*

oxygen (OCK-see-jen) The gas essential for life.

oxyhemoglobin (OCK-see-he-moh-GLOW-bin) Hemoglobin in combination with oxygen.

oxytocin (OCK-see-toe-sin) Pituitary hormone that stimulates the uterus to contract.

P

pacemaker (PACE-may-ker) Device that regulates cardiac electrical activity.

pain threshold (PANE THRESH-old) The point at which pain is first noticed.

palate (PAL-uht) Roof of the mouth.

palatine (PAL-ah-tine) Bone that forms the hard palate and parts of the nose and orbits.

palliative care (PAL-ee-ah-tiv KAIR) Care that relieves symptoms and pain without curing.

pallor (PAL-or) Paleness of the skin.

palm (PAHLM) The flat anterior surface of the hand.

palpate (PAL-pate) To examine with the fingers and hands.

palpation (pal-PAY-shun) An examination with the fingers and hands.

palpitation (pal-pih-TAY-shun) Forcible, rapid beat of the heart felt by the patient.

palsy (PAWL-zee) Paralysis or paresis from brain damage.

pancreas (PAN-kree-as) Lobulated gland, the head of which is tucked into the curve of the duodenum.

pancreatic (pan-kree-AT-ik) Pertaining to the pancreas.

pancreatitis (PAN-kree-ah-TIE-tis) Inflammation of the pancreas.

pancytopenia (PAN-site-oh-PEE-nee-ah) Deficiency of all types of blood cells.

pandemic (pan-DEM-ik) Disease attacking the population of a very large area.

panendoscopy (pan-en-DOS-koh-pee) Examination of the inside of the esophagus, stomach, and upper duodenum using a flexible fiber-optic endoscope.

panhypopituitarism (pan-HIGH-poh-pih-TYU-ih-tah-rizm) Deficiency of all the pituitary hormones.

pantothenic acid (PAN-toh-THEN-ik ASS-id) Coenzyme essential for cell function; vitamin B_5.

Pap test (PAP TEST) Examination of cells taken from the cervix.

papilla (pah-PILL-ah) Any small projection. Plural *papillae.*

papilledema (pah-pill-eh-DEE-mah) Swelling of the optic disc in the retina.

papilloma (pap-ih-LOH-mah) Benign projection of epithelial cells.

papule (PAP-yul) Small, circumscribed elevation on the skin.

para (PAH-rah) Abbreviation for number of deliveries.

paralysis (pah-RAL-ih-sis) Loss of voluntary movement.

paralytic (par-ah-LYT-ik) Pertaining to or suffering from paralysis.

paralyze (PAR-ah-lyze) To make incapable of movement.

parameter (pah-RAM-eh-ter) Evaluation or way of measuring.

paranasal (PAR-ah NAY-zal) Adjacent to the nose.

paranoia (par-ah-NOY-ah) Mental disorder with persecutory delusions.

paranoid (PAR-ah-noyd) Having delusions of persecution.

paraphimosis (PAR-ah-fi-MOH-sis) Condition in which a retracted prepuce cannot be pulled forward to cover the glans.

paraplegia (par-ah-PLEE-jee-ah) Paralysis of both lower extremities.

parasite (PAR-ah-site) An organism that attaches itself to, lives on or in, and derives its nutrition from another species.

parasitic (par-ah-SIT-ik) Pertaining to a parasite.

parasympathetic (par-ah-sim-pah-THET-ik) Pertaining to division of the autonomic nervous system; has opposite effects of the sympathetic division.

parathyroid (par-ah-THIGH-royd) Endocrine glands embedded in the back of the thyroid gland.

paraurethral (PAR-ah-you-REE-thral) Situated around the urethra.

parenchyma (pah-RENG-kih-mah) Characteristic functional cells of a gland or organ that are supported by the connective tissue framework.

parenteral (pah-REN-ter-al) Giving medication by any means other than the gastrointestinal tract.

paresis (par-EE-sis) Partial paralysis.

paresthesia (par-es-THEE-ze-ah) An abnormal sensation; for example, tingling, burning, pricking. Plural *paresthesias.*

parietal (pah-RYE-eh-tal) Pertaining to the outer layer of the pericardium and other body cavities; *or* the two bones forming the sidewalls and roof of the cranium.

parietal lobe (pah-RYE-eh-tal LOBE) Area of the brain under the parietal bone.

parity (PAIR-ih-tee) Number of deliveries.

Parkinson disease (PAR-kin-son DIZ-eez) Disease of muscular rigidity, tremors, and a masklike facial expression.

paronychia (par-oh-NICK-ee-ah) Infection alongside the nail.

parotid (pah-ROT-id) Parotid gland is the salivary gland beside the ear.

paroxysmal (par-ock-SIZ-mal) Occurring in sharp, spasmodic episodes.

particle (PAR-tih-kul) A small piece of matter.

particulate (par-TIK-you-late) Relating to a fine particle.

pasteurization (PAS-tyur-ih-ZAY-shun) The heating of fluids to moderate temperatures to destroy microorganisms.

patella (pah-TELL-ah) Thin, circular bone in front of the knee joint and embedded in the patellar tendon. Also called the *kneecap.*

patent (PAY-tent) Open.

patent ductus arteriosus (PAY-tent DUK-tus ar-TER-ee-oh-sus) An open, direct channel between the aorta and the pulmonary artery.

pathogen (PATH-oh-jen) A disease-causing microorganism.

pathologic fracture (path-oh-LOJ-ik FRAK-chur) Fracture occurring at a site already weakened by a disease process, such as cancer.

pathologic gambling (path-oh-LOJ-ik GAM-bling) Morbid, constant, uncontrollable, destructive gambling.

pathologist (pa-THOL-oh-jist) A specialist in pathology. (study of disease or characteristics of a particular disease).

pathology (pa-THOL-oh-jee) Medical specialty dealing with the structural and functional changes of a disease process; *or* the cause, development, and structural changes in disease.

pectin (PEK-tin) Plant fiber with the ability to thicken and solidify to a gel.

pectoral (PEK-tor-al) Pertaining to the chest.

pectoral girdle (PEK-tor-al GIR-del) Incomplete bony ring that attaches the upper limb to the axial skeleton.

pedal (PEED-al) Pertaining to the foot.

pediatrician (PEE-dee-ah-TRISH-an) Medical specialist in pediatrics.

pediatrics (pee-dee-AT-riks) Medical specialty of treating children during development from birth through adolescence.

pediculosis (peh-dick-you-LOH-sis) An infestation with lice.

peer (PEER) A person at the same level or standing.

pellagra (peh-LAG-rah) Disease due to dietary deficiency of niacin.

pelvic (PEL-vic) Pertaining to the pubic bone.

pelvis (PEL-vis) A cup-shaped cavity, as in the pelvis of the kidney; *or* a cup-shaped ring of bone.

penile (PEE-nile) Pertaining to the penis.

penis (PEE-nis) Conveys urine and semen to the outside.

pepsin (PEP-sin) Enzyme produced by the stomach that breaks down protein.

pepsinogen (pep-SIN-oh-jen) Converted by HCl in stomach to pepsin.

peptic (PEP-tik) Relating to the stomach and duodenum.

percentile (per-SEN-tile) One of a hundred groups in a distribution of variables.

perforated (PER-foh-ray-ted) Punctured with one or more holes.

perforation (per-foh-RAY-shun) Erosion that progresses to become a hole through the wall of a structure.

perfuse (per-FYUSE) To force blood to flow through a lumen or a vascular bed.

perfusion (per-FYU-shun) The act of perfusing.

pericarditis (PER-ih-kar-DIE-tis) Inflammation of the pericardium, the covering of the heart.

pericardium (per-ih-KAR-dee-um) Structure around the heart.

perimeter (peh-RIM-eh-ter) An edge or border.

perimetrium (per-ih-ME-tree-um) The covering of the uterus; part of the peritoneum.

perinatal (per-ih-NAY-tal) Around the time of birth.

perineal (PER-ih-NEE-al) Pertaining to the perineum.

perineum (PER-ih-NEE-um) Area between the thighs, extending from the coccyx to the pubis.

periodontal (PER-ee-oh-DON-tal) Around a tooth.

periodontics (PER-ee-oh-DON-tiks) Branch of dentistry specializing in disorders of tissues around the teeth.

periodontist (PER-ee-oh-DON-tist) Specialist in periodontics.

periodontitis (PER-ee-oh-don-TIE-tis) Inflammation of tissues around a tooth.

periorbital (per-ee-OR-bit-al) Pertaining to tissues around the orbit.

periosteum (PER-ee-OSS-tee-um) Fibrous membrane covering a bone.

peripheral (peh-RIF-er-al) Pertaining to the periphery or external boundary.

peripheral vision (peh-RIF-er-al VIZH-un) Ability to see objects as they come into the outer edges of the visual field.

periphery (peh-RIF-eh-ree) Outer part of a structure away from the center.

peristalsis (per-ih-STAL-sis) Waves of alternate contraction and relaxation of the intestinal wall to move food along the digestive tract.

peritoneal (PER-ih-toe-NEE-al) Pertaining to the peritoneum.

peritoneum (per-ih-toe-NEE-um) Membrane that lines the abdominal cavity.

peritonitis (PER-ih-toe-NIE-tis) Inflammation of the peritoneum.

peritubular (PER-ih-too-BYU-lar) Surrounding the small renal tubules.

permeable (PER-me-ah-bull) Allows passage of substances through a membrane.

pernicious anemia (per-NISH-us ah-NEE-me-ah) Chronic anemia due to lack of vitamin B_{12}.

pertussis (per-TUSS-is) Infectious disease with a spasmodic, intense cough ending on a whoop (stridor). Also known as *whooping cough.*

pes planus (PES PLAY-nuss) A flat foot with no plantar arch.

pessary (PES-ah-ree) Appliance inserted into the vagina to support the uterus.

pesticide (PES-tih-side) Agent for destroying flies, mosquitoes, and other pests.

petechia (peh-TEE-kee-ah) Pinpoint capillary hemorrhagic spot in the skin. Plural *petechiae.*

petit mal (peh-TEE MAL) Old name for an absence seizure.

Peyronie disease (pay-ROH-nee DIZ-eez) Penile bending and pain on erection.

phacoemulsification (fake-oh-ee-MUL-sih-fih-KAY-shun) Technique used to fragment the center of the lens into very tiny pieces and suck them out of the eye.

phagocyte (FAG-oh-site) Blood cell that ingests and destroys foreign particles and cells.

phagocytic (fag-oh-SIT-ik) Pertaining to phagocytes or phagocytosis.

phagocytize (FAG-oh-site-ize) Ingest foreign particles and cells.

phagocytosis (FAG-oh-sigh-TOE-sis) Process of ingestion and destruction.

phalanx (**FAY**-lanks) A bone of a finger or toe. Plural *phalanges.*

pharmacist (**FAR**-mah-sist) Person licensed by the state to prepare and dispense drugs.

pharmacology (far-mah-**KOLL**-oh-jee) Science of the preparation, uses, and effects of drugs.

pharmacy (**FAR**-mah-see) Facility licensed to prepare and dispense drugs.

pharyngitis (fair-in-**JIE**-tis) Inflammation of the pharynx.

pharynx (**FAIR**-inks) Air tube from the back of the nose to the larynx.

phenotype (**FEE**-noh-type) A visible trait.

phenylalanine (fen-il-**AL**-ah-neen) An amino acid.

phenylketonuria (**FEN**-il-**KEE**-toe-**NYU**-ree-ah) Hereditary disease with accumulation of phenylalanine and urinary excretion of its metabolites; leads to mental retardation if not controlled.

pheochromocytoma (fee-oh-**KRO**-moh-sigh-**TOE**-muh) Adenoma of the adrenal medulla secreting excessive catecholamines.

pheomelanin (**FEE**-oh-mel-ah-nin) The lighter form of melanin.

pheromone (**FER**-oh-moan) Substance that carries and generates a physical attraction for other people.

phimosis (fi-**MOH**-sis) Condition in which the prepuce cannot be retracted.

phlebitis (fleh-**BIE**-tis) Inflammation of a vein.

phlebotomist (fleh-**BOT**-oh-mist) Person skilled in taking blood from veins.

phlebotomy (fleh-**BOT**-oh-me) Taking blood from a vein.

phlegm (**FLEM**) Abnormal amounts of mucus expectorated from the respiratory tract.

phobia (**FOH**-be-ah) Pathologic fear or dread.

phonophoresis (foh-noh-for-**EE**-sis) Transport of one substance across the skin through the use of ultrasound.

phosphatase (**FOS**-fah-tase) Enzyme that liberates phosphorus.

photocoagulation (foh-toe-koh-ag-you-**LAY**-shun) The use of light (laser beam) to form a clot.

photodynamic (foh-toe-die-**NAM**-ik) Use of a light-sensitive drug with a laser beam to destroy cells.

photophobia (foh-toe-**FOH**-bee-ah) Fear of the light because it hurts the eyes.

photoreceptor (foh-toe-ree-**SEP**-tor) A photoreceptor cell receives light and converts it into electrical impulses.

photosensitivity (foh-toe-**SEN**-sih-tiv-ih-tee) Condition in which light produces pain in the eye.

phototherapy (foh-toe-**THAIR**-ah-pee) Treatment using light rays.

physiatrist (fih-**ZIE**-ah-trist) Specialist in physical medicine.

physiatry (fih-**ZIE**-ah-tree) Physical medicine.

physical medicine (**FIZ**-ih-cal **MED**-ih-sin) Diagnosis and treatment by means of remedial agents, such as exercises, manipulation, and heat.

physical therapy (**FIZ**-ih-cal **THAIR**-ah-pee) Use of remedial processes to overcome a physical defect. Also known as *physiotherapy.*

physiotherapy (**FIZ**-ee-oh-**THAIR**-ah-pee) Another term for *physical therapy.*

phytic acid (**FIE**-tik **ASS**-id) Component of fiber that can limit absorption of some minerals.

phytochemical (fie-toe-**KEM**-ih-kal) Biologically active, nonnutrient plant chemical.

pia mater (**PEE**-ah **MAY**-ter) Delicate inner layer of the meninges.

pica (**PIE**-kah) Eating substances not considered to be food.

pineal (**PIN**-ee-al) Pertaining to the pineal gland.

pink eye (**PINK EYE**) Conjunctivitis.

pinna (**PIN**-ah) Another name for *auricle.* Plural *pinnae.*

pinworm (**PIN**-worm) Intestinal parasite.

pitting edema (ee-**DEE**-mah) Edema that maintains for a time indentations made by applying pressure to the area.

pituitary (pih-**TOO**-ih-tary) Pertaining to the pituitary gland.

placebo (plah-**SEE**-boh) An inert compound with no innate therapeutic value.

placenta (plah-**SEN**-tah) Organ that allows metabolic interchange between the mother and the fetus.

plague (**PLAYG**) Infectious disease causing excessive mortality.

plantar reflex (**PLAN**-tar re-**FLEKS**) Neurologic response to stimulation of the sole of the foot.

plaque (**PLAK**) Patch of abnormal tissue.

plasma (**PLAZ**-mah) Fluid, noncellular component of blood.

plasma cell (**PLAZ**-mah **SELL**) Cell derived from B lymphocytes and active in formation of antibodies.

Plasmodium (plaz-**MOH**-dee-um) Causal agent for malaria.

platelet (**PLAYT**-let) Cell fragment involved in the clotting process. Also called *thrombocyte.*

pleura (**PLUR**-ah) Membrane covering the lungs and lining the ribs in the thoracic cavity. Plural *pleurae.*

pleurisy (**PLUR**-ih-see) Inflammation of the pleura.

plexus (**PLEK**-sus) A weblike network of joined nerves. Plural *plexuses.*

plica (**PLEE**-cah) Fold in a mucous membrane. Plural *plicae.*

pneumatic (new-**MAT**-ik) Pertaining to a structure filled with air.

pneumococcal (new-moh-**KOK**-al) Pertaining to the *Pneumococcus.*

pneumococcus (new-moh-**KOK**-us) Gram-positive cocci associated with respiratory infection. Plural *pneumococci.*

pneumoconiosis (new-moh-koh-nee-**OH**-sis) Fibrotic lung disease caused by the inhalation of different dusts.

pneumonectomy (**NEW**-moh-**NEK**-toe-me) Surgical removal of a whole lung.

pneumonia (new-**MOH**-nee-ah) Inflammation of the lung parenchyma.

pneumonic (new-**MON**-ik) Relating to pneumonia.

pneumothorax (new-moh-**THOR**-ax) Air in the pleural cavity.

podiatrist (po-**DIE**-ah-trist) Practitioner of podiatry.

podiatry (po-DIE-ah-tree) Specialty concerned with the diagnosis and treatment of disorders and injuries of the foot.

poikilocytic (POY-key-low-SIT-ik) Pertaining to an irregular-shaped RBC.

polarity (po-LAR-ih-tee) Possession of opposite characteristics.

poliomyelitis (POE-lee-oh-MY-eh-lie-tis) Inflammation of the gray matter of the spinal cord, leading to paralysis of the limbs and muscles of respiration.

pollutant (poh-LOO-tant) Substance that makes an environment unclean or impure.

pollution (poh-LOO-shun) Condition that is unclean, impure, and a danger to health.

polycystic (pol-ee-SIS-tik) Composed of many cysts.

polycythemia vera (POL-ee-sigh-THEE-me-ah) Chronic disease with bone marrow hyperplasia and an increase in the number of RBCs and blood volume.

polydipsia (pol-ee-DIP-see-ah) Excessive thirst.

polyhydramnios (POL-ee-high-DRAM-nee-os) Too much amniotic fluid.

polymenorrhea (POL-ee-men-oh-REE-ah) More than normal frequency of menses.

polymorphonuclear (POL-ee-more-foh-NEW-klee-ar) White blood cell with a multi-lobed nucleus.

polymyalgia rheumatica (poll-ee-my-AL-jee-ah rue-MAT-ick-ah) Pain in several muscle groups with systemic symptoms.

polyneuropathy (POL-ee-nyu-ROP-ah-thee) Disorder affecting many nerves.

polyp (POL-ip) Mass of tissue that projects into the lumen of the bowel.

polypectomy (pol-ip-ECK-toh-mee) Excision or removal of a polyp.

polyphagia (pol-ee-FAY-jee-ah) Excessive eating.

polyphenol (pol-ee-FEE-nol) Antioxidant found in grapes and tea.

polyposis (pol-ih-POH-sis) Presence of several polyps.

polysaccharide (pol-ee-SACK-ah-ride) A combination of many saccharides; for example, starch.

polysomnography (pol-ee-som-NOG-rah-fee) Test to monitor brain waves, muscle tension, eye movement, and oxygen levels in the blood as the patient sleeps.

polyuria (pol-ee-YOU-ree-ah) Excessive production of urine.

pons (PONZ) Part of the brainstem.

popliteal (pop-LIT-ee-al) Pertaining to the back of the knee.

popliteal fossa (pop-LIT-ee-al FOSS-ah) The hollow at the back of the knee.

portal; portal vein (POR-tal VANE) The vein that carries blood from the intestines to the liver.

postcoital (post-KOH-ih-tal) After sexual intercourse.

posterior (pos-TER-ee-or) Pertaining to the back surface of the body; situated behind.

postictal (post-IK-tal) Occurring after a seizure.

postmature (post-mah-TYUR) Infant born after 42 weeks of gestation.

postmaturity (post-mah-TYUR-ih-tee) Condition of being postmature.

postpartum (post-PAR-tum) After childbirth.

postpolio syndrome (PPS) (post-POE-lee-oh SIN-drome) Progressive muscle weakness in a person previously affected by polio.

postprandial (post-PRAN-dee-al) Following a meal.

postpubescent (post-pyu-BESS-ent) After the period of puberty.

posttraumatic (post-traw-MAT-ik) Occurring after and caused by trauma.

posture (POSS-chur) The carriage of the body as a whole and the position of the limbs.

Pott fracture (POT FRAK-chur) Fracture of the lower end of the fibula, often with fracture of the tibial malleolus.

prana (PRAH-nah) Vital power.

precancerous (pree-KAN-sir-us) Lesion from which a cancer can develop.

precipitate (pree-SIP-ih-tate) Very rapid and sudden, as labor and delivery.

precision (pree-SIH-zhun) Quality of being clearly defined or stated.

precursor (pree-KUR-sir) Cell or substance formed earlier in the development of the cell or substance.

prednisone (PRED-nih-zohn) A synthetic corticosteroid.

preeclampsia (pree-eh-KLAMP-see-uh) Hypertension, edema, and proteinuria during pregnancy.

preemie (PREE-me) Slang for *premature baby*.

pregnancy (PREG-nan-see) State of being pregnant.

pregnant (PREG-nant) Having conceived.

prehypertension (pree-HIGH-per-TEN-shun) Precursor to hypertension.

premature (pree-mah-TYUR) Occurring before the expected time; for example, an infant born before 37 weeks of gestation.

prematurity (pree-mah-TYUR-ih-tee) Condition of being premature.

premenstrual (pree-MEN-stru-al) Pertaining to the time immediately before the menses.

prenatal (pree-NAY-tal) Before birth.

prepatellar (pree-pah-TELL-ar) In front of the patella.

prepuce (PREE-puce) Fold of skin that covers the glans penis.

presbyopia (prez-bee-OH-pee-ah) Difficulty in nearsighted vision occurring in middle and old age.

preterm (PREE-term) Baby delivered before 37 weeks of gestation. Also called *premature.*

prevention (pree-VEN-shun) Process undertaken to prevent occurrence of a disease or health problem.

previa (PREE-vee-ah) Anything blocking the fetus during its birth; for example, an abnormally situated placenta, *placenta previa.*

priapism (PRY-ah-pizm) Persistent erection of the penis.

primary care (PRY-mah-ree KAIR) Comprehensive and preventive health care services that are the first point of care for a patient.

primigravida (pree-mih-GRAV-ih-dah) First pregnancy.

primipara (pree-**MIP**-ah-ruh) Woman who has given birth for the first time.

prion (**PREE**-on) Small infectious protein particle.

proctitis (prok-**TIE**-tis) Inflammation of the lining of the rectum.

proctoscopy (prok-**TOSS**-koh-pee) Examination of the inside of the anus by endoscopy.

prodromal (pro-**DRO**-mal) Beginning of disease, before the signs become overt.

progenitor (pro-**JEN**-it-or) Founder; beginning of an ancestry.

progesterone (pro-**JESS**-ter-own) Hormone that prepares the uterus for pregnancy.

progestin (pro-**JESS**-tin) A synthetic form of progesterone.

prognathism (**PROG**-nah-thizm) Condition of a forward-projecting jaw.

prognosis (prog-**NO**-sis) Forecasting of the probable course of a disease.

prolactin (pro-**LAK**-tin) Pituitary hormone that stimulates the production of milk.

prolactinoma (pro-lak-tih-**NO**-muh) Prolactin-producing tumor.

prolapse (pro-**LAPS**) The falling or slipping of a body part from its normal position.

proliferate (pro-**LIF**-eh-rate) To increase in number through reproduction.

pronate (**PRO**-nate) Rotate the forearm so that the surface of the palm faces posteriorly in the anatomical position.

pronation (pro-**NAY**-shun) Process of lying face-down or of turning a hand or foot with the volar (palm or sole) surface down.

prone (**PRONE**) Lying face-down, flat on your belly.

prophylactic (pro-fih-**LAK**-tik) The act or the agent that prevents a disease.

prophylaxis (pro-fih-**LAX**-is) Prevention of disease.

prostaglandin (**PROS**-tah-**GLAN**-din) Hormone present in many tissues, but first isolated from the prostate gland.

prostate (**PROS**-tate) Organ surrounding the beginning of the urethra.

prostatectomy (pross-tah-**TEK**-toe-me) Surgical removal of the prostate.

prostatic (pros-**TAT**-ik) Pertaining to the prostate.

prostatitis (pross-tah-**TIE**-tis) Inflammation of the prostate.

prosthesis (**PROS**-thee-sis) A manufactured substitute for a missing or diseased part of the body.

protease (**PRO**-tee-aze) Group of enzymes that break down protein.

protection (pro-**TEK**-shun) Defense against attack or invasion.

protein (**PRO**-teen) Class of food substances based on amino acids.

proteinuria (pro-tee-**NYU**-ree-ah) Presence of protein in urine.

prothrombin (pro-**THROM**-bin) Protein formed by the liver and converted to thrombin in the blood-clotting mechanism.

protocol (**PRO**-toe-kol) Detailed plan; for example, protocol for a regimen of therapy.

proton pump inhibitor (PPI) (**PRO**-ton **PUMP** in-**HIB**-ih-tor) Agent that blocks production of gastric acid.

protooncogene (pro-toe-**ON**-koh-jeen) A normal gene involved in normal cell growth.

provisional diagnosis (pro-**VISH**-un-al die-ag-**NO**-sis) A temporary diagnosis pending further examination or testing. Also called *preliminary diagnosis*.

proximal (**PROK**-sih-mal) Situated nearest to the center of the body.

pruritic (proo-**RIT**-ik) Itchy.

pruritus (proo-**RYE**-tus) Itching.

Pseudomonas (soo-doh-**MOH**-nas) Gram-negative aerobic rods.

psoriasis (so-**RYE**-ah-sis) Rash characterized by reddish, silver-scaled patches.

psychedelic (sigh-keh-**DEL**-ik) Agent that intensifies sensory perception.

psychiatric (sigh-kee-**AH**-trik) Pertaining to psychiatry.

psychiatrist (sigh-**KIGH**-ah-trist) Licensed medical specialist in psychiatry.

psychiatry (sigh-**KIGH**-ah-tree) Diagnosis and treatment of mental disorders.

psychoactive (sigh-koh-**AK**-tiv) Able to alter mood, behavior, and/or cognition.

psychoanalysis (sigh-koh-ah-**NAL**-ih-sis) Method of psychotherapy.

psychoanalyst (sigh-koh-**AN**-ah-list) Practitioner of psychoanalysis.

psychologic (sigh-koh-**LOJ**-ik) Pertaining to psychology.

psychological (sigh-koh-**LOJ**-ik-al) Pertaining to psychology.

psychologist (sigh-**KOL**-oh-jist) Licensed specialist in psychology.

psychology (sigh-**KOL**-oh-jee) Scientific study of the human mind and behavior.

psychopath (**SIGH**-koh-path) Person with antisocial personality disorder.

psychopharmacotherapy (**SIGH**-koh-**FAR**-mah-koh-**THAIR**-ah-pee) Drug treatment of mental disorders.

psychosis (sigh-**KOH**-sis) Disorder causing mental disruption and loss of contact with reality.

psychosocial (sigh-koh-**SOH**-shal) Involving both the mind and various social and community aspects of life.

psychosomatic (sigh-koh-soh-**MAT**-ik) Pertaining to disorders of the body usually resulting from disturbances of the mind.

psychotherapist (sigh-koh-**THAIR**-ah-pist) Practitioner of psychotherapy.

psychotherapy (sigh-koh-**THAIR**-ah-pee) Treatment of mental disorders through communication.

psychotic (sigh-**KOT**-ik) Pertaining to or affected by psychosis.

pterygoid (**TER**-ih-goyd) Pterygoid muscles are two wing-shaped muscles that open and close the mouth.

ptosis (**TOE**-sis) Sinking down of an eyelid or an organ.

pubarche (pyu-**BAR**-key) Development of pubic and axillary hair.

puberty (**PYU**-ber-tee) Process of maturing from child to young adult capable of reproducing.

pubic (**PYU**-bik) Pertaining to the pubis.

pubis (**PYU**-bis) Bony front arch of the pelvis of the hip. Also called *pubic bone.*

puerperium (pyu-er-**PEE**-ree-um) Six-week period after birth in which the uterus involutes.

pulmonary (**PULL**-moh-**NAR**-ee) Pertaining to the lungs and their blood supply.

pulmonologist (**PULL**-moh-**NOL**-oh-jist) Medical specialist in pulmonary disorders.

pulmonology (**PULL**-moh-**NOL**-oh-gee) Study of the lungs; *or* the medical specialty of disorders of the respiratory tract.

pulp (**PULP**) Dental pulp is the connective tissue in the cavity in the center of the tooth.

pupil (**PYU**-pill) The opening in the center of the iris that allows light to reach the lens. Plural *pupillae.*

purge (**PURJ**) Consciously throw up or cause bowel evacuation.

purging (**PURJ**-ing) The act of throwing up or evacuating the bowel.

purification (**PYUR**-if-ih-kay-shun) Make free from pathogens.

Purkinje fibers (per-**KIN**-jee fi-**BERS**) Network of nerve fibers in the myocardium.

purpura (**PUR**-pyu-rah) Skin hemorrhages that are red initially and then turn purple.

purulent (**PURE**-you-lent) Showing or containing a lot of pus.

pustule (**PUS**-tyul) Small protuberance on the skin that contains pus.

pyelitis (pie-eh-**LYE**-tis) Inflammation of the renal pelvis.

pyelogram (**PIE**-el-oh gram) X-ray image of the renal pelvis and ureters.

pyelonephritis (**PIE**-eh-loh-neh-**FRY**-tis) Inflammation of the kidney and renal pelvis.

pyloric (pie-**LOR**-ik) Pertaining to the pylorus.

pylorus (pie-**LOR**-us) Exit area of the stomach.

pyogenic (**PIE**-o-**JEN**-ik) Pus-producing.

pyorrhea (pie-oh-**REE**-ah) Purulent discharge.

pyrexia (pie-**REK**-see-ah) An abnormally high body temperature or fever.

pyridoxine (pir-ih-**DOK**-seen) Vitamin B_6.

pyromania (pie-roh-**MAY**-nee-ah) Morbid impulse to set fires.

Q

Qigong (**CHEE**-gong) Exercises and breathing routines performed daily.

quadrant (**KWAD**-rant) One-quarter of a circle.

quadrantectomy (kwad-ran-**TEK**-toe-me) Surgical excision of a quadrant of the breast.

quadriceps femoris (**KWAD**-rih-seps **FEM**-or-is) An anterior thigh muscle with four heads.

quadriplegia (kwad-rih-**PLEE**-jee-ah) Paralysis of all four limbs.

quantum physics (**KWAHN**-tum **FIZ**-iks) The study of subatomic particles.

quiescent (kwi-**ESS**-ent) Latent, dormant.

quinoa (kee-**NO**-ah) Plant with edible seeds high in protein.

R

rabid (**RAB**-id) Suffering from rabies.

rabies (**RAY**-beez) Highly fatal infectious disease transmitted by the bite of infected animals.

radial (**RAY**-dee-al) Pertaining to the forearm.

radiation (ray-dee-**AY**-shun) A spreading out, as of anatomical parts.

radical (**RAD**-ih-cal) Extensive, as in complete removal of a diseased part.

radioactive (**RAY**-dee-oh-**AK**-tiv) Spontaneously emitting alpha, beta, or gamma rays.

radioactive iodine (**RAY**-dee-oh-**AK**-tiv **EYE**-oh-dine) Any of the various tracers that emit alpha, beta, or gamma rays.

radiologist (ray-dee-**OL**-oh-jist) Medical specialist in the use of x-rays and other imaging techniques.

radiology (ray-dee-**OL**-oh-jee) The study of medical imaging.

radionuclide (**RAY**-dee-oh-**NYU**-klide) Radioactive agent used in diagnostic imaging.

radiotherapy (**RAY**-dee-oh-**THAIR**-ah-pee) Treatment using radiation.

radius (**RAY**-dee-us) The forearm bone on the thumb side.

rale (**RAHL**) Crackle heard through a stethoscope when air bubbles through liquid in the lungs. Plural *rales.*

raphe (**RAY**-fee) Line separating two symmetrical structures.

rash (**RASH**) Cutaneous eruption.

reabsorption (ree-ab-**SORP**-shun) The taking back into the blood of substances that had previously been filtered out from it.

recessive gene (ree-**SESS**-iv **JEEN**) Allele that does not manifest as a trait or characteristic.

recombinant DNA (ree-**KOM**-bin-ant dee-en-a) DNA (deoxyribonucleic acid) altered by inserting a new sequence of DNA into the chain.

rectocele (**REK**-toe-seal) Hernia of the rectum into the vagina.

rectum (**RECK**-tum) Terminal part of the colon from the sigmoid to the anal canal.

recurrent (ree-**KUR**-ent) Symptoms or lesions returning after an intermission.

reduction (ree-**DUCK**-shun) The restoration of a structure to its normal position.

reflex (**REE**-fleks) An involuntary response to a stimulus.

reflexology (ree-flek-SOL-oh-jee) Stimulation of reflexes in the feet and hands, which correspond to other parts of the body.

reflux (REE-fluks) Backward flow.

refract (ree-FRACT) Make a change in the direction of, or bend, a ray of light.

regenerate (ree-JEN-eh-rate) Reconstitution of a lost part.

regimen (REJ-ih-men) Program of treatment.

regulate (REG-you-late) To control the way in which a process progresses.

regulation (reg-you-LAY-shun) Control of the way in which a process progresses.

regurgitate (ree-GUR-jih-tate) To flow backward; for example, through a heart valve.

regurgitation (ree-gur-jih-TAY-shun) Expel contents of the stomach into the mouth, short of vomiting.

rehabilitation (REE-hah-bill-ih-TAY-shun) Therapeutic restoration of an ability to function as before.

Reiki (RAY-kee) A healing method using the transfer of energy by placing hands on or near a patient.

remission (ree-MISH-un) Period in which there is a lessening or absence of the symptoms of a disease.

remit (ree-MIT) To diminish in intensity.

renal (REE-nal) Pertaining to the kidney.

renin (REE-nin) Enzyme secreted by the kidney that causes vasoconstriction.

replication (rep-lih-KAY-shun) Reproduction to produce an exact copy.

reproductive (ree-pro-DUC-tiv) Relating to the process by which organisms produce offspring.

resection (ree-SEK-shun) Removal of a specific part of an organ or structure.

resectoscope (ree-SEK-toe-skope) Endoscope for transurethral removal of lesions.

residual (re-ZID-you-al) Pertaining to anything left over.

resistance (ree-ZIS-tants) Ability of an organism to withstand the effects of an antagonistic agent.

resistant (ree-ZIS-tant) Able to resist.

resorption (ree-SORP-shun) Loss of substance, such as bone.

respiration (RES-pih-RAY-shun) Fundamental process of life used to exchange oxygen and carbon dioxide.

respirator (RES-pir-AY-tor) Another name for *ventilator*.

restorative rehabilitation (ree-STOR-ah-tiv REE-hah-bill-ih-TAY-shun) Promote renewal of health and strength.

rete testis (REE-teh TES-tis) Network of tubules between the seminiferous tubules and the epididymis.

retention (ree-TEN-shun) Holding back in the body what should normally be discharged (e.g., urine).

reticulum (reh-TIK-you-lum) Fine network of cells in the medulla oblongata.

retina (RET-ih-nah) Light-sensitive innermost layer of the eyeball.

retinaculum (ret-ih-NACK-you-lum) Fibrous ligament that keeps the tendons in place on the wrist so that they do not "bowstring" when the forearm muscles contract.

retinoblastoma (RET-in-oh-blas-TOE-mah) Malignant neoplasm of primitive retinal cells.

retinoid (RET-ih-noyd) A class of keratolytic agents.

retinopathy (ret-ih-NOP-ah-thee) Degenerative disease of the retina.

retraction (ree-TRAK-shun) A pulling back, as a pulling back of the intercostal spaces and the neck above the clavicle.

retrograde (RET-roh-grade) Reversal of a normal flow; for example, back from the bladder into the ureters.

retroversion (reh-troh-VER-shun) The tipping backward of the uterus.

retroverted (REH-troh-vert-ed) Tilted backward.

retrovirus (REH-troh-vie-rus) Virus that replicates in a host cell by converting its RNA core into DNA.

Reye syndrome (RAY SIN-drome) Encephalopathy and liver damage in children following an acute viral illness; linked to aspirin use.

rhabdomyolysis (RAB-doh-my-oh-LIE-sis) Destruction of muscle to produce myoglobin.

rhabdomyosarcoma (RAB-doh-MY-oh-sar-KOH-mah) Cancer derived from skeletal muscle.

rheumatism (RU-mat-izm) Pain in various parts of the musculoskeletal system.

rheumatoid arthritis (RA) (RHU-mah-toyd ar-THRI-tis) Disease of connective tissue, with arthritis as a major manifestation.

rhinitis (rye-NI-tis) Inflammation of the nasal mucosa. Also called *coryza.*

rhinoplasty (RYE-no-plas-tee) Surgical procedure to change the size or shape of the nose.

rhonchus (RONG-kuss) Wheezing sound heard on auscultation of the lungs; made by air passing through a constricted lumen. Plural *rhonchi.*

riboflavin (RYE-boh-flay-vin) Vitamin B_2.

ribonucleic acid (RNA) (RYE-boh-nyu-KLEE-ik ASS-id) Information carrier from DNA in the nucleus to the ribosome to produce protein molecules.

ribosome (RYE-bo-sohm) Structure in the cell that assembles amino acids into protein.

rickets (RICK-ets) Disease due to vitamin D deficiency, producing soft, flexible bones.

rigidity (ri-JID-ih-tee) Increased muscle tone at rest.

Rinne test (RIN-eh TEST) Test for conductive hearing loss.

ritual (RITCH-you-al) An activity or set of activities established and repeated.

Rolfing (ROLF-ing) Manipulation of connective tissue to realign and balance the whole body.

root (ROOT) Fundamental or beginning part of a structure.

rooting (rue-TING) A neonatal reflex to turn toward the nipple and open the mouth when a nipple is placed on the cheek.

rosacea (roh-ZAY-she-ah) Persistent erythematous rash of the central face.

roseola infantum (roh-ZEE-oh-lah in-FAN-tum) Skin rash in infants and young children caused by a herpesvirus.

rotator cuff (roh-**TAY**-tor CUFF) Part of the capsule of the shoulder joint.

Roux-en-Y (**ROO**-on-Y) Surgical procedure to reduce the size of the stomach.

ruga (**ROO**-ga) A fold, ridge, or crease. Plural *rugae.*

rumination (**ROO**-min-ay-shun) To bring back food into the mouth to chew over and over.

rupture (**RUP**-tyur) Break or tear of any organ or body part.

S

sacral (**SAY**-kral) In the neighborhood of the sacrum.

sacroiliac joint (say-kroh-**ILL**-ih-ak JOINT) The joint between the sacrum and the ilium.

sacrum (**SAY**-crum) Segment of the vertebral column that forms part of the pelvis.

sagittal (**SAJ**-ih-tal) Pertaining to the vertical plane through the body, dividing it into right and left portions.

saliva (sa-**LIE**-vah) Secretion in the mouth from salivary glands.

Salmonella (sal-moh-**NELL**-ah) Pathogenic Gram-negative rods causing dysentery.

salpingectomy (sal-pin-**JECT**-oh-me) Surgical removal of fallopian tube(s).

salpingitis (sal-pin-**JIE**-tis) Inflammation of the uterine tube.

sanitization (**SAN**-ih-tih-**ZAY**-shun) Process of using chemicals to remove pathogens from surfaces.

saphenous (**SAPH**-ih-nus) Relating to the saphenous vein in the thigh.

saponins (**SAP**-oh-nins) Phytochemicals that can prevent cancer cell replication.

sarcoidosis (sar-koy-**DOH**-sis) Granulomatous lesions of the lungs and other organs; cause is unknown.

sarcoma (sar-**KOH**-mah) A malignant tumor originating in connective tissue.

sarcopenia (sar-koh-**PEE**-nee-ah) Progressive loss of muscle mass and strength in aging.

saturated fatty acid (satch-you-**RAY**-ted **FAT**-ee **ASS**-id) Incapable of absorbing any more hydrogen, and is solid at room temperature.

scab (SKAB) Crust that forms over a wound or sore during healing.

scabies (**SKAY**-bees) Skin disease produced by mites.

scapula (**SKAP**-you-lah) Shoulder blade. Plural *scapulae.*

scapular (**SKAP**-you-lar) Pertaining to the shoulder blade.

scar (SKAR) Fibrotic seam that forms when a wound heals.

schizoid (**SKITZ**-oyd) Withdrawn, socially isolated.

schizophrenia (skitz-oh-**FREE**-nee-ah) Disorder of perception, thought, emotion, and behavior.

Schwann cell (SHWANN SELL) Connective tissue cell of the peripheral nervous system that forms a myelin sheath.

sciatic (sigh-**AT**-ik) Pertaining to the sciatic nerve or sciatica.

sciatica (sigh-**AT**-ih-kah) Pain from compression of L5 or S1 nerve roots.

scintigraphy (sin-**TIG**-rah-fee) Recording of radioactivity with a special camera.

sclera (**SKLAIR**-ah) Fibrous outer covering of the eyeball and the white of the eye.

scleritis (sklair-**RI**-tis) Inflammation of the sclera.

scleroderma (sklair-oh-**DERM**-ah) Thickening and hardening of the skin due to new collagen formation.

sclerose (skleh-**ROZE**) To harden or thicken.

sclerosis (skleh-**ROH**-sis) Thickening or hardening of a tissue.

sclerotherapy (**SKLAIR**-oh-**THAIR**-ah-pee) To collapse a vein by injecting a solution into it to harden it.

scoliosis (skoh-lee-**OH**-sis) An abnormal lateral curvature of the vertebral column.

scrotal (**SKRO**-tal) Pertaining to the scrotum.

scrotum (**SKRO**-tum) Sac containing the testes.

scurvy (**SKUR**-vee) Deficiency of vitamin C.

seasonal affective disorder (see-**ZON**-al af-**FEK**-tiv dis-**OR**-der) Depression that occurs at the same time every year, often in winter.

sebaceous glands (se-**BAY**-shus GLANZ) Glands in the dermis that open into hair follicles and secrete an oily fluid called sebum.

seborrhea (seb-oh-**REE**-ah) Excessive amount of sebum.

sebum (**SEE**-bum) Waxy secretion of the sebaceous glands.

secrete (se-**KREET**) To release or give off, as substances produced by cells.

secretin (se-**KREE**-tin) Hormone produced by the duodenum to stimulate pancreatic juice.

sedation (seh-**DAY**-shun) State of being calmed.

sedative (**SED**-ah-tiv) Agent that calms nervous excitement.

sedentary (sed-en-**TER**-ee) Accustomed to little exercise or movement.

sediment (**SED**-ih-ment) Insoluble material that settles to the bottom of a liquid.

sedimentation (**SED**-ih-men-**TAY**-shun) Formation of a sediment.

segment (**SEG**-ment) A section of an organ or structure.

segmentectomy (seg-men-**TEK**-toe-me) Surgical excision of a segment of a tissue or organ.

seizure (**SEE**-zhur) Event due to excessive electrical activity in the brain.

self-examination (self-ek-zam-ih-**NAY**-shun) The examination of part of one's own body.

self-mutilation (self-myu-tih-**LAY**-shun) Injury or disfigurement made to one's own body.

semen (**SEE**-men) Penile ejaculate containing sperm and seminal fluid.

semilunar (sem-ee-**LOO**-nar) Appears like a half moon.

seminal vesicle (**SEM**-in-al **VES**-ih-kull) Sac of the ductus deferens that produces seminal fluid.

seminiferous (sem-ih-**NIF**-er-us) Pertaining to carrying semen.

seminiferous tubule (sem-ih-NIF-er-us TU-byul) Coiled tubes in the testes that produce sperm.

seminoma (sem-ih-NO-mah) Neoplasm of germ cells of a testis.

semipermeable (sem-ee-PER-me-ah-bull) Freely permeable to water but not to solutes.

semipermeable membrane (sem-ee-PER-me-ah-bull MEM-brain) A membrane that allows only certain substances to pass through it.

senescence (seh-NES-ens) The state of being old.

senile (SEE-nile) Characteristic of old age.

senility (seh-NIL-ih-tee) Old age.

sensation (sen-SAY-shun) The conscious feeling of the effects of a stimulation.

sensorineural hearing loss (SEN-sor-ih-NYUR-al) Hearing loss caused by lesions of the inner ear or the auditory nerve.

sensory (SEN-soh-ree) Having the function of sensation; relating to structures of the nervous system that carry impulses to the brain.

sepsis (SEP-sis) Presence of pathogenic organisms or their toxins in blood or tissues.

septicemia (sep-tih-SEE-mee-ah) Microorganisms circulating in, and infecting, the blood (blood poisoning).

septum (SEP-tum) A wall dividing two cavities. Plural *septa.*

sequence (SEE-kwens) The succession of one event after another.

sequential (see-KWEN-shal) One event following after another.

serosa (seh-ROH-sa) Outermost covering of the alimentary tract.

serotonin (ser-oh-TOE-nin) A neurotransmitter in the central and peripheral nervous systems.

serous (SEER-us) Thicker and less transparent than water.

serum (SEER-um) Fluid remaining after removal of cells and fibrin clot.

sewage (SOO-aje) Waste matter from populated areas.

sharps (SHARPS) Any medical instrument capable of puncturing skin.

sharps container (SHARPS kon-TAY-ner) Puncture-resistant container for disposal of sharps.

Shigella (she-GEL-ah) Genus of Gram-negative rods.

shigellosis (shig-eh-LOH-sis) Dysentery caused by *Shigella.*

shock (SHOCK) Sudden physical or mental collapse or circulatory collapse.

shunt (SHUNT) A bypass or diversion of fluid, such as blood.

sibling (SIB-ling) Brother or sister.

sigmoid (SIG-moyd) Sigmoid colon is shaped like an "S."

sigmoidoscopy (sig-moi-DOS-koh-pee) Endoscopic examination of the sigmoid colon.

sign (SINE) Physical evidence of a disease process.

silicosis (sil-ih-KOH-sis) Fibrotic lung disease from inhaling silica particles.

simian crease (sih-ME-an KREES) Single crease across the palm of the hand; found in monkeys.

simulate (SIM-you-late) To imitate a disease process.

sinoatrial (SA) node (sigh-noh-AY-tree-al NODE) The center of modified cardiac muscle fibers in the wall of the right atrium that acts as the pacemaker for the heart rhythm.

sinus (SIGH-nus) Cavity or hollow space in a bone or other tissue.

sinus rhythm (SIGH-nus RITH-um) The normal (optimal) heart rhythm arising from the sinoatrial node.

sinusitis (sigh-nyu-SIGH-tis) Inflammation of the lining of a sinus.

Sjögren syndrome (SHOW-gren SIN-drome) Autoimmune disease that attacks the glands that produce saliva and tears.

Skene glands (SKEEN GLANZ) Paraurethral glands in the anterior wall of the vagina. Also called *paraurethral glands.*

smegma (SMEG-mah) Oily material produced by the glans and prepuce.

Snellen letter chart (SNEL-en) Test for acuity of distant vision.

snore (SNOR) Noise produced by vibrations in the structures of the nasopharynx.

sociopath (SO-see-oh-path) Person with antisocial personality disorder.

soleus (SO-lee-us) Large muscle of the calf.

somatic (soh-MAT-ik) Relating to the body in general; *or* pertaining to a division of the peripheral nervous system serving the skeletal muscles.

somatoform (soh-MAT-oh-form) Physical symptoms occurring without identifiable physical cause.

somatostatin (SO-mah-toh-STAT-in) Hormone that inhibits release of growth hormone and insulin.

somatotropin (SO-mah-toh-TROH-pin) Hormone of the anterior pituitary that stimulates growth of body tissues. Also called *growth hormone.*

sonogram (SON-oh-gram) Image obtained by using a sonograph.

sonograph (SON-oh-graf) Instrument that uses sound waves to create images of structures.

sonographer (so-NOG-rah-fer) The technician who performs a sonogram.

sorbitol (SOR-bih-tol) Alcohol derivative of glucose.

spasm (SPASM) Sudden involuntary contraction of a muscle group.

spasmodic (spaz-MOD-ik) Having intermittent spasms or contractions.

spastic (SPAZ-tik) Increased muscle tone on movement.

species (SPEE-sheez) A group of organisms with certain common characteristics.

specific (speh-SIF-ik) Relating to a particular entity.

specificity (spes-ih-FIS-ih-tee) State of having a fixed relation to a particular entity.

sperm (SPERM) Mature male sex cell. Also called *spermatozoon.*

spermatic (SPER-mat-ik) Pertaining to sperm.

spermatid (SPER-mah-tid) A cell late in the development process of sperm.

spermatocele (SPER-mat-oh-seal) Cyst of the epididymis that contains sperm.

spermatogenesis (SPER-mat-oh-JEN-eh-sis) The process by which male germ cells differentiate into sperm.

spermatozoa (SPER-mat-oh-ZOH-ah) Sperm (plural of *spermatozoon*).

spermicidal (SPER-mih-side-al) Pertaining to sperm.

spermicide (SPER-mih-side) Agent that destroys sperm.

sphenoid (SFEE-noyd) Wedge-shaped bone at the base of the skull.

spherocyte (SFEAR-oh-site) A spherical cell.

spherocytosis (SFEAR-oh-site-oh-sis) Presence of spherocytes in the blood.

sphincter (SFINK-ter) Band of muscle that encircles an opening; when it contracts, the opening squeezes closed.

sphygmomanometer (SFIG-moh-mah-NOM-ih-ter) Instrument for measuring arterial blood pressure.

spina bifida (SPY-nah BIH-fih-dah) Failure of one or more vertebral arches to close during fetal development.

spina bifida cystica (SIS-tik-ah) Meninges and spinal cord protruding through the absent vertebral arch and having the appearance of a cyst.

spina bifida occulta (OH-kul-tah) The deformity of the vertebral arch is not apparent from the skin surface.

spinal tap (SPY-nal TAP) Placement of a needle through an intervertebral space into the subarachnoid space to withdraw CSF.

spine (SPINE) Vertebral column; *or* a short projection from a bone.

spiral fracture (SPY-ral FRAK-chur) A fracture in the shape of a coil.

spirituality (SPEAR-ih-choo-AL-ity) Meaning to life that comes from the spirit or soul rather than the physical body.

spirochete (SPY-roh-keet) Spiral-shaped bacterium causing a sexually transmitted disease (syphilis).

spirometer (spy-ROM-eh-ter) An instrument used to measure respiratory volumes.

spirometry (spy-ROM-eh-tree) Use of a spirometer.

spirulina (spy-roo-LEE-nah) Commercial product of blue-green algae containing 60% to 70% protein.

spleen (SPLEEN) Vascular, lymphatic organ in the left upper quadrant of the abdomen.

splenectomy (sple-NECK-toe-me) Surgical removal of the spleen.

splenomegaly (sple-noh-MEG-ah-lee) Enlarged spleen.

spondylosis (spon-dih-LOH-sis) Degenerative osteoarthritis of the spine.

spongiform (SPON-jih-form) Looking like a sponge.

spongiosum (spun-jee-OH-sum) Spongelike tissue.

spore (SPOR) Generic term for any tiny compact cell produced during reproduction by bacteria.

sprain (SPRAIN) A wrench or tear in a ligament.

sputum (SPYU-tum) Matter coughed up and spat out by individuals with respiratory disorders.

squamous cell (SKWAY-mus SELL) Flat, scalelike epithelial cell.

stage (STAYJ) Definition of the extent and dissemination of a malignant neoplasm.

staging (STAY-jing) Process of determination of the extent of the distribution of a neoplasm.

stapes (STAY-peas) Inner (medial) one of the three ossicles of the middle ear; shaped like a stirrup.

Staphylococcus (STAF-ih-loh-KOK-us) Genus of Gram-positive bacteria that divide in more than one plane to form clusters. Plural *staphylococci*.

starch (STARCH) Complex carbohydrate made of multiple units of glucose attached together.

status (STAT-us) A state or condition

status epilepticus (STAT-us ep-ih-LEP-tik-us) A recurrent state of seizure activity lasting longer than a specific time frame (usually 30 minutes).

stem cell (STEM SELL) Undifferentiated cell found in a differentiated tissue that can divide to yield the specialized cells in that tissue.

stenosis (steh-NOH-sis) Narrowing of a canal or passage, as in the narrowing of a heart valve.

stent (STENT) Wire mesh tube used to keep arteries open.

stereopsis (ster-ee-OP-sis) Three-dimensional vision.

stereotactic (STER-ee-oh-TAK-tic) Pertaining to a precise three-dimensional method to locate a lesion.

stereotype (STER-ee-oh-tipe) An image held in common by members of a group.

sterile (STER-isle) Free from all living organisms and their spores; *or* unable to fertilize or reproduce.

sterility (steh-RIL-ih-tee) Inability to reproduce.

sterilization (STER-ih-lih-ZAY-shun) Process of making sterile.

sterilize (STER-ih-lize) To make sterile.

sternum (STIR-num) Long, flat bone forming the center of the anterior wall of the chest.

steroid (STER-oyd) Large family of chemical substances found in many drugs, hormones, and body components.

stethoscope (STETH-oh-skope) Instrument for listening to cardiac and respiratory sounds.

stimulant (STIM-you-lant) Agent that excites or strengthens functional activity.

stimulation (stim-you-LAY-shun) Arousal to increased functional activity.

stoma (STOW-mah) Artificial opening.

strabismus (strah-BIZ-mus) A turning of an eye away from its normal position.

strain (STRAIN) Overstretch or tear in a muscle or tendon.

stratum basale (STRAH-tum ba-SAL-eh) Deepest layer of the epidermis, from which the other cells originate and migrate.

streptococcal (strep-toe-KOK-al) Pertaining to the *Streptococcus*.

Streptococcus (strep-toe-KOK-us) Genus of Gram-positive bacteria that grow in chains. Plural *streptococci*.

streptokinase (strep-toe-KI-nase) An enzyme that dissolves clots.

striated muscle (STRI-ay-ted MUSS-el) Another term for *skeletal muscle.*

striation (stri-AY-shun) Stripes.

stricture (STRICK-shur) Narrowing of a tube.

stridor (STRY-door) High-pitched noise made when there is a respiratory obstruction in the larynx or trachea.

stroke (STROHK) Acute clinical event caused by an impaired cerebral circulation.

stroma (STROH-mah) Connective tissue framework that supports the parenchyma of an organ or gland.

subarachnoid space (sub-ah-RACK-noyd SPASE) Space between the pia mater and the arachnoid membrane.

subclavian (sub-CLAY-vee-an) Underneath the clavicle.

subcutaneous (sub-kew-TAY-nee-us) Below the skin. Also known as *hypodermic.*

subdural (sub-DUR-al) Located in the space between the dura mater and the arachnoid membrane.

sublingual (sub-LING-wal) Underneath the tongue.

subluxation (sub-luck-SAY-shun) An incomplete dislocation in which some contact between the joint surfaces remains.

submandibular (sub-man-DIB-you-lar) Underneath the mandible.

submucosa (sub-mew-KOH-sa) Tissue layer underneath the mucosa.

substernal (sub-STER-nal) Under the sternum or breastbone.

sucrose (SUE-krose) Table sugar.

suction (SUK-shun) Use of a catheter to clear the upper airway or other tubes.

sugar (SHUH-gar) Basic carbohydrate; term sometimes used for glucose or sucrose.

suicidal (SOO-ih-SIGH-dal) Wanting to kill oneself.

suicide (SOO-ih-side) The act of killing oneself.

sulcus (SUL-cuss) Groove on the surface of the cerebral hemispheres that separates gyri. Plural *sulci.*

superior (soo-PEE-ree-or) Situated above.

supinate (SOO-pih-nate) Rotate the forearm so that the surface of the palm faces anteriorly in the anatomical position.

supination (soo-pih-NAY-shun) Process of lying face-upward or turning an arm or foot so that the palm or sole is facing up.

supine (soo-PINE) Lying face-up, flat on your spine.

supplement (SUH-pleh-ment) Substance taken to remedy or prevent a deficiency.

suprapubic (SOO-prah-pyu-bik) Above the symphysis pubis.

surfactant (ser-FAK-tant) A protein and fat compound that creates surface tension to hold lung alveolar walls apart.

susceptible (suh-SEP-tih-bill) Capable of being affected by.

suture (SOO-chur) Place where two bones are joined together by a fibrous band continuous with their periosteum, as in the skull; *or* a stitch to hold the edges of a wound together. Plural *sutures.*

swab (SWOB) Wad of cotton used to remove or apply something from or to a surface.

sympathetic (sim-pah-THET-ik) Pertaining to the part of the autonomic nervous system operating at the unconscious level.

sympathy (SIM-pa-thee) Appreciation and concern for another person's mental and emotional state.

symphysis (SIM-feh-sis) Two bones joined by fibrocartilage. Plural *symphyses.*

symptom (SIMP-tum) Departure from normal health experienced by the patient.

symptomatic (simp-toe-MAT-ik) Pertaining to the symptoms of a disease.

synapse (SIN-aps) Junction between two nerve cells, or a nerve fiber and its target cell, where electrical impulses are transmitted between the cells.

synchondrosis (sin-kon-DROH-sis) A rigid articulation (joint) formed by cartilage. Plural *synchondroses.*

syncope (SIN-koh-peh) Temporary loss of consciousness and postural tone due to diminished cerebral blood flow.

syncytial (sin-SISH-ee-al) Pertaining to the syncytium.

syncytium (sin-SISH-ee-um) A multinucleated mass not separated into cells.

syndesmosis (sin-dez-MOH-sis) A rigid articulation (joint) formed by ligaments. Plural *syndesmoses.*

syndrome (SIN-drohm) Combination of signs and symptoms associated with a particular disease process.

synergist (SIN-er-jist) Agent or process that aids the action of another.

synovial (si-NOH-vee-al) Pertaining to synovial fluid and synovial membrane.

synthesis (SIN-the-sis) The process of building a compound from different elements.

synthetic (sin-THET-ik) Built up or put together from simpler compounds.

syphilis (SIF-ih-lis) Sexually transmitted disease caused by a spirochete.

syringomyelia (sih-RING-oh-my-EE-lee-ah) Abnormal longitudinal cavities in the spinal cord that cause paresthesias and muscle weakness.

systemic (sis-TEM-ik) Relating to the entire organism.

systemic lupus erythematosus (sis-TEM-ik LOO-pus er-ih-THEE-mah-toe-sus) Inflammatory connective tissue disease affecting the whole body.

systole (SIS-toe-lee) Contraction of the heart muscle.

T

tachycardia (tak-ih-KAR-dee-ah) Rapid heart rate (above 100 beats per minute).

tachypnea (tak-ip-NEE-ah) Rapid breathing.

tactile (TAK-tile) Relating to touch.

tai chi (tie-CHEE) Defined series of postures performed in fluid movement.

talipes (TAL-ip-eze) Deformity of the foot involving the talus.

talus (TAY-luss) The tarsal bone that articulates with the tibia to form the ankle joint.

tampon (TAM-pon) Plug or pack in a cavity to absorb or stop bleeding.

tamponade (tam-po-NAID) Pathologic compression of an organ such as the heart.

tangent (TAN-jent) Sudden change of course.

tangentiality (tan-jen-she-AL-ih-tee) Disturbance in thought processes, which move rapidly from one topic to another.

tapeworm (TAPEWORM) Intestinal parasitic worm.

tarsus (TAR-sus) The collection of seven bones in the foot that form the ankle and instep; *or* the flat fibrous plate that gives shape to the outer edges of the eyelids.

tartar (TAR-tar) Calcified deposit at the gingival margin of the teeth. Also called *dental calculus.*

taste (TAYST) Sensation from chemicals on the taste buds.

Tay-Sachs disease (TAY-SAKS DIZ-eez) Congenital fatal disorder of fat metabolism.

temperament (TEM-per-ah-ment) Predisposition to character or personality.

temporal (TEM-por-al) Bone that forms part of the base and sides of the skull.

temporal lobe (TEM-por-al LOBE) Posterior two-thirds of the cerebral hemispheres.

temporalis muscle (tem-poh-RAHL-is MUSS-el) Muscle attached to the temporal bone that opens and closes the jaw.

temporomandibular joint (TMJ) (TEM-por-oh-man-DIB-you-lar JOYNT) The joint between the temporal bone and the mandible.

tendinitis (ten-dih-NYE-tis) Inflammation of a tendon. Also spelled *tendonitis.*

tendon (TEN-dun) Fibrous band that connects muscle to bone.

tenosynovitis (TEN-oh-sine-oh-VIE-tis) Inflammation of a tendon and its surrounding synovial sheath.

teratogen (TER-ah-toe-jen) Agent that produces fetal deformities.

teratogenesis (TER-ah-toe-JEN-eh-sis) Process involved in producing fetal deformities.

teratogenic (TER-ah-toe-JEN-ik) Capable of producing fetal deformities.

teratoma (ter-ah-TOE-mah) Neoplasm of a testis or ovary containing multiple tissues from other sites in the body.

testicle (TES-tih-kul) One of the male reproductive glands. Also called *testis.*

testicular (tes-TICK-you-lar) Pertaining to the testicle.

testis (TES-tis) A synonym for testicle. Plural *testes.*

testosterone (tes-TOSS-ter-own) Powerful androgen produced by the testes.

tetanus (TET-ah-nuss) A disease with painful, tonic, muscular contractions caused by the toxin produced by *Clostridium tetani.*

tetany (TET-ah-nee) Severe muscle twitches, cramps, and spasms.

tetralogy (teh-TRAL-oh-jee) A set of four congenital heart defects.

tetralogy of Fallot (TOF) (teh-TRAL-oh-jee OF fah-LOW) Set of four congenital heart defects occurring together.

thalamus (THAL-ah-mus) Mass of gray matter underneath the ventricle in each cerebral hemisphere.

thalassemia (thal-ah-SEE-mee-ah) Group of inherited blood disorders that produce a hemolytic anemia.

thelarche (thee-LAR-key) Onset of breast development.

thenar (THAY-nar) The thenar eminence is the fleshy mass at the base of the thumb.

therapeutic (THAIR-ah-PYU-tik) Relating to the treatment of a disease or disorder.

therapist (THAIR-ah-pist) Professional trained in the practice of a particular therapy.

therapy (THAIR-ah-pee) Systematic treatment of a disease, dysfunction, or disorder.

thermotherapy (THER-moh-THAIR-ah-pee) The use of heat in treatment.

thiamine (THIGH-ah-min) Vitamin B_1.

thoracentesis (THOR-ah-sen-TEE-sis) Insertion of a needle into the pleural cavity to withdraw fluid or air. Also called *pleural tap.*

thoracic (THOR-ass-ik) Pertaining to the chest (thorax).

thoracoscopy (thor-ah-KOS-koh-pee) Examination of the pleural cavity with an endoscope.

thoracotomy (thor-ah-KOT-oh-me) Incision through the chest wall.

thorax (THO-racks) The part of the trunk between the abdomen and the neck.

thrombin (THROM-bin) Enzyme that forms fibrin.

thrombocyte (THROM-boh-site) Another name for *platelet.*

thrombocytopenia (THROM-boh-site-oh-PEE-nee-ah) Deficiency of platelets in circulating blood.

thromboembolism (THROM-boh-EM-boh-lizm) A piece of detached blood clot (embolus) blocking a distant blood vessel.

thrombolysis (throm-BOL-ih-sis) Dissolving a thrombus (clot).

thrombophlebitis (THROM-boh-fleh-BY-tis) Inflammation of a vein with clot formation.

thrombosis (throm-BOH-sis) Formation of a thrombus.

thrombus (THROM-bus) A clot attached to a diseased blood vessel or heart lining.

thrush (THRUSH) Infection with *Candida albicans.*

thymectomy (thigh-MEK-toe-me) Surgical removal of the thymus gland.

thymine (THIGH-meen) Chemical base found in, and comprising the sequence of, DNA but not RNA.

thymoma (thigh-MOH-mah) Benign tumor of the thymus.

thymus (THIGH-mus) Endocrine gland located in the mediastinum.

thyroid (THIGH-royd) Endocrine gland in the neck; *or* a cartilage of the larynx.

thyroid hormone (THIGH-royd HOR-mohn) Collective term for the two thyroid hormones, T3 and T4.

thyroid storm (THIGH-royd STORM) Medical crisis and emergency due to excess thyroid hormones.

thyroidectomy (thigh-roy-DEK-toe-me) Surgical removal of the thyroid gland.

thyroiditis (thigh-roy-DIE-tis) Inflammation of the thyroid gland.

thyrotoxicosis (THIGH-roe-toks-ih-KOH-sis) Disorder produced by excessive thyroid hormone production.

thyrotropin (thigh-roe-TROH-pin) Hormone from the anterior pituitary gland that stimulates function of the thyroid gland.

thyroxine (thigh-ROCK-sin) Thyroid hormone, T4, tetraiodothyronine.

tibia (TIB-ee-ah) The larger bone of the lower leg.

tic (TIK) Sudden, involuntary, repeated contraction of muscles.

tic douloureux (TIK duh-luh-RUE) Painful, sudden, spasmodic involuntary contractions of the facial muscles supplied by the trigeminal nerve. Also called *trigeminal neuralgia.*

tinea (TIN-ee-ah) General term for a group of related skin infections caused by different species of fungi.

tinnitus (TIN-ih-tus) Persistent ringing, whistling, clicking, or booming noise in the ears.

tissue (TISH-you) Collection of similar cells.

titer (TIE-ter) The strength of a substance in a solution as compared to a standard.

tolerance (TOL-er-ants) The capacity to become accustomed to a stimulus or drug.

tomography (toe-MOG-rah-fee) Radiographic image of a selected slice of tissue.

tone (TONE) Tension present in resting muscles.

tongue (TUNG) Mobile muscle mass in the mouth; bears the taste buds.

tonic (TON-ik) In a state of muscular contraction.

tonic-clonic (TON-ik-KLON-ik) The body alternates between excessive muscular rigidity (tonic) and jerking muscular contractions (clonic).

tonic-clonic seizure (TON-ik-KLON-ik SEE-zhur) Generalized seizure due to epileptic activity in all or most of the brain.

tonometer (toe-NOM-eh-ter) Instrument for determining intraocular pressure.

tonometry (toe-NOM-eh-tree) The measurement of intraocular pressure.

tonsil (TON-sill) Mass of lymphoid tissue on either side of the throat at the back of the tongue.

tonsillectomy (ton-sih-LEC-toh-me) Surgical removal of the tonsils.

tonsillitis (ton-sih-LIE-tis) Inflammation of the tonsils.

topical (TOP-ih-kal) Medication applied to the skin to obtain a local effect.

torsion (TOR-shun) The act or result of twisting.

Tourette syndrome (tur-ET SIN-drome) Disorder of multiple motor and vocal tics.

toxic (TOK-sick) Pertaining to a toxin.

toxicity (toks-ISS-ih-tee) The state of being poisonous.

toxin (TOK-sin) Poisonous substance formed by a cell or organism.

toxoid (TOK-soyd) Toxin treated to destroy its toxic capability but retain its antigenic capability.

toxoplasmosis (TOK-soh-plaz-MOH-sis) Parasitic infection acquired from undercooked meat from infected animals.

trachea (TRAY-kee-ah) Air tube from the larynx to the bronchi.

trachealis (tray-kee-AY-lis) Pertaining to the trachea.

tracheostomy (tray-kee-OST-oh-me) Incision into the windpipe, usually so that a tube can be inserted to assist breathing.

tracheotomy (tray-kee-OT-oh-me) Incision made into the trachea to create a tracheostomy.

tract (TRAKT) Bundle of nerve fibers with a common origin and destination.

traction (TRAK-shun) A pulling or dragging force.

trait (TRAYT) A discrete characteristic that has a known quality.

tranquilizer (TRANG-kwih-lie-zer) Agent that calms without sedating or depressing.

trans fatty acid (TRANZ FAT-ee ASS-id) Solid or semisolid product of hydrogenation of unsaturated plant oils.

transcatheter (trans-KATH-eh-ter) Catheter with a self-expanding mushroom device that is placed and left inside a PDA.

transcript (TRAN-skript) An exact copy or reproduction.

transcription (tran-SCRIP-shun) The action of making a copy of dictated material.

transcriptionist (tran-SCRIP-shun-ist) One who makes the copy of dictated material.

transdermal (trans-DER-mal) Going across or through the skin.

transducer (trans-DYU-sir) Device that converts energy from one form to another.

transfusion (trans-FYU-zhun) Transfer of blood or a blood component from donor to recipient.

transient (TRANZ-ee-ent) Lasting only a short time.

transplant (TRANZ-plant) The tissue or organ used; *or* the act of transferring tissue from one person to another.

transplantation (TRANZ-plan-TAY-shun) The moving of tissue or an organ from one person or place to another.

transverse (trans-VERS) Pertaining to the horizontal plane dividing the body into upper and lower portions.

transverse fracture (trans-VERS FRAK-chur) A fracture perpendicular to the long axis of the bone.

tremor (TREM-or) Small, shaking, involuntary, repetitive movements of hands, extremities, neck, or jaw.

triceps brachii (TRY-sepz BRAY-key-eye) Muscle of the arm that has three heads or points of origin.

trichinosis (trik-ih-NOH-sis) Disease from ingestion of undercooked pork containing a roundworm.

Trichomonas (trik-oh-MOH-nas) A parasite causing a sexually transmitted disease.

trichomoniasis (TRIK-oh-moh-NIE-ah-sis) Infection with *Trichomonas vaginalis.*

tricuspid (try-KUSS-pid) Having three points; a tricuspid heart valve has three flaps.

trigeminal (try-GEM-in-al) Fifth (V) cranial nerve, with its three different branches supplying the face.

triglyceride (tri-GLISS-eh-ride) Any of a group of fats containing three fatty acids.

triiodothyronine (tri-EYE-oh-doh-THY-roh-neen) Thyroid hormone T3.

trimester (TRY-mes-ter) One-third of the length of a full-term pregnancy.

triplegia (tri-PLEE-jee-ah) Paralysis of three limbs.

trisomy (TRI-so-me) Presence of an extra chromosome.

trochanter (troh-KAN-ter) One of two bony prominences near the head of the femur.

trochlear (TROHK-lee-are) Fourth (IV) cranial nerve; supplies one muscle of the eye.

tropic (TROH-pik) Tropic hormones stimulate other endocrine glands to produce hormones.

trypsin (TRIP-sin) Enzyme that breaks down protein.

tuberculosis (too-BER-kyu-LOW-sis) Infectious disease that can infect any organ or tissue.

tumor (TOO-mor) Any abnormal swelling.

tunica (TYU-nih-kah) A layer in the wall of a blood vessel or other tubular structure.

tunica vaginalis (TYU-nih-kah vaj-ih-NAHL-iss) Covering, particularly of a tubular structure. The tunica vaginalis is the sheath of the testis and epididymis.

turbinate (TUR-bin-ate) Another name for the nasal conchae on the lateral walls of the nasal cavity.

turmeric (ter-MER-ik) Spice used in Ayurvedic medicine.

Turner syndrome (TER-ner SIN-drome) Syndrome associated with a chromosome count of 45 and only one X chromosome.

tympanic (tim-PAN-ik) Pertaining to the tympanic membrane or tympanic cavity.

tympanostomy (tim-pan-OS-toe-me) Surgically created new opening in the tympanic membrane to allow fluid to drain from the middle ear.

typhoid (TIE-foyd) Acute infectious disease caused by *Salmonella typhi*.

U

ulcer (ULL-cer) Erosion of an area of skin or mucosa.

ulceration (ull-cer-A-shun) Formation of an ulcer.

ulcerative (UL-sir-ah-tiv) Marked by an ulcer or ulcers.

ulna (UL-na) The medial and larger bone of the forearm.

ulnar (UL-nar) Pertaining to the ulna or any of the structures (artery, vein, nerve) named after it.

ultrasonography (UL-trah-soh-NOG-rah-fee) Delineation of deep structures using sound waves.

ultrasound (UL-trah-sownd) Use of very high frequency sound waves.

ultraviolet (ul-trah-VIE-oh-let) Electromagnetic rays at higher frequency than the violet end of the spectrum.

umbilical (um-BIL-ih-kal) Pertaining to the umbilicus or the center of the abdomen.

umbilicus (um-BIL-ih-kus) Pit in the abdomen where the umbilical cord entered the fetus.

unconscious (un-KON-shus) Not conscious, lacking awareness.

unessential (un-ee-SEN-shal) Not of importance.

unipolar disorder (you-nih-POLE-ar dis-OR-der) Depression.

unsaturated fatty acid (un-SATCH-you-ray-ted FAT-ee ASS-id) Other atoms can be added to it.

uracil (YUR-ah-sil) Chemical found in RNA.

uranium (you-RAY-nee-um) Radioactive metallic element.

urea (you-REE-ah) End product of nitrogen metabolism.

uremia (you-REE-me-ah) The complex of symptoms arising from renal failure.

ureter (you-RET-er) Tube that connects the kidney to the urinary bladder.

ureteroscope (you-REE-ter-oh-scope) Endoscope to view the inside of the ureter.

ureteroscopy (you-REE-ter-os-koh-pee) Examination of the ureter.

urethra (you-REE-thra) Canal leading from the bladder to outside.

urethritis (you-ree-THRI-tis) Inflammation of the urethra.

urethrotomy (you-ree-THROT-oh-me) Incision of a stricture of the urethra.

urinalysis (you-rih-NAL-ih-sis) Examination of urine to separate it into its elements and define their kind and/or quantity.

urinary (YUR-in-ary) Pertaining to urine.

urinate (YUR-in-ate) To pass urine.

urination (yur-ih-NAY-shun) The act of passing urine.

urine (YUR-in) Fluid and dissolved substances excreted by the kidney.

urological (yur-oh-LOJ-ih-kal) Pertaining to urology.

urologist (you-ROL-oh-jist) Medical specialist in disorders of the urinary system.

urology (you-ROL-oh-jee) Medical specialty of disorders of the urinary system.

urticaria (ur-tee-KARE-ee-ah) Rash of itchy wheals (hives).

uterus (YOU-ter-us) Organ in which an egg develops into a fetus.

uvea (YOU-vee-ah) Middle coat of the eyeball—includes the iris, ciliary body, and choroid.

uveitis (you-vee-I-tis) Inflammation of the uvea.

uvula (YOU-vyu-lah) Fleshy projection of the soft palate.

V

vaccinate (VAK-sin-ate) To administer a vaccine.

vaccination (vak-sih-NAY-shun) Administration of a vaccine.

vaccine (VAK-seen) Preparation to generate active immunity.

vagina (vah-JIE-nah) Female genital canal extending from the uterus to the vulva.

vaginal (VAJ-in-al) Pertaining to the vagina.

vaginitis (vah-jih-NIE-tis) Inflammation of the vagina.

vaginosis (vah-jih-NOH-sis) Any disease of the vagina.

vagus (VAY-gus) Tenth (X) cranial nerve; supplies many different organs throughout the body.

varicocele (VAIR-ih-koh-seal) Varicose veins of the spermatic cord.

varicose (VAIR-ih-kos) Characterized by or affected with varices.

varicosities (vair-ih-KOS-ih-tees) Collection of varicose veins.

varix (VAIR-iks) Dilated, tortuous vein. Plural *varices.*

vasectomy (vah-SEK-toe-me) Excision of a segment of the ductus deferens.

vasoconstriction (VAY-soh-con-STRIK-shun) Reduction in diameter of a blood vessel.

vasodilation (VAY-soh-di-LAY-shun) Increase in diameter of a blood vessel.

vasopressin (vay-soh-PRESS-in) Pituitary hormone that constricts blood vessels and decreases urine output. Also called *antidiuretic hormone (ADH).*

vasovasostomy (VAY-soh-vay-SOS-toe-me) Reanastomosis of the ductus deferens to restore the flow of sperm. Also called *vasectomy reversal.*

vector (VEK-tor) A virus or other molecule used to carry a gene to target cells; *or* an animal or insect capable of transmitting an infection.

vegan (VEE-gan) One who eats plants and no animal or dairy products.

vegetative (VEJ-eh-tay-tiv) Functioning unconsciously as plant life is assumed to do.

vein (VANE) Blood vessel carrying blood toward the heart.

vena cava (VEE-nah KAY-vah) One of the two largest veins in the body. Plural *venae cavae.*

venogram (VEE-noh-gram) Radiograph of veins after injection of radiopaque contrast material.

venous (VEE-nuss) Pertaining to venous blood or the venous circulation.

ventilation (ven-tih-LAY-shun) Movement of gases into and out of the lungs.

ventilator (VEN-tih-LAY-tor) Device that breathes for the patient.

ventral (VEN-tral) Pertaining to the belly or situated nearer to the surface of the belly.

ventricle (VEN-trih-kel) A cavity of the heart or brain.

ventricular (ven-TRIK-you-lar) Pertaining to a ventricle.

venule (VEN-yule) Small vein leading from the capillary network.

vermiform (VER-mih-form) Worm shaped; used as a descriptor for the appendix.

vernix caseosa (VER-nicks kay-see-OH-sah) Cheesy substance covering the skin of the fetus.

verruca (ver-ROO-cah) Wart caused by a virus.

vertebra (VER-teh-brah) One of the bones of the spinal column. Plural *vertebrae.*

vertex (VER-teks) Topmost point of the vault of the skull.

vertigo (VER-tih-go) Sensation of spinning or whirling.

vesicle (VES-ih-kull) Small sac containing liquid; for example, a blister or semen.

vestibule (VES-tih-byul) Space at the entrance to a canal.

vestibulectomy (ves-tib-you-LEK-toe-me) Surgical excision of the vulva.

vestibulocochlear (ves-TIB-you-loh-KOK-lee-ar) Eighth (VIII) cranial nerve; carrying information for the senses of hearing and balance.

villus (VILL-us) Thin, hairlike projection, particularly of a mucous membrane lining a cavity. Plural *villi.*

viral (VIE-ral) Pertaining to a virus.

virilism (VIR-ih-lizm) Development of masculine characteristics by a woman or girl.

virulence (VIR-you-lence) The power of a toxin or pathogen.

virulent (VIR-you-lent) Extremely toxic or pathogenic.

virus (VIE-rus) Group of infectious agents that require living cells for growth and reproduction.

viscera (VISS-er-ah) Internal organs, particularly in the abdomen.

visceral (VISS-er-al) Pertaining to the internal organs.

viscosity (vis-KOS-ih-tee) The resistance of a fluid to flowing.

viscous (VISS-kus) Sticky; resistant to flow.

viscus (VISS-kus) Hollow, walled, internal organ.

visual acuity (VIH-zhoo-wal ah-KYU-ih-tee) Sharpness and clearness of vision.

visualization (VIH-zhoo-wah-lih-ZAY-shun) The forming of mental images or pictures.

vital signs (VI-tal SIGNS) A procedure during a physical examination in which temperature (T), pulse (P), respirations (R), and blood pressure (BP) are measured to assess general health and cardiorespiratory function.

vitamin (VYE-tah-min) Essential organic substance necessary in small amounts for normal cell function.

vitiligo (vit-ill-EYE-go) Nonpigmented white patches on otherwise normal skin.

vitreous humor (VIT-ree-us HEW-mor) A gelatinous liquid in the posterior cavity of the eyeball with the appearance of glass.

vocal (VOH-kal) Pertaining to the voice.

void (VOYD) To evacuate urine or feces.

voluntary muscle (VOL-un-tare-ee MUSS-el) Muscle that is under the control of the will.

vomer (VOH-mer) Lower nasal septum.

vulva (VUL-vah) Female external genitalia.

vulvodynia (vul-voh-DIN-ee-uh) Chronic vulvar pain.

vulvovaginal (VUL-voh-VAJ-ih-nal) Pertaining to the vulva and vagina.

vulvovaginitis (VUL-voh-vaj-ih-NIE-tis) Inflammation of the vagina and vulva.

W

warfarin (WAR-fuh-rin) Anticoagulant; also used as rat poison, trade name Coumadin.

Weber test (VA-ber TEST) Test for sensorineural hearing loss.

wheal (WHEEL) Small, itchy swelling of the skin. Wheals raised by an injection do not itch. Also called *hives.*

whiplash (WHIP-lash) Symptoms caused by sudden, uncontrolled extension and flexion of the neck, often in an automobile accident.

white matter (WITE MATT-er) Regions of the brain and spinal cord occupied by bundles of axons.

whooping cough (WHO-ping KAWF) Infectious disease with spasmodic, intense cough ending on a whoop (stridor). Also called *pertussis.*

Wilms tumor (WILMZ TOO-mor) Cancerous kidney tumor of childhood. Also known as *nephroblastoma.*

wound (WOOND) Any injury that interrupts the continuity of skin or a mucous membrane.

X

xenograft (ZEN-oh-graft) A graft from another species. Also known as *heterograft.*

Y

yeast (YEEST) Microscopic fungus.

yoga (YOH-gah) A system of lifestyle measures.

yolk sac (YOKE SACK) Source of blood cells and future sex cells for the fetus.

Z

zeaxanthin (ZEE-ah-ZAN-thin) Carotenoid found in pepper, corn, and spinach.

zygoma (zye-GOH-mah) Bone that forms the prominence of the cheek.

zygote (ZYE-goat) Cell resulting from the union of the sperm and egg.

Photos

Welcome Chapter

Opener: Image © 2014 Nucleus Medical Media; **W.2**: © Tony Freeman/PhotoEdit Inc.; **W.3-W.7**: © The McGraw-Hill Companies, Inc./Rick Brady, photographer; **W.8**: © David Young-Wolff/PhotoEdit Inc.; **W.9**: © The McGraw-Hill Companies, Inc./Rick Brady, photographer; **W.11-W12**: © The McGraw-Hill Companies, Inc./Rick Brady, photographer; **W.13**: Vol. 115 PhotoDisc/Getty RF; **W.14**: Vol. 66 PhotoDisc/Getty RF; **W.15**: © Vstock LLC/Tetra Images/Corbis RF; **W.16**: Dynamicgraphics/Jupiter RF; **W.17**: Image © 2014 Nucleus Medical Media; **W.19**: © A. J. Photo/Photo Researchers, Inc.; **W.20**: © The McGraw-Hill Companies, Inc./Tim Vacula, photographer.

Chapter 1

Opener: Image © 2014 Nucleus Medical Media.

Chapter 2

Opener: Image © 2014 Nucleus Medical Media; **2.1-2.2**: © Dr. P. Marazzi/Photo Researchers, Inc.; **2.3**: © VEM/Photo Researchers, Inc.; **2.4**: © Custom Medical Stock Photo; **2.5**: © Medical Media/Photo Researchers, Inc.

Chapter 3

Opener: Image © 2014 Nucleus Medical Media;

Chapter 4

Opener: Image © 2014 Nucleus Medical Media; **4.2**: © Francis Leroy, Biocosmos/Photo Researchers Inc.; **4.6**: © The McGraw-Hill Companies, Inc./Photo by Alvin Telser; **4.8-4.10**: © The McGraw-Hill Companies/Joe DeGrandis, photographer; **4.13**: © The McGraw-Hill Companies/Joe DeGrandis, photographer.

Chapter 5

Opener: Image © 2014 Nucleus Medical Media; **5.8**: © Photo Network Stock/Grant Heilman Photography Inc.; **5.9**: © ISM/Phototake; **5.10**: © Medical-on-line/Alamy; **5.11**: © Mediscan/VisualsUnlimited; **5.18**: © CNRI/SPL/Photo Researchers Inc.; **5.22**: © ISM/Phototake; **5.23**: © Custom Medical Stock Photo; **5.25**: © Phototake; **5.27**: © SIU Biomedical/Photo Researchers, Inc.; **5.32**: © Collection CNRI/Phototake/Alamy; **5.33**: © CNRI/Photo Researchers, Inc.; **5.35**: © Susan Leavine/Photo Researchers Inc.; **5.36**: © SPL/Photo Researchers, Inc.

Chapter 6

Opener: Image © 2014 Nucleus Medical Media; **6.1b**: © CNRI/SPL/Photo Researchers, Inc.; **6.6**: © Medical-on-Line/Alamy; **6.9**: © Saturn Stills/SPL/Photo Researchers, Inc.

Chapter 7

Opener: Image © 2014 Nucleus Medical Media; **7.6**: © Nucleus Medical Art, Inc./Phototake; **7.7**: © Brian Evans/Photo Researchers, Inc.; **7.9a**: © Phototake; **7.9b**: © The McGraw-Hill Companies, Inc./Photo by Alvin Tesler; **7.10**: © SPL/Photo Researchers, Inc.; **7.13**: © Wellcome Photo Library; **7.14**: © English/Custom Medical Stock Photo.

Chapter 8

Opener: Image © 2014 Nucleus Medical Media; **8.3**: © CNRI/Photo Researchers, Inc.; **8.4-8.5**: © Biophoto Associates/Photo Researchers, Inc.; **8.6**: © Kenneth Greer/Visuals Unlimited; **8.7**: © Scott Camazine/Kallista Images/Visuals Unlimited, Inc.; **8.13**: © Dr. Landrum Shettles; **8.15**: © The William Boyd Museum, Dept. of Pathology and Laboratory Medicine, The Univiersity of British Columbia; **8.16**: © Scott Camazine/Phototake; **8.17**: © The William Boyd Museum, Dept. of Pathology and Laboratory Medicine, The University of British Columbia; **8.18**: © Parviz M. Pour/Photo Researchers, Inc.; **8.20**: © Sovereign/ISM/Phototake; **8.21**: © Corbis RF; **8.23**: © Getty RF; **8.27**: © BrandX Pictures/Punchstock RF; **8.29**: © Photo Researchers; **8.32**: © Susan Leavines/Photo Researchers, Inc.; **8.33**: © Biophoto Associates/Photo Researchers, Inc.; **8.35**: EP Vol. 90/Getty Images RF; **8.36**: © Wellcome Photo Library; **8.37**: © ALIX/Phanie/Photo Researchers Inc.; **8.38**: © TSI/Getty Images.

Chapter 9

Opener: Image © 2014 Nucleus Medical Media; **9.17a-9.17b**: © Phototake Inc./Alamy; **9.18a**: © Wellcome Photo Library; **9.18b**: © R. Spencer Phippen/Phototake Inc.; 9.19: © Ellen B. Senisi/Photo Researchers, Inc.; **9.20**: © James Prince/Photo Researchers, Inc.; **9.21**: © David Grossman/Photo Researchers, Inc.; **9.22**: © The Washington Post/Getty; **9.23**: © Simon Fraser/Photo Researchers, Inc.; **9.26a**: © ISM/Phototake Inc.; **9.26b**: © Scott Camazine/Alamy; **9.27**: © NIH/Phototake Inc.; **9.28**: © Mediscan; **9.29**: © James Cavallini/Photo Researchers Inc.; **9.30a**: © Wellcome Photo Library; **9.30b**: © Simon Fraser/Newcastle Hospitals NHS/Science Photo Library/Photo Researchers, Inc.; **9.31**: © Bart Äôs Medical Library/Phototake Inc.; **9.32**: © O. J. Staats/Custom Medical Stock Photography; **9.33**: © Dr. M. A. Ansary/Custom Medical Stock Photography; **9.35b**: © NMSB/Custom Medical Stock Photo; **9.37a**: © NMSB/Custom Medical Stock Photo; **9.37b**: © Phototake Inc./Alamy; **9.38**: © Marcus E. Raichle.

Chapter 10

Opener: Image © 2014 Nucleus Medical Media; **10.10**: © The McGraw-Hill Companies, Inc./Rick Brady, photographer; **10.12a-10.12b**: © Ed Reschke; **10.13**: © Pasieka/SPL/Photo Researchers, Inc.; **10.15**: © Time & Life Pictures/Getty Images; **10.16**: © SPL/Photo Researchers, Inc.; **10.17**: © Clouds Hill Imaging Ltd./Photo Researchers, Inc.; **10.24**: © Dr. P. Marazzi/Photo Researchers Inc.

Chapter 11

Opener: Vol.40/PhotoDisc/Getty RF; **11.1**: The McGraw-Hill Companies, Inc./Eric Wise, photographer; **11.2b**: © Bill Longcore/Photo Researchers, Inc.; **11.4a-11.4b**: © Ed Reschke; **11.5**: © Meckes/Ottawa/Photo Researchers, Inc.; **11.6-11.10**: © Ed Reschke; **11.11**: © Andrew Syred/SPL/Photo Researchers, Inc.; **11.13a**: © Medical-on-line/Alamy; **11.13b**: © Dr. P. Marazzi/Science Photo Library, Photo Researchers, Inc.; **11.13c**: © Paul Cox/Alamy.

Chapter 12

Opener: Image © 2014 Nucleus Medical Media; **12.4**: © The McGraw-Hill Companies, Inc./Dennis Strete, photographer;

C

E